The U.S. RDA (used on food labels)

Nutrient	RDA for an Adult Man (1968)	RDA for an Adult Woman (1968)	U.S. RDA
Nutrients that *must* appear on the label[a]			
Protein (g), PER $\geq$ casein[b]	45	—	45
Protein (g), PER $<$ casein	65	55	65
Vitamin A (RE)	1,000[c]	800[c]	1,000[c]
Vitamin C (ascorbic acid) (mg)	60	55	60
Thiamin (vitamin B_1) (mg)	1.4	1.0	1.5
Riboflavin (vitamin B_2) (mg)	1.7	1.5	1.7
Niacin (mg)	18	13	20
Calcium (g)	0.8	0.8	1.0
Iron (mg)	10	18	18
Nutrients that *may* appear on the label			
Vitamin D (IU)	—	—	400
Vitamin E (IU)	30	25	30
Vitamin B_6 (mg)	2.0	2.0	2.0
Folate (folic acid, folacin) (mg)	0.4	0.4	0.4
Vitamin B_{12} (μg)	6	6	6
Phosphorus (g)	0.8	0.8	1.0
Iodine (μg)	120	100	150
Magnesium (mg)	350	300	400
Zinc (mg)	—	—	15
Copper (mg)	—	—	2
Biotin (mg)	—	—	0.3
Pantothenic acid (mg)	—	—	10

[a]Whenever nutrition labeling is required.
[b]PER is an index of protein quality explained in Appendix J.
[c]1,000 RE was originally expressed as 5,000 IU. 800 RE was originally expressed as 4,000 IU.

Source: Adapted from U.S. Department of Health and Human Services, Public Health Service, Food and Drug Administration, Office of Public Affairs, 5600 Fishers Lane, Rockville, Maryland 20857, HHS publication no. (FDA) 81-2146, revised March 1981.

The U.S. RDA numbers used on labels are those taken from the 1968 RDA. The circled numbers are those chosen for the U.S. RDA from the adult male and female recommendations. In each case, the higher number is chosen.

In the case of thiamin, niacin, iodine, and magnesium, the RDA for an adolescent boy is used, because this is even higher than the adult RDA. In the case of calcium and phosphorus, 1 gram per day is used, more than the adult RDA. Pregnant and lactating women and rapidly growing teenagers have RDA even higher than this, but 1 gram was considered generous enough for use as a standard for labels.

In the case of the last four nutrients—zinc, copper, biotin, and pantothenic acid—RDA had not been set as of 1968, but these nutrients are known to be essential. The agency set "guestimates" for these so that percent-of-U.S.-RDA labels could include them. These four nutrients are now included in the RDA tables, but the U.S. RDA values have not changed to correspond; they are considered close enough already.

Understanding Normal and Clinical Nutrition

THIRD EDITION

Eleanor Noss Whitney
Corinne Balog Cataldo
Sharon Rady Rolfes

WEST PUBLISHING COMPANY

St. Paul
New York
Los Angeles
San Francisco

To my mother Edith Noss, my father Henry Noss, my children Lynn, Kara, and Russ, and my special friends Tonya and Sally, who enhance my world with their wisdom, compassion, goodness, and love—my gratitude always.

Ellie

To health care professionals every-where, who work small miracles by applying their knowledge to prevent disease, to restore health, and to ease suffering.

Corkie

To my family and friends, who comfort me in times of sadness and celebrate with me in times of joy—especially to Tom and Linda DeBruyne, whose gen-erosity, love, and support exemplify the meaning of friendship.

Sharon

Copyright © 1983,
1987
COPYRIGHT © 1991

By WEST PUBLISHING COMPANY
By WEST PUBLISHING COMPANY
50 West Kellogg Boulevard
P.O. Box 64526
St. Paul, MN 55164–0526

Printed in the United States of America.

98 97 96 95 94 93 92   8 7 6 5 4 3 2 1

Library of Congress Cataloging-in-Publication Data

Whitney, Eleanor Noss.
  Understanding normal and clinical nutrition / Eleanor Noss
Whitney, Corinne Balog Cataldo, Sharon Rady Rolfes.—3rd ed.
    p. cm.
  Includes bibliographical references and index.
  ISBN 0-314-87426-7 (hard)
    1. Nutrition. 2. Diet in disease. 3. Nutrition disorders.
I. Cataldo, Corinne Balog. II. Rolfes, Sharon Rady. III. Title.
    [DNLM: 1. Diet Therapy. 2. Nutrition. QU 145 W618ua]
QP141.W458 1991
613.2—dc20
DNLM/DLC
for Library of Congress   91-10348
                                                    ∞   CIP

COPYEDITING Maggie Jarpey
COMPOSITION Carlisle Communications
DUMMY ARTIST David Farr, Imagesmythe, Inc.
TEXT AND COVER DESIGN Diane Beasley
ILLUSTRATIONS Rolin Graphics; Kidd & Company
COVER IMAGE Ascorbic acid (Vitamin C) crystals, photographed un-der a polarizing photomicroscope. A 40 milligram sample of ascorbic acid was sandwiched between a coverslip and a microscope slide and heated until melted with a bunsen burner. After recrystallization the sample was photographed with 4x objective after a 540 nm retardation plate had been inserted between the sample and the analyzer. Color correction was 20cc magenta and the exposure time was 0.07 sec-onds. © M. Davidson/Custom Medical Stock Photo

PHOTO CREDITS

1,2 From D.W. Fawcett, *The Cell*, 2nd. ed. (Phila-delphia: Saunders, 1981); color by Kidd & Com-pany; **3** © Richard Hutchings/PhotoEdit; **5** Ray Stanyard; **7, 8** © Charles Gupton/Stock, Boston; **16, 17** Thomas Tottleben/BPS; **22** © Williams & Edwards/The Image Bank; **25, 26** Courtesy of U.S. Department of Agriculture; **28, 30, 31** Ray Stanyard; **36, 37** Felicia Martinez/PhotoEdit; **41** Marilyn Herbert; **43, 44** From D.W. Fawcett, *The Cell*, 2nd. ed. (Philadelphia: Saunders, 1981); color by Kidd & Company; **55** Courtesy of Dr. Susumu Ito; **71, 72** From D.W. Fawcett, *The Cell*, 2nd. ed. (Philadelphia: Saunders, 1981); color by

Kidd & Company; **73** © Peter Miller/The Image Bank; **77** © Michael Skott/The Image Bank; **82** © Tony Freeman/PhotoEdit; **87, 95** Ray Stanyard; **98** Felicia Martinez/PhotoEdit; **105, 106** From D.W. Fawcett, *The Cell*, 2nd. ed. (Philadelphia: Saunders, 1981); color by Kidd & Company; **122** © Bob Daemmrich/Stock, Boston; **124, 125** Ray Stanyard; **126** Felicia Martinez/PhotoEdit; **127** Ray Stanyard; **133, 134** From D.W. Fawcett, *The Cell*, 2nd. ed. (Philadelphia: Saunders, 1981); color by Kidd & Company; **137** Human Hemo-globin model constructed by Dr. Makio Mu-rayama, NIH, Bethesda, Maryland (scaled to ½

inch to angstrom). Atomic coordinates were sup-plied for the model by Dr. Max F. Perutz, Cam-bridge, England; **152** © Steve Maines/Stock, Bos-ton; **156** Ray Stanyard; **157** Felecia Martinez/PhotoEdit; **158** © Michael Grecco/Stock, Boston; **159 (top three photographs)** Tony Freeman/PhotoEdit; **(bottom left)** Leslye Borden/Photo-Edit; **(bottom middle and right)** Tony Free-man/PhotoEdit; **165** © Richard Hutchings/Photo-Edit; **169, 170** Woodfin Camp & Associates/Tore Johnson; **193, 194** From D.W. Fawcett, *The Cell*, 2nd. ed. (Philadelphia: Saunders, 1981); color by

(continued following index)

Contents in Brief

APPENDIXES

Contents

5 The Lipids: Fats, Oils, Phospholipids, and Sterols   105

6 Protein: Amino Acids   133

7 Metabolism: Nutrient Transformations and Interactions   169

8 The Water-Soluble Vitamins: B Vitamins and Vitamin C   193

9 The Fat-Soluble Vitamins: A, D, E, and K   237

10 Water and the Major Minerals   271

11 The Trace Minerals   314

28 *Nutrition and Disorders of the Blood Vessels, Heart, and Lungs* 853

29 *Nutrition and Disorders of the Kidneys* 893

30 *Nutrition and Wasting Disorders: Cancer and AIDS* 923

Appendixes

About the Authors

Eleanor Noss Whitney, Ph.D., R.D., received her B.A. in biology from Radcliffe College in 1960 and her Ph.D. in biology with an emphasis on genetics from Washington University, St. Louis, in 1970. Formerly an associate professor at the Florida State University, she now devotes full time to research, writing, and consulting on nutrition, health, and the environment. Her earlier publications include articles in *Science, Genetics,* and other journals. Her textbooks include *Nutrition: Concepts and Controversies, Understanding Nutrition, Nutrition and Diet Therapy, Life Choices, Life Span Nutrition,* and *The Fitness Triad.* She is editor of *Nutrition Clinics,* a bimonthly monograph series published by J. B. Lippincott, and she serves as president of the Nutrition and Health Associates, an information resource center in Tallahassee.

Corinne Balog Cataldo, M.M.Sc., R.D., L.D., C.N.S.D., received her B.S. in Community Health Nutrition from Georgia State University in 1976 and her M.M.Sc. in Clinical Dietetics from Emory University in 1979. She has worked in private practice in Atlanta, as a clinical dietitian and metabolic support nutritionist at Georgia Baptist Medical Center in Atlanta, as a faculty member and dietetic internship coordinator at Emory University, and as a nutritionist with the Infant Formula Council. She has made numerous presentations, and in addition to this book, she has written a manual on tube feeding and the book *Nutrition and Diet Therapy.* She has recently became a certified nutrition support dietitian and continues to do consulting work.

Sharon Rady Rolfes, M.S., R.D., received her B.S. in psychology and criminology in 1974 and her M.S. in nutrition and food science in 1982 at the Florida State University. She is a founding member of the Nutrition and Health Associates and serves on the board of directors. Her publications include *Understanding Nutrition, Life Span Nutrition, Life Cycle Nutrition,* and several *Nutrition Clinics* on topics such as the role of high-fat diets in obesity, cancer, heart disease, vegetarian diet planning, hypoglycemia, and dental health. She is currently working on the preparation of *Understanding Clinical Nutrition,* the clinical portion of this book, to be published separately.

Preface

 When we wrote the first edition of *Understanding Normal and Clinical Nutrition,* our goal was to provide an up-to-date and accurate textbook that included both normal and clinical nutrition. We wanted the book to hold the reader's attention—to provide more than just facts. We also wanted readers to understand how the facts apply to people and to everyday life. Our goals for this third edition of the book are basically unchanged. However, we have revised the book substantially to reflect the many changes that have taken place in the field of nutrition over the years.

This book presents the core information of an introductory nutrition course for students entering the health care profession. Based on the principles of chemistry and molecular biology, the first eleven chapters describe the nutrients and how the body handles them. Chapter 1 provides an overview of the nutrients, and Chapter 2 presents current recommendations and guides for diet planning. In Chapter 3, readers follow the journey of digestion and absorption as the body transforms foods into nutrients. Chapters 4 through 6 describe carbohydrates, fats, and proteins—their chemistry, their health effects, their roles in the body, and their place in the diet. Then Chapter 7 shows how the body yields energy from these three nutrients. Chapters 8 through 11 complete the introductory lessons by describing water, the vitamins, and the minerals—their roles in the body, their deficiency and toxicity symptoms, and their sources.

The next six chapters weave that basic information into pieces that illustrate how nutrition influences people's lives. Several of these chapters are new to this edition and reflect the trend toward promoting optimal health through optimal nutrition. Chapter 12 looks at the energy balance equation and explores the possible causes and treatments of obesity and underweight. Chapter 13 recognizes that the partnership of nutrition with fitness enhances health, and shows how the nutrients work together to support physical activity. Chapters 14 and 15 show the special nutrient needs of people through the life span—pregnancy, infancy, childhood, adolescence, and adulthood. Chapter 16 addresses consumer concerns about the safety of the food supply, and Chapter 17 displays the problems of domestic and world hunger and environmental degradation, together with some approaches to the solutions.

The clinical portion of the book begins with Chapter 18, which introduces the relationships between nutrition and illness, including the body's responses to severe stress, to attacks on the immune system, and to drug therapy. More complete than previous editions, Chapter 19 describes the methods commonly used to assess nutrition status, and Chapter 20 shows how nutrition care providers develop, implement, and evaluate nutrition care plans to meet their clients' needs. Chapters 21 and 22 focus on enteral and parenteral nutrition. The remaining eight chapters examine the specific dietary care required for clients with particular medical conditions—conditions that involve trauma, upper and lower GI dysfunctions, liver disease, diabetes, heart and blood abnormalities, lung disorders, kidney disease, and the wasting disorders of cancer and AIDS.

To the person reading this text, it will be obvious that, like even the most exact sciences, nutrition possesses no absolute certainties. Nutrition scientists simply do not have all the answers yet; in some cases, we have not even asked all the questions yet. This is true in many areas of nutrition; it is a growing, young science dating only from around the turn of the century. One of the missions of this text is to show readers how researchers and health care providers ascertain the "facts." Scattered throughout this edition's chapters, are "Nutrition Detective Work" boxes, which step behind the scenes to explain the workings of research; and "Clinical Detective Work" boxes, which ask the reader to search through the facts of case studies looking for clues to the best care for clients.

Many of the chapters in this edition also include skill boxes that guide readers through problem-solving tasks. For example, one shows readers how to calculate a person's niacin intake from a given protein consumption; another shows how to determine the energy needs of a client with burns.

Each chapter closes with study questions and a self-study exercise. Study questions offer readers an opportunity to review the major concepts presented in the chapter. In the normal nutrition chapters, the self-study sections ask readers to examine their own diets; for example, to calculate nutrient intakes for a day's meals. The clinical self-studies ask readers to experience therapeutic diets first-hand; for example, one instructs them to plan and follow a pureed diet for a day.

Highlights on current issues of interest alternate with the chapters. Each highlight provides readers with a brief look at a topic that relates to its companion chapter. The new highlights in this edition address such subjects as nutrition experts, artificial fats, the health aspects of vegetarian diets, dental health, lead toxicity in children, supplements used by athletes to enhance performance, fetal alcohol syndrome, the aging brain, and relationships between nutrition and the environment. Several of the new highlights in the clinical portion of the book describe how clients live with their diseases and treatments. Other new clinical highlights include health messages on food labels, healthful ethnic food choices, and cost containment in nutrition care.

The appendixes are valuable references for a number of purposes. Appendix A summarizes background information on the hormonal and nervous systems, complementing Appendixes B and C on basic chemistry, the chemical structures of nutrients, and major metabolic pathways. Appendix D assists readers with calculations and conversions. Appendix E contains supplemental information on nutrition assessment, and Appendix F lists nutrition resources, including book and journal recommendations as well as addresses. Appendix G presents the U.S. Four Food Group Plan, the U. S. Exchange System, and the Canadian Food Group System. Appendix H is a 1600-item food composition table made from the latest nutrient data base assembled by ESHA Research, Inc., of Salem, Oregon. Appendix I presents the Recommended Dietary Allowances (1989 RDA) and the Canadian Recommended Nutrient Intakes (1990 RNI). Appendix J describes measures of protein quality and Appendix K provides the forms needed to complete the self-study exercises presented at the ends of chapters. Appendix L offers the latest product information on enteral formulas.

We have tried to keep the number of footnotes to a minimum. Most statements that have appeared in previous editions with footnotes now appear without them, but every statement is backed by evidence, and the authors will supply references upon request.

We hope our informal, conversational writing style makes the study of nutrition an enjoyable experience. Nutrition is a fascinating subject, and we hope our enthusiasm for it comes through on every page.

Eleanor Noss Whitney
Corinne Balog Cataldo
Sharon Rady Rolfes
April 1991

Acknowledgments

To produce a book requires the coordinated effort of a team of people—and, no doubt, each team member has another team of support people as well. We salute, with a big round of applause, everyone who has worked so diligently to ensure the quality of this book.

Our thanks to Elisa Malo and Nancie Hopkins for their patient attention to manuscript preparation, permissions, and other office tasks. To Linda Patton, a special thank you for her skilled assistance in library research. We also appreciate the work of Lori Turner, Jana Kicklighter, and Wayne Billon in preparing the Instructor's Manual, Test Bank, Student Study Guide, and Case Study Manual that accompany this text. Thanks to Betty Hands, Bob Geltz, and their staff at ESHA for their meticulous effort in creating the food composition appendix and the computerized diet analysis program that accompanies this book. Our special thanks to the editorial team of Peter Marshall, Jane Bacon, and Sharon Kavanagh for their conscientious coordination of reviews and production. To the many others involved in designing, drawing, photographing, copyediting, indexing, typesetting, dummying, and marketing, we tip our hats in appreciation.

A special thank you to our associates, friends, and family members for their continued encouragement and support. We also thank our many reviewers for their comments and contributions.

Reviewers of *Understanding Normal and Clinical Nutrition*

Connie Elliff
Lamar University

Martha Erickson
Indiana University

Pam Fletcher
Albuquerque Vocational-
Technical Institute

Sally Fletcher
Kansas City Kansas Community
College

Sareen Gropper
Auburn University

Mary Jane Hamilton
Del Mar College

Annamarie Herndon
Purdue University-North Central

Margaret James
University of Wisconsin-Stout

Marilyn Murphy
George Mason University

Mary Ann Neeley
University of Texas Health
Science Center at Houston

Penni Nielsen
Eastern Washington University

Annette Peel
Eastern Michigan University

Nancy Rexrode
York College of Pennsylvania

Mary Sandall
Spokane Community College

Rani Singh
Emory University

Joanne Spaide
University of Northern Iowa

Reviewers of *Understanding Nutrition* (Fifth Edition)

Liz Applegate
University of California at Davis

Andrea Arquitt
Oklahoma State University

George Bates
Texas A & M University

Margaret Behme
University Hospital,
London, Ontario

Carolyn Campbell
University of New Mexico

Dorothy Coltrin
DeAnza College

James Daugherty
Glendale Community College

Jodee Dorsey
Florida State University

Norma Jean Downes
San Jose State University

Evelyn Farriar
East Carolina University

Gayle Gess
Fullerton College

Barbara Gilpin
Mesa Community College

Betsy Haughton
University of Tennessee-
Knoxville

Michael Houston
University of Waterloo

Jean Humphrey
Johns Hopkins University
School of Medicine

Elaine Johnson
City College of San Francisco

Catherine Justice
Purdue University

Michael Keenan
Louisiana State University

Elizabeth Kunkel
Clemson University

Roseann Kutschke
University of Texas-Austin

Richard Machemer, Jr.
St. John Fisher College

Michael McBurney
University of Alberta

Stella Miller
Mt. San Antonio College

Sandra Mitchell
California State University-Chico

Peggy Morrison
Pensacola Jr. College

Pat Munyon
Mesa College

Irvin Plitzuweit
Rochester Community College

Roseann Poole
Tallahassee Community College

Bruce Rengers
Florida State University

Carol Reynolds
California Polytechnic State
University-Pomona

Robert Sargent
University of South Florida

Genevieve Chung Schickler
Broward Community College

Lou Schutt
Western Washington University

Harry Sitren
University of Florida

Sam Smith
University of New Hampshire

Arlene Spark
New York Medical College

Joanne Steiner
Indiana University

Jody Yates-Taylor
Portland Community College

Junia Wager
Sacramento City College

Lauretta Wasserstein
California State University-
Northridge

Elise West
Cornell University

Janet White
Rochester Institute of
Technology

1

An Overview of Nutrition

Macrophage →

Lymphocytes →

Contents

The body's cells are highly sensitive and energetic, and require many nutrients to sustain their activities. Shown here are three white blood cells—the body's defenders against disease.

You are a collection of moving parts—atoms, molecules, cells, tissues, and organs—all arranged in order. These parts are continually changing, even though the overall arrangement remains constant, and they are continually using nutrients. Your skin, which seems to have covered you without changing from when you were born, is not the same skin that covered you seven years ago; it has been replaced entirely by new cells since then. The fat beneath your skin is not the same fat that was there a year ago. Your oldest red blood cell is only 120 days old, and the entire lining of your digestive tract is renewed every three days. To maintain your "self," you must continually replenish the energy you burn and replace the pieces you lose.

All the pieces you are made of have come from the nutrients contained in the foods you have eaten. Amazingly, though, you can eat foods entirely different from those someone else eats and still construct a normal human body from the nutrients in them. The secret is in the genetic information you inherited from your parents—which gives the instructions for raw materials to be assembled into the structures of your body. As long as the nutrients you need are all there in sufficient amounts, your genetic blueprint and assembly machinery will ensure that you are constructed according to plan and working as you should. The science of nutrition is the study of how this takes place—the study of the nutrients in foods and the body's handling of those nutrients.

The Nutrients

The complete chemical analysis of a food such as the green leafy vegetable spinach shows that it is composed of a number of different kinds of material, but its primary component is water (95 percent). Most of the solid materials are the compounds carbohydrate, fat, and protein. If you could remove these materials, you would find a tiny residue of minerals, vitamins, and other items. Water, carbohydrate, fat, protein, vitamins, and some of the minerals found in foods are nutrients—substances the body uses for the growth, maintenance, and repair of its tissues. (Nutrients that the body cannot make for itself in sufficient quantity to meet its needs, and so must obtain from the diet, are called *essential nutrients*.)

While a look in the mirror would not convince you, a complete chemical analysis of your body would show that it is made of materials similar to those in foods. A healthy 150-pound person's body contains about 90 pounds of water and about 30 pounds of fat. The other 30 pounds are mostly protein and carbohydrate, related organic compounds made from them, and the major minerals of the bones: calcium and phosphorus. Vitamins, other minerals, and incidental extras constitute a fraction of a pound. Thus the human body, like spinach, is composed largely of nutrients.

If you burn a food such as spinach in air, it seems to disappear. The water evaporates, and all the organic compounds are oxidized to gas (carbon dioxide) and water vapor, leaving only a residue of ash (minerals). An organic compound contains carbon atoms, usually bonded to other carbon atoms, hydrogen atoms, or both. The first organic compounds known were natural

science of nutrition: the study of nutrients in foods and of the body's handling of them (including ingestion, digestion, absorption, transport, metabolism, interaction, storage, and excretion). A broader definition includes the study of the environment and of human behavior as it relates to these processes.

food: nutritive material taken into the body for the maintenance of life and the growth and repair of tissues (**nutritive**: containing nutrients).

nutrient: a substance obtained from food and used in the body to promote growth, maintenance, and/or repair. The **essential nutrients** are those the body cannot make for itself in sufficient quantity to meet physiological need, and which must therefore be obtained from food.

The six classes of nutrients:
- Carbohydrate.
- Fat.
- Protein.
- Vitamins.
- Minerals.
- Water.

products synthesized by plants or animals; indeed, it used to be thought that only living things contributed organic compounds to our world. The term has since been expanded to include all carbon compounds, whatever their origin. Four of the six classes of nutrients (carbohydrate, fat, protein, and vitamins) are organic, whereas the other two (minerals and water) are inorganic.

This book is devoted mostly to the nutrients, but other constituents are also found in foods and in your body—alcohols, organic acids, pigments, additives, and others. Some are beneficial, some are neutral, and a few are harmful. Later sections of the book focus on some of these constituents and their significance.

organic: a substance or a molecule containing carbon or, more strictly, containing carbon-carbon bonds or carbon-hydrogen bonds.*

The organic nutrients:
- Carbohydrate.
- Fat.
- Protein.
- Vitamins.

The inorganic nutrients:
- Minerals.
- Water.

The Energy-Yielding Nutrients

During metabolism, three of the four classes of organic nutrients (carbohydrate, fat, and protein) provide energy the body can use. (In contrast, vitamins, minerals, and water do not yield energy in the human body.) The energy-yielding nutrients—nutrients that can break down to yield energy the body can use—are vital to life, for without continual replenishment of the energy you spend daily, you would soon die. When the body metabolizes the energy-yielding nutrients, the bonds between their atoms break, and the carbon and hydrogen atoms combine with oxygen to yield carbon dioxide and water. As these nutrients break down, they release energy. Some of this energy is released as heat, some is transferred into other compounds (including fat) that compose the structures of your body cells, and some is used as fuel for your activities.

The amount of energy the energy-yielding nutrients release can be measured in calories (or more properly, kilocalories or kcalories), which are familiar to everyone as a measure of food energy and of the energy the body spends during exercise. People think of "kcalories" as a constituent of foods, but strictly speaking, they are not; they are a *measure* of the energy in foods.** Thus to speak of the kcalories in an apple or a cookie is technically incorrect, just as to speak of the inches in a person is incorrect. It is correct to speak of the *energy* available from a food (and of the *height* of a person), and that is what this book will do.

When completely broken down in the body, a gram of carbohydrate provides about 4 kcalories; a gram of protein also provides 4; and a gram of fat provides 9 kcalories. The energy content of a food thus depends on how much carbohydrate, fat, and protein it contains. If your body doesn't use these nutrients to fuel metabolic and physical activities, it rearranges them (and the energy they contain) into storage compounds such as body fat, and puts them away for use between meals and overnight. If you take in more energy than

The energy-yielding nutrients:
- Carbohydrate.
- Fat.
- Protein.

energy-yielding nutrients: the nutrients that break down to yield energy the body can use.

Metabolism, the processes by which nutrients are broken down to yield energy or rearranged into body structures, is defined and described in Chapter 7.

calorie: a unit by which energy is measured. Technically, a calorie is the amount of heat necessary to raise the temperature of 1 g of water 1°C. Food energy is measured in **kilocalories** (thousands of calories), abbreviated **kcalories** or **kcal**. A capitalized version is also sometimes used: **Calories**. Most people, even nutritionists, speak of these units simply as calories, but on paper they are prefaced by a *k*. (The pronunciation of *kcalories* ignores the *k*, but some people, when speaking, pronounce it "KAY-calories" or "KAY-cal.") We will use *kcalories* and *kcal* throughout this book.

---

*This definition excludes coal and a few carbon-containing compounds that contain only a single carbon and no hydrogen, such as carbon dioxide (CO_2), calcium carbonate ($CaCO_3$), magnesium carbonate ($MgCO_3$), and sodium cyanide ($NaCN$).
**Food energy can also be measured in kilojoules (kJ). A kilojoule is the amount of energy expended when 1 kg is moved 1 meter by a force of 1 newton. It is thus a measure of work energy, whereas the kcalorie is a measure of heat energy. Both are metric measures.

One kcalorie equals 4.2 kJ. The kilojoule is the international unit of energy. The United States and Canada are slowly switching over to it, but it is not in popular use yet. This book uses the kcalorie. For those using kilojoules: 1 g carbohydrate = 17 kJ; 1 g protein = 17 kJ; 1 g fat = 37 kJ; and 1 g alcohol = 29 kJ.

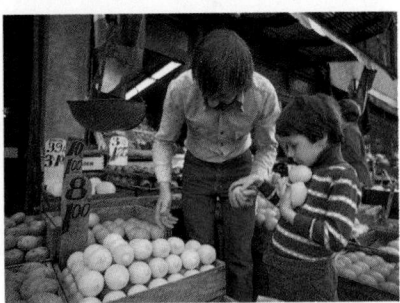

When people shop for foods, they are buying nutrients.

- 1 g carbohydrate = 4 kcal.
- 1 g protein = 4 kcal.
- 1 g fat = 9 kcal.

(In light of current research, fat kcalories may be revised upwards; see Chapter 12.)

- 1 g alcohol = 7 kcal.

A huge molecule, composed of hundreds or thousands of atoms, is a **macromolecule**. A molecule of water (H_2O), by contrast, is composed of only three atoms: two hydrogens and one oxygen.

Appendix B summarizes basic chemistry facts and provides definitions of atoms, elements, molecules, and compounds.

Compound

vitamin: an essential (organic) nutrient required in small amounts.
  vita = life
  amine = containing nitrogen (the first vitamins discovered contained nitrogen)

Vitamins yield no energy.

you expend, no matter from which of the three energy-yielding nutrients, the result is a weight gain as body fat. Too much meat (a protein-rich food) is just as fattening as too many potatoes (a carbohydrate-rich food).

One other substance contributes food energy: alcohol. Alcohol is not a nutrient, because it supports no growth, maintenance, or repair in the body. Still, people do consume alcohol, and it shares several characteristics with the energy-yielding nutrients. Like them, alcohol is metabolized in the body to yield energy (7 kcalories per gram). When taken in excess of energy need, alcohol, too, is converted to body fat and stored. However, when alcohol contributes a substantial portion of the energy in a person's diet, it is harmful. (Highlight 7 is devoted to alcohol and nutrition.)

Practically all foods contain mixtures of all three energy-yielding nutrients, although they are sometimes classified by the predominant nutrient. Thus it is inaccurate to speak of meat as a protein or of bread as a carbohydrate; they are *foods* rich in these nutrients. A protein-rich food like beef actually contains a lot of fat as well as protein; a carbohydrate-rich food like bread also contains a trace of fat and a little protein. Only a few foods are exceptions to this rule, the common ones being sugar (which is almost pure carbohydrate) and oil (which is almost pure fat).

The energy-yielding nutrients are (by molecular standards) tremendous in size. For example, a single molecule of carbohydrate may be composed of 300 smaller molecules, each containing 24 atoms, for a total of some 7,000 atoms.

Furthermore, you eat (by molecular standards) tremendous quantities of the three energy-yielding nutrients—50 to 200 grams or more a day of each. If you could extract and purify the carbohydrate, fat, and protein from your daily diet, they would fill two or three measuring cups. The foods they come in weigh much more and occupy much more volume. A hundred grams of food may contain only ten or so grams of energy-yielding nutrients, the rest being water, fiber, and other non-kcaloric materials. (The accompanying box provides a few examples of food portion sizes using metric measures.)

Your body's use (metabolism) of the energy-yielding nutrients can be summarized, simply, as follows. First, food protein, fat, and carbohydrate are broken down to simpler compounds. The process yields energy and small fragments of the original materials. The energy may:

- Help build new compounds (and some energy may be stored in them).
- Help move the body (do work).
- Escape as heat.

Then, the fragments may be:

- Used to build new compounds (contributing to fat, muscle, or other tissues).
- Excreted as waste materials.

The Vitamins

The vitamins, the next class of nutrients, differ profoundly from the first three classes (carbohydrate, fat, and protein) in almost every way: in their size and shape, in the roles they play, and in the amounts you consume. Perhaps the only characteristics the vitamins share with the first three classes of nutrients are that they are vital to life, they are organic, and they are available in food.

A Note about Metric Measures

Most people think of foods and beverages in terms of cups, quarts, and teaspoons, not milliliters, liters, and grams. It's easy to learn to think in metric measures, though, and a good idea for those who plan to work with foods in the future. A standard portion (a half cup) of most vegetables or a half cup of milk or juice has a volume of about 125 ml and weighs roughly 100 g. A quart of liquid is approximately 1 liter (1,000 ml). A teaspoon of dry powder such as sugar or salt weighs roughly 5 g. For accurate conversion factors and other units of measure, see Appendix D.

Half-cup vegetable servings are about 125 ml (close to 100 g if weighed).

A half-cup of juice or milk is also about 125 ml and weighs just over 100 g.

One teaspoon of granular powder is about 5 g.

The vitamins are generally much smaller than the energy-yielding nutrients. The body may break them down but does not extract usable energy from them; their role is to serve as helpers, making possible the processes by which the other nutrients are digested, absorbed, and metabolized to body compounds or excreted. There are 13 different vitamins, each with its own special roles to play (see Table 1–1).

That vitamins are organic has a significant consequence—they are destructible. They can be broken down and altered, and so the body must handle them with care. The body makes special provisions to absorb and transport vitamins, providing many of them with custom-made protein carriers. A vitamin may be useful in one form here and in another there, so special metabolic processes subtly alter the characteristics of a vitamin to allow it to perform a particular task.

The vitamins are divided into two classes: some are soluble in water (the B vitamins and vitamin C) and others are soluble in fat (vitamins A, D, E, and K). This fact has many implications for the kinds of foods that contain them; their potential for destruction; and the ways the body absorbs, transports, stores, and excretes them. The water-soluble vitamins are the subject of Chapter 8 and the fat-soluble vitamins, of Chapter 9.

The Minerals

Minerals are inorganic elements, even smaller than vitamins. They can occur in the simplest of chemical forms, as single atoms, tiny in comparison with the energy-yielding nutrients, which may be composed of thousands of atoms. Some minerals may be put together into orderly arrays in such structures as

■ TABLE 1–1
The Vitamins → "HELPERS"

The Fat-Soluble Vitamins

Vitamin A
Vitamin D
Vitamin E
Vitamin K

The Water-Soluble Vitamins

B vitamins
  Thiamin
  Riboflavin
  Niacin
  Vitamin B_6
  Vitamin B_{12}
  Folate
  Biotin
  Pantothenic acid
Vitamin C

Source: The names given here for the vitamins are those agreed on by the International Union of Nutritional Sciences Committee on Nomenclature, in Nomenclature policy: Generic descriptors and trivial names for vitamins and related compounds, *Journal of Nutrition* 117 (1987): 7–15.

mineral: a small, ~~inorganic~~ atom or molecule; some minerals are essential nutrients required in small amounts.

ELEMENT

Minerals yield no energy.

■ **TABLE 1–2**
The Minerals[a]

The Major Minerals

Calcium
Phosphorus
Potassium
Sodium
Chloride
Magnesium
Sulfur

The Trace Minerals

Iron
Iodine
Zinc
Chromium
Selenium
Flouride
Molybdenum
Copper
Manganese

[a]Requirements for boron, nickel, silicon, and arsenic have been established for animals; proof of a human dietary need is still lacking. Diets extremely low in cadmium, lead, lithium, tin, and vanadium cause deficiency symptoms in animals, but the evidence for essentiality is weak. No RDA for cobalt is necessary as it is an integral part of vitamin B_{12}.

Water is inorganic.
Water yields no energy.

bones and teeth—but only with the help of the body's lively metabolic machinery (which itself is composed of protein and assisted by vitamins and some minerals). When minerals float about in the fluids of the body, they give the fluids certain characteristics, but they are not metabolized nor do they yield energy. You consume small amounts of most minerals daily, slightly greater than the amounts of vitamins in your diet. Some minerals are essential in human nutrition (see Table 1–2). Other minerals are still being studied; their functions have not yet been determined. Still others are important to nutrition because they are *not* nutrients, but may displace the minerals needed in the body, causing deranged body functions. The problems caused by one of the contaminant minerals, lead, are detailed in Highlight 11.

The minerals are elements, whereas the other nutrients are all compounds. This means the minerals cannot lose their identity; they exist "forever." When you cook a food containing vitamins and minerals, the elements that make up the vitamins can undergo rearrangement, and so the vitamins can lose their chemical identity; the minerals, however, remain unchanged. Because they are indestructible, minerals in foods need not be handled with the very special care that vitamins need. They can, however, be bound by substances that make them difficult to absorb or lost in water during cooking. If minerals are scarce in your diet, you have to choose food sources of them with care. Chapters 10 and 11 are devoted to the minerals.

Water

Water, indispensable and abundant, forms the major part of almost every body tissue. It is often ignored—because, like air, it is everywhere, and we take it for granted. Water is inorganic, being composed of two atoms of hydrogen bound to one atom of oxygen (H_2O). The amounts you must consume relative to the other nutrients are enormous: 2 to 3 liters (about 2 to 3 quarts) a day. That's 2,000 to 3,000 grams, compared with 50 or so grams of protein each day, and 200 or so grams of carbohydrate.

Water provides the medium in which nearly all the body's activities are conducted. It participates in many metabolic reactions and supplies the medium for transporting vital materials to cells and waste products away from them.

In addition to the obvious dietary source—water itself—water comes abundantly in foods and beverages. In addition, water is generated from the energy-yielding nutrients in foods during metabolism (the hydrogen in these nutrients combines with oxygen during metabolism to yield water). Water from these three sources normally balances perfectly with daily water losses. Water is discussed fully in Chapters 10 and 16, but it is mentioned in every chapter. If you watch for it, you cannot help but be impressed by water's participation in all life processes.

■ Why Do We Eat As We Do?

Eating involves more than people's simply delivering nutrients to their bodies. Food choices are personal and not always sensible. To a great extent, they resist change. Among the reasons why you choose the foods you eat today may be any of the following:

- ■ Personal preference (you like their flavor).
- ■ Habit or tradition (they are familiar; you always eat them).
- ■ Social pressure (they are offered; you feel you can't refuse them).
- ■ Availability (they are there and ready to eat).
- ■ Convenience (you are too rushed to prepare anything else).
- ■ Economy (they are within your financial means).
- ■ Nutritional value (you think your body requires them).

People enjoy companionship while eating.

Food does not become nutrition until it passes the lips.—Ronald M. Deutsch

Of these seven possible reasons, only one has to do with nutrition directly. Even people who pride themselves on eating nutritious foods will admit that the other six factors also influence their food choices. No matter how nutritious a meal is, it cannot benefit your health until you eat it.

Have you ever wondered why you like your mother's soup when you are sick or why a hot dog tastes best at a ballgame? One reason people like certain foods, of course, is preferences for certain tastes. Two of these preferences are widely shared: the tastes for sugar and salt. People tend to like foods with which they have happy associations—those they eat in the midst of a warm family gathering on traditional holidays, those given to them as children by someone who loved them, or those eaten by people whom they admire. By the same token, people can attach an intense and unalterable dislike to foods that they ate when they felt sick, or that were forced on them when they weren't hungry, or that are eaten by people they don't respect. Parents may have taught their children to like and dislike certain foods for similar reasons of their own, without even being aware of it.

Social pressure is another powerful influence on food behavior. How can you refuse when your friends are going out for pizza (or ice cream or doughnuts)? Such pressure operates in all circles and across cultural lines. An almost necessary element of etiquette and politeness is to accept food or drink being shared by a group or being offered by a host; you are not a member of the social gathering until you do.

The influence of availability, convenience, and economy on your food selections is clear. Obviously, you cannot eat foods if they are not available, if you cannot prepare them, or if you cannot afford them. Convenience is a major factor in the purchasing decisions of many people. Consumers look for speed in preparation, recipes with few ingredients, and products that can be cooked in a microwave oven.[1] Apparently, the days of "three square home-cooked meals from scratch" are disappearing.

Although the nutritional value of food is only one of many factors influencing people's food choices, nutrition has grown in importance for many consumers.[2] Some people are interested in nutrition as a way to avoid illness; others seek nutrition to improve their physical well-being. Food manufacturers have responded to the scientific findings linking health and nutrition with an abundant selection of grocery-store foods and beverages advertised as low-kcalorie, low-cholesterol, low-fat, low-sodium, sugar-free, caffeine-free, high-fiber, and calcium-enriched items. Consumers accept these new, health-promoting foods in their diets, provided that the foods are easy to identify (clearly labeled), easy to find in the grocery store, fast and convenient to prepare, and that they taste good—as good as the traditional choices.

Sometimes consumers choose products they *perceive* to offer a benefit—such as an association with luxury and wealth, an image of slimness and weight loss, an association with a concern for health, or with convenience that allows more time for fun and leisure. With the right image, foods low in fat and high in nutrients would be well-accepted. Foods without labels such as nonfat milk, fruits, vegetables, lean meats, legumes, and whole grains might benefit from some trendy publicity.[3] The revival of the California raisin is an example of just how effective food image campaigns can be. Raisin growers spent millions to change their product's image in 1988, and while the product remained the same, consumers rewarded the growers' efforts with greatly increased sales. This book has much to say in the chapters to come about purchasing and preparing nutritious foods.

■ *Assessment of Nutrition Status*

What happens when people don't get enough or get too much of a nutrient? If the deficiency or excess is significant, they get sick, one way or another, and they exhibit signs of malnutrition. Assessment techniques have been developed to detect nutrient imbalances.

Malnutrition can be detected by analyzing the combined findings from a number of assessment techniques. One method of evaluating nutrition status is to obtain information about a person's diet. The assessor analyzes a record of all the foods the person has eaten over a period of days or weeks. (The days have to be fairly typical of the person's diet, and the record has to pay special attention to portion sizes.) To determine the amounts of nutrients consumed, the assessor looks up each food in a table of food composition such as Appendix H in this book or enters the food portions into a computer and uses a diet analysis program. Then the assessor compares the calculated nutrient intakes with recommended intakes. This kind of diet assessment is recommended for you, the reader, in the self-study exercises at the ends of the chapters in this book. To interpret these exercises correctly, you have to be aware that nutrient values are not absolute (different oranges vary in vitamin C content, for example), and that the exercises assume that reasonable care was taken in the preparation of foods (for example, they weren't so seriously overcooked that vitamins were lost).

A second technique that may reveal nutrition problems is the taking of anthropometric measures such as height, weight, and limb circumferences (*anthropos* means "person"; *metric* means "measuring"). These measures alert the assessor to such serious problems as growth failure in children, wasting or swelling of body tissue in adults, and obesity—conditions that reflect nutrient deficiencies or excesses.

A third nutrition assessment technique is a physical examination that looks for clues to poor nutrition status. Every part of the body that can be inspected can offer such clues: the hair, eyes, skin, posture, tongue, fingernails, and others. This technique can detect evidence pointing to deficiencies, imbalances, and toxicity states.

A fourth way to detect a developing deficiency, imbalance, or toxicity state is to take samples of body tissues (like blood or urine) and analyze them in the

malnutrition: an imbalance of nutrient intakes—either an underconsumption or an overconsumption of energy or nutrients.
  mal = bad

Nutrition assessment techniques:
  • Dietary data.
  • Anthropometric measures.
  • Physical examination.
  • Laboratory tests.

A health care provider uses weight and height measures to help evaluate nutrition status.

laboratory. In cases of malnutrition problems that are just beginning, body changes may not be obvious, but laboratory tests may reveal them. Many more details of nutrition assessment techniques are offered in Chapter 19 and in Appendix E.

The mineral iron can be used to illustrate the stages in the development of a nutrient deficiency. The appearance of an overt iron deficiency is the last of a long sequence of events, as shown in Figure 1–1. First, too little iron gets into the body—either because there is not enough iron in the person's food (a primary deficiency) or because the person's body can't absorb enough of the iron taken in or use it normally (a secondary deficiency). (A diet history would provide clues.) The body then begins to use up its own stores of iron, so there is a period of declining stores. (Laboratory tests might be able to detect these.) At this point, the deficiency might be said to be subclinical— that is, to exist already as a covert condition, before outward signs appear. Finally, iron stores are used up, and the body can't make enough of the iron-containing protein hemoglobin to fill the developing new red blood cells that carry oxygen to all the body's cells and enable them to get energy. At this point, the number of red blood cells declines, the new ones made are smaller than normal and pale, and every part of the body feels the effects of an oxygen lack. The overt symptoms of an iron deficiency—weakness, fatigue, pallor, and headaches—ensue, reflecting the internal state of the blood. (Physical examination would reveal these symptoms.)

This overview of nutrition assessment illustrates the principles that under-lie the chapters on the vitamins and minerals. For one, internal changes precede outward signs of deficiencies or excesses. As a corollary, signs of sickness need not appear before a person takes corrective measures. Tests can either reveal that there are problems in the early stages or confirm that nutrient stores are adequate.

overt (oh-VERT): out in the open and easy to observe.
  ouvrir = to open

primary deficiency: a nutrient deficiency caused by inadequate dietary intake of a nutrient.

secondary deficiency: a nutrient deficiency caused by something other than diet, such as a disease condition that reduces absorption, increases excretion, or causes destruction of the nutrient.

subclinical deficiency: a deficiency in the early stages, before the outward signs have appeared.

covert (KOH-vert): hidden, as if under covers.
  couvrir = to cover

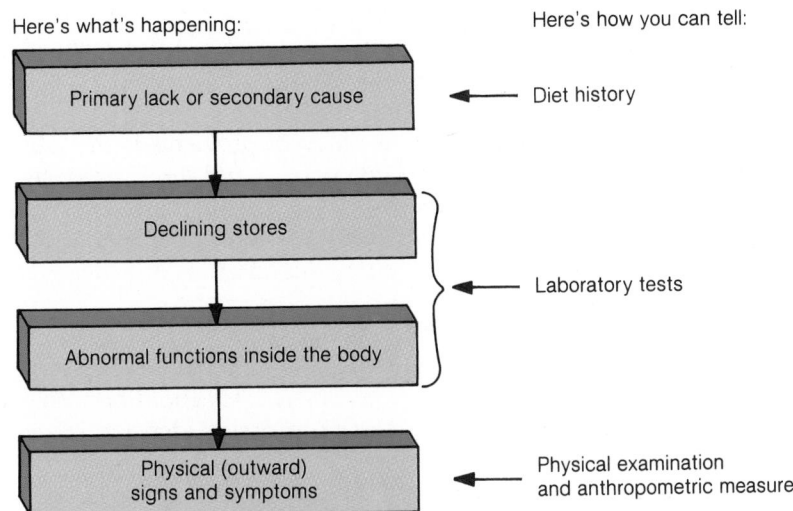

Here's what's happening:

Here's how you can tell:

Primary lack or secondary cause ← Diet history

Declining stores

Abnormal functions inside the body

← Laboratory tests

Physical (outward) signs and symptoms ← Physical examination and anthropometric measures

■ FIGURE 1–1
Stages in the Development of a Nutrient Deficiency
Notice that attention to diet can prevent problems at the earliest possible time.

Source: Adapted from H. H. Sandstead and W. N. Pearson, Clinical evaluation of nutrition status, in *Modern Nutrition in Health and Disease*, ed. R. S. Goodhart and M. E. Shils (Philadelphia: Lea and Febiger, 1973), p. 585.

■ *Nutrition Surveys*

To assess the nutrition status of a population, researchers use surveys. One kind of survey—a food consumption survey—determines what foods people eat, calculates or measures the nutrients in them, and compares the amounts of nutrients consumed with a standard such as the Recommended Dietary Allowance, or RDA. Another kind of survey—a nutrition status survey—assesses the nutrition status of the people themselves, using the techniques described in the previous section: a combination of diet histories, anthropometric measures, physical examinations, and laboratory tests.

Both kinds of surveys have been conducted in the United States and Canada, and the same general impressions have been confirmed. Many people are overconsuming foods, underexpending energy, or both. While the majority of the people are adequately nourished with respect to most individual nutrients, deficiencies and marginal intakes of nutrients do exist. The remedies for these nutrition problems can be stated in three recommendations:

- ■ Consume less fat, sugar, and salt.
- ■ Choose more foods high in fiber and nutrients relative to their kcalories.
- ■ Exercise regularly so as to afford a food energy intake sufficient to convey the needed nutrients.

The next chapter will focus on nutrient recommendations and dietary guidelines. The following chapters will describe how your body receives the nutrients from the foods you eat and will show what nutrients you need, what foods supply them, and how your body uses them. All that knowledge is not enough to support your nutritional health, however. You need to work out a way to combine foods into a healthful eating plan tailored to your individual or family lifestyle. To integrate all that you know into a way of life in which meals yield all the benefits you want from them—social enjoyment, sensory pleasure, ease of preparation, economy, *and* good health—is to serve yourself well.

food consumption survey: a survey that measures the amounts and kinds of foods people consume, estimates the nutrient intakes, and compares them with a standard such as the RDA.

nutrition status survey: a survey that evaluates people's nutrition status using diet histories, anthropometric measures, physical examinations, and laboratory tests.

SELF STUDY *Record What You Eat*

How well do you eat? Our purpose in providing these self-study exercises is to encourage you to study your own diet. Your reaction to the exercises may be that they contain both good news and bad news. The bad news is that they will require your time and attention. Like your checkbook, they have to be done carefully, with frequent checking of arithmetic and tidy handwriting, so that they will be accurate and meaningful.

The good news, however, may well outweigh the drawbacks. Most students who do these activities with thoughtful attention report that unlike income tax returns, they are intriguing, informative, and often reassuring. They are also rewarding—in direct proportion to your honesty.

In this first exercise you are to make a record of your typical days' food intake; in the next one, you will analyze the record for the nutrients it contains. You are undertaking this analysis before you have learned very much about the nutrients, but there's

an advantage in that: having the results in front of you as you read will make the reading more meaningful. As you learn about each nutrient and ask yourself how much of it you consume, you will already have the answer in front of you, ready for interpretation and action.

Use three copies of Form 1 (Appendix K), and record on them all the foods you eat for a three-day period. If, like most people, you eat differently on weekdays than on weekends, then to get a true average you should probably record for two weekdays and one weekend day. Better still, make seven copies of Form 1, and record your food intakes for a week.

As you record each food, make careful note of the amount. Estimate the amount to the nearest ounce, quarter cup, tablespoon, or other common measure. In guessing at the sizes of meat portions, it helps to know that a piece of meat the size of the palm of your hand weighs about 3 or 4 ounces. If you are unable to estimate serving sizes in cups, tablespoons, or teaspoons, try measuring out servings the size of a cup, tablespoon, and teaspoon onto a plate or into a bowl to see how they

look. It also helps to know that a slice of cheese (such as sliced American cheese) or a 1½-inch cube of cheese weighs roughly 1 ounce.

You may have to break down mixed dishes to their ingredients. However, many mixed dishes, including soups, are listed in Appendix H. Other mixtures are simple to analyze. A ham and cheese sandwich, for example, can be listed as 2 slices of bread, 1 tablespoon of mayonnaise, 2 ounces of ham, 1 ounce of cheese, and so on. If you can't discover all the ingredients, estimate the amounts of only the major ones, like the beef, tomatoes, and potatoes in a beef-vegetable soup.

You will, of course, make errors in estimating amounts. In calculations of this kind, errors of up to 20 percent are expected and tolerated. Still, you will have a rough approximation that will enable you to compare your nutrient intakes with the recommended ones.

Do not record any nutrient supplements you take. It will be interesting to discover whether your food choices alone deliver the nutrients you need. If they do not, you will know better after analyzing your diet what supplement to choose.

▮ Study Questions

1. What is a nutrient?
2. Name the nutrients found in foods.
3. Which nutrients are organic and which are inorganic? Discuss the significance of that distinction.
4. Which nutrients yield energy? How is energy measured?
5. Why do people eat certain foods and avoid others?
6. What happens when people don't get enough of the nutrients? How are nutrient deficiencies and excesses detected?
7. What methods are used in nutrition surveys, and what kinds of information can these surveys provide?

▮ Notes

1. C. Jackson, Today's food consumers: What they are looking for in a supermarket, *Cereal Foods World* 32 (1987): 417–419.
2. D.T. Farr, Consumer attitudes and the supermarket, *Cereal Foods World* 32 (1987): 413–415.
3. F.S. Sizer, *U.S. Food Choices: Recommendations and Realities,* a monograph (1989) available from J.B. Lippincott Co., East Washington Sq., Philadelphia, PA 19105.

The Body's Stress Response

Anyone interested in nutrition needs not only to study nutrients and foods, but also to acquire an understanding of the human body.* The interactions among foods, nutrients, and the body are not as simple as one might expect.

This highlight introduces the principle of homeostasis, the body's ability to adapt when internal conditions change, and to maintain equilibrium. Imagine for a moment that the body is a machine with millions of moving parts. The functioning of the whole depends on each part's doing its job exactly when needed and stopping when appropriate. The machine has a fabulous central control system—the central nervous system—that can evaluate information about conditions both within the machine and outside it. The machine can call into play whatever parts can best respond to any situation. It gets its information and transmits its instructions by way of a vast system of wiring. The system carries messages in both directions: signals about conditions from the parts to the center, and messages signaling work or rest from the center to the parts. The smooth functioning that results from the system's adjustments to changing conditions is homeostasis.

Homeostasis underlies wise nutrition judgment and competent diet advice; most misguided nutrition behavior neglects this principle. Throughout all your body systems, all processes are precisely and automatically regulated by hormone and nerve activity, without your conscious efforts. This leaves you free to compose a symphony or to gaze at the stars

instead of tying up your energy in worrying about how much calcium to store in your bones or when to contract your heart muscle. This remarkable arrangement once prompted the physiologist Claude Bernard to remark, "Stability of the internal environment is the condition of free life." Walter Cannon, another physiologist, wrote a whole book about these processes, aptly entitled *The Wisdom of the Body.*

The stress response illustrates vividly how the whole body reacts to anything that you experience as a threat to your stability or equilibrium. Both physical and psychological stressors elicit the body's stress response. Major physical stressors such as surgery, burns, and infections are discussed in more detail in Chapter 23; other physical stressors include, a very hot or humid climate, toxic compounds, radiation, and pollution. Table H1–1 lists major psychological stressors; change and threats constitute psychological stress. (Note that being busy is not necessarily stressful, as long as the busyness does not threaten your equilibrium.)

The stress response begins when your brain perceives a threat to your equilibrium. The sight of a car hurtling toward you; the terror that an enemy is concealed around a nearby corner; the excitement of planning for a party, a move, or a wedding; the feeling of pain; or any other such disturbance perceived by the brain serves as an alarm signal. There follows a chain of events that acts through both nerves and hormones to bring about a state of readiness in every body part. The effects all favor physical action (fight or flight). Notice the tremendous array of target organs in the description of the stress response that follows.

The pupils of your *eyes* widen so that you can see better; your *muscles*

tense up so that you can jump, run, or struggle with maximum strength; breathing quickens to bring more oxygen into your *lungs,* and your *heart* races to rush this oxygen to your muscles so that they can burn the fuel they need for energy. Your *liver* pours forth the needed fuels from its stored supply, and *fat cells* release alternative fuels. Body *protein tissues* break down to back up the fuel supply and to be ready to heal wounds if necessary. The *blood vessels* of your muscles expand to feed them better, whereas those of your *gastrointestinal tract* constrict; and gastrointestinal tract glands shut down (digestion is a low-priority process in time of danger). Less blood flows to your *kidney* so that fluid is conserved, and less flows to your *skin* so that blood loss will be minimized at any wound site. More *platelets* form, to allow your blood to clot faster if need be. *Hearing* sharpens, and your *brain* produces local opiumlike substances, dulling its sensation of pain, which during an emergency might distract you from taking the needed action. Your *hair* may even stand on end—a reminder that there was a time when our ancestors had enough hair to bristle, look bigger, and frighten off their enemies.

This tightly synchronized, adaptive reaction to threat provides superb support for emergency physical action. You probably remember having had to take such action; you may have performed an amazing feat of strength or speed for a few minutes, and only after it was over noticed that your heart was hammering, your breathing was fast, your fingers were cold, your skin was tingling, your mouth was dry, and the sensation of pain or exhaustion was just beginning to come through as the stress hormone epinephrine drained away.

---

*Appendix A presents the basic details of how cells work, and of the body's hormonal and nervous regulatory systems.

■ TABLE H1–1
Psychological Stressors

People ranked these events, according to how stressful they perceived them to be, on a scale from 1 to 100. Note that some "happy" events are included here. Individual people may score these events higher or lower than they are here. We have added in brackets events that might be comparable to these in the lives of students.

Life Event	Stress Points
Death of spouse	100
Divorce	73
Marital separation [breakup with boyfriend/girlfriend]	65
Jail term	63
Death of a close family member (except spouse)	63
Major personal injury or illness	53
Marriage	50
Being fired from a job [expulsion from school]	47
Marital reconciliation	45
Retirement	45
Change in health of a family member (not self)	44
Pregnancy	40
Sex difficulties	39
Gain of a new family member [change of roommate]	39
Business readjustment	39
Change in financial state	38
Death of a close friend	37
Change to a different line of work [change of major]	36
Change in number of arguments with spouse	35
Taking on a large mortgage [financial aid]	31
Foreclosure of a mortgage or loan	30
Change in responsibilities at work [change in course demands]	29
Son or daughter leaving home	29
Trouble with in-laws [trouble with parents]	29
Outstanding personal achievement	28
Spouse beginning or stopping work	26
School beginning or ending [final exams]	26
Change in living conditions	25
Revision of personal habits (self or family)	24
Trouble with boss [trouble with professor]	23
Change in work [or school] hours or conditions	20
Change in residence [moving to school, moving home]	20
Change in schools	20
Change in recreation	19
Change in church activities	19
Change in social activities [joining new group]	18
Taking on a small mortgage or loan	17
Change in sleeping habits	16
Change in number of family get-togethers	15
Change in eating habits	13
Vacation	13
Christmas	12
Minor violations of the law	11

Check the list, and identify the events that you have experienced in the past year or that you expect within the next year. Use the number system to determine how many stress points you are experiencing in this period of your life. Then score yourself as follows: over 200—urgent need of intelligent stress management; 150–199—careful stress management indicated; 100–149—stressful life, keep tabs on your mental health; under 100—no present cause for concern about stress.

Source: Adapted with permission from *Journal of Psychosomatic Research* 11, T. H. Holmes and R. H. Rahe, The social readjustment rating scale, 1967, Pergamon Journals, Ltd., as presented in Lifescore: Holmes scale, *Family Health*, January 1979, p. 32.

Anyone can respond in this magnificent fashion to sudden physical stress for a short time. But if the stress is prolonged, and especially if physical action is not a permitted response to the stress, then it can drain the body of its reserves and leave it weakened, worn, and susceptible to illness. Much of the disability imposed by prolonged stress is nutritional: you can't eat, can't digest your food or absorb nutrients, and so can't store them in reserve for periods of need.

All three energy fuels—carbohydrate, fat, and protein—are drawn upon in increased quantities during stress. If the stress requires vigorous physical action, and if there is injury, all three are used. While the body is busy responding and not eating, the fuels must be drawn from internal sources.

The conservation of water at such a time is of utmost importance. The body sends several hormonal messages to conserve water (described in Chapter 10).

As for the other nutrients, they are taken from storage for as long as supplies last, but supplies for some are exhausted within a day. Thereafter, body tissues break down to provide energy and needed nutrients (see Figure H1–1). The body uses not only *dispensable* supplies (those that are there to be used up, so to speak, like stored fat), but also functional tissue that we don't want to lose, like muscle tissue. Two questions come to mind. First, How can we prepare for these nutrient losses? Second, What measures can we take to minimize them?

The best nutritional preparation for stress is a balanced and varied diet as part of a lifestyle in which exercise plays a constant part. No supplements or gimmicks will benefit you. Just eat well to obtain the nutrients you need and exercise regularly to promote their storage, and your body will be as well prepared as it can be to withstand the impact of periods of unavoidable stress.

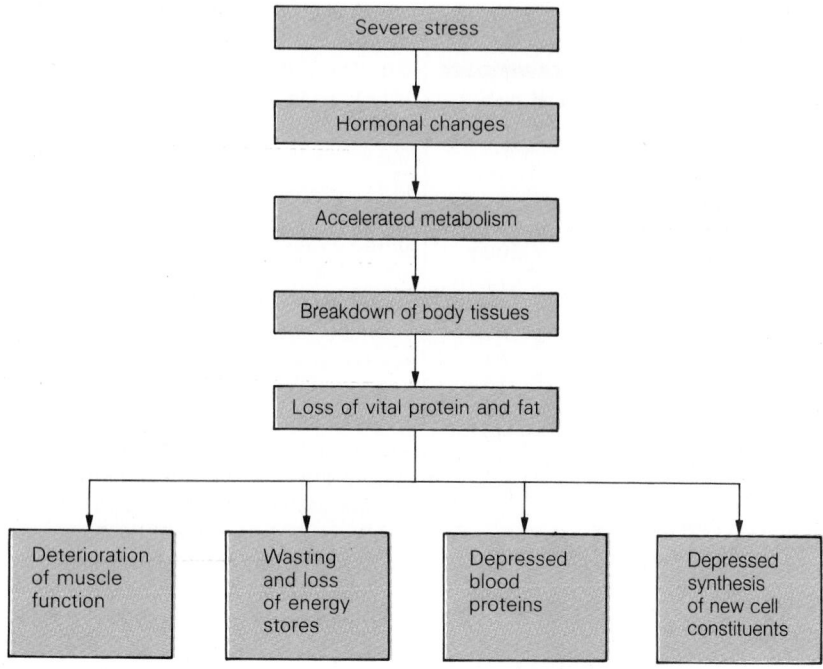

■ FIGURE H1–1
Metabolic Response to Stress
The degree to which the body is affected by stress depends on the severity and duration of stressor.

person goes without eating, the harder it can be to get started again. So it can be a no-win situation. It is frightening to see the downward spiral people can get into once they have let stress affect them to the point where they can't eat, and not eating makes it harder for them to handle the stress. It is therefore desirable not to let stress become so overwhelming that eating becomes impossible. Managing stress so that it does not overwhelm is a psychological task, and may require the help of a counselor.

If you can eat under stress, do so, of course. Take only a little if that's all you can handle, and eat more often to keep meeting your energy and nutrient needs. Choose a variety of foods. Drink fluids, too. Although the body conserves fluids during stress, it will excrete what it does not need, and by taking in water you enable your kidneys to return blood concentrations of the minerals to their equilibrium.

Whenever you can't eat, your body will inevitably lose nutrients. If you are at risk of marginal deficiencies, supplements may be a beneficial option—but not just vitamin supplements and not a fancy "stress" supplement. A vitamin-mineral preparation that supplies a balanced assortment of all the nutrients that might be needed—not in megadoses, but in amounts comparable to the RDA—is most appropriate (see Highlight 9 for a more complete discussion). And don't forget: the energy nutrients you need don't come in pill form. More importantly, supplements cannot prevent or resolve stress; only you can do that by modifying your lifestyle.

When the stressful time is over and your body can recover, the opportunity comes to replenish

During severe stress, the appetite is suppressed. (In times of less severe stress, a person may respond by overeating.) We've already said why: it's an adaptive reaction to a *physical* threat, the kind of threat that our ancestors experienced during their evolution. Energy at such a time is needed for fight or flight; it would be wasteful and risky to spend energy looking for or eating food. The blood supply has been diverted to the muscles to maximize strength and speed; so even if

food is swallowed, it may not be digested or absorbed efficiently. (In a severe upset, the stomach and intestines will even reject solid food; vomiting, diarrhea, or both are these organs' way of disposing of a burden they can't handle.) All of this means that to tell people under severe stress to eat is poor advice. They can't; and if they force themselves to eat, they can't assimilate what they've eaten.

On the other hand, fasting is itself a stress on the body, and the longer a

◢◢ NUTRITION DETECTIVE WORK

For each nutrition-related problem, researchers have learned what to do about diet by first studying the body's internal regulation and control systems. Then they design experiments to learn the effects that changes in diet will have, not only on the body's structural systems (like muscle, fluids, or bones), but also on its regulatory systems (the hormones, enzymes, and nervous system). Because researchers are still in the process of learning how the body responds to different diet therapies, their conclusions have to be revised from time to time. Even advice from authorities can change as knowledge changes; you will continue to update your nutrition knowledge throughout your lifetime.

Miniglossary

epinephrine (EP-ih-NEFF-rin): a hormone of the adrenal gland that modulates the stress response; formerly called **adrenaline**.

homeostasis (HOME-ee-oh-STAY-sis): the maintenance of relatively constant internal conditions in body systems by corrective responses to forces that, unopposed, would cause unacceptably large changes in those conditions. A homeostatic system is not static, or fixed. It is constantly changing, but within tolerable limits.

> *homeo* = the same
> *stasis* = staying

stress: any threat to a person's well-being. The threat may be physical or psychological, desired or feared, but the reaction is always the same.

stress response: the body's response to stress, mediated by both nerves and hormones initially; begins with an *alarm reaction*, proceeds through a stage of *resistance*, and then leads to *recovery* or, if prolonged, to *exhaustion*. This three-stage response has also been termed the **general adaptation syndrome**.

stressor: a demand placed on the body to adapt.

---

depleted stores. If you have lost weight, you may need to gain it back—not just by eating and putting on fat, but by eating and exercising to restore both lean and fat tissue. If you have responded to stress by overeating and have gained weight, you may need to lose it with a combination of diet and exercise. Just as important as nutrition techniques is the learning of stress-management skills to prevent the next stressful event from being so overwhelming and debilitating.

Notice that the advice offered in the previous paragraph did not suggest that you eat a certain food or follow a certain kind of diet to alleviate stress. Nutrients do not work as drugs might to cure an illness. Nutrients delivered from foods work with one another under the body's directions. The nourished, healthy body best keeps itself well. The well body—the body that best resists disease, lives the longest, and enjoys the highest quality of life in the later years—is a body that receives all of the nutrients necessary for optimum living. This kind of thinking is an example of the attitude of preventive nutrition, which supports a person's well-being. Nutrition as a preventive strategy is our focus throughout most of this book; later chapters consider the benefits of nutrition as a therapeutic strategy as well.

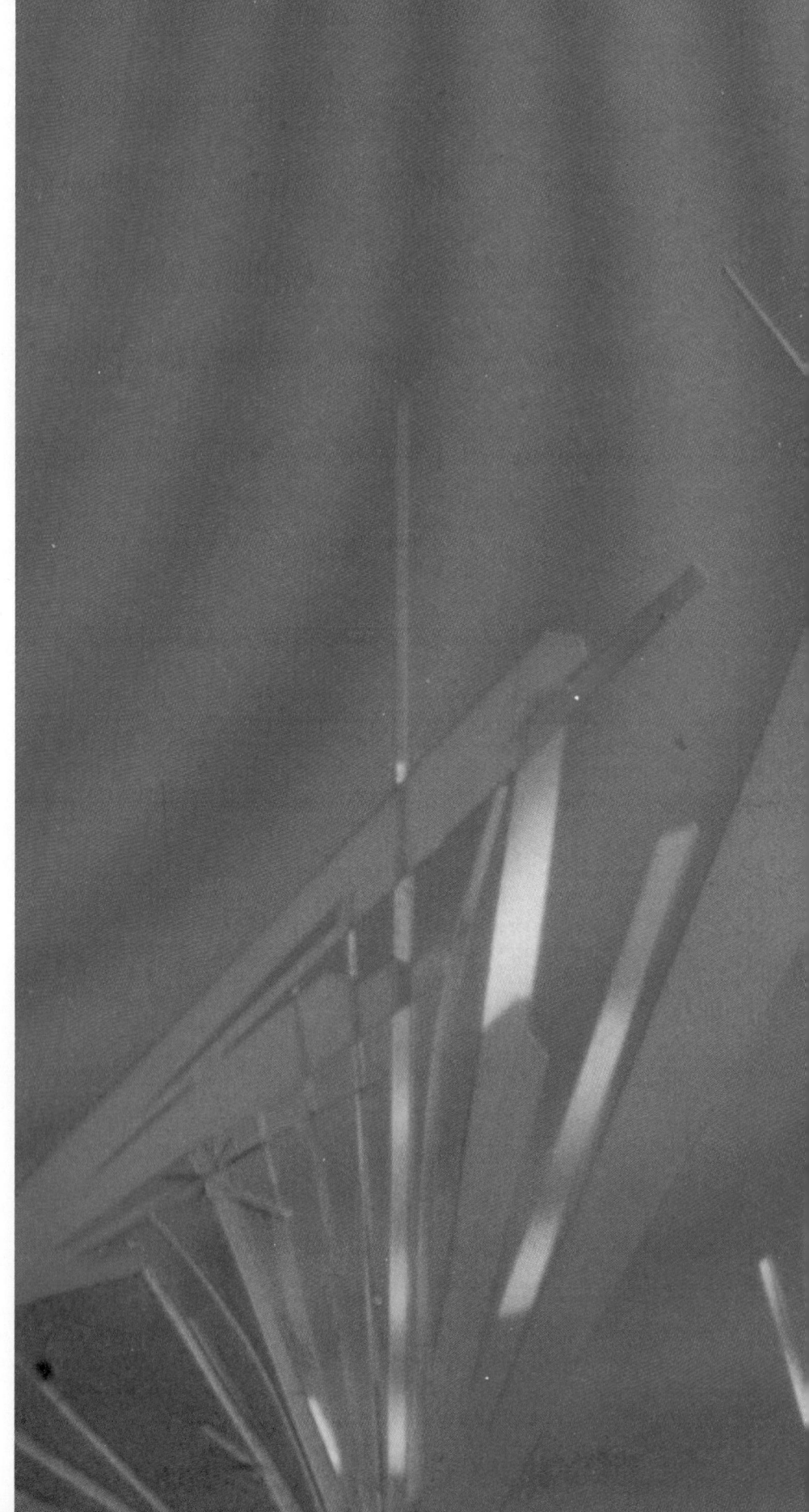

2

Recommended Nutrient Intakes and Diet-Planning Guides

The nutrients themselves are beautiful when viewed in crystalline form under the microscope. These are crystals of vitamin C.

Among the most important questions asked by nutrition scientists are how much of each nutrient the body needs and how people can make sure they get enough. This chapter shows how nutrition experts arrive at recommended nutrient intakes and how diets can be planned to deliver them.

Recommended Nutrient Intakes

Many countries have developed nutrient standards. Typical are the United States' Recommended Dietary Allowances, or RDA, and Canada's Recommended Nutrient Intakes, or RNI. The RDA are presented on the inside front cover (left) of this book and in Appendix I; the Canadian recommendations, in Appendix I.

The RDA are the best estimate of how much of a nutrient intake is required to adequately meet the known nutrient needs of practically all healthy people.[1] Much misunderstanding surrounds them. Perhaps the following facts will help put the RDA in perspective:

- The development of the RDA is funded by the federal government, but the committee that determines the RDA is composed of highly qualified scientists selected by the National Academy of Sciences for their special competencies. The committee's work is subject to approval by the National Research Council.
- The RDA are based on available scientific evidence to the greatest extent possible and are revised periodically. With each edition, a new committee reexamines the data, concepts, and assumptions that underlie the RDA, reaffirms the relationships between the observations and their conclusions, and describes how the recommendations were reached.[2] The latest edition was published in 1989.
- The RDA are recommendations, not requirements, and certainly not minimum requirements. They include a substantial margin of safety that provides for variation in requirements among individuals and in the availability of a nutrient from different food sources. Therefore, individuals whose needs are higher than the average are included within the RDA.
- The RDA are for healthy persons only. Under the stress of illness or malnutrition, a person may require a much higher intake of certain nutrients.

The RDA for nutrients (protein, vitamins, and minerals) are set differently from the RDA for energy, as the following sections show.

The Setting of the Nutrient RDA

It is important to understand how the RDA and other such recommendations are set. A theoretical discussion based on the way the Committee on Dietary

RDA: Recommended Dietary Allowances. The RDA are daily recommended intakes of nutrients intended to provide for individual variations among most normal, healthy people in the United States under usual environmental stresses.

RDA are set for:
- Energy.
- Protein.
- Vitamins—A, C, D, E, K, folate, niacin, riboflavin, thiamin, B$_6$, and B$_{12}$.
- Minerals—calcium, phosphorus, iodine, iron, magnesium, zinc, and selenium.

Minimum requirements are set for:
- Sodium.
- Chloride.
- Potassium.

Estimated Safe and Adequate Daily Dietary Intakes are set for:
- Vitamins—biotin and pantothenic acid.
- Minerals—copper, manganese, fluoride, chromium, and molybdenum.

The RDA are different from the U.S. RDA, which are used on labels (see p. 21 and the inside front cover, right).

balance study: a laboratory study in which a person is fed a controlled diet and the intake and excretion of a nutrient are measured and compared.
- Balance: intake = excretion.
- Positive balance: intake > excretion.
- Negative balance: intake < excretion.

requirement: the amount of a nutrient that will just prevent the development of specific deficiency signs in an individual; distinguished from the RDA, which is a recommended allowance for populations that includes a safety factor to provide for variability among individuals.

Allowances makes its recommendations for nutrients will illustrate the limitations and qualifications you must keep in mind when dealing with the RDA.

Suppose we were the Committee on Dietary Allowances and we had the task of setting an RDA for nutrient X (any nutrient). Ideally, our first step would be to try to find out how much of that nutrient each person needs. We would review and select the most valid studies of deficiency states, of the body's nutrient stores and their depletion, of nutrient intakes of apparently healthy people, and of many other relevant factors (such as findings from animal research). We could also measure the body's intake and excretion of nutrient X (in the case of nutrients that aren't changed before they are excreted) and find out how much of an intake is required to achieve balance between intake and excretion (this is called a balance study). For each individual subject, we could determine a *requirement* for nutrient X. Below the requirement, that person would slip into negative balance (that is, more would be excreted than was consumed) and experience declining stores.

We would find that different individuals have different requirements. Mr. A might need 40 units of the nutrient each day to maintain balance; Ms. B might need 35; Mr. C, 65. If we looked at enough individuals, we might find that their requirements fell into an even distribution—that most were near the midpoint, and only a few were at the extremes. Figure 2–1 depicts this situation.

Then we would have to decide what intake to recommend for everybody; that is, we would have to set the RDA. Should we set it at the mean (shown in Figure 2–1 at 45 units)? This is the average requirement for nutrient X; it is the closest to everyone's need. But if people took us literally and consumed exactly this amount of nutrient X each day, half of the population would develop deficiencies, Mr. C among them.

Perhaps we should set the RDA for nutrient X at or above the extreme—say, at 70 units a day—so that everyone would be covered. (Actually, we didn't study everyone, so we would have to worry that some individual we didn't happen to test would have a still higher requirement.) This might be a good idea in theory, but what if nutrient X is expensive or scarce? A person like Ms. B, who needs only 35 units a day, would then try to consume twice that, an unnecessary strain on her diet plan and on her pocketbook. Or she might overeat as a consequence, or overemphasize foods containing nutrient X to the exclusion of foods containing other valuable nutrients.

The choice we would finally make, with some reservations, would be to set the RDA at a reasonably high point so that the bulk of the population would be covered. In this example, a reasonable choice might be to set it at the point where nearly everyone's needs are covered—say, at 63 units (see Figure 2–1). The point can be chosen mathematically so that it covers 98 or 99 percent of the population. By moving the RDA further toward the extreme, we would pick up very few additional people but inflate the recommendation as it applies to most people (including Mr. A and Ms. B).

It is this kind of choice that the committee members make in setting the RDA for nutrients. They set it well above the mean requirement as best they can determine it from the available information. (Actually, they don't usually have enough data to be sure that the population's requirements are evenly distributed for every nutrient under consideration.) Relatively few people's requirements, then, are not covered by the RDA.

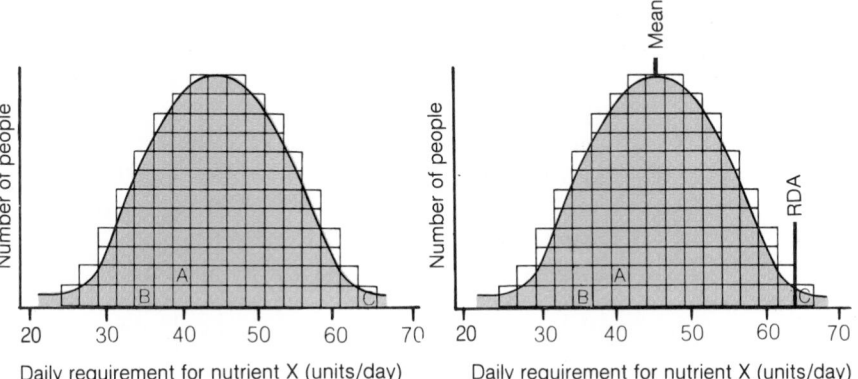

■ **FIGURE 2–1**
Setting the RDA for a Nutrient
Different individuals have different requirements. Each square represents a person. A, B, and C are Mr. A, Ms. B, and Mr. C. The second figure superimposes the recommended intake (RDA) on these data.

The RDA are generous, and although they do not necessarily cover every individual for every nutrient, they should not be exceeded by much. Some nutrients can be toxic at intakes only slightly above the RDA, and people's tolerances for high doses of nutrients vary. It is naive to think of the RDA as minimum amounts. A more accurate view is to see your nutrient needs as falling within a range, with danger zones both below and above it (see Figure 2–2). The recommendations reflect this consideration especially clearly in the tables that state recommended intakes in terms of "safe and adequate" ranges, "safe" meaning "not too high" and "adequate" meaning "not to low."

The Setting of the Energy (kCalorie) RDA

In setting allowances for energy intakes, the Committee on Dietary Allowances took a different approach than for protein, the vitamins, and the minerals. Committee members had reasoned that it would be sensible to set generous allowances for these nutrients—that small amounts of a *nutrient* in excess of the minimum required to maintain freedom from deficiency symptoms would be less harmful than small deficits. However, *energy* intakes either above or below actual need are undesirable, because obesity is as unhealthy as underweight. The Committee on Dietary Allowances therefore set the energy RDA at the mean—halfway between the lowest and highest needs of the individuals it studied. Figure 2–3 illustrates the difference between the nutrient and energy RDA. As the figure shows, most people's energy needs fall close to the mean, but few fit the mean exactly. The latest version of the RDA energy table provides recommended energy intakes for each age-sex group based on the median heights and weights of the U.S. population (see Appendix I). They cover the body's energy needs, assuming light to moderate physical activity. The best way to determine what your energy requirement may be is to monitor your food energy intake over a period of time during which your activities are typical and your weight remains constant.

Protein is the only energy-yielding nutrient for which an RDA has been established. In setting the protein RDA, an assumption is made that people

■ **FIGURE 2–2**
Naive versus Accurate View of Nutrient Needs
The RDA represent a point within a range of appropriate and reasonable intakes that lies between toxicity and deficiency. It is high enough to provide reserves in times of short-term dietary inadequacies, but not so high as to approach toxicity. Nutrient intakes above or below these ranges might be equally harmful.

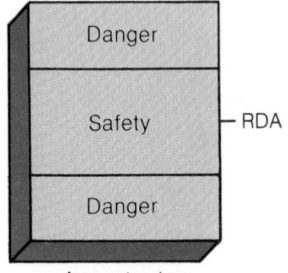

■ **FIGURE 2–3**
The Nutrient RDA and the Energy RDA
The nutrient RDA are set so that only a few people's requirements will exceed them. The energy RDA are set so that half the population's requirements will fall below and half above them.

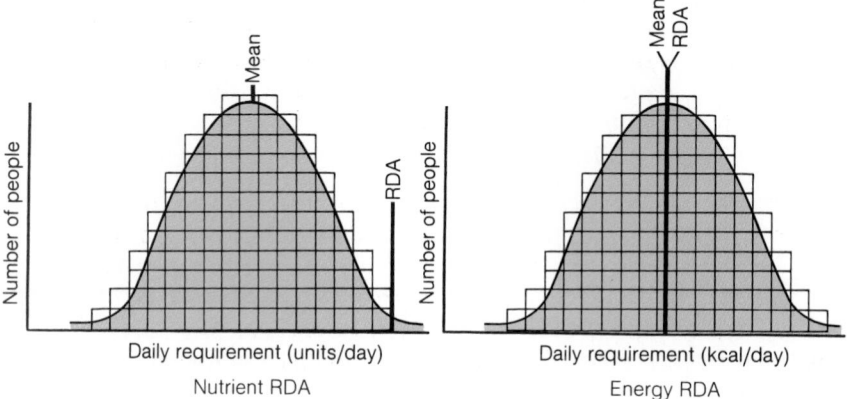

Nutrient RDA

Energy RDA

will receive energy from carbohydrate and fat (and possibly some from alcohol, according to personal preference) and only a certain minimum amount of energy from their protein intake.

Using the RDA

The widespread use of the RDA requires an awareness of their appropriate applications and limitations. With the understanding that the RDA are approximate, flexible, and generous, we can use them as a yardstick to assess the adequacy of diets. Most appropriately, diet planners use them as guidelines to aid in evaluating and planning diets for groups of people—for example, all the children in a certain school or all the people in a certain county. The RDA have been used as a standard in many surveys and research studies to evaluate people's nutrition status.

The RDA can also be used to estimate the probable risk of deficiency for an individual *when intakes are averaged over a sufficient length of time*. After all, "if the recommended levels meet the needs of essentially all members of a group, then, by definition, those levels can be applied to individuals within that group as long as it can be assured that *typical* intake is compared with the RDA."[3] For while the RDA for every nutrient can be met from a variety of foods with careful planning, this is a difficult goal to achieve on a daily basis. Even though the RDA are expressed in terms of *per day*, they should be interpreted as *average* intakes over time. The length of time varies for each nutrient, depending on the body's use and storage of the nutrient. For most nutrients, the RDA covers average intakes over at least three days; for others, the average might be several months.

When using the RDA, keep these three points in mind:

■ The RDA are intended to be met through diets composed of a variety of foods. In this way, all other nutrients for which RDA have not been established will also be covered.

- The RDA are not minimal requirements, nor are they necessarily optimal levels of intake for all individuals. They are safe and adequate recommendations that include a generous margin of safety.
- The RDA are most appropriately used for populations, but can be used to estimate probable risk of deficiency for individuals if comparison is made over a sufficient length of time.[4]

Finally, remember that the RDA derive from human judgment based on human knowledge—they are not etched on stone tablets, and they are not perfect. Still, a comparison of the RDA, from the first edition (in 1943) to the one currently used, reveals more similarities than differences.[5] Even more striking is that over these past several decades, no healthy human being who was receiving the RDA of a nutrient has suffered symptoms of a nutrient deficiency. Clearly, the safety margins used in setting the nutrient RDA cover "nearly all" the population.

Other Recommendations

As mentioned, different nations and international organizations have published different sets of standards similar to the RDA. The Canadian RNI differ from the RDA in some respects, and some of the differences between the two sets of recommendations will be explained as the nutrients are discussed in the coming chapters.

Among the most widely used recommendations is a set developed by two international groups: the Food and Agriculture Organization (FAO) and the World Health Organization (WHO). The FAO/WHO recommendations are considered sufficient for the maintenance of health in "nearly all people." They are sometimes higher, but usually lower, than the RDA, not because the RDA are wrong, but because different judgment factors apply to each. Consider that protein quality varies greatly from country to country and that the human requirement for protein depends on its quality. To avoid misinterpretation, FAO/WHO states recommendations in terms of high-quality protein. The RDA states recommendations in terms of mixed proteins (both high- and low-quality) common in the United States diet. Therefore, the FAO/WHO protein values are lower than the RDA even though each bases its recommendation on the same human requirement for protein. Nevertheless, the various recommending agencies have arrived at figures that are all within the same range.

Chapter 6 introduces the concept of protein quality and Appendix J provides details of its measurement.

■ *The U.S. RDA*

The U.S. RDA are a set of figures designed specifically for use on food labels. A food label would be most meaningful to you as an individual if it expressed the food's nutrient contents as a percentage of your need, but of course it can't do that. The makers of the product don't know who you are: a 10-year-old

U.S. RDA: United States Recommended Daily Allowances. The U.S. RDA are used on labels, and in most instances, they are the highest RDA for any age and sex group for each nutrient (see inside front cover, right).

Highlights 16 and 18 discuss food labels in detail.

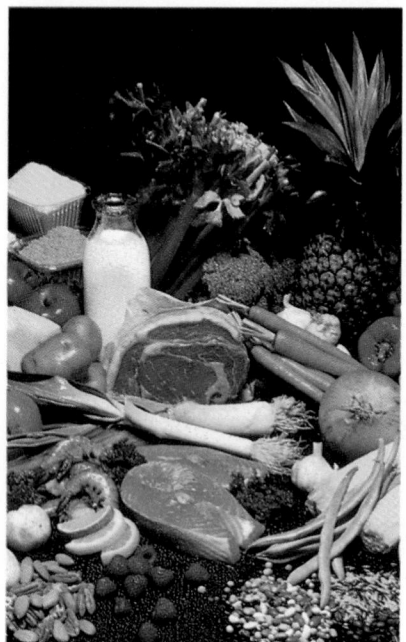

Variety helps to ensure an adequate and balanced diet.

Diet-planning principles:
- **A**dequacy.
- **B**alance.
- k**C**alorie control.
- **M**oderation.
- **V**ariety.

dietary balance: providing foods of a number of types in balance with one another, such that foods rich in one nutrient do not crowd out of the diet foods that are rich in another nutrient.

boy, a 70-year-old woman, or a pregnant teenage girl. Even if they did, they wouldn't know your particular requirements. To standardize labels, four sets of U.S. RDA were developed for different groups of people—infants, children, adults, and pregnant and lactating women. The most commonly used of these is the U.S. RDA for adults, and this is the one referred to here. The idea behind the U.S. RDA for adults was to develop a single set of standards for a sort of generalized adult human being whose nutrient needs are high—as high as people's needs generally go. So if you read on a label that a serving of cereal provides 10 percent of the U.S. RDA of a nutrient, you can be fairly sure that it will also provide at least a tenth of *your* RDA for that nutrient.

The U.S. RDA are about equal to the highest numbers for each nutrient that you can find in the RDA table. For most nutrients, they are the same as the 1968 RDA for adolescent boys or adult men, whichever are higher. For iron, the women's RDA is greater than the men's (see inside front cover, left), so the women's RDA is used. The U.S. RDA have not been revised to agree exactly with new editions of the RDA since 1968, because they still would be judged generous by any standard, and because the confusion and expense involved in converting labels to a slightly different set of numbers would not be justified by the small benefits that would result from doing so. (Further details on the U.S. RDA appear in Highlight 16 and with the table on the inside front cover, right.)

◼ Diet-Planning Guides

Knowing the individual nutrients and their recommended intakes, you can now ask how you can juggle the available foods to create a diet that supplies all the needed nutrients in the appropriate amounts for good health. The principle is simple enough: just select a variety of foods that present the nutrients you need. In practice, how does this work out? It helps to keep in mind the basic diet-planning principles, listed in the margin in alphabetical order to help you to remember them. Let's begin by discussing dietary balance.

The minerals calcium and iron illustrate the importance of dietary balance. Iron is one of the essential nutrients. You can only get it into your body by eating foods that contain it. If you miss out on these foods, you may experience symptoms of iron deficiency. You may feel weak, tired, and unenthusiastic; may have frequent headaches; and can do little muscular work without disabling fatigue. If you had added iron-rich foods to your diet, you might have prevented these symptoms. Some foods are rich in iron; others are notoriously poor. Meats, fish, poultry, and legumes are in the iron-rich category, and an easy way to obtain the needed iron is to include these foods in your diet regularly.

Calcium is another essential nutrient. A diet lacking calcium may result in poor bone development during the growing years and a gradual bone loss in adults that can totally cripple a person in later life. The iron-rich foods just named are poor sources of calcium; you can get enough calcium only by frequently consuming milk and milk products or carefully selected milk substitutes.

Just as foods that are rich in iron are poor in calcium, so is the reverse true. In fact, milk (except breast milk) and milk products are so low in iron that the overuse of these foods, by displacing iron-rich foods from the diet, can actually cause iron-deficiency anemia. And yet no one could accuse milk of being a nutrient-poor food. It is the single most nutritious food for infants and can be an important calcium contributor in the diet of people of all ages.

This discussion illustrates the need for dietary balance. Use enough—but not too many—servings of meat or meat alternates for iron; use enough—but not too many—servings of milk and milk products for calcium. Save some space for other foods needed for other nutrients.

Iron and calcium are only two of some 40-odd essential nutrients, and meat and milk are their most outstanding food sources in most people's diets. Yet there are other nutrients that are not abundant in either milk or meat; a diet consisting of milk and meat would be far from adequate. To obtain the other nutrients, you have to eat vegetables, fruits, grains, and other foods; variety in the diet helps to ensure adequacy. The task of designing an adequate, balanced diet therefore requires some thought and skillful planning. The real challenge is to incorporate kcalorie control—to eat an adequate, balanced diet without overeating.

Part of the secret to eating well without overeating is to select foods that deliver the most nutrients at the lowest kcalorie cost. Take foods containing calcium, for example: 1½ ounces of cheddar cheese and 8 ounces of nonfat milk each provide about 300 milligrams of calcium, but the cheese contributes about twice as many kcalories as the nonfat milk.* Both are nutritious, but based on the amount of calcium they offer for a given kcalorie amount, the nonfat milk has higher nutrient density than the cheese. To evaluate foods this way is to employ the concept of nutrient density.

The concept of nutrient density can help the health-conscious consumer make informed choices. The food industry has enthusiastically endorsed the selling of the nutritional *adequacy* concept. The dairy people proclaim, "Drink milk—it's good for you." The meat people boast that meat is rich in protein and iron, as indeed it is. Aware consumers realize, though, that whole milk and meat can also contribute many fat kcalories, and they use those products that are lowest in fat, thereby obtaining more nutrients for the kcalories. By selecting small quantities of low-fat foods a person practices moderation, a necessary ingredient to controlling kcalories.

Another principle necessary to successful diet planning is variety. It is generally agreed that people should not eat the same foods day after day, except for staple foods such as milk—and even for staple foods, some people recommend switching brands from time to time. Variety permits you to take advantage of the fact that some foods are better sources of some nutrients than other foods are. Also, a monotonous diet may deliver unwanted amounts of undesirable food constituents, such as contaminants (see Chapter 16). In a diet with variety, each food's ingredients are diluted by the bulk of

dietary adequacy: providing all the essential nutrients and energy necessary to maintain health and body weight. Ideally, a diet will be more than just adequate; it will be **optimal**, providing an assortment and balance of nutrients and energy to maintain appropriate body weight and the best possible state of health.

kcalorie control: management of energy intake.

nutrient density: a characteristic of a food. A nutrient-dense food provides a high quantity (relative to need) of one or (preferably) several essential nutrients, with a small quantity (relative to need) of kcalories.

↑ quantity of essential nutrients
↓ quantity of calories

moderation: providing no unwanted constituent in excess.

dietary variety: using different foods for the same nutrients on different occasions.

staple foods: foods used frequently or daily—for example, potatoes (in Ireland) or rice (in the Far East).

The principle of variety being referred to here could also be called the principle of **dilution**.

---

* These figures were taken from items 37 and 98 in Appendix H.

all the other foods eaten and even further diluted if several days are skipped before it is eaten again.

Several approaches to diet planning are possible. Two of the guides most widely used by nutrition-conscious people today are food group plans and exchange patterns. The person who understands and appreciates both is in a good position to design an optimal diet.

Food Group Plans

One of the most familiar ways of grouping foods in the United States fits the major foods into four groups, as shown in Figure 2–4. Each of the four groups contains foods that are similar in origin and nutrient content. The nutrients named in the table are representative of all the nutrients. The assumption is that once you have adequate amounts of these, you'll probably have enough of the other two dozen or so essential nutrients as well, because they occur in the same groups of foods. This is not an entirely safe assumption, but with the precaution that primarily unprocessed foods be used, the Four Food Group Plan provides a reasonable foundation for diet planning.

The Four Food Group Plan specifies that a certain quantity of food must be consumed from each group. For the adult, the recommended number of servings from the vegetables and fruits, breads and cereals, milk and milk products, and meat and meat alternates groups is four, four, two, and two, respectively (see Figure 2–4).

Many foods—such as butter, margarine, cream, sour cream, salad dressing, mayonnaise, potato chips, jelly, broth, coffee, tea, alcoholic beverages, and others—don't fit into any of the four food groups. Some of them do contribute some nutrients, and most contribute energy, to the day's intake. They are grouped together into a miscellaneous category, because their nutrient content is not significant in the nutrients characteristic of a food group, or their nutrient content has been greatly diluted by fat, sugar, alcohol, or water.

The beauty of the Four Food Group Plan lies in its simplicity and ease in learning. It may appear quite rigid, but it can be used with great flexibility once its intent is understood. For example, cheese can be substituted for milk because both supply protein, calcium, and riboflavin in about the same amounts. Legumes and nuts are alternative choices for meats (see Figure 2–5). The plan can be adapted to casseroles and other mixed dishes, as well as to different national and cultural cuisines.

The Four Food Group Plan has been criticized. It is easy for people who follow it to overconsume food energy, especially from fat. Food selections within each group must be made carefully. Large kcalorie differences exist, for example, between nonfat milk and ice cream, fish and peanut butter, green beans and sweet potatoes, and bread and biscuits.

Critics say that half of the food classes (two of the four groups) are animal products—milk and meat—which leads many people to think that half of the foods they consume should be milk and meat. (Actually, though, the plan recommends *two* milk items, *two* meat items, and *eight* food items from the plant food groups.) Also, a person can follow all of the plan's rules and still

Milk and Milk Products

Calcium, riboflavin, protein, vitamin B$_{12}$, (vitamin D and vitamin A, when fortified).

2 servings per day for adults.
3 servings per day for children.
4 servings per day for teenagers, pregnant/lactating women, women past menopause.
5 servings per day for pregnant/lactating teenagers.

Serving = 1 c milk or yogurt; ¼ c Parmesan cheese or process cheese spread; 2 c cottage cheese; 1½ c ice cream or ice milk; 2 oz process cheese food; 1⅓ oz cheese.
■ Nonfat milk, buttermilk, low-fat milk, plain yogurt.
■ Whole milk, cheese, fruit-flavored yogurt, cottage cheese.
■ Custard, milk shakes, pudding, ice cream.

Breads and Cereals

Riboflavin, thiamin, niacin, iron, protein, magnesium, folate, fiber.

4 servings per day.

Serving = 1 slice bread; ½ to ¾ c cooked cereals, rice, or pastas; 1 oz ready-to-eat cereals.
■ Whole grains (wheat, oats, barley, millet, rye, bulgur) enriched breads, rolls, tortillas.

■ Rice, cereals, pastas (macaroni, spaghetti), bagels.
■ Pancakes, muffins, cornbread, biscuits, presweetened cereals.

Vegetables and Fruits

Vitamin A, vitamin C, riboflavin, folate, iron, magnesium, low in fat, no cholesterol.

4 servings per day.

Serving = ½ c or typical portion (such as 1 medium apple, ½ grapefruit, or 1 wedge lettuce).

■ Apricots, bean sprouts, broccoli, brussels sprouts, cabbage, cantaloupe, carrots, cauliflower, cucumbers, grapefruit, green beans, green peas, leafy greens (spinach, mustard, and collard greens), lettuce, mushrooms, oranges, orange juice, peaches, strawberries, tomatoes, winter squash.
■ Apples, bananas, canned fruit, corn, pears, potatoes.
■ Avocados, dried fruit, sweet potatoes.

Meat and Meat Alternates

Protein, phosphorus, vitamin B$_6$, vitamin B$_{12}$, zinc, magnesium, iron, niacin, thiamin.

2 servings per day for adults, children, teenagers.
3 servings per day for pregnant/lactating women/teenagers.

Serving = 2 to 3 oz lean, cooked meat, poultry, or fish; 1 oz meat, poultry, or fish = 1 egg, ½ to ¾ c legumes, 2 tbsp peanut butter, ¼ to ½ c nuts or seeds.
■ Poultry, fish, lean meat (beef, lamb, pork), dried peas and beans, eggs.
■ Beef, lamb, pork, refried beans.
■ Hotdogs, luncheon meats, peanut butter, nuts.

Miscellaneous Group

Sugar, fat (vitamin E), salt, alcohol, kcalories.

No serving sizes are provided because servings of these foods are not recommended. Concentrate on the four food groups that provide nutrients; the foods in the miscellaneous group will find their way into your diet as ingredients in prepared foods, or added at the table, or just as "extras." Note that some of the following items could be placed in more than one group or in a combination group. For example, potato chips are high in both salt and fat; doughnuts are high in both sugar and fat.

■ Miscellaneous foods, not high in kcalories, include spices, herbs, coffee, tea, and diet soft drinks.
■ Foods high in fat include margarine, salad dressing, oils, mayonnaise, cream, cream cheese, butter, gravy, and sauces.
■ Foods high in salt include potato chips, corn chips, pretzels, pickles, olives, bouillon, prepared mustard, soy sauce, steak sauce, salt, and seasoned salt.
■ Foods high in sugar include cake, pie, cookies, doughnuts, sweet rolls, candy, soft drinks, fruit drinks, jelly, syrup, gelatin desserts, sugar, and honey.
■ Alcoholic beverages include wine, beer, and liquor.

Key:
■ Foods generally lowest in kcalories.
■ Foods moderate in kcalories.
■ Foods highest in kcalories.

■ **FIGURE 2–5**
Legumes
Legumes have long been scorned by the middle class as "the poor man's meat," but they are an inexpensive, health-promoting, land-sparing, nutritious food. They are used in many kinds of cooking: Orientals' bean curd (tofu) and soy sauce, Americans' peanut butter and baked beans, vegetarians' bean sprouts, and Mexicans' bean paste, among others.

Legumes include:
- Black beans.
- Black-eyed peas.
- Garbanzo beans.
- Great northern beans.
- Kidney beans.
- Lentils.
- Navy beans.
- Peanuts.
- Pinto beans.
- Soybeans.

The seeds of legumes are high in protein.

The roots of legumes "fix" nitrogen, contributing to the soil more nitrogen than the plants take out.

Many terms describe vegetarian foodways. **Ovovegetarians** eat eggs; **lactovegetarians** use milk; "pure" vegetarians, or **vegans** (VEJ-ans, VEG-ans), use neither animal flesh nor any animal products.

Highlight 6 explores the benefits of a vegetarian diet.

fail to meet the day's needs for some nutrients—especially vitamin B_6, vitamin E, iron, magnesium, and zinc.

Few would argue that the Four Food Group Plan is perfect. Other plans offering six, seven, and eight groups have auditioned for the spotlight. Each plan has its strengths and weaknesses. The Four Food Group Plan continues to serve its users because of its strengths and is capable of serving well when its users are aware of its weaknesses and make the necessary modifications. (Table 2–1 offers two alternative food group plans.)

Some people choose to exclude certain foods or food classes from their diets for religious, philosophical, cultural, or other reasons. Some exclude red meat only, while eating poultry and fish. Some eat only fish among these foods. Some exclude all animal flesh, but eat products produced by animals such as eggs, cheese, and milk. Some are "pure" vegetarians, eating plant foods only, and some go to the extreme of eating only fruit, not vegetables or grains. Each of these foodways presents a challenge to the planner—that of obtaining the needed nutrients from fewer foods or food groups.

The person who excludes meat and poultry has a nutritionally similar food to rely on—fish. In contrast, the person who eats no animal flesh, not even fish, needs an alternative source of iron, zinc, and some of the vitamins offered by meat; for this person, the liberal use of legumes is recommended. The person who uses only plant foods has to plan with still more care. For example, one nutrient, vitamin B_{12}, is found *only* in animal foods, so this person has to take a vitamin B_{12} supplement or use vitamin B_{12}–fortified soy milk or similar products daily. (As for people who attempt to eat fruit only, in no way can they maintain their health for long.) The vegetarian needs to learn much more, and later chapters offer more information. Table 2–1 presents a foundation for diet planning without meat.

■ **TABLE 2–1**
Alternative Food Group Plans

Canada's Food Guide	Vegetarian Four Food Group Plan
Milk and milk products—2 servings[a]	Milk and milk products—2 servings[d]
Meat, fish, poultry, and alternates—2 servings[b]	Protein-rich foods—2 servings[e]
	Legumes—2 servings[f]
Fruits and vegetables—4 to 5 servings[b,c]	Fruits and vegetables—4 servings[g]
Breads and cereals—3 to 5 servings[b]	Breads and cereals (whole grain only)—4 servings

[a]A serving is 250 ml, or about 1 c. See Appendix G for equivalents in the Canadian exchange system. Milk group servings differ for children up to age 11—2 to 3 servings; adolescents—3 to 4 servings; pregant and lactating women—3 to 4 servings.
[b]See Appendix G for equivalents in the Canadian exchange system.
[c]Include at least two vegetables.
[d]If not using milk or milk products, use soy milk fortified with calcium and vitamin B$_{12}$.
[e]Examples of protein-rich foods: cheeses, tofu (see meat alternates in Appendix G).
[f]Women should eat legumes (2 c daily) in addition to protein-rich foods to help meet iron requirements; count 4 tbsp peanut butter as 1 serving.
[g]Women should include 1 c dark greens daily to help meet iron requirements.
Source: *Canada's Food Guide Handbook*, revised (Helath and Welfare Canada, 1985); adapted from *Vegetarian Food Choices* (Gainesville: Shands Teaching Hospital and Clinics, Food and Nutrition Service, University of Florida, 1976).

Exchange Patterns

Whereas food group plans help most with dietary adequacy, balance, and variety, exchange systems help with kcalorie control and moderation. The person who learns to use an exchange system can gain mastery over food energy intakes, and especially fat kcalories. Originally developed for people with diabetes, exchange systems proved so useful that they are now in general use for diet planning. Weight Watchers, a well-known organization that helps people control their weight while eating a nutritious diet, bases its eating plans on the exchange system. Appendix G gives complete details of the U.S. and Canadian exchange systems.

Unlike the Four Food Group Plan, which sorts foods by their protein, vitamin, and mineral contents, the exchange system pays special attention to kcalories; proportions of carbohydrate, fat, and protein; and portion sizes. All of the food portions in a list provide approximately the same number of kcalories and the same amounts of energy nutrients (protein, fat, and carbohydrate).

The exchange system is based on six lists of foods. To remember them, it is convenient to keep in mind a typical item from each list, with portion size specified. Each food has an associated number of kcalories—which is not exact, but is an average number of kcalories for the group. The lists and their typical representatives are:

- ■ Milk—1 cup nonfat milk (90 kcalories).
- ■ Vegetables—½ cup cooked carrots or green beans (25 kcalories).
- ■ Fruits—½ banana or 1 small orange (60 kcalories).

■ Starch/bread—1 slice bread or 1 small potato (80 kcalories).

■ Meat—1 ounce lean meat (55 kcalories).

■ Fat—1 teaspoon butter (45 kcalories).

Table 2–2 shows the carbohydrate, protein, fat, and energy values that pertain to each list, and Figure 2–6 shows the foods that belong together in the exchange lists.

Foods are not always where you might first expect them to be in the exchange system, because they are grouped according to their energy nutrient contents rather than by their outward appearances. Notice that cheese is classed as a meat in this system, because its protein and fat contents are similar to those of meat. In the Four Food Group Plan, cheese is classed with milk because of its calcium content; in Canada's Food Group System (see Appendix G), it is permitted to serve either role, but not both at any one time. Corn is not a "vegetable" in the exchange system; it is listed with starch/breads as a "starchy vegetable." Similarly, olives are not a "vegetable"; they are classified as a "fat," and so is bacon. These groupings permit you to see among foods resemblances that are significant to nutrition.

The user of the exchange system is encouraged to think of nonfat milk as milk and of whole milk as milk with added fat. The vegetable list includes only low-kcalorie vegetables, so a half cup of any of them will provide about 25 kcalories. The fruit list specifies "no added sugar or sugar syrup"—not necessarily to forbid you to eat fruits with sugar, but to help you keep track of sugar consumption. Portion sizes are adjusted so that fruit portions are

Nuts and olives are so high in fat that they are listed with butter, mayonnaise, and bacon in the fat exchange list.

■ TABLE 2–2
The Six Exchange Lists

List	Portion Size	Carbohydrate (g)	Protein (g)	Fat (g)	Energy (kcal)
Starch/bread[a]	1 slice	15	3	Trace	80
Meat[b]	1 oz				
Lean		—	7	3	55
Medium-fat		—	7	5	75
High-fat		—	7	8	100
Vegetable[c]	½ c	5	2	—	25
Fruit	1 portion	15	—	—	60
Milk	1 c				
Nonfat		12	8	Trace	90
Low-fat		12	8	5	120
Whole		12	8	8	150
Fat	1 tsp	—	—	5	45

Note: This is the U.S. exchange system. The complete details, and those of the Canadian system, are shown in Appendix G.

[a]This list includes starchy vegetables such as lima beans and corn, as well as cereal, bread, pasta, and other grain products. For portion sizes see Appendix G.
[b]This list includes cheese and peanut butter as well as meat.
[c]This list includes low-kcalorie vegetables only.

Energy Values of Carbohydrate, Fat, and Protein

If you know the number of grams of carbohydrate, fat, and protein in a food, you can derive the number of kcalories. Simply multiply the carbohydrate grams times 4, the fat grams times 9, and the protein grams times 4, and add them all together.

The energy values for the exchange list items were derived this way. For example, a slice of bread contains 15 g carbohydrate (that's 60 kcal), 3 g protein (that's another 12 kcal), and a trace of fat—rounded up to 80 kcal for ease in calculating. A half cup of vegetables (not including starchy vegetables) contains 5 g carbohydrate (20 kcal) and 2 g protein (8 more), which has been rounded down to 25 kcal. At 25 kcal a half cup, you could eat 4 c of vegetables for less than the kcalorie cost of a single 3-oz hamburger patty—which is 3 medium-fat meat exchanges (225 kcal). A person who eats large quantities of vegetables is unlikely to consume as many kcalories as a person who eats the servings of fatty meat that many people think of as reasonable.

> 1 g carbohydrate = 4 kcal.
> 1 g fat = 9 kcal.
> 1 g protein = 4 kcal.

---

equal in kcalories. One small banana counts as two fruits. But a piece of cherry pie is *not* a fruit. It *includes* a fruit if it contains ten large cherries, but it also includes bread and fat exchanges, and added sugar. (Thus it might be counted as one fruit, two bread, and three fat, with two tablespoons added sugar.) The starch/bread list also clearly specifies portion sizes and makes clear which grain products contain added fat (such as biscuits). Lima beans, potatoes, and other starchy vegetables are listed with the breads, not the vegetables, because they are similar to breads in kcalorie and carbohydrate content.

Perhaps most important of all, meats and cheeses are separated into three categories—lean, medium-fat, and high-fat—and the fat list, by including items like bacon and avocados, alerts the consumer to foods that are unexpectedly high in fat kcalories. A warning: meat list items are calculated in ounces, not in servings. That is, 1 unit of meat is only 1 ounce, whereas a serving is usually 3 or 4 or more ounces, or several exchanges. Calculating meat by the ounce encourages the planner to keep close track of its portion sizes, which make significant differences in energy and fat intakes.

In contrast with the Four Food Group Plan, the exchange system facilitates kcalorie control because foods grouped within each list provide about the same amount of carbohydrate, fat, and protein, and therefore, energy. Critics of the system note that the nutrient similarities end there. Foods within each list can vary greatly in their amounts of vitamins and minerals. For example, iron-rich and calcium-poor meats are grouped together with iron-poor and

■ **FIGURE 2–6**
The Exchange System

1. Starch/breads
1 slice bread is like:
¾ c ready-to-eat cereal.
⅓ c cooked beans.
½ c corn.
1 small (3-oz) potato.
(1 bread = 15 g carbohydrate, 3 g protein, trace of fact, and 80 kcal.)

2a. Meats (lean)
1 oz lean meat is like:
1 oz chicken meat without the skin.
1 oz any fish.
¼ c canned tuna.
1 oz low-fat cheese.[a]
(1 lean meat = 7 g protein, 3 g fat, and 55 kcal.)
(One 3-oz portion of meat (such as a hamburger patty) = 3 meat exchanges. One meat exchange = ⅓ of a 3-oz hamburger patty.)

[a]Cheeses are grouped with milk in food group plans because of their calcium content but with meats in this system because, like meat, they contribute kcalories from protein and fat and have negligible carbohydrate content.

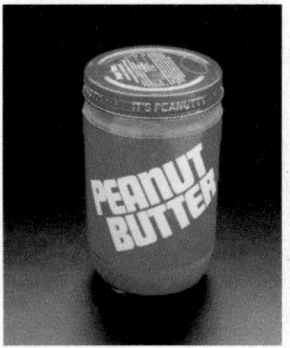

2e. Peanut butter
Peanut butter is like a meat in terms of its protein content. It is estimated as:
1 tbsp peanut butter = 1 high-fat meat
(1 tbsp peanut butter = 7 g protein, 8 g fat, and 100 kcal.)

(Don't stop reading now, and don't swear off peanut butter, necessarily. You'll need to read about the polyunsaturated character of its fat in Chapter 5, and the B vitamin contributions it makes in Chapter 8, before deciding how much of a place it should have in your diet.)

3. Vegetables
½ c carrots is like:
½ c greens.
½ c brussels sprouts.
½ c beets.
(1 vegetable = 5 g carbohydrate, 2 g protein, and 25 kcal.)

2b. Meats (medium-fat)
1 oz medium-fat meat is like 1 oz lean meat in protein content, but has 5 g fat (2 g more fat than lean meat).
Examples:
1 oz pork loin.
1 egg.
¼ cup creamed cottage cheese[a]
(1 medium-fat meat = 7 g protein, 5 g fat, and about 75 kcal.)

2c. Meats (high-fat)
1 oz high-fat meat is like 1 oz lean meat in protein content but is estimated to have an **extra "1 fat"**—that is, to have the 3 g fat of a lean meat and 5 g additional fat.
Examples:
1 oz country-style ham.
1 oz cheddar cheese.[a]
1 small hotdog (frankfurter).[b]
(1 high-fat meat = 7 g protein, 8 g fat, and 100 kcal.)

[b]The frankfurter counts as 1 high-fat meat exchange plus 1 fat exchange.

2d. Legumes
Legumes are an odd kind of plant food. They are like meats because they are rich in protein and iron, but many are lower in fat than meat. Besides, they contain a lot of starch. They can be treated as follows:
1 c legumes = 1 lean meat + 2 starch.
(1 c legumes = 30 g carbohydrate, 13 g protein, 3 + g fat, and 215 kcal.)
Legumes can also be considered similar to breads in being rich in complex carbohydrate, and the additional protein can be ignored. However, this treatment underestimates their kcalorie value, especially that of the higher-fat legumes such as peanuts.

Whatever you do with legumes on paper, however, use them often in cooking. You will learn many more reasons why they are an inexpensive, nutritious, high-quality, and health-promoting food.

4. Fruits
½ small banana is like:
1 small apple.
½ grapefruit.
½ c orange juice.
(1 fruit = 15 g carbohydrate and 60 kcal.)

5. Milks
1 c nonfat milk is like:
1 c nonfat yogurt, plain.
1 c nonfat buttermilk.
½ c evaporated nonfat milk.
(1 milk = 12 g carbohydrate, 8 g protein, trace of fat, and 90 kcal.)

6. Fats
1 tsp butter is like:
1 tsp margarine.
1 tsp any oil.
1 tbsp salad dressing.
1 strip crisp bacon.
5 large olives.
10 whole Virginia peanuts.
(1 fat = 5 g fat and 45 kcal.)

calcium-rich cheeses. However, with practice, users can learn to make selections from the exchange list that will meet vitamin and mineral requirements, as well as energy needs.

Combining Food Group Plans and Exchange Patterns

If you are a diet planner who wants to choose foods that contain all the nutrients you need, you may find both the food group plan and the exchange system useful. The food group plan promotes adequacy and balance, helping you to avoid overemphasizing one class of food. The exchange system provides the lists from which to make your food selections; by following it, you can employ moderation and control kcalories without effort.

The demonstration in Table 2–3 shows that when you use the Four Food Group Plan as a pattern and the exchange system as a guide for choosing the items to eat, you can get by with a surprisingly small food energy intake. All recommended items can total about 1,000 kcalories while providing adequacy for most of the major nutrients. An average adult would still have 500 to 1,000 more kcalories to spend. A wise choice would be to invest many of those additional kcalories in additional vegetables, fruits, and whole-grain foods, or in large servings of legumes or nuts in place of, or in addition to, some of the meat. Some of the extra kcalories could be spent adding more starch-containing foods (such as starchy vegetables or snacks like unbuttered popcorn). Others could be invested in occasional sweet desserts; some butter, margarine, or oil; or even alcohol. If these additions were made, they would be made by choice rather than through the unintentional use of high-kcalorie foods.

At the same time, you can exercise to "earn" additional kcalories. Clearly, the person interested in good health, fitness, and weight control will not just eat an adequate diet, but will combine diet and exercise into a daily pattern that supports optimal health.

■ TABLE 2–3

Diet Planning with Exchange System using Four Food Group Pattern

Pattern from Four Food Group Plan	Selections Made Using the Exchange System	Example	Energy Cost (kcal)
Milk—2 c	Milk list—select 2 exchanges	2 c nonfat milk	180
Meat—2 servings (2 to 3 oz each)	Meat list—select 6 exchanges[a]	6 oz lean meat	330
Fruits and vegetables—4 servings	Fruit and vegetable lists—select 4 exchanges	2 vegetable exchanges; 2 fruit exchanges	50 120
Grains (breads and cereals)—4 servings	Starch/bread list—select 4 exchanges	2 bread exchanges; 2 starchy vegetable exchanges	320
Total			1,000

[a]In the Four Food Group Plan, 1 serving is 2 to 3 oz. In the exchange system, 1 exchange is 1 oz.

With judicious selections, the diet can meet the need for all the nutrients and provide some luxury items as well. Adequacy and balance would be achieved, not necessarily at each meal, but within each day. The planner could achieve variety by selecting different foods each day from the exchange lists. The final plan might be like that outlined in Table 2–4 (one of many possible examples).

Diet planners use different patterns of exchanges for different energy levels. A person eating 3,000 kcalories per day could use considerably more bread exchanges, for example, than a person eating 1,500 kcalories per day. Table 2–5 shows diet plans for different energy intakes.

■ TABLE 2–4
A Sample Diet Plan

Exchange	Energy (kcal)[a]
7 starch/bread	560
6 medium-fat meat	450
2 vegetable	50
3 fruit	180
2 nonfat milk	180
4 fat	180
	1,600

[a]This diet derives about 20% of its kcalories from protein, about 30% from fat, and nearly 50% from carbohydrate.

■ *Dietary Guidelines*

Having planned a diet using the principles of adequacy, balance, kcalorie control, moderation, and variety, you can now ask how it compares with recommended nutrient intakes. You will find that the RDA and RNI make specific recommendations for protein, vitamins, and minerals, but only make general statements about energy intakes and do little to protect people from overnutrition.

Research has identified excess intakes of sugar, fat, cholesterol, salt, and alcohol as contributing factors to many illnesses, including heart disease, cancer, diabetes, and liver disease. Many nutrition scientists therefore feel that the public should be urged to curtail their intakes of these substances. However, while some feel justified in offering concrete advice, others feel uncomfortable about offering any advice at all. The two points of view might be characterized as the preventive approach and the medical approach.

The preventive approach emphasizes everyone's health, and if it errs, it does so on the side of urging more people to make more changes than may be necessary. The object is to help everyone forestall or prevent any disease whose onset or severity may be affected by diet. Proponents believe that since we can't predict just which individuals may be responsive to dietary factors related to diseases, we should offer the same advice to all.

■ TABLE 2–5
Diet Patterns for Different Energy Intakes

Exchange	Energy Level (kcal)						
	1,200	1,500	1,800	2,000	2,200	2,600	3,000
Starch/bread	4	6	8	9	11	13	15
Meat	5	5	5	6	6	7	8
Vegetable	3	3	4	5	5	6	6
Fruit	3	3	4	4	4	5	6
Milk	2	3	3	3	3	3	3
Fat	4	5	6	7	8	10	12

[a]These patterns of exchanges supply about 30% of the kcalories as fat, in accordance with the view that a moderate fat intake is desirable.

The medical approach is the more conservative, traditional position. It urges each person who needs to make a dietary change to do so. The problem is that usually, by the time the person can be identified, symptoms of the disease are already appearing. This approach waits until cure is needed rather than emphasizing prevention, and it puts the physician in the role of treating an already-existing disease rather than promoting health.

■ TABLE 2–6
Dietary Recommendations for the General Public

Year	Agency[b]	Publication	Variety	Maintain Ideal Body Weight	Include Starch and Fiber	Limit Sugar[c]	Limit Fat[c]	Limit Cholesterol	Limit Salt	Limit Alcohol
1977	U.S. Senate	*Dietary Goals for the U.S.*		+	+	+	+	+	+	
1979	DHEW	*Healthy People: The Surgeon General's Report on Health Promotion and Disease Prevention*	+	+	+	+	+	+	+	+
1979	DHEW/NCI	*Statement on Diet, Nutrition, and Cancer—Prudent Interim Principles*	+	+	+		+			+
1980	USDA/DHHS	*Dietary Guidelines for Americans*	+	+	+	+	+	+	+	+
1980	DHHS	*National 1990 Nutrition Objectives*	+	+	+	+	+	+	+	+
1984	DHHS/NHLBI	*Recommendations for Control of High Blood Pressure*		+			+		+	+
1985	USDA/DHHS	*Dietary Guidelines for Americans, 2nd edition*	+	+	+	+	+	+	+	+
1986	DHHS/NCI	*Cancer Control Nutrition Objectives for the Nation: 1985–2000*		+	+		+			+
1987	DHHS/NHLBI	*National Cholesterol Education Program Guidelines*	+	+	+		+	+		+
1988	DHHS/NCI	*Dietary Guidelines for Cancer Prevention*	+	+	+		+		+	+
1988	DHEW	*The Surgeon General's Report on Nutrition and Health*	+	+	+	+	+	+	+	+
1989	NRC	*Diet and Health: Implications for Reducing Chronic Disease Risk*	+	+	+	+	+	+	+	+

[a]Other recommendations include: increase consumption of foods containing vitamins and minerals (DHHS/NCI, 1986); increase physical activity (USDA/DHHS, 1980, 1985; DHHS, 1980); reduce intake of salt-cured or smoked foods (DHHS/NCI, 1988); use appropriate sources of fluoride, limit consumption and frequency of use of foods high in sugar, increase consumption of foods high in calcium, and consume foods that are good sources of iron (DHEW, 1988); maintain adequate calcium intake, avoid supplements in excess of RDA, and maintain optimal fluoride intake (NRC, 1989).

[b]U.S. Senate = U.S. Senate Select Committee on Nutrition and Human Needs; DHEW = Department of Health, Education, and Welfare; NCI = National Cancer Institute; USDA = United States Department of Agriculture; DHHS = Department of Health and Human Services; NHLBI = National Heart, Lung, and Blood Institute; NRC = National Research Council.

[c]Recommendations prior to 1977 were for *inclusion* in the daily diet, as opposed to subsequent recommendations to *limit* intake.

Source: Adapted from *The Surgeon General's Report on Nutrition and Health: Summary and Recommendations*, DHHS (PHS) publication no. 88–50211 (Washington, D.C.: Government Printing Office, 1988), Appendix C.

Choosing the preventive approach, government agencies and other organizations have published dietary guidelines that favor moderation. Table 2–6 lists some of the dietary guideline publications and their recommendations, including the 1988 *Surgeon General's Report on Nutrition and Health* and the 1989 National Academy of Sciences' report, *Diet and Health: Implications for Reducing Chronic Disease Risk*. This latter report was produced by the Committee on Diet and Health of the Food and Nutrition Board of the National Research Council (NRC). As you can see, there is more agreement than disagreement among these guidelines. Table 2–7 summarizes the dietary recommendations from the 1989 *NRC Report*.

From Guidelines to Groceries

To demonstrate the different influences that food selections have on a person's meeting the dietary recommendations, we've contrasted two days' meals in Figure 2–7, slightly exaggerated to make a point. One day, labeled "Monday's Meal Selections," contains fruit, vegetables, whole grains, nonfat milk, and modest amounts of seafood and legumes. The other day, labeled "Tuesday's Meal Selections," emphasizes meat or eggs at every meal. Look for the similarities and differences in these two ways of eating. You may notice that

■ TABLE 2–7
NRC Dietary Recommendations

• Reduce total *fat* intake to 30 percent or less of kcalories. Reduce saturated fatty acid intake to less than 10 percent of kcalories, and the intake of cholesterol to less than 300 milligrams daily.[a]

• Increase intake of starches and other *complex carbohydrates*.[b]

• Maintain *protein* intake at moderate levels.[c]

• Balance food intake and physical activity to maintain appropriate *body weight*.

• For those who drink *alcoholic beverages*, limit consumption to the equivalent of less than 1 ounce of pure alcohol in a single day.[d] Pregnant women should avoid alcoholic beverages.

• Limit total daily intake of *salt* (sodium chloride) to 6 grams or less.[e]

• Maintain adequate *calcium* intake.

• Avoid taking dietary *supplements* in excess of the RDA in any one day.

• Maintain an optimal intake of *fluoride*, particularly during the years of primary and secondary tooth formation and growth.

Note: Italics added to highlight the areas of concern.

[a]The intake of fat and cholesterol can be reduced by substituting fish, poultry without skin, lean meats, and low-fat or nonfat dairy products for fatty meats and whole-milk products; by choosing more vegetables, fruits, cereals, and legumes; and by limiting oils, fats, egg yolks, and fried and other fatty foods.
[b]Every day eat five or more servings of a combination of vegetables and fruits, especially green and yellow vegetables and citrus fruits, and six or more daily servings of a combination of breads, cereals, and legumes.
[c]Meet at least the RDA for protein; do not exceed twice the RDA.
[d]The committee does not recommend alcohol consumption. One ounce of pure alcohol is the equivalent of two cans of beer, two small glasses of wine, or two average cocktails.
[e]Limit the use of salt in cooking, and avoid adding it to food at the table. Salty, highly processed salty, salt-preserved, and salt-pickled foods should be consumed sparingly.

Source: Adapted from the National Academy of Sciences report, *Diet and Health: Implications for Reducing Chronic Disease Risk* which was produced by the Committee on Diet and Health of the Food and Nutrition Board of the National Research Council and partially reprinted verbatim in *Nutrition Reviews* 47 (1989): 142–149.

■ FIGURE 2–7
Two Days' Meal Selections Compared

Monday's Meal Selections

A student rises early and prepares breakfast before heading off to classes:
- 1 c coffee
- 1 c oatmeal with ¼ c raisins
- 1 c nonfat milk
- 1¼ c strawberries

The student grabs a handful of dried fruits and nuts to snack on between morning classes:
- 2 tbsp raisins
- 2 tbsp sunflower seeds

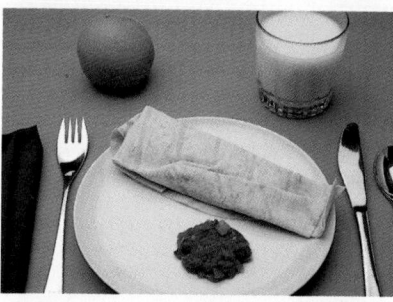

and an orange to eat with lunch. Lunch is fast-food fare:
- 1 bean burrito
- 1 c nonfat milk
- 1 orange

After classes, the student plays a quick game of racquetball and heads home. Later that evening, the student visits a friend for dinner. The friend serves:
A salad made with:
- 1 c raw spinach leaves
- 1 tbsp sesame seeds
- ¼ c fresh mushroom slices
- ¼ c water chestnuts
- ⅓ c garbanzo beans
- 1 tbsp vinaigrette dressing

A dinner of:
- 4 oz shrimp garnished with ⅛ lemon
- 1 c broccoli
- ½ c spinach noodles tossed with 2 tsp butter and ¼ c parsley
- ¼ tomato
- A glass of iced tea with 1 tsp sugar and ⅛ lemon

And, for dessert:
- ½ c sherbet

Total kcal: 1,759
57% kcal from carbohydrate
24% kcal from fat
19% kcal from protein

Tuesday's Meal Selections

Before biking off to campus, the student starts the day with a breakfast of:
  1 c coffee
  ½ c orange juice
  2 scrambled eggs
  2 pieces whole-wheat toast with 2 tsp butter

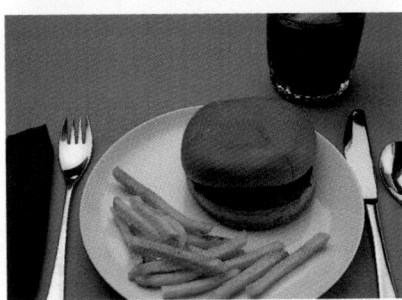

Between classes, the student grabs a fast-food meal:
  1 hamburger
  15 french fries
  12 oz diet cola

The student rides by a friend's house on the way home, and they decide to have dinner together. They prepare:
A salad made with:
  1 c iceberg lettuce
  1 tbsp ranch salad dressing
A main course of:
  6 oz steak
  ½ baked potato with 2 tsp butter
  A glass of iced tea with 1 tsp sugar and ⅛ lemon

Total kcal: 1,732
33% kcal from carbohydrate
44% kcal from fat
23% kcal from protein

Notice the similarities in these days' meals (both include a fast-food lunch and provide a similar number of kcalories) and the differences (apparent from the different food groups included). Monday's meal selections offer more food, including a snack and a dessert, and a greater variety than Tuesday's choices. Monday's meals provide less than 30% of the kcalories from fat, while Tuesday's choices supply a whopping 44% of the kcalories from fat. As

Chapter 12 will discuss, the contribution fat makes to the diet may be a greater factor in controlling body weight than is total energy intake. Wherever appropriate, the chapters will revisit these meals and see how they score with respect to individual nutrients. As you will see, neither day lacks for protein, but Monday does much better in terms of most vitamins and minerals, fiber, fat, and cholesterol than does Tuesday.

a person can eat a lot of fat without consuming much food and that a person can eat a lot of food without having to consume too much food energy or fat. You can see that even a nutritious diet has room for a sweet treat and a fast-food meal now and then, too.

People make different meal selections daily. Some days may look like Monday's choices, while other days might more closely resemble Tuesday's fare. Still others will look entirely different from either of those represented in Figure 2–7. Later chapters will discuss the contributions the foods in these meals make toward a day's intake. The chapters will show that most foods have something of value to offer. Much of the art of balancing the diet is a matter of learning appropriate frequencies with which to eat various foods.

■ Study Questions

1. What factors are considered in setting nutrient and energy intake recommendations?
2. What is the difference between the RDA and the U.S. RDA?
3. Describe the diet-planning guides and how they are used. What are each of their strengths and weaknesses?

■ Notes

1. Food and Nutrition Board, *Recommended Dietary Allowances*, 10th ed. (Washington, D.C.: National Academy Press, 1989), p. 1.
2. H. Kamin, Status of the 10th edition of the Recommended Dietary Allowances—prospects for the future, *American Journal of Clinical Nutrition* 41 (1985): 165–170.
3. H. A. Guthrie, The Recommended Dietary Allowance Committee: An overview, *Journal of the American Dietetic Association* 85 (1985): 1646–1648.
4. Food and Nutrition Board, 1989, pp. 8–9.
5. Kamin, 1985.

SELF STUDY *Calculate Your Nutrient Intakes*

This self-study exercise directs you to calculate your nutrient intakes for the three-day period in which you wrote down what foods you ate (Self Study from Chapter 1). Appendix K provides the necessary forms.

1. If you are using a computer to analyze your diet, follow program instructions for entering dietary data. If you are analyzing your diet manually, use Appendix H to calculate, for each day, your total intakes of energy, protein, fat, fatty acids, carbohydrate, fiber, and all of the nutrients listed in Appendix H.

   If the foods you have eaten are not included in the appendix or computer program, read the label on the package, or use your inge-nuity to guess their composition, using the most similar food you can find as a guide. For example, if you ate halibut (which is not listed), you would not be far off in using the values for haddock or perch. If you ate cream of celery soup, you might substitute the values for cream of mushroom soup.

   Be careful in recording the nutrient amounts in odd-sized portions. For example, if you used a quarter cup of milk, then you will have to record a fourth of the amount of every nutrient listed for a cup of milk. (Computer programs will do this mathematical calcula-tion automatically; be careful to enter the appropriate amount.)

   Note the units in which the nutrients are measured:

- Energy is measured in kcalories (kcal).
- Protein, fat, fatty acids, and carbohydrate are measured in grams (g).
- Calcium, iron, zinc, thiamin, riboflavin, niacin, vitamin C (ascorbic acid), and cholesterol are measured in milligrams (mg). Folate is measured in micrograms (mcg or μg). Thus "800 milligrams calcium" is the same as "0.8 grams calcium," and "400 micrograms folate" is the same as "0.4 milligrams folate." Be sure to convert all calcium amounts to milligrams and all folate amounts to micrograms before calculating.
- Vitamin A can be measured in international units (IU) or retinol equivalents (RE);* 1 RE equals 3 IU of vitamin A from animal foods or 10 IU of vitamin A from plant foods. Appendix H lists vitamin A in RE to ease comparison with the RDA, which is also in RE. (For more details, see Chapter 8.) If you eat a packaged food whose label lists vitamin A in IU, be sure to convert to RE before calculating.

   If you eat a packaged food whose label lists nutrient amounts as "percent of U.S. RDA," use the table on the inside front cover (right) to convert to grams, milligrams, micrograms, or RE. Suppose a food portion contains "25 percent of the U.S. RDA of iron," for example. The table shows that the U.S. RDA for iron is 18 milligrams. The food portion therefore contributes a fourth of 18 milligrams, or 4.5 milligrams of iron.

2. Now total the amount of each nutrient you've consumed for each day, and transfer your totals to Form 2. Form 2 provides a convenient means of deriving and keeping on record an average intake for each nutrient.

3. As a final step, transfer your average intakes to Form 3 for future reference. For comparison, enter the intakes recommended for a person of your age and sex, using either the RDA (on the inside front cover, left) or the Canadian RNI (in Appendix I), whichever you prefer. Note that no recommendations are made for intakes of fat or carbohydrate. Guidelines for these nutrients and for others, like cholesterol and fiber, will be presented and discussed later. Succeeding self-studies will guide you in focusing on each of the nutrients provided by your diet.

   Suspend judgment about the adequacy of your diet for the moment. You have much to learn about your individuality, the nutrients, and the recommendations before you can reach any reasonable conclusions.

4. What percentage of the kcalories you consumed comes from protein, fat, and carbohydrate? (Use Form 4 to calculate.)

5. You can get an indication of whether your diet is balanced by using the Food Group Plan Scorecard (Form 5—one copy for each day). How does your diet score by these criteria?

* One IU of vitamin A is equal to 0.344 μg of crystalline vitamin A acetate or 0.6 μg of all-*trans* beta-carotene.

Who Speaks on Nutrition?

When you need nutrition advice, whom can you ask? Many people will say you should ask your physician, for "the doctor" is supposed to be an expert on everything related to health. But can you rely on your physician to give you accurate information on nutrition? If not, on whom can you rely? The answer, as you will see, is that registered dietitians are usually the best-qualified experts on nutrition.

The dietitian is educated specifically to understand nutrition needs and to deliver counsel and care. A dietitian who is the genuine article—that is, a registered dietitian—has an undergraduate degree requiring some 60 or so semester hours in nutrition and food science, has completed a year's clinical internship or the equivalent, has passed a national examination administered over six competency areas by the American Dietetic Association or the Canadian Dietetic Association, and maintains up-to-date knowledge obtained through required continuing education activities (attending seminars, taking courses, or writing professional papers). Dietitians who have met these criteria may display the credential R.D., indicating registration with the American Dietetic Association (ADA), should a consumer want to check on their credentials.

Dietitians work in a variety of settings performing a multitude of duties. Dietitians can assume roles in clinical, administrative, consultant, public health, foodservice, research, and education settings. An example of the competencies of a clinical dietitian is provided in Table H2–1.

Why, in talking about the dietitian, did we specify that the person had to be "the genuine article"? For reasons no one quite understands, of all fields, nutrition is the most riddled with quack practitioners. Literally

■ TABLE H2–1
Competencies of the Clinical Dietitian

- Assesses nutrition status.
- Develops and individualizes care plans.
- Implements, monitors, and evaluates care plans.
- Educates clients and families.
- Develops policies and procedures.
- Communicates effectively with physicians, nurses, and pharmacists regarding clients' nutrition status, needs, and treatment.
- Interfaces with foodservice personnel.
- Supervises dietetic staff.
- Participates in professional activities to enhance knowledge and skill.
- Serves the profession politically.
- Educates dietetics students and interns.

Source: Adapted from P. M. Kris-Etherton and coauthors, A profile of clinical dietetics practice in Pennsylvania, *Journal of the American Dietetic Association* 83 (1983): 654–660.

thousands of people possess fake nutrition degrees. A well-known quack fighter says, "I am aware of no other field in which this phenomenon has ever taken place."[1]

The documents many of these people display claim that they are dietitians (without the ADA-sanctioned R.D. credentials), or nutritionists, or dietists, or other such. These titles are promoted as if they were equivalent in meaning to established credentials, but they are not.[2] That being the case, if we are to turn to dietitians for our diet advice, we have two tasks on our hands: first, to tell the real ones from the fake ones, and second, to tell the good ones from the poor ones—for, as with other professionals, the possession of even a legitimate credential does not necessarily make a person a

high-quality professional, or even an honest human being.

A person who wants to visit a dietitian and obtain nutrition advice needs to know that in many states the title *dietitian* is no guarantee of professionalism. Many states allow use of the title by anyone who wants to use it, just as people can call themselves counselors. Some states have passed laws to allow only qualified individuals to call themselves dietitians, and have specified that R.D.s or people with certain graduate degrees are the only ones who qualify. Many states now provide a further guarantee: the license to practice.[3] Licensing does not offer complete protection against nutrition quackery, but it makes it difficult for unqualified people to advertise widely that they are experts.

Some states also regulate the use of the title nutritionist—a welcome development, for that title has enticed thousands of consumers into scams where they have lost their health, their lives' savings, or both. If the term is to be meaningful, it should apply only to people who have an M.S. (master of science) or Ph.D. (doctor of philosophy) degree in nutrition or related fields from accredited colleges or universities, not other forms of education. An M.S. or Ph.D. in nutrition requires two to seven years of training in an accredited graduate school. A course of (for example) six to nine months at a correspondence school is simply not the same. Some schools are not even legitimate correspondence schools, but diploma mills—places that, essentially, sell certificates of competency to anyone who pays the fees.

Evidence of *accreditation* is important in the description of the institution from which the education comes. The most rampant abuse of credentials is

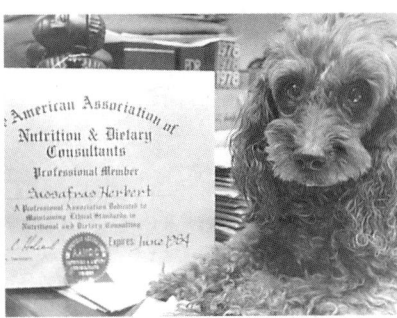

Charlie and Sassafras display their professional credentials.

Miniglossary

accreditation: approval; in the case of hospitals or universities, approval by a professional organization qualified to judge the quality of the service or educational program offered.

dietitian: a person trained in nutrition, food science, and diet planning. A **registered dietitian (R.D.)** is a dietitian who has graduated from an accredited program of dietetics, has passed the professional American Dietetic Association registration examination, and has served in an internship program to practice the necessary skills. Some states require licensing for dietitians; others do not.

license to practice: permission under state or federal law to use a certain title (such as medical doctor, osteopath, attorney, etc.) and to offer certain services. The procedure by which a license is granted involves passing a state-administered examination.

nutritionist: a person who specializes in the study of nutrition. Some nutritionists are registered dietitians, whereas others are self-described experts whose training may be minimal or nonexistent. If the term is to be meaningful, it should apply only to people who have master's (M.S.) or doctoral (Ph.D.) degrees from institutions accredited to offer such degrees in nutrition or related fields, not to those who have other forms of education.

R.D.: see *dietitian*.

registration: listing; specifically with respect to health professionals, a listing with a professional organization signifying that the professional has satisfied certain requirements, such as course work, experience, and the passing of an examination, and so may use the title and practice the profession.

in the display of master's and doctoral degrees. According to the *New York Times*, doctorates are available for around $2,300; master's degrees, for $1,250; and bachelor's, for $800—with discounts for all three together. To obtain them, a candidate need not read any books or pass any exams. They are available from "accredited" schools, too, for there are 30 phony accrediting agencies.[4]

To dramatize the situation, one writer enrolled for $82 in a nutrition diploma mill that billed itself as a correspondence school offering nutrition degrees. She made every attempt to fail the course, even answering all the examination questions wrong on purpose. Even so, she received a "Nutritionist" certificate at the end of the course, together with a letter from the "school" explaining that they were sure she must have just misread the test.[5]

In a similar stunt, Ms. Sassafras Herbert has been named a "professional member" of a professional association. For her efforts, Sassafras has received a wallet card and the privilege of being listed in a sort of fake Who's Who in nutrition that is distributed at health fairs and trade shows nationwide. Sassafras is a poodle; her master, Victor Herbert, M.D., paid $50 to prove that she could win these honors merely by sending in her name. Mr. Charlie Herbert also is a professional member of such an organization; Charlie is a cat.

To check a recommended provider's credentials, first look for the degrees listed by the person's titles. Then find out what you can about the reputations of the institutions where the degrees were obtained. One of the best sources of information as to whether a school or other institution is legitimate or not is the National Council Against Health Fraud, whose address is in Appendix F. Then call and ask your state's health-licensing agency if dietitians are licensed in your state and (if so) if the person you are interested in has met licensure criteria.

If you set about researching whether an institution is a genuine graduate school, you may find yourself pursuing a fascinating detective story:

- The university should have an address, some buildings, and a faculty consisting of people with bona fide degrees. If you ask to speak to the dean of graduate studies, such a person should exist. A post office box number without a street address is practically a guarantee that the degree-granting institution is a fraud.

- The university should show evidence of accreditation by the appropriate professional associations, membership in which constitutes a seal of approval to practice—for example, the American Medical Association (AMA) for a medical school or the American Dietetic Association (ADA) for a program in dietetics. (Read about the associations in the library's *Encyclopedia of Associations*.)

- The accrediting agency itself should be recognized by the U.S. Department of Education. (Look up the department under "United States" in the telephone book.)

Once you have found a *true* nutritionist (or preferably, a registered dietitian), you still need to find a competent one. You may have to shop around and try appointments with more than one before you are satisfied on all counts.

NOTES

1. S. Barrett, Why licensing of "nutritionists" is needed, *Nutrition Forum,* May 1985, p. 40.

2. Barrett, 1985.

3. M. B. Haschke, President's page: Licensure for dietitians: The issue in context, *Journal of the American Dietetic Association* 84 (1984): 454–457.

4. *New York Times* Service story in the *San Bernardino* (Calif.) *Times,* 6 August 1985, as cited in *National Council against Health Fraud Newsletter,* August 1985, p. 1.

5. V. Aronson, Bernardean University: A nutrition diploma mill, *ACSH News and Views,* March–April 1983, pp. 7, 11.

Digestion, Absorption, and Transport

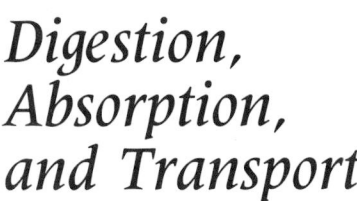

Contents

Digestion

Absorption

The Circulatory Systems

Regulation of Digestion and Absorption

Highlight: Common Digestive Problems

The cells of the gastrointestinal tract lining display an intricate architecture that supports their function. Part of one cell is shown here with microvilli at the top. The round, dark bodies are lipid droplets (chylomicrons) forming within the cell from recently absorbed lipid fragments. These will be coated with protein and released into the body for transport elsewhere. The slim, striped bodies inside the cell are mitochondria, busily producing energy to fuel the cell's work.

Have you ever wondered where the food you eat goes and what happens to it after you swallow it? Or how your body extracts nutrients from food? Have you ever marveled at how it all just seems to happen? This chapter takes you on the journey that transforms the foods you eat into the nutrients that highlight the following eight chapters. Then it follows the nutrients as they travel across the intestinal cells and into the body to do their work.

■ Digestion

The digestive system solves many problems for you without your having to make any conscious effort. In fact, the digestive tract is the body's ingenious way of getting the nutrients ready for absorption. Let's consider the problems that are involved:

Miniglossary of Digestive Enzymes appears on p. 49.

1. Human beings breathe as well as eat and drink through their mouths. Air taken in through the mouth must go to the lungs; food and liquid must go to the stomach. The throat must be arranged so that food and liquid do not travel to the lungs.
2. Below the lungs lies the diaphragm, a dome of muscle that separates the upper half of the major body cavity from the lower half. Food must be conducted through this wall to reach the abdomen.
3. To pass smoothly through the system, food must be lubricated with water and ground to a paste. Too much water would cause the paste to flow too rapidly; too little would compact it too much, which could cause it to stop moving. The amount of water should be regulated to keep the intestinal contents at the right consistency.
4. For digestive enzymes to break down food, they need it in finely divided form, suspended in a watery solution so that every particle will be accessible. Once digestion is complete and the needed nutrients have been absorbed out of the tract into the body, only a residue remains, which is excreted. It would be both wasteful and messy to excrete large quantities of water with this residue, so some water should be withdrawn, leaving a paste just solid enough to be smooth and easy to pass.
5. The materials within the tract should be kept moving, slowly but steadily, at a pace that permits all reactions to reach completion. The materials should not be allowed to back up, except when a poison or like substance has been swallowed. At such a time, the flow should reverse, to get rid of the poison by the shortest possible route (upward). If infection sets in farther down the tract, the flow should be accelerated, to speed its passage out of the body (downward).
6. The enzymes of the digestive tract are designed to digest carbohydrate, fat, and protein. The walls of the tract, composed of living cells, are also made of carbohydrate, fat, and protein. These cells need protection against the action of the powerful juices that they secrete.
7. Once waste matter has reached the end of the tract, it must be excreted, but it would be inconvenient and embarrassing if this function occurred

continuously. Provision must be made for periodic, voluntary evacuation when convenient.

The following sections show how the body elegantly and efficiently handles these situations.

Anatomy of the Digestive Tract

The gastrointestinal (GI) tract is a flexible muscular tube measuring about 26 feet in length from the mouth to the anus. Figure 3–1 traces the path followed by food from one end to the other, and the accompanying miniglossary defines GI anatomy terms. In a sense, the human body surrounds the GI tract. Only things that penetrate the tract's wall ever enter the body proper; many things pass through unabsorbed.

When you swallow a mouthful of food, it first slides across your epiglottis, bypassing the entrance to your lungs. This is the body's solution to problem 1: the epiglottis closes off your air passages so that you don't choke when you swallow. After a mouthful of food has been swallowed, it is called a bolus.

Next, the bolus slides down the esophagus, which conducts it through the diaphragm (problem 2) to the stomach. The stomach cells produce secretions to both break down food particles and protect themselves from such action (problem 6). The cardiac sphincter at the entrance to the stomach closes behind the bolus so that it can't slip back (problem 5). The stomach retains the bolus for a while, adds water to it, and grinds it to a suspension of particles in liquid called chyme. Then, bit by bit, the stomach releases the chyme through the pylorus into the small intestine, and the pylorus, too, closes behind it.

At the top of the small intestine the chyme bypasses an opening (entrance only—no exit) from a duct (the common bile duct), which is dripping fluids (problem 3) into the small intestine from two organs outside the GI tract—the gallbladder and the pancreas. The chyme travels on down the small intestine through its three segments—the duodenum, the jejunum, and the ileum—a total of 20 feet of tubing coiled within the abdomen.

Having traveled through these segments of the small intestine, the chyme arrives at another sphincter (problem 5 again): the ileocecal valve, at the beginning of the large intestine (colon) in the lower right-hand side of the abdomen. As the chyme enters the colon, it passes another opening. Had it slipped into this opening, it would have ended up in the appendix, a blind sac about the size of your little finger. The chyme bypasses this opening, however, and travels along the large intestine up the right-hand side of the abdomen, across the front to the left-hand side, down to the lower left-hand side, and finally below the other folds of the intestines to the back side of the body, above the rectum.

During chyme's passage to the rectum, the colon withdraws water from it, leaving semisolid waste (problem 4). The strong muscles of the rectum hold back this waste until it is time to defecate. Then the rectal muscles relax (problem 7), and the last sphincter in the system, the anus, opens to allow passage of the waste.

To sum up, the path followed is as shown in Figure 3–1. This is a remarkably simple route, considering all that happens on the way.

GI tract: the gastrointestinal tract or digestive tract; the principal organs are the stomach and intestines.
gastro = stomach

Choking is discussed on p. 65.

bolus (BOH-lus): the portion of food swallowed at one time.

chyme (KIME): the semiliquid mass of partly digested food expelled by the stomach into the duodenum.
chymos = juice

■ **FIGURE 3–1**
The Gastrointestinal Tract
Route followed by food: MOUTH past epiglottis to ESOPHAGUS through cardiac sphincter to STOMACH through pylorus to SMALL INTESTINE (duodenum, with entrance from gallbladder and pancreas; then jejunum; then ileum) through ileocecal valve to LARGE INTESTINE past appendix to RECTUM ending at ANUS.

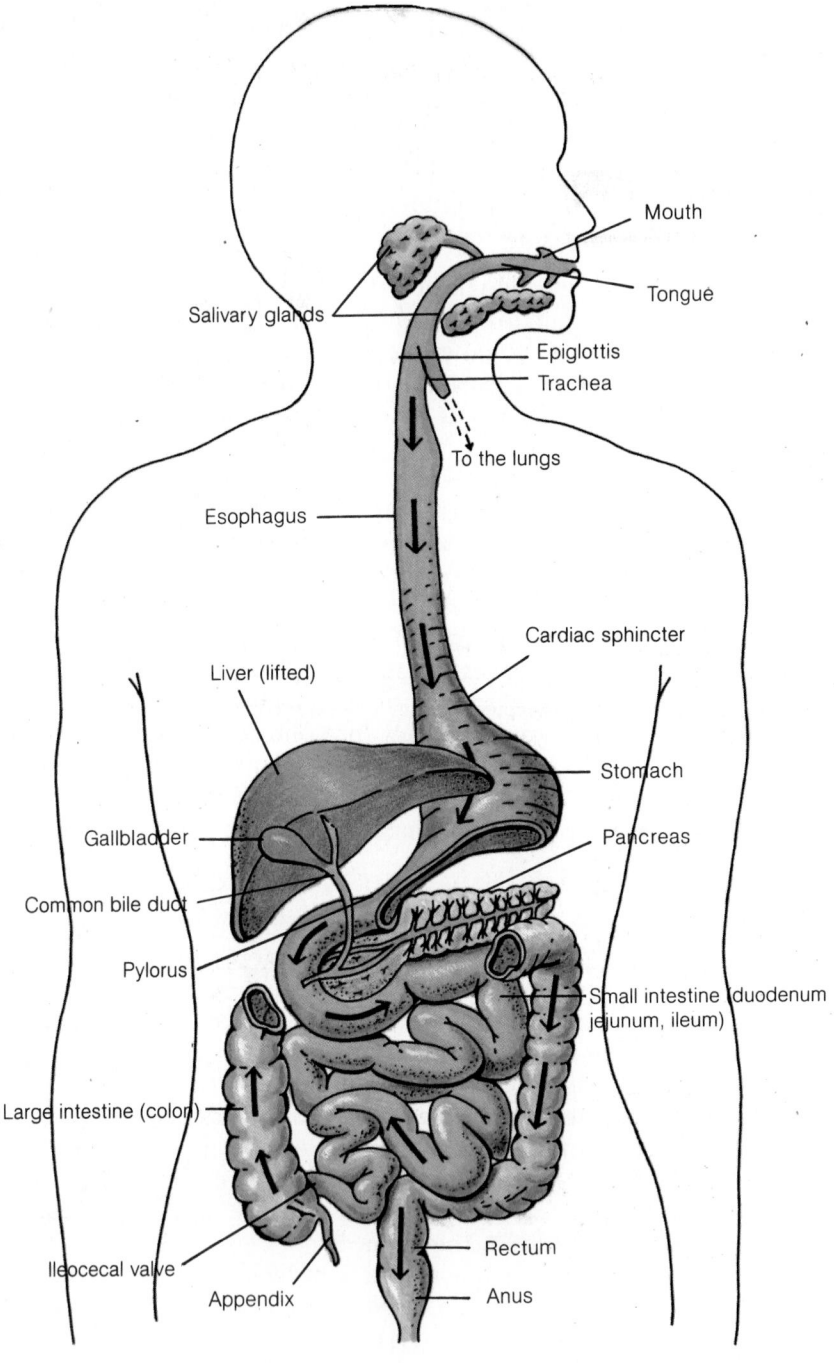

gland: a cell or group of cells that secretes materials for special uses in the body. Glands may be **exocrine glands**, secreting their materials "out" (into the digestive tract or onto the surface of the skin), or **endocrine glands**, secreting their materials "in" (into the blood).

exo = outside
endo = inside
krine = to separate

The Involuntary Muscles and the Glands

You are usually unaware of all the activity that goes on between the time you swallow and the time you defecate. As is the case with so much else that goes on in the body, the muscles and glands of the digestive tract meet internal needs without your having to exert any conscious effort to get the work done.

Miniglossary of Gastrointestinal Terms

epiglottis (epp-ee-GLOTT-iss): cartilage in the throat that guards the entrance to the trachea and prevents fluid or food from entering it when a person swallows (see p. 65).

epi = upon (over)

glottis = back of tongue

trachea (TRAKE-ee-uh): the windpipe; the passageway from the mouth and nose to the lungs.

esophagus (e-SOFF-uh-gus): the food pipe; the conduit from the mouth to the stomach.

cardiac sphincter (CARD-ee-ack SFINK-ter): the sphincter muscle at the junction between the esophagus and the stomach.

cardiac = the heart

sphincter: a circular muscle surrounding, and able to close, a body opening.

sphincter = band (binder)

pylorus: (pie-LORE-us): the sphincter muscle separating the stomach from the small intestine (also called **pyloric sphincter**).

pylorus = gatekeeper

gallbladder: the organ that stores and concentrates bile. When it receives the signal that fat is present in the duodenum, the gallbladder contracts and squirts bile down the bile duct into the duodenum.

pancreas: a gland that secretes digestive juices into the duodenum.

duodenum (doo-oh-DEEN-um, doo-ODD-num): the top portion of the small intestine (about "12 fingers' breadth" long, in ancient terminology).

duodecim = twelve

jejunum (je-JOON-um): the first two-fifths of the small intestine beyond the duodenum.

ileum (ILL-ee-um): the last segment of the small intestine.

ileocecal (ill-ee-oh-SEEK-ul) **valve:** the sphincter muscle separating the small and large intestines.

colon (COAL-un): the large intestine. Its segments are the ascending colon, the transverse colon, the descending colon, and the sigmoid colon.

sigmoid = shaped like the letter *S* (sigma in Greek)

appendix: a narrow blind sac extending from the beginning of the colon; a vestigial organ with no known function.

rectum: the muscular terminal part of the intestine, from the sigmoid colon to the anus.

anus (AY-nus): the terminal sphincter muscle of the GI tract.

You consciously control your chewing and swallowing, but even in your mouth there are some automatic processes over which you have no control. The salivary glands squirt just enough saliva to moisten each mouthful of food so that it can pass easily down your esophagus (problem 3).

At the top of the esophagus, peristalsis begins. The entire GI tract is ringed with muscles that can squeeze it tightly. Outside these rings of muscle lie longitudinal muscles. Whenever the rings tighten and the long muscles relax, the tube is constricted. Whenever the rings are relaxed and the long muscles

peristalsis (peri-STALL-sis): successive waves of involuntary muscular contraction passing along the walls of the GI tract.

peri = around

stellein = wrap

are tight, the tube bulges. These actions follow each other continuously, and push along the intestinal contents (problem 5). (If you have ever watched a lump of food pass along the body of a snake, you have a good picture of how these muscles work.) The waves of contraction ripple through the GI tract all the time, at the rate of about three a minute, whether or not you have just eaten a meal. Peristalsis, along with the sphincter muscles that surround the tract at key places, keeps things moving forward (Figure 3–2).

The intestines not only push, but also periodically squeeze, their contents at intervals—as if you had put a string around the intestines and pulled it

■ **FIGURE 3–2**
Peristalsis

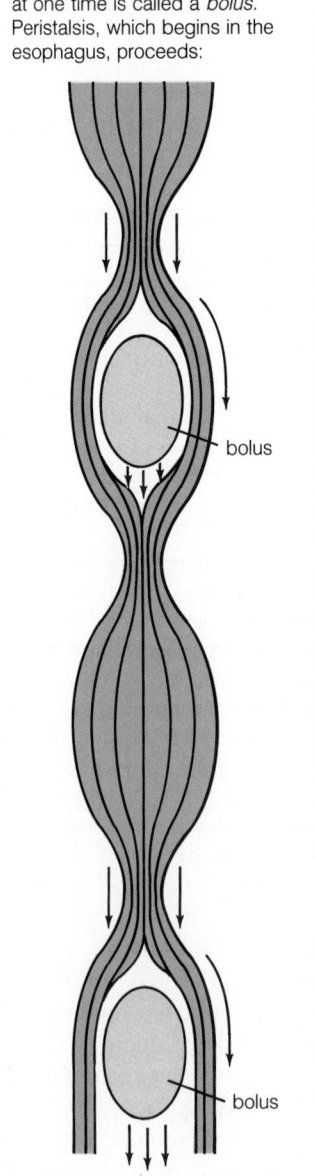

The portion of food swallowed at one time is called a *bolus*. Peristalsis, which begins in the esophagus, proceeds:

bolus

bolus

Longitudinal muscles   Circular muscles

Cross section of the GI tract muscles. Circular muscles are inside; longitudinal muscles are outside. When the inner circular muscles contract, the tube tightens. When the outer longitudinal muscles contract, the circular muscles relax and so the tube is loose.

The liquefied mass of partly digested food that travels through the intestines is called *chyme*. As the circular and longitudinal muscles tighten and relax, the chyme moves ahead of the constriction.

① ② ③

tight. This motion, called segmentation, momentarily forces the intestinal contents backward a few inches, mixing them and allowing the digestive juices and the absorbing cells of the walls to make better contact with them.

Four major sphincter muscles divide the GI tract into its principal divisions. The cardiac sphincter prevents reflux of the stomach contents into the esophagus. The pylorus, which stays closed most of the time, prevents backup of the intestinal contents into the stomach and also holds the bolus in the stomach long enough so that it can be thoroughly mixed with gastric juice and liquefied. At the end of the small intestine, the ileocecal valve performs a similar function, emptying the contents of the small intestine into the large intestine. Finally, the tightness of the rectal muscle is a kind of safety device; together with the anus, it prevents elimination until you choose to perform it voluntarily (problem 7).

Besides forcing the bolus along, the muscles of the GI tract help to liquefy it to chyme so that the digestive enzymes will have access to all the nutrients in the bolus. The first step in this process takes place in the mouth, where chewing, the addition of saliva, and the action of the tongue reduce the food to a coarse mash suitable for swallowing. A further mixing and kneading action then takes place in the stomach.

Of all parts of the GI tract, the stomach has the thickest walls and strongest muscles; in addition to the circular and longitudinal muscles, it has a third layer of diagonal muscles that also alternately contract and relax (see Figure 3–3). While these three sets of muscles are all at work forcing the chyme downward, the pylorus usually remains tightly closed, preventing the chyme from passing into the duodenum. Meanwhile, the gastric glands release juices—a mixture of hydrochloric acid and enzymes—that mix with the chyme. (The accompanying miniglossary defines some of the digestive enzymes.) As a result, the chyme is

segmentation: a periodic squeezing or partitioning of the intestine by its circular muscles.

reflux: a backward flow.
  re = back
  flux = flow

Miniglossary of Digestive Enzymes

digestive enzymes: proteins found in digestive juices that act on food substances, causing them to break down into simpler compounds.

-ase: a word ending denoting an enzyme. The first part of the word usually identifies the compound the enzyme works on.

amylase (AM-ih-lace): a carbohydrase; an enzyme that hydrolyzes amylose (a form of starch).

catalyst (CAT-uh-list): a compound that facilitates chemical reactions without itself being changed in the process.

carbohydrase: an enzyme that hydrolyzes carbohydrates.

hydrolysis (high-DROL-ih-sis): a chemical reaction in which a major reactant is split into two products, with the addition of H to one and OH to the other (from water).
  hydro = water
  lysis = breaking

lipase (LYE-pase): an enzyme that hydrolyzes lipids.

pepsin: a gastric protease. It circulates as a precursor, pepsinogen, and is converted to pepsin by the action of stomach acid.

protease (PRO-tee-ase): an enzyme that hydrolyzes proteins.

■ **FIGURE 3–3**
Stomach Muscles
The stomach has three layers of muscles.

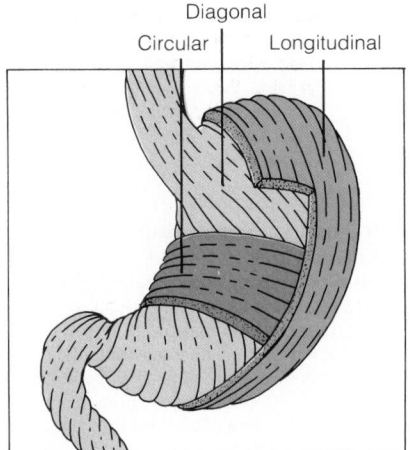

churned and forced down, hits the pylorus, and remains in the stomach. When the chyme is completely liquefied, the pylorus opens briefly, about three times a minute, to allow small portions through. At this point, the chyme no longer resembles food in the least.

The Process of Digestion

One person eats nothing but vegetables, fruits, and nuts; another, nothing but meat, milk, and potatoes. How is it that they wind up with essentially the same body composition? It all comes down to the body's rendering food—whatever it is to start with—into the basic units that make up carbohydrate, fat, and protein. The body absorbs these units and builds its tissues from them. To digest the food, five different body organs promote the breakdown of food to small units of nutrients that the body can absorb: the salivary glands, the stomach, the pancreas, the liver (via the gallbladder), and the small intestine (see Figure 3–4). (The accompanying miniglossary defines some of the digestive glands and their juices.)

Saliva The salivary glands secrete saliva, which contains water, salts, and enzymes, including salivary amylase (see Figure 3–5). Amylase breaks the bonds in the chains of starch, and thus digestion of starch begins in your mouth. In fact, you can taste the change if you choose. If you hold a piece of starchy food like white bread in your mouth without swallowing it, you can taste it getting sweeter as the enzyme acts on it. Saliva also protects the tooth surfaces and the linings of the mouth, esophagus, and stomach from attack by molecules that might harm them.[1]

pH: the unit of measure expressing a substance's acidity or alkalinity.

Highlight 3 discusses heartburn and other common digestive problems.

Gastric Juice Gastric juice is composed of water, enzymes, and hydrochloric acid. The acid is so strong (pH 2 or below—see Figure 3–6) that if it chances to reflux into the upper esophagus, it causes heartburn. The strong acidity of the stomach prevents bacterial growth and kills most bacteria that enter the body with food. It would destroy the cells of the stomach as well, but for their natural defenses. To protect themselves from gastric juice, the cells of the

■ **FIGURE 3–4**
Organs that Secrete Digestive Juices and Enzymes
The salivary glands, the stomach, the pancreas, the liver, and the small intestine produce secretions that promote the breakdown of food to small units that can be absorbed into the body. The pancreatic and bile ducts conduct secretions from the pancreas and the gallbladder into the small intestine.

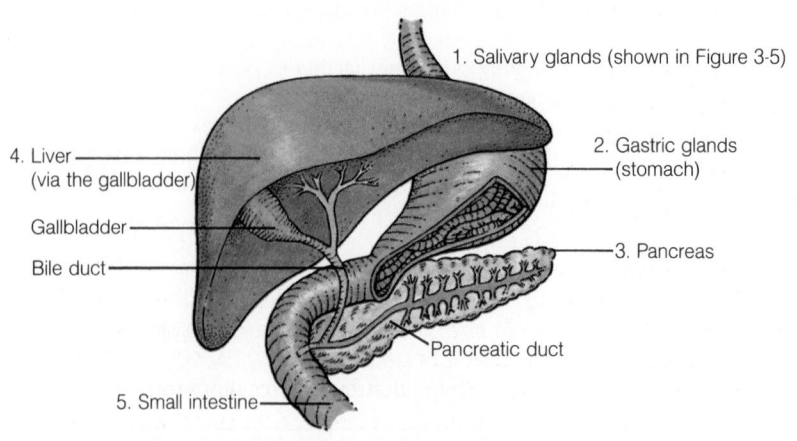

1. Salivary glands (shown in Figure 3-5)
2. Gastric glands (stomach)
3. Pancreas
4. Liver (via the gallbladder)
Gallbladder
Bile duct
Pancreatic duct
5. Small intestine

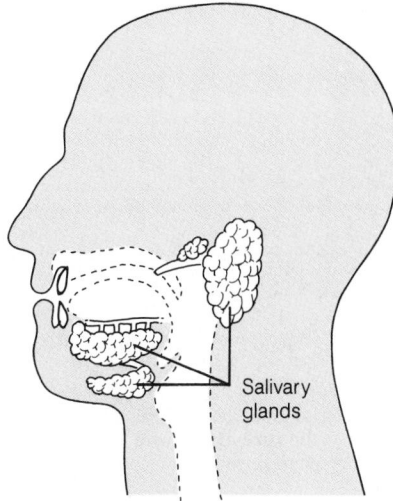

■ **FIGURE 3–5**
The Salivary Glands
The salivary glands secrete saliva into the mouth and begin the digestive process.

■ **FIGURE 3–6**
The pH Scale
A substance's acidity or alkalinity is measured in pH units. The pH is the negative logarithm of the hydrogen ion concentration. Each increment presents a tenfold increase in concentration of hydrogen particles. For example, a pH of 2 is 1,000 times stronger than a pH of 5.

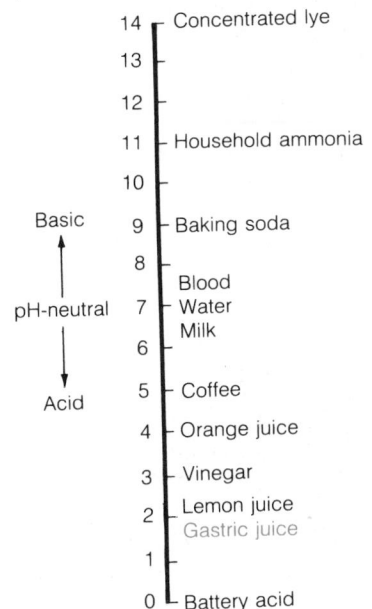

stomach wall secrete mucus, a thick, slimy, white substance that coats the cells, protecting them from the acid and enzymes that would otherwise digest them.

The stomach enzymes work most efficiently in a fluid of pH 2 or lower. However, the salivary amylase swallowed with a food does not work in acid this strong, so the digestion of starch ceases as the acid penetrates the bolus. In fact, salivary amylase becomes just another protein to be digested.

The only significant digestive event in the stomach is the partial hydrolysis of proteins. Both the enzyme pepsin and the stomach acid itself act as catalysts for this reaction. A gastric lipase accesses and hydrolyzes a very little fat in the stomach; the stomach acid hydrolyzes some carbohydrate to a very small extent; and the attachment of a protein carrier to vitamin B_{12} takes place in the stomach (discussed further in Chapter 8).

Pancreatic Juice and Intestinal Enzymes By the time food has left the stomach, digestion of all three energy nutrients has begun, but the action really gets going in the small intestine. There, the pancreas and liver contribute additional digestive juices by way of ducts leading into the duodenum (see Figure 3–4). The pancreatic juice contains enzymes (proteases, lipases, and amylases) that act on all three energy nutrients, and the cells of the intestinal wall also possess digestive enzymes on their surfaces.

In addition to enzymes, the pancreatic juice contains sodium bicarbonate, which is basic or alkaline in contrast to the stomach's acid. The pancreatic juice neutralizes the acidic chyme as it leaves the stomach to enter the small intestine. From this point on, the chyme remains at the neutral or slightly alkaline pH at which the enzymes of both the intestine and the pancreas work best.

Bile Bile also flows into the duodenum. Bile is secreted by the liver continuously, and it is concentrated and stored in the gallbladder, which squirts it into the duodenum when fat is present there. Bile is not an enzyme, but an emulsifier (described in Chapter 5); it brings fats into suspension in water so that enzymes can break them down into their component parts. Thanks to all these secretions, the three energy-yielding nutrients are digested in the small intestine.

The bacterial inhabitants of the GI tract are known as the **intestinal flora**.
flora = plant growth

The intestine, being neutral in pH, permits the growth of bacteria. In fact, a healthy intestinal tract supports a thriving bacterial population that normally does the body no harm, and may actually do some good. Provided that the normal intestinal flora are thriving, infectious bacteria have a hard time getting established and launching an attack on the system. Bacteria in the GI tract produce a variety of vitamins, but the extent of benefit to the person is unclear because nutrient absorption from the large intestine is poor.[2] However, nutrient absorption from bacterial synthesis in the small intestine is better, and may be a significant source of vitamin K. Even so, bacteria alone cannot meet the total need for vitamin K.[3]

The small intestine—and, in fact, the entire GI tract—also manufactures and maintains a strong arsenal of defenses against foreign invaders. Several different kinds of defending cells are present there and confer specific immunity against intestinal diseases.

Some vitamins and minerals are slightly altered during digestion. See "Vitamin B_{12}" in Chapter 8 and "Iron" in Chapter 11.

Chapter 4 discusses fiber in more detail.

stools: waste matter discharged from the colon; also called **feces**.

The story of how food is broken down into nutrients that can be absorbed is now nearly complete. All that remains is to recall what is left in the GI tract. The three energy-yielding nutrients—carbohydrate, fat, and protein—are the only ones that must be disassembled to basic building blocks before they are absorbed. The other nutrients—vitamins, minerals, and water—are mostly absorbable as is. Undigested residues, such as some fibers, are not absorbed, but continue through the digestive tract, providing a semisolid mass that help keep the muscles strong enough to perform peristalsis efficiently. Fiber also retains water, keeping the stools soft, and carries unwanted compounds out of the body.

The process of absorbing the nutrients into the body presents its own problems, to be discussed in the next section. For the moment, assume that the digested nutrients simply disappear from the GI tract as soon as they are ready. Most are gone by the time the contents of the GI tract reach the end of the small intestine. Little remains but water, a few dissolved salts and body secretions, and undigested materials such as fiber. These enter the large intestine (colon).

In the colon, intestinal bacteria degrade some of the fiber to simpler compounds. The colon itself actively retrieves from its contents the materials that the conservative body is designed to recycle—much of the water and the dissolved salts (see Figure 3–7). The remaining waste matter is excreted periodically.

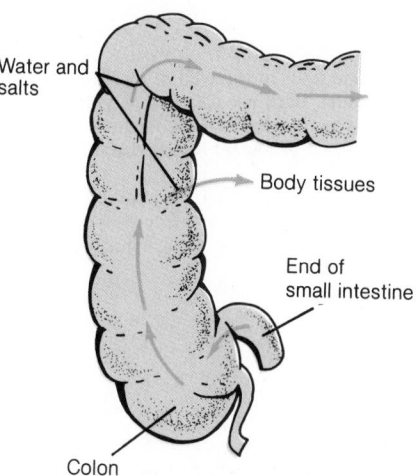

■ **FIGURE 3–7**
The Colon
The colon reabsorbs water and salts.

■ *Absorption*

Problem: Given an elaborate production in which 1,000 actors are on stage at once, provide a means by which all can exit simultaneously. This is the problem of absorption. Within three or four hours after you have eaten a dinner of beans and rice (or spinach lasagna, or steak and potatoes) with vegetable, salad, beverage, and dessert, your body must find a way to absorb—one by one—some two hundred thousand million, million, million molecules derived from carbohydrate digestion; an equivalent number of molecules derived from protein and fat digestion; and many vitamin and mineral molecules as well.

For the stage production, the manager might design multiple wings that all the actors could crowd into, a dozen at a time. A mechanical genius might somehow design conveyor-belt wings that would actively sweep up the actors as they approached. The absorptive system is no such fantasy; in 20 feet of small intestine, it provides a surface whose extent compares with a quarter of a football field in area, which engulfs and absorbs the nutrient molecules. To remove the molecules rapidly and provide room for more to be absorbed, a rush of circulating blood continuously washes the underside of this surface, carrying the absorbed nutrients away to the liver and other parts of the body.

Anatomy of the Absorptive System

The small intestine is a tube about 20 feet long and an inch or so across. Its inner surface looks smooth and slippery, but viewed through a microscope, it turns out to be wrinkled into hundreds of folds. Each fold is covered with thousands of nipplelike projections, as numerous as the hairs on velvet fabric. Each of these small intestinal projections is a villus. A single villus, magnified still more, turns out to be composed of hundreds of cells, each covered with its own microscopic hairs, the microvilli (see this chapter's opening art, and Figures 3–8 and 3–9).

The villi are in constant motion. Each villus is lined by a thin sheet of muscle, so it can wave, squirm, and wriggle like the tentacles of a sea anemone. Any nutrient molecule small enough to be absorbed is trapped among the microvilli that coat the cells and then drawn into the cells. Some partially digested nutrients are caught in the microvilli, digested further by enzymes there, and then absorbed into the cells.

Once a molecule has entered a cell in a villus, the next problem is to transport it to its destination elsewhere in the body. Everyone knows that the bloodstream performs this function, but you may be surprised to learn that there is a second transport system—the lymphatic system. Both of these systems supply vessels to each villus, as shown in Figure 3–8. When a nutrient molecule has crossed the cell of a villus, it may enter either the lymph or the blood. Eventually, all nutrients end up in the blood.

villus: a fingerlike projection from the folds of the small intestine; plural **villi** (VILL-ee, VILL-eye).

microvilli (MY-cro-VILL-ee, MY-cro-VILL-eye): projections from the membranes of the cells of the villi; singular **microvillus.**

lymphatic system: a loosely organized system of vessels and ducts that convey the products of digestion toward the heart.

lymph (limf): the body fluid found in lymphatic vessels. Lymph consists of all the constituents of blood except red blood cells.

■ **FIGURE 3–8**
The Small Intestinal Villi
A. Five folds in the wall of the small intestine. Each is covered with villi.
B. Two villi (detail of A). Each villus is composed of several hundred cells.
C. Three cells of a single villus (detail of B). Each cell is coated with microvilli. A photograph of part of two cells like these, on neighboring villi, is shown in Figure 3–10.

Villi

Microvilli

Capillaries

Lymph vessel

Vein

Artery

Lymph duct

A.

B.

C.

The problem of food contaminants, which may be absorbed defenselessly by the body, is the subject of Chapter 16.

A Closer Look at the Intestinal Cells

One of the beauties of the digestive tract is that it is selective. Materials that are nutritive for the body are broken down into particles that can be assimilated into the bloodstream. Most of the materials that are not nutritive are left undigested and pass out the other end of the digestive tract. The cells of the villi are among the most amazing in the body, for they recognize, select, and regulate the absorption of the nutrients the body needs. A close look at these cells is worthwhile, because it will help to explode a number of common misconceptions about nutrition.

Each cell of a villus is coated with thousands of microvilli, which project from the cell's membrane (see Figure 3–9). In these microvilli and in the membrane lie hundreds of different kinds of enzymes and "pumps," which recognize and act on different nutrients. (Descriptions of specific enzymes and "pumps" for each nutrient are presented in the following chapters where appropriate.)

A common misconception about digestion is that people should not eat certain food combinations (for example, fruit and meat) at the same meal,

Fluid in intestine

SURFACE COAT

Mucous coat

Microvilli on cell surface

boundaries of a single cell

■ FIGURE 3–9
Electronmicrograph of Cells of Two Adjacent Intestinal Villi
The microvilli and mucous coat are sometimes called the brush border of the intestinal cells. This photograph was taken through an electron microscope at a magnification of 51,000 times. Think how many of these cells there are in the small intestine (refer to Figure 3–8, and notice that even [A] represents but a tiny section of the intestinal wall). The photograph at the start of this chapter represents an even closer view of the one of these cells.

because the digestive system cannot handle more than one task at a time. The art of "food combining" (which actually emphasizes "food separating") is based on this idea, and it represents a gross underestimation of the body's capabilities. In fact, the contrary is often true; foods eaten together can enhance each other's use by the body. For example, the vitamin C in a pineapple enhances the absorption of some of the iron from chicken and rice eaten with it. Many other instances of mutually beneficial interactions are presented in later chapters.

As you can see, the cells of the intestinal tract wall are beautifully designed to perform their functions. A further refinement of the system is that the cells of successive portions of the tract are specialized for different absorptive functions. The nutrients that are ready for absorption early are absorbed near the top of the tract; those that take longer to be digested are absorbed farther down. Medical and health professionals who deal with digestion learn the specialized absorptive functions of different parts of the GI tract so that when one part becomes dysfunctional, the diet can be adjusted accordingly.

The rate at which the nutrients travel through the GI tract is finely adjusted to maximize their availability to the appropriate absorptive segment of the tract when they are ready. The lowly "gut" turns out to be one of the most elegantly designed organ systems in your body.

Once inside the intestinal cells, the products of digestion must be released for transport to the rest of the body. (Figure 3–10 shows the various ways in which the nutrients get into cells.) The water-soluble nutrients (including the smaller products of fat digestion) are released directly into the bloodstream via the capillaries. For the larger fats and the fat-soluble vitamins, however, access directly into the capillaries is impossible, because these nutrients are insoluble in water (and blood is mostly water). The intestinal cells assemble many of the products of fat digestion into larger molecules. These larger molecules cluster together, and special proteins are inserted into their surfaces, forming chylomicrons. Finally, the cells release these chylomicrons into the lymphatic system. The chylomicrons can then glide through the lymph spaces until they enter the bloodstream at a point near the heart.

Chylomicrons are one kind of lipoprotein. The lipoproteins are described in Chapter 5.

■ *The Circulatory Systems*

Once a nutrient has entered the bloodstream or the lymphatic system, it may be transported to any part of the body and thus become available to any of the cells, from the tips of the toes to the roots of the hair. The circulatory systems are arranged to deliver nutrients anywhere they are needed.

The Vascular System

The vascular, or blood circulatory, system is a closed system of vessels through which blood flows continuously in a figure eight, with the heart serving as a pump at the crossover point. The vascular system is diagrammed in Figure 3–11. As the blood circulates through this system, it picks up and delivers materials as needed.

All the body tissues derive oxygen and nutrients from the blood and deposit carbon dioxide and other wastes into it. The lungs are the place for the exchange of carbon dioxide (which leaves the blood to be breathed out) and oxygen (which enters the blood to be delivered to all cells). The digestive system is the place for nutrients to be picked up. The kidneys are the place where wastes other than carbon dioxide are filtered out of the blood to be excreted in the urine (see Figure 3–12).

Blood leaving the right side of the heart circulates by way of arteries into the lung capillaries and then back through veins to the left side of the heart. The left side of the heart then pumps the blood out through arteries to all systems of the body. The blood circulates in the capillaries, where it exchanges material with the cells, and then collects into veins, which return it again to the right side of the heart. In short, blood travels this simple route:

■ Heart to arteries to capillaries to veins to heart.

artery: a vessel that carries blood away from the heart.

capillary (CAP-ill-ary): a small vessel that branches from an artery. Capillaries connect arteries to veins. Exchange of oxygen, nutrients, and waste materials takes place across capillary walls.

vein: a vessel that carries blood back to the heart.

■ **FIGURE 3–10**
How Things Get into Cells

Cell membrane

Water

Small lipids

Diffusion. Some substances cross membranes freely; water is an example. The concentration of water tends to equalize on the two sides of a membrane; as long as it is higher outside the cell, water flows in; if it is higher inside the cell, water flows out. The cell cannot regulate the entrance and exit of water directly, but can control it indirectly by concentrating some other substance to which water is attracted, such as protein or sodium. Thus the cell can pump in sodium, and water will follow passively. This is the way the cells of the wall of the large intestine act to retrieve water for the body. Since nearly all the sodium is taken into these cells before waste is excreted, nearly all the water is absorbed, too. Small lipids also cross cell membranes by diffusion.

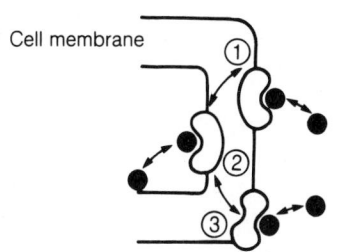

Cell membrane

Facilitated diffusion. Other compounds cannot cross the membranes of the intestinal wall cells unless there is a specific carrier or facilitator in the membrane. The carrier may shuttle back and forth from one side of the membrane to the other, carrying its passengers either way, or it may affect the permeability of the membrane in such a way that the compound is admitted. The end result is the same as for diffusion; equal concentrations are reached on both sides. By providing carriers only for the desired compounds, the cell effectively bars all others (except those to which it is freely permeable). Facilitated diffusion is also termed carrier-mediated diffusion or passive transport.
1. Carrier loads particle on outside of cell.
2. Carrier releases particle on inside of cell.
3. Or the reverse.

Cell membrane

Energy

Active transport. For compounds that must be absorbed actively, the two types of diffusion systems mentioned above will not suffice. The best a cell can do using only diffusion is to move a compound across its membrane until the concentration inside the cell is equal to that outside. An effective means of concentrating a substance inside or outside the cell is to pump it across the membrane, consuming energy in the process. Glucose, amino acids, and other nutrients are absorbed by intestinal wall cells in this manner. Energy for active transport may be supplied by ATP (see Chapter 7) or by cotransport—a process in which the movement of one substance into the cell somehow facilitates the simultaneous uptake of another. Sodium is known to facilitate glucose uptake this way.
1. Carrier loads particle on outside of cell.
2. Carrier releases particle on inside of cell.
3. Carrier returns to outside to pick up another particle. (Cells can concentrate substances inside or outside their membranes this way.)

Cell membrane

Pinocytosis. Pinocytosis involves a large area of the cell membrane, which actively engulfs liquids and "swallows" them into the cell. An occasional whole protein can get into the body this way. This can confer benefits (for example, an infant may receive antibodies from her mother this way) or hazards (allergens can enter this way, on occasion).
1. Liquid contacts cell membrane.
2. Membrane wraps around droplet.
3. Portion of membrane surrounding droplet separates into cell.

Head

Capillaries

Vein

Artery

Lungs

Vein

Heart

Aorta*

Liver

Vein

Capillaries

Digestive tract

Capillaries

Pelvis

Veins

Kidneys

Arteries

Legs

Heart (anatomically correct)

From lungs

From body

Aorta (to body)

Heart

To lungs

Key:

Arterial blood.
Venous blood.
Merging of arterial and venous blood.
Lymph.

■ **FIGURE 3–11**

The Vascular System

Blood leaves the right side of the heart, picks up oxygen in the lungs, and returns to the left side of the heart. Blood leaves the left side of the heart; goes to the head, or to the digestive tract and then the liver, or to the lower body; then returns to the right side of the heart.

*The aorta is the main artery that launches blood on its course through the body. The picture is not anatomically correct but is drawn this way for clarity. The aorta arises behind the left side of the heart and arcs upward, then divides.

■ **FIGURE 3–12**

A Nephron, One of the Kidney's Many Functioning Units
Blood flows into the entranceway (glomerulus), and some of its fluid, with dissolved substances, is filtered into the tubules (1). Then the blood passes alongside the tubules, which return fluid and substances needed by the body (2). The tubule passes waste materials (urine) on to the bladder (3).

The cleansing of blood in the nephron is roughly analogous to the way you might have your car cleaned up at the service station. First you remove all your possessions and trash so that the car can be vacuumed (1). Then you put back in the car what you want to keep (2) and throw away the trash (3).

Blood vessel carrying blood into glomerulus

Glomerulus

Capillaries of glomerulus

Blood vessel carrying blood away from glomerulus

Tubules

Blood vessel carrying blood back to body

Blood vessel carrying blood alongside tubule

To the bladder

The routing of the blood past the digestive system is unique. The blood is carried to the digestive system (as to all organs) by way of an artery, which (as in all organs) branches into capillaries to reach every cell. However, blood leaving the digestive system goes by way of a vein, not back to the heart, but to another organ: the liver. This vein *again* branches into capillaries, so that every cell of the liver also has access to the blood carried by the vein. (Blood leaving the liver then returns to the heart by way of a vein.) The route is:

■ Heart to arteries to capillaries (in intestines) to vein to capillaries (in liver) to vein to heart.

An anatomist studying this system knows there must be a reason for this special arrangement. The liver is placed in the circulation at this point so that it will have the first chance at the materials absorbed from the GI tract. In fact, the liver has many jobs to do in preparing the absorbed nutrients for use by the body. It is the body's major metabolic organ (see Figure 3–13).

You might guess that in addition, the liver may stand as gatekeeper to waylay intruders that might otherwise harm the heart or brain. Perhaps this

The blood arriving at the intestines flows through the **mesentery** (MEZ-en-terry), a strong, flexible membrane that surrounds and supports the abdominal organs.

The vein that collects blood from the mesentery and conducts it to capillaries in the liver is the **portal vein**.
portal = gateway

The vein that collects blood from the liver capillaries and returns it to the heart is the **hepatic vein**.
hepat = liver

■ **FIGURE 3–13**
The Liver
The routing of the blood ensures that the liver has first crack at all the nutrients absorbed into the bloodstream from the digestive tract:
1. Vessels gather up nutrients and reabsorbed water and salts from all over the digestive tract.
2. These vessels merge into the portal vein, which conducts all absorbed materials to the liver.
3. The hepatic artery brings a supply of freshly oxygenated blood (not loaded with nutrients) from the lungs, to offer oxygen to the liver's own cells.
4. Capillaries branch out all over the liver, making nutrients and oxygen available to all its cells, and giving the cells access to blood from the digestive system.
5. Hepatic veins gather up blood leaving the liver to return it to the heart.

In contrast, nutrients absorbed into lymph do *not* go to the liver first. They go to the heart, which pumps them to all the body's cells. The cells can remove the nutrients they want, and the liver then has to deal only with the remnants.

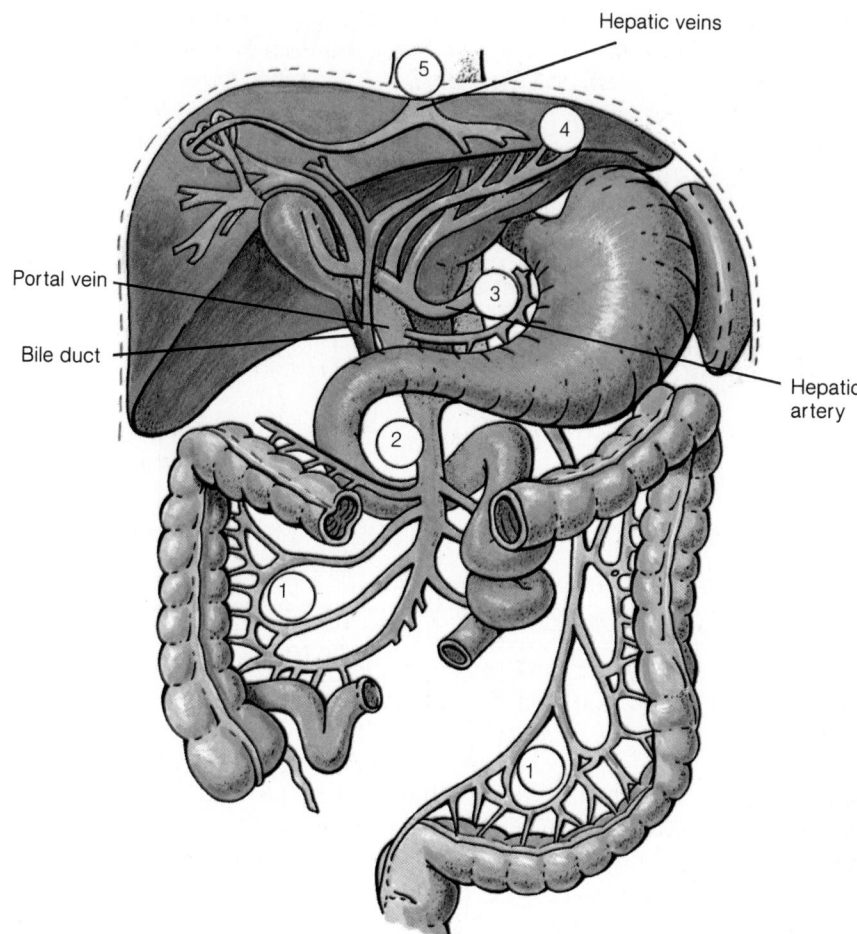

Hepatic veins
Portal vein
Bile duct
Hepatic artery

Chapter 26 describes the catastrophic consequences of liver disorders.

The duct that conveys lymph toward the heart is the **thoracic** (thor-ASS-ic) **duct**. The **subclavian vein** connects this duct with the right upper chamber of the heart, providing a passageway by which lymph can be returned to the vascular system.

is why, when people ingest poisons that succeed in passing the first barrier (the intestinal cells) and in entering the blood, it is quite often the liver that suffers the damage—from the hepatitis virus, from drugs such as barbiturates, from alcohol, from poisons, and from contaminants such as mercury. Perhaps, in fact, you have been undervaluing your liver, not knowing what heroic tasks it quietly performs for you.

The Lymphatic System

The lymphatic system provides a one-way route for fluid from the tissue spaces to enter the blood. Lymph fluid circulates between the cells of the body and collects into tiny capillary-like vessels. Lymph is almost identical to blood, except that it contains no red blood cells or platelets, because they cannot escape through the blood vessel walls.

The lymphatic system has no pump; like water in a sponge, lymph "squishes" from one portion of the body to another as muscles contract and create pressure here and there. Ultimately, much of the lymph collects in a large duct behind the heart. This duct terminates in a vein that conducts the lymph toward the heart. Thus materials from the GI tract that enter lymphatic vessels (large fats and fat-soluble vitamins) in the villi ultimately enter the blood circulatory system and then circulate through arteries, capillaries, and veins like the other nutrients, with a notable exception—they bypass the liver at first.

Once inside the vascular system, the nutrients can travel freely to any destination and can be taken into cells and used as needed. What becomes of them is described in Chapter 7.

Regulation of Digestion and Absorption

There is nothing random about digestion and absorption; they are coordinated. The GI tract's structure and functions guarantee both the dismantling of food and the delivery of its products into the body. This section details some of the ways the digestive tract routinely handles its ever-changing contents.

Gastrointestinal Hormones and Nerve Pathways

Two marvelous systems coordinate all the digestive and absorptive processes: the hormonal (or endocrine) system and the nervous system. The contents of the GI tract either stimulate or inhibit digestive secretions by way of messages that are carried from one section of the GI tract to another by both hormones and nerve pathways. Notice that the kinds of regulation that will be described are all examples of *feedback* mechanisms. A certain condition demands a response to change that condition. The change produced becomes itself the signal to cut off the response; thus the system is self-corrective. The examples that follow illustrate the principles of the body's regulation of its internal environment.

The stomach normally maintains a pH between 1.5 and 1.7. How does it stay that way? One of the regulators of the stomach pH is the hormone gastrin, secreted by cells in the stomach wall. The entrance of food into the stomach stimulates these cells to release gastrin, which, in turn, stimulates other stomach glands to secrete the components of hydrochloric acid. When pH 1.5 is reached, the gastrin-producing cells stop releasing the hormone. The acid itself turns them off. The acid-producing glands, lacking the hormonal stimulus, then stop secreting hydrochloric acid. Thus the system adjusts itself.

Another regulator consists of nerve receptors in the stomach wall. These receptors respond to the presence of food and stimulate activity by both the gastric glands and muscles. As the stomach empties, the receptors are no longer stimulated, the flow of juices slows, and the stomach quiets down.

The pylorus opens to let out a little chyme. How does it know when to close? When the pylorus relaxes, acidic chyme slips through. The cells of the pylorus muscle on the far side sense the acid, causing the pylorus to close tightly. Only after the chyme has been neutralized by pancreatic bicarbonate and the

A **hormone** is a chemical messenger. Hormones are secreted in response to altered conditions by a variety of glands in the body. Each hormone affects one or more specific target tissues or organs and elicits specific responses to restore normal conditions. Gastrointestinal hormones in general are called **enterogastrones.*** Appendix A provides more information about hormones.

Each nerve pathway is called an **enterogastric reflex**. A sensory nerve detects a changed condition and conducts a signal to a target organ such as a muscle or gland. The target organ responds to change the condition appropriately, and the sensory nerve stops firing.

gastrin: a hormone secreted by cells in the stomach wall. Target organ: the stomach. Response: secretion of gastric juice.

---

*The term *enterogastrone* refers specifically to any hormone that inhibits gastric secretions, including secretin, cholecystokinin (CCK), and gastric-inhibitory peptide; more broadly, the term refers to any hormone released from the intestine.

medium surrounding the pylorus has become alkaline can the muscle relax again. This process ensures that the chyme will be released slowly enough to be neutralized as it flows through the small intestine. This is important, because the small intestine has less of a mucous coating than the stomach does and so is not as well protected from acid.

As the chyme enters the intestine, the pancreas adds bicarbonate to it, so that the intestinal contents always remain at a slightly alkaline pH. How does the pancreas know how much to add? The presence of chyme stimulates the cells of the duodenum wall to release the hormone secretin into the blood. As this hormone circulates through the pancreas, it stimulates the pancreas to release its juices. Thus whenever the duodenum signals that acidic chyme is present, the pancreas responds by sending bicarbonate to neutralize it. When the need has been met, the secretin cells of the duodenal wall are no longer stimulated to release the hormone, the hormone no longer flows through the blood, the pancreas no longer receives the message, and it stops sending pancreatic juice. Nerves also regulate pancreatic secretions.

When fat is present in the intestine, the gallbladder contracts to squirt bile into the intestine, to emulsify the fat. How does the gallbladder get the message that fat is present? Fat in the intestine stimulates cells of the intestinal wall to release the hormone cholecystokinin (CCK). This hormone, reaching the gallbladder by way of the blood, stimulates it to contract, releasing bile into the small intestine. Once the fat in the intestine is emulsified and enzymes have begun to work on it, it no longer provokes release of the hormone, and the message to contract is canceled.

The digestion of fat takes longer than that of carbohydrate. When fat is present, intestinal motility slows to allow time for its digestion. How does the intestine know when to slow down? Cholecystokinin and gastric-inhibitory peptide slow GI tract motility, thus keeping food in the stomach longer. By slowing the digestive process, fat helps to maintain a pace that will allow all reactions to reach completion and provides a feeling of satiety. Gastric-inhibitory peptide also inhibits gastric acid secretion. Hormonal and nervous mechanisms like these account for much of the body's ability to adapt to changing conditions.

Once you have begun asking questions like these, you may not want to stop until you have become a full-fledged physiologist. For now, however, these few examples will be enough to make the point. Throughout the digestive system, all processes are precisely and automatically regulated, without your conscious efforts.

secretin (see-CREET-in): a hormone produced by cells in the duodenum wall. Target organ: the pancreas. Response: secretion of pancreatic juice.

cholecystokinin (coal-ee-sis-toe-KINE-in), or **CCK**: a hormone produced by cells of the intestinal wall. Target organ: the gallbladder. Response: release of bile and slowing of GI motility.

gastric-inhibitory peptide: a hormone produced by the intestine. Target organ: the stomach. Response: slowing of the secretion of gastric juices and of GI motility.

motility: ability to move.

The System at Its Best

We have described the anatomy of the digestive tract on several levels: the sequence of digestive organs, the structures of the villi and of the cells that compose them, and the selective machinery of the cell membranes. The intricate architecture of the GI tract makes it sensitive and responsive to conditions in its environment. Knowing what the optimal conditions are will help you to promote the best functioning of the system.

One indispensable condition is good health of the digestive tract itself. This health is affected by such factors of lifestyle as sleep, exercise, and state of

NUTRITION DETECTIVE WORK

You might have expected that the GI hormones would finely coordinate the many activities of food digestion. The sophistication of their actions has surprised and pleased scientists, even so. Even more surprising have been the GI tract hormones' connections with behavior.

Behaviorists have long known that a reward presented after a given behavior reinforces the learning of that behavior. Offer a dog biscuit each time a dog sits on command, and the dog will learn to sit on command. Scientists have pondered the following questions: *How* does the reward of food facilitate learning? Might the GI hormone cholecystokinin (CCK) have anything to do with it?[4] It is known that CCK, the hormone that, in the GI tract, causes bile release in response to feeding, also appears in the brain after a meal.

One group of researchers began to answer these questions by training three groups of mice to run a maze—one group of fed mice and two groups of hungry mice. The researchers fed the well-fed mice and one of the hungry groups immediately after training; they fed the other hungry group three hours later. All groups ate freely over the next week and then were tested again for retention. The two groups that ate immediately after the learning test performed much better on the retention test than did the group that had remained hungry. Was the enhanced learning due to the release of hormones that followed the meal? Might CCK be responsible for enhancing memory retention?

To test this possibility, researchers injected CCK into mice at low, moderate, and high doses within the first minute following training. The moderate dose of CCK—most like the natural dose that follows a meal—best facilitated learning retention (the low dose had a minimal effect and the high dose had none).

Now researchers knew that both feeding and CCK would directly enhance learning, and that the normal dose of CCK was most effective. Next, they wanted to know what, exactly, CCK was doing. They found that when they cut the vagus nerve, the major nerve pathway connecting all of the digestive system's organs with the brain, the effect of CCK on memory retention disappeared. With that bit of information, researchers concluded that CCK enhances memory by activating the vagus nerve.

mind. Adequate sleep allows for repair, maintenance of tissue, and removal of wastes that might impair efficient functioning. Exercise promotes healthy muscle tone. Mental state profoundly affects digestion and absorption through the activity of regulatory nerves and hormones; for healthy digestion, you should be relaxed and tranquil at mealtimes.

Another factor is the kind of meals you eat. Among the characteristics of meals that promote optimal absorption of nutrients are balance, variety, adequacy, and moderation. Balance means having neither too much nor too little of anything. For example, some fat is needed; fat slows down intestinal motility, permitting time for absorption of some of the nutrients that are slow to be absorbed. Too much fat is harmful, however; excess fat consumption contributes to obesity and a number of diseases. A well-planned meal presents you with no more than 30 percent of its energy as fat energy.

Chapters 24 and 25 describe how GI disorders impair ingestion, digestion, and absorption.

Chapters 4, 10, and 11 mention the compounds that bind with minerals to prevent absorption.

Variety is important for many reasons, but partly because some food constituents interfere with the absorption of others. For example, compounds that often accompany fiber in foods interfere with the absorption of minerals. Such compounds are found in whole-grain cereals and legumes, so the minerals in those foods may be to some extent "unavailable." This does not mean that whole-grain cereals are undesirable; they are rightly praised for their nutrient contributions. It does mean, though, that people who rely too heavily on cereals and legumes may be deriving less of certain minerals from their diets than they would if they were to vary their choices. They might want to exercise moderation in their use of high-fiber foods.

As for adequacy—in a sense, this entire book is about dietary adequacy. But here, at the end of this chapter, is a good place to underline the interdependence of the nutrients. It could almost be said that every nutrient depends on every other. All the nutrients work together and are all present in the cells of a healthy digestive tract. To maintain health and promote the functions of the GI tract, you should make balance, variety, adequacy, and moderation features of every day's menus.

Study Questions

1. Describe the problems involved with digesting food and the solutions offered by the human body.
2. Describe the anatomy of the GI tract, and explain how it facilitates absorption of nutrients.
3. What is the route of blood through the digestive system? Which nutrients enter the bloodstream directly? Which are first absorbed into the lymph?
4. Describe the actions of the GI hormones in digestion.

Notes

1. R. J. Gibbons and I. Dankers, Inhibition of lectin-binding to saliva-treated hydroxyapatite, to buccal epithelial cells, and to erythrocytes by salivary components, *American Journal of Clinical Nutrition* 36 (1982): 276–283.
2. D. C. Savage, Gastrointestinal microflora in mammalian nutrition, *Annual Reviews of Nutrition* 6 (1986): 155–178.
3. Food and Nutrition Board, *Recommended Dietary Allowances*, 10th ed. (Washington, D.C.: National Academy of Sciences, 1989), pp. 108–109.
4. J. F. Flood, G. E. Smith, and J. E. Morley, Modulation of memory processing by cholecystokinin: Dependence on the vagus nerve, *Science* 236 (1987): 832–834.

Common Digestive Problems

Chapter 3's discussion of the GI tract permits easy understanding of some common problems, so a few practical applications are presented here. Everyone, at one time or another, deals with choking, vomiting, diarrhea, constipation, gas, and heartburn; and everyone is familiar with ulcers. (See Chapters 24 and 25 for more details about GI disorders.)

Choking

When someone chokes on food, it is because the food has slipped into the air passage and cut off breathing (see Figure H3–1). Food can lodge so securely in the trachea that it cuts off all air. No sound can be made, because the larynx is in the trachea and makes sounds only when air is pushed across

it. This choking has happened often enough so that the event has been given a name: cafe coronary. The scenario reads like this. A person is dining in a restaurant with friends. A chunk of food, usually meat, becomes lodged in his trachea so firmly that he cannot make a sound. Often he chooses to suffer alone rather than "make a scene in public." If he tries to communicate distress to friends, he must depend on pantomime. The friends are bewildered by his antics and become terribly worried when the victim "faints" after a few minutes without air. They call a doctor or an ambulance. However, by the time the victim arrives at the hospital, he is usually dead—from suffocation. In the past, many of these cases were diagnosed as "death by coronary

thrombosis"—thus the name cafe coronary.

To help a person who is choking, first ask this critical question: "Can you make any sound at all?" If the victim makes a sound, relax. You have time to continue with your questioning to see what you can do to help; you are not going to have to make a quick decision. But whatever you do, don't hit him on the back. If you do, the particle may become lodged more firmly in his air passage.

If the choking victim is an infant, lay her face down on your lap, with her head firmly supported and held lower than her body. Administer four blows rapidly with the heel of your hand high between her shoulder blades. If that doesn't work, turn her over and deliver four rapid thrusts over her sternum using two fingers. If all else fails, open her mouth by grasping both her tongue and lower jaw and lifting. Then, and only if you can see the object, use your finger to sweep it out.

If the choking victim is a child or adult, the strategy most likely to succeed is the Heimlich maneuver. Get behind the victim, and put your arms around the lower part of her rib cage. Make a fist with one hand, and place the fist over the spot shown in Figure H3–2. Grasp the wrist of your balled-up hand with your other hand, and give a sudden strong hug inward and upward. What you are hoping to accomplish with this quick bear hug is to push the diaphragm upward, because this will expel air from the lungs. The hope is that the air will be effective in dislodging the stuck food particle in the same way that built-up gas pressure in a bottle of wine can push the cork out of the bottle. One word of caution: be certain that your fist is in the correct position and is snugly against the person's body, and that you proceed with the hug from

■ **FIGURE H3–1**
Normal Swallowing and Choking

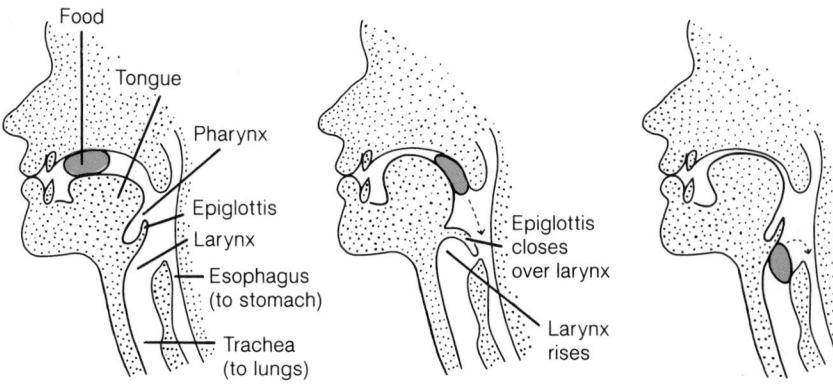

Food in mouth.

Swallowing. Food cannot enter trachea when the epiglottis closes over the larynx. The dotted arrow shows that the food is heading down the esophagus normally.

Choking.
Food is lodged in trachea. The dotted arrow points to where the food should have gone to prevent choking.

■ **FIGURE H3–2**
The Heimlich Maneuver

Source: Adapted from H. J. Heimlich and M. H. Uhley, The Heimlich maneuver, *Clinical Symposia* 31 (1979): 1–32.

Rescuer positions fist directly against victim's abdomen as shown. Rescuer grasps fist with other hand and presses into abdomen with a *quick upward thrust.*

1. Rescuer stands behind victim and wraps his arms around victim's waist.
2. Rescuer makes a fist with one hand and places the thumb side of the fist against the victim's abdomen, slightly above the navel and below the rib cage.
3. Rescuer grasps fist with other hand and presses into victim's abdomen with a *quick upward thrust.*
4. Rescuer repeats thrust several times if necessary.

Victim may attempt self administration of the standard Heimlich technique. Alternatively, victim positions herself over edge of fixed horizontal object such as a chair back, railing, or table edge, and presses abdomen into edge with quick movement. Movement should be repeated several times as necessary.

that position. Do not slam your fist against the rib cage; this might cause the food to become more securely lodged in the trachea. It would be well to practice this technique at home, for there is no time to hesitate once you are called on to perform this death-defying act.

If the Heimlich maneuver fails and the person becomes unconscious, position him on his back with his arms by his side. Open his mouth by performing the tongue-jaw lift described earlier, use your finger to remove the foreign body, and begin rescue breathing.

You can also administer the Heimlich maneuver to yourself, if need be. Make a fist with one hand, place the thumb side on the spot shown in Figure H3–2, grasp the fist with your other hand, and then press inward and upward with a quick motion.[1] If this is unsuccessful, quickly press your upper abdomen over any firm surface, such as the back of a chair, a

countertop, or a porch railing (see Figure H3–2).

Vomiting

Another common digestive mishap is vomiting. Vomiting can be a symptom of many different diseases or may come from any situation that upsets the body's equilibrium, such as air or sea travel. For whatever reason, the waves of peristalsis reverse direction, and the contents of the stomach are propelled up through the esophagus to the mouth and expelled. If vomiting continues long enough or is severe enough, the reverse peristalsis will carry the contents of the duodenum, with its green bile salts, into the stomach and then up the esophagus. Simple vomiting is certainly unpleasant and wearying for the nauseous person, but it is no cause for alarm. Vomiting is one of the body's adaptive mechanisms to rid itself of something irritating.

Vomiting can be serious, however, and a doctor's care may be needed in some cases. When large quantities of fluid are lost from the GI tract, all of the body fluids redistribute themselves so that, eventually, fluid is taken from every cell of the body. Leaving the cells with the fluid are salts that are absolutely essential to the life of the cells, and they must be replaced, which is difficult while the vomiting continues. Intravenous feedings of saline and glucose are frequently necessary while the doctor is diagnosing the cause of the vomiting and instituting corrective therapy.

In an infant, vomiting is especially serious; a doctor should be contacted soon after onset. Babies have more fluid between their body cells than adults do, so it is more critical when their body water becomes depleted and their body salt balance upset than it is with adults.

Self-induced vomiting, such as that seen in bulimia, also has serious consequences. (Bulimia is the subject of Highlight 12.) In addition to fluid and salt imbalances, repeated vomiting causes irritation and infection of the pharynx, esophagus, and salivary glands; erosion of the teeth; and dental caries. The esophagus may rupture or tear, as may the stomach. Sometimes the eyes become red from pressure on vomiting. Such behavior reflects underlying problems that require attention.

Projectile vomiting is another kind of vomiting that is not the simple type associated with nausea. In this type, the contents of the stomach are expelled with such force that they leave the mouth in a wide arc like a bullet leaving a gun. This type of vomiting can arise from a number of causes, and all of them require immediate medical care.

Diarrhea

Diarrhea, like vomiting, can incur considerable fluid and salt losses. Diarrhea is the name given to the condition characterized by frequent, loose, watery stools. This sort of stool indicates that the intestinal contents have moved too quickly through the intestines for fluid absorption to have taken place, or that water has been drawn from the cells lining the intestinal tract and added to the food residue. Diarrhea can become serious if it continues (see Chapter 25). In an infant, it may quickly lead to dehydration so severe as to require emergency medical treatment.

Constipation

Unlike diarrhea, constipation may not be such a cause for concern. Each person's GI tract responds to food in its own way, with its own rhythm, the fecal matter arriving at the rectal area in a fairly constant number of hours. Each GI tract thus has its own cycle, which depends on its owner's physical makeup and such environmental considerations as the type of food eaten, when it was eaten, and when

the person's schedule allows time to defecate. If several days pass between movements, but these movements take place without discomfort, then the person is not constipated, nor did she absorb any "toxins" that would cause irritable behavior. Nor does anyone need to worry about an inability to have daily movements—television commercials notwithstanding.

What, then, is constipation? When a person receives the signal that says to defecate and ignores it, the signal may not return for quite a few hours. In the meantime, water will continue to be withdrawn from the fecal matter, so that when the person does defecate, the bowel movement will be drier and harder. If the movement is hard and is passed with difficulty, discomfort, or pain, then it can be said that the person is constipated. (Note that in this definition of constipation, no mention has been made of the amount of time that has elapsed since the previous bowel movement; that is irrelevant.)

Careful review of daily habits may reveal the causes of the constipation. Being too busy to respond to the defecation signal is a common complaint. A person's daily regimen may need to be reexamined with the idea of instituting regular eating and sleeping times that will allow time in the day's schedule to have a bowel movement at the dictate of the person's body. This may mean going to bed earlier in order to rise earlier, so that ample time is allowed for a leisurely breakfast and a movement. If discomfort is associated with passing fecal matter, a doctor's help should be sought in order to rule out the presence of organic disease. Once this has been done, dietary or other measures for correction can be considered.

Laboratory research into the laxative quality of foods is scarce. It has been shown, however, that prunes contain a laxative substance.* If a morning defecation is desired, prune juice

*This substance is dihydroxyphenyl isatin.

Large intestine (colon)

Diverticula

■ FIGURE H3–3
Diverticula
The outpocketings of intestinal linings that balloon through weakened intestinal wall muscles are known as diverticula. Chapter 25 includes a discussion on diverticular disease.

should be drunk at bedtime; if the evening is preferred, prune juice could be taken at breakfast.

Another appropriate measure may be to increase the fiber content of the diet. Some kinds of fibers in the GI tract attract water, thus softening the stools. Dietary fibers exercise the intestinal muscles so that they retain their health and tone. The major impact of dietary fiber is on the colon, the last part of the GI tract, where colon cancer and diverticula can develop (see Figure H3–3); however, the addition of fibrous foods to the diet increases the bulk of food all along the intestine.

Some constipation may be relieved by the addition of fat to the diet. The success of this regimen was once thought due to its lubricating effect, but it is now ascribed to the stimulation of cholecystokinin, which summons bile into the duodenum. The bile acts in the same way that a saline laxative does; that is, its high salt content draws from the intestinal wall an abundance of water, which stimulates peristalsis and softens the fecal matter.

Another recommendation for helping to overcome constipation is to increase fluid intake. Apparently, the physical stimulation caused by the increased bulk on the upper GI tract promotes peristalsis throughout.

Another cause of constipation that requires some rearrangement of lifestyle is the lack of physical activity. In modern society many people drive cars or ride buses to work, stand at assembly lines or sit behind desks, and then sit in front of television sets in the evening. People who do not have the time or money to work out in spas or health clubs are finding that they can park their cars a distance from the office and walk the extra blocks, or they can walk up several flights of stairs rather than take an elevator. With such planning, people can incorporate much exercise into their days. Any activity that increases the muscle tone of the entire body also improves the muscles that are responsible for peristalsis.

These suggested changes in diet or lifestyle should correct chronic constipation without the use of laxatives. One of the fallacies often perpetrated by television commercials is that one person's successful use of a laxative product is a good recommendation for another person to use that product. As a matter of fact, even diet changes that relieve constipation for one person may increase the constipation of another. For instance, if a person has a spastic type of constipation, in which peristalsis promotes strong contractions that close off a segment of the colon and prevent passage, then increasing fiber intake would be exactly the wrong thing to do. A good rule is that if laxatives seem to be indicated, a doctor's advice should be sought.

Gas

Many people complain of problems that they attribute to excessive gas. For

---

Miniglossary

constipation: the condition of having painful or difficult bowel movements (elapsed time between movements is not relevant).

defecate (DEF-uh-cate): to move the bowels and eliminate waste.
   defaecare = to remove dregs

diarrhea: the frequent passage of watery bowel movements.

diverticula (dye-ver-TIC-you-la): outpocketings of weakened areas of the intestinal wall (like blowouts in a tire). The term **diverticulosis** (DYE-ver-tic-you-LOH-sis) describes the condition of having diverticula. The danger of diverticulosis is that it can give rise to **diverticulitis** (DYE-ver-tic-you-LYE-tis), in which the pockets become infected or inflamed and may rupture. About one in every six people in Western countries develops diverticulosis in middle or later life.
   divertir = to turn side
   osis = disease
   itis = infection or inflammation

glucose: blood sugar.

intravenous (in-tra-VEEN-us): into a vein.

larynx: the voice box (see Figure H3–1).

peptic ulcer: an erosion in the mucous membrane of the stomach or duodenum.

saline (SAY-leen): a salt solution.

---

some, belching is the complaint. Others blame intestinal gas for abdominal discomforts and embarrassment. Most people believe that the problems occur after they eat certain foods. This may be the case with intestinal gas, but belching is not caused by gas formed from any particular foods in the stomach. Rather, belching results when air that has been swallowed or sucked in is expelled. All of us swallow a little bit of air with each mouthful of food, but people who belch excessively may be eating too fast. Ill-fitting dentures, carbonated beverages, and chewing gum can also contribute to excessive belching. Occasionally, belching can be a sign of a more serious disorder, such as gallbladder pain, colonic distress, or an impending obstruction of a coronary blood vessel.

Little is known about intestinal gas, but new techniques to collect gas directly from the abdomen have allowed researchers to gain new

knowledge. While expelling gas can be a humiliating experience, it is quite normal. (People experiencing painful bloating from malabsorption diseases, however, require medical treatment.) Healthy people expel several hundred milliliters of gas several times a day. Almost all (99 percent) of the gases expelled—nitrogen, oxygen, hydrogen, methane, and carbon dioxide—are odorless. The remaining "volatile" gases are the infamous ones.

Researchers have learned that different gases reside in different parts of the GI tract. For example, nitrogen and oxygen from swallowed air are found in the stomach. Carbon dioxide from the reaction of bile acids with bicarbonate is found in the upper intestine. Hydrogen from bacterial breakdown of food by-products is found in the lower intestine.

One-third of the population produces methane gas, most likely reflecting the type of bacteria present in the intestine. An interesting association has been observed in methane-producing people that may help in the early diagnosis of colon cancer. Twice as many people with colon cancer produce methane as members of the general population. Researchers believe that this methane production is a response to the presence of the tumor, and not that cancer is more prevalent in people who produce methane.[2]

Fully understanding intestinal gas is problematic for researchers for several reasons. For one, odors are subjective; for another, volatile gases are present in small quantities (less than 1 part per billion); and for still another, gases differ depending on the individual's diet, intestinal structure, and intestinal flora.

Foods that produce gas usually must be determined individually. People can test foods suspected of forming gas by omitting them individually for a trial period and seeing if there is any improvement. The best advice seems to be to eat slowly, chew thoroughly, and relax while eating.

Heartburn and "Acid Indigestion"

Heartburn is the sensation felt when the cardiac sphincter cannot prevent the stomach contents from reentering the esophagus. Almost everyone has experienced this at one time or another, usually after a meal. If the heartburn is not caused by a physiological disorder, treatment is fairly simple. Tips for people suffering from heartburn include the following: eat small meals; eat the last meal of the day several hours before bedtime to avoid lying down immediately after a meal; lose weight, if overweight; avoid tight clothing and frequent bending after a meal; elevate the head of the bed by 4 to 6 inches; and avoid food, beverages, and medicines that are irritating (see Table H3–1). Use antacids infrequently for occasional heartburn; they may mask or cause problems if used regularly.

As far as "acid indigestion" is concerned, it should be noted here that the strong acidity of the stomach is a desirable condition—television commercials for antacids notwithstanding. People who overeat or who eat their food too quickly are likely to suffer from indigestion. The muscular reaction of the stomach to unchewed lumps or to being overfilled may be so violent that it causes regurgitation (reverse peristalsis, another solution to problem 5 at the beginning of Chapter 3). When this happens, overeaters may taste the stomach acid and feel pain. Responding to television commercials, they may take antacids to neutralize the "acid indigestion."

Antacids will provide quick relief, but they are not, in fact, the appropriate response for the stomach's discomfort. An antacid places a demand on the stomach to secrete more acid to counteract the neutralizer and enable the digestive enzymes to do their work. So the person ends up with the same amount of acid in the stomach, but the stomach has had to work against the antacid to produce it. Antacids are designed to help relieve symptoms from abnormal conditions, such as the pain felt by an ulcer patient whose stomach or duodenal lining has been attacked by acid. The person who overeats or swallows unchewed food needs to sit upright until the unhappy stomach has had a chance to cope with the problem it faces. Then, to avoid such misery in the future, the person needs to learn to eat less at a sitting, chew food more thoroughly, and eat it more slowly.

■ **TABLE H3–1**
Heartburn Irritants

To ease heartburn pain, avoid:
Alcoholic beverages.
Caffeine beverages.
Chocolate.
Cigarette smoking.
High-fat foods.
Peppermint and spearmint.

Ulcers

Another common digestive problem is ulcers of the stomach (gastric ulcers) or duodenum (duodenal ulcers). The term *peptic ulcer* includes both of these. An ulcer is an erosion of the top layer of cells from an area, such as the wall of the stomach or duodenum, leaving the second and succeeding underlying layers of cells exposed, without protection. These exposed cells exude fluid, and anything that touches the eroded area causes pain. The erosion may proceed until the capillaries that feed the area are exposed and bleeding, or until there is a perforation (a hole) in the wall.

Some people naively believe that an ulcer is caused by the secretion of stomach acid, but this is not the case—at least not at first. The stomach lining of a healthy person is well protected by its mucous coat, as you learned in Chapter 3. Why, then, do ulcers sometimes form? Two factors are required: first, a weakness in the stomach or duodenal wall; then, the secretion of gastric acid to erode the weak spot. We are in the dark with respect to the cause of the initial weakness; it may be poor nutrition, lack of rest, or any other condition (including a genetic flaw) that hinders the maintenance of healthy tissue. But once an ulcer has started to form, the secretion of stomach acid can rapidly make it worse.

People with ulcers need to seek medical treatment aimed at relieving pain, healing the ulcer, and reducing the likelihood of recurrence. At one time, milk was considered the cornerstone of dietary treatment for ulcer, but this is no longer the case; the rationale for its inclusion was not supported by scientific evidence. Treatment includes elimination of irritating foods, beverages, and medicines; use of prescribed medicines; elimination of cigarette smoking; and reduction of stress.

What is of interest about ulcers—and the reason why they are included here—is that their origin and development seem to be related more closely to stress than to diet. Remember that the secretion of digestive juices is regulated by the master coordinators, the hormones and the nerves. Both hormonal secretions and nerve activity are profoundly influenced by a person's mental state. The brain, after all, is composed of nerves, including many that impinge on the endocrine glands. Excessive anxiety and worry may or may not be the cause of the initial lesion of an ulcer, but they are clearly related to the excessive acid secretion that makes an ulcer worse.

Sue Rodwell Williams, the author of a widely used textbook on diet therapy, puts it this way: "The individual's particular emotional make-up and his manner of dealing with life's day-to-day problems and challenges, will often be reflected in the functions of his digestive tract. . . . It is not what he eats, it's what is eating him that is important." Williams also reminds her readers to remember that "surrounding every stomach there is a person."[3]

NOTES

1. H. J. Heimlich, Self-application of the Heimlich maneuver, *New England Journal of Medicine* 318 (1988): 714–715.

2. J. M. Pique, Methane production and colon cancer, *Gastroenterology 87* (1987): 601–605.

3. S. R. Williams, *Nutrition and Diet Therapy*, 3rd ed. (St. Louis: Mosby, 1977), p. 530.

The Carbohydrates: Sugar, Starch, and Fiber

Within a single cell lie hundreds of coils of membranes enfolding materials the cell makes and uses. Shown here is part of a liver cell. The clusters of dark beads are glycogen—the form in which the cell stores carbohydrate energy.

CHO → glucose "bld. sugar"
(except fibers)

most fibers are also carbs.
Carbs supply ENERGY

When someone speaks of *carbohydrate*, what comes to mind? People correctly associate the word with sugars and starches, but many do not realize that most fibers are also carbohydrates. Some people think of carbohydrates as "fattening," but they aren't—unless, of course, you eat too much of them. The primary role of carbohydrates in human nutrition is to supply an indispensable commodity—energy. When carbohydrates yield energy, they spare proteins from being used for energy so that proteins can do the jobs they are uniquely suited for. Carbohydrates appear in virtually all plant foods and in only one food taken from animals—namely, milk.

All carbohydrates are composed of simple sugars. Carbohydrates come in three main sizes: sugars whose atoms are arranged in a single circular configuration, a ring (see p. 74); sugars made from pairs of rings; and large molecules of long chains of the single-ring carbohydrates. The chemist's terms for these three types of carbohydrates are monosaccharides, disaccharides, and polysaccharides, respectively. The monosaccharides and disaccharides are known as the simple carbohydrates; the polysaccharides are known as the complex carbohydrates. The body almost invariably converts carbohydrates, whatever form they come in (except fibers), to its own energy currency, "blood sugar" (properly termed *glucose*).

carbohydrate: a compound composed of sugars—monosaccharides or multiples of monosaccharides.
　carbo = carbon (C)
　hydrate = with water (H_2O)

sugars

simple carbohydrates: monosaccharides and disaccharides; also called sugars.

STARCH

complex carbohydrates: the polysaccharides.

■ The Chemist's View of Carbohydrates

One way to understand the structure of carbohydrates is in terms of the next smaller units of which they are made. An understanding of how energy is contained in glucose molecules and how it is released when these molecules are metabolized in the body will provide the basis for understanding how the body needs and uses carbohydrate as an energy nutrient.

Chemists describe the sugar molecules most important in nutrition as molecules composed of 6 carbon atoms, 12 hydrogens, and 6 oxygens. These atoms are symbolized by the letters C, H, and O. Each type of atom has a characteristic amount of energy available for forming chemical bonds with other atoms. A carbon atom can form four such bonds; a nitrogen atom, three; an oxygen atom, two; and a hydrogen atom, only one. Chemists represent the bonds as lines between the letters that stand for the atoms (see Figure 4–1).

Atoms are put together to form molecules in ways that satisfy the bonding requirements of each atom. The structure of ethyl alcohol, the active ingredient of alcoholic beverages, is shown in Figure 4–1 as an example. You

Appendix B presents basic chemistry terms and relationships.

 FIGURE 4–1
Atoms and Their Bonds
The four main types of atoms found in nutrients are hydrogen, oxygen, nitrogen, and carbon. (Nitrogen doesn't appear in carbohydrates or lipids, but it is important in proteins and B vitamins; see Chapters 6 and 8.)

A. Each atom has a characteristic number of bonds it can form with other atoms.

B. Ethyl alcohol, a simple molecule showing bonding.

can see that the bonding requirements of each atom are met. The two carbons each have four bonds represented by lines; the oxygen has two; and each hydrogen has one bond connecting it to other atoms. In any drawing of a chemical structure these conditions must be met, not because a scientist made them up, but because they are what nature demands. Let's begin with the simple carbohydrates.

The Simple Carbohydrates

Practically all your energy comes from the food you eat—about half from carbohydrate and half from protein and fat. In fact, as mentioned in the introduction to this chapter, one of the principal roles of carbohydrate in the diet is to supply energy in the form of blood glucose. Starch (a complex carbohydrate) is the most significant contributor of glucose to people's diets, but any of the sugars (simple carbohydrates) can also be converted to glucose.

Food chemists have studied sugars and other sweet-tasting substances and have identified the exact arrangement of the atoms in that portion of the molecule that stimulates the sweet-taste receptors in the tongue. All sweet-tasting substances share this feature, including the artificial sweeteners saccharin, cyclamate, and aspartame, which are the focus of Highlight 4. Table 4–1 ranks the sugars according to their sweetness relative to table sugar (sucrose).

Monosaccharides

Table 4–2 shows the six sugars most important in nutrition and symbolizes them simply as circles, triangles, squares, and combinations of these. Three are single sugars, the monosaccharides—glucose, fructose, and galactose. Three are double sugars, the disaccharides—sucrose, lactose, and maltose.

Glucose Glucose is not as sweet tasting as sucrose (see Table 4–1); a pinch of the purified sugar on your tongue gives only a mild sweet flavor. The chemical formula for glucose is $C_6H_{12}O_6$. The complete structure of a glucose molecule is shown in Figure 4–2. Glucose is a larger and more complicated molecule than ethyl alcohol, but it obeys the same rules—as do all chemical compounds. Again, each carbon atom has four bonds; each oxygen, two bonds; and each hydrogen, one bond.

■ TABLE 4–2
The Major Sugars (simple)

Monosaccharides	Disaccharides
Glucose ●	Maltose ●–●
Fructose ▲	Sucrose ●–▲
Galactose ■	Lactose ●–■
(found only as part of lactose)	

■ Table 4–1
Sweetness of Sugars

Sugar	Relative Sweetness[a]
Fructose	170[b]
Sucrose	100
Glucose (dextrose)	70
Maltose	46
Lactose	35
Galactose	32

{from plants} — Fructose, Sucrose, Glucose, Maltose
{From milk & milk prod.} — Lactose, Galactose

[a] Sucrose is the standard by which the approximate sweetness of other sugars is compared.

[b] The sweetness of fructose depends on the temperature and acidity of the foods in which it occurs.

Source: Adapted from H. L. Sipple and K. W. McNutt, *Sugars in Nutrition* (New York: Academic Press, 1974), pp. 44–46, as cited in *Sugars and Your Health—A Report by the American Council on Science and Health* (Summit, N.J.: American Council on Science and Health, May 1986), p. 7.

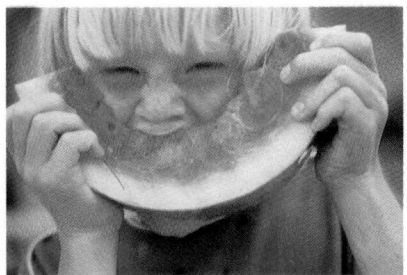

Fruits are naturally sweet because they contain simple sugars.

monosaccharide (mon-oh-SACK-uh-ride): a carbohydrate of the general formula $C_nH_{2n}O_n$ that consists of a single ring. The monosaccharides important in nutrition are all **hexoses** (n = 6) with the formula $C_6H_{12}O_6$.
 mono = one
 saccharide, ose = sugar
 hex = six

disaccharide: a pair of monosaccharides linked together.
 di = two

glucose: a monosaccharide; sometimes known as blood sugar, **dextrose**, or grape sugar.
 ose = carbohydrate
 ● = Glucose.

■ **FIGURE 4–2**
Chemical Structure of Glucose
On paper, it has to be drawn flat, but in nature the five carbons and oxygen are roughly in a plane, with the darkened bonds extending out of the paper toward you. The atoms attached to the ring carbons extend above and below the plane of the ring.

The diagram of a glucose molecule shows all the relationships between the parts and proves simple on examination. Since you will be viewing other complex structures (not necessarily to memorize them, but rather to understand certain things about them), let us adopt a simpler way to depict them. Figure 4–3 shows that a number of letters can be left out of a chemical structure without losing the information it conveys. You can easily reconstruct the complete structure, with all its details, from such a picture, just by filling in the missing carbons and hydrogens. Put a *C* for carbon wherever lines intersect and an *H* for hydrogen at the end of each single line.

fructose: a monosaccharide; sometimes known as fruit sugar or **levulose**. It is found abundantly in fruits, honey, and saps.
fruct = fruit
▲ = Fructose.

Fructose   If you have ever sampled pure, powdered fructose, you will not be surprised to learn that it is the sweetest of the sugars (see Table 4–1). Curiously, fructose has exactly the same chemical formula as glucose—$C_6H_{12}O_6$—but its structure is different (see Figure 4–4). The different arrangements of the atoms in these two sugars stimulate the taste buds on your tongue in different ways. Manufacturers sweeten many of their products with high-fructose corn syrup (HFCS), a corn product in syrup form.

galactose: a monosaccharide; part of the disaccharide lactose.
■ = Galactose.

Galactose   Galactose is seldom found free in nature but occurs as part of the disaccharide lactose. Like glucose and fructose, galactose is a hexose with the

■ **FIGURE 4–3**
Simplified Diagrams of Glucose

A. The carbons at the corners are not shown and the atoms on the flagpole carbon are written as a partial formula, CH_2OH.

B. The letters H circled in (A) are now not shown, but lines still extend upward or downward from the ring to show where they belong. This is the traditional chemical shorthand used for carbohydrates.

C. Another way to look at glucose is to notice that its six carbon atoms are all connected.

FIGURE 4–4
Two Monosaccharides: Glucose and Fructose
Can you see the similarities? If you learned the rules in Figure 4–3, you will be able to "see" 6 carbons (numbered), 12 hydrogens, and 6 oxygens in both these compounds.

formula $C_6H_{12}O_6$. It is shown in Figure 4–5 beside a molecule of glucose for comparison.

Disaccharides

The other three common sugars are disaccharides—pairs of monosaccharides linked together. Glucose is found in all three; the second member of the pair is either fructose, galactose, or another glucose. First, we'll examine how these units are put together and taken apart.

When a disaccharide is formed, a chemical reaction known as condensation links two monosaccharides together (see Figure 4–6). A hydrogen atom (H) is removed from one monosaccharide, and an oxygen-hydrogen (OH) group is removed from the other. This creates a molecule of water (H_2O) and links the two originally separate units together with a single oxygen (O).

When a disaccharide is taken apart to form two monosaccharides, a molecule of water is broken apart to obtain the H and OH needed to complete the separated structures. This reaction is called a hydrolysis reaction (Figure 4–7). Water is always used in condensation and hydrolysis reactions. In fact, the term *hydrolyze* says so; its roots are "water" and "to break." It is by condensation and hydrolysis reactions that all of the carbohydrates are put together and taken apart.

In living systems, condensation and hydrolysis reactions almost always require enzymes to facilitate them. Enzymes are discussed in Chapter 6, but for the moment, let us adopt a simple definition. An enzyme is a protein molecule that provides a surface on which other molecules react with one another. Since the making and breaking of chemical bonds is required to produce molecules that are needed for growth, maintenance, and repair in all

Appendix B describes basic chemical reactions.

condensation: a chemical reaction in which two reactants combine to yield a larger product.

hydrolysis (high-DROL-ih-sis): a chemical reaction in which a major reactant is split into two products, with the addition of H to one and OH to the other (from water).
hydro = water
lysis = breaking

Enzymes facilitate the making and breaking of chemical bonds. An enzyme is not a hormone; hormones act as master controllers, often regulating enzymes. Digestive enzymes were introduced in Chapter 3; Chapter 6 provides more details on enzymes.

FIGURE 4–5
Two Monosaccharides: Glucose and Galactose
Notice the similarities and the differences.

■ FIGURE 4–6
Condensation

A. Water is being removed from two glucoses.

B. The disaccharide maltose, with a new bond between the two glucose pieces, is the product.

living creatures, the enzymes that facilitate these reactions are indispensable to life.

sucrose: a disaccharide composed of glucose and fructose; commonly known as table sugar, beet sugar, or cane sugar. Actually, sucrose occurs in many fruits and some vegetables and grains.
  sucro = sugar
  ●—▲ = Sucrose.

Sucrose   Sucrose, or table sugar, is the most familiar of the three disaccharides. Sugarcane and sugar beets are two sources from which sucrose is purified and granulated to various extents to provide the brown, white, and powdered sugars available in the supermarket. Because the fructose part is in an accessible position for taste receptors, sucrose tastes very sweet, and it accounts for some of the sweetness of sweet fruits. It is one of the main energy-nutrient ingredients of candy and other concentrated sweets.

lactose: a disaccharide composed of glucose and galactose; commonly known as milk sugar.
  lact = milk
  ●—■ = Lactose.

Lactose   Lactose is the principal carbohydrate of milk, making up about 5 percent of its weight. Known as milk sugar, lactose contributes 30 to 50 percent of milk's energy, depending on the milk's fat content.

maltose: a disaccharide composed of two glucose units; sometimes known as malt sugar.
  ●—● = Maltose.

Maltose   The third disaccharide, maltose, is found at only one stage in the life of a plant. When the seed is formed, it is packed with starch—glucose units strung together in long arrays—to be used as fuel for the germination process. When the seed begins to sprout, an enzyme cleaves the bonds between pairs of glucose units, making maltose. Another enzyme then splits the maltose units into glucose units, and other enzymes degrade these still further, releasing energy for the sprouting of the plant's shoot and root. Once the leaves have unfolded, they can capture light from the sun, obtaining

A. The disaccharide maltose.

B. Two glucose units.

■ FIGURE 4–7
Hydrolysis
Hydrolysis of disaccharides occurs during digestion.

additional energy for growth. Maltose is also found in the GI tract when longer chains of polysaccharides are hydrolyzed.

In summary, then, the major simple carbohydrates, or sugars, are those shown earlier in Table 4–2. Glucose, fructose, maltose, and sucrose are from plants; lactose and its component galactose, from milk and milk products.

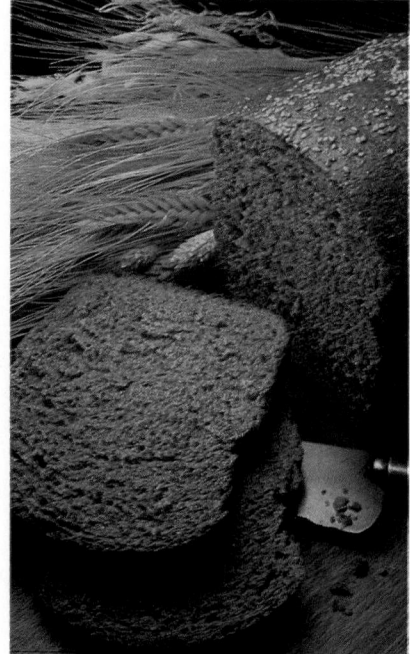

Starch supplies most of the energy in a healthful diet.

The Complex Carbohydrates

The sugars contain three monosaccharides in different combinations. In contrast, the polysaccharides important in nutrition, chiefly starch and glycogen, are composed almost entirely of only one monosaccharide—glucose. The differences between starch and glycogen have to do with the ways glucose is condensed together to form them.

Starch

As the chemist sees it, starch is a long, straight or branched chain of hundreds of glucose molecules connected together (see Figure 4–8). These units would have to be magnified more than 10 million times to appear at the size shown in this figure. However, as molecules go, starches are rather large. A single starch molecule may contain 3,000 or more glucose units linked together. These giant molecules are packed side by side in the rice grain or potato tuber—as many as a million in a cubic inch of food.

In the plant, starch serves as a storage form of the glucose that is needed for the plant's first growth. When you eat the plant, your body hydrolyzes the starch to glucose and uses the glucose for its own energy purposes.

All starchy foods are in fact plant foods. Grains are the richest food source of starch. Many human societies have a staple grain from which much of their people's food energy is derived—rice in Asia; wheat in Canada, the United States, and Europe; corn in much of Central and South America; and millet, rye, barley, and oats elsewhere.

A second important source of starch is the legume (bean and pea) family, including peanuts and such dry beans found in the supermarket as butter beans, kidney beans, "baked" beans, black-eyed peas (cowpeas), chick-peas

polysaccharide: many monosaccharides linked together.
poly = many

starch: a plant polysaccharide composed of glucose and digestible by humans. For the structures of starch's two forms, amylose (straight chain) and amylopectin (branched chain), see Appendix C.

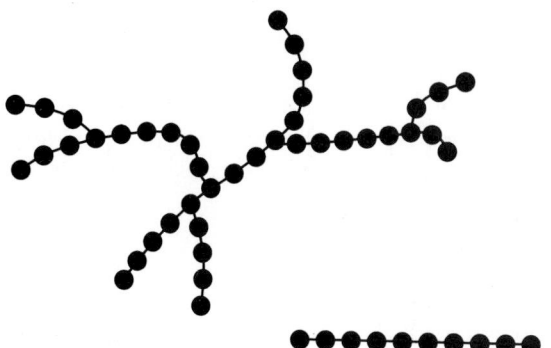

■ **FIGURE 4–8**
Starch Molecule
Starch is a long, straight or branched chain of hundreds of glucose molecules connected together. For details of the chemical structure, see Appendix C.

(garbanzo beans), and soybeans. These legumes are not only rich in starch and dietary fibers but also contain a significant amount of protein. A third major source of starch is the tuber, such as the potato, yam, and cassava of many non-Western societies.

Glycogen

Glycogen serves a function in animals similar to that served by starch in plants. Glycogen is not found in plants and is found in meats only to a limited extent. It is not, therefore, of importance as a nutrient, although it performs an important role in the body. The glycogen molecule is more complex and more highly branched than the starch molecule; its structure permits rapid hydrolysis. When the hormonal message "Release energy" arrives at a liver or muscle cell, enzymes can attack all the branches of glycogen simultaneously, producing a surge of available glucose for emergency energy. The electron micrograph at the start of this chapter shows part of a single liver cell, in which a multitude of glycogen packages await such a call.

glycogen (GLI-co-gen): an animal polysaccharide composed of glucose, manufactured and stored in liver and muscle; a storage form of glucose. For its structure, see Appendix C.

glyco = glucose
gen = gives rise to

◼ *The Fibers*

Plant foods contain many fibers, predominantly as constituents of the plant's cell walls. These fibers consist of compounds that are not digested by the enzymes in the human GI tract. Fibers include the polysaccharides cellulose, hemicellulose, pectins, gums, and mucilages, as well as the nonpolysaccharide lignins.*

Cellulose, like starch, is found abundantly in plants and is composed of glucose units connected in long chains. However, unlike the bonds in starch, the bonds holding together the glucose units of cellulose are not broken by human enzymes. Although cellulose and other dietary fibers are not hydrolyzed by human enzymes, some fibers can be digested by bacteria in the human digestive tract. This process produces lipid fragments, known as short-chain fatty acids (Chapter 5 will tell you more about them). These short-chain fatty acids are absorbed in the colon and yield energy when metabolized.[1] Food fibers are therefore not totally energy-free, although they vary in energy contribution depending on the extent to which they are broken down. For the most part, the energy contribution is negligible, although it can be as high as 15 percent of the daily intake on a high-fiber diet.[2]

Dietary fibers can be classified according to several characteristics, including their solubility in water, their chemical structure, and their digestibility by bacterial enzymes (see Table 4–3). These distinctions influence the effects fibers have on health (see p. 88).

fiber: a general term denoting in plant food the polysaccharides cellulose, hemicellulose, pectins, gums, and mucilages, as well as the nonpolysaccharide lignins, that are not digested by human digestive enzymes.

dietary fiber: the residue of plant food resistant to hydrolysis by human digestive enzymes; that is, the fiber that remains from food after passage through the small intestine prior to bacterial digestion in the colon.

A fiber that yields energy by way of bacterial digestion is a **digestible**, but **unavailable, carbohydrate**. In the body such a fiber *would* normally be digested, because there are always abundant bacteria in the normal, healthy human digestive tract.

---

*The terms *crude fiber, neutral-detergent fiber,* and *dietary fiber* identify different methodologies used to estimate the fiber contents of foods, not different types of fiber.

■ TABLE 4–3
Characteristics of Fiber

	Water Soluble	Water Insoluble
Polysaccharides	Gums Hemicellulose[a] Mucilages Pectins	Cellulose Hemicellulose[a]
Nonpolysaccharides		Lignins
Food Sources	Fruits Oats Barley Legumes	Vegetables Wheat Grains
Health Effects	Lower blood cholesterol Lower rate of glucose absorption	Softened stools Acceleration of intestinal transit time

Dietary fibers are classified according to a number of characteristics, including their solubility in water and whether they are a polysaccharide. These differences influence their physiological effect on the body (see p. 88).
[a]Some hemicelluloses are water soluble and others are water insoluble.

Digestion and Absorption

The ultimate goal of carbohydrate digestion and absorption is to render all available carbohydrates into small compounds that the body can use—chiefly glucose and fructose. The initial splitting of the larger carbohydrates begins in the mouth; the final splitting and absorption occurs in the small intestine; and conversion to a common energy currency is the task of the liver. The details follow.

The carbohydrates (starch and sugar) made available to the body by human digestive enzymes are **available carbohydrates** (in contrast to the fibers, which are **unavailable carbohydrates**).

The Processes of Digestion and Absorption

Figure 4–9 traces the digestion of carbohydrates through the GI tract. Most of the carbohydrates in foods cannot pass into the body through the intestinal cells until they are hydrolyzed to monosaccharides. As mentioned in Chapter 3, this process begins in the mouth with the secretion of saliva. The salivary enzyme amylase starts to work, hydrolyzing starch into smaller pieces (polysaccharides and the disaccharide maltose), but because the food is soon swallowed, the job is not completed. The stomach's acid and enzymes inactivate and digest the salivary enzymes, thus halting starch digestion. To a small extent, the stomach's acid continues the breakdown, but its juices contain no enzymes to digest carbohydrate. Carbohydrate digestion becomes active again when the chyme enters the small intestine.

In the intestines, a major carbohydrate-digesting enzyme continues the work. Pancreatic amylase, which has entered the intestine via the pancreatic duct, continues the hydrolysis of polysaccharides to shorter glucose chains

The short chains of glucose units that result from starch breakdown are known as **dextrins**. The word sometimes appears on food labels, because dextrins can be used as thickening agents in foods.

■ **FIGURE 4–9**
Carbohydrate Digestion through the GI Tract

Fiber	Carbohydrate

Mouth

The mechanical action of the mouth crushes and tears fiber in food and mixes it with saliva to moisten it for swallowing.

The salivary glands secrete a watery fluid into the mouth to moisten the food. The salivary enzyme amylase begins digestion:

Starch $\xrightarrow{\text{amylase}}$ small polysaccharides, maltose

Esophagus

Fiber is undigested.

The digestion of starch continues as swallowed food moves down the esophagus.

Stomach

Fiber is undigested.

Stomach acid and enzymes inactivate salivary enzymes, halting starch digestion.

Small intestine

Fiber is undigested.

The pancreas produces carbohydrases and releases them through the pancreatic duct into the small intestine:

Polysaccharides $\xrightarrow[\text{amylase}]{\text{pancreatic}}$ dextrins

Then enzymes on the surfaces of the small intestinal cells hydrolyze these into monosaccharides and the cells absorb them:

Maltose $\xrightarrow{\text{maltase}}$ glucose

Sucrose $\xrightarrow{\text{sucrase}}$ fructose

Lactose $\xrightarrow{\text{lactase}}$ galactose

Large Intestine

Most fiber passes intact through the digestive tract to the large intestine. Here, bacterial enzymes digest some fiber:

Some fiber $\xrightarrow[\text{enzymes}]{\text{bacterial}}$ fatty acids, gas

Fiber holds water; regulates bowel activity; and binds cholesterol and some minerals, carrying them out of the body.

A. Digestion of maltose. B. Digestion of sucrose. C. Digestion of lactose.

Key: ● Glucose.

▲ Fructose.

■ Galactose.

■ FIGURE 4–10
Digestion of Disaccharides

and disaccharides. The final step takes place on the outer membranes of the intestinal mucosal cells. There, specific enzymes hydrolyze specific disaccharides. Maltase hydrolyzes maltose to yield two molecules of glucose; sucrase hydrolyzes sucrose to yield one molecule of glucose and one of fructose; and lactase hydrolyzes lactose to yield one molecule of glucose and one of galactose (see Figure 4–10). Thus all disaccharides contribute glucose to the body. Within one to four hours after a meal, all the available carbohydrates—the sugars and starches—have been digested.

Most of the carbohydrate digestion and absorption activity is completed in the small intestine. Only the indigestible fibers remain in the digestive tract. These fibers function like a sponge, holding water, binding minerals, and binding acidic materials such as the bile used by the body to prepare fat for digestion.

Monosaccharides are absorbed into the bloodstream from the intestines. (Glucose is unique in that it can also be absorbed to some extent through the lining of the mouth.) When the blood circulates past the liver, the liver cells take up monosaccharides and convert them to other compounds, most often to glucose, as shown in Figure 4–11. Fructose and glucose are not used in

maltase: an enzyme that hydrolyzes maltose.

sucrase: an enzyme that hydrolyzes sucrose.

lactase: an enzyme that hydrolyzes lactose.

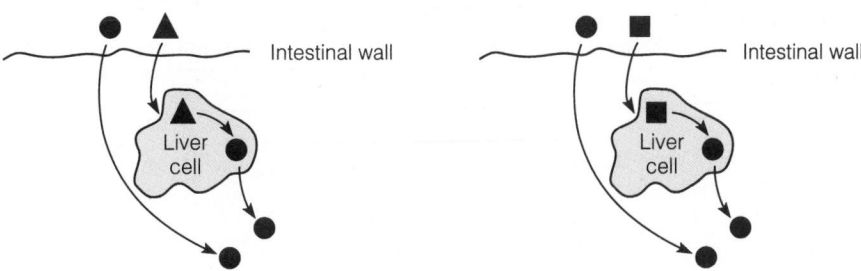

The digestion of sucrose yields one glucose and one fructose; lactose yields one glucose and one galactose. The body absorbs these monosaccharides into the bloodstream from the intestine. When they travel past the liver, liver cells take them up and can convert them to glucose. In effect, all disaccharides can ultimately contribute two glucose molecules.

Key: ● Glucose.

▲ Fructose.

■ Galactose.

■ FIGURE 4–11
Absorption of Monosaccharides and Conversion to Glucose

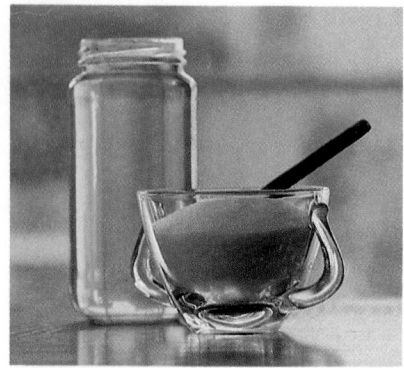

1 tsp honey = 22 kcal.
1 tsp sugar = 16 kcal.

1 tsp honey = 22 kcal.
1 tsp fruit = 2 kcal with vitamins,
minerals, and fiber.

exactly the same ways in the body, but for purposes of the discussion of metabolism in this book, they are handled in essentially the same way and are treated as being metabolically identical.

People sometimes wonder whether table sugar and honey differ in any important way. Honey, like table sugar, contains glucose and fructose. The primary difference is that in table sugar they are bonded together, and in honey some of them are not. However, the facts of digestion just presented show that whether you eat these monosaccharides linked together or individually, they will end up as monosaccharides in your body. Honey does contain a few vitamins and minerals, but to say that it is nutritious is misleading. Honey, being a liquid, is more dense than its crystalline sister and so provides more energy per spoon. However, as Table 4–4 shows, honey is not significantly more nutritious than sugar.

To say that honey is no more nutritious than sugar, however, is not to say that there are no differences among sugar sources. Consider a fruit, like an orange. From the fruit you could receive the same monosaccharides and the same energy as from sugar or honey, but the packaging is different. The fruit's sugars are diluted in a large volume of water that contains valuable trace minerals and vitamins, and the flesh and skin of the fruit are supported by fibers that also offer health value.

From these two comparisons you can see that the really significant difference between sugar sources is not between "natural" honey and "purified" sugar but between concentrated sweets and the dilute, naturally occurring sugars that sweeten foods. You can suspect an exaggerated nutrition claim when you hear the assertion that one product is more nutritious than another because it contains honey.

■ TABLE 4–4
Sample Nutrients in Sugars and Other Foods
The indicated portion of any of these foods would provide approximately 100 kcal. Notice what nutrients the eater receives along with the energy.

Food	Size of 100-kcal Portion	Carbohydrate (g)	Percentage of U.S. RDA[a]				
			Protein	Calcium	Iron	Vitamin A	Thiamin
Milk, low-fat	¾ c	9	17	26	—	3	5
Kidney beans	½ c	21	12	4	13	< 1	9
Watermelon	4-by-8-inch wedge	23	3	3	12	50	9
Bread, whole wheat	1½ slices	19	7	4	7	—	9
Sugar, white	2 tbsp	24	0	0	0	0	0
Molasses, blackstrap	2 tbsp	22	0	27	35	0	3
Cola beverage	1 c	26	0	0	0	0	0
Honey, strained or extracted	1 ½ tbsp	26	—	< 1	1	0	—

[a]Percentages are rounded to the nearest whole number. A dash means the percentage has not been determined and is not significant. The U.S. RDA are recommended adult intakes (see inside front cover, right).

Lactose Intolerance

For some people, the digestion and absorption of disaccharides do not go smoothly. Most often the problem involves the enzyme lactase, which hydrolyzes the disaccharide lactose. Normally, the presence of lactase within the intestinal cell's microvilli ensures that lactose is both split and absorbed efficiently. As soon as lactose is hydrolyzed into glucose and galactose, they are easily contacted by the nearby pumps, which move them into the interior of the cell. In the liver, galactose is converted to glucose, so each molecule of lactose eventually yields two molecules of glucose (see Figure 4–11).

Lactose intolerance departs from this norm. In rare cases, a person is simply born with a deficiency of lactase. More often, lactase deficiency develops as a consequence of another disease; any condition that changes the intestinal villi, such as prolonged diarrhea or use of some medicines, can lead to lactose intolerance. In most of the world's population, normal lactase activity gradually declines with age. Lactose intolerance is not the same as the commonly observed milk allergy, which is caused by an immune reaction to the protein in milk.

lactose intolerance: an inherited or acquired inability to digest lactose, due to failure to produce the enzyme lactase.

When lactose in the intestine is not rapidly hydrolyzed and absorbed, numerous small lactose molecules remain in the intestine undigested, attracting water and causing fullness, discomfort, cramping, nausea, and diarrhea. The lactose also becomes food for intestinal bacteria, which multiply and produce irritating acid and gas, further contributing to the discomfort and diarrhea.

A lactose-restricted diet is a highly individualized diet, because people vary widely in the amount of lactose they can tolerate. The person sensitive to even small amounts of lactose must follow a lactose-free diet. This diet can be difficult to follow, because lactose is a hidden ingredient in many foods. The person on a lactose-free diet needs to be a label reader, avoiding foods that include these ingredients: milk, milk solids, whey, and casein. Even some drugs contain lactose as fillers. Fortunately, not all people with lactose intolerance must avoid lactose completely. The amount of lactose allowed depends on the person's tolerance. Many times only milk, milk beverages, creamed foods, and ice cream have to be avoided. An enzyme preparation (Lact-Aid) can be added to milk; the enzyme hydrolyzes much of the lactose in milk to glucose and galactose, and people with lactose intolerance can then drink it without ill effects.

Chapter 25's discussion on disaccharidase deficiencies includes a table of foods to avoid on a lactose-free diet and a sample menu.

A word of caution: people who consume little or no milk or too few milk products often have diets that are calcium deficient. Chapter 10 offers help with finding other sources of calcium.

▮ Health Effects of Carbohydrates

This section focuses on the health effects of sugars, complex carbohydrates, and fibers. To give you a preview of the conclusions, for the most part, sugars add sweetness to food, which makes it appetizing, and they are neutral to health unless consumed in excess. Complex carbohydrates and fibers might also be harmful when consumed in excess, but few people attain such high levels of consumption. More likely, people will receive many health benefits when their diets contain plenty of foods rich in complex carbohydrates and fibers.

Health Effects of Sugars

The sugars are all quite similar in their effects on health. Anything true of sucrose is probably true of the other sugars as well. Many accusations have been made against sucrose:

- *It's unnatural. It isn't a nutrient; it's an additive, and so it's dangerous.* (This is largely unfounded.)
- *It causes malnutrition.* (This is overstated, but it can contribute.)
- *It causes obesity.* (This is overstated, but it can contribute.)
- *It causes diabetes (Type II).* (This is not well supported.)
- *It causes high blood lipid levels and cardiovascular disease.* (This has little support.)
- *It causes dental caries.* (This is confirmed.)
- *It causes hyperactivity.* (This is not well supported; Chapter 15 provides information on hyperactivity and diet.)

With respect to the first accusation, it is true that pure, refined sucrose is relatively new in our environment. Our cave ancestors did not have such a source of refined, concentrated sugar. In the United States, sucrose consumption was only about 20 pounds per person per year in 1820, but it had reached over 100 pounds per person per year in the 1970s. Since then, sucrose consumption has declined steadily to about 60 pounds in 1985. This decline reflects some changes in consumer habits, including the use of sugar substitutes and increases in the use of other sweeteners, such as high-fructose corn syrup (HFCS), by the food and beverage industry. All in all, *total* sugar intake continues to rise.

Sugar is the leading food additive; only about one-third of the sugar you eat is added to foods by you. The average North American eats at least 100 pounds of sugar a year, and two-thirds of this is found in common products to which it has been added by manufacturers. Sugar is not a poison, however; sucrose is just glucose plus fructose linked together. It's not dangerous—at least not in the sense that true poisons are dangerous, and it is undeniably delicious.

As for the second accusation, it is partly true. Sugar can displace needed nutrients from the diet. Starch usually comes in foods with other nutrients, but sugar contains no other nutrients—no protein, vitamins, or minerals— and so can be termed an empty-kcalorie food. If you have 200 kcalories to "spend" on something, and you spend them on pure sugar, you get nothing of value for your outlay. If you spend your 200 kcalories on three slices of whole-wheat bread instead, you get 14 percent of the protein, 24 percent of the thiamin, and 17 percent of the niacin U.S. RDA for a day, as well as comparable amounts of many other nutrients. Perhaps a reasonable compromise would be to have two slices of bread with a teaspoon of your favorite jam on each. The point is that the amount of sugar you can afford to eat depends on how many kcalories you have to spend beyond those needed to deliver valuable vitamins and minerals.

It is theoretically possible, with careful food selection, to obtain all the needed nutrients within an allowance of about 1,500 kcalories—but this is not easy for most people. An active teenage boy may need as many as 4,000 kcalories to get all the energy he needs; if he eats mostly nutritious foods, then the "empty kcalories" of cola beverages are probably an acceptable addition to his diet. On the other hand, many women consume 1,200 kcalories or even

empty-kcalorie food: a popular term used to denote foods that contribute energy but that are relatively empty of the nutrients protein, vitamins, and minerals. The most notorious empty-kcalorie foods are sugar, fat, and alcohol.

Miniglossary of a Few Representative Sweeteners

brown sugar: sugar crystals contained in molasses syrup with natural flavor and color; 91 to 96% pure sucrose. (Refiners add syrup to refined white sugar to make brown sugar.)

confectioners' sugar: finely powdered sucrose; 99.9% pure.

corn sweeteners: corn syrup and sugars derived from corn.

corn syrup: a syrup produced by the action of enzymes on cornstarch, containing mostly glucose. See also *high-fructose corn syrup (HFCS)*.

dextrose: an older name for glucose.

fructose, galactose, glucose: defined on p. 73–74.

granulated sugar: crystalline sucrose; 99.9% pure.

high-fructose corn syrup (HFCS): the predominant sweetener used in processed foods and beverages. HFCS is mostly fructose; glucose makes up the balance.

honey: sugar formed from nectar (mostly sucrose) gathered by bees. An enzyme splits the sucrose into glucose and fructose. Composition and flavor vary, but honey always contains a mixture of sucrose, fructose, and glucose.

invert sugar: a mixture of glucose and fructose formed by the hydrolysis of sucrose in a chemical process. Sold only in liquid form, and sweeter than sucrose, invert sugar is used as an additive to help preserve food freshness and prevent shrinkage.

lactose: defined on p. 76.

levulose: an older name for fructose.

maltose: defined on p. 76.

maple sugar: a sugar (mostly sucrose) purified from concentrated sap of the sugar maple tree. Maple sugar is expensive compared with other sweeteners.

molasses: a thick brown syrup, left over from sugarcane juice during sugar refining. It retains residual sugar and other by-products and a few minerals; blackstrap molasses contains significant amounts of calcium and iron—the iron from the machinery used to process sugar.

raw sugar: the first crop of crystals harvested during sugar processing. Raw sugar cannot be sold in the United States because it contains too much filth (dirt, insect fragments, and the like). Sugar sold as "raw sugar" domestically has actually gone through over half of the refining steps.

sucrose: defined on p. 76.

turbinado (ter-bih-NOD-oh) **sugar:** raw sugar from which the filth has been washed; legal to sell in the United States.

white sugar: pure sucrose, produced by dissolving, concentrating, and recrystallizing raw sugar.

less, so they can't afford any but the most nutrient-dense foods. Sugar can clearly cause malnutrition, then—not by any positive action of its own, but by displacing nutrients that prevent malnutrition. Some of the effects sugar is thought to have on behavior probably come about indirectly, by way of poor nutrition. The appropriate attitude to take is not that sugar is "bad" and that we must avoid it, but that nutritious foods must come first. If the nutritious foods end up crowding sugar out of the diet, that is fine—but not the other way around.

The third accusation, that sugar causes obesity, can be answered as follows. Excess energy from any food source, even protein, is stored in body fat. Evidence from population studies shows that in many countries obesity rises as sugar consumption increases, but sugar cannot be singled out as the sole cause. In these populations, increases in fat intake are often much more significant, and they occur simultaneously with declines in physical activity. Obesity occurs sometimes where sugar intake is low, too, and in some instances, fat people eat less sugar than thin people. Sugar can contribute to obesity, then, but does not cause obesity by itself—and obesity can occur without it.

On diabetes, the evidence is conflicting and interesting. In vast areas of the world, as the diet has changed in the direction of increased sugar consumption, a profound increase—by as much as tenfold—in the incidence of adult-onset (Type II) diabetes has occurred. (This is true for the Japanese, Israelis, Africans, Native Americans, Inuits, Polynesians, and Micronesians.) Yet in other populations, no relation has been found between sugar intake and diabetes. Wherever starch is a major part of the diet, diabetes is rare; however, this may not be an effect of the starch itself but of the nutrients, such as trace minerals and fiber, that accompany it in foods. Wherever obesity is rare, diabetes is also rare, suggesting that sugar alone is, in any case, not enough to cause the disease.

In animals, however, diets very high in sugar can cause a diabeteslike disease even if the animals do not become obese. The fairest conclusion is that obesity is a major factor in the causation of Type II diabetes, and that sugar may be a special factor.

Diabetes receives full attention in Chapter 27.

Does sugar raise blood lipid levels and cause cardiovascular disease? No simple answer is available. The blood lipid of greatest interest in connection with cardiovascular disease is cholesterol, and it is discussed in the next chapter, which shows that dietary fat exerts by far the most influence on it. Another blood lipid, not conclusively linked with heart disease, is triglycerides (also discussed in Chapter 5); moderate amounts of sugar may raise blood triglyceride levels in a special subgroup of the population—"carbohydrate-sensitive" individuals. Sugar in the amounts usually consumed seems to have no discrete influence on lipid levels in most people, however. Deaths from heart disease correlate most closely with high blood cholesterol levels, next most closely with obesity, and only loosely with sugar intake; a moderate amount of sugar has not been shown to affect the disease process.

Does sugar cause dental caries? Here the evidence is strongly positive. Dental caries develop as acid produced by bacterial growth in the mouth eats into tooth enamel. (Dental caries are discussed in detail in Highlight 10.) Bacteria thrive on carbohydrate, and so it is logical to implicate sugar as the cause of dental caries. However, any carbohydrate-containing foods, including bread, bananas, or milk, as well as sugar—can support bacterial growth. In this matter, as in the others, sugar may not be the extreme villain that some have made it out to be. Still, if sugar is guilty of any of the seven accusations listed at the start, it is guilty of contributing to tooth decay.

In summary, there is no reason to believe that a moderate consumption of sugar (5 to 10 percent of total energy intake) is in any way dangerous to healthy human beings. Clearly, however, it may be associated with other factors that are harmful: obesity, the displacement of needed nutrients and fiber, and dental caries. If on these grounds you decide to limit the sugar you eat, it is important to recognize that all kcaloric sweeteners—including fructose, honey, and the rest—are sugars, too.

This raises the problem of how food labels should declare sugar contents. Consumers want, and are entitled to, this information, but food producers are concerned that the labels not put them at an unfair disadvantage; so the exact requirements for labeling still have to be worked out. What should be called "sugar," for example? All monosaccharides and disaccharides, including those found naturally in the food? or only added sugars, including honey, corn syrup, and the like? or only added sucrose? How should sugar contents be listed? If given in grams per serving, then the amount of sugar in a cola beverage will be seen to be more than that in a serving of sugar-coated cereal; but if sugar is stated as a percentage by weight, then the amount in the cereal will appear very high, because it is not diluted by water. These questions have not been resolved, so you cannot tell how much sugar is in the products you buy unless the manufacturer has listed the amount voluntarily.

The presence of sugar does have to be revealed in the ingredient list, however, and if sugar is the first ingredient named there, you know it is the predominant substance in the product. Each of sugar's different forms may be listed separately— for example, "corn starch, sucrose, corn syrup," and so on—so even though sugar is the main ingredient, it may not appear first on the label. Be aware. Your acquaintance with the terminology presented in the accompanying miniglossary should enable you to recognize sugar in all its forms.

Because sugars add sweetness to foods, and because eating delicious foods is one of life's primary pleasures, the sensible way to use them is to enjoy them in moderation. When their presence in foods does nothing for you, leave them out, but use them, in small quantities and in strategic places, to add zest to meals.

Health Effects of Complex Carbohydrates

Dietary guidelines offered to the public by various agencies in the United States and Canada agree that reducing concentrated sweets and increasing complex carbohydrates in the diet would benefit the health of most people. Not all sugars need to be restricted, just *concentrated* sweets, relatively empty of nutrients and high in kcalories. Sugars that occur naturally in foods such as fruits, vegetables, and milk are acceptable. The trade is between relatively pure sugar on the one hand and whole foods that contain both complex and simple carbohydrates on the other.

Guidelines typically recommend that carbohydrates contribute 55 to 60 percent of the total energy intake. Concentrated sweets should represent only about one-sixth of this, or 10 percent or less of total kcalories. For most people, total carbohydrate intake should increase, and sugar intake should decline. The major additions to the diet would be foods containing starch and fiber—vegetables, grains, legumes, and fruits.

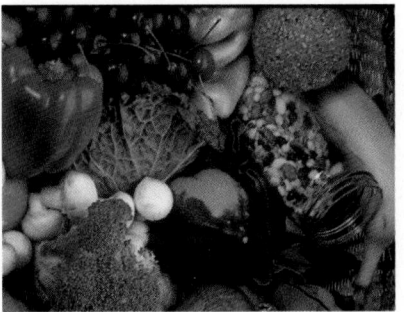

Foods rich in starch and fiber offer many health benefits.

The health benefits to be expected from such a change would be many. A diet lower in pure sugars and higher in foods containing complex carbohydrates would almost certainly be lower in fat; lower in energy; and higher in fiber, vitamins, and minerals, as well. The constellation of all these factors working together might be expected to bring about, or to contribute to, lower rates of obesity, cardiovascular disease, diabetes, cancer, malnutrition, and tooth decay. It is difficult to sort out just what dietary factors might contribute to each health benefit. Starch and fiber almost invariably appear together in foods (except refined foods), so it is especially hard to separate their effects. The next section discusses the health effects that appear to be especially closely associated with fibers.

Health Effects of Fibers

Based on the observations of physicians in Africa, the "fiber hypothesis" suggests that consumption of unrefined, high-fiber, carbohydrate foods protects against many Western diseases, such as colon cancer and cardiovascular disease. Rural Africans naturally consume a diet very high in fiber and show a low incidence of many chronic conditions. Some researchers, however, stress that it may be the higher Western intake of animal fat, sugar, and salt rather than the absence of fibrous foods that should be credited for these conditions.

High-fiber foods may also play a role in weight control. According to the fiber hypothesis, obesity is not seen in those parts of the world where people eat large amounts of fiber-rich foods. Foods high in fiber tend to be low in fat and simple sugars. High-fiber breads provide less energy per pound than refined breads. High-fiber foods, because of their water-holding capacity,

 NUTRITION DETECTIVE WORK

When researchers collect and interpret data on the incidence and distribution of disease among populations, they are conducting an epidemiological (ep-ih-DEE-me-oh-LODGE-ick-al) study. In the case of fiber, physicians collected data on the diet of a group of people in Africa and noted that it was high in fiber. They also noted that the people had a low incidence of many chronic diseases that plague Western societies.

Epidemiological data allow researchers to demonstrate a correlation between variables—a high-fiber diet correlates with a low incidence of colon cancer. Such data cannot, however, prove a cause—that is, we cannot conclude that a low-fiber diet causes colon cancer. To attribute the difference in disease incidence between developed and developing countries to differing intakes of fiber is to ignore many other possible variables. Other dietary factors such as excess fat, protein, and alcohol may also play a role, not to mention the many nondietary differences such as the urban life and lack of exercise common to developed countries. Indeed, lifestyles differ in many respects, and any one or combination of factors may be responsible. When you read epidemiological studies, remember to ask whether the researchers considered all the variables.

provide a feeling of fullness. Many of the weight-loss products on the market are composed of bulk-inducing fibers such as methylcellulose. If you wish to apply this principle in adopting a weight-loss diet, you need to select fresh fruits, vegetables, legumes, and other high-fiber foods that represent both an economic and a nutritious means of adding bulk to your diet. Foods containing fiber are thought to be beneficial with respect to the following:

- *Weight control.* A diet high in fibrous foods can promote weight loss, if those foods displace concentrated fats and sweets. This is possible because fibrous foods offer less energy per bite than concentrated fats and sweets, thus providing fullness before too much energy is taken in.
- *Constipation and diarrhea relief.* Some fibers attract water into the digestive tract, thus softening the stools. Others help to solidify watery stools. By the one mechanism, they help relieve constipation, and by the other, they help relieve diarrhea.
- *Hemorrhoid prevention.* Softer and larger stools ease elimination for the rectal muscles and reduce the pressure in the lower bowel, creating less likelihood that rectal veins will swell.
- *Appendicitis prevention.* Fiber helps prevent compaction of the intestinal contents, which could obstruct the appendix and permit bacteria to invade and infect it.
- *Diverticulosis prevention.* Fiber exercises the muscles of the digestive tract so that they retain their health and tone and resist bulging out into the pouches characteristic of diverticulosis (described in Highlight 3 and Chapter 25).
- *Colon cancer prevention.* Some fibers speed up the passage of food materials through the digestive tract, thus shortening the "transit time" and helping to prevent exposure of the tissue to cancer-causing agents in food. Some fibers bind bile (described in Chapter 5) and carry it out of the body; this is also thought to reduce cancer risk.
- *Blood lipid and cardiovascular disease control.* Some fibers bind lipids such as bile and cholesterol and carry them out of the body with the feces so that the blood lipid concentrations are lowered, and possibly the risk of heart and artery disease as a consequence.
- *Blood glucose and insulin modulation.* Monosaccharides absorbed from some complex carbohydrates, in the presence of fiber, produce a moderate insulin response and an even rise in blood glucose concentrations. Insulin levels are high in obesity, cardiovascular disease, and diabetes (Type II), so this effect of fiber may be beneficial in all three diseases.
- *Diabetes control.* Thanks to its effects on blood glucose concentrations, high-fiber foods help to manage diabetes. Persons with mild cases of diabetes, given high-fiber diets, have been able to reduce their insulin doses.

Not all the fibers have similar effects. For example, wheat bran, which is an insoluble fiber, has no cholesterol-lowering effect, whereas oat bran and some of the fibers in apples (soluble fibers) do lower blood cholesterol. On the other hand, wheat bran seems to be one of the most effective stool-softening fibers, especially if larger particle sizes are used. Water-soluble fibers (pectin and guar) delay the time of transit of materials through the intestine, whereas insoluble fibers (cellulose and hemicellulose) tend to accelerate transit time, thus alleviating or preventing constipation.

Most clinical reports are concerned with the influence of the lack of fibrous foods in the diet on health and disease. The questions of whether *excessive* fiber might be harmful, and what the ideal range of fiber intakes may be, remain to be answered.

A person who eats bulky foods, and who has only a small capacity, may not be able to take in enough food energy or nutrients. Vegetarian children are especially vulnerable to this problem. People who increase their intakes of high-fiber foods too rapidly may experience intestinal discomfort and gas. To avoid these side effects, increase dietary fiber intake gradually, and be sure fluid intake is adequate.

Insoluble fibers limit absorption of minerals and possibly vitamins.[3] Animals given *pure* fiber, apart from food, under experimental conditions excrete more minerals in their feces than otherwise—including calcium, potassium, iron, zinc, and others. Whether people experience significant mineral losses with ordinary high-fiber foods is not known. People who have marginal or inadequate intakes of the vitamins and trace minerals— including elderly people, people on low-kcalorie diets, and children—may develop nutrient deficiencies on high-fiber diets.

Clearly, though, fiber is probably like all the nutrients in that "more" is only "better" up to a point. Too much is no better for you than too little. Also, pure fiber is not as beneficial as the fiber of foods; the pure version is empty of nutrients, while the food version is loaded with them.

A compound not classed as a fiber but often found with it in foods is phytic acid. On a high-fiber diet, losses of minerals may occur if they become bound to phytic acid. Most of the phytic acid in our diet comes from seeds such as the cereal grains. (The role of phytate in the plant seed may be to store these minerals and hold them in plant tissue during germination.)

phytic acid: a nonnutrient component of plant seeds; also called **phytate** (FYE-tate). Phytic acid occurs in the husks of grains, legumes, and seeds and is capable of binding minerals such as zinc, iron, calcium, magnesium, and copper in insoluble complexes in the intestine.

Regulation of the Blood Glucose Level

A certain amount of glucose in the blood is indispensable to our functioning and feeling well. For this reason, physiologists concern themselves with how the body regulates its blood glucose, and nutritionists are particularly interested in the effects of foods on blood glucose concentrations.

The Constancy of Blood Glucose

If your blood glucose concentration falls below normal, you may become tired, hungry, and shaky; if it goes above normal, you may become sleepy. If either extreme is pushed far enough, you go into a coma. Optimal functioning is only possible when blood glucose is within a certain range of values.

Every body cell depends on glucose to a greater or lesser extent. Ordinarily, the cells of your brain and nervous system depend *primarily* on glucose for their energy. The brain cells are continually active, even while you're asleep, so they are continually drawing on the supply of glucose in the fluid

For the chief exception to this rule, ketosis, see Chapter 7.

surrounding them. To maintain the supply, a steady stream of blood moves past these cells, replenishing the glucose as the cells use it up.

What do you have to do to maintain a normal blood glucose level? Your body normally does it for you, as part of its job of maintaining homeostasis, but you can help by attending to your eating habits, as we shall show in a moment.

homeostasis (HOME-ee-oh-STAY-sis): defined on p. 15.

When you wake up in the morning, your blood probably contains between 70 and 120 milligrams of glucose in each 100 milliliters. This range, which is known as the fasting blood glucose concentration, is normal and is accompanied by a feeling of alertness and well-being (provided that nothing else is wrong, of course—that you do not have the flu, for example). If you do not eat, your blood glucose level gradually falls as the cells all over your body keep drawing on the diminishing supply. Most people experience a feeling of hunger at 60 or 65 milligrams per 100 milliliters, the low end of the normal range. The normal response to this sensation is to eat; then the blood glucose level rises again.

A **milligram (mg)** is 1/1,000 of a gram; a **milliliter (ml)** is 1/1,000 of a liter. Blood concentrations of many substances are measured in milligrams per 100 milliliters (mg/100 ml).
milli = 1,000; prefix denotes 1/1,000.

It is important that the blood glucose level not rise too high, and the body works to prevent this. The first organ to respond to raised blood glucose is the pancreas, which detects the excess and sends a hormonal message to correct it; then liver and muscle cells receive the message, remove the glucose from the blood, and store it as glycogen.

Special cells of the pancreas are sensitive to the blood glucose concentration.* When blood glucose rises, these pancreatic cells respond by secreting more of the hormone insulin into the blood. As the circulating insulin contacts the receptors on the body's other cells, these receptors respond by taking up glucose from the blood. Most of the cells can only use the glucose for energy right away, but the liver and muscle cells have the ability to store it for later use: they assemble the small glucose units into long, branching chains of glycogen. The liver cells can also convert the glucose to fat for export to other body cells (see Figure 4–12). Thus the blood glucose concentration returns to normal, and any excess glucose is put in storage as glycogen (which can return the glucose) and fat (which cannot return the glucose).

insulin (IN-suh-lin): a hormone secreted by the pancreas in response to (among other things) increased blood glucose concentration.

Between meals, a hormone that opposes insulin's action—glucagon—works to bring glucose back out of storage as needed.** Thus the stored liver glycogen (but not the muscle glycogen† or fat) can keep replenishing the blood glucose as the brain and other body cells keep drawing on it to meet their energy needs.

glucagon (GLOO-ka-gon): a hormone secreted by the pancreas in response to low blood glucose concentration that elicits release of glucose from storage.

Another hormone that elicits release of glucose from the liver cells is the famous "fight-or-flight" hormone, epinephrine. Epinephrine acts quickly when you are under stress, ensuring that all your body cells have energy fuel in emergencies. Like glucagon, epinephrine works to return glucose to the blood from liver glycogen.

epinephrine (EP-ih-NEFF-rin): defined on p. 15.

---

*These special cells are the *beta* (BAY-tuh) *cells*, one of several types of cells in the pancreas. The beta cells secrete insulin in response to increased blood glucose concentration.

**Glucagon is produced by the *alpha cells* of the pancreas.

†Normally, only glycogen from the liver, not from muscle, can return glucose units *directly* to the blood; muscle cells only use glycogen internally. Muscle cells can restore the blood glucose level *indirectly*, however: when they are oxidizing glucose for energy, they can release a breakdown product, lactic acid, into the blood, and the liver can pick this up and reconvert it to glucose. This is the so-called Cori cycle. For more about lactic acid, see Chapter 13.

■ **FIGURE 4–12**
Regulation of Blood Glucose Concentration

1. High blood glucose stimulates the pancreas to release insulin.
2. Insulin stimulates the uptake of glucose into cells. Liver and muscle cells store the glucose as glycogen.
3. Liver cells also convert glucose into fat and release it. The fat cells pick up the fat and store it.
4. Later, low blood glucose stimulates the pancreas to release glucagon into the bloodstream.
5. Glucagon stimulates liver cells to break down glycogen and release glucose into the blood.

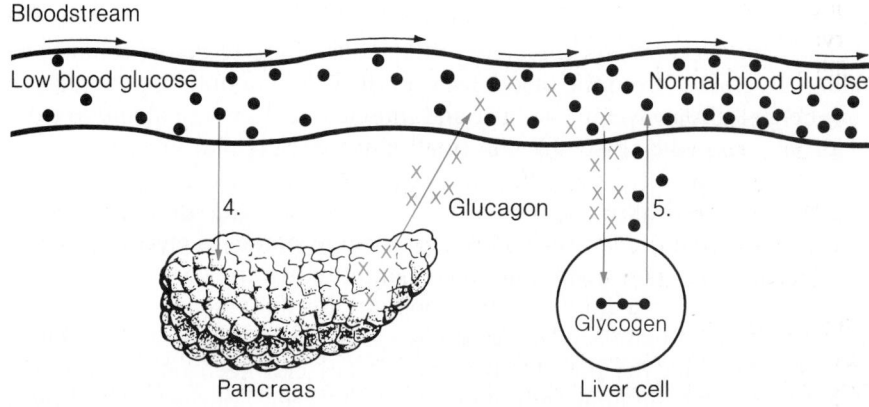

gluconeogenesis: the making of glucose from a noncarbohydrate source (described in more detail in Chapter 7).

Muscle glycogen, too, can be dismantled to glucose, but this glucose is used primarily within the muscle cells themselves, where it serves as an important fuel for muscle action. Long-distance runners know that adequate stores of muscle glycogen can make a crucial difference in their endurance toward the end of a race (as Chapter 13 details).

The maintenance of a normal blood glucose level thus depends ordinarily on two processes. When the level gets too low, it can be replenished quickly either from liver glycogen stores or from food. (If you do not eat carbohydrate, your body devours its own protein to generate glucose—a process called gluconeogenesis. The body needs its protein for other vital purposes. The "protein-sparing effect" of carbohydrate is important and will come up again in Chapters 6 and 7.) When the blood glucose concentration gets too high, insulin is secreted to siphon the excess into storage.

The way you eat can help your body keep a happy medium between the extremes. Two guidelines apply. First, when you are hungry, you should eat without waiting until you are famished. Second, when you do eat, you should eat a balanced meal, including some protein and fat as well as complex carbohydrate. The fat slows down the digestion and absorption of carbohydrate, so that it trickles gradually into the blood, providing a steady, ongoing supply. The protein elicits the secretion of glucagon, whose effects are generally opposite to those of insulin; and this damps insulin's effect, maintaining blood glucose concentrations within the normal range for a longer time.

In some people, blood glucose regulation fails for one reason or another. Two groups of conditions are especially common: hypoglycemia and diabetes. Both are surrounded by many myths and misconceptions, including much misguided advice on diet. Chapter 27 focuses on diabetes and hypoglycemia.

The Glycemic Effect of Foods

The glycemic effect of a food is the effect that food has on a person's blood glucose and insulin response—how fast and how high the blood glucose rises, and how quickly the body responds by bringing it back to normal. Most people have had the impression that simple sugars produce a major surge in blood glucose, whereas complex carbohydrates produce a flatter response curve—but now we know that the case is not so simple. The effects of different foods on blood glucose apparently depend on many factors:

- The digestibility of the starch in the food.
- Interactions of the starch with the protein in the food.
- The amounts and kinds of fat, sugar, and fiber in the food.
- The presence of other constituents, such as molecules that bind starch.
- The form of the food (dry, paste, or liquid; coarsely or finely ground; how thoroughly cooked; and so forth).

All these factors working together produce the food's glycemic effect, and it is not always what a person might expect.[4] Ice cream, for example, produces less of a response than potatoes. More important, a food's glycemic effect differs when it is eaten alone or as part of a mixed meal. To the above list of factors that influence a food's glycemic effect, add:

- The *combination* of foods consumed at a given time.

This one factor is actually quite significant, considering that most people eat a variety of foods in a meal.

The glycemic effect of a food may be important to people with abnormalities of blood glucose regulation, notably diabetes or hypoglycemia; these people may benefit from avoiding foods that produce too great a rise, and too sudden a fall, in blood glucose. For their use, researchers are attempting to produce a "glycemic index" that would rank foods according to their effects on blood glucose. For *practical* use, however, the glycemic index is of little value in meal planning. Food combinations do not yield predictable blood glucose responses. To control blood glucose, dietitians employ other methods of meal planning, such as controlling energy intake.

◼ *The Carbohydrates in Foods*

You need some carbohydrate daily as a source of glucose. How much carbohydrate is enough?

Recommended Carbohydrate Intake

Because all monosaccharides, most protein fragments, and even some fat fragments can be converted to glucose, there is no dietary recommendation for carbohydrates.[5] (The minimum amount of carbohydrate necessary to spare protein is 50 to 100 grams a day.)[6] To be safe, you should probably aim for at least 125 grams, and 300 grams might be an ideal intake for many people. (At 4 kcalories per gram, that would be 1,200 kcalories from carbohydrate.)

Another way to view carbohydrate intake is as a percentage of total energy intake. Most guidelines suggest an intake of 55 to 60 percent of the total energy intake from carbohydrate (starch and sugar) to support long-term health. A person consuming 1,500 kcalories a day should therefore have 825 to 900 kcalories of carbohydrate, or about 200 to 225 grams. A person consuming 3,000 kcalories a day should have twice that, or 400 to 450 grams. Most of this would be from foods rich in starch, with accompanying fiber; some would be the naturally occurring sugars of fruits, vegetables, and milk; only 10 percent or less would be from other sugars.

The exchange system described in Chapter 2 provides a convenient way to estimate the amount of carbohydrate in your lunchbox or on your dinner plate. In exchange systems, foods are sorted into lists in such a way that the carbohydrate contents of foods on any one list are similar. To use such a system, you need to know the carbohydrate value for the list and the members of that list with their portion sizes (see Figure 4–13). All the foods containing carbohydrate are identified in five categories. Some practice with estimating portion sizes and a familiarity with the gram amounts give you a command of the total carbohydrate content of any diet. The example given in Figure 4–14 demonstrates the system's usefulness.

This kind of calculation provides only an estimate, but it is close enough for most purposes. A more accurate way to determine the carbohydrate composition of foods is to refer to Appendix H or use a computer diet analysis program. Adding the individual carbohydrate amounts for the meals shown in Figure 4–14 yields 258 grams of carbohydrate.

The difference between the 264 gram estimate and the 258 gram amount obtained by the more accurate calculation may be disconcerting. Rough estimates are often more valuable than close calculations, however, because of the time saved and because often only a ballpark figure is needed. In this example, we know that 264 and 258 grams are both comfortably above the recommended minimum of 125 grams, and both are in the same range. The difference between them becomes insignificant from this perspective.

Most estimates of the nutrient contents of foods are rough but serviceable approximations. If we refer to a "90-kcalorie potato," you should understand this to mean "90 plus or minus about 20 percent," which makes it not

12 g in 1 c milk (lactose)

15 g in 1 slice bread (starch)

15 g in 1 fruit portion (sugars)

5 g in 1 tsp sugar (sugars)

5 g in ½ c vegetables (sugars and starch)

Four of the six exchange lists contain carbohydrate, so you need only know four values and learn a value for concentrated sugar (which is not on the exchange lists).

■ **FIGURE 4–13**
Exchange Lists Containing Carbohydrate

Milk List

1 c nonfat milk (or any other portion of food in the milk list) provides 12 g carbohydrate as lactose, a naturally occurring sugar. Cheeses have negligible carbohydrate and so are not included with milk in this system. (See Appendix G for Canadian values, which are different.)

Starch/Bread List

1 slice bread (or any other portion of food on the starch/bread list) provides 15 g carbohydrate, mostly in the form of starch. All grain foods, such as cereal and pasta, and starchy vegetables such as corn, lima beans, and potatoes, are included on this list.

Fruit List

1 fruit portion (portion sizes are shown on the fruit list) provides 15 g carbohydrate, mostly as the naturally occurring sugars glucose, fructose, and sucrose.

Vegetable List

½ c carrots (or any other portion of food on the vegetable list) provides 5 g carbohydrate, partly as the naturally occurring sugars fructose, glucose, and sucrose, and partly as starch. Starchy vegetables (those whose carbohydrate is predominantly starch) are not included on this list. (See Appendix G.)

Sugar

1 tsp white sugar provides 4 g carbohydrate as sucrose, which for most purposes can be rounded off to 5 g. The other concentrated sweets provide sucrose, fructose, glucose, and other hexoses, or mixtures of these.

significantly different from a 100-kcalorie potato. In general, for most purposes, a variation of about 20 percent is expected and is considered perfectly reasonable.

It takes only a few calculations of this kind to give you a feel for the carbohydrate content of your diet. Once you are aware of the major carbohydrate-contributing foods you eat, you can return to thinking simply in terms of the foods, developing a sense of how much of each is enough.

Sugar Intake

Sugary foods like candy, jam, and soft drinks are not considered desirable in diet plans, but people do consume them, and they certainly contain carbohydrate. To estimate an accurate total of the carbohydrate you consume, you may need a "sugar list," and we have invented one for the purpose. Among the concentrated sweets equivalent to 1 teaspoon of white sugar are:

- 1 teaspoon brown sugar.
- 1 teaspoon candy.

■ 1 teaspoon corn sweetener.

■ 1 teaspoon corn syrup.

■ 1 teaspoon honey.

■ 1 teaspoon jam.

■ 1 teaspoon jelly.

■ 1 teaspoon maple sugar.

■ 1 teaspoon maple syrup.

■ 1 teaspoon molasses.

■ 1 ounce carbonated soda.

These sugars can all be assumed to provide *about* 20 kcalories per teaspoon. Some are closer to 15 kcalories (for example, 16 kcalories for sucrose), while some are over 20 (22 kcalories for honey); so an average figure of 20 kcalories is an acceptable rough approximation. For a person who uses catsup liberally, it may help to remember that 1 tablespoon of catsup supplies about 1 teaspoon of sugar.

1 tbsp catsup = 1 tsp sugar.
1 tbsp is equivalent to 3 tsp.

The exchange system does provide for the moderate consumption of some foods that are high in sugar and fat, such as cakes and cookies. Table 4–5 lists exchanges for these concentrated sweets; notice their small portion sizes.

Fiber Intake

The amounts of dietary fiber in food are hard to estimate. (Appendix H offers dietary fiber contents of foods.) About 20 to 35 grams of dietary fiber daily is a desirable intake.[7] This is two to three times higher than the average intake in the United States.[8] The diet can supply that amount, given ample choices of whole foods, as Table 4–6 demonstrates. It involves eating more fruits, vegetables, legumes, and grains and fewer meats and dairy products than most people are accustomed to eating, but this change is not hard to make. The meals shown in Figure 4–14 provide 40 grams of dietary fiber, with significant contributions from the strawberries and orange; the broccoli; the bean burrito and garbanzo beans; and the oatmeal.

■ **TABLE 4–5**
Exchange List for Concentrated Sweets

Food	Amount	Exchanges
Angel food cake	1/12 cake	2 starches
Cake, no icing	1/12 cake, or a 3-inch square	2 starches, 2 fats
Cookies	2 small (1 3/4 inches across)	1 starch, 1 fat
Frozen fruit yogurt	1/3 c	1 starch
Gingersnaps	3	1 starch
Granola	1/4 c	1 starch, 1 fat
Granola bars	1 small	1 starch, 1 fat
Ice cream, any flavor	1/2 c	1 starch, 2 fats
Ice milk, any flavor	1/2 c	1 starch, 1 fat
Sherbet, any flavor	1/4 c	1 starch
Snack chips, all varieties	1 oz	1 starch, 2 fats
Vanilla wafers	6 small	1 starch, 1 fat

■ TABLE 4–6
Foods to Provide 25 Grams Dietary Fiber per Day

Fruits: about 2 to 4 g of fiber per serving.

Apple, 1 small	Orange, 1 small
Apricots, 3	Peach, 1 medium
Banana, 1 small	Pear, ½ small
Blackberries, ½ c	Pineapple, 1 c
Blueberries, ½ c	Plums, 2 small
Cantaloupe, ½	Prunes, 2
Dates, 5	Raspberries, ½ c
Figs, 2	Strawberries, ½ c

Grains and Cereals: about 2 to 4 g of fiber per serving.

All-Bran, ½ oz	Raisin Bran, ½ c
Barley, ½ c	Rice, 1 c
Bulgur, ½ c	Rye bread, 1 slice
Cracked wheat bread, 1 slice	Shredded Wheat, ½ c
Granola, ½ c	Wheat bran, ¼ c
Grape-Nuts, ½ c	Whole-wheat bread, 1 slice
Oatmeal, ½ c	

Vegetables: about 2 to 4 g of fiber per serving.

Artichoke, 1	Green beans, 1 c
Broccoli, ½ stalk	Lettuce, 2 c
Brussels sprouts, ½ c	Potato, 1 small
Carrots, 1 c	Spinach, 1 c
Celery, 1 c	Squash, 1 c
Corn on the cob, 2-inch piece	Tomato, 1 medium

Legumes: about 8 g of fiber per portion.

Baked beans, ½ c	Lentils, 1 c
Black beans, ½ c	Lima beans, 1 c
Blackeyed peas, 1 c	Navy beans, ½ c
Garbanzo beans, 1 c	Pinto beans, ½ c
Kidney beans, ½ c	

Miscellaneous: about 1 g of fiber per portion.

Nuts, ½ oz	Peanut butter, 1 tbsp
Olives, 5	Pickle, 1 large

This chapter showed you how important a constant blood glucose level is for the functioning of the brain and the body's other tissues, how the body can derive glucose from all foods containing starches and sugars, and which foods those are. Armed with this information, you can explode some of the myths perpetrated by advertisers of carbohydrate-containing foods and beverages. Sugar is "quick energy"—so when you need quick energy, you should reach for a candy bar and a cola beverage, right? Wrong. The best pick-me-ups are not concentrated sugars. True, sugars offer energy, but you now can see that any food containing carbohydrate can offer that to you. How about a delicious peanut butter and banana sandwich; a tall, cool glass of milk; and a fresh, juicy orange for your pick-me-up?

■ **FIGURE 4–14**
Estimating Carbohydrate Intake using the Exchange System

	Carbohydrate Grams	
	Exchange	Actual
Breakfast		
1 c oatmeal = 2 starch exchanges	30	25
¼ c raisins = 2 fruit exchanges	30	29
1 c nonfat milk = 1 milk exchange	12	12
1 ¼ c strawberries = 1 fruit exchange	15	13
Morning Snack		
2 tbsp raisins = 1 fruit exchange	15	15
2 tbsp sunflowers seeds = 2 fat exchanges	—	3
Lunch		
1 bean burrito		
(1 lg tortilla = 2 starch exchanges	30 ⎤	
½ c beans = 1 starch exchange	15 ⎬	47
+ ½ lean meat exchange)	— ⎦	
1 c nonfat milk = 1 milk exchange	12	12
1 orange = 1 fruit exchange	15	15
Dinner		
4 oz shrimp = 4 lean meat exchanges	—	0
1 c broccoli = 2 vegetable exchanges	10	9
½ c spinach noodles = 1 starch exchange	15	17
2 tsp butter = 2 fat exchanges	—	0
¼ c parsley = ¼ vegetable exchange	⎤	1
¼ tomato = ¼ vegetable exchange	5	1
¼ c mushrooms = ¼ vegetable exchange	⎬	1
¼ c water chestnuts = ¼ vegetable exchange	⎦	4
1 c fresh spinach = 1 vegetable exchange	5	2
1 tbsp sesame seeds = 1 fat exchange	—	2
1 tbsp vinaigrette and oil dressing = 1 fat exchange	—	0
⅓ c garbanzo beans = 1 starch exchange	15	15
½ c sherbet = 2 starch exchanges	30	29
1 packet sugar	10	6
Day's total	264 g	258 g

A dietitian, looking at the foods in the figure, might estimate the cup of oatmeal as "2 starch exchanges," because a 1-starch portion is ½ c of any cooked cereal. She would figure the 2 tablespoons of raisins as "1 fruit," because 2 tbsp raisins is a fruit exchange. The ways she would view each food portion as exchanges are shown. The novice would have to become familiar with the exchange system before this technique would save time, but with practice, a person can learn to estimate carbohydrate grams quite closely. The actual carbohydrate grams are shown at the right.

SELF STUDY *Examine Your Carbohydrate Intake*

Having read Chapter 4, you are in a position to study your carbohydrate intake. From the forms you filled out in the previous self-study exercises, answer the following questions:

1. How many grams of carbohydrate do you consume in a day?
2. How many kcalories does this represent? (Remember, 1 gram of carbohydrate contributes 4 kcalories.)
3. It is estimated that you should have 125 grams or more of carbohydrate in a day. How does your intake compare with this minimum?
4. What percentage of your total kcalories is contributed by carbohydrate (carbohydrate kcalories ÷ total kcalories x 100)?
5. How does this figure compare with the dietary goal that states that 55 to 60 percent of the kcalories in your diet should come from carbohydrate? (Note: If you are on a diet to lose weight, then this goal does not apply to you. See the exercises in Chapter 12's Self-Study: Diet Planning.)
6. Another dietary goal is that no more than 10 percent of total kcalories come from refined and other processed sugars and foods high in such sugars. To assess your intake against this standard, sort the carbohydrate-containing food items you ate into three groups:

   - Foods containing complex carbohydrate (foods found on the bread and vegetable exchange lists).
   - Nutritious foods containing simple carbohydrate (foods on the milk and fruit lists).
   - Foods containing mostly concentrated simple carbohydrate (sugar, honey, molasses, syrup, jam, jelly, candy, cakes, doughnuts, sweet rolls, cola beverages, and so on).

   How many grams of carbohydrate did you consume in each of these three categories? How many kcalories (grams times 4)? What percentage of your total kcalories comes from concentrated sugars? From other simple carbohydrates? Does your concentrated sugar intake fall within the recommended maximum of 10 percent of total kcalories?
7. Estimate how many pounds of sugar (concentrated simple carbohydrate) you eat in a year (1 pound = 454 grams). How does your yearly sugar intake compare with the estimated U.S. average of about 125 pounds per person per year?
8. You may be interested in computing fiber intake as well. Use Appendix H or a computer diet analysis program to determine the amount of fiber you consume. Then compare your fiber intake with the recommendation of 20 to 35 grams of dietary fiber per day.

Study Questions

1. What three monosaccharides are important in nutrition? What three disaccharides are important in nutrition? What are their component monosaccharides? Where are they found?
2. What happens in a condensation reaction? In a hydrolysis reaction?
3. What are differences between simple and complex carbohydrates?
4. What are the health effects of complex carbohydrates and fiber?
5. How is blood glucose concentration maintained? What happens when it gets too high or too low?
6. What are the dietary recommendations regarding carbohydrate intake?
7. Demonstrate how the exchange system can help you to estimate the carbohydrate content of a meal.

Notes

1. M. J. Koruda and coauthors, Effect of parenteral nutrition supplemented with short-chain fatty acids on adaptation to massive small bowel resection, *Gastroenterology* 95 (1988): 715–720.
2. M. I. McBurney and L. U. Thompson, Dietary fiber and energy balance: Integration of the human ileostomy and in vitro fermentation models, *Animal Feed Science and Technology* 23 (1989): 261–275.
3. J. L. Slavin, Dietary fiber: Classification, chemical analyses, and food sources, *Journal of the American Dietetic Association* 87 (1987): 1164–1171.
4. G. M. Reaven, Parma Symposium: Current controversies in nutrition, *American Journal of Clinical Nutrition* 47 (1988): 1078–1082.
5. Food and Nutrition Board, *Recommended Dietary Allowances*, 10th ed. (Washington, D.C.: National Academy of Sciences, 1989), p. 41.
6. Food and Nutrition Board, 1989, p. 41.
7. Position of the American Dietetic Association: Health implications of dietary fiber, *Journal of the American Dietetic Association* 88 (1988): 216.
8. F. Lanza and coauthors, Dietary fiber intake in the U.S. population, *American Journal of Clinical Nutrition* 46 (1987): 790–797.

Sugar Alternatives

People who want to avoid sugar or cut down on their use of it may encounter two sets of alternative sweeteners. One set is the sugar alcohols, which are energy-yielding sweeteners sometimes referred to as nutritive sweeteners; the other is the artificial sweeteners, which provide virtually no energy, also referred to as nonnutritive sweeteners. The sugar alcohols are sugar relatives and begin this discussion; the artificial sweeteners are sugar substitutes and follow.

Sugar Alcohols

The sugar alcohols are familiar to people who use special dietary products. Among them are mannitol, sorbitol, xylitol, and maltitol. The body either absorbs these carbohydrates more slowly or metabolizes them to glucose more slowly than most of the other sugars. For this reason, they were once used by people with diabetes who could not handle large amounts of glucose efficiently and so had to restrict their intakes of ordinary sweets (which provide glucose from the glucose portion of sucrose). However, the associated side effects of sugar alcohol products and their energy contribution make them less attractive than their sucrose counterparts for managing diabetes. The real benefit of sugar alcohols is that ordinary mouth bacteria cannot metabolize them as rapidly as sugar, so they do not contribute as much to dental caries. All the sugar alcohols provide as much energy as sucrose (4 kcalories per gram).

Mannitol is the least satisfactory of the sugar alcohols just named. Because it is less sweet than sucrose, larger amounts have to be used when it substitutes for sucrose (see Table H4-1). It lingers unabsorbed in the intestine for a long time, available to intestinal bacteria for their energy. As the bacteria consume the mannitol,

they multiply, they attract water, and they produce irritating waste, which causes diarrhea. Mannitol is therefore little used as an alternative sweetener.

Sorbitol is popular as a sweetener for sugar-free gums and candies, but it, too, has drawbacks. It is only half as sweet as sucrose, so twice the amount of sorbitol (with twice as much energy) has to be used to deliver an equivalent amount of sweetness. Also, like mannitol, it causes diarrhea; its threshold for causing diarrhea is higher than mannitol's, so of the two, sorbitol is preferred.

Xylitol is also popular, especially in chewing gums, because of reports that it helps to prevent dental caries. (It not only doesn't support caries-producing bacteria; it actually inhibits their growth, as described in Highlight 10.) Xylitol occurs in foods, and the body produces some xylitol during normal metabolic processes; it is not a foreign substance. Xylitol is widely used in many Western European countries and in Canada; however, reports that it may cause tumors in animals have led to the voluntary curtailing of its use by U.S. food producers.

Maltitol has a sweetness equal to about 75 percent that of sucrose. It is used in some carbonated beverages and canned fruits, as well as in Japanese bakery products and other sweets intended not to cause tooth decay. The manufacture of maltitol from maltose is expensive and limits its use; using maltose directly costs less.

The person who wishes to reduce energy intake should be aware that the sugar alcohols *do* provide as much energy per gram as sucrose. In spite of this, products that contain them are labeled "sugar-free." The reason they are suitable for people who must limit their intakes of ordinary sugars is because the body handles them differently, not because they are kcalorie-free. The person who is limiting energy intake must limit sugar alcohols just as carefully as sugars. For this person, artificial sweeteners may offer a reasonable alternative.

Artificial Sweeteners

The food industry adds artificial sweeteners to foods and beverages primarily to meet consumers' demands for sweet products that will not add to

■ TABLE H4-1
Sweetness of Sugar Alternates

Sugar Alternate	Relative Sweetness[a]
Sucrose	100
Sorbitol	50
Mannitol	70
Maltitol	75
Xylitol	100
Cyclamate	1,500–5,000
Aspartame	15,000–25,000
Acesulfame-K	20,000
Saccharin	24,000–50,000

[a]The relative sweetness depends on the temperature and acidity of the foods in which the substance occurs. Sucrose is the standard by which the approximate sweetness of sugar substitutes is compared.

Source: Adapted from D. B. Drucker, Sweetening agents in food, drinks and medicine: Cariogenic potential and adverse effects, *Journal of Human Nutrition* 33 (1979): 114–124.

energy intake or contribute to dental caries. Some consumers have challenged the safety of using artificial sweeteners. Considering that all compounds are toxic at some dose, it is little surprise that large doses of artificial sweeteners (or their components or metabolic by-products) have toxic effects. The question to ask is whether their ingestion is harmful to human beings at normal use (and potential abuse) concentrations.[1]

The big three synthetic sweeteners are saccharin, cyclamate, and aspartame. Table H4–1 shows that their sweetness per unit of weight far exceeds that of the sugar alcohols. Saccharin has been around since before 1900, and it has dominated the market ever since, except for a brief two decades, the 1950s and 1960s, when cyclamate was in wide use. Aspartame was approved by the Food and Drug Administration (FDA) in 1981 and rapidly began gaining the ascendancy over saccharin.[2]

The cases of saccharin and cyclamate illustrate some general points about additives and food safety that are worth a moment's attention here. Saccharin, used for nearly 100 years in the United States, is presently used by some 50 million Americans—primarily in soft drinks, secondarily as a tabletop sweetener. Questions about its safety surfaced in 1977, when experiments suggested it caused bladder tumors in rats, and the FDA proposed banning it as a result. The public outcry in favor of retaining it was so loud, however, that Congress placed a moratorium on any action, and the moratorium has since been repeatedly renewed. Products containing saccharin are required to carry the warning label, now familiar to all consumers of diet beverages, that "use of this product may be hazardous to your health. This product contains saccharin, which has been determined to cause cancer in laboratory animals."

Does saccharin cause cancer? The evidence that it does so in animals is

> ## Miniglossary
>
> **acesulfame** (AY-see-sul-fame) **potassium**: a low-kcalorie sweetener recently approved by the FDA.
>
> **aspartame:** a compound of phenylalanine and aspartic acid that tastes like the sugar sucrose but is much sweeter. It provides 4 kcal/g, as does protein, but because so little is used, it is virtually kcalorie-free. In powdered form it is mixed with lactose, however, so a 1-g packet contains 4 kcal. It is used in both the United States and Canada.
>
> **cyclamate:** a 0-kcal sweetener banned in the United States and used restrictively in Canada.
>
> **diketopiperazine** (dye-KEY-toe-pie-PER-a-zeen), or **DKP:** a product to which aspartame breaks down during metabolism.
>
> **maltitol**, **mannitol, sorbitol, xylitol:** sugar alcohols, which can be derived from fruits or commercially produced from dextrose; absorbed more slowly and metabolized differently than other sugars in the human body, and not readily utilized by ordinary mouth bacteria.
>
> **saccharin:** a 0-kcal sweetener used in the United States but banned in Canada.

as follows. When male and female rats are fed diets containing saccharin from the time of weaning to adulthood and then mated, and their offspring are also fed saccharin throughout life, the offspring have a higher incidence of bladder tumors than comparable animals not fed saccharin. The question was raised for a while whether an impurity in the saccharin used in the tests might be causing the tumors, but this was resolved: the saccharin itself was responsible.[3] It wasn't clear whether the tumors were cancerous. In Canada, on the basis of these findings and in the face of public outcry as loud as that in the United States, all uses of saccharin were banned except use as a tabletop sweetener to be sold in pharmacies, and Canada permits those sales only with a warning label.

One large-scale population study, involving 9,000 people, showed a distinctly *greater risk* of cancers in some groups such as women who drank two or more diet sodas a day and people who both smoked heavily and used artificial sweeteners heavily. Another study involving over 1,000 people showed little or no excess risk

of bladder cancers, but of course could not conclude that there was no risk at all. As of now, two alternative conclusions are possible:

1. Saccharin causes tumors, possibly cancerous, in rats but not in people.
2. Saccharin is a weak carcinogen in people, and its effects will take more years of exposure to become apparent.

Cyclamate has had a shorter life than saccharin, dominating the artificial sweetener market for only 20 years. The 1970 ban on its use in the United States, although repeatedly appealed, has been continued even though, like saccharin, cyclamate has never been conclusively proven guilty of causing cancer in human beings. In Canada, saccharin is banned, and cyclamate is restricted to use as a tabletop sweetener on the advice of a physician and as a sweetening additive in medicines.

As for aspartame, within only a few years of receiving the FDA's approval it has appeared in dozens of familiar food products and in some totally new ones as well. Worldwide, people have gratefully accepted aspartame as

NutraSweet in diet drinks, chewing gum, presweetened cereal, gelatins, and pudding, and as Equal, a powder to use at home in place of sugar. As of 1984, aspartame sales had already surpassed the sales of saccharin and were also encroaching on sugar sales in some markets.

This amazing popularity is mostly due to aspartame's flavor, which is almost identical to that of sugar. Another lure drawing people to aspartame: the hope that it may be completely harmless, unlike the other sweeteners, whose laboratory records are tarnished. Too, aspartame is touted as safe for children, so families wishing to limit sugar are turning to it. Finally, as a sweet-toothed, overweight population, many people perceive sugar substitutes as the only way to cheat the scales.

Aspartame is a simple chemical compound: two protein fragments (the amino acids phenylalanine and aspartic acid) and a methyl group (CH_3) joined together (see Figure H4–1). In the digestive tract, the two protein fragments are split apart, absorbed, and used to build protein or burned for energy, just as they would be if they had come from protein in food. The flavors of the components give no clue to the combined effect; one of them tastes bitter, and the other is tasteless. But aspartame is incredibly

■ **FIGURE H4–1**
Structure of Aspartame

Aspartic Acid   Phenylalanine   Methyl Group

sweet—200 times sweeter than sucrose.

The disease phenylketonuria (PKU) poses some interesting problems with regard to aspartame. As Highlight 26 explains, people with PKU have the hereditary inability to dispose of phenylalanine when it is eaten in excess of the need for building proteins. Therefore, they cannot use unlimited amounts of the sweetener. They can use some, but there is a compelling reason why PKU children should not get their phenylalanine from this source. Phenylalanine occurs in such protein-rich and nutrient-rich foods as milk and meat, and the PKU child is allowed only a limited amount of these foods. Such a child can obtain only with difficulty the many essential nutrients—such as calcium, iron, and the B vitamins—found along with phenylalanine in these foods. To suggest that this child squander any of the limited phenylalanine allowance on the purified phenylalanine of aspartame, with none of the associated vitamins or minerals essential for good health and normal growth, would be to invite nutritional disaster. People with PKU need to know which old, familiar products now contain aspartame, and how to avoid them. Product labels offer a special warning for people with PKU.

Another concern about aspartame's safety has to do with its chemical structure (see Figure H4–2). During metabolism, the methyl group becomes methyl alcohol (methanol) momentarily—a toxic compound. Then it is converted to formaldehyde, another toxic compound, and finally to carbon dioxide. The quantities generated from normal use of aspartame are below the threshold at which these compounds cause harm, but in the testing of aspartame, that threshold had to be determined and its acceptability evaluated.

Still another concern is about the product that aspartame breaks down to—diketopiperazine, or DKP for short. Long-term studies using animals have directly tested this product and

■ **FIGURE H4–2**
Metabolism of Aspartame

eliminated it as a source of concern. Still another concern was over the effect aspartame use might have on the brain. Experiments with rats, monkeys, and human beings were performed, and none showed any cause for concern. The monkey study involved infant monkeys given up to 3,000 milligrams of aspartame per kilogram of body weight for nine months and showed no ill effects on growth, development, health, or behavior either during the test or on the withdrawal of aspartame.[4] The conclusion reached was that aspartame is safe except for people with PKU. Some 500 individual complaints received after its approval were reviewed by the Centers for Disease Control, which concluded that some individuals may exhibit vague, but not dangerous, symptoms due to unusual sensitivity to aspartame, but that the product is considered generally safe.[5]

The FDA has approved aspartame based on the assumption that no one

NUTRITION DETECTIVE WORK

Every day, millions of people use artificial sweeteners. Every day, millions of people have headaches. What can you conclude from this information? Very little, actually. Anyone who claimed, on this basis, that artificial sweeteners caused headaches would be riding for a fall. The reason, of course, is that only a correlation, not a cause, has been shown.

An analogy may help to make clear the distinction between correlations and causal relationships. Suppose that there is an outbreak of arson, and the police are searching for the suspect. Police observe that a certain person, Mr. Adams, is always in the neighborhoods when the fires start, and they accuse him of arson. However, another sneaky individual, Ms. Brown, is the real arsonist; Mr. Adams is only following her around. Mr. Adams is associated with, but is not a causal agent in, the setting of fires. The evidence against him is only circumstantial (correlational). If the police can show that whenever Mr. Adams is in jail there are no fires and that whenever he is let out the fires start again, the evidence against him will strengthen. Better yet, if they catch him pouring gasoline and lighting the match, they will know for sure.

To return to the case at hand—suppose there is an outbreak of headaches, and researchers are searching for the suspect. They observe that some of the people with headaches use artificial sweeteners. It would be premature, though, to accuse the artificial sweeteners of causing the headaches. Some of the headache sufferers might indeed be reacting to the artificial sweeteners, but they might also be reacting to another substance in the same foods. The evidence against artificial sweeteners is, at most, only correlational.

As it happens, even the correlation does not hold up. It turns out that some people with headaches do not use artificial sweeteners and that some people use artificial sweeteners without getting headaches. The sweeteners still might be causing some headaches, of course, but until researchers can show that these headaches come and go with sweetener use, they have no consistent correlation: researchers can show the evidence remains weak. Once a correlation is found to be consistent, the clincher is still to come—demonstration of the *mechanism* by which the agent causes the effect. Be careful when you interpret data that imply a causal relationship between factors linked only by association. It's a long way from such a loose connection to a proven cause-and-effect relationship.

will consume more than 50 milligrams per kilogram of their body weight in a day. This maximum daily intake is indeed a lot: for a 132-pound person, it adds up to 80 packets of Equal. About 15 soft drinks sweetened only with aspartame provide this maximum amount. The company that produces aspartame estimates that if all the sugar and saccharin in the U.S. diet were replaced with aspartame, 1 percent of the population would be consuming the FDA maximum.[6] Some people actually do consume this amount, however. A child who drinks a quart of Kool-Aid on a hot day, and who also has pudding, chewing gum, cereal, and other products with aspartame that day, packs in more than the FDA maximum level.

In an attempt to give a guideline for a safe level of aspartame, an advisory group to the World Health Organization has recommended a maximum of 40 milligrams per kilogram of body weight for adults.[7] A much more conservative limit of three to four packets of Equal per day is suggested by the Canadian Diabetes Association as a safe and useful level.[8] The newsletter for physicians *Nutrition and the M.D.* states that it is not known if aspartame is safe for children under two years old, and it points out that there are "very few if any reasons to use a sugar substitute in infants and young children."[9] It is unfortunate, but not uncommon, to see infants' bottles filled with drinks like Kool-Aid. Until aspartame has been around for a longer time, it would be best not to let infants be unwitting "testers" of aspartame's safety.

The FDA has recently approved the artificial sweetener acesulfame potassium (or acesulfame K), which has been available for use in several other countries. Marketed under the trade name Sunette, this sweetener is about as sweet as aspartame but seems to be more stable and less expensive. It will be used as an ingredient in chewing gum, beverages, instant coffee and tea, gelatins, and puddings. Like its predecessors, acesulfame potassium is being challenged by consumer groups concerned about its safety. Further research and consumer acceptance will determine its place on the grocery shelves.

Current evidence seems to suggest that artificial sweeteners ingested at normal-use concentrations pose no health risks. For persons choosing to use them, the American Dietetic Association wisely advises that their use be moderate and as a part of a well-balanced nutritious diet.[10] The dietary principles of both moderation and variety are useful in diluting any possible risks.

NOTES

1. L. D. Stegink, The aspartame story: A model for the clinical testing of a food additive, *American Journal of Clinical Nutrition* 46 (1987): 204–215.

2. C. Lecos, The sweet and sour history of saccharin, cyclamate, aspartame, *FDA Consumer,* September 1981, pp. 8–11.

3. Council on Scientific Affairs, American Medical Association, Saccharin: Review of safety issues, *Journal of the American Medical Association* 254 (1985): 2622–2624.

4. Council on Scientific Affairs, American Medical Association, Aspartame, review of safety, *Journal of the American Medical Association* 254 (1985): 400–402.

5. Council on Scientific Affairs, Aspartame, 1985.

6. *A Health Care Practitioner's Guide,* a pamphlet (1987): available from The NutraSweet Company, P.O. Box 1111, Skokie, Illinois 60076.

7. Joint FAO/WHO Expert Committee on Food Additives, International Programme on Chemical Safety, Toxicological evaluation of certain food additives, WHO technical report series no. 669 (Geneva: World Health Organization, 1981), pp. 25–32.

8. G. S. Wong, Aspartame and its safe use, *Diabetes Dialog* 29 (1982): 3.

9. Questions readers ask, *Nutrition and the M.D.,* January 1984.

10. Position of the American Dietetic Association: Appropriate use of nutritive and non-nutritive sweeteners, *Journal of the American Dietetic Association* 87 (1987): 1689–1690.

5

The Lipids: Fats, Oils, Phospholipids, and Sterols

Contents

The Chemist's View of Lipids

Digestion, Absorption, and Transport

The Roles of Lipids in the Body

The Health Effects of Lipids

The Lipids in Foods

Highlight: Artificial Fats

Muscle cells derive their energy from both fat and carbohydrate. Here, a lipid droplet nestles close to a muscle fiber (bottom), while a mitochondrion snuggles up to the droplet and gathers energy from it. Much of the cell's metabolic activity takes place inside the mitochondria. Millions of enzyme molecules are mounted on their internal membranes, in the order in which the enzymes perform their reactions.

itochondrion

Lipid

lipids: a family of compounds that includes fats and oils (triglycerides), phospholipids, and sterols.

Lipids:
- • Triglycerides (fats and oils).
  - ▪ Glycerol.
  - ▪ Fatty acids.
    - ▪ Saturated.
    - ▪ Monounsaturated.
    - ▪ Polyunsaturated.
      - • Omega-6.
      - • Omega-3.
- • Phospholipids (example: lecithin).
- • Sterols (example: cholesterol).

lipid profile: the results of blood tests that reveal a person's total cholesterol and triglycerides and the amounts of cholesterol in the various lipoproteins. For test results and their relationships to heart disease, see Table 28–2 in Chapter 28.

High blood cholesterol is a risk factor for heart disease. Others are:
- • Cigarette smoking.
- • Hypertension.
- • Obesity.
- • Glucose intolerance (diabetes).
- • Lack of exercise.
- • Stress.
- • Family history (genetics).
- • Gender (being male).

Food lipids are 95% fats and oils (that is, triglycerides) and 5% other lipids (phospholipids and sterols). In the body, 99% of the stored body fats are triglycerides.

■ **FIGURE 5–1**
Glycerol

```
        H
        |
    H-C—O-H
        |
    H-C—O-H
        |
    H-C—O-H
        |
        H
```

■ **FIGURE 5–2**
Acetic Acid (a two-carbon organic acid)

```
      H O
      | ||
  H-C—C—O-H
      |
      H
```

Most people think that the less fat you have on your body, and the less you eat, the better. This is not true. Surprised? Like all the nutrients, fat is beneficial in appropriate quantities—and it is harmful to ingest either too much or too little of it. It is true, though, that in our society of abundance, people are more likely to encounter too much fat than too little.

Fat is actually a subset of the class of compounds known as lipids. The lipids include triglycerides (fats and oils), phospholipids, and sterols, each important to nutrition.

■ The Chemist's View of Lipids

"Your blood lipid profile looks fine." If a physician says this, the client may be reassured. Most of us are aware that the amounts of lipids in the blood reflect the probability of heart disease. Some people know, too, that the amounts of fats they eat may affect their susceptibility to cancer and other diseases. A closer look at the lipids will lay the foundation for an understanding of these relationships, which are described in Chapter 28.

When people speak of fats and oils, they are usually speaking of triglycerides (the miniglossary on page 114 defines related terms). The triglycerides predominate in quantity, both in the diet and in the body; the following section focuses on them.

The Triglycerides

To understand the fats and the beneficial and harmful effects they have on your body, you must understand their molecular structure. Triglycerides come in many sizes and several varieties, but they all share a common structure; all have a "backbone" of glycerol to which three fatty acids are attached (see Figure 5–1). All glycerol molecules are alike, but the fatty acids may vary in two ways: length of the carbon chain and degree of unsaturation.

The Fatty Acids

A fatty acid is an organic acid. An organic acid consists of a chain of carbon atoms with hydrogens attached and with an acid group (COOH) at one end. The organic acid shown in Figure 5–2 is acetic acid, the compound that gives vinegar its sour taste. This is the simplest such acid; the "chain" is only two carbon atoms long. A longer acid chain may have four, six, eight, or more carbon atoms (naturally occurring fatty acids mostly come in even numbers). Common in dairy products are fatty acids that are six to ten carbons long. Butyric acid, found in butter, is a four-carbon fatty acid. Fatty acids that predominate in meats and fish are 14 or more carbon atoms long.

To illustrate the characteristics of these fatty acids, let us look at the 18-carbon ones. Stearic acid is the simplest of the 18-carbon fatty acids (see Figure 5–3):

H H H H H H H H H H H H H H H H H O
H-C—C—C—C—C—C—C—C—C—C—C—C—C—C—C—C—C—C—O-H
H H H H H H H H H H H H H H H H H

A. The structure with all details.

■ FIGURE 5–3
Stearic Acid (an 18–carbon fatty acid)

B. A simpler way to depict the same structure. Each "corner" on the zigzag line represents a carbon atom with two attached hydrogens.

C. Still more simply, the lines representing bonds to the hydrogens can be left out. It you count the "corners," you will see that this still represents an 18-carbon fatty acid. This is the way fatty acids will be represented in many of the following diagrams.

When three fatty acids attach to a glycerol molecule, the resulting structure is a triglyceride. Figure 5–4 illustrates three stearic acids attached to a glycerol molecule:

■ FIGURE 5–4
Formation of a Triglyceride
To make a fat (triglyceride), three fatty acids are attached to glycerol.

A. The first fatty acid approaches the glycerol, a condensation reaction occurs (water is eliminated), and a bond is formed between an O on the glycerol and the C at the acid end of the fatty acid.

B. Two more fatty acids can be attached to the glycerol by the same means, resulting in a triglyceride. This is tristearin (all three fatty acids are stearic acid). Most triglycerides are mixed, as shown in Figure 5–8.

The triglyceride shown in Figure 5–4 is a saturated fat, because the fatty acids are saturated fatty acids. Fatty acids are saturated when they are loaded, or saturated, with all the hydrogen (H) atoms they can carry. If hydrogens were to be removed, the carbons would form double bonds with one another in order to satisfy their bonding needs. The result would be an unsaturated, or even a polyunsaturated, fat.

A closer look shows how this transition from saturation to unsaturation can occur. Consider stearic acid once more: if two hydrogens are removed from the middle of the carbon chain, the structure that remains looks like that in Figure 5–5:

■ **FIGURE 5–5**
A Simplified Diagram of Stearic Acid without Two Hydrogens
A fatty acid lacking two hydrogens is an impossible structure, since two of the carbons have only three bonds each.

Such a compound cannot exist, however. To satisfy nature's requirement that every carbon have four bonds connecting it to other atoms, the two carbons form an extra bond between them, creating a double bond as shown in Figure 5–6:

■ **FIGURE 5–6**
Oleic Acid (an 18–carbon fatty acid)
Because it has one point of unsaturation, oleic acid is monounsaturated.

Above is a simplified diagram. The actual shape is bent at the double bond:

Note: Rotation can occur around single bonds. These molecules, although we draw them straight, are constantly twisting and bending. At any given moment, they may be coiled, horseshoe-shaped, or straight.

The resulting structure is an unsaturated fatty acid; in this case, it is the *mono*unsaturated fatty acid oleic acid, which is found abundantly in the triglycerides of olive oil.

The degree of unsaturation among fats is of interest because of health implications. Most people should probably control their *total* fat intake. However, people threatened with heart trouble may be told to reduce their intake of *saturated* fats in particular; evidence seems to indicate that *monounsaturated* fats, *polyunsaturated* fats, and low-fat diets are about equal in their ability to control blood lipid concentrations.[1] On the other hand, people whose families show a susceptibility to cancer may be told to restrict *poly*unsaturated fats as well (see Chapter 30 for more details on cancer).

A *poly*unsaturated fat contains triglycerides in which the fatty acids have two or more points of unsaturation (that is, carbon-to-carbon double bonds). An example is linoleic acid, which lacks four hydrogens and has two double bonds, as shown in Figure 5–7. Linoleic acid is the most common of the polyunsaturated fatty acids (PUFA) in foods, and one of the most important.

The ratio between polyunsaturated and saturated fat in the diet is the P:S ratio. In light of research indicating the benefits of monounsaturated fats, it might be more meaningful to calculate a P:M:S ratio. In case you want to do this, Appendix D offers help.

linoleic acid: an essential fatty acid with 18 carbons and two double bonds (18:2).

H H H H H   H   H H H H H H H O
H–C–C–C–C–C–C=C–C–C=C–C–C–C–C–C–C–C–C–O–H
H H H H H H H H H H H H H H H H H

Above is a simplified diagram. The actual shape is bent at the double bond:

■ **FIGURE 5–7**
Linoleic Acid (an 18–carbon fatty acid)
The two points of unsaturation in linoleic acid make it polyunsaturated. Linoleic acid is one of the essential fatty acids.

Having looked at three of the most common fatty acids in foods, you can probably anticipate what the others look like. A fourth 18-carbon fatty acid is linolenic acid, which has three double bonds (see Table 5–1). A similar series of 20-carbon fatty acids exists, as well as a series of 22-carbon fatty acids. The 16- to 22-carbon fatty acids are the long-chain fatty acids. In smaller amounts, medium-chain (10- to 14-carbon) and short-chain (4- to 8-carbon) fatty acids are also present in foods.

linolenic acid: an essential fatty acid with 18 carbons and three double bonds (18:3).

To sum up what has been said to this point, the fats and oils are mostly (95 percent) triglycerides: glycerol backbones with fatty acids attached. Those that are fully loaded with hydrogens are the saturated fats; those that have double bonds are unsaturated (monounsaturated and polyunsaturated) fats. To add to the picture, a fat or oil may contain any combination of fatty acids. A mixed triglyceride, one that contains more than one type of fatty acid, is shown in Figure 5–8. The vast majority of triglycerides are mixed.

The body's cells are equipped with many enzymes that can convert one compound to another. To make triglycerides, all the enzymes need is a usable food source containing the atoms that triglycerides are composed of: carbon, hydrogen, and oxygen. Glucose does perfectly well. In fact, given an excess of blood glucose (and filled glycogen stores), this is precisely what the cells do. Enzymes cleave the glucose to make 2-carbon fragments, and then combine these fragments with the appropriate alterations, to make long-chain fatty acids. (This is why most fatty acid carbon chains come in even numbers.)

Two Families of Polyunsaturated Fatty Acids

Not only do the fatty acids come in three categories (saturated, monounsaturated, and polyunsaturated), but the polyunsaturates belong to families—two of which are particularly important in nutrition. Researchers have long

■ **TABLE 5–1**
18-Carbon Fatty Acids

Name	Notation[a]	Number of Double Bonds	Saturation
Stearic acid	18:0	0	Saturated
Oleic acid	18:1	1	Monounsaturated
Linoleic acid	18:2	2	Polyunsaturated
Linolenic acid	18:3	3	Polyunsaturated

[a]Chemists use a shorthand notation to describe fatty acids. The first number indicates the number of carbon atoms; the second, the number of double bonds.

Highlight 8 defines a blind experiment and describes its role in nutrition research.

 NUTRITION DETECTIVE WORK

When linoleic acid is missing from the diet, the skin reddens and becomes irritated, infections and dehydration become likely, and the liver develops abnormalities. In infants, growth failure also occurs. Adding linoleic acid back to the diet clears up these symptoms.

The relief of a skin rash by linoleic acid might suggest to the unwary observer that all skin rashes indicate a deficiency of this nutrient. Not so! More than a hundred body compounds besides linoleic acid are needed to ensure the health of the skin, including other oils, vitamins, minerals, and hormones. A deficiency of any of these or an imbalance among them can cause a rash. The lack of some compound might be at fault, but the compound might also be present in excess, or it might be mishandled by the skin cells. Bacterial and viral infections, allergies, physical agents such as radiation, and chemical irritants also cause rashes. There can even be a psychosomatic cause, as when excessive nervous activity in the brain generates a hormone imbalance that affects the skin. For these reasons, when you notice a symptom such as a rash, you can only know that a problem exists; you have no clue as to the cause.

In dealing with nutrition, it is important to remember the distinction being made here—the distinction between a symptom and a disease. A symptom can be alleviated (soothing oils can be applied to irritated skin to make it feel better, for example), but until you have diagnosed the disease, you cannot achieve a cure. The rule for nutritional deficiency symptoms is that if a certain nutrient clears up the symptom, then a deficiency of that nutrient *may* have been the cause. To be certain, you would have to remove the nutrient and see the symptom reappear, then reintroduce the nutrient and see the symptom disappear; and you would have to do the experiment "blind"—that is, not knowing whether the treatment was given.

The field of nutrition is littered with misunderstandings about the interpretations of symptoms. People mistakenly think that if you are going bald, you need biotin; that if you have wrinkles, you need vitamin E; that if your hair is turning gray, you need pantothenic acid; and that if you have a skin rash, you need linoleic acid. None of these statements is true. When someone tries to persuade you of any such relationships between symptoms and nutrients, beware. Chances are, the person either doesn't see the distinction or is intentionally trying to deceive you. What you need is a correct diagnosis.

The same fallacious reasoning sometimes links *foods* with symptoms. Some people think that for prevention of colds, you need to eat oranges; for health of the digestive tract, yogurt; for protection against heart attacks, fish; for sexual potency, oysters; for weight loss, grapefruits; for physical strength, beefsteak; for good eyesight, carrots; to keep the doctor away, apples; and for health of the skin, safflower oil. Actually, of course, these foods are not essential at all, although the *nutrients* in them may be, and the foods may be good sources of those nutrients. In any case, to avoid a deficiency of linoleic acid, all you need is to eat an ordinary mixed diet; it will inevitably include some oils containing polyunsaturated fat.

■ FIGURE 5–8
Mixed Triglyceride
Mixed triglycerides are typical of those found in foods. The fat in a food is a mixture of many different mixed triglycerides. (The shape of the fatty acids is shown straight for ease of viewing.)

known and appreciated the importance of the omega-6 fatty acid family.* New on the scene, and attracting much interest, are the omega-3 fatty acids.

The body's cells do not possess enzymes that can make the omega-6 and omega-3 fatty acids, so people must obtain them from foods. Researchers consider some or all of them essential.

You have already been introduced to the first member of the omega-6 family—linoleic acid, which has 18 carbons. The body cannot make linoleic acid, but given dietary linoleic acid, it can synthesize its 20-carbon relative, arachidonic acid, although this is a slow process. Arachidonic acid occurs primarily in membrane phospholipids. Any diet that contains vegetable oils and meats supplies enough of these fatty acids to meet the body's needs.

You are also familiar with the 18-carbon member of the omega-3 family—linolenic acid. Until recently, linolenic acid was the only omega-3 fatty acid considered even somewhat important in human nutrition, because its roles seemed only to overlap those of linoleic and arachidonic acid. Now researchers recognize distinct roles for linolenic acid and the 20- and 22-carbon members of the omega-3 series, eicosapentaenoic acid (EPA) and docosahexaenoic acid (DHA). Their presence is evident in many tissues. DHA is especially active in the retina of the eye and the cerebral cortex of the brain.

The human body cannot make linolenic acid, but given dietary linolenic acid, it can synthesize EPA and DHA, although this, too, is a slow process.[2] To effectively increase body stores of EPA and DHA, we must consume them; we cannot depend on linolenic acid to contribute enough of them. People probably receive plenty of omega-6 lipids in their diets, but may lack optimal amounts of omega-3 lipids.[3] The dietary imbalance is primarily due to our high intakes of vegetable oils and limited intakes of fish. Probably, for each 4 to 10 grams of omega-6 fatty acids, about 1 gram of omega-3 fatty acids is needed.[4] Table 5–2 mentions the chief dietary sources of omega fatty acids.

omega-6 fatty acid: long recognized as important in nutrition, a polyunsaturated fatty acid with its endmost double bond six carbons from its methyl (CH_3) end.

omega-3 fatty acid: relatively newly recognized as important in nutrition, a polyunsaturated fatty acid with its endmost double bond three carbons away from its methyl (CH_3) end.

arachidonic (a-RACK-ih-DON-ic) **acid:** a polyunsaturated fatty acid with 20 carbons and 4 double bonds (20:4).

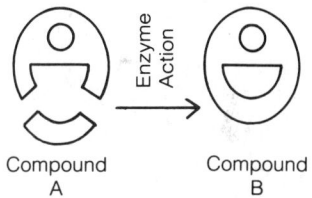

Compound A is the **precursor** of compound B; that is compound A can be converted into compound B. Linoleic acid is the precursor of arachidonic acid.

eicosapentaenoic (EYE-cossa-PENTA-ee-NO-ick) **acid** (**EPA**): an omega-3 fatty acid with 20 carbons and 5 double bonds (20:5), synthesized from linolenic acid.

docosahexaenoic (DOE-cosa-HEXA-ee-NO-ick) **acid** (**DHA**): an omega-3 fatty acid with 22 carbons and six double bonds (22:6).

*A fatty acid has two ends, designated the methyl (CH_3) end and the acid (COOH) end. Organic acids are usually numbered beginning at the acid end, but polyunsaturated fatty acids are an exception. Fatty acid chains are lengthened by adding carbons at the acid end of the chain. By numbering them from the methyl end, which does not change, chemists ease the task of keeping track of their identities: when an omega-3 acid is lengthened, the derivative is also an omega-3 acid.

phospholipid: a compound similar to a triglyceride but having choline (or another compound) and a phosphorus-containing acid in place of one of the fatty acids.

lecithin (LESS-uh-thin): one of the phospholipids; a compound of glycerol to which are attached two fatty acids, a phosphate group, and a choline molecule. The food industry uses lecithin as an emulsifier to combine two ingredients that do not ordinarily mix, such as water and oil.

The Phospholipids

The preceding pages have been devoted to one of the three classes of lipids, the triglycerides and their component parts, the fatty acids. The other two classes of lipids, the phospholipids and sterols, make up only 5 percent of the

■ **TABLE 5–2**
Dietary Sources of Omega Fatty Acids

Omega-6	
Linoleic acid	Vegetable oils
Arachidonic acid	Meat
Omega-3	
Linolenic acid	Leafy vegetables
	Vegetable oils
EPA and DHA	Fish and seafoods[a]

[a]Particularly good sources are herring, sardines, mackerel, tuna, trout, and salmon. These "fat fish" store most of their fat in muscle; in contrast, lean fish (such as cod) store their fat in their livers, which people generally do not eat.

lipids in the diet, but they are nonetheless interesting and important. Among the phospholipids, the best known is lecithin (actually, there are several lecithins).

Like the triglycerides, the lecithins and some other phospholipids have a backbone of glycerol; they are different from the triglycerides because they have only two fatty acids attached to them. In place of the third fatty acid is a phosphate group to which is attached a molecule of choline or a similar compound containing nitrogen (N) atoms. A diagram of a lecithin molecule is shown in Figure 5–9; other lecithin molecules differ in the nature of the attached fatty acids.

Choline: see Chapter 8.

Lecithin periodically receives noisy attention in the popular press, being credited with many good deeds. You may hear that it is a major constituent of cell membranes (true), that the functioning of all cells depends on the integrity of their membranes (true), and that you must therefore purchase bottles of lecithin and give yourself daily doses (false). You might as well believe that in order to grow healthy hair or to maintain the brain you must eat hair or brains! The enzyme lecithinase in the intestine hydrolyzes most of the lecithin before it passes into the body fluids, so the lecithin you eat does not reach the body tissues intact. The lecithin you need for building cell

■ **FIGURE 5–9**
A Lecithin
This is one of the lecithins. Others have other fatty acids at the upper two positions. (The plus charge on the N is balanced by a negative ion—usually chloride.)

Miniglossary of Fat Terms

fat: a mixture of triglycerides.

triglyceride (try-GLISS-er-ride): a compound composed of carbon, hydrogen, and oxygen arranged as a molecule of glycerol with three fatty acids attached. Triglycerides are also called **triacylglycerols** (try-ay-seel-GLISS-er-ols).

   tri = three
   glyceride = a compound of glycerol
   acyl = a carbon chain

glycerol (GLISS-er-ol): an organic alcohol composed of a three-carbon chain with an alcohol group attached to each carbon. An alcohol group is a reactive -OH group.

   ol = alcohol

fatty acid: an organic compound made up of a carbon chain with hydrogens attached and an acid group at one end.

acid group: the COOH group of an organic acid, which can also be represented this way:

$$\begin{array}{cc} \overset{\displaystyle O}{\overset{\|}{-C-O-H}} & \text{or} \quad \overset{\displaystyle O}{\overset{\|}{-C-O^- }}+ H^+ \end{array}$$

Notice that the O is double-bonded to the C, meeting the requirements that C have four bonds and O have two.

acid: a compound that tends to ionize (separate into charged particles) in water solution, releasing H^+ ions. The more H^+ ions that are free in the water, the stronger the acid (see Appendix B).

saturated fatty acid: a fatty acid carrying the maximum possible number of hydrogen atoms—for example, stearic acid. A **saturated fat** is composed of triglycerides in which all or virtually all of the fatty acids are saturated.

unsaturated fatty acid: a fatty acid that lacks hydrogen atoms and has at least one double bond between carbons (includes monounsaturated and polyunsaturated fatty acids).

monounsaturated fatty acid: a fatty acid that lacks two hydrogen atoms and has one double bond between carbons—for example, oleic acid.

   mono = one

polyunsaturated fatty acid (PUFA): a fatty acid that lacks four or more hydrogen atoms and has two or more double bonds between carbons—for example, linoleic acid (two double bonds) and linolenic acid (three double bonds). Thus a **polyunsaturated fat** is composed of triglycerides containing a high percentage of PUFA.

   poly = many

---

membranes and for other functions is made from scratch by the liver. In other words, the lecithins are not needed in the diet; they are not essential nutrients. Furthermore, although once thought to be harmless, large doses of lecithin may cause GI upsets, sweating, salivation, and loss of appetite.[6] Perhaps these symptoms are beneficial, because they serve to warn people to stop self-dosing with lecithin.

■ **FIGURE 5–10**
Cholesterol
Cholesterol is a member of the cy-
clopentanoperhydrophenanthrene
family, whose particular designation
is 3-hydroxy-5,6-cholestene. The fat
soluble, vitamin D is synthesized
from cholesterol. Notice the similarities.

The Sterols

A student observing the chemical structure of cholesterol for the first time once remarked, "Would you believe pentamethyl hydroxy chicken wire?" He was not far wrong; chemists do create horrendous names. It is not necessary to memorize a chemical name or structure as complex as cholesterol's (shown in Figure 5–10). But once having viewed it, you can see that it is quite different from the triglycerides and phospholipids.

Cholesterol is not at all an unusual type of molecule. Dozens of similar ones appear in the body; all are interesting and important. Among them are the bile acids, the sex hormones (such as testosterone), the adrenal hormones (such as cortisol), and vitamin D.

sterol: a compound composed of C, H, and O atoms arranged in rings like those of cholesterol, with any of a variety of side chains attached.

cholesterol: one of the sterols.

■ Digestion, Absorption, and Transport

The body has a problem in digesting and using fats—how to get at them. Substances that are soluble in fat are called hydrophobic, or water fearing. Among these substances are, of course, the fats themselves. Fats are neutral; that is, they carry no net charge. In any compartment of the digestive tract they tend to separate themselves from the watery digestive juices. Water molecules, although they too have no net charge, are polar; that is, they have a positive side and a negative side. Enzymes have positively and negatively charged groups on their surfaces, and so they mix comfortably with the polar water—enzymes are hydrophilic, or water loving. What the body needs to help mix fats and water together is a substance that is friendly with both water-fearing and water-loving substances. The bile acids and phospholipids meet that need.

The liver manufactures bile acids from cholesterol. The gallbladder stores the bile and releases it into the intestine whenever fat arrives there. Each molecule of bile acid has at one end an ionized group that is attracted to water and at the other end a fatty acid chain that is attracted to fat. Molecules of bile acid surround fat droplets and draw parts of them into the surrounding solution, where they can meet the pancreatic lipase enzymes. The process is known as emulsification (see Figure 5–11).

Now, after all of this preparation, the enzymes can get at the triglycerides and hydrolyze them. As Figure 5–12 shows, most of this action occurs in the small intestine. The enzymes digest each triglyceride by removing one, then

hydrophobic: a term referring to water-fearing, or non-water-soluble substances; also known as **lipophilic**.
hydro = water
phobia = fear
lipo = lipid
phile = friend

hydrophilic: a term referring to water-loving, or water-soluble substances.

bile: a compound made from cholesterol, composed of a lipophilic portion and a hydrophilic portion. Bile is not an enzyme, but an emulsifier; it comes in both salt and acid form and is referred to as "bile salts" or "bile acids." For our purposes, no distinction need be made between these.

emulsify (ee-MULL-sih-fye): to disperse and stabilize fat droplets in a watery solution. Bile is one emulsifier; lecithin and other phospholipids are others.

■ **FIGURE 5–11**
Emulsification of Fat by Bile
Detergents work the same way (they are also emulsifiers), which is why they are so effective in removing grease spots from clothes. Molecule by molecule, the grease is dissolved out of the spot and suspended in the water, where it can be rinsed away. You can guess where the manufacturers of "detergents with enzymes" got their idea.

Key:

Water.

Fat.

Enzyme.

Emulsifier.

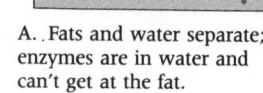

A. Fats and water separate; enzymes are in water and can't get at the fat.

B. Bile (emulsifier) has affinity for fats and for water, so it can bring them together.

C. Emulsified fat. The enzymes now have access to the fat, which is mixed in the water solution.

monoglyceride: a molecule of glycerol with one fatty acid attached.

micelles (MY-cells): tiny spherical complexes, each containing about 20 fatty acids and/or monoglycerides. They are so small that they can fit between the tiny, hairlike microvilli of a single intestinal cell. (Emulsified fat particles are 100 times larger in diameter and contain tens of thousands of molecules.)

lipoprotein (LIP-oh-PRO-teen): a cluster of lipids associated with proteins that serve as transport vehicles for lipids in the lymph and blood.

chylomicron (kye-lo-MY-cron): the lipoprotein formed in the intestinal wall cells following digestion and absorption of fat. Released from these cells, chylomicrons transport ingested fats to all cells of the body, which remove the ones they need, leaving chylomicron remnants to be picked up by the liver cells. The liver cells dismantle the chylomicron remnants and construct other lipoproteins for further transport.

the other, of its outer fatty acids, leaving a monoglyceride. (Rarely, enzymes remove all three fatty acids, leaving a molecule of glycerol.) As with the carbohydrates, the digestive process requires water, as shown in Figure 5–13.

After the triglycerides have been hydrolyzed, the monoglycerides and long-chain fatty acids merge into tiny spherical complexes, known as micelles, and easily move into the intestinal cells. (Unlike the long-chain fatty acids, glycerol and the short- and medium-chain fatty acids do not form micelles; they are absorbed directly into the blood at the portal vein.) The intestinal cells reassemble the monoglycerides and long-chain fatty acids into triglycerides.

The body has the same problem transporting lipids as it did in digesting them—the lipids are not soluble in water. The body must provide special vehicles to transport them—lipoproteins, of which there are several kinds. The newly made triglycerides and the other large lipids (cholesterol and the phospholipids) within the intestinal cells cluster together with special proteins, forming the first of these lipid-transport vehicles, chylomicrons. Finally, the intestinal cells release the chylomicrons into the lymphatic system. The

Transport of Lipids into Blood	
Glycerol	Directly into blood
Short-chain fatty acids	Directly into blood
Medium-chain fatty acids	Directly into blood
Long-chain fatty acids	Made into triglycerides
Monoglycerides	Made into triglycerides
Triglycerides	Assembled into chylomicrons, then to lymph, then blood
Cholesterol	Assembled into chylomicrons, then to lymph, then blood
Phospholipids	Assembled into chylomicrons, then to lymph, then blood

■ **FIGURE 5–12**
Triglyceride Digestion through the GI Tract

Fat

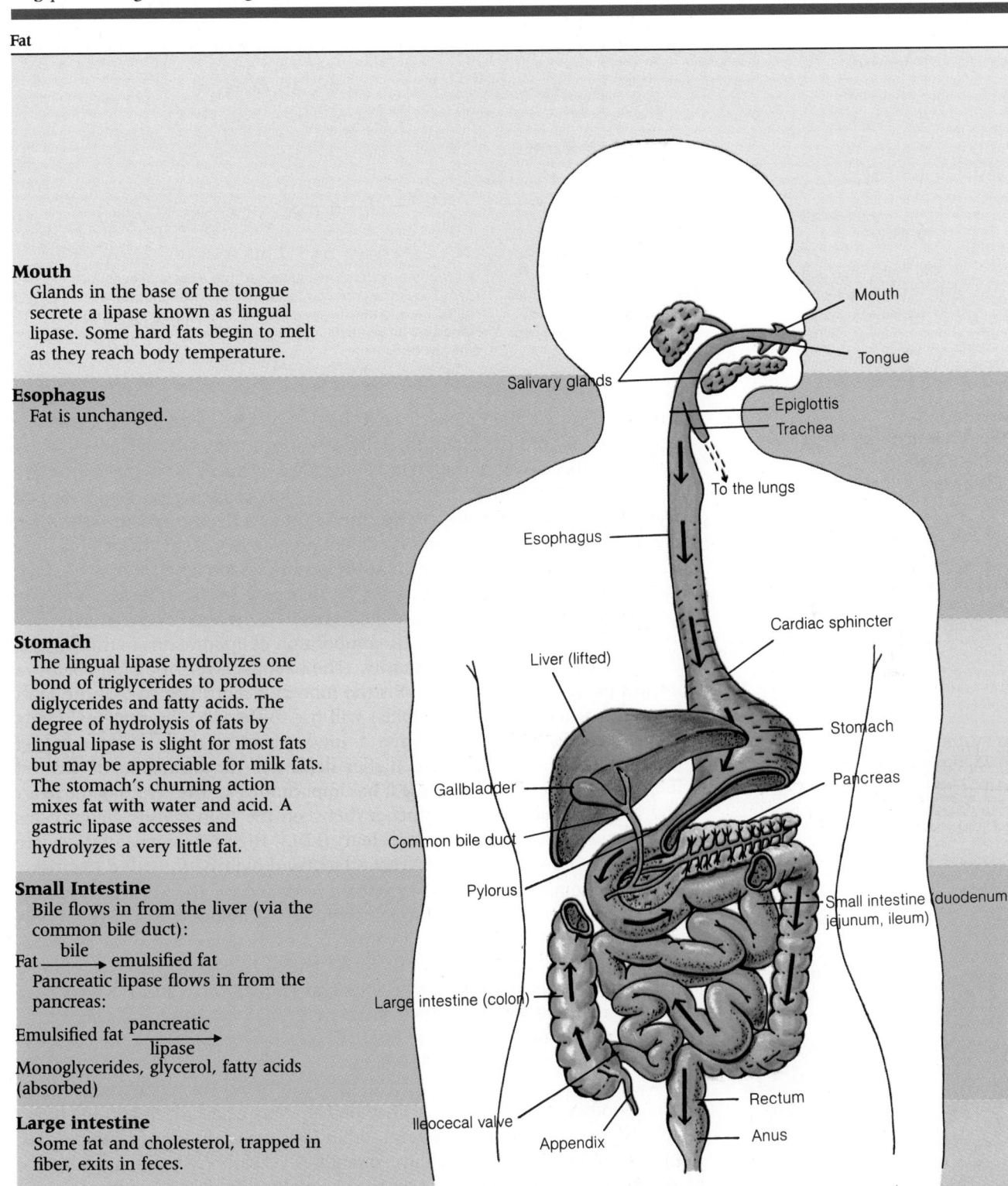

Mouth
Glands in the base of the tongue secrete a lipase known as lingual lipase. Some hard fats begin to melt as they reach body temperature.

Esophagus
Fat is unchanged.

Stomach
The lingual lipase hydrolyzes one bond of triglycerides to produce diglycerides and fatty acids. The degree of hydrolysis of fats by lingual lipase is slight for most fats but may be appreciable for milk fats. The stomach's churning action mixes fat with water and acid. A gastric lipase accesses and hydrolyzes a very little fat.

Small Intestine
Bile flows in from the liver (via the common bile duct):

$$Fat \xrightarrow{bile} emulsified\ fat$$

Pancreatic lipase flows in from the pancreas:

$$Emulsified\ fat \xrightarrow[lipase]{pancreatic}$$

Monoglycerides, glycerol, fatty acids (absorbed)

Large intestine
Some fat and cholesterol, trapped in fiber, exits in feces.

Mouth

Tongue

Salivary glands

Epiglottis

Trachea

To the lungs

Esophagus

Cardiac sphincter

Liver (lifted)

Stomach

Pancreas

Gallbladder

Common bile duct

Pylorus

Small intestine (duodenum, jejunum, ileum)

Large intestine (colon)

Ileocecal valve

Appendix

Rectum

Anus

A. The triglyceride and two molecules of water are split, and the pieces combine to give two fatty acids and a monoglyceride.

Triglyceride

B. These products may pass into the intestinal cells, but sometimes the monoglyceride is split with another molecule of water to give a third fatty acid and glycerol. Absorbed into intestinal cells: fatty acids, monoglycerides, and glycerol.

Monoglyceride + 2 fatty acids

■ FIGURE 5–13
Digestion (hydrolysis) of a Fat (triglyceride)

To help you remember, think of **HDL** as **H**ealthy, and **LDL** as **L**ess-healthy.

■ FIGURE 5–14
A Lipoprotein

Source: Adapted from D. Kritchevsky, An update on lipids, lipoproteins and fat metabolism, in *The Medicine Called Nutrition*, Medical Education (Meded) Programs, Ltd. (Englewood Cliffs, N.J.: Best Foods, 1979), p. 61.

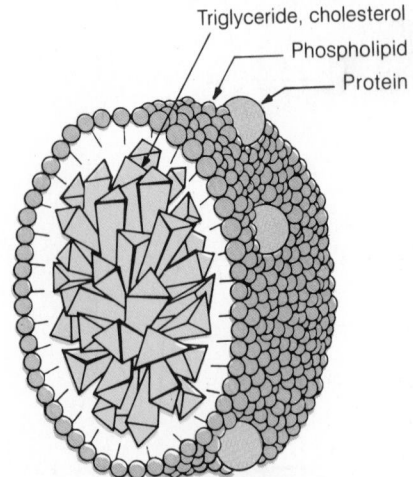

Triglyceride, cholesterol

Phospholipid

Protein

chylomicrons can then glide through the lymph spaces until they move to a point of entry into the bloodstream near the heart.

Within the circulatory system, lipids always travel from place to place wrapped in hydrophilic protein coats, as lipoproteins (see Figure 5–14). Lipoproteins are very much in the medical news these days. In fact, when physicians measure a person's blood lipid profile, they are interested not only in the types of lipid present, such as triglycerides and cholesterol, but also in the types of proteins in their coats. To help you picture the four types of lipoproteins, Figure 5–15 depicts their relative sizes and composition.

In the scientist's laboratory, the composition of lipoproteins in the blood is determined by their size and density. (The scientist layers the blood below a thick fluid in a test tube and spins the tube in a centrifuge so that the most buoyant particles (highest in lipids) will rise to the top. Lipoproteins with a higher percentage of lipids have a lower density; those with a higher percentage of proteins have a higher density.) The distinction of greatest interest for the rest of us, because it has implications for the health of the heart and blood vessels, is the distinction between the high-density lipoproteins (HDL) and the low-density lipoproteins (LDL). High LDL concentrations are associated with a high risk of heart attack, and high HDL, with a low risk.

As mentioned earlier, newly absorbed lipids leaving the intestinal cells are mostly packaged in large lipoproteins known as chylomicrons. Cells all over the body remove fat from the chylomicrons as they pass by, so the chylomicrons get smaller and smaller until, by the end of 14 hours, little is left of them but protein remnants and a few odds and ends of fat. The liver cells have special protein receptors on their membranes that recognize and remove the remnants from the blood. Once the liver cells have gathered in the chylomicron remnants, they dismantle them.

Meanwhile, the liver cells have the task of metabolizing many other compounds for the body's use. They pick up fatty acids arriving in the blood and use them to make cholesterol, other fatty acids, and other compounds. (At the same time, if they have quantities of carbohydrates, proteins, or alcohol to deal with, the liver cells may be making lipids from some of these.) The liver is the most active site of lipid synthesis. Ultimately, some of the

Review 4 types of Lipoproteins

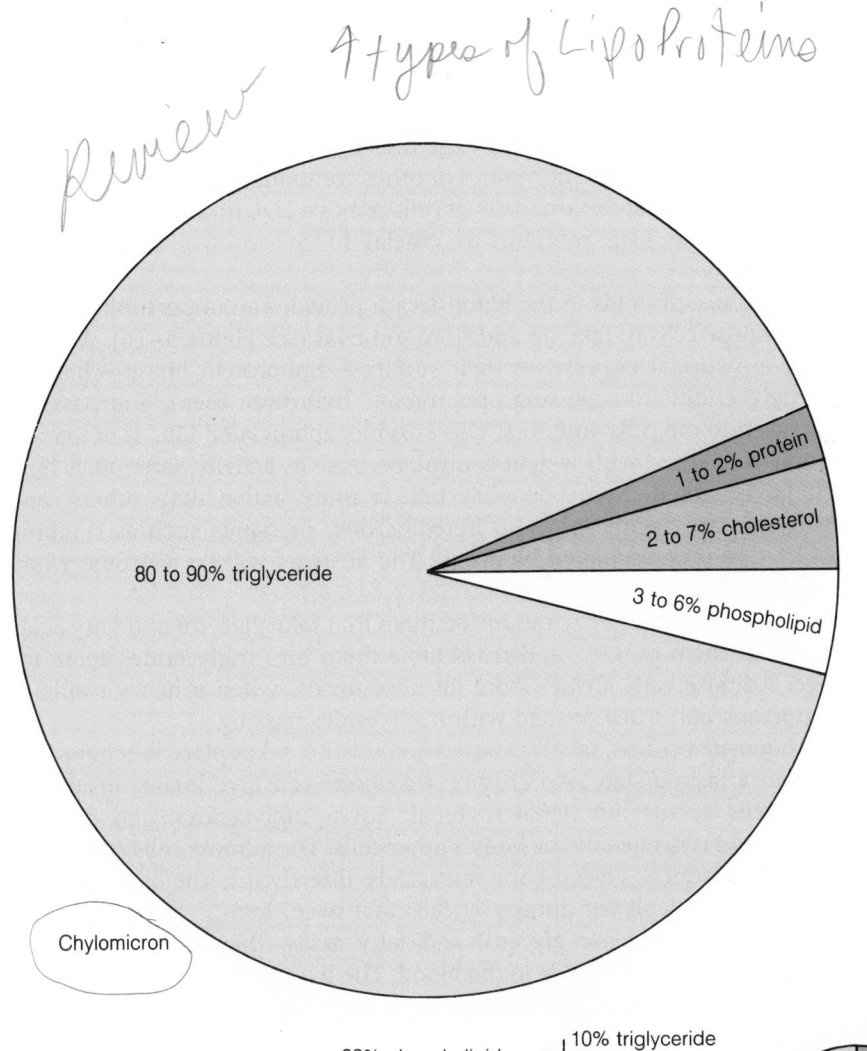

■ **FIGURE 5–15**
The Lipoproteins
A chylomicron. The density of these particles is very, very low because they contain so little protein and so much triglyceride. You can see how the laboratory report that a person has "high blood triglycerides" might easily reflect a high concentration of chylomicrons in the blood.
High-density lipoprotein (HDL). These particles are denser than the others because they contain such a high percentage of protein.
Very-low density lipoprotein (VLDL) and low-density lipoprotein (LDL). Compare these particles with the chylomicrons and HDL. Note that "high blood cholesterol" might easily reflect a high LDL concentration.

Protein amt. affects DENSITY
↑ proteins → ↑ density

↑ % Lipids → ↓ density

↑ % of Proteins
HDL *High Density Lipoprotein*
Healthy

↑ % of Lipids
LDL *Low density Lipoprotein*
Less-Healthy

VLDL *Very Low Density Lipoprotein*

triglycerides the liver cells manufacture will need to be used or stored in other parts of the body. To send them there, the liver packages them with proteins, cholesterol, and phospholipids, and ships them out as very-low-density lipoproteins (VLDL).

The VLDL made by the liver carry all three classes of lipids—triglycerides, phospholipids, and cholesterol. As the body's cells remove triglycerides from the VLDL, the VLDL become LDL. The LDL contain few triglycerides but are about half cholesterol (see Figure 5–15). These lipoproteins circulate throughout the body, making their contents available to all the cells—muscle, including the heart muscle; adipose tissue; the mammary glands; and others. The body cells select not only triglycerides but also cholesterol and phospho-

VLDL (very-low-density lipoprotein): type of lipoprotein made primarily by liver cells to transport lipids to various tissues in the body.

LDL (low-density lipoprotein): type of lipoprotein derived from very-low-density lipoproteins (VLDL) as cells remove triglycerides from them.

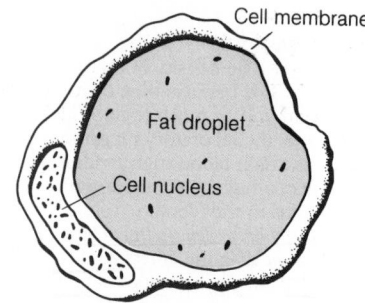

■ FIGURE 5–16
An Adipose Cell
Within the fat cell, lipid is stored in a globule. This globule can enlarge, and the fat cell membrane will grow to accommodate its swollen contents.

adipose(ADD-ih-poce) **cells**: the body's fat cells.

lipoprotein lipase (**LPL**): an enzyme mounted on the surface of fat cells (and other cells) that hydrolyzes triglycerides passing by in the bloodstream and directs their parts into the cells, where they can be metabolized or reassembled for storage.

hormone-sensitive lipase: an enzyme inside adipose cells that responds to the body's need for fuel by hydrolyzing triglycerides so that their parts (glycerol and fatty acids) will escape into the general circulation and thus become available to other cells as fuel. The signals to which this enzyme responds include epinephrine and glucagon, which oppose insulin (see Chapter 4).

HDL (high-density lipoprotein): type of lipoprotein that transports cholesterol back to the liver from peripheral cells.

lipids from these lipoproteins. They use the latter two kinds of lipids to build new membranes, to make hormones or other compounds, or to store for later use. Special LDL receptors on the liver cells remove LDL from circulation. This clearance by the LDL receptors is crucial in the control of cholesterol concentrations.[7]

The presence of lipids in the bloodstream provides an opportunity for the body's adipose cells to take up and store some fat (see Figure 5–16). Adipose cells have a special enzyme on their surfaces—lipoprotein lipase—that can seize triglycerides from passing lipoproteins, hydrolyze them, and pass the fatty acids into the cells' interiors. This enzyme, abbreviated LPL, is of interest to people concerned with weight control, because its activity determines how much fat is stored. Some people's LPL is more active than others' and investigators are asking why. Do heredity, diet, or habits such as smoking affect it? Can it be regulated by drugs? The answers will be welcome when they yield to research.

The cells have other enzymes inside them that take glycerol and fatty acids delivered to them by LPL, and reassemble them into triglycerides again for storage. Adipose cells always store fat after meals, when a heavy traffic of chylomicrons and VLDL loaded with triglycerides pass by.

The opposite process, fat breakdown and release, takes place whenever the body is in a fasting state. An enzyme (hormone-sensitive lipase) inside the adipose cells awaits the signal to break down triglycerides, and does so whenever fuel is needed by the body's other cells. The adipose cells release the breakdown products, glycerol and fatty acids, directly into the blood, so that they become available for uptake by cells that need them.

When fat cells release glycerol and fatty acids, they may also return cholesterol and phospholipids to the blood. The liver makes HDL packages to carry cholesterol and phospholipids from the cells back to the liver for recycling or disposal.

Cholesterol gets around in more ways than this, though. Not only does it shuttle back and forth between the liver and the body cells in lipoproteins; cholesterol also visits the intestinal tract in the form of bile made by the liver and stored in the gallbladder. As bile, cholesterol has two possible destinations. One is to enter the intestine, emulsify fat, and get reabsorbed from the intestine and recycled, as illustrated in Figure 5–17. The second possibility is that, once out in the intestine, some of the bile can be trapped by certain kinds of dietary fibers (notably, pectin and gums), which carry it out of the body with the feces. The excretion of bile reduces the total amount of cholesterol remaining in the body.

Knowing that fiber binds cholesterol and carries it out of the body, people have for years been buying pure fiber to sprinkle onto their foods in the hope of improving their health. Unfortunately, the pure fiber they most often buy is wheat bran, the type with the least cholesterol-lowering effect. As Chapter 4 pointed out, the fibers most effective at lowering blood cholesterol include pectin and gums—found in abundance in fruits, oats, and legumes, but this does not mean that people should buy these in purified form, either. Foods, not purified nutrients or other food components, are likely to offer the greatest benefits to those who seek good health—and not so much any particular foods as a variety of foods. You may recall that other nutrition knowledge points in the same direction.

The Roles of Lipids in the Body

Lipids in the body provide many services that would be hard to do without. Perhaps most importantly, fats provide energy. An uninterrupted flow of energy is so vital to life that in a pinch, any other function is sacrificed to maintain it. To go totally without an energy supply, even for a few minutes, would be to die. The urgency of the need for energy has ensured, over the course of evolution, that all creatures have built-in reserves to protect themselves from ever being deprived of it.

Chapter 4 described one provision against this sort of emergency—the stores of glycogen in the liver that can return glucose to the blood whenever the supply runs short. However, the liver cells can store only a limited amount of energy as glycogen; once this is depleted, the body must receive new food or start degrading body protein to continue making glucose.

The body's adipose cells contain large stores of triglycerides, specifically to meet moment-to-moment needs for energy; it is these cells that people refer to when they speak of their body fat. Unlike the liver's glycogen stores, the body's fat mass has a virtually unlimited storage capacity, and fat supplies 60 percent of the body's ongoing energy need during rest.[8]. During exercise or prolonged periods of food deprivation, fat stores may make an even greater contribution to energy needs.

A person who fasts (drinking only water) will rapidly metabolize body fat. A pound of body fat provides 3,500 kcalories;* so you might think a fasting person who expended 2,000 kcalories a day could lose more than ½ pound of body fat each day. Actually, the person has to obtain some energy from lean tissue because of the brain's need for glucose, which fat cannot supply; fat cannot be lost this rapidly, even when nothing is eaten. Still, in conditions of enforced starvation—say, during a siege or a famine—the fatter person survives longer than the thinner person thanks to this energy reserve.

If you happen to be acquainted with a polar bear, you may be aware that the same thing is true for him. As he lumbers about on his iceberg, great masses of fat ripple beneath his thick fur coat. During the long winter hours when he hibernates, he metabolizes that fat, extracting energy (tens of thousands of kcalories) from it to maintain his body temperature and to fuel other metabolic processes. Come spring, he is a hundred or more pounds thinner than when he went to sleep.

Although fat provides energy during a fast, it cannot provide enough in the form of glucose to provide the energy needed by the brain and nerves. After prolonged glucose deprivation, brain and nerve cells develop the ability to derive about two-thirds of their energy from a special form of fat known as ketone bodies. This is not enough, however, and as Chapter 7 will explain, death will occur even in a fat person who fasts too long.

Fat serves other roles in the body, in addition to providing energy. A layer of fat tissue beneath the skin, being a poor conductor of heat, insulates the

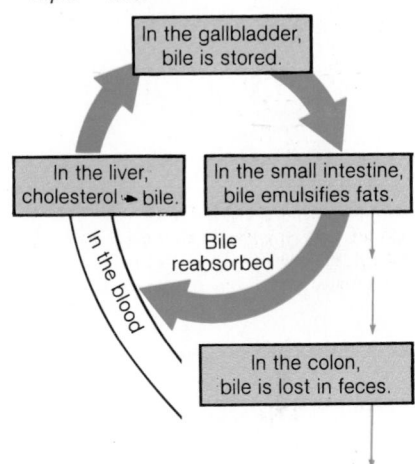

■ FIGURE 5–17
Enterohepatic Circulation
The recycling of cholesterol and bile through the intestine and liver is known as the **enterohepatic circulation** of bile.
enteron = intestine
hepat = liver

1 lb body fat = 3,500 kcal.

The small contribution that fat can make to the body's glucose is detailed in Chapter 7.

ketone (KEE-tone) **bodies:** a product of fat metabolism produced when carbohydrate is not available (see Chapter 7).

---

*The reader who knows that 1 pound = 454 grams and that 1 gram fat = 9 kcalories may wonder why a pound of body fat does not equal 9 × 454 kcalories. The reason is that body fat contains some cell water and other materials; it is not quite pure fat.

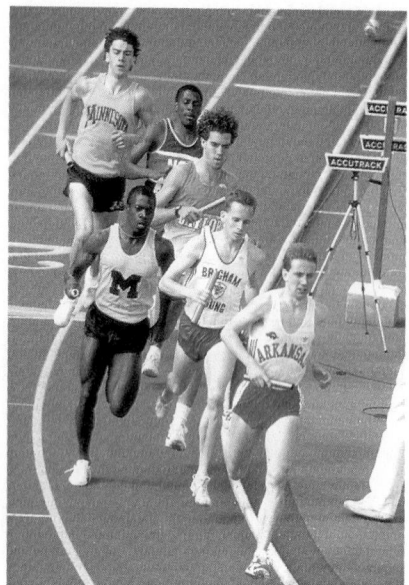

Fat supplies most of the energy for these exercising muscles.

All the carbons in cholesterol come from acetyl CoA (see Chapter 7), which in turn can be derived from many other body compounds, glucose and fatty acids among them.

atherosclerosis (ath-er-oh-scler-OH-sis): a type of artery disease characterized by accumulations of lipid-containing material on the inner walls of the arteries (see Chapter 28).

body from extremes of temperature. A pad of hard fat beneath each kidney protects it from being jarred and damaged, even during a motorcycle ride on a bumpy road. The soft fat in the breasts of a woman protects her mammary glands from heat and cold and cushions them against shock.

Lecithins and other phospholipids are important cell membrane constituents that allow the easy passage of fat-soluble substances, including vitamins and hormones, in and out of cells. The phospholipids also act as emulsifying agents, helping to keep other fats in solution in the blood and body fluids. The structure of lecithin reveals how the phospholipids can do this (review Figure 5–9); the choline part of the molecule is water soluble, while the fatty acid part is fat soluble. (Food chemists take advantage of lecithin's properties and use it as an emulsifier in foods. When you read on a food label that lecithin is present, as on a chocolate bar, that's probably why it's there.)

Cholesterol forms part of the multitude of external and internal membranes that make up the cells' structure and perform their work.[9] That is where you will find more than nine-tenths of all the body's cholesterol. In addition to serving as a component of cell membranes, cholesterol can be transformed into related compounds like hormones, bile, and vitamin D. Impressed? That's right. Cholesterol is not a villain lurking in some evil foods—it is a compound your body makes and uses. It does have some saving graces, in spite of all its bad press. Your liver is manufacturing cholesterol now, as you read, at the rate of perhaps 5×10^{16} (50,000,000,000,000,000) molecules per second. The raw materials that the liver uses to make cholesterol can be derived from carbohydrate, protein, or fat.

Cholesterol does exert one negative influence in the body, however. On its way into the cells from the bloodstream, some cholesterol is deposited in the artery walls. It is the depositing of cholesterol in arteries, atherosclerosis, that creates disease conditions leading to heart attacks and strokes. Chapter 28 describes how this occurs and how diet and exercise can help prevent it.

To sum up the roles of body fat, it provides a continuous fuel supply, protects body organs from temperature extremes and mechanical shock, and helps maintain the structure and health of all cells. When body fat is being used for fuel in the absence of glucose, it forms ketone bodies that can meet about two-thirds of the energy needs of the brain and nervous system. The phospholipids and sterols contribute to the cells' structures; cholesterol also serves as the raw material for hormones, vitamin D, and bile.

▪ *The Health Effects of Lipids*

Of all the nutrients, fat is implicated most often as a contributing factor to disease. Many diseases are linked to excessive intakes of dietary fat or to excess body fat; fat contributes to obesity, diabetes, cancer, hypertension, and atherosclerosis. The one change that most people should make in their diets is to limit their intake of total fat, which would moderate energy intake. (A second change might be to limit saturated fat and cholesterol, specifically, as well. Many current guidelines suggest these changes in that priority order: avoid excess fat, saturated fat, and cholesterol.)

In contrast to the negative impacts of fats on health are those of moderate intakes of the omega-3 fatty acids. Omega-3 fatty acids arrived on the news scene when researchers learned that the Inuit peoples of Alaska and Greenland, despite their high-energy, high-fat, high-cholesterol diets, enjoy relative freedom from heart diseases—particularly atherosclerosis. Analysis of the foods common in Inuit diets, which are taken from marine animals, revealed that they were rich in omega-3 fatty acids, particularly EPA and DHA.

What effects do EPA and DHA have on the cardiovascular system? For one, they lower blood cholesterol and triglyceride concentrations. For another, they reduce the tendency of the blood to clot. Researchers speculate that some protective effects of omega-3 fatty acids are mediated by a class of hormone-like compounds known as eicosanoids. The 20-carbon fatty acids of both omega series (arachidonic acid and EPA) serve as starting material for the synthesis of eicosanoid compounds such as prostaglandins and thromboxanes. Eicosanoids regulate many of the body's systems—not only blood lipid concentrations and blood clot formation, but also blood pressure, the immune response, and the inflammation response to injury and infection. (Chapter 28 provides more details of how omega-3 fatty acids and eicosanoids protect against heart disease.)

How much fish do we need to eat to receive the beneficial effects of omega-3 fatty acids? The answer is unknown, although the American Heart Association currently recommends two to three fish meals a week. Fish oil supplements are not recommended, for a number of reasons. Their effectiveness is unproven. Too much fish oil might cause excessive bleeding or interfere with wound healing. Fish oil supplements are made from fish livers, which may have accumulated toxic concentrations of pesticides, heavy metals, and other environmental contaminants. They also contain large amounts of vitamins A and D, which can have toxic effects. Lastly, they are expensive.

In addition to being excellent sources of omega-3 fatty acids, fish contain many valuable nutrients. They are leaner than most other animal-protein sources and rich in many minerals (with the exception of iron) and vitamins. In an effort to improve our health, we are well advised to eat fish periodically, for they provide us with an excellent way to obtain nutrients and help forestall heart disease.

eicosanoids (eye-COSS-uh-noyds): derivatives of 20-carbon fatty acids; hormonelike compounds that regulate blood pressure, clotting, and other body functions.

prostaglandins (PROS-tah-gland-ins): eicosanoid compounds with a multitude of diverse effects on the body, including blood vessel contractions, nerve impulses, and hormone responses; synthesized from the 20-carbon fatty acids.

thromboxanes: eicosanoid compounds with effects on the blood-clotting system; synthesized from the 20-carbon fatty acids.

The Lipids in Foods

Not only is fat important in the body, it is also important in foods. Many of the compounds that give foods their flavor, aroma, and tenderness are found in fats and oils; they are fat soluble. Whenever a fatty liquid and a watery liquid separate, the fat-soluble compounds go along with the fat, and the water-soluble compounds, with the water. When the fat is removed from a food, many of the fat-soluble compounds are also removed. Significant among these are flavors and vitamins. Four vitamins—A, D, E, and K—are soluble in fat.

By carrying both flavor and aroma, fat lends palatability to foods. It is the fat that makes the delicious aromas associated with bacon, ham, hamburger, and other meats, as well as onions being fried, french fries, and stir-fried vegetables. The attractiveness of fat is responsible for the popularity of fast

palatability: pleasing taste. The *palate* (PAL-ut) is the roof of the mouth, against which the tongue presses foods when tasting them.

Pork chop with a half inch of fat (275 kcal).

Potato with 1 tbsp butter and 1 tbsp sour cream (350 kcal).

Whole milk, 1 c (150 kcal).

Pork chop with fat trimmed off (165 kcal).

Plain potato (220 kcal).

Nonfat milk, 1 c (90 kcal).

■ **FIGURE 5–18**
Comparison of Fat in Common Foods

satiety (sat-EYE-uh-tee): the feeling of satisfaction and fullness that food brings.
  sate = to fill

Fortification of milk actually involves adding back more vitamin D than was in the whole milk originally.

Remember, fat is a more concentrated energy source than the other energy nutrients: 1 g carbohydrate or protein = 4 kcal, but 1 g fat = 9 kcal or even more (see Chapter 12).

foods, which, critics say, are too palatable for our own good. Fat also adds satiety to foods—another reason why fast foods are so popular.

Milk, when skimmed, loses flavor, and more importantly, loses all its vitamins A and D. To provide nonfat milk with the desired amounts of these nutrients, manufacturers add vitamins A and D to it; hence the "vitamin A and D fortified" label you see on nonfat milk. (Vitamin D is also added to whole milk, because its natural vitamin D level is low.)

An additional feature is lost when fat is removed: energy (see Figure 5–18). A small pork chop with the fat trimmed to within a half inch of the lean provides 275 kcalories; with the fat trimmed off completely, it provides 165 kcalories. A large baked potato with butter and sour cream (1 tablespoon each) has 350 kcalories; plain, it has 220.* So it goes. The single most effective step you can take to reduce the energy value of a food is to eat it with less fat. Learning the fat contents of foods and managing the diet so as to meet recommendations is an important goal for nutrition-conscious consumers.

Recommended Fat Intake

Generally, guidelines recommend that *total* fat intake should not exceed 30 percent of the day's total energy intake. Saturated fats should contribute less than 10 percent; polyunsaturated fats should not exceed 10 percent. Such guidelines easily cover the minimum intakes suggested for the essential fatty acids—3 percent of energy from linoleic acid and 0.3 percent of energy from

---

*These figures were taken from items 622, 623, 159, 80, 899, 93, and 98 in Appendix H.

linolenic acid.[10] (Most diets provide 6 to 8 percent of the kcalories from linoleic acid and 1 percent from linolenic acid.) Guidelines for cholesterol intake generally suggest an upper limit of 300 milligrams daily.

Limiting dietary fat energy intake to 30 percent of total energy intake may be sound, but according to research on people's food habits, people are eating about 37 percent of their energy intake as fat. That is more than at the turn of the century, and certainly more than they need, even though still commendably less than in the recent past. Those who wish to adjust their dietary fat intakes need to know where the fats are found in foods. Let's consider, first, the total fat in foods; then, the degree of unsaturation of that fat; and, finally, the accompanying cholesterol.

The exchange system presented in Chapter 2 provides a useful means of learning how much fat is present in foods (see p. 27). Three of the six lists in the exchange system—the milk list, the meat list, and the fat list—include foods containing appreciable amounts of fat:

- Items on the milk list contain protein, carbohydrate, and fat.
- Items on the meat list contain protein and fat (legumes contain carbohydrate as well).
- Items on the fat list contain fat only.

Figure 5–19 shows the lists that contain fat, with their portion sizes. Figure 5–20 shows how the exchange system can be used to estimate the amount of fat in a meal or in a day's meals.

The listing of milk's three fat levels emphasizes the importance of being aware of the fat content of milk. Users of the exchange system learn to think of nonfat milk as milk, and of low-fat and whole milk as milk with added fat.

A person studying the meat list for the first time may be surprised to note how many fat kcalories come from the meats and some of their relatives. An ounce of lean meat supplies about half of its energy from fat (28 protein kcalories and 27 fat kcalories). An ounce of high-fat meat supplies 72 percent of its energy from fat (28 protein kcalories and 72 fat kcalories). Two tablespoons of peanut butter supplies 72 percent of its energy from fat (56 protein kcalories and 144 fat kcalories). Thus many meats, which are often thought of as protein-rich foods, actually contain more fat energy than protein energy, and excess consumption of meat often accounts for excess weight gain.

Note that the unit by which meat is measured in this system is a single ounce. To use the system, you need to be aware of the number of ounces in typical servings. An egg, in this system, is equivalent to 1 ounce of meat. A hamburger is usually 3 or 4 ounces. A dinner steak may be 6 or 8 ounces or even more.

As for the members of the fat list, everyone knows that butter, margarine, and oil belong there, but it can be a surprise to discover that bacon, olives, avocados, and many kinds of nuts are also on the list. These foods are listed together because the amount of fat they contain makes them essentially equivalent to pure fat. An eighth of an avocado, a slice of bacon, or a little handful of peanuts can contain as much fat as a pat of butter, and like butter, offers negligible protein and carbohydrate. Hence, when you eat them, you are eating fat-rich foods.

Some foods not on the exchange lists are also significant contributors of fat to the diet. It can be surprising to see how much of the energy in foods comes

■ **FIGURE 5–19**
Exchange Lists Containing Fat

Milk List

1 c non fat milk contains	trace of fat
1 c 2% milk contains	5 g fat
1 c whole milk contains	8 g fat

Meat List

1 oz lean meat contains	3 g fat
1 oz medium-fat meat contains	5 g fat
1 oz high-fat meat contains	8 g fat
1 tbsp peanut butter contains	8 g fat

Fat List

1 tsp butter or margarine (or any other serving of food on the fat list) contributes	5 g fat

8 g in 1 c whole milk

3 g 1 oz lean meat

5 g in 1 part butter or margarine

■ **FIGURE 5–20**
Estimating Fat Intake Using the Exchange System

	Fat Grams	
	Exchange	Actual
Breakfast		
1 c oatmeal = 2 starch exchanges	Trace	2
¼ c raisins = 2 fruit exchanges	—	0
1 c nonfat milk = 1 milk exchange	Trace	0
1¼ c strawberries = 1 fruit exchange	—	1
Morning Snack		
2 tbsp raisins = 1 fruit exchange	—	0
2 tbsp sunflower seeds = 2 fat exchanges	10	8
Lunch		
1 bean burrito		
(1 lg tortilla = 2 starch exchanges	Trace	
½ c beans = 1 starch exchange +	Trace	10
½ lean meat exchange)	1½	
1 c nonfat milk = 1 milk exchange	Trace	0
1 orange = 1 fruit exchange	—	0
Dinner		
4 oz shrimp = 4 lean meat exchanges	12	1
1 c broccoli = 2 vegetable exchanges	—	0
½ c spinach noodles = 1 starch exchange	Trace	1
2 tsp butter = 2 fat exchanges	10	8
¼ c parsley = ¼ vegetable exchange	—	0
¼ tomato = ¼ vegetable exchange	—	0
¼ c mushrooms = ¼ vegetable exchange	—	0
¼ c water chestnuts = ¼ vegetable exchange	—	0
1 c fresh spinach = 1 vegetable exchange	—	0
1 tbsp sesame seeds = 1 fat exchange	5	4
1 tbsp vinaigrette dressing = 1 fat exchange	5	8
⅓ c garbanzo beans = 1 starch exchange	Trace	1
½ c sherbet = 2 starch exchanges	Trace	2
1 packet sugar	—	0
Day's Total	43.5 g	46 g

To estimate the amount of fat eaten at a meal or in a day, two reminders are needed. First, fat is often hidden in cooked vegetables; as a rule of thumb, vegetables served with butter or margarine contain about 1 tsp (1 exchange) of fat per half-cup serving. Second, meats and milks come in low-, medium-, and high-fat categories; be sure to count the fat in meats and milks.

An estimate of the amounts of fat in these meals reveals that these meals are low in fat and fit the NRC recommendations. (These are the same meals used as examples in Chapters 2 and 4.) Vegetables, fruit, and starchy vegetables and breads can be assumed to contain no fat, so the only foods to inspect are the meats, milks, and fats.

from fat—even when you can't see it—that is, from *invisible* fat. Anything fried contains abundant fat: potato chips, french fries, fried wonton, fried fish, and many other of people's favorite foods. Many baked goods, too, are high in fat: pie crusts, pastries, biscuits, cornbread, doughnuts, Danish sweet rolls, cookies, and cakes. (Table 4–5 on p. 96 provides an exchange list for some of these items.) Chocolate bars contain even more fat energy than sugar energy. Even cream-of-mushroom soup prepared with water has 66 percent of its energy from fat. Surprisingly, abundant fat lurks even on salad bars; you can construct a plate bearing 50 percent of its energy from fat without even trying. Not only the salad dressings, but also the mixed salads—the potato salad, the macaroni salad, the coleslaw, and the marinated beans—are largely fat or oil. This is not to condemn the salad bar, but to remind you to choose items with an awareness of their fat contents.

The fat on your plate includes *visible fats* and oils, such as butter, the oil in salad dressing, and the fat you trim from meat. It also includes *invisible fat*—it is present, but not very apparent to people—such as the fat that "marbles" a steak or that is hidden in foods like nuts, cheese, crackers, avocados, olives, fried foods, bakery items, and chocolate.

Fatty Acids and Cholesterol in Foods

In addition to knowing which foods are high in fat, a person would benefit from studying the fatty acid contents of foods. Foods that present the most fat altogether will have the greatest impact on the fatty acid balance of the diet. The fatty acid contents of some typical dietary fats are shown in Figure 5–21. The figure is arranged so that you can easily see the contribution each type of fat makes. The fat and fatty acid contents of many other foods are shown in Appendix H.

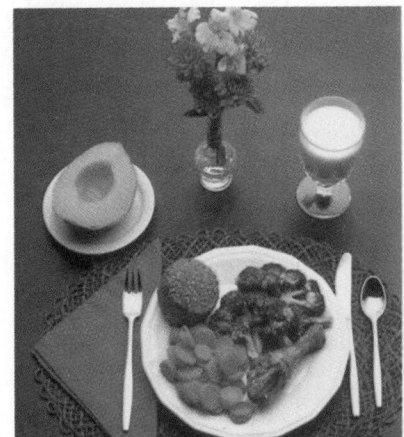

Fat hides in unexpected places. In this meal, no butter is used and the beverage is nonfat milk, but 30 percent of the kcalories come from fat.

DIETARY FAT	CHOLESTEROL mg/Tbsp	SATURATED FAT	Linoleic Acid (omega-6)	Linolenic Acid (omega-3)	MONOUNSATURATED FAT	OTHER FATS
Canola (Rapeseed) Oil	0	6%	22%	10%	62%	
Safflower oil	0	10%	77%	Trace	13%	
Sunflower oil	0	11%	69%		20%	
Corn oil	0	13%	61%	1%	25%	
Olive oil	0	14%	8%	1%	77%	
Soybean oil	0	15%	54%	7%	24%	
Margarine	0	17%	32%	2%	49%	
Peanut oil	0	18%	33%		49%	
Chicken fat	11	31%	21%	1%	47%	
Lard	12	41%	11%	1%	47%	
Palm oil*	0	51%	10%		39%	
Beef fat	14	52%	3%	1%	44%	
Butterfat	33	66%	2%	2%	30%	
Coconut oil*	0	77%	2%	6%	15%	

POLYUNSATURATED FATS:

■ **FIGURE 5–21**
Comparison of Dietary Fats
*Data on linoleic and linolenic acids for palm and coconut oils not available.

Source: Canola oil: data on file, Procter & Gamble. All others: J. B. Reeves and J. L. Weihrauch, *Composition of Foods*, Agriculture Handbook No. 8–4.(Washington, D.C.: U. S. Department of Agriculture, 1979). Reprinted with permission from Procter & Gamble © 1987.

The length of the carbon chain and the degree of saturation of a fat determine how hard it is at a given temperature. A clue to whether a fat is more or less saturated than another is its hardness at room temperature. Chicken fat, for example, is softer than pork fat, which is softer than beef tallow. Of the three, beef tallow is the most saturated and chicken fat, the least saturated. Polyunsaturated fats melt more readily. Generally speaking, vegetable and fish oils are rich in polyunsaturates, whereas the harder fats—animal fats—are more saturated. Coconut and palm oils are *saturated* even though they are of *vegetable* origin; it is their short carbon chains that make them liquid.

Cholesterol is found only in animal foods, and these generally are also major sources of saturated fats. Some animal foods without much total fat can also contain appreciable cholesterol. Table 5–3 lists the cholesterol content of selected foods. Many more foods, with their cholesterol contents, appear in Appendix H.

The foods that contain the highest amounts of cholesterol are organ meats such as liver and kidneys, as well as eggs. Lower but still detectable levels of cholesterol are contained in cheeses and meats. Shellfish have been thought to contain high concentrations of cholesterol, but the findings on which this idea was based have been called into question. Shellfish contain sterols, but possibly not the kind that have metabolically negative effects, and they contain much less cholesterol than has been thought in the past.

As a general rule, anyone wishing to reduce both saturated fat and cholesterol intake could accomplish these objectives by selecting fish, poultry without skin, lean meats, and nonfat milk products; choosing vegetables, fruits, cereals, and legumes; and limiting oils, fats, egg yolks, and fried foods. A vegetarian who uses milk, eggs, and cheese could shift to nonfat milk and low-fat cheese, as well as limiting butter and egg intake. Vegetarians who avoid all foods derived from animals eat a diet relatively low in fat (unless they eat large quantities of nuts) and consume no cholesterol, because plant foods do not contain it.

Eggs contain just over 200 milligrams of cholesterol each, all of it in the yolk. This is 24 percent less than measurements first indicated. For a person trying to adhere strictly to a low-cholesterol diet, the use of eggs, or at least egg yolks, has to be curtailed. For most people trying to lower blood cholesterol, however, it is not as effective to limit cholesterol intake as to limit saturated fat intake. Thus some eggs may still be a valuable part of the diet, because they are inexpensive, useful in cooking, and a source of high-quality protein. An American Heart Association guideline limits eggs to four a week.

Each culture has its own favorite food sources of fats and oils. In Canada, canola oil is widely used. Peoples of the Mediterranean (Greeks, Italians, and Spaniards) rely heavily on olive oil, and Asians use the polyunsaturated oil of soybeans. Jewish cookery traditionally employs chicken fat, whereas U.S. southerners rely heavily on pork fat (lard and bacon).* Elsewhere in the United States, butter and margarine are widely used, and the popularity of fast foods has increased the use of hydrogenated vegetable oil.

Enjoy low-fat foods for good heart health.

*The saturated fat consumption of blacks is cause for concern among health authorities, who note a high incidence of heart disease—both atherosclerosis and high blood pressure—among these people. This high rate of heart disease may be diet related, genetically caused, or both. High blood pressure is related to fat intake and in some people, to salt (sodium) intake (see Chapter 28).

■ TABLE 5–3
Cholesterol Content of Common Foods

Foods	Cholesterol (mg)
Fruits/vegetables	0
Grains	0
Milks (1-c serving)	
Whole milk	33
Yogurt (whole milk)	30
Low-fat milk	22
Low-fat yogurt	14
Buttermilk	9
Nonfat milk	4
Cheeses (1-oz serving)	
Cheddar	30
American processed	27
Swiss	26
Ice creams and puddings (½-c serving)	
Ice cream	29
Pudding	15
Butter (1 tsp)	11
Margarine, all vegetable (1 tsp)	0
Creams (1 tsp)	
Whipping	20
Sour	6
Half and half	6
Meats (3-oz serving)	
Veal cutlet	100
Lamb chop	83
Pork chop	83
Chicken	75
Beef steak	70
Hotdogs	43
Organ meats (3-oz serving)	
Brains	1,696
Liver	410
Kidneys	329
Eggs (1 large egg)	
Yolk	213
White	0
Fish (3-oz serving)	
Shrimp	166
Lobster	61
Clams	57
Fish fillets	54
Oysters	47

Source: Food Processor computer diet analysis program, ESHA, Salem, OR 97302.

Processed Fat

When researchers began to realize that saturated fats were linked to heart disease and that polyunsaturated fats might not be, advertisers began proclaiming their oils and margarines as "high in polyunsaturates." Indeed,

For some questions and answers about antioxidants, see Chapter 16.

hydrogenation (high-dro-gen-AY-shun): a chemical process by which hydrogens are added to unsaturated or polyunsaturated fats to reduce the number of double bonds, making them more saturated (solid) and more resistant to oxidation.

■ **FIGURE 5–22**
Hydrogenation
Hydrogen is added at the double bond, yielding a saturated fatty acid.

Monounsaturated fatty acid   Saturated fatty acid

margarines made from vegetable oils and plant foods such as peanut butter do contain unsaturated fatty acids, and this is why they spread and melt more easily than foods that contain saturated fats.

Unfortunately polyunsaturated fats do not resist spoilage well. The more double bonds in a fatty acid, the more easily oxygen can destroy it. When oxygen attacks the double bond, a chain reaction occurs, yielding a variety of products that smell bad; the product has spoiled. (Other types of spoilage, due to microbial growth, can occur, too.) In general, unsaturated fatty acids are less stable than their saturated counterparts.

Marketers of fat-containing products have three alternative ways of dealing with the problem of spoilage—none perfect. They may keep their products tightly sealed away from oxygen and under refrigeration—an expensive storage system. The consumer then has to do the same, and most people prefer to buy products they can store on the shelf. Marketers may also protect their products by adding preservatives such as antioxidants, but additives are unpopular with some consumers. Finally, manufacturers may increase the products' stability by processing the fat (hardening or hydrogenating it). Figure 5–22 shows hydrogens being added at a carbon-to-carbon double bond to hydrogenate a fat molecule.

Hydrogenation makes fat more solid, which is often desirable. Margarine made from vegetable oils is solid at room temperature because the oils have been partially hydrogenated, and this makes it easy to work with. Hydrogenation, however, diminishes the margarine's polyunsaturated fat content and possibly, therefore, its health value. As with all such trade-offs, the choice of which products to use, and in what quantities, is up to you, the consumer.

With respect to fat, an old expression seems to require new wording: "Everything I like is either unsafe, unhealthy, or fattening." True, while dietary fats help make foods delicious, the consequences of excessive fat to your health can be severe. Does this really mean that in order to eat healthful meals you must eat without pleasure? Not at all. Use fat, but use it with respect. Use it where you will really notice its taste benefits. Substitute other foods for it where they will not detract from your pleasure. Use fat substitutes (see Highlight 5) and where you can, learn to enjoy foods with less fat in or on them. This chapter has described the many forms lipids come in, the important roles they play in the body, and the qualities they bring to foods. With this information, you can appreciate the energy and the enjoyment that fat provides, but take care not to exceed your needs.

SELF STUDY *Examine Your Fat Intake*

These exercises make use of the information you recorded on Forms 1 to 3. (Appendix K provides the necessary forms.)

1. How many grams of fat do you consume in a day?
2. How many kcalories does this represent? (Remember, 1 gram of fat contributes 9 kcalories.)
3. What percentage of your total energy is contributed by fat? (To figure this, divide fat kcalories by total kcalories, then multiply by 100.)
4. A dietary guideline says fat should contribute not more than 30 percent of total kcalories. How does your fat intake compare with this recommendation? If it is higher, look over your food records: what specific foods could you cut down on or eliminate, and what foods could you add to your diet, to bring your total fat intake into line?
5. How much linoleic acid do you consume? Remembering that linoleic acid is a lipid (energy value, 9 kcalories per gram), calculate the number of kcalories it gives you. What percentage of your total kcalories comes from linoleic acid? The guideline recommends a generous 3 percent.
6. How much cholesterol do you consume daily? How does your cholesterol intake compare with the suggested limit of 300 milligrams a day? If your intake is high, you might want to read Chapter 28 before arriving at any conclusions regarding the importance of this limit.

Study Questions

1. Describe the structure of a triglyceride. What are the differences between saturated, unsaturated, monounsaturated, and polyunsaturated fats?
2. How do phospholipids differ from triglycerides in structure? How does cholesterol differ in structure from the other lipids?
3. What are the special problems of fat digestion, and how are they solved?
4. What is the basic structure and purpose of a lipoprotein? What are the differences between the chylomicrons, VLDL, LDL, and HDL?
5. What are the possible roles and destinations of cholesterol in the body?
6. What services do the fats in the body provide?
7. What features do fats bring to food?
8. What are the dietary recommendations regarding fat and cholesterol intake? Which food lists of the exchange system supply fat in abundance? In moderation? Not at all?

Notes

1. F. H. Mattson, A changing role for dietary monounsaturated fatty acids, *Journal of the American Dietetic Association* 89 (1989): 387–391.
2. A. Leaf and P. C. Weber, Cardiovascular effects of n-3 fatty acids, *New England Journal of Medicine* 318: (1988): 549–555.
3. L. D. McBean, Nutritional and health effects of unsaturated fatty acids, *Dairy Council Digest* 59 (1988): 1–6.
4. P. J. Nestel, Polyunsaturated fatty acids (n-3, n-6), *American Journal of Clinical Nutrition* 45 (1987): 1161–1167; M. Neuringer, G. J. Anderson, and W. E. Connor, The essentiality of N-3 fatty acids for the development and function of the retina and brain, *Annual Review of Nutrition* 8 (1988): 517–541.
5. G. J. Anderson and W. E. Connor, On the demonstration of ω-3 essential-fatty-acid deficiency in humans, *American Journal of Clinical Nutrition* 49 (1989): 585–587.
6. J. L. Wood and R. G. Allison, Effects of consumption of choline and lecithin on neurological and cardiovascular systems, *Federation Proceedings* 41 (1982): 3015–3021.
7. S. M. Grundy, Cholesterol and coronary heart disease, *Journal of the American Medical Association* 256 (1986): 2849–2858.
8. M. H. Williams, *Nutritional Aspects of Human Physical and Athletic Performance*, 2nd ed. (Springfield, Ill.: Thomas Books, 1985) p. 110.
9. M. S. Brown and J. S. Goldstein, Lowering plasma cholesterol by raising LDL receptors (editorial), *New England Journal of Medicine* 305 (1981): 515–517.
10. K. S. Bjerve, S. Fischer, and K. Alme, Alpha-linolenic acid deficiency in man: Effect of ethyl linolenate on plasma and erythrocyte fatty acid composition and biosynthesis of prostanoids, *American Journal of Clinical Nutrition* 46 (1987): 570–576.

Artificial Fats

Given that heart disease and obesity are two major health problems linked to dietary fat, artificial fats offer hope for the prevention and treatment of both. Imagine being able to enjoy the rich flavor and creamy texture that fats and oils impart to foods without suffering the consequences of ingesting excess fat and food energy. Food chemists have been working on artificial fats since the 1960s, but only recently have manufacturers filed petitions with the FDA for approval of their products. This explains the sudden spate of reports currently appearing in popular magazines and on television news programs. One product the FDA has had under consideration for the past year is a kcalorie-free fat replacement formerly known as sucrose polyester; its generic name is now olestra. Olestra is a synthetic combination of sucrose and fatty acids, but unlike either, it is indigestible. Because the body cannot digest it, olestra passes through the digestive tract unabsorbed. Its presence in the digestive tract reduces blood cholesterol concentrations by interfering with the absorption of both dietary cholesterol and cholesterol recycled through the enterohepatic pathway.

Olestra looks, feels, and tastes like dietary fat and can substitute for fats and oils in meals without diminishing flavor, adding energy, or raising blood lipid concentrations. It has the same cooking properties as fats and oils and can be used in products such as shortenings, oils, margarines, snacks, ice creams, and other desserts.

Scientific research on animals and human beings seems to support the safety of olestra as a partial replacement for dietary fats and oils. An undesirable side effect of olestra is its interference with vitamin E absorption. One proposed solution to this problem is to supplement olestra products with vitamin E. Studies suggest that, for people routinely using olestra, an intake of two times the RDA of vitamin E might be appropriate. Early formulations of olestra caused diarrhea in some people, but this seems to have been corrected by improving the composition of olestra.

Another fat substitute, named Simplesse, is also being considered for approval by the FDA. Simplesse is fabricated in a process called microparticulation, which heats and blends proteins from egg whites or milk into tiny round particles. This method counters the normal changes that occur when a protein is subjected to heat. The company that developed Simplesse has altered naturally occurring proteins to create the *perception* of fat; the tongue perceives creaminess because of the extremely small size of the protein particles.

Olestra and Simplesse differ in that olestra is a sucrose polyester, while Simplesse is made of protein. However, Simplesse is like olestra in that its mistlike protein particles feel and taste like fat and can replace fat in foods, thus lowering the fat and energy contents of meals. The differences in the chemical structures of olestra and Simplesse become evident in both the body's and the chef's use of the product. In the body, Simplesse is digested and absorbed, contributing to energy intake. Simplesse provides 1⅓ kcalories per gram—a substantial reduction from fat's 9 kcalories per gram. In the kitchen, Simplesse is unsuitable for frying or baking, because it gels when heated. Simplesse is not available for home use. Instead, manufacturers can use it in dairy products such as ice cream, yogurt, and sour cream and in oil-based products such as salad dressing, mayonnaise, and margarine.

Food manufacturers are trying to reproduce the functional and taste properties of fats and oils for less than fat's 9 kcalories per gram. The task for food chemists is complex, as they attempt to juggle the needs of the human body with those for food preparation. To satisfy the body, researchers must develop a low-energy, nontoxic compound without negative side effects that will be completely excreted itself, but will not rob the body of fat-soluble vitamins. The compound must also have the right mouthfeel and flavor for consumer acceptability. When added to a food item, the compound must remain stable while meeting the particular food product's requirements for temperature and moisture. That is a tall order, but it looks as if food chemists are mastering the task, and artificial fats will soon be as commonplace as artificial sweeteners.

Miniglossary

microparticulation: a process in which egg white proteins are heated and blended into mistlike particles.

olestra: a 0-kcalorie artificial fat made from a combination of sucrose and fatty acids; formerly known as **sucrose polyester**.

Simplesse: a low-kcalorie artificial fat made from proteins.

Protein:
Amino Acids

Contents

Enzymes work rapidly and systematically. Part of a cell is shown here, in which about 12 genes (segments of DNA, or deoxyribonucleic acid) are being copied into RNA, or ribonucleic acid. About 50 enzymes are at work in each gene, creating a Christmas-tree-like formation. Each enzyme is moving along the DNA, making an RNA copy. Those that have moved the farthest have made the longest RNA branches.

protein: a compound composed of C, H, O, and N atoms, arranged into amino acids linked in a chain. Some amino acids also contain S (sulfur) atoms.

Everybody knows that protein is the material of muscles, and that it is important in the diet. The word *protein* suggests strength and power, and people eat steak to obtain it. In fact, as you will see, protein and meat have been so overvalued that many people eat more than enough, sometimes at the expense of other nutrients and foods that are equally important. An understanding of the quantity and quality of protein people need will help put it in its proper place as only one—although an important one—of the nutrients needed in correct proportions to achieve a balanced diet.

This chapter begins with a description of the chemical structure of protein. The extraordinary structure of proteins enables them to play far more versatile roles in the body than either carbohydrates or lipids. Researchers who have worked on elucidating the chemical structure of protein have been rewarded with a profound insight into the elegance of nature's designs.

■ The Chemist's View of Protein

A protein is a chemical compound that contains the same atoms as carbohydrate and lipid—carbon, hydrogen, and oxygen—but protein is different in that it also contains nitrogen atoms. These C, H, O, and N atoms are arranged into amino acids, which are linked into chains to form proteins. It is easy to construct a protein once an amino acid is understood, for amino acids are the building blocks of proteins.

amino (a-MEEN-oh) **acid**: a building block of protein; a compound containing an amino group and an acid group attached to a central carbon atom, which also carries a distinctive side chain.
amino = containing nitrogen

```
    -N-H            O
     |              ‖
     H           —C—O-H

  Amino group    Acid group
```

Recall that C forms 4 bonds with other atoms; O, 2; and H, 1. N forms 3 bonds.

Amino Acid Structure

The structures of all amino acids have three things in common: connected to a central carbon is an amino group (NH_2), an acid group (COOH), and a hydrogen (H). These three parts of the molecule are identical in all amino acids. The central carbon atom also has another atom or group of atoms attached to it, which varies from one amino acid to another. Figure 6–1 illustrates the structure of an amino acid.

The side chains on amino acids are what make proteins so varied in comparison with either carbohydrates or lipids. A polysaccharide (starch, for example) is composed entirely of glucose units one after the other. The polysaccharide may be several thousand units long, but every unit in the chain is a glucose molecule just like all the others. In a protein, on the other hand, 20 different amino acids may appear, each differing from the others in the nature of its side chain.* Table 6–1 lists the amino acids; Appendix C presents their chemical structures.

■ FIGURE 6–1
Amino Acid Structure
The asterisk denotes the central carbon.

*Amino acids sometimes occur in related forms (for example, proline can add an OH group to become hydroxyproline; two cysteines in a protein chain can bind to make cystine), and others occur individually (for example, taurine and ornithine). Chemists can make still other amino acids. We have elected to present (in Appendix C) the structures of the most common amino acids, as in Nomenclature policy: Abbreviated designations of amino acids, *Journal of Nutrition* 117 (1987): 15.

■ TABLE 6–1
Amino Acids

These are the 20 amino acids important to human nutrition. The first column presents the *essential* amino acids (those the body cannot make—that must be provided in the diet).

Histidine	(HISS-tuh-deen)	Alanine	(AL-ah-neen)
Isoleucine	(eye-so-LOO-seen)	Arginine[a]	(ARJ-ih-neen)
Leucine	(LOO-seen)	Asparagine	(ah-SPAR-ah-geen)
Lysine	(LYE-seen)	Aspartic acid	(ah-SPAR-tic acid)
Methionine	(meh-THIGH-oh-neen)	Cysteine[a]	(SIS-teh-een)
Phenylalanine	(fen-il-AL-ah-neen)	Glutamic acid	(GLU-tam-ic acid)
Threonine	(THREE-oh-neen)	Glutamine	(GLU-tah-meen)
Tryptophan	(TRIP-toe-fan, TRIP-toe-fane)	Glycine	(GLY-seen)
Valine	(VAY-leen)	Proline	(PRO-leen)
		Serine	(SEER-een)
		Tyrosine[a]	(TIE-roe-seen)

[a] A conditionally essential amino acid.

The simplest amino acid, glycine, has a hydrogen atom in the side chain position. A slightly more complex amino acid, alanine, has an extra carbon with three attached hydrogen atoms. Other amino acids have still more complex side chains. For example, one amino acid may have an acid group, whereas another may have a basic amino group. Still others may have neutral side chains, including some complicated ring structures. These acidic, basic, and neutral groups confer different characteristics on the amino acids. Thus, although the amino acids all share a common starting structure, their properties differ (see Figure 6–2 for examples of amino acids).

Amino Acid Sequence

Amino acids may be linked together in a great variety of ways to form proteins. They connect by means of a condensation reaction, (see p. 76). An OH is removed from the acid end of one amino acid, and an H is removed from the amino group of another. A bond forms between the two amino acids, and the H and OH join to form a molecule of water. The resulting

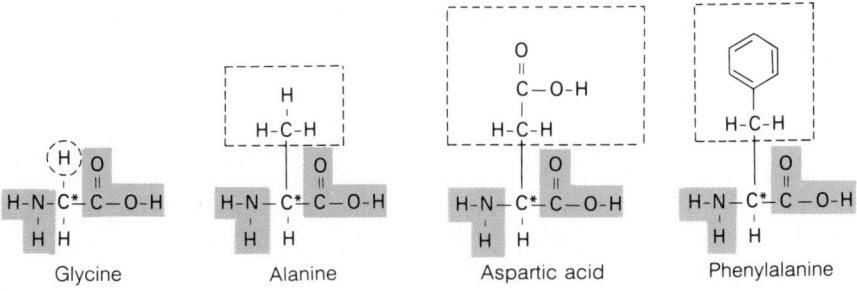

Glycine   Alanine   Aspartic acid   Phenylalanine

■ FIGURE 6–2
Examples of Amino Acids
Note that the side chains are different in each. The asterisk denotes the central carbon.

■ FIGURE 6–3
Formation of a Dipeptide
A dipeptide forms as two amino acids are condensed, with the removal of water. Condensation reactions have already been shown twice before (Figure 4–6 and Figure 5–4). The shaded area highlights the peptide bond.

dipeptide: two amino acids bonded together. The bond between two amino acids is a **peptide bond**.
di = two
peptide = amino acid

tripeptide: three amino acids bonded together by peptide bonds.
tri = three

polypeptide: many (ten or more) amino acids bonded together by peptide bonds. An intermediate string of between four and ten amino acids is an **oligopeptide**.
poly = many
oligo = few

structure is a dipeptide (see Figure 6–3). By the same reaction, the OH can be removed from the acid end of the second amino acid and an H from the amino group of a third to form a tripeptide. As additional amino acids are added to the chain, a polypeptide is formed. Most proteins are polypeptides, 100 to 300 amino acids long. Figure 6–4 shows the amino acid sequence of insulin, a relatively small protein.

It would be misleading, however, to end the description here, because in showing the structures on paper, we have drawn straight, flat chains. Actually, polypeptide chains fold and tangle so that they look like crazy jungle gyms. The sequence of amino acids in a protein determines which specific way the chain will fold.

Folding of the Chain

You can best visualize the structure of a protein by keeping in mind that each amino acid side chain has special characteristics that attract it to other side chains. Some side chains are charged, or polar, and are attracted to the charges around water molecules (hydrophilic). Other side chains are neutral and are repelled by water (hydrophobic). As amino acids are added to a growing polypeptide, the charged hydrophilic side chains are attracted to positions on the outer surface of the completed protein. The neutral hydrophobic groups tend to tuck themselves inside, away from water. The shape the polypeptide finally assumes is either roughly spherical or fibrous—whichever gives it the maximum stability in water. Finally, two or more of these giant molecules may associate to form a still larger working aggregate. Thus the completed protein is a tangled, complicated chain of amino acids, bristling on the surface with positive and negative charges. Sometimes two, three, or four such chains tangle together to make a giant protein molecule. Hemoglobin, shown in Figure 6–5, is a big protein containing four associated chains.

The change in a protein's shape brought about by heat, acid, or other conditions is known as **denaturation**. Past a certain point, denaturation is irreversible.

Large protein molecules are fragile; their conformation depends on constant conditions in their surroundings. When they are subjected to heat, acid, or other conditions that disturb their stability, they uncoil or change their shapes, losing their functions. You have seen many examples of this—in the hardening of an egg when it is cooked, in the curdling of milk when it is heated or made acid, and in the stiffening of egg whites when they are whipped.

The Completed Protein

If you could step onto a carbohydrate molecule like starch and walk along it, the first stepping stone would be a glucose. The next stepping stone would be glucose again, and then glucose, and then glucose, and then glucose. But if you were to walk along a polypeptide chain, your first stepping stone might be a methionine. Your second might be an alanine. The third might be a glycine, and the fourth a tryptophan, then another alanine, and so on. In other words, the units in a protein are varied in both their nature and the sequence in which they appear.

Another analogy compares the amino acids to letters in an alphabet. If you were to try to make a sentence using only the letter *G*, you could only speak gibberish: G-G-G-G-G-G-G. But with 20-odd different letters available, you can say, ''To be, or not to be: that is the question''—or, on a different plane, ''The way to a man's heart is through his stomach.'' The Greek alphabet contains only 24 letters, and all of Homer's work was written with it.

The variety of sequences in which the 20 amino acids can be linked together is even greater than that possible for letters in a sentence, because proteins do not have to be pronounced, as words do. This gives them a tremendous range of possible surface structures, which in turn enables them to perform distinct, individual, and specialized functions. The human body

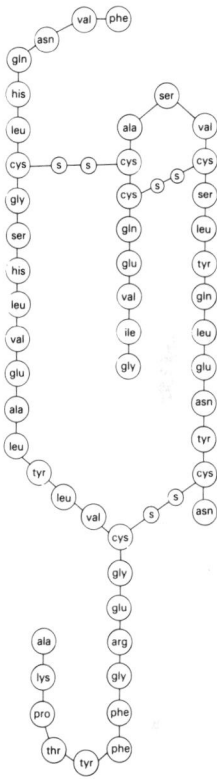

■ FIGURE 6–4
Amino Acid Sequence of Insulin
Insulin is a small protein. S-S represents the cross-links between cysteine molecules, known as disulfide bridges. (For structures and abbreviations of individual amino acids, see Appendix C.)

■ FIGURE 6–5
Hemoglobin
This model represents the intricate structure of one molecule of hemoglobin, magnified 27 millon times.

contains an estimated 10,000 to 50,000 different kinds of proteins. Of these thousands, only about 1,000 have been identified,[1] and only about ten are described in this chapter.

Digestion, Absorption, and Metabolism

The hydrolysis of proteins begins in the stomach. The cells lining the stomach secrete a gastric protease in its inactive form (pepsinogen). The hydrochloric acid of the stomach activates pepsinogen, creating pepsin, which can cleave whole proteins—large polypeptides—into smaller polypeptides.

When these small polypeptides enter the small intestine, pancreatic and intestinal proteases hydrolyze them into short oligopeptides, tripeptides, dipeptides, and amino acids. Then peptidases on the surfaces of the intestinal cells hydrolyze the dipeptides and tripeptides into amino acids—the final products of protein digestion. Amino acids are transferred to pumps, which carry them into the interior of the intestinal cells for passage into the blood. Figure 6–6 illustrates the digestion of protein through the GI tract.

Knowing that most proteins are broken down to amino acids before they are absorbed puts you in a position to refute certain untrue claims made about foods—for instance, "Don't eat food A. It contains enzyme B, which will harm you." Or "Eat enzyme C. It will help you digest your food." Any enzyme you eat becomes but one among thousands of different proteins in your digestive tract. Except for the digestive enzymes, whose design prevents them from being digested while they work, enzymes you eat are simply proteins that are broken down to fragments identical to those from the other proteins you eat. Your body cannot tell the source of a particular fragment. Don't be fooled by claims that imply that enzymes you eat will not be digested by the body.

Some people believe that eating predigested protein (amino acid preparations such as the "liquid protein" products sold to body builders and dieters) saves the body the work of having to digest protein and keeps the digestive system from "wearing out" so easily. Nothing could be further from the truth. As a matter of fact, the amino acids from whole proteins are better absorbed and utilized than are hydrolyzed amino acid mixtures, because they are released at the rate and in the order that the body can best use them. (Amino acid supplements will be discussed in a later section.)

Besides serving as units of proteins, amino acids assume many individual roles in the body. For example, the amino acid tyrosine serves as the precursor to the neurotransmitters norepinephrine and epinephrine; the skin pigment melanin; and the hormone thyroxin. Tryptophan serves as the precursor to the neurotransmitter serotonin and the vitamin niacin.

Amino acids also serve as a source of energy, more so when other energy sources are limited. The body assigns top priority to meeting its energy need, and when no energy from other sources is limited, it will break down body protein to meet this need. After stripping off the amino nitrogen (deamination), the body metabolizes the carbon skeletons of the amino acids just as it does for glucose or fatty acids. However, because proteins perform a long list of amazing tasks, energy production is a low-priority use of proteins. An

---

pepsin: a gastric protease. Pepsin is secreted in an inactive form, **pepsinogen,** which is activated by stomach acid.

peptidase: a digestive enzyme that hydrolyzes peptide bonds. *Tripeptidases* cleave tripeptides; *dipeptidases* cleave dipeptides.

neurotransmitter: a substance that is released at the end of one nerve cell when a nerve impulse arrives there, diffuses across the gap to the next cell, and alters the membrane of that cell in such a way that it becomes either less or more likely to fire (or does fire).

deamination: removal of the amino (NH_2) group from a compound such as an amino acid.

■ **FIGURE 6–6**
Protein Digestion through the GI Tract

Protein

Mouth

Chewing and crushing moistens protein-rich foods and mixes them with saliva to be swallowed.

Esophagus

No action.

Stomach

Stomach acid uncoils protein strands and activates stomach enzymes:

$$\text{Protein} \xrightarrow[\text{HCl}]{\text{pepsin}} \text{smaller polypeptides}$$

Small Intestine

Pancreatic and small intestinal enzymes split polypeptides further:

$$\text{Polypeptides} \xrightarrow[\text{intestinal proteases}]{\text{pancreatic and}} \text{dipeptides, tripeptides, and amino acids}$$

Then enzymes on the surface of the small intestinal cells hydrolyze these peptides, and the cells absorb them:

$$\text{Peptides} \xrightarrow[\text{and tripeptidases}]{\text{intestinal dipeptidases}} \text{amino acids (absorbed)}$$

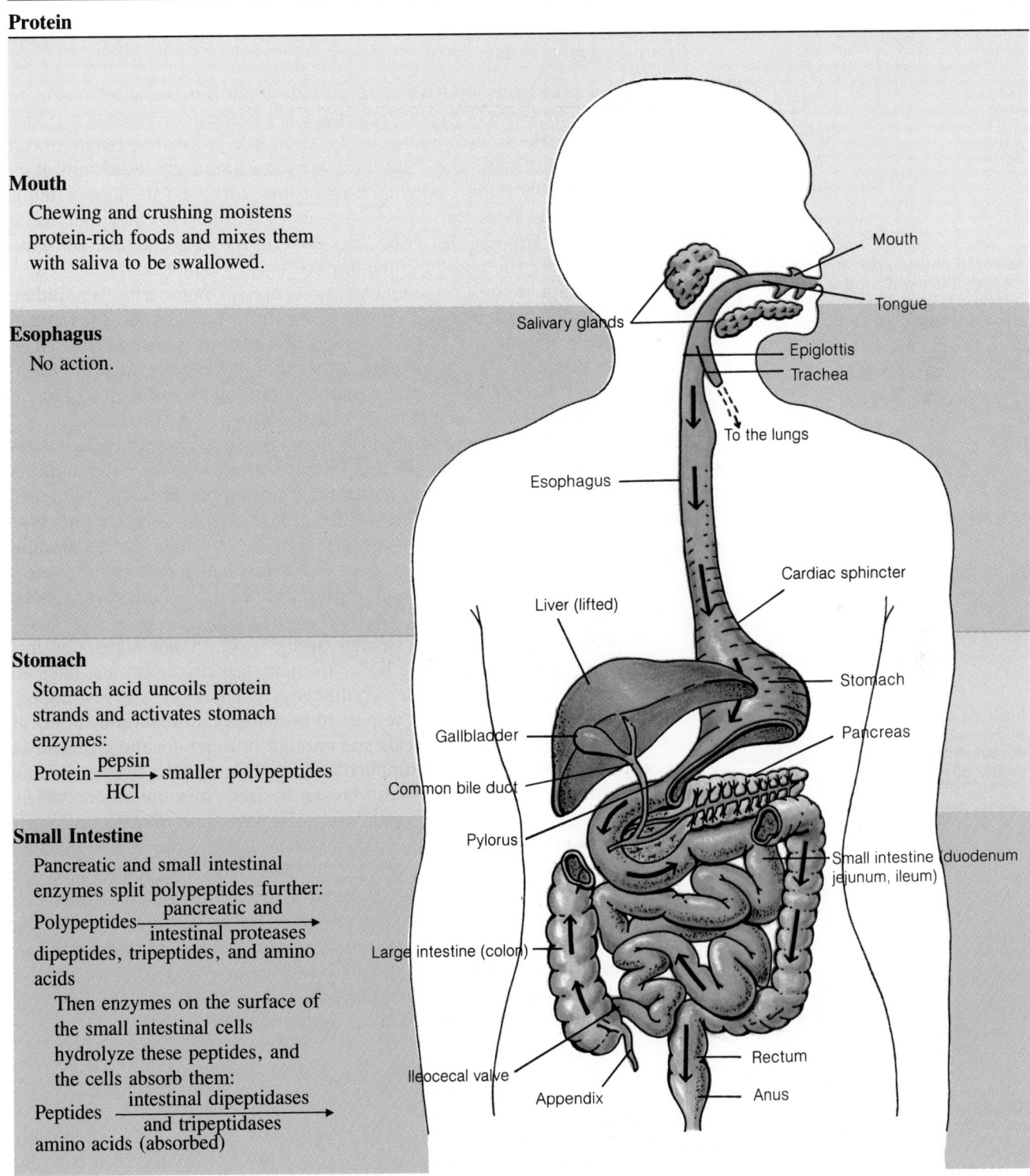

Mouth
Tongue
Salivary glands
Epiglottis
Trachea
To the lungs
Esophagus
Cardiac sphincter
Liver (lifted)
Stomach
Gallbladder
Pancreas
Common bile duct
Pylorus
Small intestine (duodenum, jejunum, ileum)
Large intestine (colon)
Ileocecal valve
Appendix
Rectum
Anus

Carbohydrate and fat allow amino acids to be used to build body proteins. This is known as the **protein-sparing action** of carbohydrate and fat.

Protein in Food
↓
supplies AminoAcids
↓
Body makes own Proteins

essential amino acid: an amino acid that the body can't synthesize in amounts sufficient to meet physiological need. See also the definition of *essential nutrient* on p. 2.

limiting amino acid: the essential amino acid found in the shortest supply relative to the amounts needed for protein synthesis in the body.

The sign maker has run out of *L*s, so he can't complete his sign (LEFT TURN ONLY). Similarly, if one essential amino acid is missing, the body can't complete its proteins.

adequate intake of carbohydrates and fats spares amino acids from being used for energy and allows them to perform their unique roles.

Essential Amino Acids

The role of protein in food is not to provide body proteins directly, but to supply the amino acids from which the body can make its own proteins. Since the body can make some amino acids for itself, the proteins in the diet need not contain these amino acids. But there are some amino acids the body can't make at all, and some it can't make fast enough to meet its need. (This is because the body does not possess the genes for the enzymes that could synthesize these amino acids, or because the enzymes it does make work too slowly.) These are the nine essential amino acids (see Table 6–1).

The distinction between essential and nonessential amino acids is not quite clear-cut. Histidine often appears not to be essential, perhaps because the diet supplies it in abundance; now, however, it has been added to the list of essential amino acids.[2] Arginine may, under some conditions, be synthesized too slowly to fully meet the human need.[3] Cysteine and tyrosine normally are not essential, because the body makes them from methionine and phenylalanine—but if there is not enough of these precursors to make them from, then they have to be supplied in the diet. Another amino acid, taurine, not found in proteins, is used to make materials important in brain and eye function and in the digestion of fat. Under special circumstances, infants may require an external dietary source of taurine; its concentration in human milk is high, but it has to be added to cow's milk in making formula. States of illness can interfere with amino acid transformations in the body and so make other amino acids essential for individual human beings.

A diet that supplies each essential amino acid in adequate amounts supports protein synthesis in the body. To make protein, cells must have all the needed amino acids available simultaneously. Therefore, the first important characteristic of a diet with respect to protein is that it should supply at least the nine essential amino acids and enough nitrogen for the synthesis of the others. If one amino acid is supplied in an amount smaller than is needed, the total amount of protein that can be synthesized from the others will be limited. Partial proteins are not made, only complete ones; there is an all-or-none law of protein synthesis. By analogy, suppose that a sign maker plans to make l00 identical signs, each saying LEFT TURN ONLY. This requires 200 *L*s, 200 *N*s, 200 *T*s, and 100 of each of the other letters. If the sign maker has only 20 *L*s, then only 10 signs can be made, even if all the other letters are available in unlimited quantities. The *L*s limit the number of signs that can be made. Furthermore, the sign maker has no place to keep leftover letters (just as the body has no storage place for extra amino acids), so without additional *L*s right away, all the other letters will have to be thrown away.

Protein Quality

A diet that contains an imbalance of amino acids so severe as to limit body protein synthesis is said to be a diet containing protein of poor quality. When the body attempts to use the amino acid supply from such a diet, it wastes many amino acids; in the absence of one, it can't use the others—and it has no place to store them. Enzymes strip off the nitrogen-containing amino groups (deaminating the amino acids) and convert them into the compound urea, which is excreted in the urine. Only the carbon chains remain, and these are used to make glucose or fat, or are metabolized for energy. Urea excreted comes partly from amino acids not retained from food proteins (not built into body proteins) and partly from the normal continuous breakdown of body protein tissues.

People usually eat many foods containing protein. Each food has its own characteristic amino acid balance, and together, they almost invariably supply more than enough nitrogen and plenty of the essential amino acids. This is true, at least, for those of us privileged to live in the developed countries today, where the food supply is reliable, abundant, and varied. It has not always been true in the past, and even today in most of the world, the protein supply and the food energy supply are the two most crucial factors determining the quality of people's diets and their nutritional health. Where protein is scarce and only one protein-rich food is eaten regularly, the quality of that particular food's protein is crucially important to children's development and all people's health. Therefore, scientists use tests of protein quality to determine the adequacy of selected food proteins in countries where people have to rely on limited amounts of single foods to meet their amino acid needs.

A complete protein is defined as a protein that contains all of the essential amino acids in relatively the same amounts as human beings require; it may or may not contain all of the other amino acids that the body can make. People generally associate complete protein with such foods as meats and eggs, not with plant foods, and the association has some validity. Generally, proteins derived from animal foods (meat, fish, poultry, eggs, and milk) are quite uniformly complete, although gelatin is an exception. Proteins derived from plant foods (vegetables, grains, and legumes) vary more. Some plant proteins are notorious for being incomplete—for example, corn protein. Some, however, are complete—for example, the proteins of rice and potatoes. A person who derives most or all of the day's food energy from rice or potatoes, and who therefore obtains enough protein to meet the day's need, will also obtain all essential amino acids in the needed amounts. Moreover, plant proteins are usually eaten in combinations. When two plant proteins, each containing the amino acids that the other lacks, are eaten at the same meal, they can make an acceptable complete protein.

Completeness is not the only issue of concern with respect to protein quality. For the highest quality, proteins must be not only complete but also digestible, so that sufficient numbers of their amino acids reach the body's cells to permit them to make the proteins they need. One of the finest proteins available by these standards is egg protein (although again, the proteins of rice and potatoes are of relatively high quality). The nitrogen of egg protein tends to be retained in the body, indicating that it is utilized with little waste. Egg protein has been designated the reference protein for purposes of measuring protein quality, and has been assigned a biological value (BV) of 100 by the Food and Agriculture Organization (FAO) of the United Nations, which sets world standards. Eggs are a highly valued protein source in less-developed nations where protein-rich foods are scarce. They offer high-quality protein, they are relatively inexpensive, and they store well.

Urea metabolism is described in Chapter 7.

complete protein: a protein containing all the amino acids essential in human nutrition in amounts adequate for human use.

Protein	Chemical score	NPU
Eggs	100	100
Milk	93	75
Rice	86	67
Beef	75	80
Fish	75	83
Corn	72	56

Different measures of protein quality produce different rank orders for animal and plant proteins. Notice that rice protein ranks above beef protein in one of them and below it in the other.

Source: Adapted from Assessment of proteins, *Nutrition and the M.D.*, June 1985, pp. 3–4.

high-quality protein: an easily digestible, complete protein.

digestibility: a measure of the amount of amino acids absorbed from a given protein intake.

reference protein: egg protein; used by FAO/WHO as a standard against which to measure the quality of other proteins.

biological value (BV): the amount of protein nitrogen that is retained from a given amount of protein nitrogen that has been digested and absorbed; a measure of protein quality (see Appendix J).

To summarize, for the body to use proteins with maximum efficiency, they must present a suitable amino acid pattern, must be digestible, must be consumed with sufficient energy from other sources so that the amino acids will not be sacrificed for energy, must be accompanied by the vitamins and minerals needed to facilitate their use, and must be received by a body that is healthy and equipped to use them. To evaluate protein quality, researchers use several measures, including chemical scoring, biological value, net protein utilization, and protein efficiency ratio; these are described in Appendix J.

Nitrogen Balance

If the body retains in its tissues the same amount of protein from day to day, it is in balance. If the body adds protein, it is in positive balance; if it loses protein, it is in negative balance. Since protein is the only major nutrient that contains nitrogen, these balance states can be detected by measuring the amounts of nitrogen entering and leaving the body.

Nitrogen balance is important, because proteins are needed for the growth and maintenance of all body tissues. Whenever you take a bath, you wash off whole cells from the surface layers of your skin, losing protein. In fact, your skin is replaced totally every seven years. The cells that manufacture hair and fingernails have to synthesize new protein constantly to go into these structures; these processes also result in a net loss of body protein. Protein losses also occur inside your body. When you swallow food, it passes down your intestinal tract. Ultimately, the undigested materials—fiber, water, and waste—leave your body, carrying with them cells that have been shed from the intestinal lining. Both inside and outside, you must constantly build new cells to replace those lost from the exposed surfaces.

In addition, proteins are continuously being dismantled in every organ and tissue inside the body. When these proteins break down, they free amino acids to join the general circulation. Some of these may be promptly recycled into body organs; some are deaminated and their amino groups excreted. The constant degradation and synthesis of body proteins is known as protein turnover; the protein that participates in this flux is endogenous protein.

Given either fat or carbohydrate as an energy source, the body can construct many of the materials needed to replace lost cells. But to rebuild protein, the body needs dietary protein for two reasons: first, because food protein is the only source of the *essential* amino acids; and second, because it is the only practical source of amino nitrogen with which to build the *non*essential amino acids.

If the body is growing, it must manufacture more cells than are lost. Children end each day with more blood cells and more skin cells than they had at the beginning of the day. So protein is needed both for routine maintenance (replacement) and growth (addition) of body tissue.

The quantity of protein a person needs depends on the amount of lean tissue in the body. Fat tissue requires relatively little protein to maintain itself, but the muscles, blood, and other metabolically active tissues must be maintained by a continuous supply of sufficient energy and essential amino acids. To determine how much protein people need, laboratory scientists

nitrogen balance: the amount of nitrogen consumed (N in) as compared with the amount of nitrogen excreted (N out) in a given period of time.

protein turnover: the degradation and synthesis of endogenous protein.

endogenous protein: the protein in the body.
  endo = within
  gen = arising

perform nitrogen balance studies.* Nitrogen balances reflect a wide variety of physiological states of the body, both in health and in disease.

Growing children and pregnant women are in positive nitrogen balance; every day they are adding to their bodies, blood, bone, and muscle cells that contain protein. (When a woman gives birth, she suddenly loses most of the protein she has helped her baby to accumulate.) When a woman is lactating, she is in nitrogen equilibrium, but it is a sort of enhanced equilibrium: she is both eating more protein and excreting more protein in her milk than before she was pregnant.

- Nitrogen equilibrium (zero nitrogen balance): N in = N out.
- Positive nitrogen balance: N in > N out.
- Negative nitrogen balance: N in < N out.

In contrast, people who are sick or in trauma are often in negative nitrogen balance; when they have to rest in bed for a long time, their muscles atrophy, and the protein-nitrogen that escapes is excreted in the urine. A circumstance in which positive nitrogen balance reflects illness is in kidney disease: an accumulation of urea nitrogen in the blood reflects a failure of excretion. Negative nitrogen balance in such a case reflects recovery.

Nitrogen balance studies enable researchers to test the quality of various food proteins. Protein from a single food source is fed (together with adequate energy from other foods) in a quantity that would be adequate to meet the body's needs if the protein's amino acid supply were similar to that of egg protein. If, under these conditions, the body starts losing nitrogen, then something is wrong with the protein. Either it isn't being well digested—so that its nitrogen is being excreted in the feces—or it has one or more limiting essential amino acids. If the problem is a limiting essential amino acid, then additional nitrogen will be lost in the urine. The body cells, lacking enough of some one amino acid to make the proteins they need, break down the other amino acids they can't use. They derive energy from the carbon skeletons, much as they do from carbohydrate or fat, but they release the amino nitrogens into the bloodstream as the compound ammonia. The liver picks up the ammonia, converts it into urea (a less toxic compound), and returns that to the blood. Finally, the kidneys filter the urea out of the bloodstream; thus the amino nitrogen ends up in the urine as urea.

Three terms are used to describe nitrogen excreted from the body: **endogenous** (en-DODGE-en-us) **nitrogen**, meaning "from inside the body"; **metabolic N**, meaning from the intestinal cells; and **exogenous** (ex-ODGE-en-us) **nitrogen**, meaning "from outside the body"—that is, from food. The nitrogen in urine is of two kinds—some from broken-down body proteins (endogenous) and some from food amino acids that got as far as the cells but then didn't get used (exogenous). The nitrogen in feces is also of two kinds—some from intestinal cells (metabolic) and some from food (exogenous).

Proteins in the Body

This chapter's introduction remarked on the variety and versatility of proteins. Now that protein structure has been explained, it is time to examine these magnificent molecules more closely.

Enzymes

Chapter 3 first introduced digestive enzymes as proteins that hydrolyze food substances into smaller pieces. Digestive enzymes have appeared in every chapter since, but digestion is only one of the many processes enzymes

enzyme: a protein that facilitates chemical reactions without itself being changed in the process; a protein catalyst.

*The average amino acid weighs about 6.25 times as much as the nitrogen it contains, so the laboratory scientist can estimate the amount of protein in a sample of food, body tissue, or excreta by multiplying the weight of the nitrogen in it by 6.25.

facilitate. They not only break down substances, they also build substances and transform one substance into another.

Enzymes and what they do are so fundamental to all life processes that it seems worthwhile to introduce an analogy to clarify two important characteristics they all share. Enzymes are comparable to the clergy and judges who make and dissolve human matrimonial bonds. When two individuals come to a minister to be married, the couple leaves with a new bond between them. They are joined together—but the minister is only momentarily involved in the process and remains unchanged. One minister can therefore perform thousands of marriage ceremonies. Similarly, a judge who facilitates the separation of married couples may decree many divorces before retiring or dying.

The minister represents enzymes that synthesize larger compounds from smaller ones—the synthetases, which build body structures. The judge represents enzymes that hydrolyze larger compounds to smaller ones; an example is the digestive enzymes.

synthetase (SIN-the-tase): an enzyme that synthesizes compounds.

Like both the minister and the judge, enzymes are not themselves altered by the reactions they facilitate. They are catalysts. Biologists and chemists define enzymes as *protein catalysts*.

What makes you different from any other human being is minute differences in your body proteins. These differences are determined by the amino acid sequences of your proteins, which are written into the genetic code of the DNA (deoxyribonucleic acid) you inherited from your parents and ancestors. Each person receives at conception a unique combination of genes (DNA codes for protein sequences). The genes direct the making of all the body's proteins, as shown in Figure 6–7. (To see how the protein synthesis machinery fits into the anatomy of a cell, turn to Appendix A.)

Perhaps you have realized by now that the protein story moves in a circle. All enzymes are proteins. All proteins are made of amino acids. Amino acids have to be put together to make proteins. Enzymes put together the amino acids. In short, some proteins make other proteins. Only living systems work with such self-renewal. A broken toaster cannot be fixed by another toaster; a car cannot make another car. Only living creatures and the parts they are composed of—the cells—can duplicate themselves.

To follow the circle in nutrition, start with a person eating food proteins. The proteins are broken down in the stomach and intestines by proteins (digestive enzymes) into amino acids. The amino acids enter the cells of the body, where proteins (synthetases) put them together in long chains with sequences specified by DNA. The chains fold and become enzymes themselves. These enzymes go to work breaking apart other compounds or putting other compounds together. Day by day, a billion reactions by a billion reactions, these processes repeat themselves, and life goes on.

Figure 6–8 provides an example of the details of an enzyme's action. In a biochemical pathway, each compound encounters an enzyme, is converted to another compound that encounters another enzyme, and so forth; the final product may be entirely different from the starting material.

The following discussion focuses on protein's other roles in the body—roles in which vitamins and minerals cooperate. Margin references in this section introduce you to these other nutrients, and later chapters then provide more details.

■ **FIGURE 6–7**
Protein Synthesis

The instructions for making every protein in a person's body are transmitted in the genetic information received at conception. This body of knowledge is filed away in the nucleus of every cell. The master file is the DNA (deoxyribonucleic acid), which never leaves the nucleus. The DNA is identical in every cell and is specific for each individual. Each specialized cell has access to the total inherited information but calls on only the instructions needed for its own functions.

1. DNA is in the nucleus of each cell.

To inform the cell of the proper sequence of amino acids for a needed protein, a "photocopy" of the appropriate portion of DNA is made. This copy is messenger RNA (ribonucleic acid), which is able to escape through the nuclear membrane.

2. DNA makes a copy of that portion of itself that has instructions for the protein the cell needs.

In the cell fluid the messenger RNA seeks out and attaches itself to one of the ribosomes (a protein-making machine, itself composed of RNA and protein).

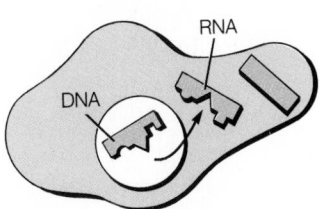

3. RNA leaves the nucleus.

Thus situated, the messenger RNA presents the sequence in which the amino acids should be linked into a protein strand. Meanwhile, another form of RNA, called transfer RNA, collects amino acids from the cell fluid and brings them to the messenger. For each of the 20 amino acids, there is a specific kind of transfer RNA.

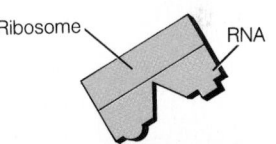

4. RNA attaches itself to the protein-making machinery of the cell.

Thousands of these transfer RNAs, with their loads of amino acids, cluster around the ribosomes, like vegetable-laden trucks around a farmers' market awaiting their turn to unload. When an amino acid is called for by the messenger, the transfer RNA carrying it snaps into position. Then the next and the next and the next loaded transfer RNAs move into place. Thus an enzyme bonds the amino acids together in the right sequence.

5. Transfer RNAs carry their amino acids to the messenger RNA, where they are snapped into place.

Finally, the completed protein strand is released, the messenger is degraded, and the transfer RNAs are freed to return for another load. It takes many words to describe the events, but in the cell, 40 to 100 amino acids can be added to a growing protein strand in only a second.

6. The completed protein strand is released, and the messenger RNA is degraded.

■ **FIGURE 6–8**

Enzyme Action

In the breakdown of glucose (a 6-carbon compound), enzymes add two phosphate groups, alter the arrangement of the atoms, and then split the molecule in half so that two 3-carbon compounds result.* One of these is compound A. The other is converted to compound A, so that the two halves derived from glucose go through an identical process from that point on. Let us look closely at the pathway for four steps thereafter, starting with compound A.

Compound A floats around until it encounters an enzyme that recognizes it. This enzyme has the specialized function of removing hydrogen atoms from molecules of compound A. The encounter results in the altered compound, compound B.

Compound A

Compound B is released from the enzyme and encounters another enzyme whose sole mission in life is to remove oxygens from compound B and to substitute amino groups in their place. What results is compound C.

Compound B

The next enzyme removes the phosphate group from the end carbon and replaces it with a hydrogen, leaving compound D.

Compound C

If you look closely at the picture of compound D, you may recognize its characteristics and not be surprised by the statements that follow. But let us take the process one more step. Another enzyme, whose function is to remove CH_2OH groups from molecules, forms compound E.

Compound D

Amazing! The cellular machinery started with a molecule of glucose (a derivative of dietary carbohydrate), made one small change after another, and transformed it into an amino acid (a member of the protein family). The lesson to learn from this sequence of events is that the body can make, from glucose and nitrogen-containing compounds, many of the amino acids needed to build body proteins. The amino acid glycine is just one example. Compound D, which precedes glycine on the pathway, is another example: it is the amino acid serine. Thus, among the thousands of tasks that enzymes perform, they even manufacture many of the amino acids they themselves are made of.

Look at this product closely; you have seen it before. It has an amino group at one end, an acid group at the other, and a central carbon carrying two hydrogen atoms. It is the amino acid glycine (Figure 6–2).

Compound E

*The enzyme that produced compound B was a dehydrogenase; enzyme that produced compound C, a transaminase; and the one that produced compound D, a phosphatase.

Fluid Balance

Proteins help maintain the body's fluid balance. Fluid is present in several body compartments. Chief among them are the space inside the blood vessels; the spaces within the cells; and the spaces between the cells, outside the blood vessels. Fluids flow back and forth between these compartments, and proteins in the fluids, together with minerals, help to maintain the needed distribution of these fluids.

Fluid and electrolyte balance is fully discussed in Chapter 10.

The reasons why proteins in fluids can help determine the fluids' distribution in living systems are that proteins are large and attracted to water (hydrophilic). Being large, they cannot pass freely across the membranes that separate compartments; they are trapped where they are. Being hydrophilic, they keep water molecules near them, which in effect makes them even larger. A cell that "wants" to keep a certain amount of water in its interior space can't move the water around, directly, but it can manufacture proteins to keep inside itself, and those proteins will hold water. Thus the cell uses protein to regulate the distribution of water indirectly. Similarly, the body makes proteins for the blood and the intercellular fluid (lymph) and these proteins help maintain the fluid volume in those spaces.

Minerals are helper nutrients. The attraction of protein and mineral particles to water is due to osmotic pressure; see Chapter 10.

Acid-Base Balance

Another balance that proteins help maintain is that between acids and bases within the body's fluids. An acid solution is one in which hydrogen ions abound; the more hydrogen ions, the more concentrated the acid. Proteins (and minerals), which have negative charges on their surfaces, and hydrogen ions, which have positive charges, attract each other. As long as the concentration of hydrogen ions—that is, the strength of the acid—stays within certain limits, the proteins maintain their integrity. If the acid becomes too strong, however, the positively charged hydrogen ions neutralize some of the negative charges on the proteins, changing the internal interactive forces. When this happens, the proteins lose their shape and can no longer function. They are denatured (see p. 136). The situation is similar when the balance tips too far toward base.

acid-base balance: the balance maintained in the body between too much and too little acid; see Chapter 10.

Of all the consequences that stem from exceeding the normal limits of the acid-base balance, the most direct and serious is protein denaturation. A disturbance of their shapes renders the proteins that carry out so many vital body functions useless. Just to give one example, hemoglobin loses its capacity to carry oxygen. Both acidosis and alkalosis can be lethal if unchecked. The proteins in the plasma, such as albumin, help to prevent these conditions from arising. In a sense, the proteins protect one another by sequestering extra hydrogen ions when there are too many in the surrounding medium and by releasing them when there are too few. This ability to regulate the acidity of the medium is known as the buffering action of proteins.

acidosis: too much acid in the blood and body fluids.

alkalosis: too much base in the blood and body fluids.

lethal: causing death.

sequester (see-KWESS-ter): to hide away or take out of circulation.

buffer: a compound that can help keep a solution's acidity or alkalinity constant; see Chapter 10.

Antibodies

Other major proteins found in the blood—the antibodies—act against disease agents. When a body is invaded by a foreign organism, such as a virus—

antibodies: large proteins of the blood and body fluids, produced in response to the invasion of the body by unfamiliar molecules (mostly proteins); antibodies inactivate the invaders and so protect the body.

A) The body is challenged by foreign invaders.

B) The body makes the code for manufacturing the antibody.

C) The code makes the antibody.

D) The antibody inactivates the foreign invader.

E) The code remains to make antibodies faster the next time a foreign invader attacks.

■ **FIGURE 6–9**
Development of Immunity

Chapter 18 focuses on the body's system of defense against disease—the immune system—and Chapter 30 on its attacker—the disease of AIDS.

The thyroid hormone contains iodine, and insulin associates with zinc; these minerals are helper nutrients (see Chapter 11). For descriptions of many hormones important in nutrition, see Appendix A.

These membrane-associated proteins are variously called **permeases**, **vectorial enzymes**, and **transferases**.

See Figure 3–10 for an illustration of active transport.

whether it is one that causes flu, smallpox, measles, or the common cold—the virus enters the cells and multiplies there. One virus may produce 100 replicas of itself within an hour or so. These burst out and invade 100 different cells, soon yielding 10,000 virus particles, which invade 10,000 cells. After several hours there may be a million viruses, then 100 million, and so on. If they were left free to do their worst, they would soon overwhelm the body with the disease they cause.

One of the body's defenses against viruses, bacteria, and other foreign organisms is to circulate antibodies, giant protein molecules, in the blood. Each type of antibody molecule is different and specific, able to combine with and inactivate a specific foreign protein, such as that in a virus coat or bacterial cell membrane. The antibodies work so efficiently that in a normal, healthy individual, the many disease agents that attempt to attack never have a chance to get started. If a million bacterial cells are injected into the skin of a healthy person, fewer than ten are likely to survive for five hours.

Once the body has manufactured antibodies against a particular disease agent (such as the measles virus), the cells never forget how to produce them (see Figure 6–9). Consequently, the next time that virus invades the body, the antibodies will respond even more quickly. Thus the body acquires immunity against the diseases it is exposed to, by virtue of the molecular memory of the antibody-producing cells.

Hormones

Hormones are messenger molecules, and some are made of amino acids. Various glands in the body secrete hormones in response to changes in the internal environment. The blood carries the hormones to their target tissues, where they elicit the appropriate response to restore normal conditions. Among hormones are the thyroid hormone, insulin, and the enterogastrones. The thyroid hormone regulates the body's metabolic rate—the rate of the chemical reactions that yield energy (more to come in Chapter 7). Insulin regulates the concentration of the blood glucose and its transportation into cells, upon which the brain and the nervous system depend (as Chapter 4 described). The enterogastrone hormones help to coordinate the digestive and absorptive processes (described in Chapter 3). Hormones have many other profound effects, which will become evident as you read further.

Transport Proteins

A special group of the body's proteins specializes in moving nutrients and other molecules into and out of cells. These proteins reside in the membranes of every cell of the body, and each is specific for a certain compound or group of related compounds. Most of these proteins are confined to the cell membranes but can rotate or shuttle from one side of the membrane to the other. Thus they act as "pumps," picking up compounds on one side of the membrane, depositing them on the other, and thereby permitting the cells to "decide" what substances to take up and what to release.

Almost every water-soluble nutrient seems to have its own transport system in cell membranes. By contrast, lipids can cross membranes without the help of pumps. A cell can regulate a lipid's distribution by trapping it once it gets where it belongs. The cell attaches the lipid to a protein or other molecule so that it *cannot* move freely across membranes any more.

The cell membranes' protein machinery can be switched on or off in response to the body's needs. Often hormones do the switching, with a marvelous precision. A familiar example is provided by insulin and glucose. When there is too much glucose in the blood, the pancreas steps up its output of the hormone insulin. The insulin stimulates the cells' transport proteins to pump glucose into the cells faster than it can leak out. (After acting on the message, the cells destroy the insulin.) Then, as the blood glucose concentration returns to normal, the pancreas reduces its insulin output. The blood concentration of calcium is regulated in a similar manner by the hormones calcitonin and parathormone. Hundreds of other body proteins maintain the distribution of hundreds of other substances in the various body spaces.

Calcium concentration is tightly controlled by hormones, as described in Chapter 10.

Other transport proteins, not attached to membranes, move about in the body fluids; they carry nutrients and other molecules from one organ to another. Foremost among these is the protein hemoglobin, which carries oxygen to the cells. Also recall the lipoproteins, which transport the cumbersome lipid molecules from place to place. In addition, the fat-soluble vitamins are carried by special proteins, and research indicates that many water-soluble vitamins also have protein carriers.

The mineral iron is a nutrient whose handling in the body illustrates especially well how precisely proteins operate. Upon moving into a cell of the intestinal wall, iron is captured by a protein residing in the cell, which will not let go of it unless the iron is needed in the body. Iron leaving the cell to enter the bloodstream is attached to a carrier protein. The carrier, in turn, can pass iron on to a storage protein in the bone marrow or other tissues, which will hold it until it is called for. Then, when it is needed, iron is incorporated into the structure of still another protein in the red blood cells, where it assists in oxygen transport, or into a muscle protein, which helps muscle cells oxidize their energy fuels.

The protein residing in the intestinal wall cells is **ferritin**; the carrier protein, **transferrin**; the storage protein, **ferritin** again; the red blood cell protein, **hemoglobin**; and the muscle cell protein, **myoglobin** (see Chapter 11).

Blood Clotting

Blood has a remarkable ability to remain a liquid tissue even though it carries many large molecules and cells through the circulatory system. But blood can also turn solid within seconds when the integrity of that system is disturbed. (If it did not clot, a single pinprick could drain your entire body of all its blood, just as a tiny hole in a bucket makes the bucket forever useless for holding water.) When you cut yourself, a rapid chain of events leads to the production of fibrin, a stringy, insoluble mass of protein fibers that plugs the cut and stops the leak. Later, more slowly, a scar forms to replace the clot and permanently heal the cut.

Vitamin K (involved in the production of prothrombin) and calcium (needed for the blood to clot) are helper nutrients; see Chapters 9 and 10.

Structural Proteins

Proteins help make scar tissue, bones, and teeth. When the construction of a bone or a tooth begins, bone-building cells first lay down a scaffolding made of the connective tissue protein collagen. Later, these cells lay down crystals

collagen: the protein material of which connective tissue such as scars, tendons, ligaments, and the foundations of bones and teeth are made.
kolla = glue
gennan = to produce

Blood Clotting

The chain of events in blood clotting is as follows:

- A phospholipid (**thromboplastin**) is released from blood platelets (small, cell-fragment-like structures in the blood).
- Thromboplastin catalyzes the conversion of **prothrombin** (a precursor protein made in the liver that circulates in the blood) to the enzyme **thrombin**.
- Thrombin then catalyzes the conversion of **fibrinogen** (another circulating precursor protein) to **fibrin**.

  thrombo = clot
  fibr = fibers
  ogen = gives rise to

Vitamin C (needed to form collagen) and minerals (to calcify bones and teeth) are helper nutrients; see Chapters 8 and 10.

of calcium, phosphorus, fluoride, and other minerals on this matrix to form the hardened bone. When a bone breaks, the bone-building cells begin mending the break by molding a collagen matrix, then laying down the bony material. Collagen is also the mending material in torn tissue, forming scars to hold the separated parts together. It is the material of ligaments and tendons and is a strengthening glue between the cells of the artery walls that helps enable them to withstand the pressure of surging heartbeats.

Proteins are also a part of the body's other lean tissues—the organs, glands, and muscles. The unique structure of the contractile proteins allows muscle action.

Visual Pigments

opsin: the protein of the visual pigments. Vitamin A is a helper nutrient, attached to opsin to form the pigment rhodopsin; see Chapter 9.

The light-sensitive pigments in the cells of the retina are molecules of the protein opsin. Opsin responds to light by changing its shape, thus initiating the nerve impulses that convey the sense of sight to the higher centers of the brain.

The list of protein functions here is by no means exhaustive, but it does give some sense of their immense variety and importance in the body. With this information as background, you are in a position to appreciate the significance of the world's most serious malnutrition problem: protein-energy malnutrition.

■ Health Effects of Protein

As you might imagine from the previous description of the many roles proteins play, a dietary deficiency wreaks havoc on the body. An excess of dietary protein has its own consequences as well. This section describes the health effects of inadequate and excessive protein intakes.

Miniglossary of Protein and Energy Malnutrition Terms

protein-energy malnutrition (PEM), also called **protein-kcalorie malnutrition (PCM)**: a deficiency of both protein and energy; the world's most widespread malnutrition problem, including kwashiorkor, marasmus, and states in which they overlap.

acute PEM: acute protein-energy malnutrition, caused by recent severe food restriction, and characterized in children by thinness for height.

chronic PEM: chronic protein-energy malnutrition, caused by long-term food deprivation, and characterized in children by short height for age.

kwashiorkor (kwash-ee-OR-core, kwash-ee-or-CORE): the deficiency disease caused by inadequate protein in the presence of adequate food energy (kcalories).

marasmus (ma-RAZ-mus): the disease of starvation; deficiency of both protein and food energy.

Protein-Energy Malnutrition

The most widespread form of malnutrition among children in the developing world today is protein-energy malnutrition, or PEM (see the accompanying miniglossary of related terms). PEM takes two forms. Children who are thin for their height may be suffering from acute PEM (recent severe food restriction), whereas children who are short for their age have experienced chronic PEM (long-term food restriction). Stunted growth due to PEM is easy to overlook, because a small child can look perfectly normal, but it may be the most common sign of malnutrition in developing countries.[4]

Chapter 18 describes the relationships between PEM and illness, and Chapter 19 shows how assessment data can identify and classify PEM.

Kwashiorkor   Inadequate protein in a diet that provides adequate food energy causes kwashiorkor. *Kwashiorkor* is the Ghanaian name for "the evil spirit that infects the first child when the second child is born."* In countries where kwashiorkor is prevalent, parents customarily give their newly weaned children watery cereal rather than the food eaten by the rest of the family. The child is suddenly switched from breast milk containing high-quality protein designed beautifully to support growth to a weak drink with scant protein of low quality. Small wonder the just-weaned child sickens when the new baby arrives.

Like the malnourished newborn, the newly malnourished older infant or young child meets this threat to life by engaging in as little activity as possible. Apathy is one of the earliest signs of protein deprivation; the body collects all its forces to meet the crisis and so cuts down on any expenditure of protein not needed for the heart, lungs, and brain. As the apathy increases, the child

---

*Research is under way to assess the impact of a food fungus common in tropical countries as the producer of aflatoxins. Remarkable similarities exist between the impairment of liver function seen in aflatoxin poisoning and kwashiorkor, and researchers are asking whether aflatoxins may be the initial cause of liver damage and the vicious infection–malnutrition cycle seen in kwashiorkor. R. G. Hendrickse and coauthors, Aflatoxins and kwashiorkor: A study in Sudanese children, *British Medical Journal*, 285 (1982): 843–846.

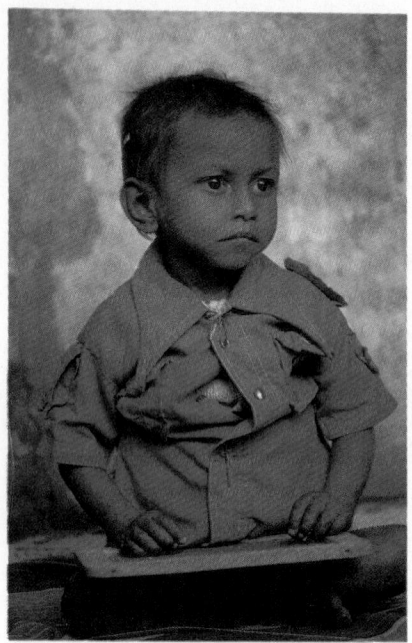

Protein malnutrition impairs learning.

edema (eh-DEEM-uh): the swelling of body tissue caused by leakage of fluid from the blood vessels, seen in (among other conditions) protein deficiency.

dysentery (DISS-en-terry): an infection of the digestive tract that causes diarrhea.

doesn't even cry for food; parental neglect then exacerbates the malnutrition problem. All growth ceases; the child is no larger at age four than at age two. New hair grows without the protein pigment that gives it its color. The skin also loses its color, and when sores open, they fail to heal. Digestive enzymes are in short supply, the digestive tract lining deteriorates, and absorption fails. The child can't assimilate what little food is eaten. Proteins and hormones that previously kept the fluid correctly distributed among the compartments of the body now are diminished, so that fluid leaks out of the blood (edema) and accumulates in the belly and legs. Blood proteins, including hemoglobin, are no longer synthesized, so the child becomes anemic; this further increases the weakness and apathy. The kwashiorkor victim often develops a fatty liver, caused by lack of the protein carriers that transport fat out of the liver. Antibodies to fight off invading bacteria are degraded to provide amino acids for other uses; the child becomes an easy target for infection. Dysentery, an infection of the digestive tract, causes diarrhea, further depleting the body of nutrients, especially minerals. Measles, which might make a healthy child sick for a week or two, kills the kwashiorkor child within two or three days.

If caught in time, a kwashiorkor child's life may be saved by careful nutrition therapy. The fluid balances are most critical. Diarrhea will have depleted the body's potassium stores and upset other electrolyte balances. Careful correction of these critical balances will prevent sudden death from heart failure about half the time. Only later can nonfat milk, providing protein and carbohydrate, be safely given; fat comes later, when body protein is sufficient to provide carriers.

Marasmus   A diet lacking both protein and food energy causes marasmus. Children with marasmus suffer symptoms similar to those of children with kwashiorkor, since both cause loss of body protein tissue, but there are also differences between the two. Kwashiorkor children retain some of their stores of body fat (because they are still consuming some food), accumulate fat in their livers (because they can't make protein to carry it away), and develop edema (from protein lack). Marasmus children experience ketosis during the body's effort to conserve protein; kwashiorkor children do not, because they are receiving some carbohydrate. Kwashiorkor is actually a less balanced state and a disease for which therapy is more difficult to manage than marasmus for children at any given age.

A marasmus child looks like a wizened little old person—just skin and bones. The child is often sick, because resistance to disease is low. All the muscles are wasted, including the weakened heart muscle. Metabolism is so slow that body temperature is subnormal. There is little or no fat under the skin to insulate against cold. Hospital workers caring for victims of this disease find that the children primarily need to be wrapped up and kept warm. They also need love, because they have often been deprived of maternal attention as well as of food.

Unlike the kwashiorkor child, who is fed milk until weaning, the marasmus child may have been neglected from early infancy. The disease occurs most commonly in children from 6 to 18 months of age in all the overpopulated city slums of the world. Since the brain grows most rapidly just prior to birth and continues growing through the first two years of life, marasmus slows brain development, permanently impairing learning ability.

Protein Excess

It is possible to consume too much protein. Animals fed high-protein diets experience a protein overload effect, exhibited in the hypertrophy of their livers and kidneys. Infants are placed at risk in many ways if fed excess protein.[5] People who wish to lose weight may be handicapped in their efforts if they consume too much protein.[6] Protein-rich foods are often fat-rich foods and contribute to obesity and its accompanying risks. Obese people can lose weight on diets that provide adequate protein, minimal fat, and ample energy from carbohydrates. The higher a person's intake of protein-rich foods such as meat and milk, the more likely it is that fruits, vegetables, and grains will be crowded out of the diet, making it inadequate in other nutrients.

Diets high in protein promote calcium excretion, depleting the bones of their chief mineral.[7] Protein from animal, as opposed to vegetable, food sources raises serum cholesterol concentrations in animals; studies to determine effects in human beings are less conclusive. Some authorities recommend an intake of at least as much vegetable as animal protein (a 1-to-1 ratio).[8] There are evidently no benefits to be gained by consuming a diet that derives more than 15 percent of its energy from protein, and there are possible risks as intakes rise to 20 percent or more when energy is adequate.[9] The *NRC Recommendations* advise a moderate protein intake—one that falls between the RDA and twice the RDA.

hypertrophy (high-PURR-tro-fee): growing too large.
hyper = too much
trophy = growth

Chapter 13 shows that excess protein doesn't help the body builder to add muscle.

■ *Protein in Foods*

The body continuously breaks down its proteins, and cannot store amino acids. Therefore, the proteins in foods provide the amino acids to replenish the stock of amino acids, especially the essential ones.

Recommended Protein Intakes

Recommendations for protein intakes can be stated in three ways—as a percentage of total energy, as grams per kilogram of body weight per day, or as an absolute number (grams per day). Dietary guidelines generally recommend that people's protein intakes contribute about 12 percent of the total energy consumed. (This allows almost 60 percent of energy or more to come from carbohydrate, and 30 percent or less to come from fat.) Most people in this country already eat this much protein, and more.

The Committee on Dietary Allowances of the Food and Nutrition Board of the National Academy of Sciences states the RDA in grams of protein per kilogram of body weight per day. They consider that a generous protein allowance for a healthy adult would be 0.8 grams per kilogram of appropriate body weight per day. Protein RDA for people of average heights at all ages are presented in the RDA table (inside front cover, left). If your height is not average, you can compute your own individualized RDA for protein by using your appropriate *weight*. Suppose your appropriate weight is 50 kilograms (110 pounds), for example; your protein RDA would then be 0.8 times 50, or

Protein RDA
0.8 g/kg/day.

>> **NUTRITION DETECTIVE WORK**

The question of what dietary protein sources might be best for human beings has been investigated, largely, using animals. Animal studies offer an excellent opportunity for examining human diseases, and in nutrition, they allow researchers to predict, among other things, the consequences of eating particular substances. Animal studies are particularly valuable when the direct study of human beings would be unethical or would take too long to be of value to the present generation. Researchers can control many variables while manipulating the one in question. However, anyone evaluating animal research must consider certain important issues before reaching conclusions as to how far, if at all, animal test results can be extended to apply to human beings.

Laboratory animals differ from human beings in many ways, including their sizes, the details of their metabolism, and their life spans. Such differences can dramatically alter the relevance of animal findings. For example, experiments using rabbits to learn about cholesterol metabolism offer little useful information, because rabbits' metabolism of cholesterol differs significantly from that of human beings.

Laboratory diets can also differ from those of human beings. In many of the studies that report high blood cholesterol concentrations in response to an animal-protein diet as compared with a vegetable-protein diet, the animals were fed purified test meals. Of course, human beings do not eat pure protein from one source. Diets usually contain a variety of foods that provide proteins from several sources, as well as a mixture of other nutrients. Results from human studies on the effects of dietary protein on blood cholesterol have been inconsistent.

Animal studies are valuable in suggesting possible relationships between diet and health and in helping researchers to explore the possible mechanisms of action, but their implications must be tested directly on human beings before conclusions can be accepted as valid. Be careful about drawing conclusions from animal studies.

40 grams of protein each day. The Canadian recommendation (RNI) for protein is similar to the RDA: 0.86 grams per kilogram for adults (see examples in Appendix I). Average protein intakes of most Canadians generally exceed this protein recommendation.

The Committee on Dietary Allowances uses an appropriate reference weight, not the actual weight, for a given height. Reference weight is more proportional to the *lean* body mass of the average person than is actual weight, which may reflect varying quantities of fat. Lean body mass determines protein need. If you gain fat, you gain weight of course, but as mentioned, fat tissue does not require much protein for maintenance.

In setting the RDA, the committee assumes that you are a healthy individual, with no unusual metabolic need for protein. The committee also

---

Recommended Protein Intakes

To calculate the percentage of energy you derive from protein:

- Use your total energy as the denominator (example: 1,900 kcal).
- Multiply your protein *grams* by 4 kcal/g to obtain kcalories from protein as the numerator (example: 70 g protein $\times$ 4 kcal/g = 280 kcal).
- Divide to obtain a decimal, multiply by 100, and round off (example: $280 \div 1,900 \times 100 = 15$ % kcalories from protein).

To figure your protein RDA:

- Look up the appropriate weight for a person of your height (inside back cover). Use this weight as your reference weight.
- Change pounds to kilograms (pounds $\div$ 2.2).
- Multiply kilograms by 0.8 g/kg.

Example (for a 5'8" medium-frame male):

- Reference weight: about 150 lb.
- 150 lb $\times$ 1 kg/2.2 lb = 68 kg (rounded off).
- 68 kg $\times$ 0.8 g/kg = 54 g protein (rounded off).

---

assumes that the protein eaten will be of mixed quality, that the efficiency of body utilization of the protein is similar to that of reference proteins, that the protein is consumed with adequate energy from carbohydrate and fat, and that other nutrients in the diet are adequate.

Note the qualification "adequate energy" in the previous statement. As mentioned earlier, a recommended protein intake can be stated as a percentage of energy intake or as an absolute number (grams per day). An absolute number, such as 50 grams per day for a 62-kilogram, moderately active person, offers a reasonable percentage of daily energy from protein—but only if the person receives an adequate *amount* of energy (say, 2,000 kcalories a day). In that case, 50 grams of protein, equal to 200 kcalories, provides 10 percent of the total energy from protein. But if the person cuts energy intake drastically—to, say, 800 kcalories a day—then 200 kcalories from protein is suddenly 25 percent of the total, yet it's still the same absolute number of grams. It's still a reasonable protein intake, too; it's the energy intake that's not reasonable. Similarly, if the person's energy intake is high—say, 4,000 kcalories—the 50 grams protein intake represents only 5 percent of the total, yet it's *still* a reasonable protein intake. Again, it's the energy intake that's unreasonable.

Be careful when judging a protein intake as a percentage of energy. Always ask what the absolute number of grams is, too, and compare it with the RDA or some such standard given in grams. A recommendation stated as a percentage of energy intake is useful only if the energy intake is within reason.

The World Health Organization has a task somewhat different from that of the U.S. and Canadian agencies, and this accounts for its lower recommendation: 0.75 grams per kilogram of body weight. WHO must find acceptable levels of nutrient intakes for a world in which poverty makes generous

For information on how the RDA was set, see Chapter 2.

intakes a luxury. WHO carefully defines its protein recommendation in terms of egg or milk protein and also publishes a set of graded recommendations for proteins of lower quality. The difference between the WHO and the Canadian and U.S. recommendations reflects the different realities in the societies for which they were designed.

Protein Intakes

The foods that supply protein in abundance are those on the milk and meat lists of the exchange system. A cup of milk provides 8 grams of protein; an ounce of the average meat, 7 grams, as shown in Table 2–2 (p. 28). A 1-cup portion of legumes, when used as a meat alternate, provides 13 grams of protein in the exchange system (counted as 2 starch and 1 lean meat exchanges). As the table also shows, the foods in the vegetable and bread lists contribute small amounts of protein to the diet, but they become significant when several servings are consumed.

The exchange system provides an easy way to estimate the amount of protein a person consumes. Figure 6–10 shows the protein contents of foods, and Figure 6–11 demonstrates the calculation of how much protein is in a day's meals.

The protein RDA represents a generous intake; it is set high enough to cover the estimated needs of most people, even those with unusually high requirements. Still, most people in developed countries such as the United States ingest much more protein than the RDA. This is not surprising when you consider that a single ounce of meat delivers about 7 grams of protein, and that the RDA for an average-sized person is only about 50 grams a day.

To illustrate this point, suppose that *your* recommended protein intake is 50 grams per day. This would divide easily into three meals: 10 grams at

8 g in 1 c milk   3 g in 1 starch portion

2 g in ½ c vegetables   7 g in 1 oz meat

■ FIGURE 6–10
Exchange Lists Containing Protein
Milk List
1 c milk contains 8 g protein

Meat List
1 oz meat contains 7 g protein

Vegetable List
½ c vegetables contains 2 g protein

Starch/Bread List
1 slice bread, 1 portion cereal, or 1 starchy vegetable contains 3 g protein

■ **FIGURE 6–11**
Estimating Protein Intake Using the Exchange System

	Protein Grams	
	Exchange	Actual
Breakfast		
1 c oatmeal = 2 starch exchanges	6	6
¼ c raisins = 2 fruit exchanges	—	1
1 c nonfat milk = 1 milk exchange	8	8
1¼ c strawberries = 1 fruit exchange	0	1
Morning Snack		
2 tbsp raisins = 1 fruit exchange	—	0
2 tsp sunflower seeds = 2 fat exchanges	—	6
Lunch		
1 bean burrito (1 lg tortilla = 2 starch exchanges	6	
½ c beans = 1 starch exchange	3	13
+ ½ lean meat exchange)	3½	
1 c nonfat milk = 1 milk exchange	8	8
1 orange = 1 fruit exchange	—	1
Dinner		
4 oz shrimp = 4 lean meat exchanges	28	24
1 c broccoli = 2 vegetable exchanges	4	5
½ c spinach noodles = 1 starch exchange	3	3
2 tsp butter = 2 fat exchanges	—	0
¼ chopped parsley = ¼ vegetable exchange		0
¼ c tomato = ¼ vegetable exchange	2	0
¼ c mushrooms = ¼ vegetable exchange		0
¼ c water chestnuts = ¼ vegetable exchange		0
1 c fresh spinach = 1 vegetable exchange	2	2
1 tbsp sesame seeds = 1 fat exchange	—	2
⅓ c garbanzo beans = 1 starch exchange	3	5
1 tbsp vinaigrette dressing = 1 fat exchange	—	0
1 packet sugar	—	0
½ c sherbet = 2 starch exchanges	6	1
Day's Total	82.5 g	86 g

Let's estimate the amounts of protein in the meals shown here. (These are the same meals used as examples in Chapters 2, 4, and 5.) The fruits and fats can be assumed to contain no protein, so the only foods to inspect are the meats, milks, grains, starchy vegetables and breads, and vegetables. Peas and beans (members of the legume family) contain more protein than other vegetables do.

breakfast, 20 grams at lunch, and 20 grams at dinner. An egg and a glass of milk at breakfast would exceed the amount allotted for breakfast by half. A chef's salad with only 3 ounces of cut-up meat or cheese would more than cover the amount allotted for lunch. A small piece of chicken would suffice for dinner. By the time you added a few vegetables, the recommended second cup of milk, and the four bread and/or cereal items suggested by the Four Food Group Plan, you would have exceeded your protein needs for the day by far. No wonder most people get more than twice as much protein as they need. Most likely, if they have an adequate *food* intake, they have an adequate protein intake.

As mentioned earlier, high protein intakes can create problems. Care must be taken to balance the energy budget and to avoid excessive intakes of fat and cholesterol (which accompany foods in the meat and milk groups). Chapter 2 introduced the <u>principles of wise diet planning: adequacy, balance, energy (kcalorie) control, moderation, nutrient density, and variety</u>. With respect to protein, the principle to emphasize is moderation.

Vegetarianism

The vegetarian has the same nutrition tasks as any other person—planning a diet that will deliver a variety of foods that will provide all the needed nutrients within an energy allowance that won't cause weight gain or loss. The added challenge comes from doing so with at least one less food group.

Some vegetarians omit meat, fish, and poultry from their diets, but use animal products such as eggs, cheese, yogurt, and milk. Others exclude eggs; the only foods of animal origin they use are milk products. Still others (vegans) allow themselves no foods that come from animals in any form, and restrict themselves to an all-plant diet. Whichever type of vegetarian, they all omit meat, and one of the nutrients that meats are famous for is protein.

Those who eat animal products such as milk and eggs are availing themselves of the highest-quality protein available and need fear no protein deficiencies. Those who eat an all-plant diet may need to give thought to their protein intakes, because plant proteins—at least individually—are of lower quality, and because plants offer less protein per unit (either weight or measure) of food than animal proteins.

Vegans have long been told that they should know how to combine plant proteins that are missing, or are low in, one or more essential amino acids in order to improve the quality of the plant proteins they eat. This strategy is called mutual supplementation, and the two protein foods chosen are complementary proteins. Mixtures that provide higher-quality protein than the individual protein foods they are made from are shown in Figure 6–12. The *amounts* of protein such mixtures provide are ample, too, as shown in Table 6–2.

Studies indicating that mutual supplementation was a necessity for the vegan were first conducted on rats. The protein requirements of human beings are different from those of rats, but the idea that plant proteins are inadequate sources of essential amino acids carried over for years. Now it appears that adequate consumption of the essential amino acids is possible without practicing mutual supplementation.[10] Plant foods can provide more

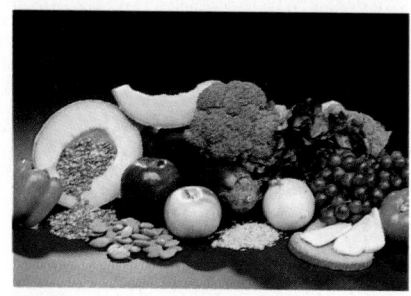

Vegetarians obtain protein from legumes, nuts, vegetables, grains, and milk products.

mutual supplementation: the strategy of combining two protein foods in a meal so that each food provides the essential amino acid(s) lacking in the other.

complementary proteins: two or more proteins whose amino acid assortments complement each other in such a way that the essential amino acids missing from each are supplied by the other.

■ FIGURE 6–12
Nonmeat Mixtures That Provide High-Quality Protein

Vegetarians who eat no foods from animal sources select foods from two or more of these columns to create high-quality protein combinations:

Grains	Legumes	Seeds and Nuts	Vegetables
Oats	Peanuts	Cashews	
Rice	Soy products	Nut butters	
Whole-grain breads			
Pasta			

Examples:

Black beans and rice, a favorite Hispanic combination.

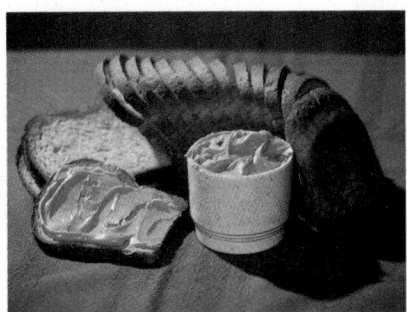

Peanut butter and wheat bread, a North American tradition.

Tofu and stir-fried vegetables with rice, an Asian dish.

Vegetarians who eat foods from animal sources may also combine any of these foods with those above to create high-quality protein combinations:

Eggs or Milk Products

Eggs
Milk
Yogurt
Cheese
Cottage cheese

Examples:

Eggplant Parmesan, a favorite Italian combination.

Cereal with milk, a traditional American breakfast.

Vegetable omelets, a nourishing meal any time of day.

■ **TABLE 6–2**
Protein Sources

Food	Amount	Protein (g)	Energy (kcal)
These are the usual foods people think of when they think of protein:			
Cheese:			
Cheddar	1 oz	7	115
Cottage	½ c	12 to 15	85 to 130
Egg	1 large	7	80
Fish, light and dark, cooked	3 oz	20 to 25	125 to 175
Meat, cooked:			
Ground beef	3 oz	20 to 23	185 to 235
Heart, kidney, liver	3 oz	23 to 28	160 to 215
Pork	3 oz	23 to 28	310
Poultry (without skin), light and dark, cooked	3 oz	25	145 to 175
Milk:			
Nonfat	1 c	9	90
Whole	1 c	9	160
These are other good sources of protein that you could use instead:			
Vegetables, cooked:			
Broccoli	1 medium stalk	6	45
Brussels sprouts	1 c	7	55
Cauliflower	1 c	3	30
Greens	1 c	3 to 7	30 to 65
Legumes:			
Dried, cooked	½ c	7 to 8	90 to 115
Mung sprouts, raw	½ c	2	20
Tofu (soybean curd)	4 oz	9	85
You can also get significant quantities of protein from these foods (if you can afford the kcalories):			
Cereal grain products:			
Barley, whole grain, cooked	½ c	4	135
Bran, unprocessed	½ c	4	55
Bran cereal (100% bran), uncooked	½ c	5	90
Breads	1 slice	2 to 3	60 to 80
Cornmeal, unrefined ground, uncooked	½ c	5	215
Millet, whole grain, cooked	½ c	3	95
Oatmeal, cooked	1 c	5	130
Pasta, enriched, cooked	1 c	5 to 7	155 to 200
Rice, cooked	1 c	4 to 5	225 to 230
Wheat, bulgur, cooked	½ c	7	225
Wheat, cracked, cooked	½ c	4	110
Wheat berries, cooked	½ c	5	110
Starchy vegetables:			
Corn	1 medium ear or ½ c	3	70
Peas, fresh	1 c	9	115
Potato, baked	1 large	4	145
Winter squash, baked	1 c	4	130
Miscellaneous:			
Nut butters[a]	1 tbsp	4	95
Nuts[a]	2 tbsp	2 to 5	80 to 115
Seeds[a]	2 tbsp	3 to 5	95 to 100
Yeast, brewer's	2 tbsp	6	40 to 45

[a]These items are high in fat and should be used in moderation.

Source: Adapted from Society for Nutrition Education materials.

than enough of all the essential amino acids, and can sustain people in good health, as long as there are not too many empty-kcalorie foods in the diet.

Assuming that the vegan consumes enough energy, the possibility of a protein deficiency is remote. Only when fruits and certain poorly chosen vegetables define the core of the diet might protein deficiency result. Fruits provide adequate energy, but most are low in protein. Even advocates of a fruitarian diet include nuts and seeds regularly. The root vegetable cassava, which is used as the diet's major staple food in many developing countries, provides another instance of adequate energy but inadequate protein.

Vegans can improve the quality of protein consumed by practicing mutual supplementation, but they should probably not be overly concerned about it. A wiser use of time and energy is to obtain, prepare, and eat a wide variety of foods from the vegetarian four food groups (see Table 2–1 in Chapter 2) to obtain adequate energy, protein, and other nutrients.

To ease obtaining a variety of foods, convenience foods and other new food products are available for vegetarians. Among them are meat replacements— textured vegetable-protein products formulated to look and taste like meat, fish, or poultry. Many of these are designed to match the known nutrient contents of animal-protein foods, but sometimes they fall short. Instead of relying on these products completely, a wise vegetarian would learn to use combinations of whole foods as suggested in Figure 6–12.

meat replacement: a textured vegetable-protein product formulated to look and taste like meat, fish, or poultry.

An advantage of vegetarian protein foods is that they are generally lower in fat than meats and are often higher in fiber and richer in certain vitamins and minerals as well. Vegetarians can therefore enjoy a nutritious diet that is low in fat, provided that they also limit other high-fat foods like butter, cream cheese, sour cream, cheese, nuts, and avocados.

Protein and Amino Acid Supplements

Health food stores advertise a wide variety of health claims to encourage people to take protein and amino acid supplements. Why do people take these supplements? Athletes take them to build muscle. Dieters take them to spare their bodies' protein while losing weight. Women take them to improve the strength of their fingernails. People take individual amino acid supplements to cure herpes, to make themselves sleep better, to lose weight, and to relieve depression. As is the case with many magic solutions to health problems, protein and amino acid supplements don't work these miracles, and they can be harmful.

Muscle work builds muscle; protein supplements do not, and athletes do not need them. Athletes need, instead, a well-balanced diet that provides sufficient dietary protein and adequate energy. Food energy spares body protein; carbohydrate and fat serve this purpose well. Fingernails remain unaffected by protein supplements, provided the diet is otherwise adequate. Normal, healthy people never need protein supplements.

Furthermore, protein supplements are expensive, less well digested than protein-rich foods, and when used as replacements for such foods, often downright dangerous. The "liquid protein" diet, advocated some years ago for weight loss, caused deaths in many users; even some physician-supervised protein-sparing modified fasts based on liquid protein have caused abnormal heart rhythms.[11] The Food and Drug Administration requires all very-low-kcalorie (below 400-kcalorie) protein diets to carry warnings that their use as a total diet without medical supervision "may cause serious illness or death."

As for amino acid supplements, they, too, are unnecessary and can be dangerous.[12] The body is designed to handle whole proteins best. It breaks proteins down into dipeptides and tripeptides, then splits these a few at a time, simultaneously absorbing amino acids into the blood. When proteins are predigested in a laboratory and served up as mixtures of single amino acids, the absorptive mechanism cannot accommodate them all at once, so fewer are digested and absorbed. When amino acids are presented singly, severe imbalances and toxicities can occur. Groups of chemically similar amino acids compete for the carriers that absorb them into the blood, and an excess of one amino acid can create such demand for a carrier that it prevents the absorption of another amino acid. The result is a deficiency. Every amino acid is toxic when taken in excess, for this and other reasons less well understood. In some cases, *excess* means not very much above normal daily intake levels.

In two cases, recommendations of amino acids have led to widespread public use—lysine to prevent or relieve the infections that cause herpes cold sores and sexually transmitted diseases; and tryptophan to relieve pain, depression, and insomnia. In both cases, enthusiastic popular reports and careful scientific experiments are at odds. Lysine does not relieve or cure herpes infections, and if long-term use helps prevent them, it does so only in some individuals and with unknown associated risks.[13] Tryptophan does have some interesting effects with respect to pain and sleep in responsive individuals.[14] Its use is still experimental, though, and requires medical supervision. Tryptophan does not affect depression, and people taking large doses may be damaging their livers.[15] It is safer to receive tryptophan and other amino acids in protein foods, taken with a little carbohydrate to facilitate uptake in the body—a turkey sandwich, for example. With all that we know about science, it is hard to improve on nature.

■ Study Questions

1. How do proteins differ from carbohydrates and fats in their chemical structure? Describe amino acids in terms of their structure, sequence, and shaping of a protein.
2. What are enzymes? What is their role in chemical reactions?
3. Describe the roles proteins serve in the human body.
4. What determines the quality of dietary protein? Define nitrogen balance, and name conditions that are associated with zero, positive, and negative balances.
5. What factors are considered in establishing recommended protein intakes?
6. Which food lists of the exchange system supply protein in abundance? In moderation? Not at all?

■ Notes

1. A. Rosenfeld, The great protein hunt, *Science 81*, January–February 1981, pp. 64–67.
2. S. A. Laidlaw, Indispensable amino acids, *Nutrition and the M.D.*, August 1986, pp. 1–3; K. C. Hayes, Taurine requirements in primates, *Nutrition Reviews* 43 (1985): 65–70.
3. W. J. Visek, Arginine needs, physiological state and usual diets: A reevaluation, *Journal of Nutrition* 116 (1986): 36–46.
4. S. N. Gershoff, Science—Neglected ingredient of nutrition policy, *Journal of the American Dietetic Association* 70 (1977): 471.
5. Infections and undernutrition, *Nutrition Reviews* 40 (1982): 119–128.

SELF STUDY *Evaluate Your Protein Intake*

These exercises make use of the information you recorded on Forms 1 to 3. (Appendix K provides the necessary forms.)

1. How many grams of protein do you consume in a day?
2. How many kcalories does this represent? (Remember, 1 gram of protein contributes 4 kcalories.)
3. What percentage of your total kcalories is contributed by protein?
4. Dietary guidelines suggest that protein should contribute about 10 to 15 percent of total kcalories. How does your protein intake compare with this recommendation? (Note: If you are on a kcalorie-restricted diet, then a higher percentage of your kcalories should come from protein. See the self-study exercise for Chapter 12.) If your protein intake is out of line, what foods could you consume more of—or less of—to bring it into line?
5. Calculate your protein RDA (0.8 grams per kilogram of body weight). Is it similar to the RDA for an "average" person of your age and sex as shown in the RDA tables (inside front cover, left)?
6. Compare your average daily protein intake with your RDA. On the average, about what percentage of your RDA for protein are you consuming each day? If you are "average" and healthy, the RDA is probably a generous recommendation for you, and yet you may be eating more than the recommendation. This means that you may be spending protein prices for an energy nutrient. What substitutions could you make in your day's food choices so that you would derive from carbohydrate, rather than from protein, the kcalories you needed for energy?
7. How many of your protein grams are from animal, and how many from plant, foods? Assuming that the animal protein is all of high quality, no more than 20 percent of your total protein need come from this source. Should you alter the ratio of plant to animal protein in your diet? If you did, what effect would this have on the total *fat* content of your diet?
8. How is your protein intake distributed through the day? (At what times do you eat how many grams of protein each time?) Do you have amino acids at breakfast time to help maintain your blood glucose supply from carbohydrate? At lunchtime, to replenish dwindling pools? At dinnertime, to sustain you through the evening?

6. Dietary protein and body fat distribution, *Nutrition Reviews* 40 (1982): 89–90.
7. M. G. Holl and L. H. Allen, Comparative effects of meals high in protein, sucrose, or starch on human mineral metabolism and insulin secretion, *American Journal of Clinical Nutrition* 48 (1988): 1219–1225; M. B. Zemel, Calcium utilization: Effect of varying level and source of dietary protein, *American Journal of Clinical Nutrition* 48 (1988): 880–883.
8. K. K. Carroll, Dietary protein and heart disease, *Nutrition and the M.D.*, June 1985.
9. High protein diets and bone homeostasis, *Nutrition Reviews* 39 (1981): 11–13.
10. K. Akers, *A Vegetarian Sourcebook* (New York: Putnam, 1983).
11. R. A. Lantigua and coauthors, Cardiac arrhythmias associated with a liquid protein diet for the treatment of obesity, *New England Journal of Medicine* 303 (1980): 735–738.
12. N. J. Benevenga and R. D. Steele, Adverse effects of excessive consumption of amino acids, *Annual Review of Nutrition* 4 (1984): 157–181.
13. Myth of the month: Lysine for herpes, *Nutrition and the M.D.*, December 1984, p. 4.
14. L. J. Fitten, J. Profita, and T. G. Bidder, L-tryptophan as a hypnotic in special patients, *Journal of the American Geriatrics Society* 33 (1985): 294–297.
15. M. E. Trulson and H. W. Sampson, Ultrastructural changes of the liver following L-tryptophan ingestion, *Journal of Nutrition* 116 (1986): 1109–1115.

Nutrition without Meat

"I eat only foods of plant origin. I'm sure that I am healthier than people who eat foods derived from animals."

"I disagree. I think that I am healthier than you because I eat foods from plants *and* dairy products such as eggs, cheese, and milk."

"No, I'm sure that I'm healthier than either of you two. I eat all foods except red meats. I include poultry and fish in my diet and I'm sure it's the best way to eat."

"Wait a minute. I eat better than all of you. I eat all foods in moderation. You can't design a truly adequate diet without using at least some red meat."

Who's right? The answer, of course, has more to do with the *nutrients* you get than with the foods you choose to get them from. Any of the four people just quoted may be well or poorly nourished depending on the amounts, balance, and variety of foods in the particular diet he or she regularly eats. For the sake of people who choose to omit red meats, all meats, or all animal-derived foods from their diets, this highlight contrasts the various foodways and offers pointers on obtaining nutrition from all of them. After all, some 2 million people in the United States eat no meat at all. If they plan their diets right, they can be perfectly healthy, and in some cases ever healthier than the average meat eater.

Meat in the Diet

Anyone who appreciates the indispensability of protein in nutrition will make conscientious efforts to get enough daily. To many people this means making sure to eat plenty of meat. The idea that dietary protein means "meat" seems reasonable at first glance. A review of the exchange lists will quickly show that among the six lists, the meats and meat alternates

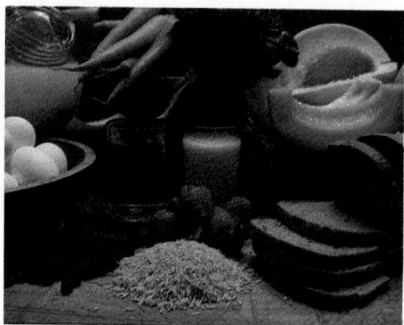
Lacto-ovo-vegetarians obtain their protein from milk, legumes, eggs, whole-grains, and vegetables.

are the only foods other than those on the milk list that provide substantial quantities of protein (7 grams per ounce of meat, as compared with 8 grams per cup of milk). Fruits and fats provide no protein, and the items from the vegetable list and the starch/bread list seem to provide only a little protein—2 to 3 grams per portion. (Withhold judgment on these latter items, however. At the end, this discussion will show that their protein contributions are highly significant.)

Many people plan their meals centered around meat. They first decide what cut of beef, ham, pork, lamb, poultry, or fish to prepare and then fill in the menu with an accompanying "starch" (potato, rice, or noodles), salad or other vegetable, and bread.

In contrast, nonmeat eaters omit meat from their diets completely. They fill their dinner plates with legumes, grains, vegetables, and fruits. Many include milk products and eggs and some may occasionally include fish or poultry. (Within the nonmeat eater category, subgroups differ in their selections of foods to include or exclude from the diet.[1] The Miniglossary defines vegetarian subgroups for your reference.)

If you were to ask a group of nonmeat eaters why they have chosen to omit meat from their diets, you would receive a variety of answers. Their answers might reflect health attitudes, taste preferences, philosophies, or religions. Regardless of the specifics, your general impression would be that these people are conscious of their food selections. This may not seem unusual until you consider that many people give little or no thought to the foods they select to eat—if they like them, they eat them. The awareness that the foods a person eats may bring benefits or harm is laudable, and everyone can adopt it, regardless of whether they eat meat.

When researchers categorize people based on their consumption of meat, they usually speak of vegetarians versus nonvegetarians, or omnivores. Because these terms are practically universally used in research, this highlight has to use them in referring to that research. However, it might be desirable to abandon the term *vegetarian*, which often connotes a philosophical or religious attitude, and to recognize that people's dietary choices fall along a continuum—from one end, where a person eats no foods from the meat list, to the other end, where a person eats generous quantities of meat items at every meal. One of the missions of this highlight is to find the *range* of meat consumption compatible with the most health benefits.

Positive Health Aspects of Meatless Diets

Researchers have studied vegetarians to further their knowledge of the relationships between diet and health. This would be an ideal research situation if the only difference between vegetarians and others was their consumption of meat. Of course, the study of people is rarely so simple. Many vegetarians have adopted lifestyles that differ from those of meat eaters in other ways that affect health besides eating a no-meat diet. Of course there are exceptions, but typically, vegetarians do not smoke; they use alcohol in moderation (if at all); they are usually physically active; and they cultivate an awareness of their bodies' well-being.

The following paragraphs provide a summary of the findings from research comparing vegetarians with nonvegetarians.[2] Many of the vegetarians in these studies are Seventh-Day Adventists, a religious group whose foodways center on a lacto-ovo-vegetarian diet (one that includes milk and eggs, but excludes meat, poultry, and fish).

Body Weight

The vegetarians who have been studied have tended to be closer to a healthy body weight than nonvegetarians. As this book repeatedly mentions, obesity impairs health in a number of ways. Thus these vegetarians may have a health advantage by virtue of their maintaining appropriate body weight.

Exactly why these vegetarians are leaner than nonvegetarians remains unclear. Perhaps it is simply because they consciously control their food intakes and exercising habits. Then again, it may be a fringe benefit of their diet, which tends to be low in fat and high in bulky foods containing complex carbohydrates and fiber, and therefore lower in kcalories than the average diet based on meat. The healthy body weight, combined with a high intake of complex carbohydrates and fiber, lowers the risk of several diseases, including diabetes.

Blood Pressure

In some studies, vegetarians have lower blood pressure than nonvegetarians; in others, there is no difference. Various combinations of lifestyle factors and diet seem to influence blood pressure. Among lifestyle factors, smoking and alcohol intake raise blood pressure, and exercise lowers it. That many vegetarians forgo smoking and alcohol and embrace exercise may explain their lower blood pressure. However, diet alone may be responsible, for in one group of volunteers, blood pressure declined during the period of a vegetarian diet and rose again during the omnivore diet.[3] The effect of a vegetarian diet on blood pressure remains apparent even when comparing vegetarians with nonsmoking nonvegetarians. Perhaps, most important, appropriate body weight helps to maintain appropriate blood pressure.

Coronary Artery Disease

Fewer vegetarians suffer from diseases of the heart and arteries than meat eaters, even when they are compared with nonsmoking meat eaters. The dietary factor most directly related to coronary artery disease is the lipids—especially saturated fat and cholesterol. When vegetarians are fed meat, which contains saturated fat and cholesterol, their lipid profiles change for the worse; when nonvegetarians are fed a low-fat vegetarian diet, their lipid profiles improve. In general, the typical vegetarian diet is lower in total fat, saturated fatty acids, and cholesterol, and higher in dietary fiber, than the typical nonvegetarian diet.

GI Disorders

Constipation and diverticular disease are less common in people who consume a vegetarian or semivegetarian diet that is high in dietary fiber than in people who consume a typical meat-based diet. The types and amounts of dietary fiber that influence the health of the digestive system were described in Chapter 4.

Cancer

Seventh-Day Adventists have a mortality rate from cancer about one-half to two-thirds that of the rest of the population, even when cancers linked to smoking and alcohol are taken out of the picture. It is possible that their low cancer mortality may be due to their low meat intakes, their high intakes of vegetables and cereal grains, or both—or to other lifestyle factors. In general, studies of populations have suggested that low cancer rates correlate with low meat and high vegetable and grain intakes.

Studies of closely matched groups of people in which researchers study dietary factors in a context relatively free of interference by nondiet variables also implicate diet in cancer causation. In various studies, for example, people with colon cancer have been seen to eat more meat, less fiber, and more saturated fat than others without cancer.[4] Researchers have begun to close in on the way high-fat, high-protein, low-fiber diets can create an unfavorable environment in the human colon which predisposes some people to colon cancer.[5]

In general, people who practice a vegetarian diet reduce their risks of several chronic degenerative diseases, including obesity, coronary artery disease, hypertension, diabetes, cancer, and others.[6] Their diets tend to be high in complex carbohydrates and fiber and low in total fat, saturated fat, and cholesterol—all practices beneficial to health.

Negative Health Aspects of Meatless Diets

For the most part, the negative health aspects of meatless diets reflect poor diet planning, for careful attention to energy intake and specific problem nutrients can ensure adequacy. Diet planning during pregnancy, lactation, infancy, childhood, and illness, in particular, must reflect the certain

---

Miniglossary

lactovegetarians: people who include milk or milk products, but exclude meat, poultry, fish, seafood, and eggs from their diets.

   lacto = milk

lacto-ovo-vegetarians: people who include milk or milk products and eggs, but exclude meat, poultry, fish, and seafood from their diets.

   ovo = egg

omnivores: people who have no formal restriction on the eating of any type or group of animal-derived foods.

semivegetarians: people who include some, but not all, groups of animal-derived foods in their diets; they usually exclude meat, and may occasionally include poultry, fish, and seafood; also called **partial vegetarians**.

vegans: people who exclude all animal-derived foods (including meat, poultry, fish, eggs, and dairy products) from their diets; also called **pure vegetarians** or **total vegetarians**.

vegetarians: a general term used to describe people who exclude meat, poultry, fish, or other animal-derived foods from their diets.

---

increases in energy and nutrient needs during those times—for the consequences of poor nutrition can be great. For example, vegetarian women may enter pregnancy too lean and fail to gain enough weight during pregnancy to support normal growth and development of their infants.

Few lactovegetarians or lacto-ovo-vegetarians, whose diets include milk products or milk products and eggs, have nutrient deficiency concerns.[7] For the vegan who excludes all animal products, achieving adequate energy and nutrient intakes may be troublesome, particularly for children. Vegan diets usually fail to provide the nourishment required to support the full growth of a child, within a small enough bulk of food for the child to eat.[8] A vegan child is likely to get full before eating enough food to meet nutrient needs. Vegan children therefore tend to be smaller in height and lighter in weight than meat-eating children.[9] Perhaps the most significant limiting factor in the rate of growth of vegan children is their low food energy intakes.[10] Meat, which

contains abundant protein, iron, and food energy in a small bulk, could significantly improve the nutritive value of such a vegan child's diet. Plant foods best suited to meet protein and energy needs in a small volume are cereals, legumes, and nuts; these should be emphasized in a vegan child's diet.

When protein is supplied only by plant foods, the standard protein recommendations may be inadequate to support the growth of a vegan child.[11] For normal growth and health, vegan children may require protein intakes even greater than the RDA.

Vegans, like all vegetarians, must pay particular attention to vitamin B_{12}, vitamin D, calcium, iron, and zinc. The next section, on diet planning, will provide suggestions to meet these nutrient needs.

Diet Planning without Meat

In Chapter 2, the watchwords for diet planning were introduced: adequacy, balance, kcalorie control, moderation, and variety. These principles work together to help a person achieve a

healthy diet. For example, variety ensures adequacy and balance and kcalorie control requires moderation. When a person overemphasizes or underemphasizes a group of foods (such as meat, fish, and poultry), careful attention to certain principles can help to keep them in harmony. For example, meat eaters might benefit their health most by attending to balance and moderation. In contrast, people who eat no meat need most to emphasize nutrient adequacy, for they are using diets that exclude at least one whole category of foods. The foods they do eat include fruits; vegetables; whole-grain breads and cereals; nuts and seeds; legumes; and for many vegetarians, low-fat milk products and a limited number of eggs. Both vegetarian and nonvegetarian diet plans have the potential to benefit health, just as both can be detrimental to health when overloaded with nutrient-poor foods, such as sweets and fatty foods.

A well-planned meatless diet can provide adequate amounts of all the nutrients a person needs for good health. The Four Food Group Plan suggests that vegetarians use legumes to the same extent that meat eaters use meat, and calcium-fortified soy milk if they don't use milk. In general, such a plan can provide an adequate intake of many of the nutrients that commonly present problems to vegetarians, but it can fall short on meeting energy needs.[12] To increase energy intake and improve the amino acid balance of the diet, a vegetarian could include a serving of nuts and seeds, an additional one to four servings of vegetables and fruits, and an additional three to five servings of grains and cereals using the Four Food Group Plan. Nutrients that commonly present problems to vegetarians include iron, zinc, calcium, and vitamins B_{12} and D.

Iron presents a problem for many people, and particularly people who exclude iron-rich meats from their diets. Vegetarians can obtain iron from plant foods such as dark green, leafy vegetables, iron-fortified cereals, and whole grains. Absorption of iron can be enhanced by eating vitamin C-rich foods with these foods.

Zinc is similar to iron in that it is difficult for many people to get enough in their diets and that its bioavailability from foods varies widely. Consider that half of the zinc in the average diet comes from meat, fish, and poultry and that zinc from plant sources such as cereals and legumes is of low bioavailability (due to the presence of fiber and the binders phytate and oxalate). In addition, soy products which are commonly used as meat substitutes, impair zinc bioavailability. Consequently, vegetarian diets are often limited in zinc quantity, quality, or both. Perhaps the best advice to vegetarians regarding zinc is to limit soy, fiber, phytate, and oxalate intake; eat a variety of nutrient-dense foods; and maintain an adequate energy intake.[13]

Calcium deficiency in vegetarians who include milk products in their diets is rare. For those who exclude milk products, calcium-fortified foods are necessary. It is worth noting that not all soy milk is rich in calcium; the calcium-fortified type is recommended.

Because the requirement for vitamin B_{12} is so small and because this vitamin is found in all animal-derived foods, lactovegetarians and lacto-ovo-vegetarians are unlikely to be vitamin B_{12} deficient. Vegans, on the other hand, risk vitamin B_{12} deficiency.[14] They must rely on vitamin B_{12}–fortified sources. Fermented plant products such as tempeh, made from soy sauce, may contain some vitamin B_{12} contributed by the bacteria that did the fermenting, but unfortunately, much of the vitamin B_{12} found in these products may be an inactive form of the vitamin.[15] Vegans may need to use soy milk that is fortified with vitamin B_{12} (as well as calcium) or breakfast cereals fortified with vitamin B_{12} (read the label). Alternatively, they can take

vitamin B_{12} supplements to ensure against vitamin B_{12} deficiency.

For people who do not use vitamin D–fortified milk and who do not receive enough sunlight exposure to produce adequate amounts of vitamin D, supplements may be warranted. This is particularly important for children and older adults.

Protein is usually not a problem nutrient for vegetarians, even though their intakes may be lower than those of meat eaters. Protein intakes are usually satisfactory when energy intakes are adequate and protein sources varied.[16] A mixture of proteins from whole grains, legumes, seeds, nuts, and vegetables can provide adequate amounts of all the needed amino acids. A protein intake somewhat lower than that most people consume may actually be beneficial in reducing the risk of osteoporosis (recall from Chapter 6 that diets high in protein promote calcium excretion, thus depleting the bones of their calcium). Meat eaters moderating their protein intakes could also lower their dietary fat intakes, since foods high in protein are often high in fat.

Some people find it easiest and most acceptable to meet current dietary recommendations by following a vegetarian diet.[17] Such diets can meet all of the *NRC Recommendations* that Chapter 2 presented as easily as, if not more easily than, a nonvegetarian diet.

The *NRC Report* suggests limiting fat intake to 30 percent of total kcalorie intake.[18] Because the meat, milk, and fat lists are the only ones to contribute fat, everyone can concentrate their efforts to limit fat on just those lists. To reduce fat and cholesterol intake:

- From the meat list, select fish, poultry without skin, and lean meats.
- From the milk list, select low-fat or nonfat dairy products.
- From the fat list, limit oils, fats, and fried and other fatty foods.

To limit fat intake, vegetarians need only be concerned with the last two lists; and vegans, with only the last list. However, a word of caution is in order: Vegetarian diets can be high in fat. Nuts, fried foods, cheeses, salad dressings, and desserts raise fat and food energy intake.

The *NRC Recommendations* advise the consumption of six servings of grains and five servings of vegetables and fruits. This recommendation is easy to meet with a vegetarian diet. Six servings from the starch/bread list would provide 18 grams of protein, and if all five servings of vegetables and fruits were from the vegetable list, they would provide 10 grams more. That's 28 grams of protein from the very items whose protein contribution seemed insignificant at the start. Two to three servings of milk (to meet calcium recommendations) provides 16 to 24 *more* grams of protein. With these choices made and selections from the meat alternate group still to go, a diet planner cannot fail to meet protein needs.

Obviously, by selecting the appropriate number of servings from the starch/bread list, the vegetable list, and the milk list, a person can meet the RDA for protein without using any meat. The *NRC Recommendations* advise limiting protein to between 0.8 and 1.6 grams per kilogram body weight. While it does not recommend against eating meat, it does suggest consuming meat in smaller and fewer portions than is typical of U.S. diets. Members of the NRC committee suggest that, in general, two 3-ounce servings of meat per day, at most, are needed.[19] Two 3-ounce servings of meat adds 42 grams of protein to the day's intake. This level of intake (86 to 94 grams protein) satisfies the RDA for a person weighing up to 250 pounds and approaches the upper limit for a 135-pound person. With the evidence pointing to the health advantages of a vegetarian diet, perhaps between 0 and 6 ounces of meat daily would best serve the needs of most people.

For the most part, it seems that vegetarians can be as healthy as, if not healthier than, nonvegetarians. However, vegetarian diets hold no magical curative powers. Meat eaters would not be wise simply to toss meat out of their diets; they can make their diets healthful by choosing foods with the dietary recommendations in mind. (Similarly, vegetarian diets are best when wise food selections are made.) Remember, too, that diet is but one factor influencing health. Whatever a diet consists of, its context is important, too: a lifestyle of no smoking; consuming alcohol in moderation, if at all; regular physical activity; adequate rest; and medical attention when needed.

NOTES

1. B. M. Calkins, Executive summary of the congress, *American Journal of Clinical Nutrition* 48 (1988): 709–711.

2. J. T. Dwyer, Health aspects of vegetarian diets, *American Journal of Clinical Nutrition* 48 (1988): 712–738.

3. L. J. Beilin and coauthors, Vegetarian diet and blood pressure levels: Incidental or causal association? *American Journal of Clinical Nutrition* 48 (1988): 806–810.

4. M. B. Grosvenor, Diet and colon cancer, *Nutrition and the M.D.*, April 1989; S. A. Bingham, Meat, starch, and nonstarch polysaccharides and large bowel cancer, *American Journal of Clinical Nutrition* 48 (1988): 762–76; B. S. Reddy and coauthors, Nutrition and its relationship to cancer, *Advances in Cancer Research* 32 (1980): 238–245.

5. M. I. McBurney, P. J. Van Soest, and J. L. Jeraci, Colonic carcinogenesis: The microbial feast or famine mechanism, *Nutrition and Cancer* 10 (1987): 23–28.

6. Position of the American Dietetic Association: Vegetarian diets, *Journal of the American Dietetic Association* 88 (1988): 351–355.

7. Position of the American Dietetic Association, 1988.

8. C. Jacobs and J. T. Dwyer, Vegetarian children: appropriate and inappropriate diets, *American Journal of Clinical Nutrition* 48 (1988): 811–818.

9. T. A. B. Sanders, Growth and development of British vegan children, *American Journal of Clinical Nutrition* 48 (1988): 822- 825.

10. Sanders, 1988.

11. P. B. Acosta, Availability of essential amino acids and nitrogen in vegan diets, *American Journal of Clinical Nutrition* 48 (1988): 868–874.

12. P. B. Mutch, Food guides for the vegetarians, *American Journal of Clinical Nutrition* 48 (1988): 913–919.

13. J. Freeland-Graves, Mineral adequacy of vegetarian diets, *American Journal of Clinical Nutrition* 48 (1988): 859–862.

14. V. Herbert, Vitamin B-12: Plant sources, requirements, and assay, *American Journal of Clinical Nutrition* 48 (1988): 852–858.

15. Position of the American Dietetic Association, 1988.

16. Dwyer, 1988.

17. Position of the American Dietetic Association, 1988.

18. National Academy of Sciences report, *Diet and Health: Implications for Reducing Chronic Disease Risk*, as partially reprinted verbatim in *Nutrition Reviews* 47 (1989): 142–149.

19. *The Nation's Health*, a newsletter published by the American Public Health Association, April 1989, p. 15.

7

Metabolism: Nutrient Transformations and Interactions

Contents

The compound acetyl CoA, central to energy metabolism, is made in part from the B vitamin pantothenic acid. These are pantothenic acid crystals viewed under a microscope.

169

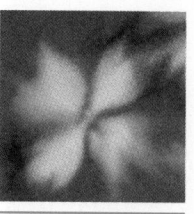

The mission of this chapter is to shed some light on how the body manages its energy supply. Along the way, it answers some of the questions people often ask about diets. What makes a person gain weight? Are carbohydrate-rich foods more fattening than other foods? What's the best way to lose weight? Is fasting safe? The answers to these questions lie in an understanding of metabolism.

metabolism: the sum total of all the chemical reactions that go on in living cells. **Energy metabolism** includes all the reactions by which the body obtains and uses the energy from food.

meta = among
bole = change

Metabolism is defined as the sum total of all the chemical reactions that go on in living cells. Energy metabolism includes all the ways the body obtains and uses energy from food. The previous three chapters laid the groundwork for the study of metabolism; a brief review may be helpful. (Protein's amino acids are not, strictly speaking, primarily energy nutrients, but they can flow into energy pathways if needed, so they are included.)

■ *Starting Points*

The energy-yielding nutrients that are found in foods—carbohydrates, fats, and proteins—are broken down during digestion into basic units that are absorbed into the blood. Four of these basic units are seen throughout the metabolic transformations that follow, and they appear again and again in this chapter (see Figure 7–1):

- From carbohydrates—glucose.
- From fats—glycerol and fatty acids.
- From proteins—amino acids.

■ **FIGURE 7–1**
Basic Units from Carbohydrates, Lipids, and Proteins after Digestion
Each square represents a carbon atom; the triangles represent nitrogen-containing amino groups.
A. *Carbohydrates*. During digestion, all available carbohydrates are broken down to monosaccharides and absorbed into the blood. Fructose and galactose are then converted by the liver to glucose (or molcules that are metabolized similarly to glucose). To follow carbohydrate through metabolism, we will simply follow glucose.
B. *Lipids*. Most of the dietary lipids are triglycerides, composed of two basic units—glycerol and fatty acids. To follow lipids through metabolism, we will follow glycerol and fatty acids.
C. *Proteins*. Proteins are ultimately digested to amino acids; these are the units we will follow through metabolism. Amino acids contain different numbers of carbon atoms.

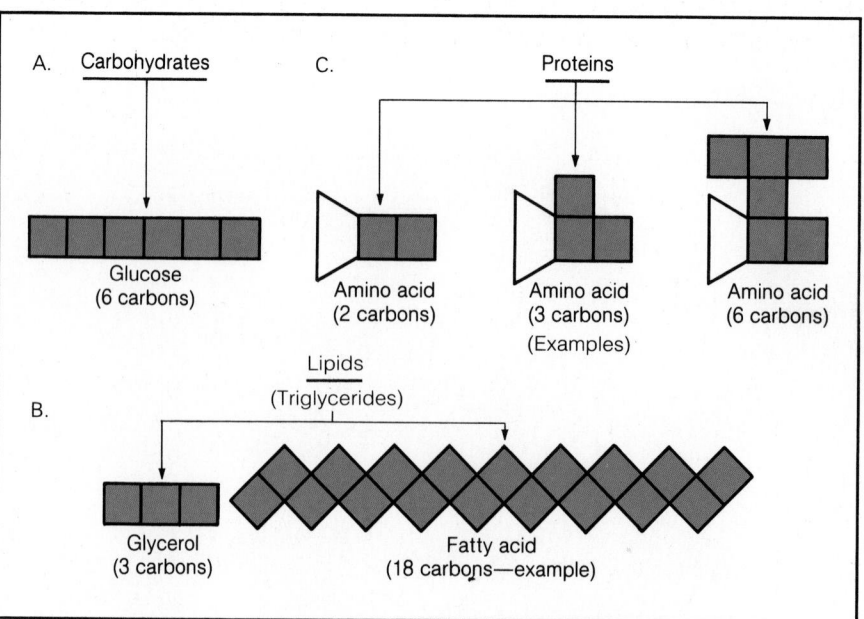

■ *Building Body Compounds*

You already know what becomes of these basic units when their energy is not needed by the cells; they are used to build body compounds. Glucose units may be joined together to make glycogen chains. Glycerol and fatty acids may be assembled into triglycerides. Amino acids may be used to make proteins. These building reactions, in which simple compounds are put together to form larger, more complex structures, involve doing work and so require energy. They are called anabolic reactions and this book represents them by ''up'' arrows in diagrams such as those in Figure 7–2.

anabolism (an-ABB-o-lism): reactions in which small molecules are put together to build larger ones. Anabolic reactions consume energy and often involve reduction (a type of chemical reaction in which a substance gains electrons; see Appendix B).

ana = up

■ *Breaking Down Nutrients for Energy*

If the body needs energy, it may break apart any or all of these four units into smaller fragments. The breakdown reactions are called catabolic reactions. They release energy and are represented by ''down'' arrows in diagrams. Much of the body's metabolic work is done with the help of enzymes in the liver cells, and all of the reactions described in this chapter can take place there (the accompanying box offers a preview). Other cells, including those in the brain, muscles, glands, and other tissues, are also metabolically active.

A special compound is almost always involved when energy transfers are taking place. This compound, available in all cells, is ATP (adenosine triphosphate), the body's quick-energy molecule. The structure of ATP includes three phosphate groups that are attached together and that can be readily broken off when energy is needed. Hydrolysis of ATP splits off one or more phosphate groups and releases energy. Figure 7–3 explains how the

catabolism (ca-TAB-o-lism): reactions in which large molecules are broken down to smaller ones. Catabolic reactions usually release energy and often involve oxidation (a type of chemical reaction in which a substance loses electrons; see Appendix B).

kata = down

ATP (adenosine triphosphate): the body's high-energy compound composed of a purine (adenine), a sugar (ribose), and three phosphates. Another high-energy compound—**phosphocreatine (PC)**, which is used by muscles—is discussed in Chapter 13.

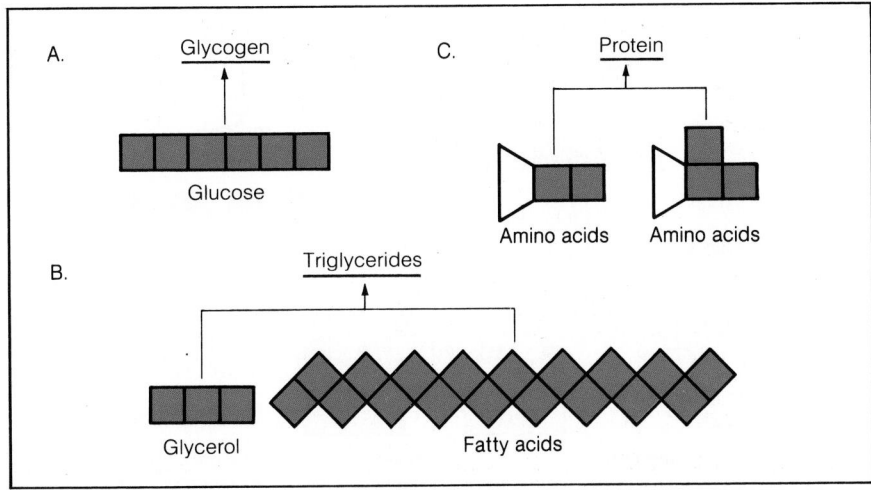

■ **FIGURE 7–2**
Anabolic Reactions
The following basic units are used to build body compounds:
A. *Carbohydrates.* Glycogen synthesis is an anabolic reaction that attaches glucose molecules into chains several thousand to hundreds of thousands of glucose molecules long, with branches at every ten or so glucose molecules. This branched structure provides numerous ends for glucose attachment and forms a dense storage system in a cell.
B. *Lipids.* Triglyceride synthesis is an anabolic reaction that attaches three fatty acids to glycerol.
C. *Protein.* Protein synthesis is an anabolic reaction that bonds amino acids together in chains.

As you read this list of liver functions, consider the multitude of problems liver dysfunction might cause. Chapter 26 describes the consequences of liver disorders and the dietary treatments for them.

Metabolic Work of the Liver

Here are *some* of the things the liver does with the nutrients that arrive there:

- *Carbohydrates.* Converts fructose and galactose to glucose. Removes excess glucose from the blood in response to insulin, and makes and stores glycogen. Releases glucose in response to glucagon.
- *Lipids.* Builds and breaks down triglycerides, phospholipids, and cholesterol as needed. Packages extra lipids in lipoproteins for export to other body organs. Manufactures bile to send to the gallbladder for use in digestion. Makes ketone bodies when called for.
- *Proteins.* Manufactures nonessential amino acids that are in short supply. Removes from circulation amino acids that are present in excess of need and deaminates them or converts them to other amino acids. Removes ammonia from the blood and converts it to urea to be sent to the kidneys for excretion. Makes other nitrogen-containing compounds the body needs (such as bases used in DNA and RNA). Makes plasma proteins such as albumin, antibodies, clotting factors, and anticlotting factors.
- *Other.* Detoxifies alcohol, drugs, wastes, and poisons. Stores vitamins, iron, and copper. Produces heat. Forms lymph.

■ **FIGURE 7–3**

ATP (adenosine triphosphate), the Body's Quick-Energy Molecule

As glucose and fat break down, some of their energy is used to build ATP molecules by attaching phosphate groups to molecules of adenosine diphosphate (ADP). ATP then releases energy when it is hydrolyzed to ADP plus phosphate. ADP is lower in energy than ATP; AMP (adenosine monophosphate) is even lower.

Note: Glycogen and fat are the body's long-term energy-storage compounds (sort of like bank accounts). ATP is the body's instant energy source, always available in every cell (like pocket money). Cell structures that ATP energy might be used to build include glycogen, fat, proteins, hormones, and others.

Half or more of the total original energy is lost as heat in all such reactions, accounting for the temperature-raising effect of metabolism. ATP can also break apart without doing work, and release all of its energy as heat, if needed.

A. Before ATP use.

A molecule of ATP with energy contained in the chemical bonds that hold its three phosphate groups in place.

An enzyme complex that can use ATP's energy to do work.

A molecule with a piece to be added to it.

B. During ATP use.

Breaking of bond to release energy

Bond formation

A phosphate group breaks off. The energy is used to attach the free piece to the growing molecule.

C. After ATP use.

A molecule of ADP and a free phosphate group produced as by-products.

The enzyme complex now ready to work again.

The growing molecule now one piece longer.

body uses ATP as its energy currency to build body structures, do other work, or generate heat from it, as needed.

At this point, it must be recalled that although glucose, glycerol, fatty acids, and amino acids are the basic units from food, they are composed of still smaller units, the atoms. During metabolism, the body actually separates these atoms from one another. To follow how this takes place, it will help to recall the structures of these compounds, introduced in earlier chapters. There is no need to remember exactly how they are put together; it is enough to remember how many carbons are in their "backbones." Figure 7–1 reviews this information.

A major point to notice in the following discussion is that compounds that have a 3-carbon skeleton can be used to make the vital nutrient glucose. Those that have 2-carbon skeletons cannot.

What happens to these compounds inside of cells can be best understood by starting with glucose. Two new names appear—pyruvate (3 C) and acetyl CoA (2 C)—and the rest of the story falls into place around them.

- Glucose has 6 C.
- Glycerol has 3 C.
- Fatty acids have multiples of 2 C.
- Amino acids have 2 or 3 or more C with N attached.
- 3 C can make glucose; 2 C cannot.

Glucose

The pathway by which glucose breaks down to smaller compounds is called glycolysis (glucose splitting). Figure 7–4 shows a simplified drawing of glycolysis, which actually involves several steps and several enzymes. At the end of this pathway, the 6-carbon glucose is split in half, releasing energy and forming two 3-carbon compounds. One is pyruvate, and the other is a 3-carbon compound that is converted to pyruvate, so that two pyruvates appear.

Should a cell "change its mind" after splitting glucose to pyruvate, it can reverse this glycolysis pathway and put the two halves back together to make glucose again.* For this reason, arrows are shown pointing both up and down between glucose and pyruvate.

glycolysis (gligh-COLL-ih-sis): the metabolic breakdown of glucose to pyruvate (see Appendix C).
glyco = glucose
lysis = breakdown

pyruvate (PIE-roo-vate): pyruvic acid, a 3-carbon compound derived from glucose and certain amino acids in metabolism. The term *pyruvate* means a salt of pyruvic acid. (Throughout this book the ending *-ate* is used interchangeably with *-ic acid*; for our purposes they mean the same thing.)

$$\begin{array}{c} CH_3 \\ | \\ C = O \\ | \\ COOH \end{array}$$

---

*The step from glucose to pyruvate is not *literally* reversible. That is, the enzyme that splits glucose can't also put it back together again. But other enzymes can make glucose from 3-carbon compounds, so in this sense it is reversible: the glucose is retrievable.

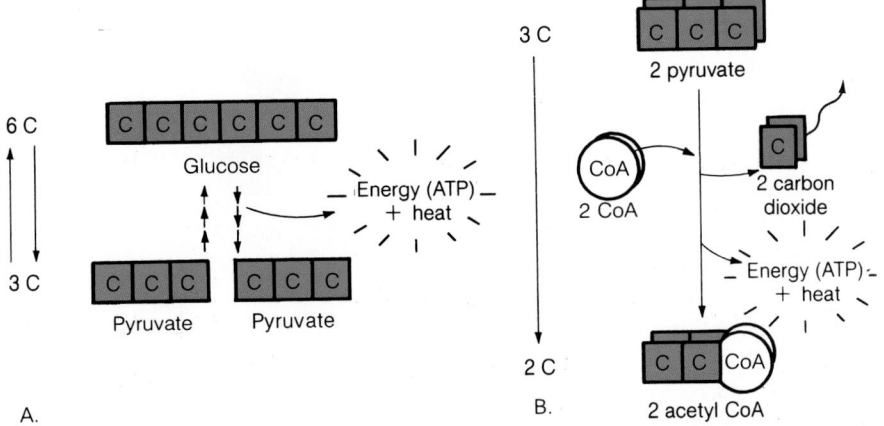

A.

B.

■ **FIGURE 7–4**
The Breakdown of Glucose to Acetyl CoA (simplified)
A. Glucose first splits to two 3-carbon compounds (pyruvate). The pathway is shown as reversible, because 3-carbon compounds such as these can be used to remake glucose. The pathway is known as glycolysis (glucose splitting).
B. Each pyruvate loses a carbon as carbon dioxide and picks up a molecule of CoA, becoming acetyl CoA. The arrow is shown as one-way (down), because the step is not reversible. Result (from 1 glucose): 2 carbon dioxide and 2 acetyl CoA.

CoA (coh-AY): the abbreviation for a compound described further in Chapter 8. As pyruvate loses a carbon and becomes a 2-carbon compound (**acetate**, or **acetic acid**), a molecule of CoA is attached to it, making **acetyl CoA** (ASS-eh-teel, or ah-SEET-il, coh-AY). For our purposes, acetyl CoA is just acetate, "a 2-carbon compound"; the CoA will not be discussed further here.

oxidation: a reaction in which electrons are removed from a molecule (see Appendix C). Often, this occurs when a molecule reacts with oxygen; hence the name. Oxidation reactions usually result in the release of energy. In chemical oxidation of nutrients, the energy released is largely chemical and mechanical; in oxidative combustion (burning), the energy released is mostly heat (and light).

In splitting glucose to pyruvate, the cell has obtained a little energy. No oxygen has been required thus far. More energy can be made available by splitting pyruvate further, but oxygen is needed for the next reaction. If the cell still needs energy and oxygen is available, it cleaves a carbon from each pyruvate.* The lone carbon is combined with oxygen obtained from water molecules to make carbon dioxide, which is released into the blood, circulated to the lungs, and breathed out. The 2-carbon compound that remains, acetate, picks up a molecule of CoA, becoming acetyl CoA.

The role of oxygen in metabolism is worth noticing, for it helps make many things understandable. As you breathe oxygen into your lungs, the oxygen is attached to a carrier (hemoglobin) in your red blood cells that brings it to the metabolizing cells to make it available for energy metabolism. You know you need to breathe harder when you are using energy faster (exercising), but you may not have realized what is happening. Energy nutrients are being broken down to provide that energy, and oxygen is always ultimately involved in the oxidation process.

Should the cell "change its mind" after splitting pyruvate and want to retrieve the shed carbons from carbon dioxide and remake glucose, it could not do so. The step from pyruvate to acetyl CoA is metabolically irreversible. It is a one-way step, and it is shown with only a "down" arrow in the diagram. Acetyl CoA is the building block for fatty acids, but it cannot be used to make glucose.

Finally, acetyl CoA may be split, yielding two more carbon dioxide molecules. This process is shown as a single step in Figure 7–5, but it actually takes place in a long sequence of reactions, known as the TCA cycle, the details of which are given in Appendix C. The energy released from acetyl CoA during the TCA cycle powers most of the cell's activities.

*If the cell still needs energy, and oxygen is not available, it converts pyruvate to lactic acid. Chapter 13 provides details.

■ **FIGURE 7–5**
The Breakdown of Acetyl CoA
In the TCA cycle, the remaining carbons are converted to carbon dioxide. Each CoA returns to pick up another acetate (coming from glucose, lipids, or protein). Net (from 2 acetate): 4 carbon dioxide.
The reactions by which the complete oxidation of acetyl CoA is accomplished are those of the **TCA** (tricarboxylic acid) **cycle,** or **Krebs cycle** (named for the biochemist who elucidated them), and **oxidative phosphorylation** (also known as the **electron transport chain**). The net result is that acetyl CoA splits, the carbons combine with oxygen, and the energy originally in the acetyl CoA is stored in ATP and similar compounds, thus becoming available for the body's use. For more details, see Appendix C.

Figure 7–6 combines Figures 7–4 and 7–5 to show the whole sequence of steps in glucose breakdown. In summary, the main steps in the metabolism of glucose are:

glucose
to
pyruvate
to
acetyl CoA
to
carbon dioxide.

Notice (again) that glucose can only be retrieved from the 3-carbon compounds in this sequence. Later steps are irreversible.

Most people spend their entire lives without ever making the acquaintance of pyruvate and acetyl CoA, yet chemists and nutritionists can become quite excited talking about them. The behavior of these two compounds explains the most interesting and important aspects of nutrition and makes it possible to answer questions that interest everyone. For example, in some athletic events the muscles use fat and glucose, while in others they absolutely depend on glucose only. The person who wants to use up body fat during exercise needs to know which kind of exercise to do (Chapter 13 provides the answers). For another example, during weight loss, the body derives energy sometimes from body fat and at other times from muscle protein. To avoid using muscle protein for energy during a weight-loss program, you have to know how to go about losing weight (Chapter 12 provides the details). Much of it hinges on which fuels can be converted to glucose and which cannot. The parts of protein and fat that can be converted to pyruvate (3 C) *can* provide glucose for the body; those that are converted to acetyl CoA (2 C) *cannot* provide glucose—and glucose is all-important.

How Fat Enters into Metabolism

Figure 7–7 shows how glycerol and fatty acids enter the pathways of metabolism. The glycerol (3 C) is easily converted to pyruvate (also 3 C, but with a different arrangement of H and OH on the C), and then may go either ''up'' to form glucose or ''down'' to form acetyl CoA and, finally, carbon dioxide. The fatty acids, however, cannot be broken down to 3-carbon compounds. They are taken apart, *2* carbons at a time, to make acetyl CoA. The arrow from pyruvate to acetyl CoA goes one way (down) only, showing that the fatty acids cannot be used to make glucose.

The significance of this is that fat, for the most part, cannot normally provide energy for the organs (brain and nervous system) that require glucose as fuel. Remember that almost all dietary lipid is triglyceride, and that the typical triglyceride consists of a molecule of glycerol (3 C) and three fatty acids (each about 18 C on the average, or about 54 C). True, the glycerol can yield glucose, but that represents only 3 out of 57 parts of the fat molecule—about 5 percent of its weight (see Figure 7–8). Thus fat is an inefficient source of glucose by itself. About 95 percent of fat cannot be converted to glucose. Only

■ **FIGURE 7–6**
Glucose Breakdown
These are the processes by which energy from glucose is made available to do the cells' work. Many chemical reactions are involved. Ultimately, glucose is completely disassembled to single-carbon fragments, and the fragments are combined with oxygen to form carbon dioxide. Much of the energy released is trapped and stored in ATP (see Figure 7–3). Details of the TCA cycle and the electron transport chain are shown in Appendix C.

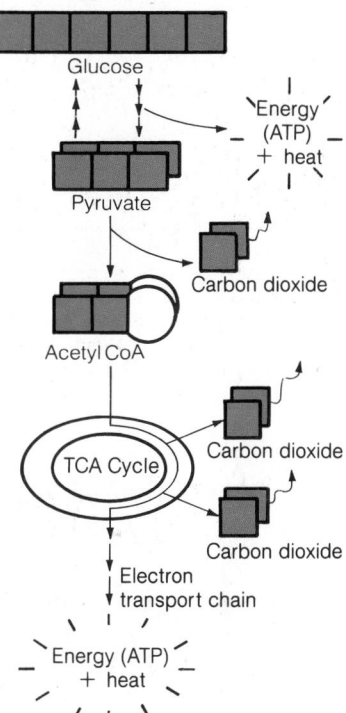

■ **FIGURE 7–7**

How Lipids Enter the Metabolic Path
Glycerol enters the metabolic path about midway between glucose and pyruvate and then is converted to pyruvate; fatty acids are converted to acetyl CoA. Net from an 18-carbon fatty acid: 9 acetyl CoA molecules, which are converted to 18 carbon dioxide molecules. Notice that you have seen the lighter part of this figure before—in Figure 7–6.

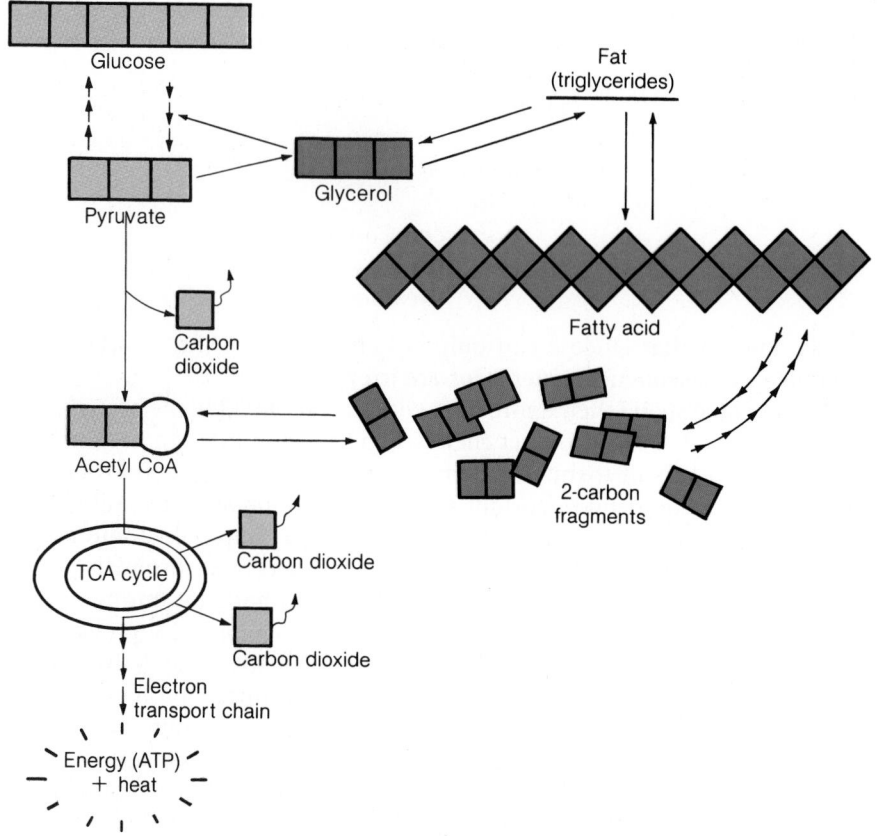

The making of glucose from protein or the glycerol portions of triglycerides is **gluconeogenesis** (gloo-co-nee-o-GEN-uh-sis). About 5% of fat (the glycerol portion of triglycerides) and most amino acids can be converted to glucose.

  gluco = glucose
  neo = new
  genesis = making

■ **FIGURE 7–8**

The Carbons of a Triglyceride
Only 3 of this triglyceride's 57 carbon atoms are in glycerol and can be converted to glucose.

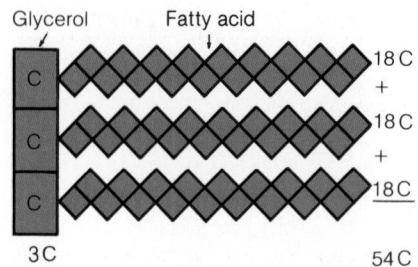

3 of this triglyceride's 57 carbon atoms are in glycerol and can be converted to glucose.

How Protein Enters the Metabolic Pathway

Amino acids will not enter the energy-yielding pathway being described here if they are used to replace needed body proteins. But if the amino acids are needed for energy, or if they are consumed in excess of the need for protein, they enter the metabolic pathway as shown in Figure 7–9. They are stripped of their nitrogen (see the next section) and then catabolized in a variety of ways.* The end result is that some of the amino acids are converted to pyruvate; others go either to acetyl CoA or directly into the TCA cycle. Those that are used to make pyruvate can provide glucose for the body. Thus protein, unlike fat, is a fairly good source of glucose when carbohydrate is not available.

Let's stop a moment to review the ways the body can use the energy-yielding nutrients (see Table 7–1). Glucose and fatty acids are the body's primary energy fuels, although amino acids can provide energy, if needed. Carbohydrates and

---

*Some of the amino acids are rearranged to form pyruvate. Others are 4-carbon compounds that are split into two acetyl CoA molecules. One, which contains only 2 carbons after the nitrogen is removed, is rearranged directly to become acetyl CoA. Still others enter the TCA cycle as compounds other than acetyl CoA.

■ **FIGURE 7–9**

How Amino Acids Enter the Metabolic Pathway

Some are converted to pyruvate (and therefore can be used to synthesize glucose); some are converted dirctly to acetyl CoA or bypass acetyl CoA completely and go directly into the TCA cycle. Net from one amino acid: the products depend on the side chain of the amino acid. (See Appendix C.) Notice that you have seen the lighter part of this figure before—in Figure 7–6. Note: The arrows from pyruvate and the TCA cycle to amino acids are possible only for *nonessential* amino acids. Remember that the body cannot make essential amino acids.

most amino acids can provide glucose, whereas only 5 percent of fat can be converted to glucose. Amino acids build body proteins, and glucose can be used to make amino acids when nitrogen is available; fats cannot be used to make body proteins. Finally, all three energy-yielding nutrients are converted to fat for storage when consumed beyond the body's needs.

The understanding of these metabolic details permits applications of interest to people concerned with down-to-earth realities such as weight control and fitness. Recall from Chapter 6 that surplus amino acids cannot be stored in the body as such; they have to be converted to other compounds. Amino acids eaten in excess of need first have their amino groups removed, then most are converted to acetyl CoA (either directly or indirectly, through

■ **TABLE 7–1**

Summary of Energy-yielding Nutrient Metabolism

Nutrient	Yields Energy	Can Yield Glucose	Can Yield Amino Acids and Body Proteins	Can Yield Fat Stores
Carbohydrates (glucose)	Yes	Yes	Yes—when nitrogen is available, can yield *nonessential* amino acids	Yes
Lipids (triglycerides)	Yes	No—glycerol provides minimal amount	No	Yes
Proteins (amino acids)	Yes—if needed	Yes—when carbohydrate is unavailable	Yes	Yes

pyruvate). This acetyl CoA is not broken down further when energy is not needed. Instead, it is used to make fatty acids and is stored in body fat. Thus even the so-called lean nutrient, protein, can add to fat stores if you eat too much of it.

The high-protein dieter objects to the previous statement, saying, "Protein makes you thin!" In fact, many weight-loss diets are based on high protein intakes, making the following claim: "Protein will give you energy but will not make you fat. Eat all you want—just stay away from fattening carbohydrates."

One secret of these diets, when they do seem to promote weight loss, is that meals without carbohydrate are in truth so unappetizing that people who ingest them eat much less total food than they normally do. Try eating your breakfast of bacon, eggs, toast, and juice without the toast and juice. Have a ham-and-cheese sandwich without the bread; try a dinner of steak, potatoes, and peas without the potatoes and peas. You'll be surprised how quickly you lose your enthusiasm for the permitted foods. (Some people report, after eating nothing but bacon, eggs, ham, cheese, and steak for a few days, that they start *dreaming* of toast and juice!)

The high-protein method of weight loss may sound inviting to the person who wants to lose pounds fast, but the next few sections of this chapter show why it is not a safe choice. Meanwhile, it should now be clear that protein, in and of itself, is not nonfattening. People who eat huge portions of meat, even lean meat, and other protein-rich foods may wonder why they have a weight problem. It may be those very foods that are causing the trouble.

There is a message for the athlete, too, in these metabolic facts about protein. *Excess* protein is not a muscle-building food but a fat-building food. To the extent that protein is used for energy, carbohydrate would do the job more efficiently. In other words, there is no point in loading up on protein for any reason. Chapter 13 elaborates on nutrition for the athlete.

Disposal of Excess Nitrogen

In describing how amino acids are degraded for energy or used to make fat, we left some amino groups dangling. The reaction that removes an amino acid's nitrogen-containing amino group is called deamination. The product is ammonia, chemically identical to the ammonia in the bottled cleaning solutions used in hospitals and industry. It is a strong-smelling poison.

A small amount of ammonia is always being produced by liver deamination reactions. Some of this ammonia is used by liver enzymes in the synthesis of nonessential amino acids, but what cannot be used is quickly combined with carbon dioxide to make urea, a much less toxic compound (see Figure 7–10). Ammonia is a base, and if the body produces larger quantities than it can handle, then the body's critical acid-base balance becomes upset.

Urea is released from the liver cells into the blood, where it circulates until it passes through the kidneys (see Figure 7–11). One of the functions of the kidneys is to remove urea from the blood for excretion in the urine. The balance between the liver's synthesis of urea and the kidneys' ability to clear urea from the blood highlights (once again) the wisdom of the body.

■ **FIGURE 7–10**
Urea Synthesis
When amino nitrogen is stripped from amino acids, ammonia is produced. The liver detoxifies ammonia by combining it with another waste product, CO_2, to produce urea before releasing it into the bloodstream. The diagram greatly oversimplifies the reactions; details are shown in Appendix C.

urea (you-REE-uh): the principal nitrogen-excretion product of metabolism. Two ammonia fragments are combined with carbon dioxide to form urea.

Urea is the body's principal vehicle for excreting unused nitrogen; water is required to keep it in solution. This is one reason why people who consume a high-protein diet must drink more water than usual, and why the hazard of dehydration attends the high-protein, low-carbohydrate diet. In fact, the weight loss from water loss is another reason why the diet *appears* to work, but water loss, of course, is of no value to the person who wants to lose body fat.

Putting It All Together

All the details this chapter has presented so far are combined in Figure 7–12. After a normal mixed meal, if you do not overeat, the body handles the nutrients as shown. The digestion of carbohydrate yields glucose; some is stored as glycogen, and some is taken into brain and other cells and broken down to pyruvate and acetyl CoA to provide energy. The acetyl CoA can then enter the TCA cycle to provide more energy. The digestion of protein yields amino acids, some of which are used to build body protein. However, if there is a surplus, or if not enough carbohydrate and fat are present to meet energy needs, some amino acids are broken down through the same pathways as glucose to provide energy. Other amino acids enter directly into the TCA cycle, and these, too, can be broken down to yield energy. The digestion of fat yields glycerol and fatty acids; some are put together and stored as fat, and others are broken down to acetyl CoA, enter the TCA cycle, and provide energy. In summary, although carbohydrate, fat, and protein enter the TCA cycle by different routes, the cycle is the energy-generating pathway common to all energy-yielding nutrients.

A few hours after the meal, when the glucose, glycerol, and fatty acids from the foods eaten have all been disposed of, the body starts using its stores. Glycogen and fat begin to be released from storage to provide more glucose, glycerol, and fatty acids to keep metabolism going. As the body shifts to a fasting mode and begins drawing energy out of storage, it signals hunger; it is time to eat again.

The average person takes in close to a million kcalories a year and expends more than 99 percent of them, maintaining a stable weight for years on end. This remarkable achievement, which many people manage without even thinking about it, could be called the economy of maintenance. The body's energy budget is balanced. Some people, however, eat too little and get thin; others eat too much and get fat. The possible reasons why they do are explored in Chapter 12; the metabolic consequences are discussed here.

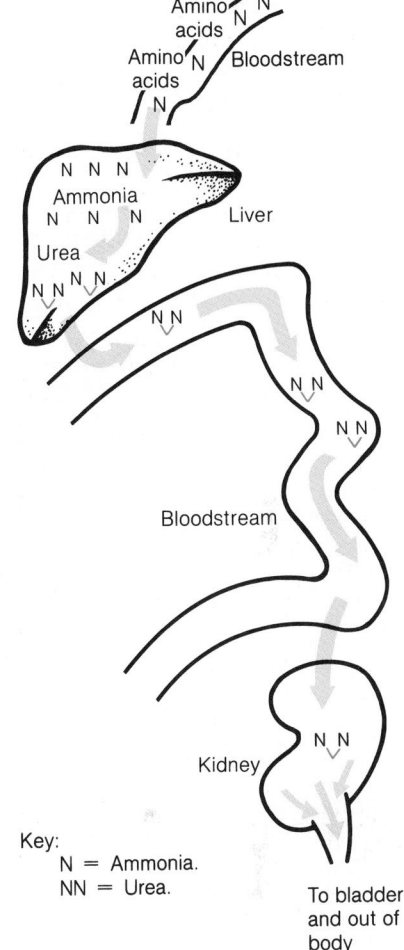

■ **FIGURE 7–11**
Urea Excretion
The liver and kidney each play a role in enabling the body to dispose of excess nitrogen. Can you see why the person with liver disease has high blood ammonia, while the person with kidney disease has high blood urea? (Figure 3–12 provides details of how the kidney works.)

■ The Economics of Feasting

Figure 7–13 shows how metabolism favors fat formation when you eat too much of any energy-yielding nutrient—carbohydrate, fat, or protein. Surplus carbohydrate (glucose) is first stored as glycogen, but there is a limit to the capacity of the glycogen-storing cells. Once glycogen stores are filled, the overflow is routed to fat (part A of the figure). Fat cells enlarge as they fill with fat, and their storage

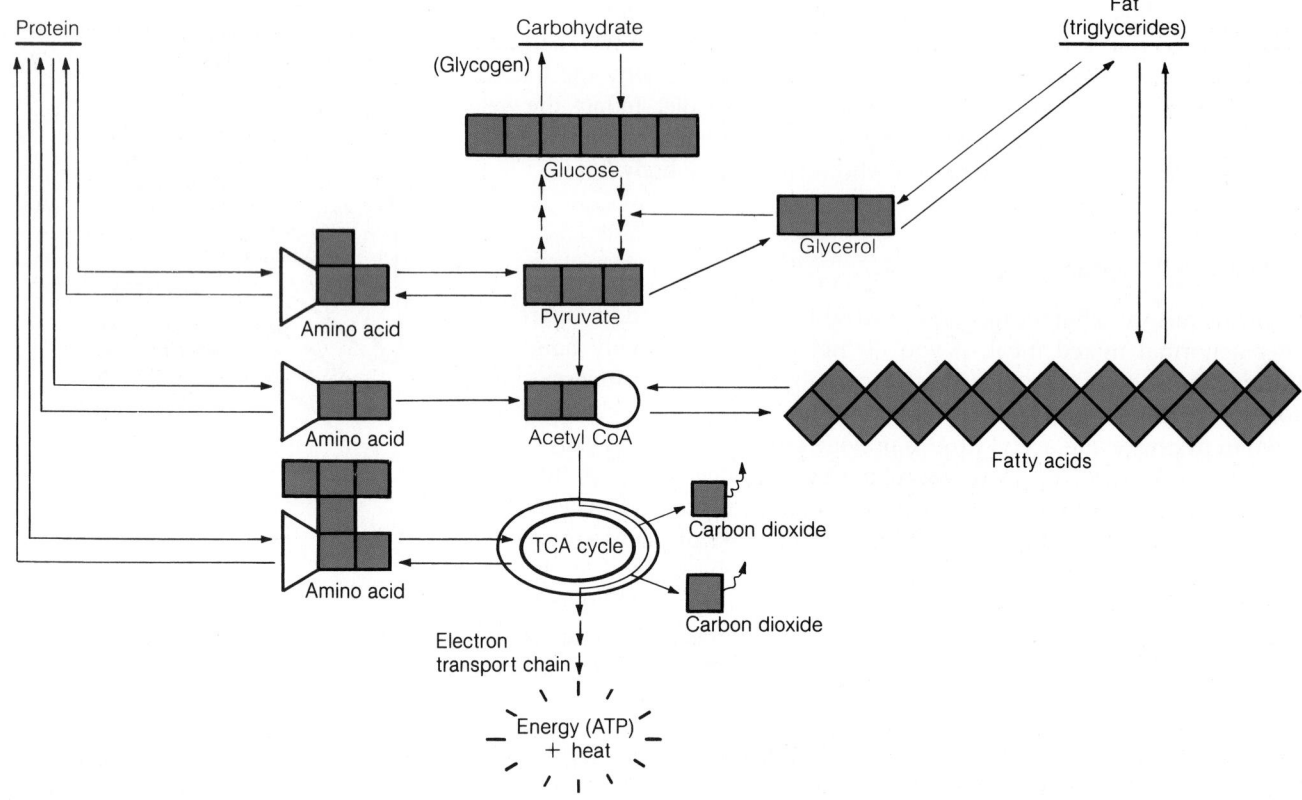

■ FIGURE 7–12
The Central Pathways of Metabolism
Details are in Appendix C.

capacity seems to be able to expand indefinitely, as diagrammed in Figure 7–14. Thus excess carbohydrate can contribute to obesity.

In the same way, surplus dietary fat can contribute to the fat stores in the body. It may break down to fragments such as acetyl CoA, but if energy flow is already rapid enough to meet the demand, these fragments will not be broken down further. Instead, they will be routed to the assembly of triglycerides and be stored in the fat cells (part B of Figure 7–13).

Finally, surplus protein may encounter the same fate (part C of Figure 7–13). If not needed to build body protein or to meet present energy needs, amino acids will be deaminated and their carbon skeletons converted through the intermediates, pyruvate and acetyl CoA, to triglycerides. These, too, swell the fat cells and increase body weight.

■ *The Economics of Fasting*

Even when you are asleep and totally relaxed, the cells of many organs are hard at work spending energy. In fact, this work, of which your are unaware, represents about two-thirds to three-fourths of the total energy you spend in a day. The other portion, which is smaller, is the work that you do with your muscles during waking hours.

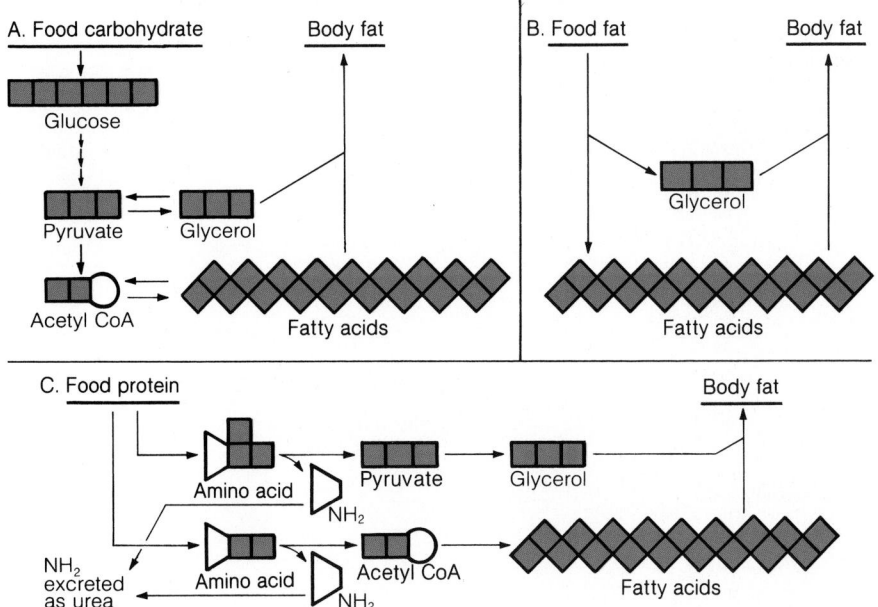

■ FIGURE 7–13

How Carbohydrate, Fat, and Protein, Eaten in Excess, Contribute to Body Fat

A. Carbohydrate, eaten in excess of need, is broken down to pyruvate and acetyl CoA; these then are built up into fat.

B. Fat, eaten in excess of need, is either stored directly or broken down to pyruvate and acetyl CoA; these then may be built up into different fat molecules.

C. Protein is broken down to amino acids. These, if not used to build body protein, are deaminated, and the nitrogen is excreted as urea; the remaining carbon skeletons are converted to pyruvate and acetyl CoA, and then to fat.

The body's top priority is to meet the cells' needs for energy, and its normal way of doing so is by periodic refueling—that is, by eating. When food is not available, the body must find other fuel sources in its own tissues. If people choose not to eat, we say they are fasting; if they have no choice (as in a famine), we say they are starving; but there is no metabolic difference between the two. In either case, the body is forced to switch to a wasting metabolism, drawing on its reserves of carbohydrate and fat and, within a day or so, on its vital protein tissues as well. Figure 7–15 shows the metabolic pathways operating in the body as it shifts from feasting to fasting.

As you can see from this figure, all paths lead to energy—fuel must be delivered to every cell. As the fast begins, glucose from the liver's stored glycogen and fatty acids from the body's stored fat are both flowing into cells, then breaking down to yield acetyl CoA, and delivering energy to power the cells' work. Several hours later, however, most of the glucose is used up—liver glycogen is exhausted. Low blood glucose concentrations serve as a signal to further promote fat breakdown.[1]

At this point, most of the cells are depending on fatty acids to continue providing their fuel. But the nervous system and brain cells cannot; they still need glucose. (It is their major energy fuel, and even if other energy fuels are available, glucose has to be present to permit the energy-metabolizing machinery of the brain cells to work.) Normally, the nervous system tissues (brain and nerve cells) consume about two-thirds of the total glucose used each day—about 400 to 600 kcalories' worth. About one-fifth of the energy the body uses when it is at rest is used for the brain.

The brain's special requirement for glucose poses a problem for the fasting body. The body can use its stores of fat, which may be quite generous, to furnish most of its cells with energy, but for the brain and nerves, it must

Brain, in its rigid vault, cannot store more than a few minutes' worth of glycogen at the most. . . . Hence, the compliant liver expands and contracts.—G. F. Cahill, T. T. Aoki, and A. A. Rossini

■ FIGURE 7–14

Fat Cell Enlargement

Fat cells enlarge when you eat too much of any energy-yielding nutrient—carbohydrate, fat, or protein.

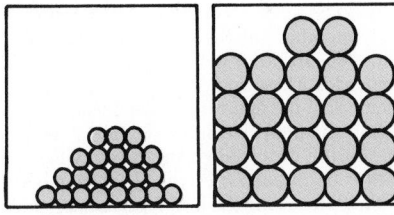

■ **FIGURE 7–15**

Feasting and Fasting

A. When a person eats in excess of energy needs, the body stores limited amounts of glycogen and larger quantities of fat.

B. When food is unavaiable to provide energy, the body draws on its glycogen and fat stores for energy.

C. When glycogen stores are depleted, the body begins to break down its protein (muscle and lean tissue) to amino acids for glucose synthesis needed for brain and nervous system energy. In addition, the liver converts fats to ketone bodies, which serve as an alternative energy source for the brain, thus slowing the breakdown of body protein.

ketone (KEE-tone) **body**: a compound formed during the incomplete oxidation of fatty acids. Ketones contain a C = O group between other carbons; when they also contain a COOH (acid) group, they are called keto-acids. These and compounds related to them, as in the figure, are ketone bodies. Small amounts of ketone bodies are a normal part of the blood chemistry; but when their concentration rises, the pH of the blood declines, upsetting the acid-base balance, and ketone bodies spill into the urine.

supply energy in the form of glucose. This is why body protein tissues, such as muscle and liver, always break down to some extent during fasting. Only those amino acids that yield 3-carbon pyruvate can be used to make glucose; and to obtain them, body proteins must be broken down. The other amino acids, which can't be used to make glucose, are used as an energy source for other body cells. This is an expensive way to gain glucose, but to extract a molecule of glycerol from a triglyceride obligates the body to dispose of some 50 or 60 carbons' worth of fatty acids, which is even more expensive. In the first few days of a fast, body protein provides about 90 percent of the needed glucose and glycerol, about 10 percent. If body protein loss were to continue at this rate, death would ensue within three weeks, regardless of the quantity of fat a person had stored.

As the fast continues, the body finds a way to use its fat to fuel the brain. It adapts by condensing together acetyl CoA fragments derived from fatty acids to produce an alternate energy source, ketone bodies (see Figure 7–16). Normally produced and used in only small quantities, ketone bodies can serve as a fuel for some brain cells. Ketone body production rises until, at the end of several weeks, it is meeting about two-thirds or more of the nervous system's energy needs. Still, many areas of the brain rely exclusively on glucose, and body protein continues to be sacrificed to produce it.

It has been thought that ketosis caused loss of appetite. The theory was that it would be an advantage to a person in a famine to have no appetite, because the search for food would be a waste of energy. When the person finds food and eats carbohydrate again, the body shifts out of ketosis, the hunger center gets the message that food is again available, and the appetite returns. This hypothetical chain of events has served as justification for weight-loss routines, such as fasting and fad diets, that cause ketosis. However, it may be that any kind of food restriction, with or without ketosis, leads a person to adapt by losing appetite. An ordinary low-kcalorie diet can induce the same effect.[2]

In any case, while the body is shifting to the use of ketone bodies, it simultaneously reduces its energy output and conserves both its fat and lean tissue. As the lean (protein-containing) organ tissue shrinks in mass, it performs less metabolic work, reducing energy expenditures. As the muscles waste, they do less work, reducing energy expenditures further. Because of the slowed metabolism, the loss of fat falls to a bare minimum—less, in fact, than the fat that would be lost on a low-kcalorie diet. Thus, although *weight* loss during fasting may be quite dramatic, *fat* loss may be less than when at least some food is supplied.

The adaptations just described—slowing of energy output and reduction in fat loss—occur in the starving child, the fasting religious person, and the malnourished hospital client, and help to prolong their lives. The physical symptoms of energy deprivation include wasting, slowed metabolism, lowered body temperature, and reduced resistance to disease.

The body's adaptations to fasting are sufficient to maintain life for a long period. Mental alertness need not be diminished, and even physical energy may remain unimpaired for a surprisingly long time. Still, fasting is not without its hazards, as physician-supervised fasting has revealed. Among the multitude of changes that take place in the body are:

- Loss of body protein.
- Sodium and potassium depletion.
- An increase in body uric acid (a by-product of lean tissue breakdown).
- A decrease in thyroid hormone.

The same alterations are seen in low-carbohydrate dieting, as will be described in the next section. Renewed food intake, especially of carbohydrate, results in dramatic changes in the body's salt and water balance. This accounts for most of the wide swings in body weight seen in people on fasts or low-carbohydrate diets.

The Low-Carbohydrate Diet

An economy similar to that of fasting prevails in the person who consumes a low-carbohydrate diet. Advocates of the low-carbohydrate diet would have you believe there is something magical about ketosis—something that promotes faster weight loss than a regular low-kcalorie diet. In fact, the low-carbohydrate diet presents the same problem as a fast. Once the body's available glycogen reserves are spent, the only significant remaining source of glucose is protein. The low-carbohydrate diet usually provides some protein

Formation of ketone bodies:

This ketone may lose a molecule of carbon dioxide to become another ketone:

Or, the keto-acid may add 2 hydrogens, becoming a related compound (a ketone body). See Appendix C for more details.

■ **FIGURE 7–16**
Ketone Body Formation

ketosis: the combination of high blood ketone bodies (ketonemia) and ketone bodies in the urine (ketonuria).

The ketone **acetone** (ASS-eh-tone) is familiar to some as the solvent used in nail-polish remover. "Acetone breath" indicates that a person is in ketosis.

Low-carbohydrate dieting = living on dietary protein and fat and on body protein and fat almost exclusively.

from food, but some is still taken from body tissue. The onset of ketosis is the signal that this wasting process has begun.

People are attracted to the low-carbohydrate diet because of the dramatic weight loss it brings about within the first few days. They would be disillusioned if they realized that much of this weight loss is a loss of glycogen and protein together with quantities of water and important minerals. A dieter who boasts of losing 7 pounds in two days on a low-carbohydrate diet must be unaware that at best, a pound or two is fat, and 5 or 6 pounds are lean tissue, water, and minerals. Once the dieter is off the diet, the body will avidly devour and retain these needed materials, and the weight will zoom back, quite often to higher than the starting point.

A warning is suggested by these facts. Beware of those who promote quick-weight-loss schemes. Learn to distinguish between loss of *fat* and loss of *weight*. Table 12–6 in Chapter 12 lists questions to ask when evaluating weight-loss diets.

The Protein-Sparing Fast

Protein-sparing fasting = living on dietary protein and on body protein and fat.

A variant on fasting is the technique of ingesting only protein. The hope is that the protein will spare lean tissue and that the person will break down body fat at a maximal rate to meet other energy needs. The protein does spare the lean tissues to some extent from being used to provide glucose, but the protein also is largely used as a glucose source itself, just as dietary carbohydrate would be. The idea sounded good when it was first suggested for use with very obese people, but it has met with mixed results. It seems effective only after considerable lean tissue has already been lost, at which time the body may be conserving itself quite efficiently anyway. The fast has not been shown more effective than a mixture of protein and carbohydrate. Furthermore, it has a low long-term success rate; most people regain the lost weight. Thus the protein-sparing fast has to be judged at best a moderate success and at worst a failure, for the ultimate criterion of success in any weight-loss program is maintenance of the new low weight.

The idea of a protein-sparing fast originated with some responsible physicians who experimented carefully with it, using whole foods naturally rich in protein, such as fish and lean beef. The results of their work are presented in Chapter 12 in a discussion on very-low-kcalorie diets. Unfortunately, the idea of such a fast was seized upon and misused with the publication of a popular book, *The Last Chance Diet*, in 1977.[3] Fad dieters, usually without any medical supervision, drank liquid protein potions prepared from low-quality sources, or they consumed very-low-kcalorie, high-protein diets and lost dramatic amounts of weight—including, of course, lean tissue, water, and vital minerals. Within the year, 11 deaths had been ascribed to the fad, and since then, many more have died. Supplements consisting of high-quality protein were used by some of the victims—so the quality of the protein was not alone responsible for the deaths.[4] Mineral deficiencies were suspected as contributing factors.

The term *protein sparing* has been used in another connection. Hospital clients enduring severe physical stresses such as certain diseases or major surgery also lose body protein. This is especially likely, and especially dangerous, if they are simultaneously fighting infection, which prevents the body from going into ketosis. Physicians make every effort to prevent the loss of vital lean tissue by supplying amino acids as well as glucose in some form—through a vein if the client can't eat. The effort to provide protein-sparing *therapy* for prevention of malnutrition circumstances should not be confused with the profiteering of faddists who promote the protein-sparing *fast* for weight loss.

Moderate Weight Loss

Your body's cells and the enzymes within them have the task of converting the energy nutrients you eat into those you need. They are extraordinarily versatile. They relieve you of having to compute exactly how much carbohydrate, fat, and protein to eat at each meal. As you have seen, the body's remarkable machinery can convert either carbohydrate (glucose) or protein to fat. To some extent, it can convert protein to glucose. To a very limited extent, it can even convert fat (the glycerol portion) to glucose. But a grossly unbalanced diet or one that is severely limited in energy imposes hardships on the body. If energy intake is too low or if carbohydrate and protein energy is undersupplied, the body is forced to degrade its own lean tissue to meet its glucose need.

Someone who wants to lose body fat must be reconciled to the hard fact that there is a limit to the rate at which fat tissue will break down. The maximum rate, except for a very large, very active person, is 1 to 2 pounds a week. To design a moderate diet requires adjusting energy balance so that energy intake is reduced, energy output is increased, or both. The most effective way to achieve a weight loss that actually reflects a loss of body fat is to adopt a balanced, low-kcalorie diet supplying all three energy nutrients in reasonable amounts while adjusting energy expended on exercise to a reasonable level. In effect, this means adjusting the energy budget so that intake is 500 to 1,000 kcalories per day less than output. A person who wants to gain weight needs to make the opposite adjustment. Energy balance and weight control are the subjects of Chapter 12.

■ Study Questions

1. Define metabolism, anabolism, and catabolism; give an example of each.
2. Name the four basic units used by the body after digestion in metabolic transformations.
3. What is the body's quick-energy molecule, and how is it used?
4. Summarize the main steps in the metabolism of glucose, fatty acids, glycerol, and amino acids.
5. Describe how a surplus of the three energy nutrients contributes to body fat stores.
6. Define ketosis. What adaptations does the body make during a fast?
7. Distinguish between a loss of *fat* and a loss of *weight* on a low-carbohydrate diet.

■ Notes

1. S. Klein and coauthors, Effect of plasma glucose concentration on the lipolytic response to fasting (abstract), *American Journal of Clinical Nutrition* 45 (1987): 856.
2. J. C. Rosen and coauthors, Mood and appetite during minimal-carbohydrate and carbohydrate-supplemented hypocaloric diets, *American Journal of Clinical Nutrition* 42 (1985): 371–379.
3. R. Linn and S. L. Stuart, *The Last Chance Diet* (New York: Bantam Books, 1977).
4. T. B. Van Itallie and M. U. Yang, Cardiac dysfunction in obese dieters: A potentially lethal complication of rapid, massive weight loss, *American Journal of Clinical Nutrition* 39 (1984): 695–702.

Alcohol and Nutrition

As people arrive at their teen and adult years, they have to choose whether or not to drink alcohol. Many of those who choose to drink manage their relationship with alcohol relatively safely, but unfortunately, about one in nine drinkers goes on to become an alcohol abuser. More than 9 million people in the United States abuse alcohol to the point that their personal relationships, jobs, and health become impaired.

One of the health hazards of alcohol abuse is malnutrition. Alcohol produces euphoria, which depresses appetite, so heavy drinkers tend to eat poorly. Alcohol also attacks the lining of the stomach, so digestion is poor. Since much of their energy fuel comes from the empty kcalories of alcohol, heavy drinkers consume too few essential nutrients. Even if a person eats well, however, large amounts of alcohol will impair nutritional health, because alcohol hinders the absorption, alters the metabolism, and increases the excretion of many nutrients. Malnutrition therefore occurs even in well-fed drinkers. With the understanding of metabolism gained from Chapter 7, you are in a position to understand just how the body handles alcohol and how alcohol affects metabolism.

Alcohol in Beverages

To the chemist, *alcohol* refers to a class of organic compounds containing hydroxyl (OH) groups. The glycerol to which fatty acids are attached in triglycerides is an example of an alcohol to a chemist. But to most people, *alcohol* refers to the intoxicating ingredient in beer, wine, and hard liquor (distilled spirits). The chemist's name for this particular alcohol is *ethyl alcohol*, or *ethanol*.

■ FIGURE H7–1
Two Alcohols: Glycerol and Ethanol

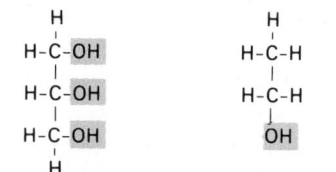

Glycerol is an alcohol.

Ethanol is the alcohol in beer, wine, and distilled spirits.

Glycerol has 3 carbons with 3 hydroxyl groups attached; ethanol has only 2 carbons and 1 hydroxyl group (see Figure H7–1). The remainder of this highlight talks about a particular alcohol—ethanol—but refers to it simply as *alcohol.*

Alcohol arises naturally from carbohydrates when certain microorganisms metabolize them in the absence of oxygen—a process called fermentation. Since all plants contain carbohydrate, all can serve as the starting material for fermentation. Different societies use different plants to produce alcoholic beverages; the most familiar are grapes and other berries (used to make wine), apples (fermented, or hard, cider), and grains (beer and various distilled liquors). Wines, ciders, and beers are used as is, after fermentation, whereas the so-called hard liquors are made by further distilling the products of fermentation, so as to concentrate the alcohol. Thus grain mashes can be distilled further to yield the whiskeys—bourbon (at least half from corn), rye (from rye), scotch (from barley), vodka (from wheat, rye, corn, or potatoes), rum (from cane products such as molasses), and brandy (from wine). Hard liquors may then be served with mixers such as carbonated beverages or fruit juices (cocktails), or

they may be sweetened with herbs and spices (liqueurs, or after-dinner drinks). Wine and beer have a relatively low percentage of alcohol, whereas whiskey, vodka, rum, and brandy may be as much as 50 percent alcohol (the accompanying miniglossary defines the term *proof*, which describes the percentage of alcohol in distilled liquor).

The alcohols affect living things profoundly, partly because they act as lipid solvents. They can dissolve the lipids right out of cell membranes, destroying the cell structures and thereby killing the cells. For this reason, most alcohols are toxic, or poisonous; by the same token, because they kill microbial cells, they are useful as disinfectants.

Ethanol, like the other alcohols, is toxic—but less so than some. Sufficiently diluted and taken in small enough doses, it produces euphoria—an effect that people seek—not with zero risk, but with a low enough risk (if the doses are low enough) to be tolerable. Used to achieve these effects, alcohol is a drug—that is, a substance that can modify one or more of the body's functions. Like all drugs, alcohol offers some benefits; it also has tremendous abuse potential.

Wine, beer, and other fermented beverages have given pleasure and relaxation to people for more than 5,000 years. People have always known that these beverages affected their moods, sensations, and behavior, but only recently has science begun to learn exactly how the little molecule ethanol acts in people's bodies. Taken in moderation, alcohol relaxes people, reduces their inhibitions, and encourages desirable social interactions. Such moderate uses of alcohol can prolong life and good health, although a person might be even better off learning how to relax in the face of life's pressures without chemical help.

The term *moderation* is important in the statement above. Just what is moderate use of alcohol? We cannot name an exact amount of alcohol per day that would be appropriate for everyone, because people differ in their tolerance levels, but authorities have attempted to set limits that are acceptable for most healthy people. They define moderation in terms of *drinks*, and then, of course, have to specify just what is meant by a drink (see the miniglossary). The general agreement defines moderate drinking for the average-sized, healthy man as taking not more than three drinks a day, and for the average-sized, healthy woman as taking not more than two drinks a day. This amount is supposed to be enough to produce euphoria without incurring any long-term harm to health. Doubtless some people could consume slightly more; others could definitely not handle nearly so much without significant risk.

You may have heard that drinking, at least moderately, improves the heart's health by raising the blood concentration of HDL (high-density lipoproteins), the indicator of a low risk of heart attack (see Chapter 16). It turns out, though, that two classes of HDL exist—one class associated with lowered heart disease risk, and another associated with moderate drinking. Alcohol raises one type of HDL, but not the type that reduces heart disease risk.[1]

Alcohol in the Body

From the moment alcohol enters the body in a beverage, it is treated as if it has special privileges. Foods sit around in the stomach for a while, but not alcohol. The tiny alcohol molecules need no digestion. About 20 percent

Miniglossary

alcohol: a class of chemical compounds containing hydroxyl (OH) groups.
alcohol dehydrogenase: a liver enzyme that converts ethanol to **acetaldehyde** (ass-et-AL-duh-hide). The MEOS also oxidizes alcohol (see *MEOS*).
antidiuretic hormone (ADH): a hormone produced by the pituitary gland in response to dehydration (or a high sodium concentration in the blood); stimulates the kidneys to reabsorb more water and so excrete less. This ADH should not be confused with the enzyme alcohol dehydrogenase, which is sometimes also abbreviated ADH.
cirrhosis (seer-OH-sis): advanced liver disease (see Chapter 26), in which liver cells have died, hardened, and turned orange; often associated with alcoholism.
  cirrhos = an orange
drink: a dose of any alcoholic beverage that delivers ½ oz of pure ethanol:

- 3 to 4 oz of wine.
- 8 to 12 oz of beer.
- 1 oz of hard liquor (whiskey, scotch, rum, or vodka).

drug: a substance that can modify one or more of the body's functions.
ethanol: a particular type of alcohol found in beer, wine, and distilled spirits; also called *ethyl alcohol* (see Figure H7−1).
euphoria (you-FORE-ee-uh): a feeling of great well-being, which people often seek through the use of drugs such as alcohol.
  eu = good
  phoria = bearing
fatty liver: an early stage of liver deterioration seen in several diseases, including protein malnutrition and alcoholic liver disease, characterized by an accumulation of fat in the liver cells (see Chapter 26).
fermentation: the oxidation of carbohydrate in the absence of atmospheric oxygen, a process that yields alcohol as the end product.
fibrosis: an intermediate stage of liver deterioration seen in several diseases, including viral hepatitis and alcoholic liver disease. In fibrosis, the liver cells lose their function and assume the characteristics of connective tissue cells (fibers).
gout (GOWT): a painful condition in which uric acid crystals form in the joints.
MEOS (microsomal ethanol-oxidizing system): a system of enzymes in the liver that oxidize not only alcohol, but also several classes of drugs. (The **microsomes** are tiny particles of membranes with associated enzymes that can be collected from broken-up cells.)
  micro = tiny
  soma = body
narcotic (nar-KOT-ic): any drug that dulls the senses, induces sleep, and becomes addictive with prolonged use.
proof: a way of stating the percentage of alcohol in distilled liquor. Liquor that is 100 proof is 50% alcohol; 90 proof is 45%, and so forth.

■ **FIGURE H7–2**
Alcohol in the Stomach
The alcohol (Alc) in a stomach filled with food has a low probability of touching the walls and diffusing through.

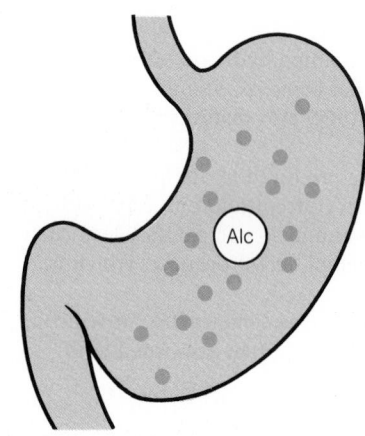

of the alcohol consumed is absorbed right through the walls of the stomach. It can reach the brain within a minute. Consequently, a drinker can feel euphoric right away when drinking, especially on an empty stomach. When the stomach is full of food, the molecules of alcohol have less chance of touching the walls and diffusing through (as illustrated in Figure H7–2), so the drinker doesn't feel the effects of alcohol so quickly. If you want to drink without becoming intoxicated at parties, then eat the snacks provided by the host. Carbohydrate snacks are best suited for slowing alcohol absorption. High-fat snacks help, too, because they slow peristalsis.[2]

When the stomach contents are emptied into the duodenum, it no longer matters that plenty of food is mixed with the alcohol. The small intestine absorbs alcohol rapidly anyway, as if it were a V.I.P. (Very Important Person).

Alcohol Arrives in the Liver

The capillaries that surround the digestive tract merge into the veins that carry the alcohol-laden blood to the liver. Here the veins branch and rebranch into capillaries that touch every liver cell. Liver cells are the only cells in the body that can make enough of the enzyme alcohol dehydrogenase to oxidize alcohol at an appreciable rate. Alcohol affects every organ of the body, but the most dramatic evidence of its disruptive behavior appears in the liver. If liver cells could talk, they would describe the alcohol of intoxicating beverages as demanding, egocentric, and disruptive of the liver's efficient way of running its business. For example, liver cells normally prefer fatty acids as their fuel, and they like to package excess fatty acids into triglycerides and ship them out to other tissues. When alcohol is present, however, the liver cells are forced to metabolize alcohol and let the fatty acids accumulate, sometimes in huge stockpiles.

There is a limit to the amount of alcohol the liver can process in a given time—about ½ ounce *ethanol* per hour, the amount in an average drink. This limit is set by the number of molecules of alcohol dehydrogenase that reside in the liver. If more molecules of alcohol arrive at the liver cells than the enzymes can handle, the extra alcohol must wait to be processed (Figure H7–3). It enters the general circulation and moves on past the liver. From the liver, the alcohol is carried to all parts of the body, circulating again and again until liver en-

■ **FIGURE H7–3**
Enzymes Limit Alcohol's Metabolic Progress
If more molecules of alcohol arrive at the liver cells than the enzymes can handle, the extra molecules must wait to be processed.

■ **FIGURE H7–4**
Alcohol Metabolism
The conversion of alcohol to acetyl CoA requires the B vitamin niacin in its role as NAD. When the enzymes oxidize alcohol, they remove H atoms and attach them to NAD. Thus NAD is used up, and NADH accumulates. (Note: More accurately stated, NAD^+ is converted to $NADH + H^+$. For simplicity's sake, the description here is stated as if one hydrogen is added to NAD, but really, two are added to NAD.)

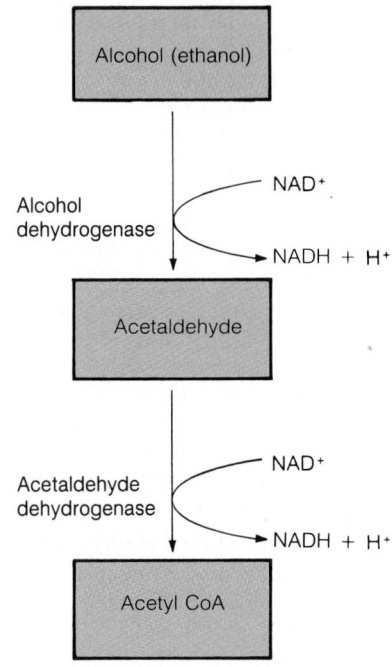

zymes are finally available to convert it to acetaldehyde (Figure H7–4).

The rate at which alcohol dehydrogenase can work limits the rate of the body's handling of alcohol. The type of enzyme produced varies with individuals, depending on the genes they have inherited. Some racial groups—for example, Asians—have genetic information that causes them to produce atypical forms of alcohol dehydrogenase and its partner enzyme acetaldehyde dehydrogenase. This difference explains why some persons are made too uncomfortable by alcohol to become addicted.[3] High concentrations of acetaldehyde in the brain and other tissues are responsible for many of the punishing effects of alcohol abuse.

The amount of alcohol dehydrogenase present in the liver depends also on how recently the person has eaten. Fasting for as little as a day causes degradation of the enzyme (a protein) within the cells, and can slow the rate of alcohol metabolism by half. Drinking on an empty stomach thus not only causes the drinker to feel the effects more promptly, but also brings about higher blood alcohol concentrations for longer times and lets alcohol anesthetize the brain more completely.

The alcohol dehydrogenase enzyme system breaks down alcohol by removing hydrogens in two steps (see Figure H7–4). In the first step, alcohol dehydrogenase oxidizes alcohol to acetaldehyde. In the second step, a related enzyme, acetaldehyde dehydrogenase, oxidizes the acetaldehyde to acetyl CoA, the "crossroads" compound that can enter the TCA cycle to generate energy. These reactions produce hydrogen ions (acid). The B vitamin niacin (in its role as a compound known as NAD) helpfully picks up these hydrogen ions (becoming NADH). Thus whenever the body breaks down alcohol, NAD diminishes and NADH accumulates.

Alcohol Disrupts the Liver

During alcohol metabolism, NAD becomes unavailable for the multitude of other jobs the body has for it to do (these are mentioned in Chapter 8). Its presence is sorely missed in the pathway from glucose to energy. Without NAD, the energy pathway is blocked. Traffic either backs up, or an alternate route will be taken. Such changes in the normal flow of traffic from glucose to available energy have striking physical consequences.

For one, the accumulation of hydrogen ions during alcohol metabolism results in a dangerous shift of the body's acid-base balance (described in Chapter 10) toward acid.

■ **FIGURE H7–5**
Alternate Route for Acetyl CoA: To Fat
Acetyl CoAs are blocked from getting into the TCA cycle by the high level of NADH. Instead of being used for energy, acetyl CoAs become building blocks for fatty acids.

For another, the accumulation of NADH depresses the TCA cycle, so pyruvate and acetyl CoA build up. Excess acetyl CoA then takes the route to fatty acid synthesis (as Figure H7–5 illustrates), and fat clogs the liver.

As you might expect, a liver clogged with fat cannot function properly. Liver cells lose efficiency in performing a number of tasks. Much of this inefficiency impairs a person's nutritional health in ways that cannot be corrected by diet alone. For example, the liver has difficulty activating vitamin D, as well as producing and excreting bile. To overcome such problems, a person needs to stop drinking alcohol.

The synthesis of fatty acids accelerates as a result of the liver's exposure to alcohol. Fat accumulation can be seen in the liver after a single night of heavy drinking. Fatty liver, the first stage of liver deterioration seen in heavy drinkers, interferes with the distribution of nutrients and oxygen to the liver cells. If the condition lasts long enough, the liver cells will die, and the area will be invaded by fibrous scar tissue—the second stage of liver deterioration, called fibrosis. Fibrosis is reversible with good nutrition and abstinence from alcohol, but the next (last) stage—cirrhosis—is not.

The fatty liver has difficulty generating glucose from protein. The lack of glucose from this source, together with the overabundance of acetyl CoA molecules blocked from getting into the TCA cycle, sets the stage for a shift into ketosis. The body uses the acetyl CoA to make ketone bodies, but some ketone bodies are acids, so they push the acid-base balance further toward acid.

Excess NADH promotes the making of lactic acid from pyruvate. The conversion of pyruvate to lactic acid helpfully uses the hydrogens from NADH and restores some NAD, but a lactic acid buildup has serious consequences of its own—it adds still further to the body's acid burden and interferes with the excretion of another acid, uric acid, causing goutlike symptoms.

The presence of alcohol alters amino acid metabolism in the liver cells. Synthesis of some proteins important in the immune system slows down, weakening the body's defenses against infection. Synthesis of lipoproteins speeds up, increasing blood triglyceride levels. Protein deficiency can develop, both from the depression of protein synthesis in the cells and from a poor diet. Normally the cells would at least use the amino acids that a person happened to eat, but the drinker's liver deaminates the amino acids and channels their carbon backbones into fat or ketones. Eating well does not protect the drinker from protein depletion. A person has to stop drinking alcohol for complete protection.

The liver's V.I.P. treatment of alcohol is reflected in its handling of drugs, as well as nutrients. In addition to the alcohol dehydrogenase enzyme system already described, the liver possesses an enzyme system that metabolizes *both* alcohol and several types of other drugs. Called the MEOS (microsomal ethanol-oxidizing system), this system handles only about one-fifth of the total alcohol a person consumes, but the MEOS enlarges if repeatedly exposed to alcohol. This may not make the drinker able to handle much more alcohol at a time than before, because the total alcohol-metabolizing ability of the MEOS is small, but the effect on the ability to metabolize drugs is considerable.

When the MEOS enlarges, it makes the body able to metabolize drugs much faster than before. This can make it confusing and tricky to work out the correct doses of medications. The physician who prescribes sedatives every four hours, for example, assumes that the MEOS will dispose of the drug at a certain predicted rate. Well and good; but in a client who is a heavy drinker, the MEOS is adapted to metabolizing large quantities of alcohol. It therefore metabolizes the sedative extra fast. The drug's effects wear off unexpectedly fast, leaving the client undersedated. Imagine the surgeon's alarm if a client wakes up on the table during an operation! A skilled anesthesiologist always asks clients about their drinking patterns before putting them to sleep.

An enlarged MEOS will oxidize drugs *faster* than expected, but only as long as there is no alcohol in the system. If the person drinks and uses another drug at the same time, the second drug will be metabolized more *slowly* and so will be much more potent. The MEOS is busy disposing of alcohol, so the drug can't be handled till later; and the dose may build up to where it greatly oversedates, or even kills, the user.

This discussion has emphasized the major way that the blood is cleared of alcohol—metabolism by the liver—but there is another way. About 10 percent of the alcohol leaves the body through the breath and in the urine. This is the basis for the breath and urine analysis tests for drunkenness. The amounts of alcohol in the breath and in the urine are in proportion to the amount still in the bloodstream. In nearly all states, legal drunkenness is set at 0.10 percent, reflecting the relationship between alcohol use and industrial and traffic accidents.

Alcohol Disrupts the Rest of the Body

Alcohol affects other tissues in other ways as well. The stomach becomes inflamed, overproduces acid, and becomes likely to develop ulcers. Intestinal cells fail to absorb the vitamins thiamin, folate, and vitamin B_{12}. Rod cells in the retina of the eye, which normally process the alcohol form of vitamin A to its aldehyde form needed in vision, find themselves processing ethanol to acetaldehyde instead. The kidney excretes increased quantities of the minerals magnesium, calcium, potassium, and zinc.

Acetaldehyde interferes with metabolism, too. For example, it dislodges vitamin B_6 from its protective binding protein so that it is destroyed, causing a vitamin B_6 deficiency and, thereby, lowered production of red blood cells.

Alcohol Arrives in the Brain

Alcohol is a narcotic. People have used it for centuries as an anesthetic because it can deaden pain. But alcohol is a poor anesthetic, because one could never be sure how much a person would need and how much would be a fatal dose. New, more

■ **FIGURE H7–6**
Alcohol's Effects on the Brain
Alcohol is rightly termed an anesthetic, because it puts brain centers to sleep in order: first, the emotion- and decision-governing centers; then the centers that govern muscular control; and finally, the deep centers that control respiration and heartbeat.

Most sensitive: judgment and reasoning

Next most sensitive: muscular control

Last to be affected: respiration and heart action

predictable anesthetics, discovered more recently, have replaced alcohol. However, alcohol continues to be used today as a kind of anesthetic on social occasions, to help people relax or to relieve anxiety. People think that alcohol is a stimulant, because it seems to make them lively and uninhibited at first. Actually, though, the way it does this is by sedating *inhibitory* nerves, which are more numerous than excitatory nerves. Ultimately, it acts as a depressant, because it affects all the nerve cells.

When alcohol flows to the brain, it sedates the frontal lobe first—the reasoning part (Figure H7–6). As the alcohol molecules diffuse into the cells of this lobe, they interfere with reasoning and judgment. If the drinker drinks too fast for the liver to keep up, then the blood alcohol concentration rises, the area that governs reasoning becomes more incapacitated, and the speech and vision centers of the brain become narcotized. At still higher concentrations, the cells of the brain responsible for large-muscle control

■ **TABLE H7–1**
Alcohol Doses and Brain Responses

Number of Drinks Consumed[a]	Blood Alcohol Concentration[b]	Effect on Brain
1 to 4	0.05	Impaired judgment, relaxed inhibitions, altered mood, increased heart rate
5 to 6	0.10	Impaired coordination, delayed reaction time, exaggerated emotions, impaired peripheral vision, impaired ability to operate a vehicle
6 to 8	0.15	Slurred speech, blurred vision, staggered walk, seriously impaired coordination and judgment
8 to 10	0.20	Double vision, inability to walk
10 to 15	0.30	Uninhibited behavior, stupor, confusion, inability to comprehend
15+	0.40 to 0.60	Unconsciousness, shock, coma, death (cardiac or respiratory failure)

[a]1 drink = 12 oz of 4.5% beer.
  4 oz of 14% wine.
  1 to 1½ oz of 50% liquor.
[b]Blood alcohol concentration depends on a number of factors, including alcohol in the beverage, the rate of consumption, the person's gender, and body weight. For example, a 100-lb female can become legally drunk, (0.10 concentration) by drinking three beers in an hour, whereas a 220-lb male consuming that amount at the same rate would have a 0.05 blood alcohol concentration.

are affected; at this point, people "under the influence" stagger or weave when they try to walk. Finally, the conscious brain is completely subdued, and the person "passes out." Now, luckily, the person can drink no more; this is lucky because a higher dose's anesthetic effect could reach the deepest brain centers, which control breathing and heartbeat, and the person could die. Table H7–1 shows the blood alcohol levels that correspond with progressively greater intoxication.

We have called it lucky that the brain centers respond to alcohol in the order just described, because one passes out before one can drink a lethal dose. It is possible, though, to drink fast enough that the effects of alcohol continue to accelerate after one has gone to sleep. The occasional death that takes place during a drinking contest is attributed to this effect: the drinker drinks fast enough to receive a lethal dose before passing out.

Liver cells are not the only cells that die with excessive exposure to alcohol; brain cells are particularly sensitive. When liver cells have died, others may later multiply to replace them, but brain cells have little or no power to regenerate. This is one reason for the permanent brain damage observed in some heavy drinkers.

Alcohol depresses production of antidiuretic hormone (ADH) by the pituitary gland in the brain. All people who drink alcoholic beverages have observed the increase in urination that accompanies drinking, but they may not realize that they can easily get into a vicious cycle as a result. Loss of body water leads to thirst, and thirst leads to more drinking. The only fluid that will relieve dehydration is water, but the thirsty drinker may choose another alcoholic beverage instead. A person who tries to use alcoholic beverages to quench thirst, however, only worsens the problem. The smart drinker, then, either drinks beer

(which contains plenty of water), or drinks mixers or chasers with wine or hard liquor. Better still, the drinker alternates alcoholic beverages with glasses of water and limits the total amount consumed.

The water loss caused by depressed ADH involves the loss of more than just water and some alcohol. With water loss there is a loss of such important minerals as magnesium, potassium, calcium, and zinc. As Chapters 10 and 11 will explain, these minerals are vital to the maintenance of the fluid balance and to many chemical reactions in the cells, including muscle contraction. For the person made sick by excessive alcohol intake and requiring detoxification, repletion therapy has to be instituted early to bring magnesium and potassium levels back to normal as quickly as possible.

As you can tell, alcohol dramatically changes normal metabolism. With these changes in mind, it may be appropriate to take a moment to discuss personal strategies for alcohol consumption.

Personal Strategies

If you choose to drink socially, sip your drinks slowly with food. The alcohol molecules should dribble slowly enough into the liver cells so that the enzymes can handle the load. Space your drinks, too. It takes about an hour and a half to metabolize one drink, depending on your body size, on previous drinking experience, on how recently you have eaten, and on how you are feeling at the time.

If you want to help sober up a friend who has had too much to drink, don't wear yourself out walking arm in arm around the block. Walking muscles have to work harder, but muscle cells can't metabolize alcohol; only liver cells can. Remember that each person has a particular amount of alcohol dehydrogenase that keeps on clearing the blood at a steady rate. In short, time alone will do the job.

Nor will it help to give your friend a cup of coffee. Caffeine is a stimulant, but it won't speed up the metabolism of alcohol. The police say ruefully, "If you give a drunk a cup of coffee, you'll just have a wide-awake drunk on your hands."

Don't drive too soon after drinking. The lack of glucose for the brain's function and the length of time needed to clear the blood of alcohol make alcohol's adverse effects linger long after alcohol's blood concentration has fallen to zero. Driving coordination is still impaired the morning *after* a night of drinking, even if the drinking was moderate.[4] Responsible aircraft pilots know that they must allow 24 hours for their bodies to clear alcohol completely, and they refuse to fly any sooner. Major airlines enforce this rule. Health care providers warn prepregnant and pregnant women to abstain from the use of alcohol, because it severely threatens the development of the fetus's central nervous system. (Highlight 14 provides more detail on fetal alcohol syndrome.)

You may have heard the story of the country woman who kept saying "Amen!" as the preacher ranted about one sin after another; but when he got to her favorite sin, she whispered to her husband that the preacher had "quit preachin' and gone to meddlin'." We've tried to stick to scientific facts, so the only "meddlin'" that we'll do is to urge you to look again at the drawing of the brain in Figure H7–6 and note that judgment is affected first when someone drinks. Judgment may tell a person to limit alcohol

consumption to two drinks at a party, but the first drink may take judgment away, so many more drinks follow. The failure to stop drinking as planned, on repeated occasions, is a danger sign that indicates that the person should not drink at all.

Ethanol interferes with a multitude of chemical and hormonal reactions in the body—many more than have been enumerated here. The point of this highlight, however, was not to summarize every effect of alcohol; the point was to offer a reward to the reader for learning the basics of metabolism explained in Chapter 7. The understandings gained permit a profound appreciation of processes like those described here.

NOTES

1. Alcohol and plasma lipids, *Nutrition and the M.D.*, August 1984.

2. A. B. Eisenstein, Nutritional and metabolic effects of alcohol, *Journal of the American Dietetic Association* 81 (1982): 247–251.

3. Alcohol dehydrogenase, although atypical, works as fast as normal in Asians, but their acetaldehyde dehydrogenase works more *slowly*, so that they suffer from a kind of acetaldehyde poisoning. D. P. Agarwal, S. Harada, and H. W. Goedde, Racial differences in biological sensitivity to ethanol: The role of alcohol dehydrogenase and acetaldehyde dehydrogenase enzymes, *Alcoholism: Clinical and Experimental Research* 5 (1981): 12–16.

4. D. Pine, Hungover driving, *Health*, May 1984, p. 12.

8

The Water-Soluble Vitamins: B Vitamins and Vitamin C

Collagen—made with the help of vitamin C—is the body's major connective material. Here, strands of collagen lie tangled near a muscle fiber membrane disrupted by freezing and chemical etching.

The last five chapters were devoted primarily to the energy-yielding nutrients—carbohydrates, lipids, and proteins—and their digestion and metabolism. The presence of these nutrients in the body accounts for what you are (you are made of these three materials and compounds derived from them) and for what you do (they supply the energy for all of your activities). The vitamins differ from the energy-yielding nutrients in several ways, and this chapter begins with an overall look at the vitamins.

vitamins: organic, essential nutrients required in minute amounts.
  vita = life
  amine = containing nitrogen (the first vitamins discovered were amines)

◼ *The Vitamins*

The vitamins differ from the carbohydrates, fats, and proteins in the following ways:

- ◼ Size (vitamins are much smaller).
- ◼ Structure (vitamins act singly; they are not strung together to make body compounds).
- ◼ Function (vitamins do not yield energy when broken down but assist enzymes with energy production and help cells multiply for growth and healing).
- ◼ Food contents (the amounts you commonly consume from foods range from a few micrograms to many milligrams or so a day, as compared with 50 to 200 grams or so for the energy-yielding nutrients).

Perhaps the only characteristics vitamins share with the energy-yielding nutrients are that they are vital to life, that they are organic, and that they are available in foods.

The consequence of being organic is that vitamins are destructible. They can be oxidized, broken down, and altered in shape. Such destruction leaves vitamins unable to perform their duties; therefore, they must be handled with care. People who handle foods must treat vitamins with respect. The body also treats vitamins respectfully, making special provisions to absorb them and providing several of them with custom-made protein carriers. Because vitamins may be useful in one form for one role and in another form for another role, the body also provides special enzymes to slightly alter their forms, thus activating them for specific roles.

As you may recall, some compounds (such as carbohydrates and proteins) are hydrophilic (water loving), and others (such as lipids) are hydrophobic (water fearing). The vitamins divide along the same lines—the hydrophilic, water-soluble ones include the B vitamins and vitamin C; and the hydrophobic, fat-soluble ones include vitamins A, D, E, and K.

Solubility has implications for the body's absorption, transport, storage, and excretion of the vitamins. The body absorbs water-soluble vitamins directly into the blood; fat-soluble vitamins must first enter the lymph before entering the bloodstream. Once in the bloodstream, many of the water-soluble vitamins travel freely; many of the fat-soluble vitamins require protein carriers for transport. Upon reaching the body cells, water-soluble vitamins freely circulate into the water-filled compartments of the body; fat-soluble vitamins tend to become trapped in the cells, associated with fat.

The kidneys, sensitive to high concentrations of substances in the blood that flows through them, detect and remove excess water-soluble vitamins. Less readily excreted are the fat-soluble vitamins, which tend to remain in fat-storage sites in the body rather than accumulate in the blood. Because of this, fat-soluble vitamins are more likely to reach toxic levels when consumed in excess.

These solubility differences also have implications for the way a person chooses foods. When a person consumes fat-soluble vitamins in excess of the body's needs, they may be stored. Later, when blood concentrations begin to decline, these vitamins may be retrieved from storage, thus maintaining the body's required supply. To put it another way, fat-soluble vitamins can be eaten in large amounts once in a while and still meet the body's needs over time. In contrast, when a person consumes water-soluble vitamins in excess of the body's needs, they will be more promptly excreted, thus reducing the blood concentrations to normal and leaving little behind. Then, when blood concentrations begin to decline, a deficiency sets in. Water-soluble vitamins are retained for varying periods in the body; a single day's omission from the diet does not bring on a dire emergency, but still, the water-soluble vitamins must be eaten more regularly than the fat-soluble vitamins.

In summary, the water-soluble vitamins are, for the most part, carried in the bloodstream; excreted in the urine; needed in frequent, small doses; and unlikely to be toxic, except when taken in unusually large quantities. The fat-soluble vitamins are, in general, absorbed into the lymph and then carried in the blood by protein carriers, stored in fat tissues, needed in periodic doses, and more likely to be toxic when consumed in excess of needs.

Exceptions to the statements just made occur, but these differences between the water- and fat-soluble vitamins are worth remembering as generalizations. This chapter focuses on the water-soluble vitamins; the next, on the fat-soluble vitamins.

■ The Water-Soluble Vitamins

As mentioned, the water-soluble vitamins include vitamin C and the B vitamins. They got their names from the labels *B* and *C* on the test tubes into which they were first collected. Later, test tube B turned out to have more than one vitamin in it; the fractions were given subscripts (B_1, B_2, and so on); and later still, most of them received names (see Table 8–1).

The discussion of B vitamins begins with an explanation of coenzymes, for most of the B vitamins serve in that role. Then it provides a brief description of each of the individual B vitamins, followed by a look at the collective whole. Thus a presentation of the "trees" is followed by a survey of the "forest," for there is much to be learned from viewing the B vitamins both as individuals and as a group.

To provide all the details now known about the absorption, metabolism, and interrelationships of the B vitamins would require more pages than remain in this book and would burden the reader with specialized knowledge beyond the level appropriate for the beginning study of nutrition. But to omit them all would be to deprive the reader, leaving the curtains closed on a colorful and dramatic theater of action that fascinates its audience. A

■ TABLE 8–1
B Vitamin Terminology

Many of the vitamins have both names and numbers, a mixture of terminologies that confuses newcomers to the study of nutrition. A single set of names for the vitamins has been agreed on and published, and those names are used in this book.[a] Still, to read the many worthwhile writings published prior to this nomenclature policy, you have to be aware of the alternative names.

Standard Vitamin Name	Other Names Commonly Used[b]
Thiamin	Vitamin B_1
Riboflavin	Vitamin B_2
Niacin	Nicotinic acid, nicotinamide, niacinamide, vitamin B_3
Vitamin B_6	Pyridoxine, pyridoxal, pyridoxamine
Folate	Folacin, folic acid, pteroylglutamic acid
Vitamin B_{12}	Cobalamin
Pantothenic acid	(None)
Biotin	(None)

[a]The vitamin names used here are those agreed on, and published by, the International Union of Nutritional Sciences Committee on Nomenclature, in Nomenclature policy: Generic descriptors and trivial names for vitamins and related compounds, *Journal of Nutrition* 117 (1987): 7–15.
[b]Also see Appendix C.

compromise is attempted here: a sneak peek at the scene in which nutritional biochemists spend their days.

■ *The B Vitamins—As Individuals*

Vitamin ads would have you believe that vitamins give you energy. They don't. The energy-yielding nutrients discussed in Chapters 4, 5, and 6 can be used as fuel, and the B vitamins help to burn that fuel, but the vitamins do not serve as fuel themselves.

It is true, though, that without B vitamins you would lack energy. Some of the B vitamins serve as helpers to the enzymes that release energy from carbohydrate, fat, and protein; they stand alongside the metabolic pathways, so to speak, and help to keep the disassembly lines moving. Some B vitamins assist in the assembly of compounds such as proteins. In an industrial plant, they would be called expediters.

B vitamins also help cells to multiply, and this is especially important in populations of cells with short life spans that must replace themselves rapidly. Such are the red blood cells and the cells lining the GI tract—both key members of the team of cells that deliver energy to all the body's tissues.

Each B vitamin plays several roles in metabolism; the roles they play as parts of coenzymes are the best understood. Coenzymes are small nonprotein molecules that associate closely with some enzymes. There are differences in the details of the relationships between coenzymes and enzymes, but one thing is true of all: without its coenzyme, an enzyme cannot function.

As you read the following sections describing individual B vitamins, note the many coenzymes and metabolic pathways mentioned. Keep in mind that a later section will put these pieces of information together to provide an overall picture of the activities of these vitamins.

coenzyme (co-EN-zime): a small molecule that works with an enzyme to promote the enzyme's activity. Many coenzymes have B vitamins as part of their structures.
co = with

To review the structures and functions of enzymes, see Chapter 6.

Thiamin

In 1937, the coenzyme form of thiamin was first discovered and isolated. Since then, the world of vitamins and enzyme action has opened up, revealing its intricacies and permitting medicine and science to put vitamins and enzymes to use in a multitude of ways.

Thiamin is the vitamin part of the coenzyme TPP which plays a significant role in energy metabolism. The TPP coenzyme participates in the conversion of pyruvate to acetyl CoA. Besides playing this pivotal role in the energy metabolism of all cells, thiamin occupies a special site on the nerve cell membrane. Consequently, processes in nerves and in their responding tissues, the muscles, depend heavily on thiamin.

thiamin (THIGH-ah-min): a B vitamin; the coenzyme form is TPP (thiamin pyrophosphate).

beriberi: the thiamin-deficiency disease; it pointed the way to discovery of the first vitamin, thiamin.

Thiamin Deficiency Prolonged thiamin deficiency can result in the disease beriberi, which was first observed in the Far East when the custom of polishing rice became widespread. Rice provided 80 percent of the energy intake of the people of those areas, and rice hulls were their principal source of thiamin. When the hulls were removed in the effort to make the rice whiter and more pleasing to the people, beriberi spread like wildfire.

Beriberi was first believed to be caused by an infectious agent. Medical researchers wasted much time and energy seeking a microbial cause before they realized that the problem was not what was present in the food, but what was absent from it. People often have to relearn this valuable nutrition lesson.

Considering thiamin's participation in nerve processes, it is not surprising that paralysis sets in when this nutrient is lacking. The symptoms of beriberi include damage to the nervous and cardiovascular systems, as well as wasting of the muscles.

Thiamin Toxicity Too much thiamin also affects the nervous system. High doses of thiamin, taken by injection, cause a nervous system hypersensitivity reaction. Table 8–2 summarizes thiamin deficiency and toxicity symptoms, as well as the vitamin's main functions and food sources.

The edema of beriberi. Thiamin deficiency also sometimes produces a "dry" beriberi, without edema, for reasons not well understood. Another marked symptom is inability to walk, manifested by collapse of the lower limbs when the person tries to stand.

■ **TABLE 8–2**
Thiamin—A Summary

Other Names	Deficiency Disease Name	
Vitamin B$_1$	Beriberi	
Chief Functions in the Body	**Deficiency Symptoms**	**Toxicity Symptoms**
Part of TPP (thiamin pyrophosphate), a coenzyme used in energy metabolism; supports normal appetite and nervous system function	**Blood/Circulatory System**	
	Edema, enlarged heart, abnormal heart rhythms, heart failure	Rapid pulse
	Nervous/Muscular Systems	
Significant Sources	Degeneration, wasting, weakness, painful calf muscles, low morale, difficulty walking, loss of ankle and knee jerk reflexes, mental confusion, paralysis	Weakness, headaches, insomnia, irritability
Occurs in all nutritious foods in moderate amounts; pork, ham, bacon, liver, whole grains, legumes, nuts		

Thiamin RDA: 0.5 mg/1,000 kcal/day
(1 mg/day minimum).
Canadian RNI: 0.4 mg/1,000 kcal/day
(0.8 mg/day minimum).

Thiamin Requirements   The RDA for thiamin is stated in terms of milligrams per 1,000 kcalories of food energy. Generally, if you are consuming enough energy to meet your needs and obtaining that energy from thiamin-containing foods, your thiamin intake will adjust to your need.

People who derive a large proportion of their energy from empty-kcalorie items like sugar or alcohol risk thiamin deficiency. A person who is fasting or who has adopted a very-low-kcalorie diet still needs to obtain the same amount of thiamin as when on a 2,000–kcalorie diet.

Thiamin Food Sources   Table 8–3 shows the thiamin amounts in different types of foods as measured against the U.S. RDA. In Table 8–3 and similar tables in this chapter and the next three chapters, colored bars will help to tell you at a glance which food groups best represent a nutrient. Notice the diversity of colors in the table. Thiamin is a nutrient that can be obtained in small quantities from any nutritious food, and you can meet your RDA by eating single servings of many different foods. A few red bars near the top of the graph represent meats that are exceptionally good thiamin sources; these are members of the pork/ham family. Large servings of these meats significantly increase a person's energy intake, however. Many other colors are apparent in the top half of the table; note, particularly, the browns (legumes) and greens (vegetables).

If you study Table 8–3 while thinking about your own food habits, you will probably conclude that many of the foods you like and eat daily contribute some thiamin, but none by itself can meet your total need for a day. A useful guideline is to keep to a minimum the empty-kcalorie foods in your diet and to include ten or more different servings of nutritious foods each day, assuming that on the average each serving will contribute about 10 percent of your need. Foods chosen from the bread and cereal group should be either whole grain or enriched.

riboflavin (RYE-boh-flay-vin): a B vitamin; the coenzyme forms are FMN (flavin mononucleotide) and FAD (flavin adenine dinucleotide).

Riboflavin

Riboflavin is another of the water-soluble B vitamins. Like thiamin, it helps enzymes to facilitate the release of energy from nutrients needed in every cell

Nutrient Density

If the foods in Table 8–3 were ranked by their nutrient density (for example, by their thiamin *per 100 kcal*), the ranking would offer a different perspective. You would discover that vegetables would rank significantly higher in a thiamin-per-100-kcal list than they do in the thiamin-per-serving list of foods, because vegetables provide more than adequate amounts of thiamin while providing less energy (fewer kcalories) and less fat than meats and other foods derived from animals. If you were to eat large quantities of vegetables, you could obtain significant amounts of thiamin from them, even though they didn't make large contributions *per serving*. The high nutrient density value of vegetables holds true for most vitamins. Vegetables offer people the best deal for their energy "dollar" (the kcalorie).

■ TABLE 8–3
Thiamin in Commonly Eaten Foods Ranked Richest to Poorest

Food, Serving Size (Energy)

U.S. RDA = 1.5 milligrams

Brewer's yeast, 1 tbsp (25 kcal)
Pork chop, 3.1 oz broiled (275 kcal)
Ham, 3 oz canned roasted (140 kcal)
Sunflower seeds, ¼ c dry (205 kcal)
Green peas, 1 c cooked (146 kcal)
Black beans, 1 c cooked (225 kcal)
Black-eyed peas, 1 c cooked (190 kcal)
Watermelon, 1 slice (152 kcal)
Canadian bacon, 2 pieces cooked (86 kcal)
Wheat germ, ¼ c raw (68 kcal)
Oysters, 1 c raw (160 kcal)
Split peas, 1 c cooked (230 kcal)
Oatmeal, 1 c cooked (145 kcal)
Acorn squash, 1 c boiled (83 kcal)
Baked potato, 1 whole (220 kcal)
Winter squash, 1 c baked (96 kcal)
Peanuts, 1 oz dried unsalted (161 kcal)
Asparagus, 1 c cooked (44 kcal)
Tofu (soybean curd), 1 block (86 kcal)
Broccoli, 1 c cooked (46 kcal)
Kidney beans, 1 c canned (230 kcal)
Orange, 1 fresh medium (60 kcal)
Sirloin steak, 3 oz lean (180 kcal)
Cantaloupe, ½ (94 kcal)
Honeydew melon, ¹⁄₁₀ (45 kcal)
Whole-wheat bread, 1 slice (70 kcal)
Millet, ½ c cooked (54 kcal)
Whole milk, 1 c (150 kcal)
Nonfat milk or yogurt, 1 c (86 kcal)
Green beans, 1 c cooked (44 kcal)
Bean sprouts, 1 c fresh (32 kcal)
Cauliflower, 1 c cooked (30 kcal)
Mushrooms, 1 c raw sliced (18 kcal)
Summer squash, 1 c cooked (36 kcal)
Zucchini, 1 c cooked (29 kcal)
Tomato, 1 whole raw (24 kcal)
Turnip greens, 1 c cooked (29 kcal)
Chicken breast, ½ roasted (142 kcal)
Mustard greens, 1 c cooked (21 kcal)
Romaine lettuce, 1 c chopped (9 kcal)
Bok choy, 1 c cooked (20 kcal)
Sole/flounder, 3 oz baked (120 kcal)
Cabbage, 1 c raw shredded (16 kcal)
Parsley, 1 c chopped fresh (20 kcal)
Miso, 3 tbsp (88 kcal)
Loose-leaf lettuce, 1 c (10 kcal)
Alfalfa seeds, 1 c sprouted (10 kcal)
Apple, 1 fresh medium (80 kcal)
Celery, 1 large outer stalk (6 kcal)
Cheddar cheese, 1 oz (114 kcal)

¼ U.S. RDA

Key:
= Milk.
= Meat.
= Vegetable.
= Fruit.
= Legumes.
= Bread.
= Miscellaneous.

The diversity of colors in this table shows that
thiamin can be obtained from many different
foods; several servings of a variety of nutritious
foods will help you to meet your RDA.

Milligrams/Serving

A Note on Looking to Foods for Single Nutrients

Table 8–3 is the first of a long series of tables that present the nutrients in foods, one by one, through the next three chapters. If you looked at only one or a few of these tables, you might get the wrong impression: that you should think in terms of single nutrients and learn which foods supply each one. Realistically, though, people cannot eat for single nutrients, and the tables are not intended to show you how to do so. Withhold judgment for a while, until you see the effect of all the tables taken together. A conclusion can be shown about how to eat, after surveying the whole array of nutrients in foods, and this will be done in Chapter 16.

For the most part, the serving sizes in these tables are those that people might realistically eat. For example, 3 oz is used for most meats, but because people who eat oysters don't eat them by the ounce, the serving for oysters is 1 c. People wanting to use the exchange system could easily convert 3 oz of sirloin steak to 3 lean meat exchanges. Similarly, the vegetable serving size is given as 1 c instead of the ½-c portion used in the exchange system.

These tables list the food, the serving size, and the food energy (kcalories) on the left and graph the milligrams of these nutrients on the right. The ¼ U.S. RDA arrow gives you a feel for about how many servings of various foods you need to eat to receive your recommended intake. The colors represent various food groups: blue for the milks and milk products; green for vegetables; purple for fruits; brown for legumes; gold for breads and cereals; red for meat, fish, and poultry; and gray for miscellaneous. Whereas the exchange system best groups foods according to their energy-yielding nutrients, the groups used in these tables better reflect the similarities in the vitamin and mineral contents of the foods within a group, and that is our focus in these chapters.

Notice that Table 8–3 is not a list of the foods highest in thiamin. The table presents an array of commonly eaten foods that range from excellent to poor sources of thiamin. Thus the bottom of the list can be as informative as the top.

In addition, foods representative of each of the food groups appear in the table. This table and all the tables that follow include some foods—such as an apple, green beans, sole/flounder, and sirloin steak—not because they are particularly rich in a nutrient but because they are commonly eaten foods of different types. Careful study of all of the tables taken together will show that variety is the key to nutrient adequacy.

Brewer's yeast, or nutritional yeast, is included in these tables because people who eat plant foods exclusively often mix it into their recipes and beverages to enhance the nutrient contributions of their meals. As you will see, brewer's yeast is high (per tablespoon) in a number of nutrients, which makes it a valuable addition to the diets of people who do not use foods derived from animals.

nutritional yeast: a preparation of yeast cells grown especially as a nutrient supplement, particularly for vegetarian diets. The type of yeast used is brewer's yeast, not baker's yeast.

of the body. The coenzyme forms of riboflavin include FMN and FAD. The FAD coenzyme plays an active role in the TCA cycle, and both coenzymes FMN and FAD are essential parts of enzyme complexes that transfer energy during the final stage of metabolism of the energy nutrients.[1]

Riboflavin Deficiency   No one disease is associated with riboflavin deficiency. Lack of the vitamin affects the facial skin (cracks and redness near the corners of the eyes and lips), eyes (inflamed eyelids and sensitivity), and GI tract (painful, smooth, purplish red tongue). Table 8–4 provides a summary of riboflavin's deficiency symptoms, as well as its chief functions and food sources.

Riboflavin Requirements   Like thiamin needs, riboflavin needs are stated in terms of milligrams per 1,000 kcalories of food energy. The variations in the riboflavin RDA primarily reflect changes in energy intake. Infant's, children's, and pregnant women's needs rise rapidly during their times of active growth.

Riboflavin RDA: 0.6 mg/1,000 kcal/day (1.2 mg/day minimum).
Canadian RNI: 0.5 mg/1,000 kcal/day (1 mg/day minimum).

Riboflavin Food Sources   Three colors dominate the top of Table 8–5, which shows the riboflavin contents in foods per serving—red for meats, fish, and poultry; green for vegetables; and blue for milk and milk products. Contrast this table with the table of thiamin, which showed no blue until halfway down. Clearly, milk, milk products such as cheese, and organ meats dominate the top of the riboflavin list, with a few other meats and exceptionally nutritious vegetables scattered among them. The need for riboflavin provides a major reason for including milk and milk products in every day's meals; no other commonly eaten food can make such a substantial contribution in a single serving.

Most people have little trouble meeting their RDA for riboflavin. On the average, they derive about half their riboflavin from milk and milk products, about a fourth from meats, and most of the rest from green vegetables (such as broccoli, turnip greens, asparagus, and spinach) and whole-grain or

■ TABLE 8–4
Riboflavin—A Summary

Other Names	Deficiency Disease Name	
Vitamin B$_2$	Ariboflavinosis	

Chief Functions in the Body	Deficiency Symptoms	Toxicity Symptoms
Part of FMN (flavin mononucleotide) and FAD (flavin adenine dinucleotide), coenzymes used in energy metabolism; supports normal vision and skin health	**Mouth, Gums, Tongue** Cracks at corners of mouth,[a] magenta tongue **Nervous System and Eyes** Hypersensitivity to light,[b] reddening of cornea	
Significant Sources	**Other**	
Milk, yogurt, cottage cheese, meat, leafy green vegetables, whole-grain or enriched breads and cereals	Skin rash	Interference with anticancer medication

[a]Cracks at the corners of the mouth are termed *cheilosis* (kee-LOH-sis).
[b]Hypersensitivity to light is *photophobia*.

■ TABLE 8—5
Riboflavin in Commonly Eaten Foods Ranked Richest to Poorest

Food, Serving Size (Energy)

Braunschweiger sausage, 2 pieces (205 kcal)
Mushroom pieces, 1 c cooked (42 kcal)
Ricotta cheese, 1 c part skim (340 kcal)
Nonfat milk plus solids, 1 c (91 kcal)
Oysters, 1 c raw (160 kcal)
Cottage cheese, 1 c low-fat 2% (205 kcal)
Beet greens, 1 c cooked (40 kcal)
Spinach, 1 c cooked (41 kcal)
Milk, 1 c low-fat 1% (102 kcal)
Milk, 1 c whole (150 kcal)
Buttermilk, 1 c (99 kcal)
Milk or yogurt, 1 c nonfat (86 kcal)
Goat's milk, 1 c (168 kcal)
Brewer's yeast, 1 tbsp (25 kcal)
Mushrooms, 1 c raw sliced (18 kcal)
Broccoli, 1 c cooked (46 kcal)
Pork roast, 3 oz (187 kcal)
Peach halves, 10 dried (311 kcal)
Sirloin steak, 3 oz lean (180 kcal)
Ham, 3 oz roasted (133 kcal)
Almonds, 1 oz whole dried (167 kcal)
Asparagus, 1 c cooked (44 kcal)
Bean sprouts, 1 c stir-fried (62 kcal)
Corned beef, 3 oz canned (185 kcal)
Ground beef, 3 oz 10% fat (230 kcal)
Dandelion greens, 1 c cooked (35 kcal)
Salmon, 3 oz smoked (150 kcal)
Turkey, 3 oz (145 kcal)
Green beans, 1 c cooked (44 kcal)
Bok choy, 1 c cooked (20 kcal)
Cheddar cheese, 1 oz (114 kcal)
Strawberries, 1 c fresh (45 kcal)
Chicken breast, ½ roasted (142 kcal)
Black-eyed peas, 1 c cooked (190 kcal)
Kidney beans, 1 c canned (230 kcal)
Turnip greens, 1 c cooked (29 kcal)
Mustard greens, 1 c cooked (21 kcal)
Sole/flounder, 3 oz baked (120 kcal)
Summer squash, 1 c cooked (36 kcal)
Whole-wheat bread, 1 slice (70 kcal)
Cantaloupe, ½ (94 kcal)
Romaine lettuce, 1 c chopped (9 kcal)
Tomato, 1 whole raw (24 kcal)
Parsley, 1 c chopped fresh (20 kcal)
Oatmeal, 1 c cooked (145 kcal)
Orange, 1 fresh medium (60 kcal)
Peanuts, 1 oz dried unsalted (161 kcal)
Loose-leaf lettuce, 1 c (10 kcal)
Alfalfa seeds, 1 c sprouted (10 kcal)
Apple, 1 fresh medium (80 kcal)

U.S. RDA = 1.7 milligrams

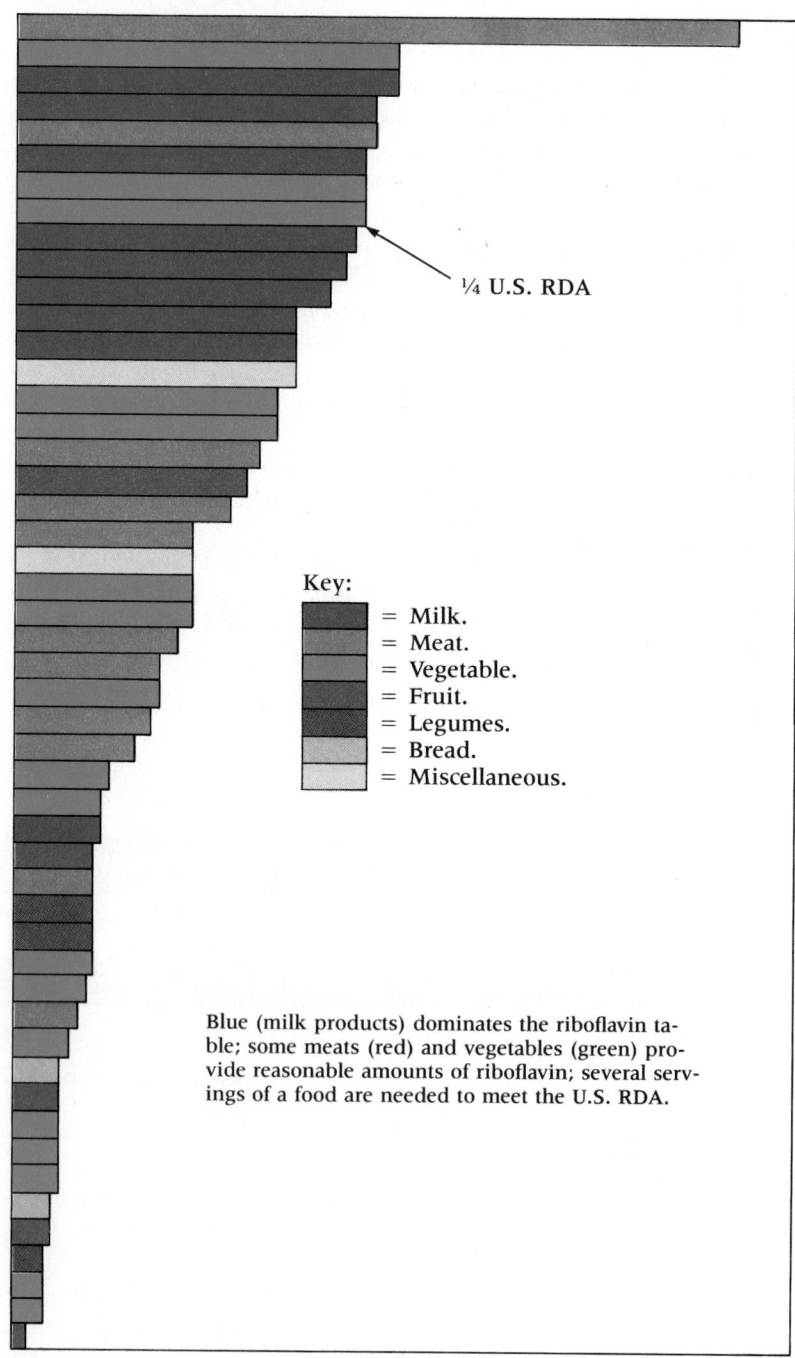

¼ U.S. RDA

Key:

= Milk.
= Meat.
= Vegetable.
= Fruit.
= Legumes.
= Bread.
= Miscellaneous.

Blue (milk products) dominates the riboflavin table; some meats (red) and vegetables (green) provide reasonable amounts of riboflavin; several servings of a food are needed to meet the U.S. RDA.

Milligrams/Serving

enriched bread and cereal products. A list of riboflavin sources ranked per 100 kcalories would include many more dark green, leafy vegetables high on the list. Vegetarians who don't use milk can meet their riboflavin needs with ample servings of dark greens. Brewer's yeast is another rich source of riboflavin for the vegetarian.

Table 8–5 illustrates another point of interest. Compare the various milk items listed, and note that the lower-fat items have the higher amounts of riboflavin. It stands to reason: riboflavin is a water-soluble vitamin. The less fat in a given volume, the more water there will be, and therefore the more water-soluble nutrient.

Light and irradiation can destroy riboflavin. For these reasons, precautions must be taken during the addition of vitamin D by irradiation and in the packaging of milk. Milk is seldom sold in transparent glass or translucent plastic containers; cardboard or opaque plastic containers protect the riboflavin in the milk from light. In contrast, riboflavin is heat stable, so ordinary cooking does not destroy it.

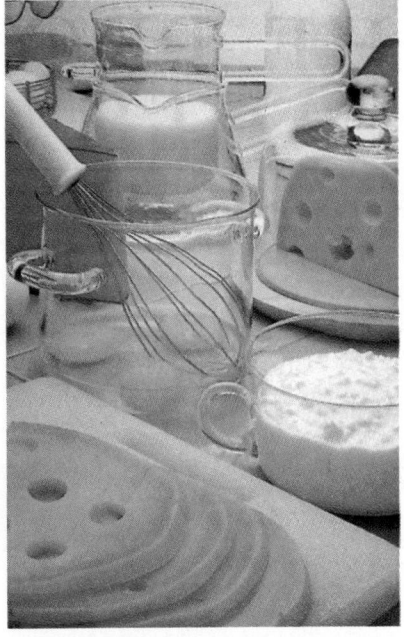

Milk and milk products provide much of the riboflavin in the diets of most people.

Niacin

The name niacin includes two forms of the vitamin, nicotinic acid and nicotinamide. The body can easily convert nicotinic acid to nicotinamide, which is the active form of niacin.[2]

The two coenzyme forms of niacin, NAD and NADP, participate in numerous metabolic activities. They are central in energy-transfer reactions and especially evident in the metabolism of glucose, fat, and alcohol. The way NAD works is shown in Figure 8–1.

niacin (NIGH-a-sin): a B vitamin. Niacin can be eaten preformed or can be made in the body from its precursor, tryptophan, one of the amino acids. The active coenzyme forms are NAD (nicotinamide adenine dinucleotide) and NADP (the phosphate form of NAD).

A. An enzyme with coenzyme NAD$^+$ encounters a molecule containing two hydrogens.

B. A complex is formed.

C. The hydrogens are removed from the molecule and attached to NAD$^+$, forming NADH + H$^+$. The enzyme releases NADH + H$^+$ and the molecule.

D. Later the NADH + H$^+$ donates the hydrogens to another compound and returns to its enzyme again as NAD$^+$.

■ **FIGURE 8–1**
Coenzyme Action
Each coenzyme is specialized for certain kinds of chemical reactions. NAD$^+$ (containing niacin), for example, can accept hydrogen atoms removed from other compounds and can lose them to compounds that ultimately pass them to oxygen. In many steps during the catabolism of glucose, hydrogens are removed and NAD$^+$ participates this way. A model of the way NAD$^+$ works with an enzyme to remove hydrogens is shown here.

Niacin is unique among the B vitamins in that the body can make it from the amino acid tryptophan. To make 1 milligram of niacin requires approximately 60 milligrams of dietary tryptophan.

Niacin Deficiency   The niacin deficiency disease, pellagra, includes the symptoms of dermatitis, diarrhea, and dementia. (See Table 8–6 for a summary of niacin's deficiency and toxicity symptoms, as well as its various names, functions, and food sources.) Pellagra became widespread in the U.S. South in the early part of this century, in people who subsisted on a low-protein diet whose staple grain was corn. This diet was unusual in that it supplied neither enough niacin nor enough of its amino acid precursor tryptophan to make up the deficiency. (Usually, tryptophan provides roughly half of the niacin requirement.)

pellagra (pell-AY-gra): the niacin-deficiency disease.
pellis = skin
agra = rough

The dermatitis of pellagra. The skin darkens and flakes away as if it were sunburned. In kwashiorkor there is also a "flaky paint" dermatitis, but the two are easily distinguishable. The dermatitis of pellagra is bilateral and symmetrical and occurs only on those parts of the body exposed to the sun.

■ TABLE 8–6
Niacin—A Summary

Other Names	Deficiency Disease Name	
Nicotinic acid, nicotinamide, niacinamide, vitamin B_3; precursor is dietary tryptophan	Pellagra	

Chief Functions in the Body	Deficiency Symptoms	Toxicity Symptoms
Part of NAD (nicotinamide adenine dinucleotide) and NADP (its phosphate form), coenzymes used in energy metabolism; supports health of skin, nervous system, and digestive system	**Digestive System**	
	Diarrhea	Diarrhea, heartburn, nausea, ulcer irritation, vomiting
	Mouth, Gums, Tongue	
		Inflammed, swollen, smooth tongue[a]
	Nervous System	
	Irritability, loss of appetite, weakness, dizziness, mental confusion progressing to psychosis or delirium	Fainting, dizziness
Significant Sources		
Milk, eggs, meat, poultry, fish, whole-grain and enriched breads and cereals, nuts, and all protein-containing foods	**Skin**	
	Bilateral symmetrical dermatitis, especially on areas exposed to sun	Painful flush and rash, itching, burning excessive sweating
	Other	
		Abnormal liver function, low blood pressure

[a]Smoothness of the tongue is caused by loss of its surface structures and is termed *glossitis* (gloss-EYE-tis).

Niacin Toxicity Large doses of nicotinic acid and nicotinamide act like drugs in the nervous system, and on blood lipids and blood glucose. Niacin in large doses (10 times the RDA or more) dilates the capillaries and causes a tingling effect that, if intense, can be painful; the effect is known as the "niacin flush." (The niacinamide form doesn't have this effect.) At one time, researchers were hopeful that large doses of niacin would help cure schizophrenia or learning disorders in children. A careful review of the evidence shows, however, that niacin is ineffective in correcting these problems.[3]

Physicians use diet and a combination of large doses of niacin and a drug to treat people with atherosclerosis. This treatment successively lowers total blood cholesterol and LDL concentrations and elevates HDL concentrations.[4] High doses of niacin may injure the liver, cause peptic ulcer, and produce laboratory evidence of diabetes, so self-dosing is ill-advised.

Niacin Requirements The RDA for niacin also relates to energy intake. Recommended niacin intakes are stated in "equivalents," reflecting the body's ability to convert the amino acid tryptophan to niacin. A food containing 1 milligram of niacin and 60 milligrams of tryptophan contains the equivalent of 2 milligrams of niacin, or 2 niacin equivalents (NE).

Niacin Food Sources Tables of food composition list only the preformed niacin in foods, although, as already stated, people actually derive the vitamin from both niacin itself and dietary tryptophan. To calculate the amount of niacin available from the diet is a complicated matter. The body first uses tryptophan to build needed body proteins, and then, if any tryptophan is left over, makes niacin. A means of obtaining a rough approximation of niacin intake is shown in the accompanying box. Step 2 assumes that protein intake above the RDA is "leftover" protein available for niacin synthesis; but the RDA already provides a generous protein allowance, so "leftover" protein may be even greater than this. On the average, diets supply enough preformed niacin to meet the daily need; additional niacin equivalents from tryptophan are available from any diet that is more than adequate in complete protein.

The predominance of red bars at the top of Table 8−7 explains why meat, poultry, and fish contribute about half the niacin equivalents consumed by

When a normal dose of a nutrient clears up a deficiency condition and gives rise to a normal blood concentration, the nutrient is having a (**physiological effect.**) When a megadose (100 times larger than normal) overwhelms some system and acts like a drug, the nutrient is having a (**pharmacological effect.**)

Niacin RDA: 6.6 mg NE/1,000 kcal/day (13 mg NE minimum).
Canadian RNI: 7.2 mg NE/1,000 kcal/day (14.4 mg NE minimum).

niacin equivalents: the amount of niacin present in food, including the niacin that can theoretically be made from its precursor, tryptophan, present in the food.

Determining Niacin Intake

To obtain a rough approximation of niacin intake:

1. Calculate total protein consumed (grams).
2. Subtract the recommended protein intake to obtain "leftover" protein available to make niacin (grams).
3. Divide by 100 to obtain the amount of tryptophan in this protein (grams).
4. Multiply by 1,000 to express this amount of tryptophan in milligrams.
5. Divide by 60 to get niacin equivalents (milligrams).
6. Finally, add the amount of niacin obtained preformed in the diet (milligrams).

■ **TABLE 8–7**
Niacin in Commonly Eaten Foods Ranked Richest to Poorest

Food, Serving Size (Energy)

Tuna, 3 oz canned (135 kcal)
Beef liver, 3 oz fried (185 kcal)
Chicken breast, ½ roasted (142 kcal)
Halibut, 3 oz broiled (140 kcal)
Mushroom pieces, 1 c cooked (42 kcal)
Pink salmon, 3 oz canned (120 kcal)
Oysters, 1 c raw (160 kcal)
Peach halves, 10 dried (311 kcal)
Salmon, 3 oz broiled/baked (140 kcal)
Lamb chop, 3 oz braised (238 kcal)
Ground beef, 3 oz 21% fat (245 kcal)
Braunschweiger sausage, 2 pieces (205 kcal)
Turkey, 3 oz (145 kcal)
Sardines, 3 oz canned (175 kcal)
Pork chop, 3.1 oz broiled (275 kcal)
Peanuts, 1 oz dried unsalted (161 kcal)
Hash brown potatoes, 1 c (340 kcal)
Sirloin steak, 3 oz lean (180 kcal)
Shrimp, 3.5 oz boiled (109 kcal)
Potato, 1 microwaved with skin (212 kcal)
Baked potato, 1 whole (220 kcal)
Brewer's yeast, 1 tbsp (25 kcal)
Mushrooms, 1 c raw sliced (18 kcal)
Crab meat, 1 c canned (135 kcal)
Wheat bran, ¼ c (19 kcal)
Asparagus, 1 c cooked (44 kcal)
Sole/flounder, 3 oz baked (120 kcal)
Cantaloupe, ½ (94 kcal)
Kidney beans, 1 c canned (230 kcal)
Broccoli, 1 c cooked (46 kcal)
Whole-wheat bread, 1 slice (70 kcal)
Summer squash, 1 c cooked (36 kcal)
Spinach, 1 c cooked (41 kcal)
Peach, 1 fresh medium (37 kcal)
Green beans, 1 c cooked (44 kcal)
Tomato, 1 whole raw (24 kcal)
Bok choy, 1 c cooked (20 kcal)
Cauliflower, 1 c cooked (30 kcal)
Mustard greens, 1 c cooked (21 kcal)
Turnip greens, 1 c cooked (29 kcal)
Parsley, 1 c chopped fresh (20 kcal)
Green pepper, 1 whole (18 kcal)
Orange, 1 fresh medium (60 kcal)
Oatmeal, 1 c cooked (145 kcal)
Romaine lettuce, 1 c chopped (9 kcal)
Nonfat milk or yogurt, 1 c (86 kcal)
Loose-leaf lettuce, 1 c (10 kcal)
Whole milk, 1 c (150 kcal)
Apple, 1 fresh medium (80 kcal)
Cheddar cheese, 1 oz (114 kcal)

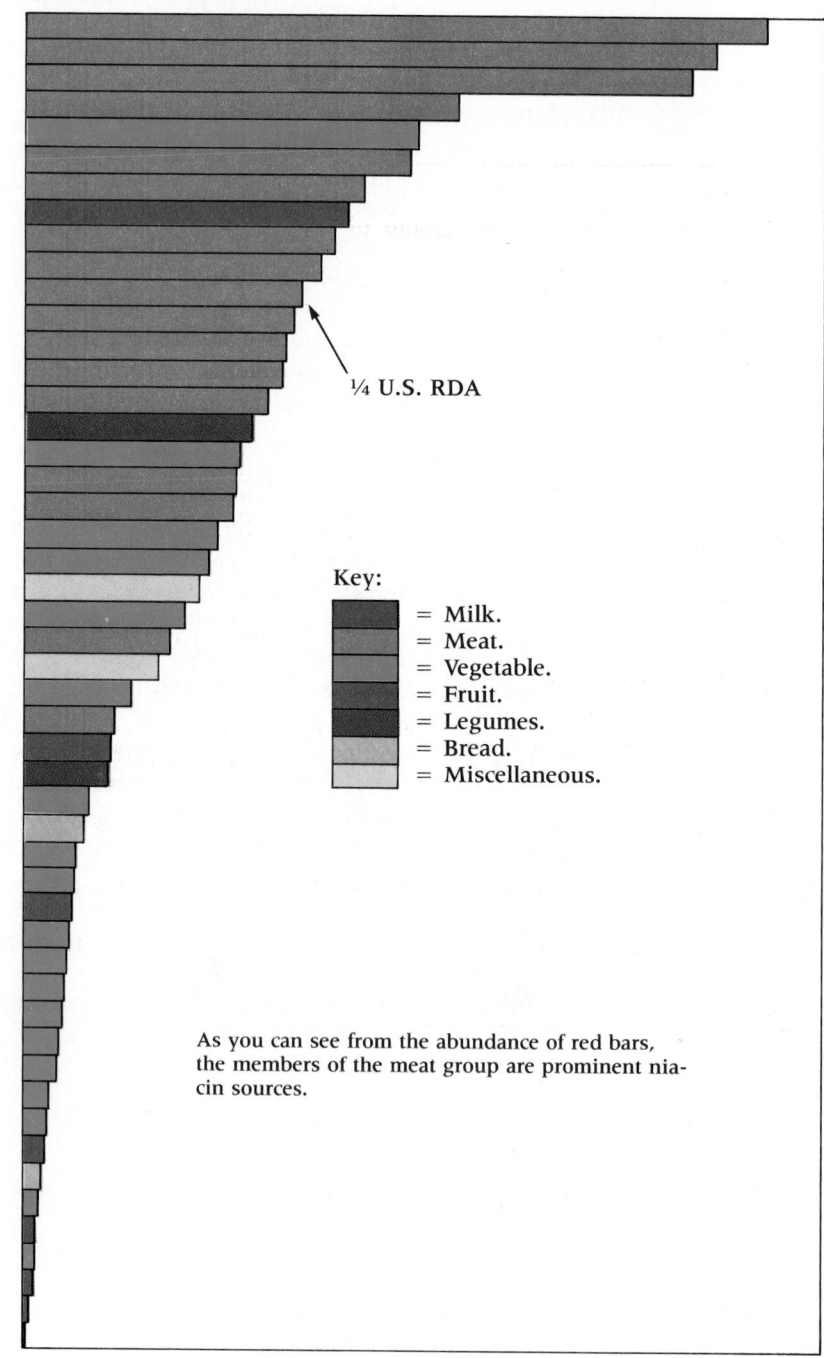

U.S. RDA = 20 milligrams

¼ U.S. RDA

Key:
= Milk.
= Meat.
= Vegetable.
= Fruit.
= Legumes.
= Bread.
= Miscellaneous.

As you can see from the abundance of red bars, the members of the meat group are prominent niacin sources.

Milligrams/Serving

most people. About a fourth of most people's niacin comes from enriched breads and cereals. As for vegetables, mushrooms, asparagus, and green leafy vegetables are among the richest vegetable sources (per kcalorie), and they can provide abundant niacin to the person who eats generous amounts of them.

Vitamin B₆

Vitamin B₆ appears in three forms—pyridoxal, pyridoxine, and pyridoxamine. All three forms can be converted to the vitamin B₆ coenzyme PLP.

The coenzyme PLP has the ability to transfer amino groups from one compound to another. Thus, with the help of this vitamin B₆ coenzyme, the body can synthesize nonessential amino acids when amino groups are available. PLP can also add free amino groups to compounds and remove amino groups from them. Thus it plays a significant role in protein and urea metabolism. The production of both niacin and the neurotransmitter serotonin from tryptophan relies on PLP.

Among the many drugs that interact with vitamin B₆, alcohol stands out. As Highlight 7 described, when the body breaks down alcohol, it first produces acetaldehyde, a toxic compound that must quickly be broken down further. Acetaldehyde knocks PLP loose from its enzymes; once loose, PLP breaks down to an excretion product; and then the kidneys dispose of it. Thus alcohol actively promotes the destruction of vitamin B₆ and its loss from the body.

Another drug that acts as a vitamin B₆ antagonist is INH, a potent inhibitor of the growth of the tuberculosis bacterium.* INH has saved countless lives, but as a vitamin B₆ antagonist, it binds and inactivates the vitamin, inducing a deficiency. Whenever INH is used to treat tuberculosis, supplements of vitamin B₆ must be given to protect the client from deficiency.

Vitamin B₆ Deficiency   When people are given a vitamin B₆–deficient diet, they experience such vague symptoms as weakness, irritability, and insomnia. More clearly defined symptoms include growth failure, impaired motor function, and convulsions.

Vitamin B₆ Toxicity   The first major report of toxic effects of vitamin B₆ appeared in 1983. Until that time, everyone (including researchers and dietitians) believed that, like the other water-soluble vitamins, vitamin B₆ could not reach toxic concentrations in the body. The first report told of seven women who had been taking more than 2 grams of vitamin B₆ daily (the RDA for women is less than 2 *milli*grams) for two months or more.

Most of these women were attempting to cure the symptoms of premenstrual syndrome (PMS). PMS is a cluster of physical, emotional, and psychological symptoms that some women experience prior to menstruation. Specific PMS symptoms and combinations of symptoms vary from woman to woman, but they share one distinguishing feature—the timing of the symptoms: they begin seven to ten days prior to menstruation and diminish with

vitamin B₆: a family of compounds—pyridoxal, pyridoxine, and pyridoxamine; the active coenzyme forms are PLP (pyridoxal phosphate) and PMP (pyridoxamine phosphate).

serotonin (SER-oh-tone-in): a neurotransmitter important in sleep and sensory perception that is synthesized from the amino acid tryptophan with the help of vitamin B₆.

alcohol destroys vit. B₆

antagonist: something that counteracts the action of another thing. When a drug displaces a vitamin from its site of action, it renders the vitamin ineffective, thus acting as a vitamin antagonist.

Common PMS symptoms:
- Headaches.
- Breast swelling and tenderness.
- Water retention.
- Weight gain.
- Irritability.
- Anxiety.
- Fatigue.
- Depression.
- Appetite changes and food cravings.
- Backaches.
- Acne.
- Constipation.

---

*INH stands for isonicotinic acid hydrazide.

menstruation. The cause or causes of PMS remain undefined, although researchers generally agree that the hormonal changes of the menstrual cycle must be responsible.[5] Without a full understanding of the ways PMS arises, medical treatments flounder, and quack treatments abound. Vitamin B_6 is a nutrient that receives much PMS attention.

Large doses of vitamin B_6 may cause irreversible nerve damage, starting with numb feet, then lost sensation in the hands, then an inability to work. Later, in some cases, the mouth becomes numb. Symptoms begin clearing up after withdrawal of the supplements, but whether they will completely disappear is uncertain.[6] (Table 8–8 lists common symptoms of both deficiency and toxicity, as well as chief functions and food sources of vitamin B_6.)

Since that first report, other cases have been reported, in which doses as low as 200 milligrams, taken for an extended time, caused "pins and needles," numbness of the hands, difficulty walking, and other symptoms reflecting severe impairment of the sensory nerves. In most cases, when the person stops taking the supplement, the condition improves; however, the symptoms may not completely disappear.

Vitamin B_6 Requirements Because the vitamin B_6 coenzymes play many roles in amino acid metabolism, dietary needs are roughly proportional to

■ TABLE 8–8
Vitamin B_6—A Summary

Other Names	Deficiency Symptoms	Toxicity Symptoms
Pyridoxine, pyridoxal, pyridoxamine	**Blood/Circulatory System**	
	Anemia (small-cell type)[a]	Bloating
	Mouth, Gums, Tongue	
	Smooth tongue,[b] cracked corners of the mouth[c]	
Chief Functions in the Body	**Nervous/Muscular Systems**	
Part of PLP (pyridoxal phosphate) and PMP (pyridoxamine phosphate), coenzymes used in amino acid and fatty acid metabolism; helps to convert tryptophan to niacin; helps to make red blood cells	Abnormal brain wave pattern, irritability, muscle twitching, convulsions	Depression, fatigue, irritability, headaches, numbness, damage to nerves leading to loss of reflexes and sensation, difficulty walking
	Skin	
	Irritation of sweat glands, dermatitis	
Significant Sources	**Other**	
Green and leafy vegetables, meats, fish, poultry, shellfish, legumes, fruits, whole grains	Kidney stones	

[a]Small-cell type anemia is *microcytic anemia*.
[b]Smoothness of the tongue is caused by loss of its surface structures and is termed *glossitis* (gloss-EYE-tis).
[c]Cracks at the corners of the mouth are termed *cheilosis* (kee-LOH-sis).

protein intakes. The RDA for vitamin B_6 is high enough to handle at least 100 grams of protein per day for men, and 60 grams of protein per day for women.

Vitamin B_6 Food Sources   Table 8–9 shows the vitamin B_6 in foods, ranked by the amounts per serving. As you can see, meats, fish, and poultry (red), potatoes and a few other vegetables (green), and fruits (purple) offer vitamin B_6. Vitamin B_6 is similar to thiamin and riboflavin in that you need to eat several servings of vitamin B_6–rich foods to meet recommended intakes.

Vitamin B_6 RDA: 0.016 mg/g protein.
2.0 mg/g (men).
1.6 mg/g (women).
Canadian RNI: 0.015 mg/g protein/day.

Folate

Folate is also known as folic acid or folacin, as well as its flying dinosaurlike name pteroylglutamic acid (or PGA, for short). Its primary coenzyme form is THF. THF is part of an enzyme complex that handles one-carbon units that arise during metabolism (see Figure 8–2). This action is critical to such processes as synthesis of the DNA required for rapidly growing cells, including those in the GI tract, blood, and all fetal tissues.

The body receives folate from foods mostly in the "bound" form—folate combined with a string of amino acids (glutamic acid), known as polyglutamate (see Appendix C for a diagram of this structure). The intestine prefers to absorb the "free" folate form—folate with only one glutamate attached (the monoglutamate form), sometimes with a methyl (CH_3) group attached, also. Enzymes on the surfaces of the intestinal cells hydrolyze the polyglutamate and then may attach the methyl group; special transport systems take up the monoglutamate either with or without a methyl group; and both travel freely in the blood.

The liver receives these two forms of folate and treats them in different ways. To the plain monoglutamate, it adds additional glutamates, thus converting it into the polyglutamate form for storage. As for the methyl form, the liver secretes most of it into bile and ships it to the gallbladder, whence it returns to the intestine again—an enterohepatic circulation route like that of bile itself (see Figure 5–17 on p. 121). Should the methyl folate be needed within the body, the methyl group would have to be removed—and the enzyme that removes it requires another B vitamin as a coenzyme: vitamin B_{12}, to be discussed next.

The cells of organs other than the liver also absorb the monoglutamate form of folate and add glutamates to it to keep it from escaping. They hydrolyze it back to the monoglutamate form to release it again.

This complicated transportation and conversion system for the folates is vulnerable to interference from a number of sources. For one, since one form of folate is actively secreted back into the intestinal tract with bile, it has to be reabsorbed repeatedly. If it is not—if something interferes with absorption, such as injury to the GI tract cells—then folate will be rapidly lost from the body. Such is the case in the person whose GI tract is injured by alcohol abuse; folate deficiency rapidly develops and, ironically, impairs the GI tract further. The folate coenzymes, remember, are active in cell multiplication—and the cells lining the GI tract are among the most rapidly renewed cells in

folate (FOLL-ate): a B vitamin; also known as folic acid, folacin, or pteroylglutamic (tare-oil-glue-TAM-ick) acid (PGA). The coenzyme forms are DHF (dihydrofolate) and THF (tetrahydrofolate).

■ FIGURE 8–2
One-Carbon Compounds Assisted by Folate
These are three one-carbon compounds, each more oxidized (having fewer hydrogens or more oxygens) than the one before. The folate coenzymes can carry all of them.

```
      H
      |
  H-C—O-H
      |
      H
   Methanol


  H-C = O
      |
      H
  Formaldehyde


  H-C = O
      |
      O-H
  Formic acid
```

■ TABLE 8–9
Vitamin B₆ in Commonly Eaten Foods Ranked Richest to Poorest

Food, Serving Size (Energy)

Navy beans, 1 c cooked (225 kcal)
Baked potato, 1 whole (220 kcal)
Watermelon, 1 slice (152 kcal)
Potato, 1 microwaved with skin (212 kcal)
Salmon, 3 oz broiled/baked (140 kcal)
Banana, 1 peeled (105 kcal)
Salmon, 3 oz smoked (150 kcal)
Chicken breast, ½ roasted (142 kcal)
Soybeans, 1 c cooked (235 kcal)
Potato, 1 microwaved without skin (156 kcal)
Sunflower seeds, ¼ c dry (205 kcal)
Spinach, 1 c cooked (41 kcal)
Tuna, 3 oz canned (135 kcal)
Figs, 10 dried (477 kcal)
Trout, 3 oz broiled (175 kcal)
Brewer's yeast, 1 tbsp (25 kcal)
Turkey, 3 oz (145 kcal)
Ground beef, 3 oz 10% fat (230 kcal)
Pork chop, 3.1 oz broiled (275 kcal)
Cantaloupe, ½ (94 kcal)
Broccoli, 1 c cooked (46 kcal)
Beef liver, 3 oz fried (185 kcal)
Bok choy, 1 c cooked (20 kcal)
Sirloin steak, 3 oz lean (180 kcal)
Sole/flounder, 3 oz baked (120 kcal)
Turnip greens, 1 c cooked (29 kcal)
Asparagus, 1 c cooked (44 kcal)
Cauliflower, 1 c cooked (30 kcal)
Mustard greens, 1 c cooked (21 kcal)
Wheat germ, ¼ c raw (68 kcal)
Zucchini, 1 c cooked (29 kcal)
Summer squash, 1 c cooked (36 kcal)
Green pepper, 1 whole (18 kcal)
Chicken liver, 1 simmered (30 kcal)
Milk, 1 c whole (150 kcal)
Parsley, 1 c chopped fresh (20 kcal)
Milk or yogurt, 1 c nonfat (86 kcal)
Tomato, 1 whole raw (24 kcal)
Peanuts, 1 oz dried unsalted (161 kcal)
Orange, 1 fresh medium (60 kcal)
Green beans, 1 c cooked (44 kcal)
Cabbage, 1 c raw shredded (16 kcal)
Apple, 1 fresh medium (80 kcal)
Mushrooms, 1 c raw sliced (18 kcal)
Collards, 1 c cooked (20 kcal)
Whole-wheat bread, 1 slice (70 kcal)
Oatmeal, 1 c cooked (145 kcal)
Kidney beans, 1 c canned (230 kcal)
Romaine lettuce, 1 c chopped (9 kcal)
Loose-leaf lettuce, 1 c (10 kcal)
Cheddar cheese, 1 oz (114 kcal)

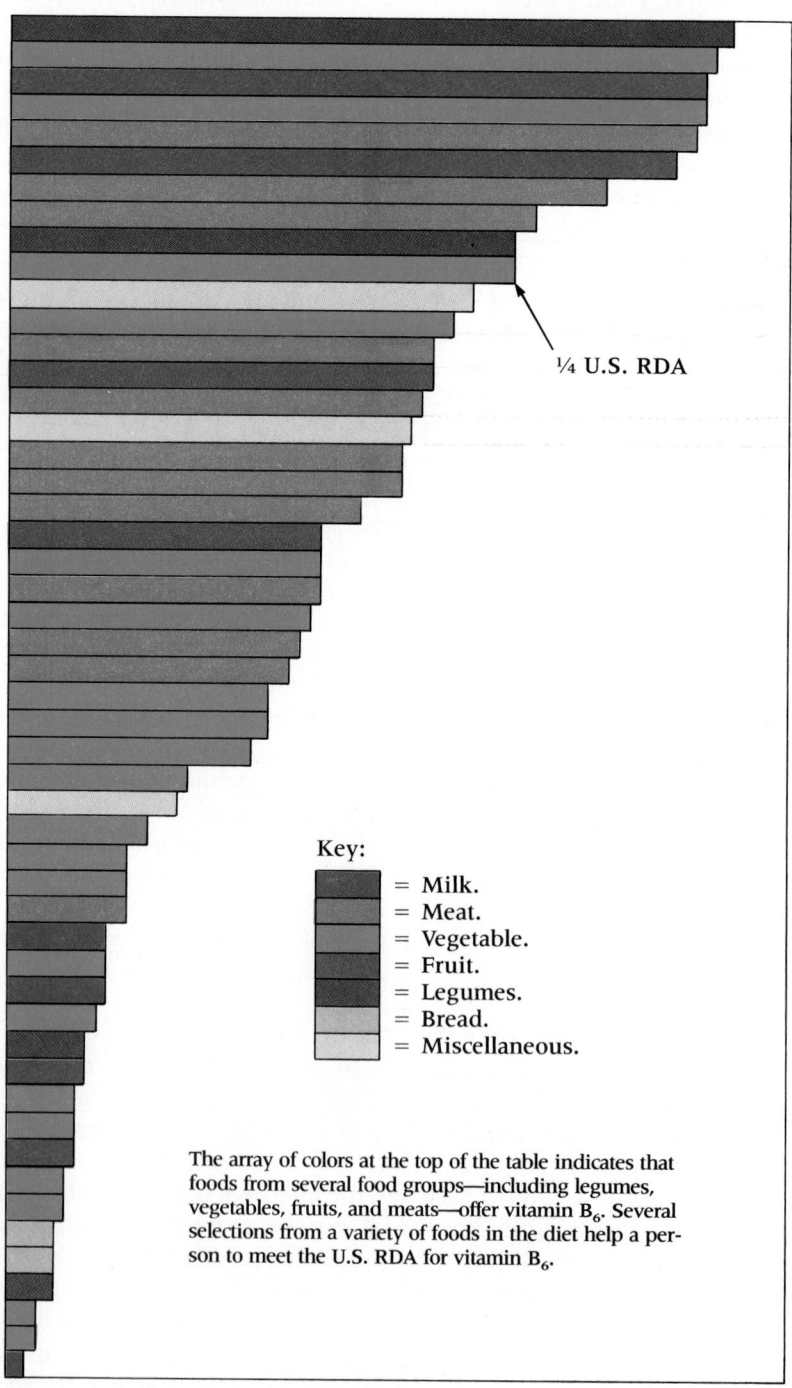

U.S. RDA = 2.0 milligrams

¼ U.S. RDA

Key:
= Milk.
= Meat.
= Vegetable.
= Fruit.
= Legumes.
= Bread.
= Miscellaneous.

The array of colors at the top of the table indicates that foods from several food groups—including legumes, vegetables, fruits, and meats—offer vitamin B₆. Several selections from a variety of foods in the diet help a person to meet the U.S. RDA for vitamin B₆.

Milligrams/Serving

the body. Without the ability to make new cells, the tract rapidly deteriorates, and it not only loses folate more rapidly, but also fails to absorb other nutrients.

Folate Deficiency A too-low intake is theoretically possible in anyone whose diet does not include generous amounts of folate-rich foods. An inadequate intake is seen in babies fed goat's milk, which is notoriously low in folate. Folate deficiency may result not only from an inadequate intake, but also from impaired absorption or an unusual metabolic need for the vitamin. Overconsumers of alcohol or other empty-kcalorie items are vulnerable, and deficiency can also be precipitated by any condition that requires cell multiplication to speed up: multiple pregnancies (twins and triplets), cancer, skin-destroying diseases, such as chicken pox and measles, burns, blood loss, GI tract damage, and more. Folate deficiency impairs cell division and protein synthesis—processes critical to growing tissues. In a folate deficiency, the replacement of red blood cells and GI tract cells falters. Not surprisingly then, two of the first symptoms of a deficiency of folate are a type of anemia and GI tract deterioration. (A summary of deficiency symptoms, as well as toxicity symptoms, common names, primary roles in the body, and food sources, appears in Table 8–10.)

anemia: literally, "too little blood." Anemia is any condition in which there are too few red blood cells, or the red blood cells are immature or too small, or they contain too little hemoglobin to carry the normal amount of oxygen to the tissues. It is not a disease itself but can be a symptom of many different disease conditions, including many nutrient deficiencies, bleeding, excessive red blood cell destruction, defective red blood cell formation, and other causes.

an = without
emia = blood

■ **TABLE 8–10**
Folate—A Summary

Other Names	Deficiency Symptoms	Toxicity Symptoms
Folic acid, folacin, pteroylglutamic acid (PGA)	**Blood/Circulatory System** Anemia (large-cell type)[a]	
Chief Functions in the Body	**Digestive System**	
Part of THF (tetrahydrofolate) and DHF (dihydrofolate), coenzymes used in new cell synthesis	Heartburn, diarrhea (loss of villi and their enzymes), constipation	Diarrhea
	Immune System	
	Suppression, frequent infections	
Significant Sources	**Mouth, Gums, Tongue**	
Leafy green vegetables, legumes, seeds, liver	Smooth, red tongue[b]	
	Nervous System	
	Depression, mental confusion, fainting, fatigue	Insomnia, irritability
	Other	
		Masking of vitamin B$_{12}$–deficiency symptoms

[a]Large-cell type anemia is *macrocytic* or *megaloblastic anemia.*
[b]Smoothness of the tongue is caused by loss of its surface structures and is termed *glossitis* (gloss-EYE-tis).

Folate appears to be particularly vulnerable to interactions with drugs. Drugs that have a chemical structure similar to folate can displace the vitamin from an enzyme and block normal metabolic pathways. Many drugs used to treat cancer are of this type. Cancer cells, like normal cells, need the real vitamin to grow; when the vitamin is not available, they die. Unfortunately, other cells in the body also need folate, and deficiency results with the use of these anticancer drugs. Aspirin also interferes with the body's handling of folate by displacing it from its carrier protein, thus increasing its excretion. Deficiencies from all these causes are common.

Folate Toxicity   High doses of folate have been reported to have adverse effects, but research reports are inconsistent. Perhaps the greatest risk of overdosing with folate arises from its close relationship with vitamin B_{12}. The next section explains how, without enough vitamin B_{12}, folate can be trapped inside of cells—unavailable for the body's use. Therefore, some of the symptoms of vitamin B_{12} deficiency can be masked by the presence of adequate folate.

Folate RDA: 3 μg/kg body weight.
             180 μg/day (women).
             200 μg/day (men).
Canadian RNI: 3.1 μg/kg body weight/day.
Note: A microgram (μg) is one-thousandth of a milligram, or a millionth of a gram.

Folate Requirements   Recommendations for daily intake are stated in terms of total folate. About half of dietary folate is available for use in the body. The need for folate rises considerably during pregnancy and whenever cells are multiplying, so the recommendations for pregnant women are considerably higher than for other adults.

Folate Food Sources   Although estimates of folate in foods are less reliable than those for some other nutrients, you can still tell from tables of food composition which foods are likely to be the best sources. The abundance of green bars in Table 8–11 shows that folate is especially abundant in vegetables. (The vitamin's name reminds us of the word *foliage* and that green leafy vegetables are outstanding sources.) In contrast, the infrequent appearance of red and blue bars illustrates that meats, milk, and milk products are not notable for their folate contents.

Among the poor in the United States and in other parts of the world, folate deficiency due to inadequate intake is probably the most common of all vitamin deficiencies. Folate-deficiency anemia is especially common among pregnant women. Even with the increased need during pregnancy, women can meet their folate RDA without supplements.

Vitamin B_{12}

vitamin B_{12}: a B vitamin; the active forms of coenzyme B_{12} are methylcobalamin and deoxyadenocobalamin.

The distinction between vitamin B_{12} and folate was blurry until the middle of this century. Their roles intertwine, but each serves a specific function that the other cannot perform. They share a special relationship: vitamin B_{12} assists the enzyme that removes the methyl group from methyl folate, thus regenerating the folate coenzyme THF. Its action is evident whenever cells are rapidly dividing. Vitamin B_{12} also maintains the sheath that surrounds and protects nerve fibers and promotes their normal growth. In addition to these two primary roles of vitamin B_{12}, bone cell activity and metabolism seem to depend on its presence.[7]

■ **TABLE 8–11**
Folate in Commonly Eaten Foods Ranked Richest to Poorest

Food, Serving Size (Energy)

Brewer's yeast, 1 tbsp (25 kcal)
Spinach, 1 c cooked (41 kcal)
Asparagus, 1 c cooked (44 kcal)
Turnip greens, 1 c cooked (29 kcal)
Lima beans, 1 c cooked (260 kcal)
Beef liver, 3 oz fried (185 kcal)
Black-eyed peas, 1 c cooked (190 kcal)
Pinto beans, 1 c cooked (265 kcal)
Parsley, 1 c chopped fresh (20 kcal)
Spinach, 1 c fresh chopped (12 kcal)
Navy beans, 1 c cooked (225 kcal)
Broccoli, 1 c cooked (46 kcal)
Beets, 1 c cooked (52 kcal)
Sunflower seeds, ¼ c dry (205 kcal)
Kidney beans, 1 c canned (230 kcal)
Dandelion greens, 1 c cooked (35 kcal)
Cantaloupe, ½ (94 kcal)
Romaine lettuce, 1 c chopped (9 kcal)
Great northern beans, 1 c (210 kcal)
Bean sprouts, 1 c stir-fried (62 kcal)
Winter squash, 1 c baked (96 kcal)
Cauliflower, 1 c cooked (30 kcal)
Bean sprouts, 1 c fresh (32 kcal)
Wheat germ, ¼ c raw (68 kcal)
Tofu (soybean curd), 1 block (86 kcal)
Collards, 1 c cooked (20 kcal)
Grapefruit juice, 1 c fresh (96 kcal)
Green beans, 1 c cooked (44 kcal)
Orange, 1 fresh medium (60 kcal)
Cabbage, 1 c raw shredded (16 kcal)
Honeydew melon, 1/10 (45 kcal)
Summer squash, 1 c cooked (36 kcal)
Bok choy, 1 c cooked (20 kcal)
Zucchini, 1 c cooked (29 kcal)
Peanuts, 1 oz dried unsalted (161 kcal)
Strawberries, 1 c fresh (45 kcal)
Whole-wheat bread, 1 slice (70 kcal)
Milk or yogurt, 1 c nonfat (86 kcal)
Mushrooms, 1 c raw sliced (18 kcal)
Milk, 1 c whole (150 kcal)
Tomato, 1 whole raw (24 kcal)
Green pepper, 1 whole (18 kcal)
Alfalfa seeds, 1 c sprouted (10 kcal)
Milk, 1 c 2% low-fat (121 kcal)
Sole/flounder, 3 oz baked (120 kcal)
Oatmeal, 1 c cooked (145 kcal)
Sirloin steak, 3 oz lean (180 kcal)
Cheddar cheese, 1 oz (114 kcal)
Celery, 1 large outer stalk (6 kcal)
Apple, 1 fresh medium (80 kcal)
Chicken breast, ½ roasted (142 kcal)

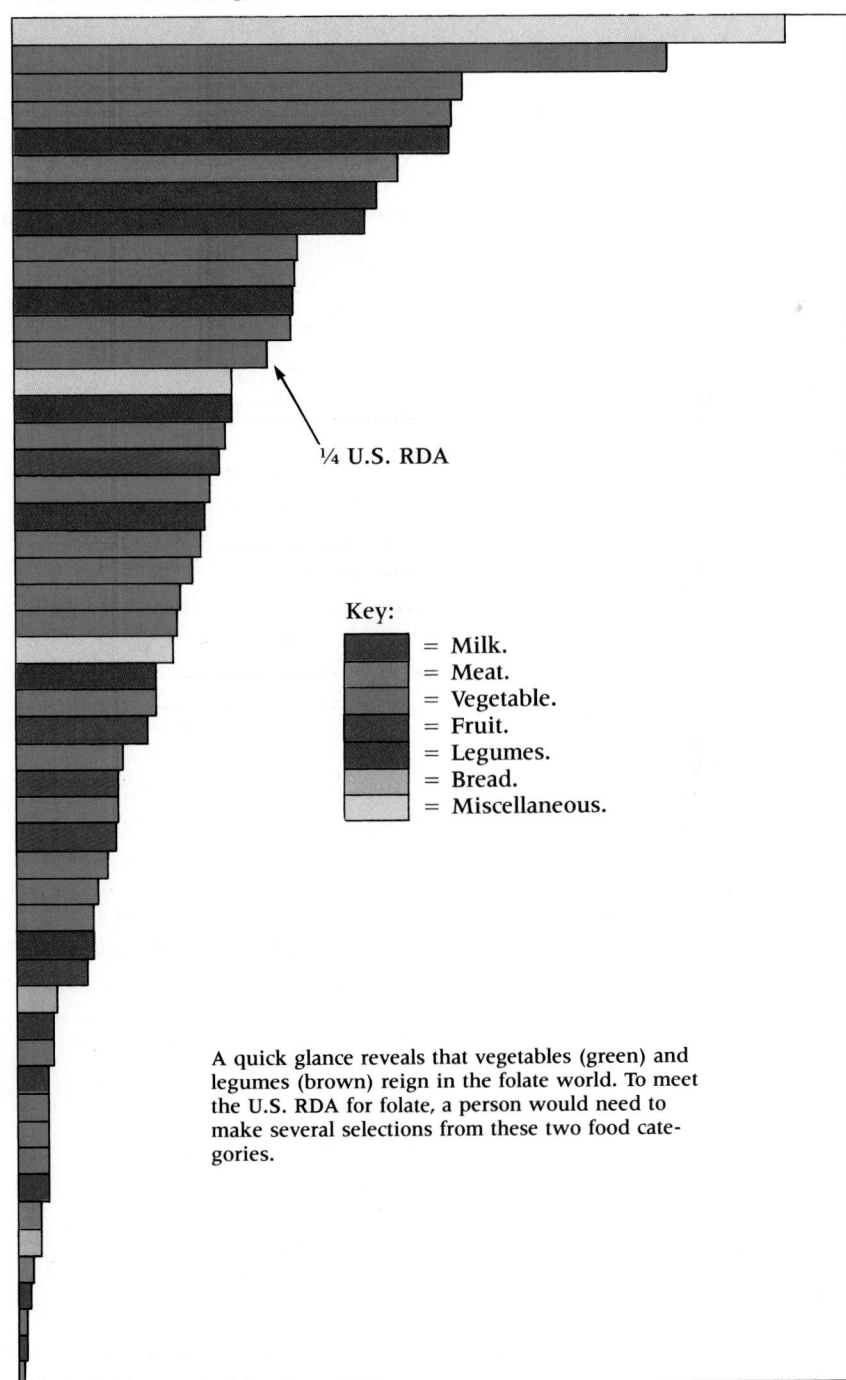

U.S. RDA = 400 micrograms

¼ U.S. RDA

Key:
= Milk.
= Meat.
= Vegetable.
= Fruit.
= Legumes.
= Bread.
= Miscellaneous.

A quick glance reveals that vegetables (green) and legumes (brown) reign in the folate world. To meet the U.S. RDA for folate, a person would need to make several selections from these two food categories.

Micrograms/Serving

intrinsic: inside the system. The **intrinsic factor** is a glycoprotein (a protein with glucose molecules attached) made in the stomach that aids in the absorption of vitamin B_{12}.

After ingestion, vitamin B_{12} requires an "intrinsic factor" for absorption from the intestinal tract into the bloodstream. The genes carry the code for this factor, which is synthesized in the stomach. There, the intrinsic factor attaches to vitamin B_{12} and passes to the small intestine, where it is gradually absorbed. Transport of vitamin B_{12} in the blood depends on specific binding proteins.

Certain people have in their genetic makeup a gene for the intrinsic factor that becomes defective, usually in midlife. Without the intrinsic factor, they can't absorb vitamin B_{12} even though they are taking enough in their diets, and so they develop deficiency symptoms. In such a case, or when the stomach has been injured and cannot produce enough of the intrinsic factor, vitamin B_{12} must be supplied to the body by injection to bypass the need for intrinsic factor in the intestinal tract. The vitamin B_{12} deficiency caused by lack of intrinsic factor is known as pernicious anemia.

pernicious anemia: vitamin B_{12} deficiency caused by lack of intrinsic factor.
pernicious = evil

Vitamin B_{12} Deficiency One of the most obvious vitamin B_{12}–deficiency symptoms is the anemia of folate deficiency, characterized by the large, immature red blood cells indicative of slow DNA synthesis (illustrated in Figure 8–3). Slow DNA synthesis is primarily due to either inadequate folate or inactive folate due to inadequate vitamin B_{12}.[8] (Remember that vitamin B_{12} is needed to free folate; without it, folate can't help manufacture red blood cells.) Either vitamin B_{12} or folate will clear up this condition. However, neurological symptoms of vitamin B_{12} deficiency can occur in the absence of this anemia.[9] (Remember that vitamin B_{12} also functions in maintaining the sheath that surrounds and protects nerve fibers and in promoting their normal growth.) A deficiency of vitamin B_{12} causes a creeping paralysis of the nerves

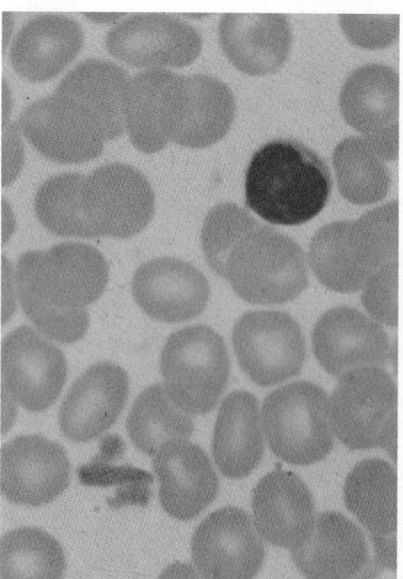

Normal blood cells. Both size and color are normal. The one large, purple cell is a normal "white" blood cell, stained purple.

Blood cells in pernicious anemia (megaloblastic). The large cells are red blood cells, arrested at an immature stage of development. When they mature, they lose their nuclei.

■ **FIGURE 8–3**
Normal and Anemic Blood Cells

■ TABLE 8–12
Vitamin B$_{12}$—A Summary

Other Names	Deficiency Disease Name
Cobalamin (and related forms)	Pernicious anemia[a]
Chief Functions in the Body	**Deficiency Symptoms**
Part of methylcobalamin and deoxyadenocobalamin, coenzymes used in new cell synthesis; helps to maintain nerve cells	**Blood/Circulatory System** Anemia (large-cell type)[b] **Mouth, Gums, Tongue** Smooth tongue[c]
Significant Sources	**Nervous System** Fatigue, degeneration of peripheral nerves progressing to paralysis
Animal products (meat, fish, poultry, shellfish, milk, cheese, eggs)	**Skin** Hypersensitivity

[a]The name *pernicious anemia* refers to the vitamin B$_{12}$ deficiency caused by lack of intrinsic factor, but not to that caused by inadequate dietary intake.
[b]Large-cell type anemia is *macrocytic* or *megaloblastic anemia.*
[c]Smoothness of the tongue is caused by loss of its surface structures and is termed *glossitis* (gloss-EYE-tis).

and muscles, which begins at the extremities and works inward and up the spine. Such paralysis cannot be remedied by administering folate—only vitamin B$_{12}$. Early detection and correction are necessary to prevent permanent nerve damage and paralysis. Table 8–12 provides a summary of deficiency symptoms, functions, and food sources.

Vitamin B$_{12}$ Requirements   According to the RDA, adults need about 2 micrograms of vitamin B$_{12}$ a day. This is the tiniest amount imaginable—two-millionths of a gram. The ink in the period at the end of this sentence may weigh about 2 micrograms. But what seems like such a tiny amount to the human eye contains billions of molecules of vitamin B$_{12}$, enough to provide coenzymes for all the enzymes that need its help.

Vitamin B$_{12}$ RDA: 2 μg/day.
Canadian RNI: 1 μg/day.
Note: 2 μg is 0.002 mg, or two-millionths of a gram.

Vitamin B$_{12}$ Food Sources   Vitamin B$_{12}$ is unique among the nutrients in being found almost exclusively in animal flesh and animal products. Anyone who eats reasonable amounts of meat is guaranteed an adequate intake, and lacto-ovo-vegetarians (if they use enough milk, cheese, and eggs) are also protected from deficiency. "Enough" means a cup of milk or 3½ ounces of cheese or one egg in a given day.[10] Vegans, however, need a reliable source, such as vitamin B$_{12}$–fortified soy "milk" or meat replacements. Yeast grown in a vitamin B$_{12}$–enriched environment can be a good source of vitamin B$_{12}$.

Vegans generally maintain normal vitamin B$_{12}$ status for prolonged periods, but eventually show some signs of vitamin B$_{12}$ deficiency disease.[11] Many hypotheses have been advanced to account for this finding. For one, deficiency takes a long time to develop, because up to four years' worth can linger in the body. For another, vegans ingest bacteria containing the vitamin with their foods or drinking water.

meat replacements: textured vegetable-protein products formulated to look and taste like meat, fish, or poultry.

■ **TABLE 8–13**
Biotin—A Summary

Chief Functions in the Body	Deficiency Symptoms
Part of a coenzyme used in energy metabolism, fat synthesis, amino acid metabolism, and glycogen synthesis	**Blood/Circulatory System** Abnormal heart action
	Digestive System Loss of appetite, nausea
Significant Sources	**Nervous/Muscular Systems** Depression, muscle pain, weakness, fatigue
Widespread in foods	**Skin** Drying, scaly dermatitis, loss of hair

Biotin

biotin (BY-oh-tin): a B vitamin that attaches to the enzymes it works with.

In comparison with the other B vitamins, little is known about biotin (a brief summary is provided in Table 8–13). Its discovery and research are relatively new.

Biotin plays an important role in carbohydrate, fat, and protein metabolism. As a cofactor for several key enzymes, it participates in many reactions, including gluconeogenesis and fatty acid synthesis and breakdown.

Biotin Deficiency Biotin deficiencies have been seen in human beings, invariably associated with artificial feeding—that is, feeding mixtures of purified nutrients, lacking biotin, into a vein in hospital clients who couldn't eat. In such cases, therapeutic doses of biotin are given to correct for the deficiency.

The protein **avidin** in egg whites binds biotin.
avid = greedy

Researchers can induce a biotin deficiency in animals or human beings by feeding them raw egg whites, which contain a protein that binds biotin. However, it takes more than two dozen raw egg whites to produce the effect; and cooking denatures the binding protein, which eliminates the problem. Occasional drinkers of eggnog need not worry.

Estimated safe and adequate intake:
- U.S.: 30 to 100 μg/day.
- Canada: 1.5 μg/kg body weight/day.

Biotin Requirements Recommendations for daily intakes of biotin have not been established; instead, "estimated safe and adequate daily dietary intakes" have been made. Biotin is needed in very small amounts.

Biotin Food Sources Biotin is widespread in foods (including egg yolks), and there seems to be no danger that people who consume a variety of foods will suffer deficiencies. (Biotin is also synthesized by GI tract bacteria, but how much of it is available for absorption remains uncertain.) Claims that biotin is needed in supplement form to prevent or cure disease conditions are at best unfounded and at worst intentionally misleading.

■ TABLE 8–14
Pantothenic Acid—A Summary

Chief Functions in the Body	Deficiency Symptoms	Toxicity Symptoms
Part of Coenzyme A, which is used in energy metabolism	**Digestive System** Vomiting, intestinal distress	Occasional diarrhea
Significant Sources	**Nervous System** Insomnia, fatigue	
Widespread in foods	**Other**	Water retention (infrequent)

Pantothenic Acid

Pantothenic acid was first recognized as a substance that stimulates growth. Its presence is evident in many metabolic reactions. It plays an important role as part of coenzyme A (or CoA, for short). You may recall from Chapter 7 that when CoA is attached to acetate, it forms acetyl CoA, the "crossroads" compound that can enter a number of metabolic pathways, including the TCA cycle. (Then, as is typical of all coenzymes, it is released, so that it can be recycled to attach to another acetate.) Coenzyme A helps shuttle acetate (as acetyl CoA) and other small molecules along pathways in glucose, fatty acid, and energy metabolism.

pantothenic (PAN-toe-THEN-ick) **acid**: a B vitamin; the principal active form is as part of coenzyme A, called "CoA" throughout Chapter 7.

Pantothenic Acid Deficiency Pantothenic acid deficiency is rare. Its symptoms involve a general failure of all the body's systems (see Table 8–14 for an overall summary of pantothenic acid). Dietary deficiency is unlikely.

Pantothenic Acid Requirements No RDA has been established for pantothenic acid. Like biotin, estimated safe and adequate intakes have been established.

Estimated safe and adequate intake:
- U.S.: 4 to 7 mg/day.
- Canada: 5 to 7 mg/day.

Pantothenic Acid Food Sources Pantothenic acid is widespread in foods. Meat, fish, poultry, whole grain cereals, and legumes are particularly good sources. Typical diets seem to provide an adequate intake.

B Vitamin Relatives

A trio of compounds sometimes called B vitamins are inositol, choline, and lipoic acid. These are not essential nutrients for human beings, although deficiencies can be induced in laboratory animals in order to study the functions of these three compounds. Like the B vitamins described above, they serve as coenzymes in metabolism. Even if they were essential for human beings, supplements would be unnecessary, because they are abundant in foods.

inositol (in-OSS-ih-tall): a nonessential nutrient.

choline (KOH-leen): a nonessential nutrient.

lipoic (lip-OH-ick) **acid**: a nonessential nutrient.

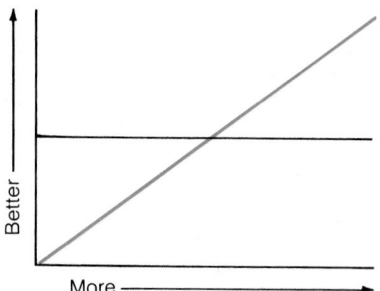

As you progress in the direction of more, the effect gets better and better, with no end in sight (real life is seldom, if ever, like this).

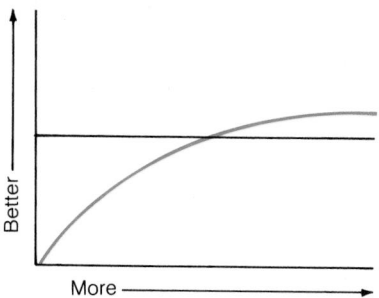

As you progress in the direction of more, the effect reaches a maximum and then a plateau, becoming no better with higher doses.

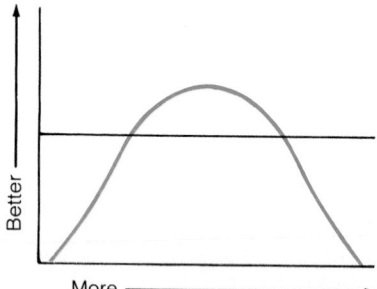

More is better up to a point and then harmful. As you progress in the direction of more, the effect reaches an optimum at some intermediate dose and then declines, showing that too much is as harmful as too little. This represents the situation with nutrients.

■ **FIGURE 8–4**
Dose Levels and Effects

> ▶▶ **NUTRITION DETECTIVE WORK**
>
> If you read or hear a report of a substance's having a beneficial or harmful effect, it is an oversimplification to conclude that the substance itself is generally beneficial or harmful. You must ask what dose was used. Two corollaries to this statement might be the following:
>
> ■ A substance that is poisonous at a high concentration may be an essential nutrient at a lower concentration.
>
> ■ A nutrient needed at a low concentration may be toxic at a high concentration.
>
> Figure 8–4 shows three possible relationships between dose levels and effects. The third diagram represents the situation with nutrients—more is better up to a point, and beyond that point, still more is harmful.

Health food purveyors make much of inositol, choline, and lipoic acid, insisting that we must supplement our diets with them. Some vitamin companies include them in their formulations in hopes that you will read the label and conclude that their vitamin pill is more "complete" than someone else's. (For a rational way to compare different vitamin-mineral supplements, read Highlight 9.) Incorrect notions about this kind of supplementation arise from an unjustified application of findings from animal studies to human beings.

Medical practitioners have witnessed and reported on the effects of overdoses of choline and its relative lecithin (which contains choline as part of its structure). These compounds can cause not only short-term discomforts such as GI distress, sweating, salivation, and anorexia, but also long-term health hazards from disturbance of the nervous and cardiovascular systems.[12]

In addition to choline, inositol, and lipoic acid, other substances have been mistaken for essential nutrients for humans because they are needed for growth by bacteria or other forms of life. These substances include:

- PABA (para-aminobenzoic acid).
- Bioflavonoids (vitamin P or hesperidin).
- Ubiquinone.

Other names you may hear are vitamin B_5 (another name for pantothenic acid), vitamin B_{15} (also called "pangamic acid," a hoax), vitamin B_{17} (Laetrile, a fake "cancer cure" and not a vitamin by any stretch of the imagination), and "vitamin B_T" (carnitine, an important piece of cell machinery, but not a vitamin, because the body can make it as it needs to).

■ *The B Vitamins—In Concert*

Figure 8–5 is intended to give you an *impression* of the ways B vitamins swarm all over the body's metabolic pathways, involving themselves in every crucial step. The details are too numerous to mention, but the message is that

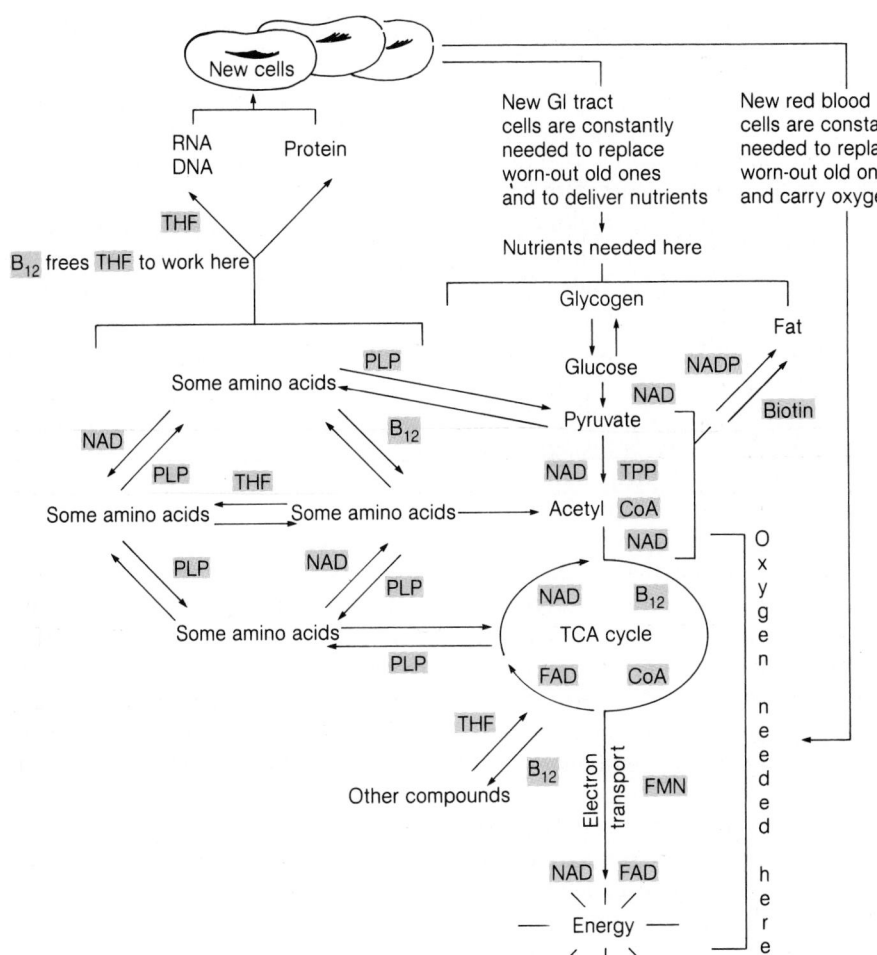

■ **FIGURE 8–5**
Metabolic Pathways Involving B Vitamins
These metabolic pathways are presented here to highlight the many coenzymes that facilitate the reactions. These coenzymes depend on the following vitamins:
- NAD and NADP: niacin.
- TPP: thiamin.
- CoA: pantothenic acid.
- B_{12}: vitamin B_{12}.
- FMN and FAD: riboflavin.
- THF: folate.
- PLP: vitamin B_6.
- Biotin.
For further details, see Appendix C.

metabolism is the body's work, and that the B vitamin coenzymes are indispensable to it. Study the pathways of metabolism depicted in the figure, and note the abbreviations for the coenzymes that keep the processes going.

Look at the first step in the now-familiar pathway of glucose breakdown. To break down glucose to pyruvate, the cells must have certain enzymes. For the enzymes to work, they must have the niacin coenzyme NAD. To make NAD, the cells must be supplied with niacin (or enough of the amino acid tryptophan to make niacin). The rest of the coenzyme they can make without outside help.

The next step in glucose catabolism is the breakdown of pyruvate to acetyl CoA. The enzymes involved in this step require NAD plus the thiamin coenzyme, TPP. The cells can manufacture the TPP they need from thiamin, but thiamin must be supplied in the diet.

Another coenzyme needed for this step is CoA. As you have no doubt anticipated, the cells can make CoA except for an essential part of it that must be obtained in the diet—pantothenic acid. Still another coenzyme requiring biotin serves the enzyme complex involved in converting pyruvate to a

The TCA cycle receives detailed attention in Appendix C.

compound that can either generate glucose or combine with acetyl CoA to enter the TCA cycle.

These and other coenzymes are involved throughout all the metabolic pathways. When the diet provides riboflavin, the body synthesizes FAD—a needed coenzyme in the TCA cycle. Vitamin B_6 is an indispensable part of PLP—a coenzyme required for a multitude of interconversions of amino acids, for a crucial step in the making of the iron-containing portion of hemoglobin for red blood cells, and for many other reactions. Folate becomes THF—the coenzyme required for the synthesis of new genetic material and therefore new cells. The vitamin B_{12} coenzyme, in turn, frees THF from a chemical form in which it tends to get stuck; so vitamin B_{12} is also necessary for the formation of new cells.

Thus each of the B vitamin coenzymes is involved, directly or indirectly, in energy metabolism. Some are facilitators of the energy-releasing reactions themselves; others help build new cells to deliver oxygen and nutrients, which permits the energy pathways to run.

Now suppose the body's cells lack one of these B vitamins—niacin, for example. Without niacin, the cells cannot make NAD. Without NAD, the enzymes involved in every step of the glucose-to-energy pathway will fail to function. Since it is from these steps that energy is made available for all the body's activities, everything will begin to grind to a halt. This is no exaggeration. The deadly disease pellagra, caused by niacin deficiency, produces the "devastating Ds": dermatitis, which reflects a failure of the skin to maintain itself; dementia (insanity), a failure of the nervous system; diarrhea, a failure of digestion and absorption; and eventually, as would be the case for any severe nutrient deficiency, death. These are only the most obvious, observable consequences of deficiency; it affects every organ in the body, because all are dependent on the energy pathways. As you can see, niacin is like the horseshoe nail for want of which a war was lost. All the vitamins are like such horseshoe nails.

In summary, the eight B vitamins play many specific roles in helping the enzymes perform thousands of different molecular conversions in the body. The B vitamins are active in carbohydrate, fat, and protein metabolism and in the making of DNA and thus new cells. They are found in every cell and must be present continuously for the cells to function as they should.

For want of a nail, a horseshoe was lost.
For want of a horseshoe, a horse was lost.
For want of a horse, a soldier was lost.
For want of a soldier, a battle was lost.
For want of a battle, the war was lost,
And all for the want of a horseshoe nail!
—Mother Goose

B Vitamin Interactions

To this point, the chapter has described some of the impressive ways that vitamins work individually, as if it were simple to disentangle their many actions in the body. In fact, oftentimes it is difficult to tell which one is truly responsible for a given effect. Often, a function of one vitamin depends on the presence of another. You have already seen this interdependence in the case of folate and vitamin B_{12}. The case of these two vitamins also showed that a deficiency of either would produce the same symptoms.

A couple of examples will illustrate other B vitamin relationships. Folate assists in thiamin absorption, although the exact site of action is not known.[13] A folate deficiency therefore can cause a thiamin deficiency, and even thiamin supplements don't correct the thiamin deficiency until after the folate deficiency has been corrected. In another case, the enzymes involved in the metabolism of many other nutrients, including vitamin B_6, folate, niacin, and vitamin K, require riboflavin.[14] Thus a riboflavin deficiency invariably tangles up with deficiencies of other nutrients.

The nutrients are interdependent; they affect one another's absorption, metabolism, and excretion, so that an apparent deficiency of one may reflect a deficiency or abnormality in the action of another. The following section will show that this is true of many of the B vitamin deficiencies.

B Vitamin Deficiencies

Oddly enough, although we know a great deal about their individual molecular functions, we are unable to say precisely why a deficiency of one B vitamin produces one disease, whereas the deficiency of another produces another disease. With the deficiency of any B vitamin, many body systems become deranged, and similar symptoms may appear. Removing a number of ''horseshoe nails'' can have such disastrous and far-reaching effects that it is difficult to imagine or predict the results.

Deficiencies of single B vitamins seldom show up in isolation. After all, people do not eat nutrients singly; they eat foods, which contain mixtures of nutrients. If a major class of foods is missing from the diet, the nutrients contributed by that class of foods will all be lacking to varying extents. Only in the two cases described earlier—beriberi and pellagra—have dietary deficiencies associated with single B vitamins been observed on a large scale in human populations. Even in these cases, the deficiencies were not pure. When foods were provided containing the one vitamin known to be needed, the other vitamins that may have been in short supply came as part of the package.

Significantly, these deficiency diseases were eliminated by supplying foods—not pills. Although both diseases were attributed to deficiencies of single vitamins, both were likely to have been deficiencies of several vitamins in which one vitamin happened to stand out above the rest. Giving a single B vitamin to a person with a multiple deficiency may make hidden deficiencies of other B vitamins become obvious.

Pushers of vitamin pills make much of the fact that vitamins are vital and indispensable to life. But human beings obtained their nourishment from foods for centuries before there were vitamin pills. If your diet lacks a vitamin, the natural solution is to adjust your intake so that food supplies that vitamin.

Pushers of so-called natural vitamins would have you believe that their pills are the best of all because they are purified from real foods rather than synthesized in a laboratory. But if you think back on the course of human evolution, you may conclude that it really is not natural to take any kind of pills at all. In reality, the finest, most complete vitamin ''supplements'' available are meat, fish, poultry, eggs, legumes, nuts, milk and milk products, vegetables, fruits, and grain products. Any time you hear the suggestion that you should meet your vitamin needs by taking pills, look out. Someone may be trying to sell you something you don't need.

Once vitamin research was well under way and several B vitamins had been discovered, the clarification of their function was often greatly helped by laboratory experiments in which animals or human volunteers were fed diets

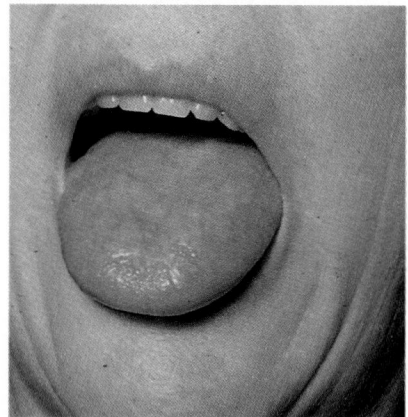

Tongue symptoms of B vitamin deficiency. The tongue is smooth due to atrophy of the tissues (glossitis).

devoid of one vitamin. The effect of the deficiency of that vitamin could then be studied to determine what functions it normally performed. Other deficiency diseases were discovered in this way and have since been observed to occur outside the laboratory.

A review of the summary tables in this chapter will make another generalization possible. Different body systems depend to different extents on these vitamins. But again, each nutrient is important in all systems, and these lists of symptoms are far from complete.

The skin and the tongue appear to be especially sensitive to vitamin B deficiencies, but you should note that the listing of these items in the summary tables gives them undue emphasis. Remember that in a medical examination, these are two body parts that are visible. If the skin is degenerating, other tissues beneath it may be, too. Similarly, the mouth and tongue are the visible part of the digestive system; if they are abnormal, there may well be an abnormality throughout the GI tract. What is really happening in a vitamin deficiency happens inside the cells of the body; what the doctor sees and reports are its outward manifestations.

⟫ NUTRITION DETECTIVE WORK

It is more and more apparent that you cannot observe a symptom and automatically jump to a conclusion regarding its cause. As you can see from the summary tables in this chapter, deficiencies of riboflavin, niacin, and vitamin B_6 can all cause rashes. A deficiency of protein, or of the phospholipid lecithin, or of vitamin A can, too. Because skin is on the outside, where you and your doctor can easily look at it, it is a useful indicator of things-going-wrong-in-cells. But by itself, a skin symptom tells you nothing about its possible cause.

The same is true of anemia. We often think of anemia as being caused by an iron deficiency, and often it is. But anemia can also be caused by a folate or vitamin B_{12} deficiency; by digestive tract failure to absorb any of these nutrients; or by such nonnutritional causes as infections, parasites, cancer, or loss of blood. So be careful. You can often recognize a false claim by the implication that a specific nutrient will always cure a given symptom.

A person who feels chronically tired may be tempted to self-diagnose iron-deficiency anemia, and self-prescribe an iron supplement. But the iron supplement will relieve tiredness only if the symptom is indeed caused by iron-deficiency anemia. If the problem is a folate deficiency, taking iron will only prolong the period in which the tiredness persists. A person who is better informed may decide to take a vitamin supplement with iron, covering the possibility of a vitamin deficiency. But there may be a nonnutritional cause of the symptom. If the cause of the tiredness is actually hidden blood loss due to cancer, the postponement of a diagnosis may be equivalent to suicide. A person who is chronically tired should see a physician rather than self prescribe.

Major, epidemiclike deficiency diseases such as pellagra and beriberi are no longer seen in the United States and Canada, but lesser deficiencies of nutrients, including the B vitamins, sometimes are observed. When they occur, it is usually in people whose food choices are poor because of poverty, ignorance, illness, or poor health habits like alcohol abuse. Don't forget, deficiencies arise not only because of deficient intakes, but also for other (secondary) reasons.

B Vitamin Toxicities

Toxicities of the B vitamins are observed when people overuse supplements. When the body's cells become oversaturated with a vitamin, they must work to reduce the excess. They remove water-soluble vitamins by excreting excesses in the urine, but sometimes they cannot eliminate the excesses fast enough to regain homeostasis. Healthy individuals who augment a well-balanced diet with supplements may be unintentionally creating problems. Toxicity reactions caused by excess B vitamins from foods alone are unknown.

B Vitamin Food Sources

The food tables presented in this chapter, taken together, sing the praises of the balanced diet. The meat and meat alternate group serves thiamin, niacin, vitamin B_6, and vitamin B_{12} well. The milk and milk products group stands out for riboflavin and vitamin B_{12}. The fruits and vegetables group excels for folate. The cereal and bread group delivers thiamin, riboflavin, and niacin. A diet that offers a variety of foods from each of the food groups, prepared with reasonable care, will provide an adequate intake of the vitamins. By emphasizing the low-fat items from each of the food groups, a person will be able to achieve kcalorie control while still receiving adequate intakes of all the vitamins.

meat, milk, fruits, veg.

■ Vitamin C

Two hundred fifty years ago, any man who joined the crew of a seagoing ship knew he had only half a chance of returning alive—not because he might be slain by pirates or die in a storm, but because he might contract the dread disease scurvy. As many as two-thirds of a ship's crew might die of scurvy on a long voyage. Only ships that sailed on short voyages, especially around the Mediterranean Sea, were safe from this disease. It was not known at the time that the special hazard of long ocean voyages was that the ship's cook used up his provisions of fresh fruits and vegetables early and relied for the duration of the voyage on cereals and meat.

The first nutrition experiment conducted on human beings was devised in 1747 to find a cure for scurvy. James Lind, a British physician, divided 12 sailors with scurvy into six pairs. Each pair received a different supplemental ration: cider, vinegar, sulfuric acid, seawater, oranges and lemons, or a purgative mixed with spices. The ones receiving the citrus fruits were cured within a short time. Sadly, it was 50 years before the British Navy made use

scurvy: the vitamin C–deficiency disease.

purgative: a strong laxative.

antiscorbutic factor: the original name for vitamin C.
anti = against
scorbutic = causing scurvy

ascorbic acid: one of the two active forms of vitamin C (see Figure 8–7 later in the chapter). Many people refer to vitamin C by this name.
a = without
scorbic = having scurvy

antioxidant: a compound that protects others from oxidation by being oxidized itself.

Chemists describe the antioxidant action of vitamin C as maintaining the "oxidation-reduction equilibrium," or "redox state."

collagen: see definition on p. 149.

■ **FIGURE 8–6**
Collagen
Collagen is unique among body proteins, because it contains large amounts of the amino acid hydroxyproline, the hydroxy derivative of proline.

Proline

Hydroxyproline

of Lind's experiment by requiring all vessels to carry sufficient lime juice for every sailor to receive some daily. British sailors are still nicknamed "limeys" as a result of this tradition.

The antiscurvy "something" in limes and other foods was dubbed the antiscorbutic factor. Nearly 200 years later, the factor was isolated from lemon juice and found to be a six-carbon compound similar to glucose. It was named ascorbic acid. Shortly thereafter, it was synthesized, and today hundreds of millions of vitamin C pills are produced in pharmaceutical laboratories each year and sold for a few dollars a bottle.

Vitamin C Roles

Vitamin C parts company with the B vitamins in its mode of action, which differs in different situations. In some settings vitamin C assists a specific enzyme in the performance of its job. In others, it acts in a more general way—for example, as an antioxidant. An antioxidant is any substance that can reduce (donate electrons to) another substance. When it reduces the other substance, it simultaneously becomes oxidized itself.

Many substances found in foods and important in the body can be altered or even destroyed by oxidation. (For example, oils turn rancid when exposed to air.) Vitamin C—because it can be destroyed itself—can protect other substances from this destruction. Vitamin C is like a bodyguard for oxidizable substances; it stands ready to sacrifice its own life to save theirs. Unemotionally, chemists call such a bodyguard an antioxidant.

Because of vitamin C's antioxidant property, manufacturers sometimes add it to food products, not to improve their nutritional value, but to protect important constituents in the foods. In the cells and body fluids, vitamin C probably helps to protect other molecules, and in the intestines, it protects iron and promotes its absorption (a function fully discussed in Chapter 11).

Vitamin C's most completely characterized specific role is that it helps to form the fibrous, structural protein collagen. (Chapter 6 briefly mentioned this single most important protein of the connective tissue.) Collagen serves as the matrix on which bone and teeth are formed. When you have been wounded, collagen glues the separated tissue faces together, forming scars. Cells are held together largely by collagen; this is especially important in the artery walls, which must expand and contract with each beat of the heart, and in the walls of the capillaries, which are thin and fragile and must withstand a pulse of blood every second or so without giving way.

The body makes all proteins by stringing together chains of amino acids. In collagen, the amino acid proline appears in abundance. During synthesis of collagen, after the addition of each proline to the growing protein chain, an enzyme hydroxylates it (adds an OH group to it), making the amino acid hydroxyproline (see Figure 8–6). This hydroxylase enzyme requires both vitamin C and iron. Iron works as a cofactor in the reaction, and vitamin C maintains iron in the state that allows it to do so. Without them, the hydroxylation step does not occur. Hydroxyproline favors the binding together of collagen fibers, thus making strong, ropelike structures.

Vitamin C operates in the metabolism of several amino acids. Some of these may end up being converted to hormones—notably, the hormones norepinephrine and thyroxin. The adrenal glands contain a higher concentration of vitamin C than any other organ in the body. During emotional or physical stress, these glands release large quantities of the vitamin, together with the hormones epinephrine and norepinephrine. What the vitamin has to do with the stress reaction is unclear, although there is some indication that it may be involved in the synthesis of these hormones. Some *physical* stresses increase vitamin C needs, but *psychological* stress alone does not appear to increase needs above the RDA.

The hormone thyroxin regulates the rate of metabolism. The metabolic rate speeds up under extreme stress and also when the body needs to produce more heat—for example, in fever or cold weather. Thus infections and exposure to cold increase needs for vitamin C. Perhaps its involvement in the fever response to infection explains the speculation surrounding the vitamin's possible effects on cold prevention and symptom reduction. (Highlight 8 explores these effects, as well as the relationship between vitamin C and cancer.)

Scorbutic gums. Unlike other lesions of the mouth, scurvy presents a symmetrical appearance without infection.

Vitamin C Deficiency

Vitamin C, like all the vitamins, is a small organic compound needed by human beings in minute amounts daily. Being an organic compound, it can convert to several different forms, two of which are active (see Figure 8–7). Because vitamin C is water soluble, the body rapidly excretes excesses. With an adequate intake, the body maintains a fixed pool of vitamin C and rapidly excretes any excess in the urine. With an inadequate intake, the pool becomes depleted at the rate of about 3 percent a day.

With an inadequate intake, the body's vitamin C pool size dwindles, and latent scurvy appears. Two of the earliest signs of a vitamin C deficiency relate to its role in maintaining the integrity of blood vessels. The gums around teeth bleed easily, and capillaries under the skin break spontaneously, producing pinpoint hemorrhages. Atherosclerotic plaques grow rapidly in the arteries. Table 8–15 provides a summary of deficiency symptoms, as well as toxicity symptoms, functions, and food sources.

When the vitamin pool falls to about a fifth of its optimal size (this may take two months or more to occur), overt scurvy symptoms begin to appear. Failure to promote normal collagen synthesis causes further hemorrhaging. Muscles, including the heart muscle, degenerate. The skin becomes rough,

latent: hidden; with reference to a disease, the period when the conditions are present but before the symptoms have begun to appear.
latens = lying hidden

overt: see definition on p. 9.

■ **FIGURE 8–7**
Active Forms of Vitamin C
The reduced form can lose two hydrogens with their electrons, becoming oxidized. The electrons may then reduce some other compound.

Ascorbic Acid (Reduced Form)   Dehydroascorbic Acid (Oxidized Form)

■ **TABLE 8–15**
Vitamin C—A Summary

Other Names	Deficiency Disease Name	
Ascorbic acid	Scurvy	

Chief Functions in the Body	Deficiency Symptoms	Toxicity Symptoms
Collagen synthesis (strengthens blood vessel walls, forms scar tissue, is a matrix for bone growth), antioxidant, thyroxin synthesis, amino acid metabolism, strengthens resistance to infection, helps in absorption of iron	**Blood/Circulatory System** Anemia (small-cell type)[a] atherosclerotic plaques, pinpoint hemorrhages	Blood cell breakage in certain racial groups[b]
	Digestive System	Nausea, abdominal cramps, diarrhea
	Immune System Depression, frequent infections	
	Mouth, Gums, Tongue Bleeding gums, loosened teeth	
	Nervous/Muscular Systems Muscle degeneration and pain, hysteria, depression	Headache, fatigue, insomnia
	Skeletal System Bone fragility, joint pain	
Significant Sources Citrus fruits, cabbage-type vegetables, dark green vegetables, cantaloupe, strawberries, peppers, lettuce, tomatoes, potatoes, papayas, mangos	**Skin** Rough skin, blotchy bruises	Hot flashes, rashes
	Other Failure of wounds to heal	Interference with medical tests, aggravation of gout symptoms, excessive urination, kidney stones,[c] (deficiency symptoms may appear at first on withdrawal of high doses)

[a]Small-cell type anemia is *microcytic anemia*.
[b]Groups susceptible to vitamin C toxicity are Sephardic Jews, black Americans and Africans, and Asians.
[c]People who have a tendency toward gout and those who have a genetic abnormality that alters the break down of vitamin C are prone to forming kidney stones. Vitamin C is inactivated and degraded by several routes, and sometimes a product along the way is oxalate, which can form stones in the kidneys. People can also have oxalate crystals in their kidneys that are not due to vitamin C overdoses.

brown, scaly, and dry. Wounds fail to heal because scar tissue will not form. Bone rebuilding falters; the ends of the long bones become softened, malformed, and painful, and fractures appear. The teeth become loose as the cartilage holding them in place weakens. Anemia and infections are common. There are also characteristic psychological signs, including hysteria and depression. Sudden death is likely, occasioned by severe atherosclerosis or by massive bleeding into the joints and body cavities.

In scurvy, protein metabolism may be altered, resulting in negative nitrogen balance. No one knows why this occurs, but the involvement of vitamin C with amino acids provides a notable example of the way nutrients of different classes cooperate with one another to maintain health.

Once diagnosed, scurvy is readily reversed by vitamin C. Moderate doses in the neighborhood of 100 milligrams per day are sufficient, curing the scurvy within about five days.

Vitamin C Toxicity

The easy availability of vitamin C in pill form and the publication of a book recommending intakes of over 2 grams a day (see Highlight 8) have led thousands of people to take vitamin C megadoses. Not surprisingly, instances have surfaced of vitamin C's causing harm.

Some of the suspected toxic effects of megadoses have not been confirmed. Vitamin C megadoses probably do not upset the body's acid-base balance; or destroy vitamin B_{12}, resulting in a deficiency; or interfere with the action of vitamin E. Research and reasoning have demonstrated that these effects are theoretically possible, but no cases of their actual occurrence in human beings have yet been seen with intakes as high as 3 grams a day.

Other toxic effects, however, have been seen often enough to warrant concern. Nausea, abdominal cramps, and diarrhea are often reported; Table 8–15 lists other common symptoms of vitamin C toxicity. Several instances of interference with medical regimens are known. The large amounts of vitamin C excreted in the urine obscure the results of tests used to detect diabetes, giving a false positive result in some instances and a false negative result in others. People taking medications to prevent their blood from clotting may unwittingly abolish the effect of these medicines if they also take massive doses of vitamin C.

People of certain genetic backgrounds are more likely to be harmed by vitamin C megadoses than others. Some black Americans and Africans, Sephardic Jews, Asians, and certain other ethnic groups have an inherited enzyme deficiency that makes them susceptible to any strong reducing agent. Megadoses of vitamin C can make their red blood cells burst, causing hemolytic anemia. Those with sickle-cell anemia may also be vulnerable to megadoses of vitamin C. In sickle-cell anemia, the hemoglobin protein is abnormal; it responds to a reducing agent by assuming a shape that distorts the red blood cells, making them clump and clog capillaries. Those who have a tendency toward gout and those who have a genetic abnormality that alters the way they break down vitamin C to its excretion products are prone to forming kidney stones if they take megadoses of vitamin C.

The body of a person who has taken large doses of vitamin C for a long time may adjust by limiting absorption and destroying and excreting more of the vitamin than usual.[15] If the person then suddenly reduces intake to normal, the accelerated disposal system may not be able to put on its brakes fast enough to avoid destroying too much of the vitamin. It has been suggested that adults who discontinue megadosing may develop scurvy on intakes that would protect a normal adult, but evidence is scanty on this point. If it occurs, it is not unlike the withdrawal reaction seen in drug and

Infant scurvy. This is the characteristic "scorbutic pose," with legs bent and thighs rotated open. The infant's joints are painful, and she will cry if made to move.

The anticlotting agents with which vitamin C interferes are such anticoagulants as warfarin, dicumarol, heparin, and coumadin. It is unclear whether vitamin C inhibits the absorption or the action of these drugs.

gout (GOWT): a metabolic disease in which crystals of uric acid precipitate in the joints.

withdrawal reaction: a reaction to withdrawal (usually of a drug) that reveals that the user has become dependent. One infant is reported to have been born of a mother who took massive doses of vitamin C. The infant developed **rebound scurvy** on an intake that would have been adequate for the average infant.

■ FIGURE 8–8
Vitamin C Intake (mg)

Vitamin C RDA: 60 mg/day.
Canadian RNI: 40 mg/day (men);
30 mg/day (women); 50% increase for
cigarette smokers.

reasons to ↑ dose of vit C

alcohol abusers when they discontinue drug use. When people discontinue their vitamic C megadose regimens they might be wise to do so gradually.[16]

Few instances warrant the taking of more than 100 to 300 milligrams of vitamin C a day. For adults who dose themselves with 1 to 2 grams a day, the risks may not be great; those taking more than 2 grams, and especially those taking amounts above 8 grams per day, should be aware of the distinct possibility of harm.

In conclusion, the range of safe vitamin C intakes seems to be broad, as is typical for water-soluble vitamins. Between the absolute minimum of 10 milligrams a day and a reasonable maximum of perhaps 1,000 milligrams, nearly everyone can find a suitable intake. People who venture outside these limits do so at a risk.

Vitamin C Requirements

How much vitamin C is enough? Allowances recommended by different nations vary from as low as 30 milligrams per day in Great Britain to 60 milligrams per day in the United States and Canada and 75 in West Germany (see Figure 8–8).

The requirement—the amount needed to prevent the appearance of the overt deficiency symptoms of scurvy—is well known to be only 10 milligrams daily. However, 10 milligrams a day apparently does not saturate all the body tissues; larger intakes increase the body's total vitamin C pool. At about 60 milligrams per day, the pool size in the average person stops responding to further increases in intake, and at 100 milligrams per day, 95 percent of the population probably reaches tissue saturation. After the tissues are saturated, all added vitamin C is excreted.

It may seem strange that of West Germany and Great Britain, two similar industrialized nations, one should recommend two and a half times the vitamin C intake of the other. In view of the wide range of possible intakes, however, the German and British recommendations are not so far apart. Both are generously above the minimum requirement, and both are well below the level at which toxicity symptoms might appear. The range of possible safe intakes is broad, as illustrated in Figure 8–8; all the different recommendations fall within it. In contrast, the recommendation by Dr. Linus Pauling and others that people should take 2 to 4 grams a day (or even 10 grams) is clearly way up in the clouds.

Remember that recommended allowances for vitamin C, like those for all the nutrients, are amounts intended to maintain health in healthy people, not to restore health in sick people. Unusual circumstances may increase nutrient needs. In the case of vitamin C, a variety of physical stresses deplete the body pool and may make intakes higher than 60 milligrams or so desirable. Among the stresses known to increase vitamin C needs are infections; burns; extremely high or low temperatures; toxic levels of heavy metals such as lead, mercury, and cadmium; cigarette smoking; and the chronic use of certain medications, including aspirin, barbiturates, and oral contraceptives. (The recommendation for people who smoke cigarettes regularly is 100 milligrams per day.) After oral surgery, dentists may prescribe supplemental vitamin C to hasten healing; after a major operation (such as removal of a breast) or extensive burns, when a tremendous amount of scar tissue must form during healing, the amount needed may be as high as 1,000 milligrams (1 gram) a day or even more. Under such medical conditions, a physician may prescribe vitamin supplementation; self-medication is not recommended under any circumstances.

Vitamin C Food Sources

The inclusion of intelligently selected fruits and vegetables in the daily diet guarantees a generous intake of vitamin C. Even those who wish to ingest amounts well above the recommendations can easily meet their goals this way. If you drink a double portion of orange juice at breakfast, choose a salad for lunch, and include a stalk of broccoli and a potato on your dinner plate, you will exceed 300 milligrams even before counting the contributions made by incidental other sources. Clearly, then, you would have no need for vitamin C pills unless you wanted to join the ranks of the megadosers.

Table 8–16 shows the amounts of vitamin C in various common foods. The overwhelming abundance of purple and green bars reveals that in addition to the citrus fruits (rightly famous for being rich in vitamin C), other fruits and vegetables are in the same league: broccoli, brussels sprouts, greens, cabbage, cantaloupe, and strawberries. You have to eat larger servings of the vegetables than of the fruits to get the same amount of the vitamin, but you can do this without an excessive energy intake. A single serving of any of these provides more than 30 milligrams of the vitamin and an array of other nutrients for less than 50 kcalories.

The humble potato is an important source of vitamin C in Western countries, not because a potato by itself meets the daily needs, but because potatoes are such a popular staple that they make significant contributions. Potatoes provide about 20 percent of all the vitamin C in the U.S. diet. Some young men report french fries as their only regular source of vitamin C, and yet because they eat so many, they receive the recommended amount.

No vitamin C is found in seeds; it appears only in growing plants. Thus grains are devoid of the vitamin. The minimal showing of blue and red bars in Table 8–16 confirms that milk (except breast milk) is a notoriously poor source, and meats in general contribute little vitamin C to the diet. Organ meats (liver, kidneys, and others) contain some vitamin C, but most people don't eat large quantities of these. Raw meats also contain small amounts of vitamin C, but again, these are rare in the U.S. diet. Raw meats and fish make enough of a contribution of vitamin C to be significant in the diets of the Inuit people of Alaska and Canada, and in Japanese cuisine; but in most of Canada and the United States, fruits and vegetables are necessary to supply vitamin C.

Vita means life. After this discourse on the vitamins, who could argue with the meaning of their name? Their regulation of metabolic processes and assistance in the transfer of energy make them vital to the normal growth, development, and maintenance of the human body—to life itself. It is remarkable that a small quantity of a substance that does not serve as an energy source or a significant part of the body's structures can be so indispensable. The wonder of the vitamins continues in the next chapter.

When nutritionists say "vitamin C," people think "oranges."

But these foods are also rich in vitamin C.

staple: a food kept on hand at all times and used daily or almost daily in meal preparation.

■ TABLE 8–16
Vitamin C in Commonly Eaten Foods Ranked Richest to Poorest

Food, Serving Size (Energy)

Papaya, 1 whole fresh (117 kcal)
Orange juice, 1 c fresh (111 kcal)
Cantaloupe, ½ (94 kcal)
Broccoli, 1 c cooked (46 kcal)
Brussels sprouts, 1 c cooked (60 kcal)
Green pepper, 1 whole (18 kcal)
Grapefruit juice, 1 c fresh (96 kcal)
Strawberries, 1 c fresh (45 kcal)
Oysters, 1 c raw (160 kcal)
Orange, 1 fresh medium (60 kcal)
Cauliflower, 1 c cooked (30 kcal)
Mango, 1 fresh (135 kcal)
Parsley, 1 c chopped fresh (20 kcal)
Asparagus, 1 c cooked (44 kcal)
Watermelon, 1 slice (152 kcal)
Pink/red grapefruit, ½ (37 kcal)
Tomato juice, 1 c canned (42 kcal)
Bok choy, 1 c cooked (20 kcal)
Turnip greens, 1 c cooked (29 kcal)
Spinach, 1 c cooked (41 kcal)
White grapefruit, ½ (39 kcal)
Tomatoes, 1 c whole canned (47 kcal)
Mustard greens, 1 c cooked (21 kcal)
Sauerkraut, 1 c canned (44 kcal)
Cabbage, 1 c raw shredded (16 kcal)
Honeydew melon, ¹⁄₁₀ (45 kcal)
Butternut squash, 1 c baked (83 kcal)
Raspberries, 1 c fresh (60 kcal)
Baked potato, 1 whole (220 kcal)
Winter squash, 1 c baked (96 kcal)
Pineapple chunks, 1 c fresh (76 kcal)
Beef liver, 3 oz fried (185 kcal)
Tomato, 1 whole raw (24 kcal)
Dandelion greens, 1 c cooked (35 kcal)
Bean sprouts, 1 c fresh (32 kcal)
Romaine lettuce, 1 c chopped (9 kcal)
Green beans, 1 c cooked (44 kcal)
Summer squash, 1 c cooked (36 kcal)
Apple, 1 fresh medium (80 kcal)
Celery, 1 large outer stalk (6 kcal)
Milk or yogurt, 1 c nonfat (86 kcal)
Milk, 1 c whole (150 kcal)
Sole/flounder, 3 oz baked (120 kcal)
Brewer's yeast, 1 tbsp (25 kcal)
Whole-wheat bread, 1 slice (70 kcal)
Kidney beans, 1 c canned (230 kcal)
Peanuts, 1 oz dried unsalted (161 kcal)
Chicken breast, ½ roasted (142 kcal)
Sirloin steak, 3 oz lean (180 kcal)
Cheddar cheese, 1 oz (114 kcal)

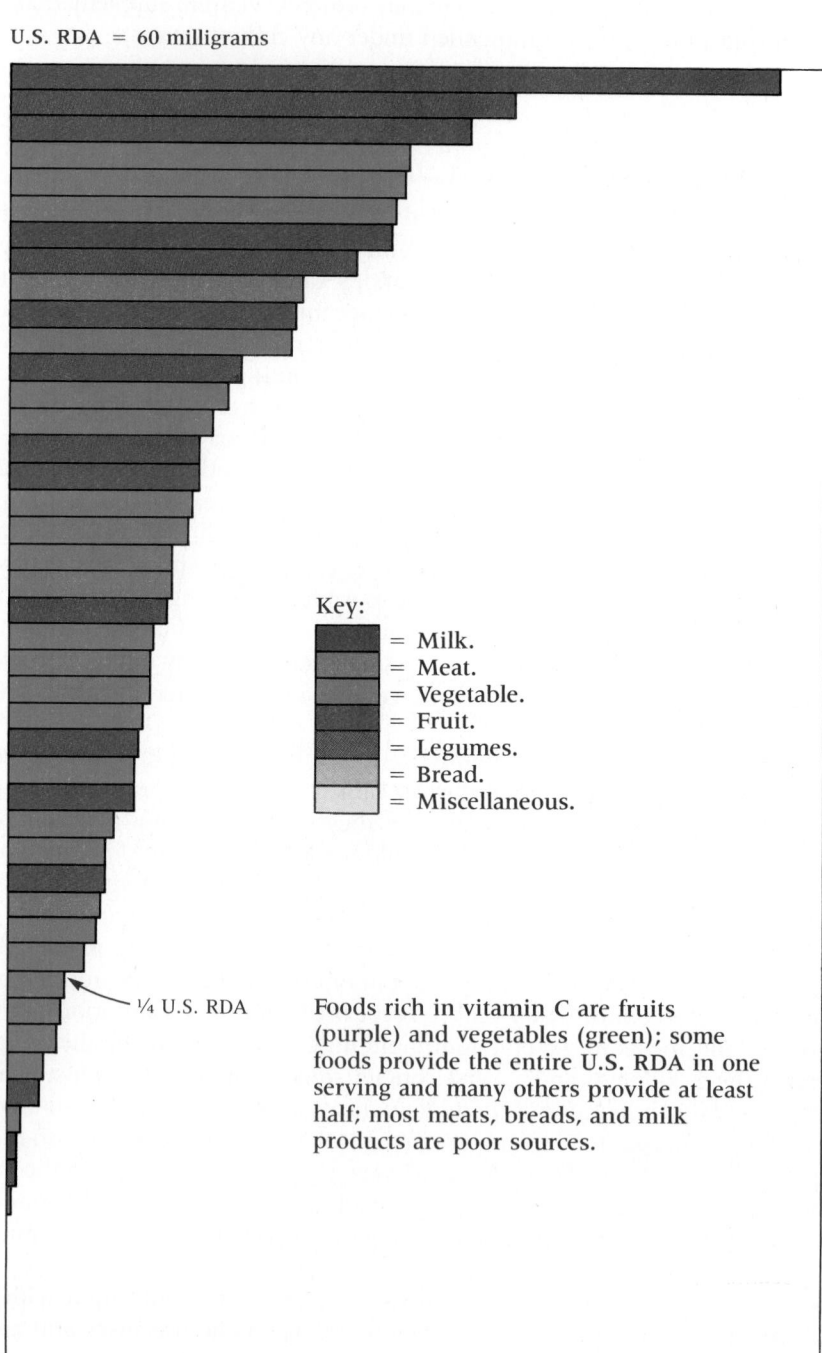

U.S. RDA = 60 milligrams

Key:
= Milk.
= Meat.
= Vegetable.
= Fruit.
= Legumes.
= Bread.
= Miscellaneous.

¼ U.S. RDA

Foods rich in vitamin C are fruits (purple) and vegetables (green); some foods provide the entire U.S. RDA in one serving and many others provide at least half; most meats, breads, and milk products are poor sources.

Milligrams/Serving

SELF STUDY *Evaluate Your Water-Soluble Vitamin Intakes*

Several of these exercises make use of the information you recorded on Forms 1 to 3.

1. Look up and record your recommended intake of thiamin (from the RDA tables on the inside front cover, left, or from the Canadian recommendations in Appendix I). Also record your actual intake, from the average derived on Form 2. What percentage of your recommended intake did you consume? Was this enough? What foods contribute the greatest amount of thiamin to your diet? If you consumed more than the recommendation, was this too much? Why or why not? In what ways would you change your diet to improve thiamin intake?

2. Repeat exercise 1 using riboflavin as the subject.

3. Estimate your niacin intake using the method outlined on p. 205. Did you consume enough niacin preformed in foods to meet your recommended intake? If not, did you consume enough extra protein to bring your intake up to the recommendation? What do you suppose are the limitations on this means of estimating niacin intake?

4. Repeat exercise 1 using each of the other B vitamins and vitamin C as the subject.

Study Questions

1. For thiamin, riboflavin, niacin, vitamin B_6, folate, vitamin B_{12}, pantothenic acid, biotin, and vitamin C, state:

   ■ Its chief function in the body.
   ■ The deficiency symptoms characteristic of it.
   ■ Significant food sources for it.

2. What is the relationship of tryptophan to niacin?
3. Which B vitamins are involved in energy metabolism? Protein metabolism? Cell division?
4. What risks are associated with megadoses of vitamin C?

Notes

1. E. M. N. Hamilton and S. A. S. Gropper, *The Biochemistry of Human Nutrition: A Desk Reference* (St. Paul, Minn.: West, 1987), pp. 242–243.
2. Hamilton and Gropper, 1987, pp. 242–243.
3. B. S. N. Rao and C. Gopalan, Niacin, in *Present Knowledge in Nutrition*, 5th ed. (Washington, D.C.: The Nutrition Foundation, 1984), pp. 318–331.
4. D. H. Blankenhorn and coauthors, Beneficial effects of combined colestipol-niacin therapy on coronary atherosclerosis and coronary venous bypass grafts, *Journal of the American Medical Association* 257 (1987): 3233–3240.
5. *Premenstrual Syndrome* (New York: American Council on Science and Health, July 1985).
6. H. Schaumberg and coauthors, Sensory neuropathy from pyridoxine abuse, *New England Journal of Medicine* 309 (1983): 445–448.
7. R. Carmel and coauthors, Cobalamin and osteoblast-specific proteins, *New England Journal of Medicine* 319 (1988): 70–75.
8. V. Herbert, The 1986 Herman Award Lecture: Nutrition science as a continually unfolding story: The folate and vitamin B–12 paradigm, *American Journal of Clinical Nutrition* 46 (1987): 387–402.
9. J. Lindenbaum and coauthors, Neuropsychiatric disorders caused by cobalamin deficiency in the absence of anemia or macrocytosis, *New England Journal of Medicine* 318 (1988): 1720–1728.
10. A. M. Immerman, Vitamin B_{12} status on a vegetarian diet: A critical review, *World Review of Nutrition and Dietetics* 37 (1981): 38–54.
11. V. Herbert, Vitamin B–12: Plant sources, requirements, and assay, *American Journal of Clinical Nutrition* 48 (1988): 852–858.
12. J. L. Wood and R. G. Allison, Effects of consumption of choline and lecithin on neurological and cardiovascular systems, *Federation Proceedings* 41 (1982): 3015–3021.
13. V. Tanphaichitr and B. Wood, Thiamin, in *Present Knowledge in Nutrition*, 5th ed. (Washington, D.C.: The Nutrition Foundation, 1984), pp. 273–281.
14. R. S. Rivlin, Riboflavin, in *Present Knowledge in Nutrition*, 5th ed. (Washington, D.C.: The Nutrition Foundation, 1984), pp. 285–302.
15. Toxicity of vitamin C megadoses, *Nutrition and the M.D.*, October 1980.
16. S. T. Omaye, J. H. Skala, and R. A. Jacob, Rebound effect with ascorbic acid in adult males (letter), *American Journal of Clinical Nutrition* 48 (1988): 379–380.

Vitamin C—Rumors versus Research

When Dr. Linus Pauling published his book *Vitamin C and the Common Cold* in 1970, he started a storm of controversy.[1] Newspaper headlines screamed, "VITAMIN C CURES COLDS"; others yelled back, "VITAMIN C NO EFFECT." One "famous scientist" said this, another that. Meanwhile, behind the scenes, teams of researchers in laboratories and hospitals across the world went to work designing and executing controlled experiments to determine whether, in fact, vitamin C has any therapeutic or preventive effect against the viruses that cause the myriad disorders collectively called the cold.

Since then some hundreds of articles have been published in the research journals, numbering several thousands of pages. Hundreds of people have been tested in a variety of experimental designs, and some conclusions have been reached. Meanwhile, Dr. Pauling has gone on to make additional claims for vitamin C; he urges that any client diagnosed as having cancer should immediately start taking 10 grams a day.[2] More research studies have followed, and the cancer question has generated nearly as much controversy as the common cold.

The purpose of this highlight is primarily to make you aware of the difficulties inherent in attempting to discover whether a nutrient (or any therapeutic approach) remedies symptoms or cures a disease. New findings on the efficacy of various treatments appear every week, but always, the same kinds of questions have to be answered before the usefulness of the findings can be evaluated. Research on vitamin C and colds illustrates particularly well what those questions are. Along the way, the relationship of vitamin C to colds

Miniglossary

blind experiment: an experiment in which the subjects do not know whether they are members of the experimental or the control group.

control group: a group of individuals similar in all possible respects to the group being experimented on, except for the experimental treatment. Ideally, the control group receives a sham treatment while the experimental group receives a real one.

double-blind experiment: an experiment in which neither the subjects nor those conducting the experiment know which subjects are members of the experimental group and which are serving as control subjects, until after the experiment is over.

experimental group: a group of individuals similar in all possible respects to the control group, except for the treatment. The experimental group receives the real treatment while the control group receives a placebo.

longitudinal study: a study in which the subjects are studied over time—for example, in 1960 and again in 1970, 1980, and 1990.

placebo (pla-SEE-bo): an inert, harmless medication given to provide comfort and hope.

  placere = to please

placebo effect: the healing effect that faith in medicine, even inert medicine, often has.

randomization: a process of choosing the members of the experimental and control groups in a random fashion.

replication: repeating an experiment and getting the same results. The skeptical scientist, on hearing of a new, exciting finding, will ask, "Has it been replicated yet?" If it hasn't, the scientist will withhold judgment regarding its validity.

validity: having the quality of being founded on fact or evidence.

will be clarified. As for cancer, more nutrients than just vitamin C are involved, and Chapter 16 attempts to put them all in perspective.

In most studies on the efficacy of vitamin C, two groups of people are selected. One group is given vitamin C, and the other is not; both are followed to determine whether the vitamin C group does better in terms of colds or cancer than the control group. A number of pitfalls are inherent in an experiment of this

kind; they must be avoided if the results are to be believed.

Controls

First, the two groups of people must be similar in all respects (except that one group receives vitamin C). Most important, both must have the same track record with respect to colds, to rule out the possibility that an observed difference might have occurred anyway. (If group A would have caught twice as many colds as group B anyway, then the fact that group B happened to receive the vitamin proves nothing.) Also, in experiments involving a nutrient, it is imperative that the diets of both groups be similar, especially with respect to that nutrient. (If those in group B were receiving less vitamin C from their diet, this fact might cancel the effects of the supplement.) Similarity of the experimental and control groups is one of the characteristics of a well-controlled experiment and is accomplished by randomization, a process of choosing the members from the same starting population by throws of the dice or some such method involving chance.

Sample Size

To ensure that chance variation between the two groups does not influence the results, the groups must be large. (If one member of a group of five people catches a bad cold by chance, he will pull the whole group's average toward bad colds; but if one member of a group of 500 catches a bad cold, she will not unduly affect the group average.) In reviewing the results of experiments of this kind, always ask whether the number of people tested was large enough to rule out chance variation. Statistical methods are useful for determining the significance of differences between groups of various sizes.

Placebos

If people take vitamin C for colds and believe it will cure them, the chances of recovery are greatly improved. The administration of anything believed to be medicine hastens recovery in about half of all cases.[3] This phenomenon, the effect of faith on healing, is known as the placebo effect. In experiments designed to determine whether vitamin C actually affects prevention of, or recovery from, colds or cancer,

this mind-body effect must be rigorously controlled.

One way experimenters control for the placebo effect is to give pills to all participants, some containing vitamin C and others, of similar appearance and taste, containing an inactive ingredient (placebos). This way, all subjects believe they are receiving the treatment, and the effects of faith will work equally in both groups. If it is not possible to convince all subjects that they are receiving vitamin C, then the extent of belief or unbelief must be the same in both groups. An experiment conducted under these conditions is called blind—that is, the subjects do not know (are blind to) whether they are members of the experimental group (receiving treatment) or the control group (receiving placebo).

Double Blind

The experimenters, too, must not know which subjects are receiving the placebo (the control group) and which are receiving the vitamin C (the experimental group). Being fallible human beings and having an emotional investment in a successful outcome, researchers may hear what they want to hear and so interpret and record results with a bias in the expected direction. This is not dishonest, but is an unconscious shifting of the experimenters' perceptions of reality to agree with their expectations. To prevent it, the pills given to the subjects must be coded by a third party, who does not reveal to the experimenters which subjects received which medication until all results have been recorded quantitatively.

Reviewing the Evidence

In 1975, Dr. Thomas C. Chalmers, a physician, reviewed the data from 14 clinical trials of vitamin C in the treatment and prevention of the common cold.[4] Of the trials, five were poorly controlled, in Chalmers's judgment; nine were reasonably well

NUTRITION DETECTIVE WORK

In discussing these subtleties of experimental design, our intent is not to make a research scientist out of you, but to show you what a far cry real scientific validity is from the experience of your neighbor Mary (sample size, one; no control group), who says she takes vitamin C when she feels a cold coming on and "it works every time." (She knows what she is taking, she has faith in its efficacy, and she tends not to notice when it doesn't work.) Before concluding that an experiment has shown that a nutrient cures a disease or alleviates a symptom, you have to ask yourself these questions:

- Was there a control group similar in all important ways to the experimental group?
- Was the sample size large enough to rule out chance variation?
- Was a placebo effectively administered (blind)?
- Was the experiment double blind?

These are a few, but not all, of the important variables involved in studying the efficacy of a "cure." With them in mind, this highlight reviews the literature to see how successfully Dr. Pauling's vitamin C theory has stood the test of experimentation.

controlled in that the subjects given vitamin C and those given placebos were randomly chosen. In addition, eight of these nine studies were double blind. When the data from these eight studies were pooled, there was a difference of one-tenth of a cold per year and an average difference in duration of one-tenth of a day per cold in favor of those subjects taking vitamin C. In two studies, the effects of vitamin C seemed to be more striking in girls than in boys.

In one study, a questionnaire given at the conclusion revealed that a number of the subjects had correctly guessed the contents of their capsules. A reanalysis of the results showed that those who received the placebo *who thought they were receiving vitamin C* had fewer colds than the group receiving vitamin C *who thought they were receiving the placebo!*

Other reviewers who have assembled and looked at all the evidence, as Dr. Chalmers did, have reached the same conclusions. At the start of the 1980s, reports of additional experiments were still coming out, and most were consistent with previous findings. The balanced picture emerging from the reviews seems to indicate that the effects of the vitamin on colds, if any, are small.

The writer of popular health articles rarely reports on such reviews of literature, because they are cold; objective; and give many viewpoints, rarely stressing one. They are not, therefore, sensational enough to sell in the marketplace. Who wants to read a scholarly, conservative, textbooklike report in a newspaper? What usually appears in the newspaper or on TV is the report of one experiment that obtained a significant result. "Professor So-and-So of the Such-and-Such Lab at the Etcetera University," the commentator may say, "has found that vitamin C does make a difference after all, at least for little girls. In a double-blind, co-twin study, in which one of each pair of twins received vitamin C and the other a placebo, the youngest girls, but not the boys, receiving vitamin C had significantly shorter and less severe illnesses than their twins. . . ."

If you chose to look up the source of the report, you would probably find that the study had been conducted as described and that the little girls had indeed had fewer colds than the little boys. But the researchers themselves did not jump to the conclusion that vitamin C makes a difference. In an admirable effort to put their finding in perspective, they pointed out that even their apparently valid result might have occurred by chance: "One should be aware that, as the number of tests increases, the possibility of obtaining a 'significant' result by chance alone is also increased."[5] In other words, their experiment would have to be repeated and the same result seen several times more before it could be accepted as real. The general public may be made uneasy by scientists who admit that their results are inconclusive, but the scientific community prefers total honesty to dogmatic statements.

The scientist who reports a "significant" finding from a single experiment is not being dishonest. The term *significant* means that *statistical* analysis suggests that the findings probably didn't arise from a chance event, but from the experimental treatment being tested. However, the *human* significance, or meaning, of the findings is apparent only after the piece of research is added into the total picture. Sources you should turn to for a broad and balanced picture of the available information are the journals, the indexes, and the reviews of literature (see Figure H8–1). If you are relying on a single source for your information, ask yourself, "Is this one viewpoint? Or is it a balanced picture?"

The statistical effect of vitamin C on the common cold in the kinds of populations studied to date has been small. Meanwhile, what has the research on vitamin C and cancer shown so far?

Vitamin C and Cancer

In 1976, Dr. Pauling and his associate Dr. Cameron reported that they had administered vitamin C to 100 cancer clients in the Vale of Leven, Scotland, and had prolonged their survival rate. As compared with 1,000 similar clients who had been in the same hospital in earlier years and who had lived only 50 days, these clients lived 210 days.[6] In response, a group of researchers at the Mayo Clinic in Rochester, Minnesota, conducted a study to test the validity of this finding. The Mayo Clinic researchers criticized the earlier study on several grounds. It was not legitimate to use former clients as controls; most important, they said the control subjects should have been chosen randomly from the *same* population as those given vitamin C, to make sure they were similar. The Mayo researchers therefore conducted a randomized, controlled, double-blind trial, giving vitamin C to 60 clients and a placebo that tasted and looked similar to vitamin C to 63 clients. Clients in both groups worsened at the same rate and died at the same times. The authors concluded, "We cannot recommend the use of high-dose vitamin C in patients with advanced cancer who have previously received radiation treatment or chemotherapy."[7]

Dr. Pauling, in turn, pointed out that the Mayo researchers had not fairly tested the original hypothesis. Pauling's clients had relatively strong immune systems, because they had not had the debilitating cancer treatments (radiation or chemotherapy) that the Mayo clients had had. The question whether large doses of vitamin C prolong survival time in cancer clients whose immune systems are not already severely damaged remains to be tested in a randomized, controlled, double-blind trial.[8]

Since the Mayo study, a few other reports have trickled in, relating to the vitamin's effect on cancer. The question remains open whether vitamin C helps with cancer at all, but

■ FIGURE H8–1
Sources of Reliable Nutrition Information

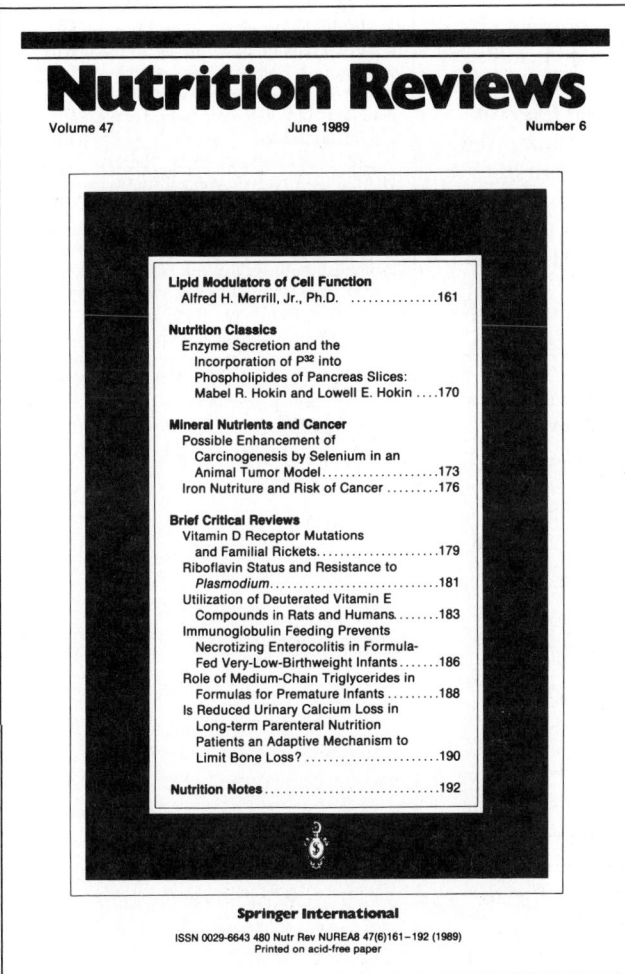

Reviews

To find a critique of all the important work on a subject, you can turn to a journal of reviews like the one shown here. One major review appears in *Nutrition Reviews* every month. It is followed by a bibliography that provides references to all of the original work reviewed.

Journals

Reports of single experiments are presented in journals like the *Journal of the American Medical Association*.

Indexes

You can look up a large number of experiments on a single topic in an index of abstracts. The part of a page shown here, from *Biological Abstracts*, lists all recently published titles containing the term *vitamin C* and gives each one a reference number. The number refers to a short summary of the reported work, which also tells exactly where it was published. The indexes will lead you to reports of experiments in many different journals. New volumes of *Biological Abstracts* come out semimonthly. *Nutrition Abstracts and Reviews*, a monthly publication, would also contain titles including the word *vitamin C*.

one result is clear from the Mayo study. Vitamin C did not help with advanced cancer clients who had received radiation or chemotherapy.

Researchers are hard at work in many labs and clinics pursuing greater understanding of what vitamin C does and doesn't do. This highlight cannot give a final answer on such a subject, but it has fulfilled its two promises: to make you aware of the difficulties inherent in this kind of research, and to show you the kinds of research questions that will have to be answered before we know what vitamin C does.

While you await reports of the next controlled, double-blind studies on carefully defined and randomized groups of clients, you may wonder what doses of vitamin C to take, yourself, in light of what is already known. The decision is entirely up to you, but in case you should choose to aim for an intake of several hundred milligrams a day (say, ten times the RDA), this reminder is in order. You can easily obtain this amount of vitamin C by including many vitamin C–rich vegetables and fruits in your daily diet. There is no need to take any kind of pills.

NOTES

1. L. C. Pauling, *Vitamin C and the Common Cold* (San Francisco: W. H. Freeman, 1970).
2. L. Pauling, Vitamin C therapy of advanced cancer (letter to the editor), *New England Journal of Medicine* 302 (1980): 694; N. Horwitz, Now Japanese report 6-fold survival jump in terminal cancer with ascorbate megadoses, *Medical Tribune,* July 22, 1981.
3. This finding is widely agreed on; it is discussed, among other places, in the debate on vitamin C in *Nutrition Today,* March–April 1978.
4. T. C. Chalmers, Effects of ascorbic acid on the common cold, *American Journal of Medicine* 58 (1975): 532–536.
5. J. Z. Miller and coauthors, Therapeutic effect of vitamin C: A co-twin control study, *Journal of the American Medical Association* 237 (1977): 248–251.
6. E. Cameron and L. Pauling, Supplemental ascorbate in the supportive treatment of cancer: Prolongation of survival times in terminal human cancer, *Proceedings of the National Academy of Science USA* 73 (1976): 3685–3689.
7. E. T. Creagan and coauthors, Failure of high-dose vitamin C (ascorbic acid) therapy to benefit patients with advanced cancer, *New England Journal of Medicine* 301 (1979): 687–690.
8. Pauling, 1980.

The Fat-Soluble Vitamins: A, D, E, and K

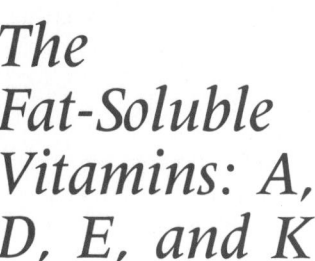

The eye's light-sensitive pigments lie in layers in the rods and cones. This is a cone cell between two rod cells. At the tip of the cone *(top)* is a stack of discs packed with pigment containing vitamin A (retinal). Beneath the tip lies a bundle of spaghetti-like mitochondria prepared, when light hits the cone, to produce the energy needed to stimulate the next cell to initiate a nerve impulse.

Has it ever occurred to you how remarkable it is that you can see things? As an infant you were enchanted with the power this gave you. You closed your eyes, and the world disappeared. You opened them and made everything come back again. Later you forgot the wonder of this, but the fact remains that your ability to see brings everything into being for you, more so than any of your other senses. Light reaching your eyes puts you in touch with things outside your body, from your friend sitting near you to stars in other galaxies.

Has it ever occurred to you how extraordinary it is that a child grows? From a mere nothing, a speck so tiny that it is invisible to the naked eye, each person develops into a full-size human being with arms and legs, teeth and fingernails, a beating heart and tingling nerves. Years go into the making of an adult human being, with each day bringing changes so gradual they seem undetectable. Only if you are absent during a part of this process do you notice it on your return and remark to a child, "My, how you've grown!"

And when did you last think about your breathing? In, out, in, out, day and night, year after year, you take in the oxygen you need and release it, disposing of the used-up carbons whose energy moves you and keeps you alive. The nutrients discussed in this chapter—vitamins A, D, E, and K—are vital for these and other processes that you may often take for granted.

The fat-soluble vitamins A, D, E, and K differ from the water-soluble vitamins in several ways. They are found in the fat and oily parts of foods. Because they are insoluble in water, they require bile for digestion and chylomicrons for transport. They enter the lymphatic system upon absorption, before entering the bloodstream. They tend to move into the liver and adipose tissue and remain there, rather than being regularly excreted, as most of the water-soluble vitamins are. Their storage in the body makes it possible to survive for days, weeks, or even months or years without eating foods containing them; an *average* daily intake is all a person has to aim for. The risk of toxicity is greater than it is for the water-soluble vitamins.

■ Vitamin A

Vitamin A has the distinction of being the first fat-soluble vitamin to have been recognized. Three different forms of vitamin A are active in the body: retinol (an alcohol), retinal (an aldehyde), and retinoic acid (an acid). In addition, plant pigments known as carotenoids can be converted to vitamin A by the liver with low efficiency. The most active of the carotenoids is beta-carotene. When beta-carotene is split, it yields two molecules, one of which is converted to retinol. Figure 9–1 illustrates the similarities and differences among these vitamin A relatives (see Appendix C for their complete structures).

Each form of vitamin A has its own special binding proteins (retinol has several) in the cells in which it works. There is also a special transport protein, retinol binding protein (RBP), to pick up vitamin A from the liver, where it is stored, and carry it in the blood. Cells that will receive and use vitamin A also have special receptors for it, as if it were fragile and had to be passed carefully from hand to hand without being dropped.

retinol (RET-ih-nol): the alcohol form of vitamin A.

retinal (RET-ih-nal): the aldehyde form of vitamin A, active in the eye.

retinoic acid: the acid form of vitamin A.

beta-carotene (BAY-tah KARE-oh-teen): a vitamin A precursor found in plants.

retinol binding protein (RBP): the specific protein responsible for transporting retinol.

Retinol, the alcohol form

Retinal, the aldehyde form

Retinoic acid, the acid form

Beta-carotene

■ FIGURE 9–1
Vitamin A and Beta-carotene
In this diagram, corners represent carbon atoms, as in all previous diagrams in this book. A further simplification, here, is that methyl groups (CH_3) are understood to be at the ends of the lines extending from corners. The arrow on beta-carotene points to where cleavage occurs, resulting in two molecules of retinal.

Each form of vitamin A triggers specific reactions in cells that are set up to respond to it. Retinol and retinoic acid, for example, act like hormones; they travel into cells, cross the nuclear membranes, and interact with DNA. This causes certain genes to express their coded instructions, which results in the making of specific proteins.

Vitamin A may be the most versatile of the fat-soluble vitamins because of its roles in several important body processes. Its roles in promoting good night vision, the health of mucous membranes and skin, and growth of the body's tissues are well known. Other roles vitamin A plays include:

■ Maintaining the stability of cell membranes.
■ Helping the adrenal glands to synthesize a hormone (cortisol).
■ Helping to ensure a normal output of the hormone thyroxin from the thyroid gland.
■ Helping to maintain nerve cell sheaths.
■ Assisting in immune reactions.
■ Helping to manufacture red blood cells.

The best known of vitamin A's roles involves vision (see the Miniglossary of Vision Terms for relevant definitions). At the place where light hits the retina of the eye, profoundly informative communication occurs between the environment and the person. The eye receives the light and transforms it into signals that travel to the interior of the brain. There a mental picture forms of what the light conveys (Figure 9–2). For this to happen, the eye must perform

■ **FIGURE 9–2**
Vision
A. As light enters the eye, pigments within the cells of the retina absorb the light.
B. Each pigment molecule (in this diagram, rhodopsin) contains retinal (the active form of vitamin A) and a protein (in this diagram, opsin).
C. When retinal absorbs light, its shape and color change, causing its release from opsin, which also changes shape, generating nerve impulses that travel into the brain.

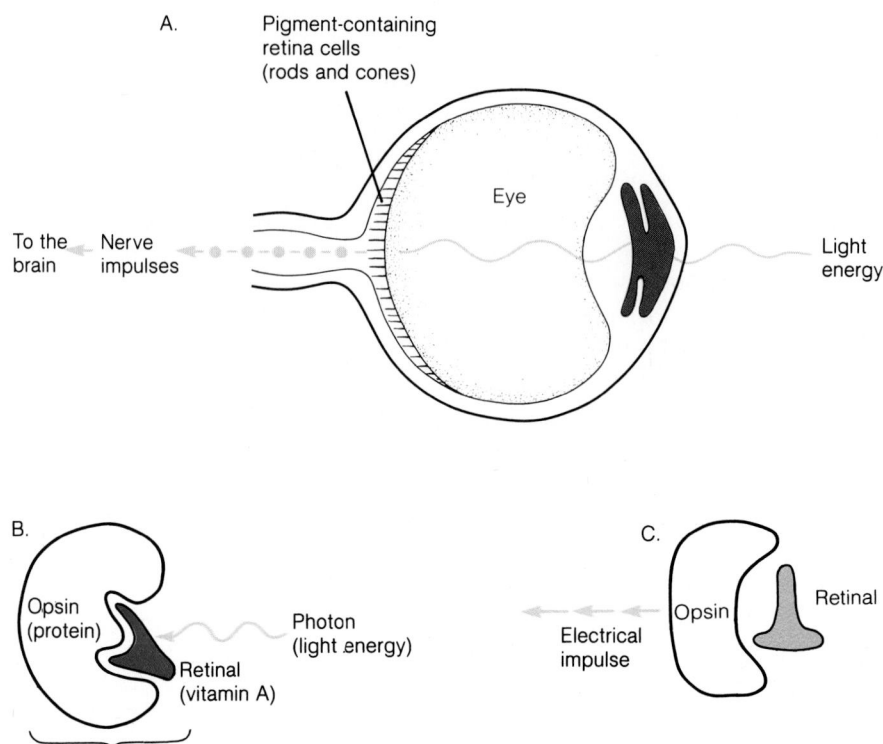

a remarkable transformation of light energy into nerve impulses. The transformers are the molecules of pigment (rhodopsin, iodopsin, and others) in the cells of the retina.

The pigment molecules inside the cells absorb the light. Each pigment molecule is composed of a protein called opsin bonded to a molecule of retinal. When a unit of light energy (a photon) enters the eye, the retinal portion of the pigment molecule absorbs it and responds by changing shape. It shifts from a *cis* to a *trans* configuration, as fatty acids do during hydrogenation (p. 130). In the process, the retinal changes color, too, becoming bleached. In its altered form, retinal cannot remain bonded to opsin and so is released. This disturbs the shape of the opsin molecule.

This shape change disturbs the membrane of the cell containing the pigment, permitting charged ions to enter and leave the cell. The cell hyperpolarizes (that is, the electrical differential across its membrane increases), and an electrical impulse travels along the cell's length. At the other end of the cell, the impulse is transmitted to a nerve cell, which conveys it deeper into the brain. Thus the message is sent.

A mechanical genius could not have designed such a system better. Light itself cannot be conducted through the solid material of the brain, so it is changed into signals transmitted by nerves. But light comes in different colors (wavelengths), which convey needed information. To keep the colors sorted out, the eye uses different light-sensitive cells (cones) to receive them. Blue light is absorbed by one set of cells, green by another, and yellow-red by a third. By day, combinations of these give the full range of color vision. By

---

Miniglossary of Vision Terms

cones: the cells of the retina that respond to bright light and are responsible for color vision.

iodopsin (eye-o-DOP-sin): the light-sensitive pigment of the cones in the retina. Both rhodopsin and iodopsin contain retinal; the protein portions of the pigments differ.

opsin (OP-sin): the protein portion of the visual pigment molecule.

photon (FOE-ton): a unit of light energy. Depending on its wavelength, a photon conveys different colors of light.

pigment: a molecule capable of absorbing certain wavelengths of light, so that it reflects only those that we perceive as a certain color.

retina (RET-in-uh): the layer of light-sensitive cells lining the back of the inside of the eye; consists of rods and cones.

rhodopsin (ro-DOP-sin): the light-sensitive pigment of the rods in the retina.

rods: the cells of the retina that respond to dim light and convey black-and-white vision.

---

night, the light entering the eye is of low intensity, and the set of cells (rods) that can receive this light are of one kind only; so by night a person can normally discern only the presence of light, not its color.

After receiving light and sending a message about it, the molecule of retinal is converted back to its original form and rejoined to opsin to regenerate the pigment rhodopsin. Many molecules of retinal are involved in this process. There are about 6 to 7 million cone cells and 100 million rod cells in the retina, and each contains about 30 million molecules of visual pigment. Repeated small losses incurred by visual activity necessitate the constant replenishment of retinal from the blood, which brings a new supply from the body stores. Ultimately, vitamin A and its relatives in food are the source of all the retinal in the pigments of the eye.

Bright light seen suddenly, when the eyes are dark-adapted, destroys much more retinal than light seen by day, a fact that is reflected in the early vitamin A-deficiency symptom of night blindness. The eye is especially vulnerable to retinal destruction at night for three reasons. First, the pupil is wide open at night, to allow as much light as possible to enter the eye. Second, a shadowing pigment that protects the rods by day withdraws at night, leaving them exposed. Third, there are many more rods than cones. Hence, if a bright light suddenly shines at night through the wide-open pupil onto the unprotected rods, much of the pigment in them is bleached and momentarily inactivated. More retinal than usual is freed, and more is lost. A moment passes before the pigments regenerate and sight returns. You no doubt remember being "blinded" on occasion by a flashlight shining directly into your eyes. This is normal, but if you didn't quickly recover your ability to see, you might suspect you had night blindness.

Vitamin A is undeniably an important nutrient, if for no other reason than that it plays a vital role in vision. But only one-thousandth of the vitamin A

mucosa (myoo-COH-suh): the membranes, composed of cells, that line the surfaces of body tissues.

urethra (you-REE-thruh): the tube through which urine from the bladder passes out of the body.

goblet cells: cells found in the epithelium of the GI tract and lungs that secrete mucus.

mucus (adjective **mucous**): a class of substances secreted by the goblet cells of the mucosa; a glycoprotein. (A **glycoprotein** consists of a carbohydrate and protein.)

epithelial (ep-i-THEE-lee-ul) **cells**: cells on the surface of the skin and mucosa.

in the body is in the retina. Much more is in the body's skin and linings. All surfaces, both inside and out, are maintained with the help of vitamin A.

It is important that each of these mucosa surfaces be smooth: the linings of the mouth, stomach, and intestines; the linings of the lungs and the passages leading to them; the linings of the urinary bladder and urethra; the linings of the uterus and vagina; the linings of the eyelids and sinus passageways. Vitamin A helps to maintain the integrity of these mucous membranes (see Figure 9–3). Within the body, the mucous membranes of the GI tract alone line an area larger than a quarter of a football field, so this function of vitamin A accounts for most of the body's vitamin A need. The cells of all these surfaces—goblet cells—synthesize and secrete a smooth and slippery substance (mucus) that coats and protects them from invasive microorganisms and other harmful particles. The mucous lining of the stomach also shields its cells from digestion by the gastric juices. In the upper part of the lungs, the epithelial cells possess little whiplike hairs (cilia), which continuously sweep the coating of mucus up and out, so that any foreign particles that chance to get in are carried away by the flow. (When you clear your throat and swallow, you are excreting this waste by way of your digestive tract.) In the vagina, similar cells sweep the mucus down and out. During an infection in any of these locations, these goblet cells secrete more mucus and become more active, so that a noticeable discharge occurs; when you cough it up, blow your nose, or wash it away, you help to rid your body of the infective agent.

As you might predict, vitamin A plays an important role in fighting infection.[1] Children with even mild vitamin A deficiency develop respiratory diseases and diarrhea at two and three times the rate of children with normal vitamin A status.[2] By maintaining strong epithelial tissues, vitamin A prevents the invasion of bacteria and viruses. In addition, vitamin A is required for the growth of many of the body's tissues, including the lymph glands where antibodies are produced. These are only two of the many ways in which vitamin A supports the immune system.

As mentioned, vitamin A supports growth. At the beginning of this century, when researchers first discovered the vitamin, they noted a steady decline in the growth of animals deprived of vitamin A. This connection now offers a solution to one of the developing world's major nutrition problems—vitamin A deficiency. When children who are vitamin A deficient are given a vitamin A supplement, they gain weight and grow taller.[3] Vitamin A–supplemented children also benefit from a stronger immune system. In a study in Indonesia of 25,000 preschool children, the distribution of two

■ **FIGURE 9–3**
Mucous Membrane Integrity

Vitamin A maintains a healthy body lining.

Without vitamin A, body lining cells are altered.

large-dose vitamin A capsules per year resulted in a 34 percent reduction in childhood deaths.[4]

The growth of bones offers a glimpse of vitamin A in action and illustrates that growth is a complex phenomenon of remodeling, not simply a matter of the body "getting bigger." The process is similar to that of enlarging the interior of a brick fireplace; the first thing you have to do is remove some of the old bricks. Similarly, as Figure 9–4 shows, to convert a small bone into a large bone, the bone-remodeling cells must "undo" some parts of the bone as they go.

Vitamin A participates in the undoing. Some of the cells involved in bone formation contain sacs of degradative enzymes that can take apart the structures of bone. With the help of vitamin A in a sensitively regulated process, these cells release their enzymes, which eat away at selected sites in the bone, removing the parts that are not needed as the bone grows longer. (A similar process occurs when a tadpole loses its tail and becomes a frog. As you know, the tail doesn't simply fall off; rather, it is resorbed, "growing" shorter and shorter until it disappears. As a fetus you also had a tail and lost it, a process that depended on vitamin A.)

Vitamin A research still in progress is yielding many new details of how this nutrient functions in the body. As you might expect of this busy vitamin, its deficiency has severe consequences.

Vitamin A Deficiency

Vitamin A deficiency commonly occurs together with protein and zinc deficiency. The details of the relationships between these nutrients remain unclear, but in general, both zinc and protein deficiency impair protein synthesis, including that of the retinol-binding protein that transports vitamin A around the body. A specific connection between zinc and vitamin A is evident in the retina of the eye, where zinc assists the enzyme that regenerates retinal from retinol.

Vitamin A deficiency depends on the adequacy of vitamin A stores and protein (to provide its carrier). Up to a year's supply of vitamin A may be stored in the body, 90 percent of it in the liver. If a healthy adult were to stop eating good food sources of the vitamin, deficiency symptoms would not begin to appear until after stores were depleted, which would take one to two years. Then, however, the consequences would be profound and severe. Table 9–1 itemizes deficiency symptoms, as well as toxicity symptoms, functions in the body, and food sources.

Night blindness is one of the first detectable signs of vitamin A deficiency and aids in diagnosis of the condition. When the blood bathing the cells of the retina does not supply sufficient retinal to rapidly regenerate visual pigments bleached by light, a person experiences night blindness. This can occur following a flash of bright light at night or simply after the lights go out. In many parts of the world, after the sun goes down, night-blind children are unable to find their way home. They sit still, afraid that they may trip or fall if they try to walk. In many developing countries, night blindness due to vitamin A deficiency is so common that the people have a special word in their vocabulary to describe it.[5] In Indonesia, the term is *buta ayan*, which means "chicken

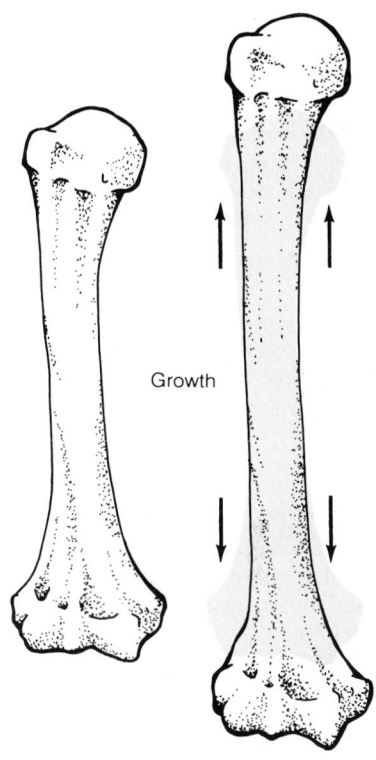

■ **FIGURE 9–4**
Growth of Bone
As bone lengthens, vitamin A helps remove old bone.

These sacs of degradative enzymes are **lysosomes** (LYE-so-zomes).
lyso = to break
soma = body

The cells that destroy bone during growth are **osteoclasts**; those that build bone are **osteoblasts.**
osteo = bone
clast = break
blast = build

night blindness: an inability to see in dim light; an early symptom of vitamin A deficiency.

■ **TABLE 9–1**
Vitamin A—A Summary

Other Names	Deficiency Disease Name	Toxicity Disease Name
Retinol, retinal, retinoic acid; precursor is provitamin A carotenoids such as beta-carotene	Hypovitaminosis A	Hypervitaminosis A[a]

Chief Functions in the Body	Deficiency Symptoms	Toxicity Symptoms
Vision; maintenance of cornea, epithelial cells, mucous membranes, skin; bone and tooth growth; reproduction; hormone synthesis and regulation; immunity; cancer protection	**Bones/Teeth[b]** Cessation of bone growth, change in shapes of bones, painful joints. Malfunctioning of enamel-forming cells, development of cracks in teeth and tendency to decay, atrophy of dentin-forming cells	Increased activity of osteoclasts[c] causing decalcification, joint pain, fragility, stunted growth, and thickening of long bones; increase of pressure inside skull, mimicking brain tumor; headaches
Significant Sources		
Retinol: fortified milk, cheese, cream, butter, fortified margarine, eggs, liver. Beta-carotene: spinach and other dark, leafy greens; broccoli; deep orange fruits (apricots, cantaloupe) and vegetables (squash, carrots, sweet potatoes, pumpkin)	**Blood** Anemia, often masked by dehydration	Loss of hemoglobin and potassium by red blood cells, cessation of menstruation, slowed clotting time, easily induced bleeding
	Eyes[d] Night blindness, changes in epithelial tissue caused by failure to secrete mucopolysaccharide (hyperkeratinization), drying (xerosis), triangular gray spots on eye (Bitot's spots), irreversible drying (keratomalacia), and degeneration of the cornea causing blindness (most severe)	
	Skin Plugging of hair follicles with keratin, forming white lumps (hyperkeratosis)	Dryness; itching; peeling; rashes; dry, scaling lips; cracking and bleeding of lips; nosebleeds; loss of hair; brittle nails

[a]A related condition, hypercarotenemia, is caused by the accumulation of too much of the vitamin A precursor beta-carotene in the blood, which turns the skin noticeably yellow. Hypercarotenemia is not, strickly speaking, a toxicity symptom.
[b]Highlight 10 describes vitamin A's role in tooth formation in more detail.
[c]Osteoclasts are the cells that destroy bone during its growth. Those that build bone are osteoblasts.
[d]The eyes' symptoms of vitamin A deficiency are collectively known as *xerophthalmia*.

eyes." (Chickens do not have rods in their eyes and therefore cannot see at night.) Sadly, mothers noticed that their children, like chickens, stumbled after dark. Figure 9–5 shows the eyes' slow recovery in night blindness.

When vitamin A is not present, the goblet cells that secrete mucus diminish in number and activity, and the epithelial cells change shape and begin to secrete the protein keratin—the hard, inflexible protein of hair and nails. These two processes contribute to the epithelial tissue's losing its integrity and becoming defenseless against infection.

keratin (KERR-uh-tin): a water-insoluble protein; the normal protein of hair and nails. Keratin-producing cells may replace mucus-producing cells in vitamin A deficiency.

■ TABLE 9–1
Vitamin A—A Summary   (continued)

Deficiency Symptoms	Toxicity Symptoms
Digestive System	
Changes in lining, diarrhea	Nausea, vomiting, abdominal pain, diarrhea, weight loss
Immune System	
Depression of immune reactions	Stimulation of immune reactions
Nervous/Muscular System	
Brain and spinal cord growth too fast for stunted skull and spine, paralysis caused by injury to brain and nerves	Loss of appetite, irritability, fatigue, insomia, restlessness, headache, blurred vision, nausea, vomiting, muscle weakness, interference with thyroxin
Respiratory Tract	
Changes in lining, infections	
Urogenital Tract	
Changes in lining that favor calcium deposition, resulting in kidney stones and bladder disorders; infections of bladder and kidney; infections of vagina	
Reproductive System	
	Amenorrhea[e]
Liver[f]	
	Jaundice,[g] enlargement, massive accumulation of fat and vitamin A
Spleen	
	Enlargement

[e]Elevated serum carotene concentrations are associated with amenorrhea.
[f]If liver impairment is severe, the "classic" signs seen in skin and hair may be masked.
[g]A symptom of liver disease, in which bile and related pigments spill into the bloodstream and the skin yellows, is *jaundice* (JAWN-diss).

In the eye, the cornea becomes dry and hard. Further changes may progress to permanent blindness. Mucous secretion in the stomach and intestines diminishes, hindering normal digestion and absorption of nutrients, and so indirectly worsening the deficiency. Infections of the respiratory tract, the GI tract, the urinary tract, the vagina, and possibly the inner ear are more likely with vitamin A deficiency. The outer body surface hardens, too. The skin becomes dry, rough, and scaly as an accumulation of hard material makes a lump around each hair follicle (see Figure 9–6).

Because growth and development of the brain and eyes are most rapid in the fetus and in the very young infant, the effects of vitamin A deficiency are most severe during pregnancy and around the time of birth. For example, in a child of one or two, stunted growth of the skull may cause crowding of the

In the eye, the symptoms of vitamin A deficiency are collectively known as **xerophthalmia** (zer-off-THAL-mee-uh). An early sign is **xerosis** (drying of the cornea); the latest and most severe stage is **keratomalacia** (total blindness).
xero = dry
ophthalm = eye
malacia = softening, weakening

cornea (KOR-nee-uh): the transparent membrane covering the outside of the front of the eye.

follicle (FOLL-i-cul): a group of cells in the skin from which a hair grows.

■ **FIGURE 9–5**
Night Blindness
These photographs illustrate the eyes' slow recovery in response to a flash of bright light at night. In animal research studies, the response rate is measured with electrodes.

brain (which is growing rapidly at that age), mimicking the signs of a brain tumor. Tooth growth may also be abnormal, because vitamin A is needed to lay the foundation for enamel.[6]

Vitamin A deficiency is the major cause of childhood blindness in the world, destroying the vision of a quarter of a million preschool children each year in Asia alone. Most likely, the problem is just as great in Africa. More than 5 million children worldwide endure less severe forms of vitamin A deficiency and suffer growth retardation and increased infections.

Vitamin A Toxicity

Vitamin A toxicity occurs when all the binding proteins for vitamin A are swamped, and free vitamin A attacks the cells. Such effects are not likely if you depend on a balanced diet for your nutrients, but if you take supplements containing the vitamin, toxicity is a real possibility. Toxicity symptoms (see Table 9–1) are likely only when excess amounts of the preformed vitamin from animal foods or supplements are taken. The precursor beta-carotene, which is available from plant foods, is not converted to vitamin A efficiently enough in the body to cause toxicity, but is instead stored in fat depots as carotene. Being yellow in color, beta-carotene may accumulate under the skin to such an extent that the overdoser actually turns yellow (hypercarotenemia).

Overdoses of vitamin A have serious effects on the same body systems that exhibit symptoms in vitamin A deficiency (see Table 9–1). Children are most

preformed vitamin A: vitamin A in its active form.

vitamin A precursor: a compound that can be converted into active vitamin A. Another name for vitamin precursors is **provitamins**.

■ **FIGURE 9–6**
Follicular Hyperkeratosis
In vitamin A deficiency, the epithelial surface hardens with keratin in a process known as *keratinization*. (In the GI tract, this doesn't occur, but mucus-producing cells dwindle, and mucus production declines.) The progression of this condition to the extreme is *hyperkeratinization* or *hyperkeratosis*. When keratin accumulates around each hair follicle it is known as *follicular hyperkeratosis*.

likely to be affected, because they need less, they are smaller and more sensitive to overdoses, and it is easy to give them too much in pill form or in other concentrates. The availability of breakfast cereals, instant meals, fortified milk, and chewable candylike vitamins—each containing 100 percent or more of the recommended daily intake of vitamin A—makes it possible for a well-meaning parent to provide several times the daily allowance of the vitamin to a child in a few hours. Serious toxicity is seen in small infants when they are given more than ten times the recommended amount every day for weeks at a time. A child may also overdose, liking vitamin pills and thinking of them as candy.

Neither deficiency nor toxicity symptoms appear over a wide range of vitamin A intakes (see Figure 9–7). Recommended intakes in both the United States and Canada are set at about double the minimum necessary to prevent deficiency. Doubtless, many people need not consume amounts this high. The exact upper limit of safety cannot be determined, because people's tolerances to overdoses vary. The National Nutrition Consortium advises that adults should avoid intakes of more than five to ten times the recommended amounts to ensure safety.

Adolescents should be warned that massive doses of vitamin A taken internally will have no beneficial effect on acne, but they may cause the miseries itemized in Table 9–1. The belief that vitamin A cures acne arises from the knowledge that it is needed for the health of the skin. As with all nutrients, however, the vitamin promotes health when enough is supplied; more than enough has no further beneficial effects and can actually be harmful.

The acne medicine Accutane is made from vitamin A but is chemically different from over-the-counter vitamin A. Taken orally, Accutane is effective against the deep lesions of cystic acne. It is highly toxic, especially during growth, and causes serious birth defects in the infants of women who have

■ **FIGURE 9–7**

Vitamin A Deficiency and Toxicity
As the dose increases from zero, normalcy is reached. A range of intakes is safe, and then toxicity is reached. For reference, 100 μg/kg body weight would equal about 7,000 RE for a 150-lb person.

Source: Adapted from J. Hathcock, Vitamin safety: A current appraisal, *Vitamin Issues* 5 (1985): 4 (Figure 1).

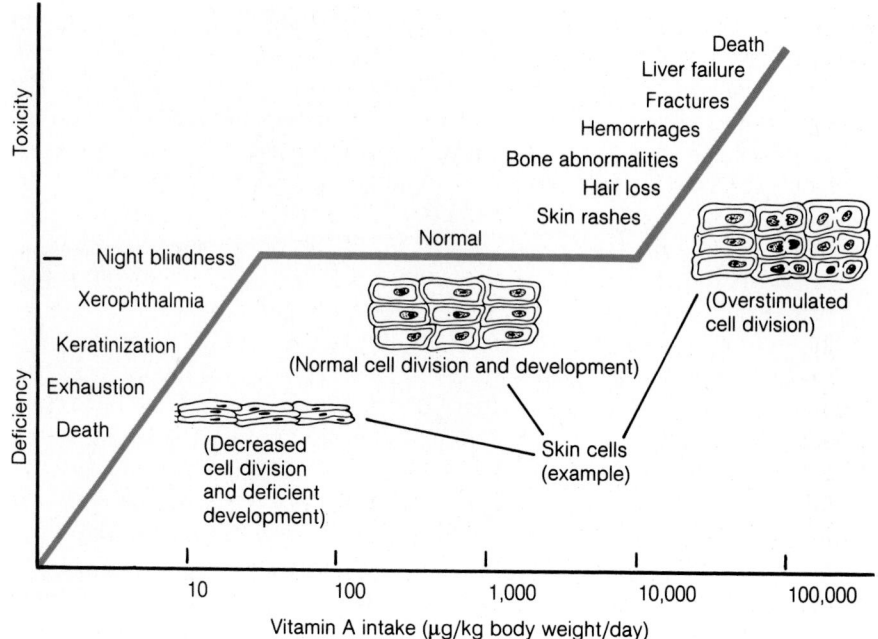

taken it during their pregnancies. For this reason, dermatologists prescribe Accutane with caution, and the label advises women to use an effective form of contraception beginning at least one month before the start, and continuing until one month after the end, of Accutane's use.

Another vitamin A relative, Retin-A, fights acne and the wrinkles of aging. Applied topically, this ointment reduces wrinkles and softens skin. The skin is particularly sensitive during the period of treatments. It becomes red and tender, and it peels. Questions remaining to be answered include, What are its long-term toxicity effects? How does it work? What is the minimum effective dose? How long will the benefits last?

Beta-carotene may play a preventive role with respect to cancer, as explained in Chapter 30. Retinol itself has not proven to be effective, but this doesn't stop gullible people from taking massive doses of vitamin A in the hope of preventing cancer. Because of this, it is expected that more cases of vitamin A toxicity will be reported in the years to come, but it is hoped that no reader of this book will be among them.[7]

Vitamin A in Foods

As mentioned earlier, vitamin A assumes a number of different forms, and these convert to the active forms in the body. The conversions to active forms take place with different efficiencies. In animal foods, vitamin A occurs as preformed vitamin A (retinol). In plant foods, no biologically active, preformed vitamin A occurs, but many contain beta-carotene, which produces vitamin A with low efficiency.

The active form of vitamin A used for reference is retinol, and the recommended amounts of vitamin A are stated in terms of retinol equivalents

RE (retinol equivalent): a measure of vitamin A activity; the amount of retinol that a vitamin A compound will yield after conversion in the body. 1 RE corresponds to the biological activity of 1 μg of retinol, 6 μg of beta-carotene, or 12 μg of other carotenes.

(RE). Both U.S. and Canadian authorities use this terminology and make the same dietary recommendation.

The amounts of vitamin A found in *foods*, however, are often still reported using an older system of measurement, international units (IU), which are based on some assumptions now known to be inaccurate. In the future, tables of food composition will report the vitamin A activity of foods in RE. Until they do, you have to do some computing if you wish to use a table of food values expressed in IU to estimate your vitamin A intake. You have to remember both terms, RE and IU, and that 1 RE is roughly equivalent to 3.33 IU of vitamin A from animal tissues or 10 IU from plant tissues.[8] This book's "Table of Food Composition" (Appendix H) presents vitamin A in RE.

To make matters still more difficult, researchers use still another unit for vitamin values when they are measured in the body, the SI. People who work in clinical laboratories are familiar with and use these units, and this book refers to them in tables presented in later chapters when discussing disease conditions.

Table 9–2 shows the vitamin A activity of various kinds of foods. The abundance of green and purple bars in the table shows vegetables and fruits to be the richest in vitamin A activity. Most foods with vitamin A activity are brightly colored—green, yellow, orange, and red. Any plant food with significant vitamin A activity must have some color, since carotene is a rich, deep yellow (almost orange) compound. The dark green, leafy vegetables contain abundant amounts of the green pigment chlorophyll, which masks the carotene in them. An attractive meal includes foods of different colors that complement one another; such a meal probably ensures a good supply of vitamin A as well.

On the other hand, a food with a yellow or orange color does not invariably provide vitamin A activity. Many of the compounds that give foods their colors, such as the yellow and red xanthophylls, are unrelated to vitamin A and have no nutritional value. Red peppers, for example, are not noted for their vitamin A activity, nor are the yellower variety of sweet potatoes, although their skins have the same orange color as the deep orange, carotene-rich sweet potatoes.

On the third hand (this chapter has three hands), if a plant food is white or colorless, you can be sure it possesses little or no vitamin A activity. Potatoes, pasta, rice, and other colorless foods are in this category.

About half of the vitamin A activity in foods consumed in the United States comes from vegetables and fruits, and half of this comes from the dark leafy greens (like spinach—not celery or cabbage) and the rich yellow or deep orange vegetables (such as winter squash, cantaloupe, carrots, and sweet potatoes—not corn or bananas). The other half of the vitamin A activity comes from milk, cheese, butter, and other dairy products; eggs; and liver. Since vitamin A is fat soluble, it is lost when milk is skimmed. To compensate, nonfat milk is often fortified so as to supply about 40 percent of the RDA per quart.** Margarine is usually fortified so as to provide the same amount of vitamin A as butter.

Vitamin A RDA and Canadian RNI: 1,000 μg RE/day (men); 800 μg RE/day (women).

IU (international unit): a measure of vitamin activity, determined by such biological methods as feeding a given compound to vitamin-deprived animals and measuring the number of units of growth produced. This system was used to measure vitamin A before chemical analysis of the vitamin A compounds and their precursors was possible.

1 RE = 3.33 IU (retinol from animal foods).
= 10.00 IU (beta-carotene from plant foods).
= 5.00 IU (on the average).

SI units (standard international units): a uniform system of reporting laboratory data.*

vitamin A activity: a term useful for referring to both the preformed vitamin A and carotene contents of foods, without having to distinguish between them.

chlorophyll: the green pigment of plants, which absorbs photons and transfers their energy to other molecules, initiating photosynthesis.

xanthophylls (ZAN-tho-fills): pigments found in plants responsible for the color changes seen in autumn leaves.

Recall that folate, too, is found most abundantly in dark green vegetables.

---

*To convert units of retinol (in blood) to SI units, use the factor 1 μg/dL retinol = 0.03491 μmol/L. The complete SI table has been published in *Annals of Internal Medicine* 106 (1987): 114–129; reprints are available.

**Fortification of milk in Canada follows a similar standard. Milks and margarines in Canada and the United States may also be fortified with vitamin D; read the label to find out.

■ **TABLE 9–2**
Vitamin A in Commonly Eaten Foods Ranked Richest to Poorest

Food, Serving Size (Energy)

Beef liver, 3 oz fried (185 kcal)
Sweet potato, 1 baked (118 kcal)
Carrot, 1 whole fresh (31 kcal)
Spinach, 1 c canned (50 kcal)
Spinach, 1 c fresh cooked (41 kcal)
Butternut squash, 1 c baked (83 kcal)
Dandelion greens, 1 c cooked (35 kcal)
Winter squash, 1 c baked (96 kcal)
Cantaloupe, ½ (94 kcal)
Mango, 1 fresh (135 kcal)
Turnip greens, 1 c cooked (29 kcal)
Papaya, 1 whole fresh (117 kcal)
Green onions, 1 c chopped (26 kcal)
Bok choy, 1 c cooked (20 kcal)
Mustards greens, 1 c cooked (21 kcal)
Tomatoes, 1 c cooked (60 kcal)
Parsley, 1 c chopped fresh (20 kcal)
Apricots, 3 fresh pitted (51 kcal)
Apricot halves, 10 dried (83 kcal)
Oysters, 1 c raw (160 kcal)
Broccoli, 1 c cooked (46 kcal)
Watermelon, 1 slice (152 kcal)
Kefir, 1 c (160 kcal)
Asparagus, 1 c cooked (44 kcal)
Milk or yogurt, 1 c nonfat (86 kcal)
Romaine lettuce, 1 c chopped (9 kcal)
Tomatoes, 1 c whole canned (47 kcal)
Tomato, 1 whole raw (24 kcal)
Loose-leaf lettuce, 1 c (10 kcal)
Cheddar cheese, 1 oz (114 kcal)
Green beans, 1 c cooked (44 kcal)
Egg, 1 poached (79 kcal)
Milk, 1 c whole (150 kcal)
Sole/flounder, 3 oz baked (120 kcal)
Summer squash, 1 c cooked (36 kcal)
Peach, 1 fresh medium (37 kcal)
Zucchini, 1 c cooked (29 kcal)
Green pepper, 1 whole (18 kcal)
Butter, 1 pat (34 kcal)
Pink/red grapefruit, ½ (37 kcal)
Orange, 1 fresh medium (60 kcal)
Apple, 1 fresh medium (80 kcal)
Chicken breast, ½ roasted (142 kcal)
Celery, 1 large outer stalk (6 kcal)
Sirloin steak, 3 oz lean (180 kcal)
Oatmeal, 1 c cooked (145 kcal)
Kidney beans, 1 c canned (230 kcal)
White grapefruit, ½ (39 kcal)
Brewer's yeast, 1 tbsp (25 kcal)
Whole-wheat bread, 1 slice (70 kcal)
Peanuts, 1 oz dried unsalted (161 kcal)

U.S. RDA = 1,000 RE

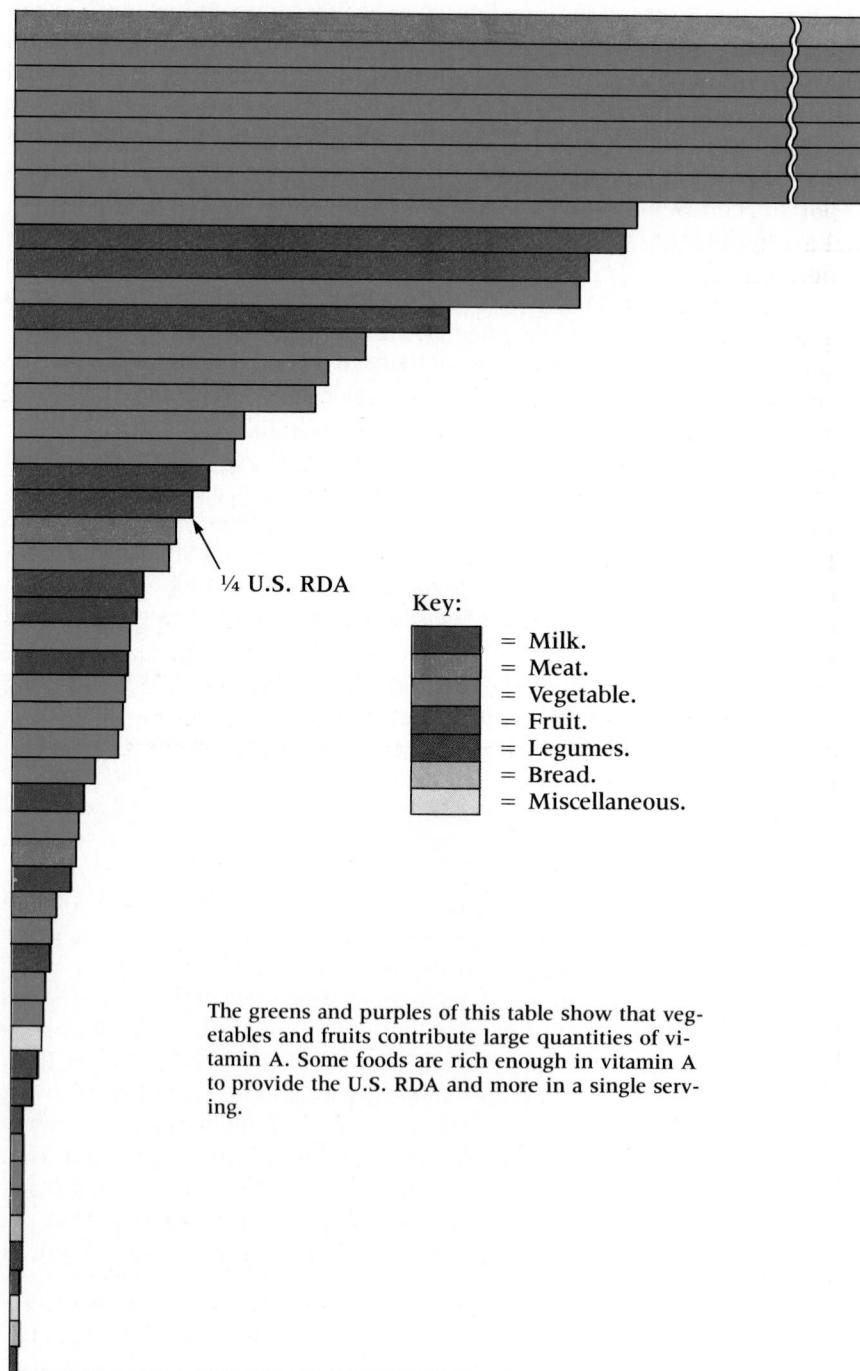

¼ U.S. RDA

Key:

= Milk.
= Meat.
= Vegetable.
= Fruit.
= Legumes.
= Bread.
= Miscellaneous.

The greens and purples of this table show that vegetables and fruits contribute large quantities of vitamin A. Some foods are rich enough in vitamin A to provide the U.S. RDA and more in a single serving.

RE/Serving

The safest and easiest way to meet your vitamin A needs, then, is to consume generous servings of a variety of dark green and deep orange vegetables and fruits. A 1-cup serving of carrots, sweet potatoes, or dark greens such as spinach would provide such liberal amounts of carotenoids that even allowing for inefficient absorption and conversion, intake would be sufficient. Alternatively, a diet including more or larger servings of medium sources would ensure an ample intake. No doubt you can find food sources of the vitamin that appeal to you and can easily calculate the minimum amounts you should eat to meet your needs.

The fruit and vegetable family is, of course, one of the four food groups. Its importance for meeting vitamin A needs is reflected in the recommendation that adults have at least four servings a day, including at least one dark green or deep orange item every other day.

Fast foods are notable for their *lack* of vitamin A. Anyone who dines frequently on hamburgers, french fries, shakes, and the like is advised to emphasize vegetables heavily—and not just salads—at other meals.

One animal food notable for its vitamin A content is liver. A moment's reflection should reveal the reason for this. Vitamin A not needed for immediate use is stored in the liver.* Some nutritionists recommend that people include a serving of liver in their diets every week or two, partly for this reason.

People sometimes wonder if vitamin A toxicity can result from eating liver too frequently. This problem has been observed in the Arctic, where explorers who have eaten large quantities of polar bear liver have become ill with symptoms suggesting vitamin A toxicity. Closer to home, vitamin A toxicity symptoms have been reported in children who had been eating chicken liver spread several times a week for weeks on end.[9] Liver offers many nutrients, and its periodic intake may serve a person well, but moderation is an important key to a healthy diet.

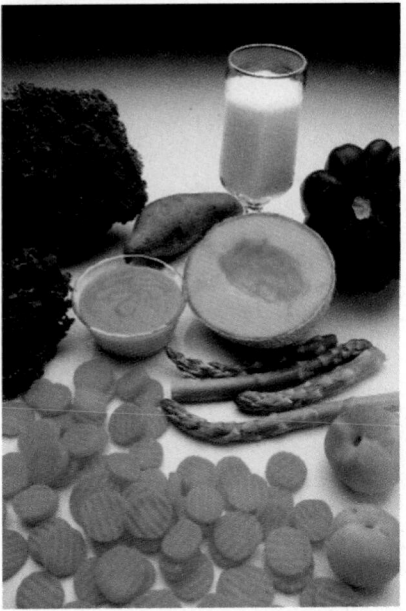

Foods rich in vitamin A add color to a meal.

Vitamin D

Vitamin D is different from all the other nutrients in that the body can synthesize it with the help of sunlight. Therefore, in a sense, vitamin D is not an essential nutrient. Given enough sun, you need consume no vitamin D at all in the foods you eat. Rather, it is like a hormone—a compound manufactured by one organ of the body that has effects on another. Like certain hormones, it can actually enter a cell, cross the nuclear membrane, attach to specific receptors on the DNA or its protein wrapping, and promote the synthesis of specific proteins.

Figure 9–8 diagrams the synthesis of vitamin D from its precursor (a relative of cholesterol) to its active form. Ultraviolet rays from the sun, hitting the precursor, convert it to previtamin D_3, which works its way back into the

The precursor of vitamin D made in the liver is 7-dehydrocholesterol, which is made from cholesterol (see Figure 5–10 on p. 115 and Appendix C). This is one of the body's many "good" uses for cholesterol.

---

*Liver is not the only organ that stores vitamin A. The kidneys, adrenals, and other organs do, too, but liver is the only one commonly eaten.

> ### ≫ NUTRITION DETECTIVE WORK
>
> The report of children's receiving too much vitamin A from eating chicken liver spread is a case history. A case history is a well-documented study of one case, reported in a reliable medical or scientific journal.
>
> In this case, three siblings regularly ate a chicken liver spread that provided them with a daily average of up to three times their recommended intake of vitamin A. One of the little boys developed symptoms of a vitamin A toxicity that eventually led to his death. His younger brother also showed signs of toxicity and was given a vitamin A–restricted diet. Their older sister remained healthy. Researchers speculate that genetic differences accounted for the differences in the children's tolerances to vitamin A.
>
> What can we learn from case histories? Each case, like a drop in the ocean, may contribute slightly to the whole, but does not describe the whole. Quite often, case histories describe the unusual, not the norm. This case provides the rare exception to the rule that vitamin A toxicity cannot occur from dietary intake alone. That is the drop it has contributed to the ocean of vitamin A research. For the rest of us, vitamin A toxicity is probably only a threat when we take supplements, but a message from this research rings clear: exercise moderation in vitamin A intake, as in all things.
>
> Sometimes several case histories tell the same story and when taken together provide a valuable lesson. As case histories of vitamin toxicities accumulate, they will help to define the upper limits of tolerance.

interior of the body. Slowly, then, over the next 36 hours, the previtamin is converted, with the help of the body's heat, to vitamin D_3. Two more steps occur before the vitamin becomes fully active. First, the liver adds an OH group, and then the kidney adds another OH group at specific locations to produce the active vitamin. (This is why diseases affecting either the liver or

■ **FIGURE 9–8**
Vitamin D Synthesis

NUTRITION DETECTIVE WORK

Vitamin D claims fame primarily for the body's ability to generate it from sunshine and its role in bone mineralization. But vitamin D may be quietly working miracles we have yet to discover. New research suggests that vitamin D may boost resistance to tuberculosis.[10] Observations that fresh air and sunshine seemed to help cure the disease intrigued researchers to look for the link between folk medicine and science. Sure enough, when the white blood cells that fight the tuberculosis-causing bacteria are armed with high concentrations of vitamin D, they can slow or stop the bacterial activity. The amount of vitamin D required to have such an effect is higher than normally found in the blood, but white blood cells can synthesize the vitamin from a precursor commonly found in the blood. Researchers speculate that the presence of the bacteria may actually stimulate such production. Curiously, blacks and Asians have a high susceptibility to tuberculosis and low concentrations of vitamin D in their blood.

This bit of information on vitamin D illustrates how bits and pieces of knowledge overlap, interlock, and in general, contribute to our understanding of nutrition and the body. Perhaps the connection between vitamin D and tuberculosis resistance will not stand up to further research and will be left as a bit of passing interest. Or perhaps additional pieces will join this one in the making of an epic body of work on vitamin D yet to be written.

the kidney exhibit symptoms of vitamin D deficiency.) As Chapter 15 mentions, the synthesis of vitamin D diminishes in later life.

Vitamin D is a member of a large and cooperative bone-making and bone-maintenance team made up of nutrients and other compounds, including vitamin A; vitamin C; the hormones parathormone and calcitonin; the protein collagen, which underlies and supports bone; and the minerals calcium, phosphorus, magnesium, and fluoride, which compose the inorganic part of bone. The special function of vitamin D is to promote normal bone mineralization. Its action helps to make calcium and phosphorus available in the blood that bathes the bones, to be deposited as the bones harden (mineralize).

Vitamin D raises blood concentrations of these minerals in three ways: by stimulating their absorption from the GI tract, by helping to withdraw calcium from bones into the blood, and by stimulating calcium retention by the kidneys. The star of the show is calcium itself; vitamin D is a director. A description of how calcium moves from food into the blood and into and out of bone is reserved for Chapter 10, where a closer view of the whole system is provided. The object here is to make you aware of the importance of vitamin D, the risks of deficiency and toxicity, and the ways in which the vitamin can be obtained.

The technical name for the final product, active vitamin D, is 1,25-dihydroxycholecalciferol.

Parathormone (also called parathyroid hormone) and calcitonin are described in Chapter 10.

Collagen: see p. 149.

mineralization: the process in which calcium, phosphorus, and other minerals crystallize on the collagen matrix of a growing bone, hardening the bone.

Vitamin D Deficiency

Both inadequate and excessive vitamin D intakes take their toll in the United States and Canada, even though the vitamin has been known for decades to be essential for growth and toxic in excess. Worldwide, the vitamin D-deficiency disease rickets still afflicts large numbers of children.

The symptoms of an inadequate intake of vitamin D are those of calcium deficiency, shown in Table 9–3. The bones fail to calcify normally and may be so weak that they become bent when they have to support the body's weight. A child with rickets who is old enough to walk characteristically develops bowed legs, often the most obvious sign of the disease (see Figure 9–9).

Adult rickets, or osteomalacia, occurs most often in women who have low calcium intakes and little exposure to sun, and who go through repeated pregnancies and periods of lactation. The bones of the legs may soften to such an extent that a young woman who is tall and straight at twenty may be condemned by repeated pregnancies to become bent, bowlegged, and stooped before she is thirty.

Any failure to synthesize vitamin D in adequate amounts will set the stage for the mobilization of calcium from the bones and retardation of bone remodeling.[11] This combination leads to a loss of bone mass, which can result in fractures. Chapter 10 describes the many factors that lead to the development of osteoporosis.

Vitamin D Toxicity

Just as vitamin D deficiency depresses calcium absorption and results in low blood calcium levels and abnormal mineralization of bone, an excess of the vitamin does the opposite, as shown in Table 9–3. It increases calcium absorption, causing abnormally high concentrations of the mineral in the blood, and it promotes return of bone calcium into the blood as well. The excess calcium in the blood tends to precipitate in the soft tissue, forming stones. This is especially likely to happen in the kidneys, which concentrate calcium in the effort to excrete it. Calcification or hardening of the blood vessels may also occur and is especially dangerous in the major arteries of the heart and lungs, where it can cause death.

The range of safe intakes of vitamin D is narrower than that of vitamin A. Half the recommended intake is too little, but over a few times the recommended intake may be too much. Intakes of 100 micrograms per day cause high blood calcium levels in infants, and some infants are sensitive to lower doses than this. Intakes of 250 micrograms per day for four months or 5,000 micrograms per day for two weeks cause toxicity in children and, if further prolonged, in adults. The amounts of vitamin D found in foods available in the United States and Canada are well within these limits, but pills containing the vitamin in concentrated form should definitely be kept out of the reach of children and used cautiously by adults.

Vitamin D from Self-Synthesis

The way to meet your vitamin D needs is to synthesize it yourself with the help of sunlight. Some foods contain the preformed vitamin—chiefly animal

rickets: the vitamin D–deficiency disease in children. A rare type of rickets, not caused by vitamin D deficiency, is known as **vitamin D–refractory rickets.**

osteomalacia (os-tee-o-mal-AY-shuh): the vitamin D–deficiency disease in adults; osteomalacia may also occur in calcium deficiency (see Chapter 10).
osteo = bone
mal = bad (soft)

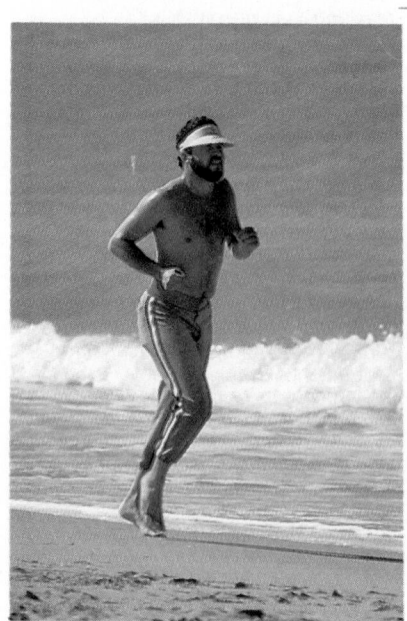

Sunlight promotes vitamin D synthesis in the skin. Exposure to sun should be reasonable; excessive exposure may cause skin cancer.

■ TABLE 9–3
Vitamin D—A Summary

Other Names	Deficiency Disease Names	Toxicity Disease Name
Calciferol, cholecalciferol, dihydroxy vitamin D; precursor is the body's own cholesterol	Rickets, osteomalacia	Hypervitaminosis D

Chief Functions in the Body	Deficiency Symptoms		Toxicity Symptoms
	Bones/Teeth		
Mineralization of bones (raises calcium and phosphorus blood levels by increasing absorption from digestive tract, withdrawing calcium from bones, stimulating retention by kidneys)	**Rickets** Faulty calcification, resulting in misshapen bones (bowing of legs) and retarded growth; enlargement of ends of long bones (knees, wrists); deformities of ribs (bowed, with beads or knobs);[a] delayed closing of fontanel, resulting in rapid enlargement of head (see accompanying figure); slow eruption of teeth; teeth not well formed, with a tendency to decay	**Osteomalacia** Softening effect: deformities of limbs, spine, thorax, and pelvis; demineralization; pain in pelvis, lower back, and legs; bone fractures	Increased calcium withdrawal

Fontanel
A fontanel is the open space in the top of a baby's skull before the bones have grown together. In rickets, closing of the fontanel is delayed.

Posterior fontanel normally closes by the end of the first year

Anterior fontanel normally closes by the end of the second year.

Significant Sources	Deficiency Symptoms		Toxicity Symptoms
	Blood		
Self-synthesis with sunlight; fortified milk, fortified margarine, eggs, liver, fish	Decreased calcium and/or phosphorus	Decreased calcium and/or phosphorus, increased alkaline phosphatase[b]	Increased calcium and phosphorus concentration
		Nervous/Muscular Systems	
	Lax muscles resulting in protrusion of abdomen; muscle spasms	Involuntary twitching, muscle spasms	Loss of appetite, headache, weakness, fatigue, excessive thirst, irritability, apathy
		Excretory System	
	Increased calcium in stools, decreased calcium in urine		Increased excretion of calcium in urine, kidney stones, irreversible renal damage
		Other	
	Abnormally high secretion of parathormone		Calcification of soft tissues (blood vessels, kidneys, heart, lungs, tissues around joints), death

[a]Bowing of the ribs causes the symptom known as *pigeon breast*. The beads that form on the ribs resemble rosary beads; thus this symptom is known as *rachitic* (ra-KIT-ik) *rosary* ("the rosary of rickets").
[b]Alkaline phosphatase is an enzyme in the blood that rises during bone resorption.

■ **FIGURE 9–9**
Rickets
As Table 9–3 points out, rickets affects many areas of the body. The child on the left has the characteristic protruding belly resulting from lax abdominal muscles. The child on the right has the bowed legs commonly seen in rickets.

ergocalciferol: the plant version of cholecalciferol.

Vitamin D activity was previously expressed in international units (IU), but is now expressed in micrograms of cholecalciferol. To convert, use the following factor: 1 IU = 0.025 µg cholecalciferol. For example:
- 100 IU = 2.5 µg.
- 400 IU = 10 µg.

Vitamin D RDA: 5 µg (200 IU)/day. Canadian RNI: 2.5 µg (100 IU)/day; increases to 5 µg/day over age 50.

foods, such as milk, fish, eggs, and liver—but unless they are fortified, they are not likely to meet the RDA. A plant version of vitamin D (ergosterol) may also yield an active compound, vitamin D_2 (ergocalciferol), on irradiation, but again, its contribution to needs is minor.

The recommendation for vitamin D in rapidly growing children is twice as high as that for mature adults. Neither cow's milk nor human breast milk supplies enough vitamin D to meet human needs reliably; hence cow's milk is fortified, and infants are given either fortified formula or supplements. The fortification of milk is the best guarantee that children will meet their vitamin D needs and underscores the importance of milk in children's diets.* The milk-drinking vegetarian is protected (provided the milk is vitamin D fortified, of course), but there is no practical source of vitamin D in plant foods. Without fortification or supplementation, diet alone cannot meet the body's vitamin D needs.

Fortunately, significant amounts of vitamin D can be made with the help of sunlight. It is generally agreed that most adults, especially in sunnier regions, need not make special efforts to obtain vitamin D in food. If children are taken out in the sun for a while each day around noon, they will receive enough light to generate a protective dose of vitamin D. However, people who are not

*Vitamin D fortification of milk in the United States is 10 µg cholecalciferol (400 IU) per quart; in Canada, 360 IU/L.

outdoors much or who live in northern or predominantly cloudy or smoggy areas are advised to make sure their milk is fortified with vitamin D, and to drink at least 2 cups a day.

Darker-skinned people make less vitamin D on limited exposure to the sun. By three hours of exposure, however, vitamin D synthesis in strongly pigmented skin arrives at the same plateau as that at 30 minutes in fair skin. The difference may account for the finding that darker-skinned people in northern, smoggy cities are more prone to rickets. These experiments also suggest that overexposure to sun cannot cause vitamin D toxicity, because synthesis of vitamin D is limited to a fixed maximum amount on each exposure.[12]

Smog filters out ultraviolet rays of the sun.

■ *Vitamin E*

Vitamin E is an antioxidant like vitamin C, but fat soluble. If there is plenty of vitamin E in the membranes of cells exposed to an oxidant, chances are this vitamin will take the brunt of the oxidative attack, protecting the lipids and other vulnerable components of the cell and its membranes. Within the mitochondria of a cell, vitamin E protects a part of the metabolic equipment that transforms energy fuels into ATP. Vitamin E is especially effective in preventing the oxidation of the polyunsaturated fatty acids (PUFA), but it protects all other lipids (for example, vitamin A) as well. Table 9–4 presents

antioxidant: see p. 224.

oxidant: a compound (such as oxygen itself) that oxidizes other compounds.

■ TABLE 9–4
Vitamin E—A Summary

Other Names	Deficiency Symptoms	Toxicity Symptoms
	Blood/Circulatory System	
Alpha-tocopherol, tocopherol, tocotrienol	Red blood cell breakage,[a] anemia	Augments effects of anticlotting medication
	Digestive System	
		General discomfort
Chief Functions in the Body	**Nervous/Muscular Systems**	
Antioxidant (detoxification of strong oxidants), stabilization of cell membranes, regulation of oxidation reactions, protection of PUFA and vitamin A	Degeneration, weakness difficulty walking, severe pain in calf muscles	Headache, weakness, dizziness, fatigue, visual abnormalties
	Other	
	Fibrocystic breast disease	
Significant Sources		
Plant oils (margarine, salad dressings, shortenings), green and leafy vegetables, wheat germ, whole-grain products, liver, egg yolk, nuts, seeds		

[a]The breaking of red blood cells is called *erythrocyte hemolysis.*

a summary of vitamin E's functions, deficiency symptoms, toxicity symptoms, and food sources.

One of the most important places in the body in which vitamin E exerts its antioxidant effect is in the lungs, where the exposure of cells to oxygen is maximal. Several kinds of cells benefit from the vitamin's protection: the red and white blood cells that pass through the lungs, and the cells of the lung tissue itself. The vitamin acts to:

- Detoxify oxidizing radicals that arise as unwanted by-products during normal metabolism.
- Stabilize cell membranes.
- Regulate oxidation reactions.
- Protect vitamin A and PUFA from oxidation.

Lungs are sometimes exposed to air pollutants that are strong oxidizing agents, such as nitrogen dioxide or ozone. Ozone causes peroxidation of the cell membrane lipids, producing a product (pentane) that can be measured in expired air. People exercising in an ozone-contaminated environment breathe out more pentane (an index of peroxidation) than do those exercising in an ozone-free environment. Taking vitamin E supplements for two weeks (about 1,000 IU per day) restores pentane production to normal, suggesting that vitamin E acts as a scavenger of free radicals. Studies using animals found that vitamin E seems to exert a protective effect not only in lungs, but also in liver and adrenal tissue.[13]

Vitamin E protects white blood cells as well as red blood cells, and thus participates in the body's immune defenses. Deficiency of vitamin E suppresses the immune system, and sufficiency benefits it in several species of animals.[14]

Vitamin E Deficiency

Studies related to vitamin E's effects have seldom revealed any carryover of animal findings to human beings. In fact, of 12 possible diseases associated with vitamin E deficiency in animals, only one has been demonstrated in human beings. When the blood concentration of vitamin E falls below a certain critical level, the red blood cells tend to break open (erythrocyte hemolysis) and spill their contents, probably due to oxidation of the PUFA in their membranes. Vitamin E treatment corrects erythrocyte hemolysis.

Claims of Vitamin E Benefits

Many extravagant claims have been made for vitamin E. It has been such a popular "miracle vitamin" that it vies with the snake-oil medicines of past times. But while research has revealed possible roles for vitamin E, it also has shown clearly some things that vitamin E does *not* do. During the 1960s and 1970s, vitamin E was said to improve athletic endurance and skill, to increase potency and enhance sexual performance, to prolong the life of the heart, and to reverse the damage caused by atherosclerosis and even heart attacks. An immense amount of experimentation has discredited these and many similar claims. Vitamin E also does *not* help with:

---

radicals: molecular intermediates that have a single, unpaired electron. Radicals are unstable and arise during oxidation reactions. They are highly reactive and readily attack other molecules with which they come in contact; see Appendix B.

peroxidation: the production of unstable molecules containing more than the usual amount of oxygen. Hydrogen peroxide, H_2O_2, for example, may be produced from water, H_2O. Appendix B explains the chemistry of free-radical formation.

pentane: a product of peroxidation reactions; a compound with the chemical formula C_5H_{12}.
pente = five

scavenger: a cleanup agent; for example, a garbage collector or an animal that feeds on refuse and waste.

Some similar roles are played by an enzyme containing the trace mineral nutrient selenium; see Chapter 11.

The breaking open of red blood cells is **erythrocyte** (eh-REETH-ro-cite) **hemolysis** (he-MOLL-uh-sis), the vitamin E–deficiency disease in human beings.

erythrocyte: red blood cell.
erythro = red
cyte = cell
hemolysis: bursting of red blood cells.
hemo = blood
lysis = breaking

- Lowering high blood lipids, including cholesterol.
- Hot flashes.
- Bladder cancer.
- Preventing scarring after a skin cut or wound.
- Preventing heart attacks.
- Restoring or improving sexual potency.
- Improving athletic ability.

Nor does it prevent or slow processes of aging, such as graying of the hair, wrinkling of the skin, or slowing of body organs' activities.

Another thing vitamin E does *not* do is prevent or cure muscular dystrophy in human beings. In animals, a deficiency of vitamin E produces muscular weakness and atrophy of the muscles. This nutritional muscular dystrophy can be cured by reintroducing vitamin E into the diet. At no time has there been any reliable evidence presented in scientific journals that links this condition to the hereditary muscular dystrophy disease that afflicts children. These children do not benefit from vitamin E treatment and usually die at an early age when their respiratory muscles deteriorate.

muscular dystrophy (DIS-tro-fee): a hereditary disease in which the muscles gradually weaken; its most debilitating effects arise in the lungs.

nutritional muscular dystrophy: a vitamin E–deficiency disease of animals, characterized by gradual paralysis of the muscles.

Vitamin E Toxicity

All kinds of people take vitamin E supplements for all kinds of reasons. As a result, some signs of toxicity are now known or suspected, but toxicity is not as common or its effects as serious as with vitamins A and D. "Possible GI disturbances" are reported in some people who consume more than 600 milligrams a day. High doses may enhance anticoagulant effects of drugs used to oppose unwanted blood clotting; people given anticoagulant therapy, therefore, should not take large amounts of vitamin E.[15]

Vitamin E Intakes and Food Sources

Vitamin E includes two classes of compounds: tocopherols and tocotrienols. The most active compound is alpha-tocopherol. Tocopherols occur in two forms, D and L, of which the D form is more active. Different forms of vitamin E differ in their activity; to reconcile them, the recommended intake is expressed in terms of "the amount of vitamin E activity equivalent to that of 10 milligrams of D-alpha-tocopherol."*

A person's need for vitamin E is higher if the amount of PUFA consumed is higher. Fortunately, vitamin E and PUFA tend to occur together in the same foods.

Vitamin E is widespread in foods. About 60 percent of the vitamin E in the diet comes directly or indirectly from vegetable and seed oils in the form of margarine, salad dressings, and shortenings; another 10 percent comes from fruits and vegetables; smaller percentages come from grains and other products. Soybean oil and wheat germ oil have especially high concentrations

tocopherol (tuh-KOFF-er-all): a kind of alcohol (see Appendix C). D-alpha-tocopherol is one of several forms of tocopherol with vitamin E activity.
tocos = life giving, birth
pherein = to carry

tocotrienol (TOE-koe-try-EEN-ol): less active forms of vitamin E.

D, L: *D* stands for *dextro*, or "right-handed," and *L*, for *levulo*, or "left-handed," referring to the shapes of the molecules, which are mirror images of each other.

Vitamin E RDA: 10 mg/day (men).
8 mg/day (women).
Canadian RNI: 10 mg/day (men, declines with age).
7 mg/day (women, declines with age).

*The RDA is expressed in milligrams of D-alpha-tocopherol equivalents. One milligram equivalent has the biological activity of 1 mg D-alpha-tocopherol. The RNI is expressed in the same units, relative to which beta- and gamma-tocopherol and alpha-tocotrienol have activities of one-half, one-tenth, and one-third the activity, respectively.

NUTRITION DETECTIVE WORK

Researchers conducting either animal and human research must fulfill certain conditions in order to show that the lack of a nutrient is causing a certain symptom. First, they must mix up a test diet that lacks that nutrient, and only that nutrient. Next, they must show that the diet results consistently in the appearance of the deficiency symptom and that when the nutrient is returned to the diet, the deficiency symptom always disappears.

If the researchers are working with animals, they must also take several preparatory steps. First, they must find an animal that does not synthesize the nutrient. For example, they could not conduct research on vitamin C deficiency on rats or dogs, because these animals synthesize their own vitamin C. Guinea pigs cannot synthesize vitamin C, so researchers could use them instead.

In mixing up a laboratory feed that contains all essential nutrients except the one under study, researchers must undertake the time-consuming task of mixing a large number of nutrients in the correct proportions—usually synthetic nutrients, since natural foods would very likely contain traces of the nutrient being excluded. They must be prepared to prove that the mixture is indeed free from the nutrient and that it is not lacking in another essential nutrient. (Alternatively, they might use an antinutrient to bind, inactivate, or compete with the nutrient in question, but then they must distinguish between the effects of the nutrient's lack and the possibility that effects may be due to the antinutrient's presence.)

In addition, researchers must employ animals with a common heredity and maintain them on similar diets for identical periods of time before starting the experiment. For certain nutrients, researchers may also have to fulfill other special conditions. For example, if other work has shown that a nutrient's absorption is under seasonal hormonal control, they will have to design their experiments with this in mind.

When the researchers have produced the deficiency symptom in the laboratory animal and alleviated it with the addition of the missing nutrient, they can make a cautious claim. They can say that in that species they have found the lack of a particular nutrient to cause a particular symptom. After other laboratories have replicated these results, the finding will be accepted,

of vitamin E; corn, cottonseed, and sunflower oils rank second, with a tablespoon of any of these supplying more than half of the RDA of the vitamin. Other oils contain less (for example, peanut oil supplies about half as much per tablespoon). Animal fats such as butter and milk fat have negligible amounts of vitamin E.

Vitamin E is readily destroyed by heat processing and oxidation, so fresh or lightly processed foods are preferable as sources of this vitamin. Processed and convenience foods do not contribute enough vitamin E to ensure an adequate intake.

but only for that species. Many more experiments are required, even to show that this relationship is true for another species of animal.

It is trickier still to apply such findings to human beings. Researchers can cage their experimental animals, thus controlling the feed, fluid, temperature, and most of the other factors in the environment. If necessary, they can continue the experiment until the animals have died, and then perform autopsies to show the effects of the nutrient deficiency on the internal organs.

In research with human beings, researchers cannot control the intakes of food and fluid except in short-term experiments. Nor can they be certain that all subjects are in a similar nutrition state at the start of the experiment. This fact necessitates the use of large numbers of human subjects so that the results can be averaged. Finding a large population hinders the launching of such an experiment and increases the cost. Experimentation on human beings must also depend on subjects who are free to break the restrictions of the diet or to drop out of the experiment at any time, even if they are being paid to be subjects.

In the case of vitamin E research on human beings, several unique obstacles have plagued researchers in addition to these. For one thing, vitamin E is so widely distributed in foods that a diet totally devoid of it is almost impossible to devise. Also, vitamin E is stored in such large quantities in the body that it may take months before a dietary deficiency produces any symptoms.

A way to conduct research on vitamin E deficiency in human beings is to pool results from many case studies, searching for a common thread. It is by these means that vitamin E has been shown to be ineffective in the treatment of such diseases as muscular dystrophy, reproductive failure, and heart disease.

In summary, even when a nutrient deficiency has clearly produced a symptom in several species of laboratory animals, this can only be used as a pointer toward the existence of the same relationship in human beings. Until the deficiency symptom is produced directly in human subjects by a diet deficient in the nutrient and then cured by the restoration of that nutrient, it cannot be concluded that the symptom, in people, results from the lack of that nutrient.

■ *Vitamin K*

Vitamin K seems to act primarily in blood clotting. There, its presence can make the difference between life and death. At least 13 different proteins and the mineral calcium are involved in making a blood clot. Vitamin K is essential for the synthesis of at least four of these proteins, among them

K stands for the Danish word *koagulation* ("coagulation" or "clotting").

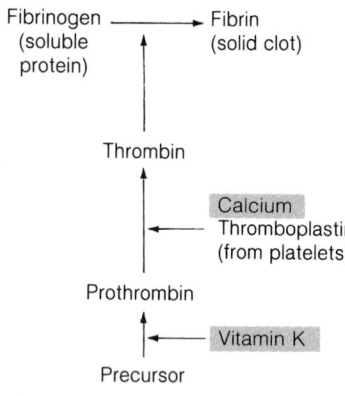

FIGURE 9–10
Blood-clotting Process

Vitamin K RDA:
   1 μg/kg body weight.
   65 μg/day (women).
   80 μg/day (men).

hemorrhagic (hem-o-RAJ-ik) **disease**: the vitamin K–deficiency disease.

hemophilia: a hereditary disease having no relation to vitamin K, but caused by a genetic defect that renders the blood unable to clot because of lack of ability to synthesize certain clotting factors.

sterile: free of microorganisms, such as bacteria.

prothrombin, made by the liver as a precursor of the protein thrombin (see Figure 9–10).

Long known only for its role in blood clotting, vitamin K is now known to have another function. A bone protein requires the presence of vitamin K for its synthesis.[16] Without vitamin K, the bones produce an abnormal protein that cannot bind to the mineral crystal deposits that normally accumulate in bones. The rate of synthesis of this protein is regulated by the more famous bone vitamin—vitamin D.

Vitamin K from Bacterial Synthesis and Foods

Vitamin K can be made within your GI tract—but not by you. In your intestinal tract there are billions of bacteria, which normally live in perfect harmony with you, doing their thing while you do yours. One of their "things" is synthesizing vitamin K that you can absorb and store in your liver. You cannot depend on bacterial synthesis alone for your vitamin K, however. Many foods contain ample amounts of the vitamin, notably liver, green leafy vegetables, and members of the cabbage family. Milk, meats, eggs, cereals, fruits, and vegetables provide smaller, but still significant amounts.

Vitamin K Deficiency and Toxicity

When any of the factors required for coagulation is lacking, blood cannot clot, and hemorrhagic disease results; if an artery or vein is cut or broken under these circumstances, bleeding goes unchecked. (As usual, this is not to say that the cause of hemorrhaging is always vitamin K deficiency. Another cause is hemophilia, which is not curable by vitamin K.) Deficiency of vitamin K may occur under abnormal circumstances when absorption of fat is impaired (that is, when bile production is faulty, or in diarrhea). The vitamin is sometimes administered before operations to reduce bleeding in surgery but is only of value at this time if a vitamin K deficiency exists. (Symptoms of vitamin K deficiency and toxicity, as well as the vitamin's functions and sources, appear in Table 9–5.)

Vitamin K deficiency is seldom seen except when an unusual combination of circumstances conspire to bring it about. When it does occur, however, it can be fatal. The scenario goes like this. A hospital client with marginal vitamin K stores is given antibiotics to prevent or overcome infection and is fed a formula diet that does not include vitamin K. The antibiotics kill intestinal bacteria, and vitamin K stores are depleted. During surgery, the blood fails to clot normally, and the client bleeds to death. The combination of antibiotics, unsupplemented formula diet, and surgery raises a warning flag and requires that clotting time be checked before surgery is performed.[17] People taking sulfa drugs, which destroy intestinal bacteria, may also become deficient in vitamin K.

Newborn babies are commonly susceptible to a vitamin K deficiency, for two reasons. First, a baby is born with a sterile digestive tract; it takes the bacteria weeks to establish themselves in the baby's intestines. Second, a baby may not be fed at the very outset (and vitamin K in breast milk is minimal).

■ TABLE 9–5
Vitamin K—A Summary

Other Names	Deficiency Symptoms	Toxicity Symptoms
Phylloquinone, naphthoquinone	**Blood/Circulatory System**	
Chief Functions in the Body	Hemorrhaging	Interference with anticlotting medication, possible jaundice caused by vitamin K analogues
Synthesis of blood-clotting proteins and a blood protein that regulates blood calcium		
Significant Sources		
Bacterial syntheseis in the digestive tract; liver; green, leafy vegetables, cabbage-type vegetables; milk		

A single dose of vitamin K (usually in a water-soluble form similar but not identical to the natural vitamin) is given at birth to prevent hemorrhagic disease of the newborn.

Sometimes people have to take drugs to oppose blood clotting—for example, when the clotting mechanism is overly active and threatens to block arteries. In such cases, anticoagulant medications are prescribed. Cases are on record in which a person's intake of vitamin K from large amounts of green, leafy vegetables was high enough to oppose the action of a prescribed anticoagulant. A person taking anticlotting drugs should not make major changes in the amounts of greens consumed without warning the physician.

Toxicity is not common but can result when water-soluble substitutes for vitamin K are prescribed, especially to infants or to pregnant women. Toxicity symptoms include red cell hemolysis, jaundice, and brain damage.

The synthetic substitute usually given for vitamin K is **menadione** (men-uh-DYE-own); see Appendix C.

jaundice: yellowing of the skin, due to spillover of bile pigments (**bilirubin**) from the liver into the general circulation (see Chapter 26); also known as **hyperbilirubinemia** (HIGH-per-BILL-eh-roo-bin-EE-me-ah). When these pigments invade the brain, the condition is **kernicterus**.

■ *The Fat-Soluble Vitamins—In Summary*

In summary, the four fat-soluble vitamins play many specific roles in the growth and maintenance of the body. Their presence affects the health and function of the eyes, skin, GI tract, lungs, bones, teeth, nervous system, and blood; consequently, their deficiencies become apparent in these areas as well (review the tables presented earlier for specific symptoms of deficiencies).

Toxicities of the fat-soluble vitamins are also possible, especially when people use supplements. When the body becomes oversaturated with a fat-soluble vitamin, it does not excrete excesses as it does with water-soluble vitamins, but rather, it stores them. Excessive concentrations of the fat-soluble vitamins can lead to symptoms of toxicity.

The roles the fat-soluble vitamins play differ from those of the water-soluble vitamins, and they appear in different foods. Yet, they are just as essential to life, and the need for them underlines the need to obtain a wide variety of nourishing foods daily.

Study Questions

1. List the fat-soluble vitamins. What characteristics do they have in common? How do they differ from the water-soluble vitamins?
2. Summarize the roles of vitamin A and symptoms of its deficiency.
3. What is meant by vitamin precursors? Name the precursors of vitamin A, and tell in what classes of foods they are located. Give examples of foods with high vitamin A activity.
4. What is the chief function of vitamin D? What are the richest sources of this vitamin?
5. What are the chief functions of vitamins E and K in the body? What are the chief symptoms of deficiency of vitamin E? Of vitamin K? What conditions may lead to vitamin K deficiency?

Notes

1. Why vitamin A may fight infections, *Science News* 132 (1987): 46.
2. A. Sommer, J. Katz, and I. Tarwotjo, Increased risk of respiratory disease and diarrhea in children with preexisting mild vitamin A deficiency, *American Journal of Clinical Nutrition* 40 (1984): 1090–1095.
3. K. P. West and coauthors, Vitamin A supplementation and growth: A randomized community trial, *American Journal of Clinical Nutrition* 48 (1988): 1257–1264; Muhilal and coauthors, Vitamin A-fortified monosodium glutamate and health, growth, and survival of children: A controlled field study, *American Journal of Clinical Nutrition* 48 (1988): 1271–1276.
4. A. Sommer and coauthors, Impact of Vitamin A supplementation on childhood mortality: A randomized controlled community trial, *Lancet* 1 (1986): 1169–1173.
5. J. Humphrey, research associate in opthalmology at the Dana Center for Preventive Opthalmology, the Johns Hopkins University, Baltimore, Maryland (personal communication, February 1989).
6. J. H. Shaw and E. A. Sweeney, Oral health, in *Nutritional Support of Medical Practice*, eds. H. A. Schneider, C. E. Anderson, and D. B. Coursin (Philadelphia: Harper & Row, 1983), pp. 517–540.
7. Masked hypervitaminosis A and liver injury, *Nutrition Reviews* 40 (1982): 303–305.
8. J. G. Bieri and M. C. McKenna, Expressing dietary values for fat-soluble vitamins: Changes in concepts and terminology, *American Journal of Clinical Nutrition* 34 (1981): 289–295.
9. T. O. Carpenter and coauthors, Severe hypervitaminosis A in siblings: Evidence of variable tolerance to retinol intake, *Journal of Pediatrics* 111 (1987): 507–512.

10. Study sheds light on TB resistance, *Science News* 133 (1988): 60.

11. M. F. Holick, Vitamin D synthesis by the aging skin, in *Nutrition and Aging*, eds. M. L. Hutchinson and H. N. Munro (New York: Academic Press, 1986), pp. 45–58.

12. M. F. Holick, J. A. MacLaughlin, and S. H. Doppelt, Regulation of cutaneous previtamin D_3 photosynthesis in man: Skin pigment is not an essential regulator, *Science* 211 (1981): 590–593.

13. F. Umeda and coauthors, Inhibitory effect of vitamin E on lipoperoxide formation in rat adrenal gland, *Tohoku Journal of Experimental Medicine* 137 (1982): 369–377.

14. Effect of vitamin E on prostanoid biosynthesis, *Nutrition Reviews* 39 (1981): 317–320.

15. Council on Scientific Affairs, Vitamin preparations as dietary supplements and as therapeutic agents, *Journal of the American Medical Association* 257 (1987): 1929–1936.

16. P. A. Price, Role of vitamin-K-dependent proteins in bone metabolism, *Annual Review of Nutrition* 8 (1988): 565–583.

17. Intestinal microflora, injury and vitamin K deficiency, *Nutrition Reviews* 38 (1980): 341–343.

Vitamin Supplements

Many people are not sure that they meet their nutrient needs using foods alone. Fully half of the population uses nutrient supplements regularly, collectively spending billions of dollars on them each year.[1] Many people take a single daily pill; others take huge quantities of single nutrients. Many are self-prescribed, taken on the advice of friends, television, or books that may or may not be reliable.

This highlight examines several questions related to supplement taking. What are the arguments for taking supplements? What are the arguments against taking them? Should people choose to do so, how should they go about choosing the ones to take?

Arguments for Supplements

Nutrition surveys on the U.S. and Canadian populations do detect deficiencies of protein, vitamins, and minerals. The incidence of these deficiencies is low, but they provide the basis for the argument that people may need to take nutrient supplements. Proponents argue that if deficiency symptoms are seen, then marginal or subclinical deficiencies must also lie undetected—states of unwellness shy of classic, obvious deficiencies. Individuals, although cloaked in fat, may be more or less subtly impaired by nutrient deficiencies. For example,

- Classic signs of the thiamin deficiency disease beriberi don't appear until the sixth week. However, within the first four weeks, as the deficiency develops, loss of appetite and weight, irritability, insomnia, and malaise appear together with a fall in a blood enzyme (transketolase), detectable only by laboratory test.

- No clinical signs of a developing riboflavin deficiency appear until the eighth week, but behavioral symptoms such as lethargy can be detected by the sixth week.
- As vitamin B_6 deficiency develops, clients complain of fatigue and headaches; only later does one see the classic small red blood cells of the anemia characteristic of vitamin B_6 deficiency.

In other words, somewhere between the adequate intake of a nutrient and the development of a physically observable deficiency, there is an in–between area—an area of marginal deficiencies—in which people don't feel well and don't function well. Since physically observable deficiencies are seen in North America, even if they are not very common, there must be people—in fact, more people—in the in-between area, too.

For people who are at risk of marginal deficiencies, supplements may be a rational and beneficial choice. The following adults are on that list:[2]

- People with low energy intakes, such as habitual dieters.*
- The elderly, especially if they are malnourished.
- People who eat bizarre or monotonous diets, such as some food faddists.
- People with illnesses that take away the appetite.*

---

*The taking of supplements by groups tagged with an asterisk is endorsed by D. Heber, W. Mertz, and R. E. Schucker, Food versus pills versus fortified foods, *Dairy Council Digest*, March–April 1987; A. E. Harper, ''Nutrition insurance''—A skeptical view, *Nutrition Forum*, May 1987, pp. 33–37.

- People with illnesses that impair absorption of nutrients—including diseases of the liver, gallbladder, pancreas, and digestive system.*
- People taking medications that interfere with the body's use of specific nutrients (such as INH, mentioned on p. 207).
- People who have diseases, infections, or injuries, or who have undergone surgery resulting in increased metabolic needs.
- Women who are pregnant or lactating, and whose metabolic needs are therefore increased.*
- Vegetarians who exclude all animal-derived foods from their diets.*
- Women who bleed excessively during menstruation.*

Most of these people would benefit from a multivitamin-mineral supplement that supplied approximately the RDA amount of every essential nutrient. Those taking drugs that interfered with specific nutrients would need individual advice. Pregnancy and lactation incur increased needs for iron, calcium, and folate in particular; vegetarians who exclude all animal-derived foods from thier diets need special provisions to meet their needs for vitamin B_{12}, calcium, iron, and zinc; and women who lose much blood during menstruation need iron supplements. Other special cases exist. For example, newborns are routinely given a single dose of vitamin K at birth. Infants may need supplements, depending on whether they are receiving formula or breast milk, and on whether their water is fluoridated (see Chapter 14). The end of this highlight will come back to the question of how to choose a general multivitamin-mineral supplement, but first, there are arguments against doing so.

Arguments against Supplements

One argument states its case not so much against supplements in general as against high-dose supplements. High doses of almost every nutrient pose dangers. People's tolerances for high doses of nutrients vary, just as their thresholds for deficiencies vary. Thus amounts that some can tolerate may not be safe for others, and no one knows who falls into which category.

Toxic overdoses of vitamins and minerals may be more common than we realize. Fruit-flavored, chewable vitamins shaped like cartoon characters entice young children to accept them eagerly, offering the potential to cause poisoning. Iron-containing supplements are especially toxic and must be kept out of reach of children. A mild overdose causes GI distress, nausea, and black diarrhea; severe overdoses result in bloody diarrhea, shock, liver damage, coma, and in some cases, death.

The extent and severity of the problem of supplement toxicity remains unclear. Even an alert health care provider who is on the lookout for nutrient toxicity cases fails to spot them. Only a few recognize the signs of short-term acute toxic doses; no doubt many cases of chronic nutrient toxicity, in which the effects develop more subtly and slowly, go unrecognized.[3] The FDA has been, as of 1987, collecting reports of adverse reactions to overdoses of nutrients from physicians and will report on them in due course. The project is titled the Adverse Reaction Monitoring System.[4] The FDA is also developing a set of safety indexes for nutrients— indexes of the safety of doses higher than the RDA. The safety index for calcium is 10, for example (up to ten times the U.S. RDA is a safe dose for an adult); that for selenium is 5.[5] The FDA monitors supplements and foods similarly; supplements are not considered drugs. Consequently, they do not receive the close regulation that drugs do, nor does FDA require manufacturers to prove their safety or effective-

ness. In view of the hazards supplements present, many authorities believe supplements should be required to bear warning labels.

In light of today's knowledge, it is impossible to say just how much of a nutrient is too much. Assuming, however, that it is best to err on the

---

Miniglossary

at risk: a term used in nutrition to describe people on the verge of developing nutrient deficiencies or toxicities.

bioavailability: absorbability; a term used to refer to the individual differences in nutrients' ease of absorption.

bonemeal: a nutrient supplement made from bone, intended to supply calcium and other bone minerals; also known as **powdered bone**.

desiccated liver: dehydrated liver, a powder sold in health food stores and supposed to contain, in concentrated form, all the nutrients found in liver. Possibly not dangerous, this supplement has no particular nutritional merit, and fresh liver is considerably less expensive.

desiccated = totally dried

garlic oil: an extract of garlic.

granola: a cereal mixed from rolled oats and other grains.

green pills: pills containing dehydrated, crushed vegetable matter. One pill contains nutrients equal to those in one small forkful of fresh vegetables—minus losses incurred in processing. Sixty pills costing $15 deliver vegetable matter worth about $1.50.

kelp: a kind of seaweed used by the Japanese as a foodstuff. Kelp tablets are made from dehydrated kelp.

marginal deficiency: see *subclinical deficiency*.

nutritional yeast: a preparation of yeast cells, often praised for its high nutrient content. Yeast is a concentrated source of B vitamins, as are many other foods. The type of yeast used is brewer's, not baker's, yeast; see items 992 and 993 in Appendix H.

optimal nutrition: the best possible nutrition; distinct from merely adequate nutrition, which characterizes the person who has no overt deficiency signs. This term describes people free of marginal deficiencies, imbalances, and toxicities, and who are not at risk for them.

powdered bone: see *bonemeal*.

safety index: a numerical statement of the safety of high doses of nutrients. A safety index of 5, for example, means that doses up to five times the U.S. RDA are safe.

spirulina: a kind of alga ("blue-green manna") said to contain large amounts of vitamin B_{12} and to suppress appetite. It does neither.

subclinical deficiency (also called a **marginal deficiency**): a nutrient deficiency that has no visible or otherwise detectable symptoms. It is possible for such a deficiency to develop, but the term is often used as a scare tactic to persuade consumers to buy nutrient supplements they don't need.

supplement: a preparation (such as a pill, powder, or liquid) containing nutrients; not a food. Breakfast cereals that contain "100 percent of the U.S. RDA" for certain nutrients are defined by law as dietary supplements, not foods.

wheat germ: the oily embryo of the wheat kernel, rich in nutrients.

■ TABLE H9–1
Vitamin and Mineral Doses for Supplements

Substance	Safe Dose (FDA, RDA)	
	Prevention	Treatment of Deficiency
Vitamins		
Vitamin A (IU)	1,250 to 2,500	5 to 10,000
Vitamin D (IU)	400 (up to age 18)	Do not use[a]
	200 (adults)	
Vitamin E (mg)	50	300
Thiamin (mg)	1 to 2	5 to 25
Riboflavin (mg)	1 to 2	5 to 25
Niacin	10 to 20	25 to 50
(as niacinamide, mg)		
Vitamin B_6 (mg)	1.5 to 2.5	7.5 to 25
Folate (mg)	0.1 to 0.4	Do not use[a]
	1.0 (pregnancy, lactation)	
Vitamin B_{12} (μg)	3 to 10	Do not use[a]
Pantothenic acid (mg)	Not recommended in supplement form	
Biotin (mg)	Not recommended in supplement form	
Vitamin C (mg)	50 to 100	300 to 500
Minerals		
Calcium (mg)	400 to 800	Do not use[a]
Phosphorus (mg)	No need to supplement	
Magnesium (mg)	No need to supplement	
Iron (mg)	10 to 30 (women)	Do not use[a]
	30 to 60 (pregnancy, lactation)	
Zinc (mg)	10 to 25 (adults)	Do not use[a]
	25 (pregnancy, lactation)	
Iodine (mg)	Iodized table salt is the accepted way to supplement dietary iodine in the United States	

[a]The FDA and the Committee on Dietary Allowances do not recommend that these nutrients be used to attempt to correct deficiencies, because deficiencies often arise from nonnutritional causes such as disease or interference by drugs. In these cases, the underlying causes of the deficiencies must be correctly diagnosed and treated; supplements may mask, but will not correct, the problems.

Source: Parts adapted from A. Hecht, Vitamins over the counter: Take only when needed, *FDA Consumer*, April 1979, pp. 17–19.

conservative side, Table H9–1 presents upper limits for vitamin and mineral doses to be obtained from supplements.

Another argument against the use of supplements is that no one knows exactly how to formulate the "ideal" supplement. What nutrients should be included? How much of each? On whose needs should the choices be based? How should an individual choose a supplement, since no individual's needs are exactly like anyone else's?

Another argument against supplements is that they may lull the taker into a false sense of security. A person might eat irresponsibly, thinking, "My supplement will cover my needs." Or, experiencing the warning sign of a disease, a person might postpone seeking a diagnosis, thinking, "I probably need a nutrient supplement to make this go away." Such self-diagnosis is always dangerous.

Other invalid reasons why people may take supplements include:

- Their feeling of insecurity about the nutrient content of the food supply.
- Their desire for additional energy or strength.
- Their belief that extra vitamins and minerals will help them cope with stress.
- Their desire to prevent, treat, or cure symptoms or diseases ranging from the common cold to cancer.

Ironically, though, one study found that supplement users actually eat more nutrient-dense diets than non-supplement users and therefore need the supplements the least.[6] In addition, little relationship exists between the nutrients individuals need and the ones they take in pills.[7]

Another problem is that of bioavailability. In general, the body absorbs nutrients best from foods, in which they are diluted and dispersed among other ingredients that may facilitate their absorption. Taken in pure, concentrated form, the nutrients are more likely to interfere with one another's absorption or with the absorption of the nutrients in foods eaten simultaneously with them. Documentation of these effects is particularly extensive for minerals: zinc hinders copper and calcium absorption, iron hinders zinc absorption, calcium hinders magnesium and iron absorption, and magnesium hinders the absorption of calcium and iron. The same interference takes place when people use foods that are fortified with added minerals; this leaves no recourse other than the use of ordinary whole foods to the consumer who wants the benefits of optimal absorption of nutrients.[8]

In view of all the negatives associated with supplement taking, several professional nutrition societies have joined to issue guidelines indicating that people should ordinarily *not* use them:

Healthy children and adults should obtain adequate nutrient intakes from dietary sources. Meeting nutrient needs by choosing a variety of foods in moderation, rather than by supplementation, reduces the potential risk for both nutrient deficiencies and nutrient excesses. Individual recommendations regarding supplements and diets should come from physicians and registered dietitians . . . .

The Recommended Dietary Allowances represent the best currently available assessment of safe and adequate intakes, and serve as the basis for the U.S. Recommended Daily Allowances shown on many product labels. There are no demonstrated benefits of self-supplementation beyond these allowances.[9]

The societies agree that supplement use may be warranted only in the instances marked with an asterisk in the list presented earlier. They urge that whenever a person's diet is reviewed and found to be inadequate, the action to take is not to begin supplementation, but to improve the person's food choices and eating patterns.[10]

From the perspective of the experts, then, it seems that supplementation is not the wisest course for most people. Still, when a supplement is needed, some pointers can assist in its selection.

Selection of Supplements

People often think in terms of "vitamin pills." However, when you go looking for an all-purpose supplement, remember that if you need vitamins, you will need minerals, too. A single, balanced vitamin-mineral supplement should do the job.[11]

If you decide to take a vitamin-mineral supplement, you may find yourself bewildered in front of a drugstore counter, reading the clever, and usually deceptive, ads on labels—"For vitality!" "Infants only!" "For those with active lives!" "What you need for stress!" or "Be more fun, sexier, smarter, and more healthy!"—the key to each quality to be found, of course, in *that* particular supplement. The first step in escaping the clutches of the health hustlers is to imagine that you have a bottle of

white paint and can simply white out the picture of the sexy people on the beach and the meaningless, glittering generalities like "new and improved." After you have whited out the label claims, all you have left is the list of ingredients, what form they are in, and the price. Here's where the truth lies, and from here you can make a rational decision based on facts.

You have two basic questions to answer. The first question: What form do you want—chewable, liquid, or pills? If you'd rather drink your vitamins and minerals than chew them, fine. (Remember, you whited out *infant* on the labels, so now those bottles are just liquid supplements.) The second question: What vitamins and minerals do *you* need? The RDA table (on the inside front cover, left) and the table for Canadians (Appendix I) are the standards appropriate for virtually all reasonably healthy people (if you aren't healthy, see your health care provider).

Generally, most people who need a supplement should choose one that provides all the RDA nutrients in amounts smaller than, equal to, or very close to the RDA. Avoid taking supplements that, in a daily dose, provide more than the RDA of any vitamin or mineral.[12] Other warnings:

- Avoid preparations with high iron concentrations (say, more than 10 milligrams per dose) except for menstruating women. People who menstruate need more iron, but people who don't, don't. Iron is hard to get rid of once it's in the body, so an excess of iron can cause problems, just as a deficiency can (Chapter 11).
- Avoid "organic" or "natural" preparations. They are no better than standard pharmacy types. The word *synthetic* may sound like "fake," but to synthesize just means to put together. The synthetic supplement is identical in every way to the vitamins that are synthesized by plants and animals. Your body can't tell the difference, but your wallet can.

- Avoid products that make "high potency" claims. More is not better. If a supplement covers your RDA, it's more than enough. You're eating foods, too, after all, so you're getting well over RDA amounts of vitamins and minerals.
- Avoid megadoses unless they are prescribed by a knowledgeable physician. Nutrients can build up and cause unexpected problems. (For example, a man who takes vitamins and begins to lose his hair may think it means he needs *more* vitamins, when in fact hair loss may be an early sign of vitamin A overdose.)
- Avoid preparations that contain items not needed in human nutrition, such as choline and inositol. It's not that these particular items will harm you, but they reveal a marketing strategy that makes the whole mix suspect. The manufacturer may want you to believe that its brand of pills contains the latest "new" nutrient that the takers of all other brands will miss out on, but in fact, for every valid discovery of this kind these days, there are "999,999" frauds.
- Avoid geriatric "tonics." They are generally poor in vitamins and minerals, and yet so high in alcohol as to threaten inebriation. The liquids designed for infants are more complete.

When shopping for supplements, remember that local or store brands may be just as good as the nationally advertised supplements. If they are less expensive, it is not because they are inferior, but because the price does not have to cover the cost of national advertising. (One full-page color ad in a national magazine costs upwards of $60,000.)

Steer clear of doses that are too high. Think of the original Stone Age person, who had to depend only on foods for life and health. If the foods available to Stone Age people *could* have supplied the amount of a nutrient being advocated by a supplement manufacturer today, then perhaps it is not unsafe for us, their descendants, to ingest that amount ourselves.

By this standard, the doses some people take are clearly excessive. To obtain 840 milligrams of vitamin E from its best food source, wheat germ, for example, you would have to eat 15 pounds of wheat germ—yet some people take supplements containing more than 840 milligrams of vitamin E every day. To obtain 5 grams of vitamin C, you would have to eat 19 pounds of oranges, yet some people consume more than that much vitamin C daily from supplements.

Our ancestors survived for centuries without nutrient supplements and arrived successfully at the point of producing us. On this basis alone, it can be argued that we must need no more vitamins or minerals than what *we* can obtain from food. That much, but not more, would be reasonable to look for in a supplement.

But, come to think of it, if all the nutrients we need can come from food, why not just get them from food? Foods have so much more to recommend them than do supplements. Nutrients in foods come in an infinite variety of combinations with a multitude of different carriers, absorption facilitators, antioxidation protectors, and other benefits. They come with water, fiber, and a host of beneficial and interesting nonnutrients. They come with kcalories. (You have to eat some kcalories each day; why not ask nutritious foods to deliver them?) They offer pleasing mouth sensations, satiety, and opportunities for socializing while eating. In no way can nutrient supplements hold a candle to foods as a means of meeting human health needs.

NOTES

1. $2.9 billion for vitamins, *FDA Consumer,* April 1987, p. 4.

2. D. Heber, W. Mertz, and R. E. Schucker, Food versus pills versus fortified foods, *Dairy Council Digest,* March–April 1987; A. E. Harper, ''Nutrition insurance''—A skeptical view, *Nutrition Forum,* May 1987, pp. 33–37.

3. Nutrient toxicity, a special report, *Nutrition Reviews* 39 (1981): 249–256.

4. Heber, Mertz, and Schucker, 1987.

5. Heber, Mertz, and Schucker, 1987.

6. N. Kurinij, M. A. Klebanoff, and B. I. Graubard, Dietary supplement and food intake in women of childbearing age, *Journal of the American Dietetic Association* 86 (1986): 1536–1540.

7. S. J. A. Bowerman and I. Harrell, Nutrient consumption of individuals taking or not taking nutrient supplements, *Journal of the American Dietetic Association* 83 (1983): 298–305.

8. Heber, Mertz, and Schucker, 1987.

9. Heber, Mertz, and Schucker, 1987.

10. Heber, Mertz, and Schucker, 1987.

11. This discussion is adapted with permission from L. K. DeBruyne and S. R. Rolfes, *Selection of Supplements* (a 1987 monograph in the *Nutrition Clinics* Series available from Stickley Publishing Co., 210 Washington Sq., Philadelphia, PA 19106).

12. National Academy of Sciences, *Diet and Health: Implications for Reducing Chronic Disease Risk,* as partially reprinted verbatim in National Academy of Sciences Report on Diet and Health, *Nutrition Reviews* 47 (1989): 142–149.

Water and the Major Minerals

The mineral phosphorus abounds in DNA. The tremendous, orderly tangle shown here is part of a chromosome consisting of long loops of DNA.

The ocean—a fluid that nourishes cells.

Salt does not refer only to sodium chloride but also to other ionic compounds, as defined later.

It was assuredly not chance that led Thales to found philosophy and science with the assertion that water is the origin of all things.—Lawrence J. Henderson

ECF has ↑ Na⁺ & Chloride

ICF has ↑ K⁺ & Phosphate

intracellular fluid: fluid within the cells, usually high in potassium and phosphate concentrations.
  intra = within

interstitial fluid: fluid between the cells, usually high in sodium and chloride concentrations; also called **extracellular fluid** (fluid outside the cells).

The body's water cannot be considered separately from the minerals dissolved in it. One can drink pure water, but in the body, that water mingles with minerals to become fluids in which all life processes take place. This chapter begins by discussing water and the minerals that give the body fluids their character; then it considers some other properties of major mineral nutrients.

The body fluids provide the medium in which all of the cells' chemical reactions take place: the fluids participate in many of these reactions and supply the means for transporting vital materials to cells and carrying waste products away from them. Every cell is bathed in a fluid of the exact composition that is best for it. Each of these fluids is constantly undergoing loss and replacement of its constituent parts as cells withdraw nutrients and oxygen from it and excrete carbon dioxide and other waste materials into it. Yet the composition of the body fluids in each compartment remains remarkably constant at all times. The lymph and blood, for example, always have high concentrations of sodium and chloride ions and lower concentrations of about eight other major ions. The intracellular fluid always has high potassium and phosphate concentrations and lower concentrations of other ions. These special fluids regulate the functioning of cells; the cells, in turn, regulate the composition and amounts of the fluids. The entire system of cells and fluids remains in a delicate but firmly maintained state of dynamic equilibrium.

The maintenance of this balance is so important that it is credited with our ability and that of other animals to live on land. It is thought that we had single-celled ancestors that depended on the seawater they lived in to provide nutrients and oxygen and to carry away their waste. We have managed, over the course of our 2-billion-year evolutionary history, to internalize the ocean—to continue bathing our cells in a warm, nutritive fluid that keeps them alive. The body fluids' salt contents and temperature are believed to be the same as in the ocean—not as it is now, but as it was at the time when our ancestors emerged onto land. The ocean has since become more salty and cooler, but we still carry the ancient ocean within us.

Water constitutes about 55 to 60 percent of an adult's body weight and a higher percentage of a child's. As for the major minerals, Figure 10–1 shows the amounts found in the body. The major minerals (those to the left of the line in the figure) are discussed in this chapter; the trace minerals (to the right of the line) are discussed in Chapter 11. All of the major minerals strongly influence the body's fluid balances and blood pressure. Individual minerals contribute to the structure of the bones, serve as cofactors to enzymes, assist in nerve impulse transmissions, and perform other roles to be discussed in more detail later.

■ *Water and the Body Fluids*

The body fluids form a river coursing through the arteries, capillaries, and veins, carrying a heavy traffic of nutrients and waste products. Fluids also fill the cells (intracellular fluid) and the spaces between them (interstitial, or extracellular, fluid).

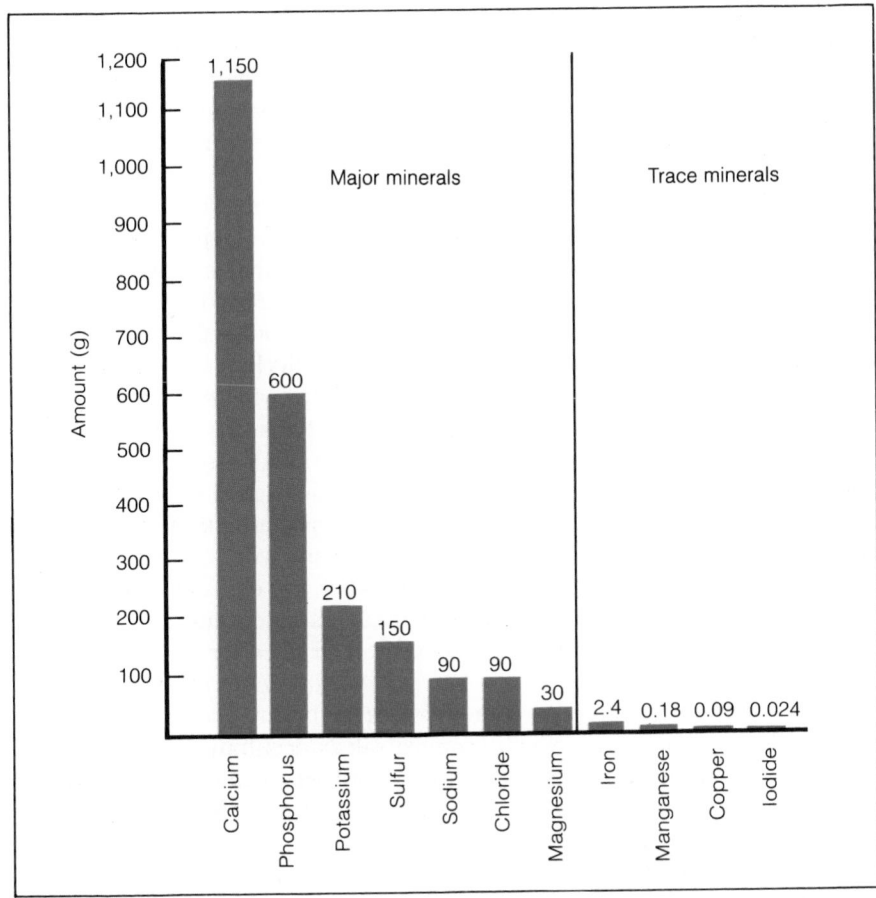

■ FIGURE 10–1
The Amounts of Minerals in a 60-Kilogram Human Body
A line separates the major minerals from the trace minerals. The major minerals are those present in amounts larger than 5 g (a teaspoon). A pound is about 454 g; thus only calcium and phosphorus appear in amounts larger than a pound. There are more than a dozen trace minerals, although only four are shown here.

Water molecules nestle around the body's giant proteins, glycogen, and other macromolecules, helping to form their structure and participating actively in many chemical reactions. In summary, fluids:

- Carry nutrients and waste products throughout the body.
- Fill the cells and the spaces between them.
- Help to form the structure of macromolecules.
- Participate in chemical reactions.

In addition, fluids:

- Serve as the solvent for minerals, vitamins, amino acids, glucose, and a multitude of other small molecules.
- Act as lubricants around joints.
- Serve as shock absorbers inside the eyes, spinal cord, and amniotic sac in pregnancy.
- Aid in the body's temperature regulation.

The total amount of fluid in the body is homeostatically regulated to remain constant, thanks to sensitive balancing mechanisms. Imbalances can occur—dehydration and water intoxication—but the body restores them to normal as promptly as it can.

dehydration: loss of too much fluid from the body.

water intoxication: the condition in which body water contents are too high.

The term **water balance** refers to the balance between water intake and excretion (conceptually similar to *nitrogen balance*).

hypothalamus (high-po-THAL-ah-mus): a brain center that controls activities such as maintenance of water balance and regulation of body temperatures.

Water follows salt and other solutes, moving in the direction of higher osmotic pressure.

ADH (antidiuretic hormone): a hormone released by the pituitary gland in response to high salt concentration in the blood. The kidney responds by reabsorbing water, thus preventing water loss. Another name for ADH is **vasopressin**, a term that refers to blood pressure.
anti = against
di = through
ure = urine
vaso = vessel
press = pressure

The amount of water you have to excrete each day is the **obligatory** water excretion—about a pint.

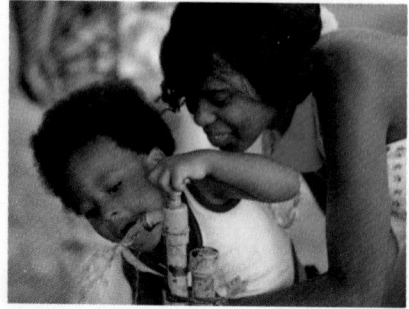

Water is the most vital nutrient.

Water Balance

The body regulates both water intake and excretion. Thirst and satiety govern water intake, apparently sensed by the mouth, hypothalamus, and stomach. When the blood is too concentrated (having lost water, but not salt and other solutes), its solutes attract water out of the salivary glands. The mouth becomes dry as a result, and you drink to wet your mouth. The hypothalamus also monitors the concentration of the blood. When the hypothalamus finds that the blood is too concentrated, it initiates impulses that stimulate drinking behavior. The stomach may also play a role: thirsty animals drink until nerves in their stomachs, known as stretch receptors, are stimulated enough to turn off the drinking. More must be learned about these mechanisms, but it is clear from what we know already that thirst adjusts to provide needed water.

Thirst lags behind water lack. A water deficiency that develops slowly can switch on drinking behavior in time to prevent serious dehydration, but one that develops fast may not. Also, thirst itself does not remedy a water deficiency; you have to notice that you are thirsty, pay attention, and take the time to get a drink. In short, the thirst mechanism works imperfectly. The long-distance runner, the gardener in hot weather, the child busy playing, or the elderly person whose attention wanders can experience serious dehydration; they need to learn to notice consciously their need for water and drink promptly in response to it.

The mechanism of water excretion involves the brain and the kidneys. The cells of the hypothalamus, which monitor salt concentration in the blood, stimulate the pituitary gland to release a hormone, antidiuretic hormone (ADH), whenever the body's salt concentration is too high. ADH stimulates the kidneys to hold back (actually, to reabsorb) water, so that it is recirculated rather than excreted. Thus the more water you need, the less you excrete. This system responds directly to water lack in the brain and promotes water reabsorption by the kidneys.

There are also cells in the kidney itself that respond to a low volume of blood passing through them by releasing a substance.* By a roundabout route, this substance also causes the kidneys to retain more water (see Figure 28−4 in Chapter 28 for more details). Again, the effect is that when more water is needed, less is excreted. This system responds to water lack in the kidneys and promotes sodium retention (and thereby water retention) indirectly.

These renal excretion mechanisms cannot work by themselves to maintain water balance unless you drink enough water. This is because the body must excrete a minimum amount of water each day—the amount necessary to carry away the waste products generated by a day's metabolic activities. Above this amount (a minimum of about 500 milliliters a day—that is, about a pint), the amounts of water you excrete can be adjusted to balance your intake. If you drink more water, the urine merely becomes more dilute. Hence drinking plenty of water is usually a good idea.

In addition to the obvious dietary source, water itself, nearly all foods contain water. In addition, water is generated from the energy nutrients in foods; recall that the carbons and hydrogens in these nutrients combine with oxygen during metabolism to yield carbon dioxide (CO_2) and water (H_2O). Daily water intake

*This substance is the enzyme *renin*. See Figure 28−4 in Chapter 28 for its action leading to the release of *aldosterone*.

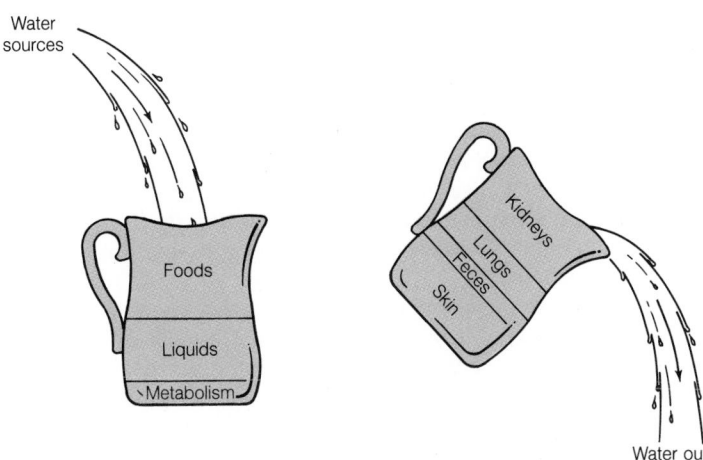

Water Source	Amount (ml)
Liquids	550 to 1,500
Foods	700 to 1,000
Metabolic water	200 to 300
	1,450 to 2,800
Water Output	
Kidneys	500 to 1,400
Lungs	350
Feces	150
Skin	450 to 900
	1,450 to 2,800

from these three sources totals, on the average, about 2½ liters (about 2½ quarts). Similarly, in addition to the water excreted via the kidneys, some water is lost from the lungs as vapor, some in feces, and some from the skin. The losses of all of these also total about 2½ liters a day, on the average. Figure 10–2 shows how intake and excretion naturally balance out.

Fluid and Electrolyte Balance

The body uses electrolytes to help regulate the distribution, composition, and acidity of its fluids. (See the Miniglossary of Electrolyte Terms for definitions of related terms.) This regulation is vital to the life of the cells, for all cells must be continuously bathed in fluid both within and without. Electrolytes are formed when mineral (or other) salts dissolve in water. When salts dissolve, their positive and negative ions separate (dissociate) and move about independently throughout the water. (Pure water conducts electricity poorly, but ions efficiently carry electrical current, hence the term *electrolyte*.) A solution of sodium chloride (NaCl)—common table salt—in water is an electrolyte solution.

The reason why the body uses electrolytes to regulate its fluid balance is that without them, water molecules move freely across cell membranes. Cells have no way to hold onto water molecules directly; these molecules slip through all barriers. However, the cells are able to move electrolytes around, and water follows them, so the cells move water by this indirect means. Informally, we say that "water follows salt."

Many salts, or electrolytes, are important in the body besides sodium chloride. Table 10–1 lists some of the most important electrolytes and reveals that some have a positive charge (cations) and others, a negative charge (anions). Many of the anions are not single atoms, but molecules that bear an overall negative charge. Table 10–1 also reveals that, of the *mineral* ions involved in electrolyte balance, some are found chiefly outside cells (notably sodium and chloride) and some, inside (notably potassium, magnesium, phosphate, and sulfate).

The phrase **fluid and electrolyte balance** refers to the maintenance of the proper concentrations of all of the electrolytes within the body fluids.

- Na = sodium.
- Cl = chloride.

Miniglossary of Electrolyte Terms

anion (AN-eye-un): a negatively charged ion.

cation (CAT-eye-un): a positively charged ion.

dissociation: the physical separation of a compound into ions.

electrolyte: a salt that dissolves in water and dissociates.

electrolyte solution: a solution that can conduct electricity.

ion (EYE-un): an atom or molecule with an electrical charge. For a closer look at ions, see Appendix B.

milliequivalent (**mEq**): the amount of a substance that contains the same number of charges as 1 mg of hydrogen. The number of milliequivalents is a useful measure when considering ions, because the number of charges reveals characteristics about the solution. If two solutions contain the same number of milliequivalents, they contain the same number of charges. To calculate mEq/L, multiply the milligrams per liter by the valence of the chemical and divide by the molecular weight of the substance.

salt: a compound composed of charged atoms or molecules (ions). An example is potassium chloride (K^+Cl^-). Exceptions: a compound in which the cations are H^+ is an acid (example: H^+Cl^-, or hydrochloric acid); a compound in which the anions are OH^- is a base (example: K^+OH^-, or potassium hydroxide).

solutes (SOLL-yutes): the substances that are dissolved in a solution.

■ TABLE 10–1
Important Body Electrolytes

Electrolyte	Extracellular Concentration (mEq/L)	Intracellular Concentration (mEq/L)
Cations		
Sodium (Na^+)	142	10
Potassium (K^+)	5	150
Calcium (Ca^{++})	5	2
Magnesium (Mg^{++})	3	40
	155	202
Anions		
Chloride (Cl^-)	103	2
Bicarbonate (HCO_3^-)	27	10
Phosphate ($HPO_4^=$)	2	103
Sulfate ($SO_4^=$)	1	20
Organic acids (lactate, pyruvate)	6	10
Proteins	16	57
	155	202

Note: This table illustrates the point that the same number of positive and negative charges occur in a given fluid. For example, in extracellular fluid, the numbers of cations and anions both equal 155 milliequivalents per liter (mEq/L). Of the cations, sodium ions make up 142 mEq/L; and potassium, calcium, and magnesium ions make up the remainder. Of the anions, chloride ions number 103 mEq/L; bicarbonate ions number 27; and the rest are provided by phosphate ions, sulfate ions, organic acids, and protein.

■ **FIGURE 10–3**
Water Follows Salt

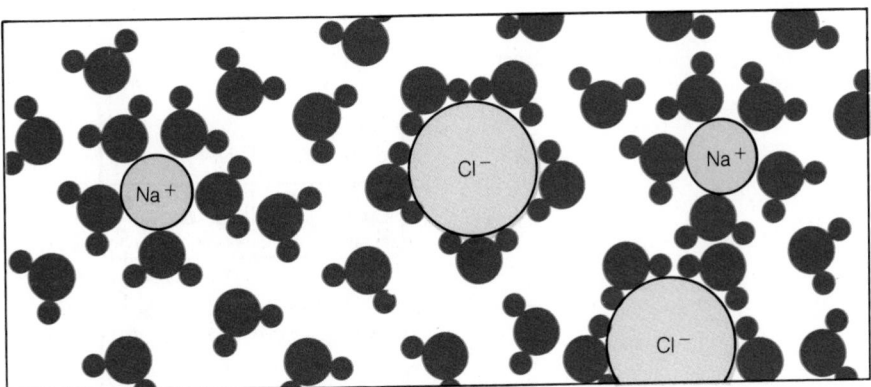

A. Water is polar, because the negatively charged electrons that bond the hydrogens to the oxygen spend most of their time near the large oxygen atom. This results in the oxygen being slightly negative and the hydrogen, slightly positive (see Appendix B).

B. In an electrolyte solution, therefore, water molecules are attracted to both anions and cations. Notice that the negative oxygen atoms of the water molecules are drawn to the sodium cation (Na^+) here, while the positive sides of the water molecules are drawn to the chloride ions (Cl^-).

In any fluid with dissolved electrolytes, as in any other substance, there will always be the same number of positive and negative charges. If an anion enters a cell, a cation must accompany it or another anion must leave so that electroneutrality will be maintained. Table 10–1 illustrates this point.

Water molecules are attracted to electrolytes because water molecules are "polar." This means that although each water molecule bears a net charge of zero, the oxygen side of the molecule is slightly negatively charged, and the hydrogens are slightly positively charged. Figure 10–3 shows the result in an electrolyte solution: both positive and negative ions attract clusters of water molecules around them.

As mentioned earlier, water follows salt. More precisely, water may move freely from one place to another, but it tends to remain wherever electrolytes such as sodium and chloride are concentrated. Water will tend to concentrate on one side of a barrier rather than another only if such solutes are concentrated on that side, and if the barrier separating the two fluid solutions is permeable to water but not permeable (or less freely permeable) to the solutes. Figure 10–4 shows this principle in operation.

You have seen this force at work if you have ever put salad dressing on lettuce an hour before eating it. When you came back to the salad, the lettuce was wilted, and there was water in the salad bowl. The high concentration of salt (and therefore low concentration of water) in the dressing caused water to move out of the lettuce cells. They collapsed (the lettuce wilted), and the water puddled in the salad dish. Sugar would have caused the same reaction. You can prevent this by coating the lettuce lightly with oil before adding the salty dressing. The oil acts as a barrier against the salt and prevents it from pulling water out of the lettuce.

The divider between the water inside and outside a cell is the cell membrane. The cell cannot pump water directly across its membrane, but it does have proteins in its membrane that can move positive sodium ions from one side of the membrane to the other. (Negative ions follow.) These proteins,

polar: having two opposite charges.

This tendency of water to follow solutes such as ions is known as the **osmotic pressure** of a solution. Water flows *toward* the higher osmotic pressure.

The cell membrane is **selectively permeable;** that is, it permits only the solvent (water) to pass freely. Solutes such as sodium ions have to be actively transported out or else cannot exit across the cell membrane easily. Osmotic pressure moves water across the membrane whenever the concentration of a **solute** (SOLL-yute), a dissolved substance, on the two sides of the membrane is not equal.

■ **FIGURE 10–4**
Osmotic Pressure
Water flows in the direction of the higher concentration of solute.

1. With equal numbers of solute particles on both sides, there are equal amounts of water.

— Solute

2. Now additional solute is added to side B. Solute cannot flow across the divider.

3. Water can flow across the divider. It moves both ways, but has a greater tendency to remain on side B, where there is more solute. The volume of water becomes greater on side B, and the concentrations on sides A and B become equal.

— Pressure

4. Now suppose that physical pressure (such as a pump) compresses the fluid on side B. The amount of pressure just sufficient to restore the original volume would equal the osmotic pressure exerted by the added particles.

concentration gradient: a difference in concentration of a solute on two sides of a semipermeable membrane.

known as sodium pumps, pump out sodium faster than it can diffuse back into the cell. Water then follows the sodium ions. Cells also have potassium pumps that pump in potassium, and water follows. By maintaining the concentrations of sodium, potassium, and other electrolytes inside and outside its boundaries in this manner, the cell can regulate the amount of water it contains.

Thanks to these pumps, a higher concentration of potassium and a lower concentration of sodium are maintained inside the cells than in the surrounding medium. Laboratory scientists know they are observing pumps at work whenever they find a cell maintaining such a concentration gradient of a substance across its membrane. If the concentrations of sodium and potassium on the outside and inside of cells were the same, we would know that no pumps were working. These gradients help cells do their work. For example, nerve cells use the sodium-potassium distribution across their membranes to generate electricity, making it possible for nerve impulses to travel—and so for you to think and act.

The maintenance of fluid and electrolyte balance requires that the amounts of various salts in the body remain nearly constant. If they are lost, they must be replaced from external sources—meaning, of course, foods and beverages.

The salt needed in the largest quantity is sodium chloride; a review of Table 10–1 will reveal the reason. Because sodium and chloride are the body's principal extracellular cation and anion, they are first to be lost when fluid is lost by sweating, bleeding, or renal or fecal excretion.

We have thirst to govern our intake of water, but do we have a salt hunger to govern our intake of sodium? Salt hunger is well known in plant-eating animals like cattle, which will travel long distances to a salt lick when they have been depleted of sodium. The tongue, in both animals and human beings, is equipped with specific taste receptors that respond only to the salty taste. Animals know instinctively when to seek this stimulus, but human beings may seek it when they have no need. Future research may determine whether a true salt hunger operates in human beings. Discussion of food sources of minerals is reserved for later in this chapter.

The body neither helplessly absorbs nor helplessly excretes electrolytes. It has highly evolved regulatory mechanisms to help ensure that its content of each mineral stays within bounds. Regulation occurs chiefly at two sites: the GI tract and the kidney.

The GI tract pours minerals continuously into its upper portions (stomach and small intestine) with the digestive juices and bile it secretes. It then reabsorbs these minerals in its lower segment (the colon) as needed. In a day, 8 liters (8 quarts) of fluids are recycled this way, providing ample opportunity for the regulation of electrolyte balance.

The kidney's control of water excretion has already been described. If you drink too little water or eat too much salt, your extracellular fluid (including your blood) becomes hypertonic (see the accompanying miniglossary). The brain receives the signal, it secretes ADH, and the kidney responds by retaining water. The urine volume is small, so the urine is a concentrated solution of excretion products. In the reverse situation, the urine becomes more dilute.

To control electrolyte excretion, the kidney depends on the adrenal glands to signal any change needed in the blood level of an electrolyte. The hormone aldosterone carries the message. Aldosterone promotes sodium reabsorption and potassium excretion from the kidney tubule, if the body's sodium level is

(handwritten margin note):
(cation)   (anion)
NA^+ CL^-
chief ECF

There are four kinds of taste receptors on the tongue: those sensitive to salty, sweet, sour, and bitter flavors.

adrenal glands: glands adjacent to, and just above, each kidney.
  ad = to
  renal = kidney

aldosterone: a hormone secreted by the adrenal glands that regulates sodium, chloride, and potassium concentrations.

Miniglossary of Terms Used to Describe Electrolyte Solutions

hypertonic: having a higher osmotic pressure than human body fluid.
  hyper = above
hypotonic: having a lower osmotic pressure than human body fluid.
  hypo = under
isotonic: having the same concentration of solute and therefore the same osmotic pressure as human body fluid. The **saline** (salt) solutions used in the hospital are made isotonic to human blood.
  iso = equal

low. (A review of how the kidney functions as illustrated in Figure 3–12 on page 60 may be helpful.)

The ability of the kidneys to regulate the sodium and water content of the body is remarkable. Sodium is absorbed easily from the intestinal tract; it then travels in the blood, where it ultimately passes through the kidneys. The kidneys filter all the sodium out, and then with great precision return to the bloodstream the exact amount of sodium needed. Normally, the amount excreted equals the amount ingested that day.

The blood concentration of sodium rises after a person eats heavily salted foods or meals very high in carbohydrate.* The high blood concentration stimulates thirst receptors in the brain, and the person drinks until the sodium-to-water ratio reaches a target level. Then the kidneys excrete the extra water together with the extra sodium.

Thus you are well protected from imbalances of water and electrolytes. However, you may encounter situations in which you lose such large amounts of fluid and electrolytes so rapidly that your kidneys, thirst instinct, and cell membranes cannot compensate. Vomiting, diarrhea, heavy sweating, burns, wounds, and the like may result in such great fluid losses that a medical emergency results.

Fluid and Electrolyte Imbalance

The details of electrolyte balance are among the most important ones that medical students must learn. These details are taught in physiology courses and in medical and nursing curricula. Everyone, however, should appreciate the importance of the balance and the principles by which it is maintained, and be aware of the situations that threaten it. When any of these gets out of control, the appropriate action is to seek medical help. We usually take water and salts for granted and ignore them, but the loss of water and salts can more rapidly result in life-threatening conditions than the lack of any of the other nutrients.

A few examples will illustrate. Suppose, for example, that the kidneys are poisoned and excrete too much potassium. Or suppose that fluid is lost by vomiting or diarrhea—a situation in which sodium is lost wholesale. Now suppose that water is pulled out of the body by a solute not normally excreted (for example, glucose, in the person with uncontrolled diabetes). All three situations bring on dehydration, but drinking water is not necessarily the solution to this problem. In each case, electrolyte imbalance must be restored by a medical professional.

Acid-Base Balance

The body uses ions not only to help maintain water balance, but also to help regulate the acidity (pH) of its fluids. The pH scale of Chapter 3 is repeated here in Figure 10–5 with the addition of normal and abnormal pH ranges in

pH: a measure of the concentration of H^+ ions (see Appendix B). The lower the pH, the stronger the acid. Thus at pH 2, a solution is a strong acid, and at pH 6, a solution is a weak acid (pH 7 is neutral). A pH above 7 is alkaline, or basic (a solution in which OH^- ions predominate).

---

*Overeating of carbohydrate results in sodium retention, probably mediated by effects of insulin and glucose on the kidney's regulatory mechanisms. Conversely, starvation, carbohydrate-free, and low-carbohydrate diets increase sodium excretion. S. F. Hull, Body fluid and electrolyte balance, *Dietetic Currents* 12 (1985): 3–4.

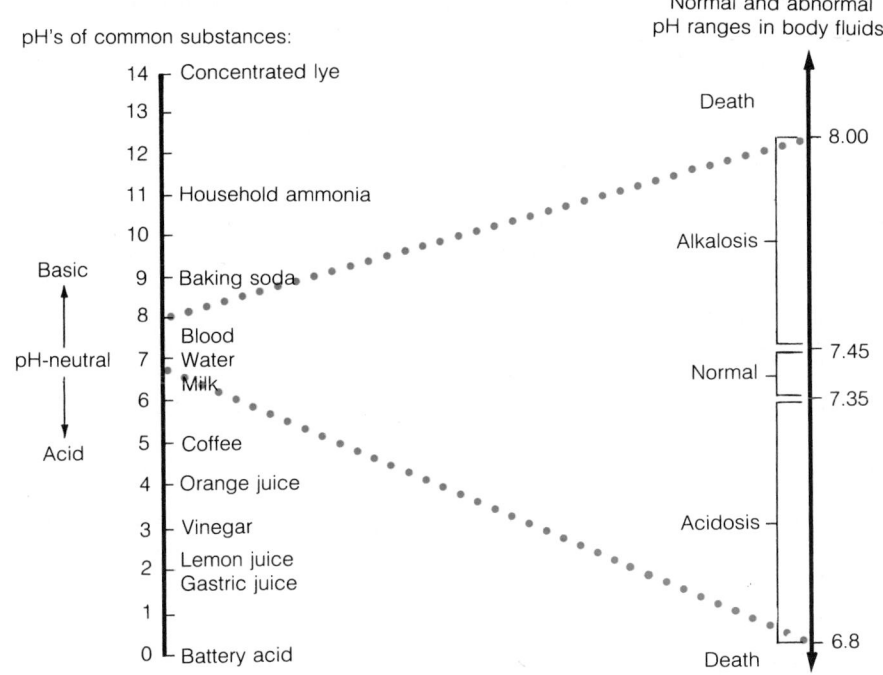

body fluids. Some of the electrolyte mixtures in the body fluids, as well as some of the proteins, protect the body against changes in acidity by acting as buffers—substances that can neutralize newly introduced acids or bases.

Chapter 6 described the buffering action of proteins; Figure 10–6 illustrates the body's most important electrolyte buffering system—the bicarbonate buffer system. The blood contains positive sodium ions (Na^+) and negative bicarbonate ions (HCO_3^-). When a strong acid is added to this solution, it forms two products: a salt, which is neutral, and a different acid, carbonic acid. It so happens that carbonic acid breaks down to carbon dioxide and water; the lungs excrete the carbon dioxide and the kidneys excrete the water, so the end products are neither acidic nor basic.

The body's buffer systems (proteins and electrolytes) serve as a first line of defense against changes in the fluids' acid-base balance. The lungs, skin, GI tract, and kidneys provide other defenses. If acid builds up, the respiration rate speeds up, and more carbon dioxide is exhaled. If base builds up, the respiration rate slows, so that carbon dioxide, which is being formed all the time by cellular respiration, will form additional carbonic acid to balance it. The skin can excrete acid in sweat, and the specialized tear ducts can alter the composition of tears. The stomach excretes acid as well. These are of minor, but not negligible, importance, but the chief regulatory organ is the kidneys.

The kidneys help to adjust the acid-base balance by selecting which ions to retain and which to excrete. Their work is so complex that whole books have been written on renal physiology, but their net effect is easy to sum up. The *body's* total acid burden remains nearly constant; and to a great extent, it is the acidity of the *urine* that is affected by what you ingest.

The bicarbonate/carbonic acid buffer system starts with sodium bicarbonate dissociated in water:

$$Na^+ \quad {}^-O-\overset{\overset{\textstyle O}{\|}}{C}-O-H$$

When an acid such as hydrochloric acid is added:

$$HCl \rightarrow H^+ + Cl^-$$

The sodium and chloride electrically balance each other (as salts always do):

$$Na^+ \quad Cl^-$$

The bicarbonate combines with the H^+ to yield carbonic acid:

$$H^+ + {}^-O-\overset{\overset{\textstyle O}{\|}}{C}-O-H \rightarrow H-O-\overset{\overset{\textstyle O}{\|}}{C}-O-H$$

Being unstable, carbonic acid releases carbon dioxide, which is expelled in the breath:

$$O=C=O$$

What's left is water:

$$H-O-H$$

■ FIGURE 10–6
An Example of a Buffer System

A Note on Acid Formers and Base Formers

In connection with the acidity of the urine, some foods have been called "acid forming" and others "base forming." This concept has won wide acceptance, but its practical implications are unclear. It is true that when foods are burnt to ash and the ashes are put in water, solutions of different pH's may result; but the acidity of the urine when these same foods are eaten cannot be predicted from that. The ashing of foods drives off gases containing nitrogen, sulfur, and other elements that, when metabolized in the body, produce compounds that dissolve in the fluids and affect their pH. To make things more complicated, the metabolic by-products of the constituents of foods differ depending on how they are metabolized. Also, the body has other ways of excreting acid than in the urine as just described. The notion that the "acid-forming" and "base-forming" effects of foods on the urine can be predicted from the composition of their ashes oversimplifies the case.

The theory that diets can be designed around such foods to produce a more acidic or basic urine seems not to have been established by actual research. Such diets have been used, however, for two chief purposes. One is to inhibit the growth of bacteria causing a bladder infection; the other is to reduce the likelihood of certain stones' forming in the kidney (some stones precipitate from acid solutions and others, from basic solutions). Acid-ash diets, intended to make the urine more acid, center on meat, cheese, eggs, whole grains, and some fruits. Alkaline-ash diets, intended to reduce the acidity of the urine, emphasize milk, vegetables, and most fruits. These diets are seldom used anymore. For bacterial infections, antibacterial drugs are preferred. For stone formation, strategies proven effective are to increase water intake so as to produce a dilute urine in which the precipitation of any kind of stone will be less likely, and to limit intake of the constituents of the stone.

■ *Sodium*

People have held salt (sodium chloride) in high regard throughout recorded history. The saying "You are the salt of the earth" means that a person is valuable. If, on the other hand, "you are not worth your salt," you are worthless. Even the word *salary* comes from the word *salt*.

Sodium in the Body

Sodium is the cation in the compound sodium chloride and in some other salts. As already mentioned, it is the chief extracellular ion, and it helps to maintain the body's fluid balance. Sodium is essential for water regulation, nerve transmission, and muscle contraction. (Table 10–2 summarizes sodium's chief functions in the body, its symptoms of deficiency and toxicity, and food sources.)

■ TABLE 10–2
Sodium—A Summary

Chief Functions in the Body	Deficiency Symptoms	Toxicity Symptoms	Significant Sources
An electrolyte that maintains normal extracellular fluid balance and acid-base balance; assists in nerve impulse transmission	Muscle cramps, mental apathy, loss of appetite	Hypertension[a]	Salt, soy sauce; moderate quantities in whole, unprocessed foods; large amounts in processed foods

[a]Chapter 16 describes the role of sodium in the development of hypertension.

Foods usually contain more sodium than the body requires, and absorption from the GI tract occurs freely. The kidneys sensitively filter excess sodium out of the blood into the urine; in the rare event of a deficiency, they conserve sodium and return it to the blood. With great precision, the adrenal hormone aldosterone maintains sodium concentration in the bloodstream at the exact amount needed.

If the blood level of sodium rises, as it will after a person eats salted foods, thirst ensures that the person will drink water until the sodium-to-water ratio is constant. Then the kidneys can excrete the extra fluid along with the extra sodium. Normally, the amount excreted equals the amount ingested that day. About 30 to 40 percent of the body's sodium is thought to be stored on the surfaces of the bone crystals, where it is easy to recover if the blood level drops.

Dieters sometimes think that eating too much salt or drinking too much water will make them gain weight, but this is not the case. Excess water is excreted immediately. Excess salt is excreted as soon as enough water is drunk to carry the salt out of the body. From this perspective, then, the way to keep body salt (and "water weight") under control is to drink more, not less, water.

If the blood level of sodium drops, both water and sodium must be replenished to avert emergency. Overly strict use of low-sodium diets in the treatment of kidney or heart disease can deplete the body of needed sodium; so can vomiting, diarrhea, or heavy sweating. Under normal conditions of sweating due to exercise, salt losses may easily be replaced later in the day with plain foods rather than salt tablets. Salt tablets are not recommended, because too much salt, especially if taken with too little water, incurs the risks of dehydration.

Sodium Requirements and Intakes

Diets rarely lack sodium. For this reason, no RDA has been set; the estimated minimum requirement for adults is 500 milligrams. The *NRC Recommendations* advise limiting daily salt intake to less than 6 grams (2,400 milligrams sodium).

A healthy person requires about 115 milligrams of sodium daily (300 milligrams of salt). Yet the average sodium intake is estimated at 4 to 6 grams daily (equivalent to 10 to 15 grams of salt, or 2 to 3 teaspoons). The American Heart Association recommends limiting sodium intake to 3 grams daily;

Estimated minimum requirement for sodium: 500 mg/day.
Canada: 115 mg/day.

5 g salt is about 2 g (2,000 mg) sodium.
5 g salt = 1 tsp.

■ TABLE 10–3
Suggestions for Avoiding Excessive Sodium Intake

Learn to enjoy the unsalted flavors of foods.
Cook with only small amounts of added salt.
Add little or no salt to food at the table.
Read labels with an eye open for salt.
Cut down on:
  Foods prepared in brine, such as pickles, olives, and sauerkraut.
  Salty or smoked meats, such as bologna, corned or chipped beef, frankfurters, ham, luncheon meats, salt pork, sausage, and smoked tongue.
  Salty or smoked fish, such as anchovies, caviar, salted and dried cod, herring, sardines, and smoked salmon.
  Snack items such as potato chips, pretzels, salted popcorn, and salted nuts and crackers.
  Bouillon cubes; seasoned salts (including sea salt); and soy, Worcestershire, and barbecue sauces.
  Cheeses, especially processed types.
  Canned and instant soups.
  Prepared horseradish, catsup, and mustard.

Chapter 28 discusses the roles of sodium and other minerals in the development and prevention of hypertension.

people with mild to moderate hypertension may benefit from restriction to 2 grams of sodium daily.[1] To restrict sodium intake, avoid highly salted foods, and remove the saltshaker from the table. Table 10–3 provides general suggestions for avoiding sodium in foods.

Three sources of sodium contribute about equally to the American diet. Some sodium naturally occurs in foods; some sodium is added to processed foods when manufacturers use salt as a preservative and flavoring agent; and some sodium is added to foods when individuals use salt from the shaker.

Processed foods do not always taste salty. Most people are surprised to learn that a ¾-cup serving of cornflakes contains more sodium than a 1-ounce serving of cocktail peanuts—and that a ½-cup serving of instant chocolate pudding contains still more.* The reason the peanuts taste saltier is because the salt is all on the surface, where the tongue's sensors immediately pick it up.

Table 10–4 shows that processed foods generally contain more sodium and less potassium than their less-processed relatives. Potassium loss may be as significant as sodium gain when it comes to blood pressure regulation, so these foods do you two ill turns.

Reading food labels provides valuable information. All foods that bear nutrition labels must state their sodium contents; sodium-conscious consumers can easily learn to read them. The serious sodium avoider must also stay away from fast-food places; order carefully at Asian restaurants whose staple sauces and flavorings are based on soy sauce and monosodium glutamate (MSG, also sold under the trade name Accent); and stop using many canned, frozen, and instant foods at home. (On the positive side, fresh foods are lower in sodium—and higher in potassium—than most people realize.)

Foods eaten without salt seem far less tasty at first. With practice, however, people can learn to enjoy the flavors of many unsalted foods and, where

*Data are taken from items #498, #740, and #138 in Appendix H.

■ TABLE 10–4
What Processing Does to the Sodium and Potassium Contents of Foods[a]

Food	Amount	Potassium (mg)	Sodium (mg)	Potassium-to-Sodium Ratio
Milk Foods				
Milk (whole)	1 c	370	120	3:1
Chocolate pudding (cooked from mix)	1 c	190	167	1:1
Chocolate pudding (instant)	1 c	352	880	1:2
Meats				
Beef roast (cooked)	3 oz	300	53	6:1
Corned beef (canned)	3 oz	116	855	1:7
Chipped beef	3 oz	378	2,952	1:8
Vegetables				
Corn (cooked)	1 c	228	8	29:1
Creamed corn (canned)	1 c	344	730	1:2
Sugar-coated cornflakes	1 c	22	284	1:13
Fruits				
Peaches (fresh)	1	171	1	171:1
Peaches (canned)	1	98	3	33:1
Peach pie	1 piece	235	423	1:2
Grains				
Whole-wheat flour	1 c	444	4	111:1
Whole-wheat bread	1 slice	50	180	1:3
Wheat crackers	4	17	69	1:4

[a]Data are taken from Items #93, #139, #138, #603, #607, #608, #847, #848, #518, #277, #282, #462, #562, #367, and #424 in Appendix H.

spices are needed, to make liberal use of sodium-free spices like those listed in Table 10–5. If you persist long enough (say, two months) in eating a low-salt diet, your taste threshold for salt will actually change so that your preferred level is lower.[2]

■ TABLE 10–5
Sodium-free Spices and Flavorings

Allspice	Mustard powder
Almond extract	Nutmeg
Basil	Onion powder
Bay leaves	Onions
Caraway seeds	Oregano
Chives	Paprika
Cinnamon	Parsley
Curry powder	Pepper
Dill	Peppermint extract
Garlic	Pimiento
Garlic powder	Rosemary
Ginger	Sage
Green peppers	Sesame seeds
Lemon extract	Tarragon
Lemon juice	Thyme
Mace	Turmeric
Maple extract	Vanilla extract
Marjoram	Vinegar
Mint	Walnut extract

Chloride

The element *chlorine* (Cl_2) occurs as a poisonous gas. Chlorine is added to public water before it flows through pipes into people's homes. It kills dangerous microorganisms that might otherwise spread disease, and then it evaporates, leaving the water safe for human consumption. The addition of chlorine to public water is one of the most important public health measures ever introduced in the developed countries and has eliminated such water-borne diseases as typhoid fever, which once ravaged vast areas, killing thousands of people.

When chlorine reacts with sodium, hydrogen, or another metal in salt, it forms the negative chloride ion (Cl^-). *Chloride* is not poisonous; on the contrary, it is a required element in the diet.

chloride: the ionic form of chlorine, Cl^-. (For metals, the same term applies to the neutral form and to the ion. For example, *sodium* refers to both Na and Na^+.) See Appendix B for a description of the chlorine-to-chloride conversion.

■ TABLE 10–6
Chloride—A Summary

Chief Functions in the Body	Deficiency Symptoms	Toxicity Symptoms	Significant Sources
An electrolyte that maintains normal fluid balance and proper acid-base balance; part of the hydrochloric acid found in the stomach, necessary for proper digestion	Growth failure in children; muscle cramps, mental apathy, loss of appetite	Vomiting	Salt, soy sauce; moderate quantities in whole, unprocessed foods; large amounts in processed foods

Chloride in the Body

The chloride ion is the major anion of the extracellular fluids, where it is found mostly in association with the sodium ion (Table 10–6 summarizes its roles and food sources). Chloride can move freely across membranes and so also associates with potassium inside the cells. Its role in balancing the pH of the blood was illustrated in Figure 10–6.*

In the stomach, the chloride ion is part of hydrochloric acid, which maintains the strong acidity of the stomach. The cells that line the stomach continuously expend energy to push chloride into the stomach fluid. One of the most serious consequences of vomiting is the loss of acid from the stomach, which upsets the acid-base balance.

Chloride Requirements and Intakes

Chloride is never naturally lacking in the diet. It abounds in foods as part of sodium chloride and other salts. The only way in which people can suffer a chloride deficiency is through human error; a case is on record in which chloride was mistakenly omitted from infant formula and caused illness before it was discovered. The Committee on Dietary Allowances has not established an RDA for chloride, but has provided an estimated minimum requirement for adults, as for sodium.

Estimated minimum requirement for chloride: 750 mg/day.
Canada: 175 mg/day.

■ Potassium

Like sodium, potassium is a cation. In contrast to sodium, it is more concentrated within the cells than outside them (review Table 10–1).

---

*The exchange of chloride and bicarbonate between intracellular and vascular fluids is known as the ''chloride shift.''

Potassium in the Body

Potassium, as mentioned earlier, is the body's principal intracellular electrolyte, important in maintaining the fluid volume inside cells, as well as the acid-base balance. Cell membranes are relatively permeable to potassium— 100 times more so than to sodium or chloride—but as it leaks out, a highly active cell membrane pump promptly shuttles it back in, in exchange for sodium. It is important that potassium remain inside cells, for if the cells were to give up to the blood only 6 percent of the potassium they contain, it would stop the heart.[3]

During nerve transmission and muscle contraction, potassium and sodium briefly exchange places across the cell membrane. The cell then quickly pumps them back into place. This makes sodium and potassium critical in the transmission of messages along nerves and from nerves to muscles, as well as in the response of muscles, including the heart muscle, to those messages. Potassium is also known to play a catalytic role in carbohydrate and protein metabolism. The role of potassium in maintaining the blood pressure is discussed in Chapter 28.

When body potassium is depleted, its concentration in the blood and in the muscle cells falls, but its concentration in the central nervous system remains unchanged.[4] The brain and nerves have a way of protecting themselves from changes they cannot tolerate; apparently potassium is too crucial to their function to be allowed to vary. Blood and muscle potassium appear to be used as stores from which potassium can be released gradually to keep the nervous system's supply constant.[5]

The pump referred to actively exchanges sodium for potassium across the cell membrane, maintaining a strong concentration gradient of each. Known as the **sodium-potassium pump,** it uses ATP (Chapter 7) as an energy source and the enzyme **sodium-potassium ATPase** (A-T-P-ace).

Potassium Requirements and Intakes

A deficiency of potassium from getting too little in the diet is unlikely, but diets low in fresh fruits and vegetables can make it a possibility. Abnormal conditions such as diabetic acidosis or dehydration can also cause potassium deficiency. One of the earliest symptoms is muscle weakness (see Table 10–7 for a summary of potassium functions, symptoms of deficiency and toxicity, and food sources).

Gradual potassium depletion might occur if a person sweated profusely day after day and failed to replenish potassium stores. However, even four days of heavy sweating and a low-potassium diet fail to deplete body potassium stores, as measured in plasma and muscle.[6] Furthermore, anyone who sweats heavily due to hard work or exercise presumably also eats more as well. Many of the selections a person makes in a day can easily be potassium-rich (see Table 10–8).

Because potassium is found inside of all living cells, both plant and animal, and because cells remain intact unless foods are processed, many of the richest sources of potassium are *fresh* foods of all kinds—especially fruits, vegetables, and legumes, as the purple, green, and brown bars of Table 10–8 show. If you were to scan the table of food composition in Appendix H, you would see that fresh foods contain much more potassium than sodium. In contrast, most processed foods such as canned vegetables, ready-to-eat

Estimated minimum requirement for potassium: 2,000 mg/day.

■ **TABLE 10–7**
Potassium—A Summary

Chief Functions in the Body	Deficiency Symptoms[a]	Toxicity Symptoms	Significant Sources
An electrolyte that maintains normal fluid balance and proper acid-base balance; facilitates many reactions, including the making of protein; supports cell integrity; assists in the transmission of nerve impulses and the contraction of muscles, including the heart	Muscular weakness, paralysis, confusion	Muscular weakness; vomiting; if given into a vein, can stop the heart	All whole foods: meats, milk, fruits, vegetables, grains, legumes

[a]Deficiency accompanies dehydration.

Fresh fruits and vegetables provide potassium in abundance.

cereals, and luncheon meats contain more sodium and less potassium (recall Table 10–4).

If you were playing a word game and said "potassium" to your partner, a likely response would be "bananas." People seem to know that bananas contain potassium. But Table 10–8 shows that their potassium content is not notable compared with that of other foods. Why did bananas get such a reputation for being high in potassium? Probably because bananas are higher in potassium than other commonly eaten fruits such as apples or oranges; they are easy to prepare and eat; and they are well-liked by many people. Other fruits have comparable or greater potassium contents, and vegetables have more potassium still, especially on a per-kcalorie basis. Advantages that fruits offer over other fresh foods, including vegetables, are that many of them are convenient to carry along and eat raw, and that they are practically sodium-free. People who have just run a marathon tend to think they must eat bananas afterward, but perhaps they should run home and eat potatoes instead.

It is hardly ever necessary to take potassium supplements, because food sources are so rich in potassium. Among healthy people, only a few groups risk depletion. One group is people who eat diets composed of heavily processed, heavily salted foods. Those people might fail to get enough potassium, but of course, rather than take supplements, they need to change their eating habits. Their nutritional health would be bound to benefit in many other ways from an improved diet. Another group is people who ingest fewer than 800 kcalories a day—for example, people on semifasts to lose weight. A physician must monitor the potassium status of these people and order supplements commensurate with the degree of depletion.[7] Physicians must also monitor the potassium status of clients who use diuretics that cause potassium loss.

Potassium toxicity is a greater concern than potassium deficiency. Toxicity could result from the overuse of potassium salt, especially in an infant or a

■ TABLE 10–8
Potassium in Commonly Eaten Foods Ranked Richest to Poorest

Food, Serving Size (Energy)

Peach halves, 10 dried (311 kcal)
Lima beans, 1 c cooked (260 kcal)
Winter squash, 1 c baked (96 kcal)
Pear halves, 1 c dried (459 kcal)
Potato, 1 microwaved with skin (212 kcal)
Pinto beans, 1 c cooked (265 kcal)
Baked potato, 1 whole (220 kcal)
Spinach, 1 c cooked (41 kcal)
Cantaloupe, ½ (94 kcal)
Kidney beans, 1 c canned (230 kcal)
Bok choy, 1 c cooked (20 kcal)
Prunes, 10 dried (201 kcal)
Split peas, 1 c cooked (230 kcal)
Butternut squash, 1 c baked (83 kcal)
Black-eyed peas, 1 c cooked (190 kcal)
Watermelon, 1 slice (152 kcal)
Asparagus, 1 c cooked (44 kcal)
Beets, 1 c cooked (52 kcal)
Tomatoes, 1 c whole canned (47 kcal)
Orange juice, 1 c fresh (111 kcal)
Apricot halves, 10 dried (83 kcal)
Zucchini, 1 c cooked (29 kcal)
Banana, 1 peeled (105 kcal)
Broccoli, 1 c cooked (40 kcal)
Milk or yogurt, 1 c nonfat (86 kcal)
Cauliflower, 1 c cooked (30 kcal)
Green beans, 1 c cooked (44 kcal)
Milk, 1 c whole (150 kcal)
Sirloin steak, 3 oz lean (180 kcal)
Summer squash, 1 c cooked (36 kcal)
Parsley, 1 c chopped fresh (20 kcal)
Apricots, 3 fresh pitted (51 kcal)
Sole/flounder, 3 oz baked (120 kcal)
Mushrooms, 1 c raw sliced (18 kcal)
Tomato, 1 whole raw (24 kcal)
Orange, 1 fresh medium (60 kcal)
Carrot, 1 whole fresh (31 kcal)
Chicken breast, ½ roasted (142 kcal)
Peanuts, 1 oz dried unsalted (161 kcal)
Cabbage, 1 c raw shredded (16 kcal)
Peach, 1 fresh medium (37 kcal)
Romaine lettuce, 1 c chopped (9 kcal)
Apple, 1 fresh medium (80 kcal)
Brewer's yeast, 1 tbsp (25 kcal)
Loose-leaf lettuce, 1 c (10 kcal)
Green pepper, 1 whole (18 kcal)
Celery, 1 large outer stalk (6 kcal)
Red radishes, 10 (7 kcal)
Wheat bran, ¼ c (19 kcal)
Whole-wheat bread, 1 slice (70 kcal)
Cheddar cheese, 1 oz (114 kcal)

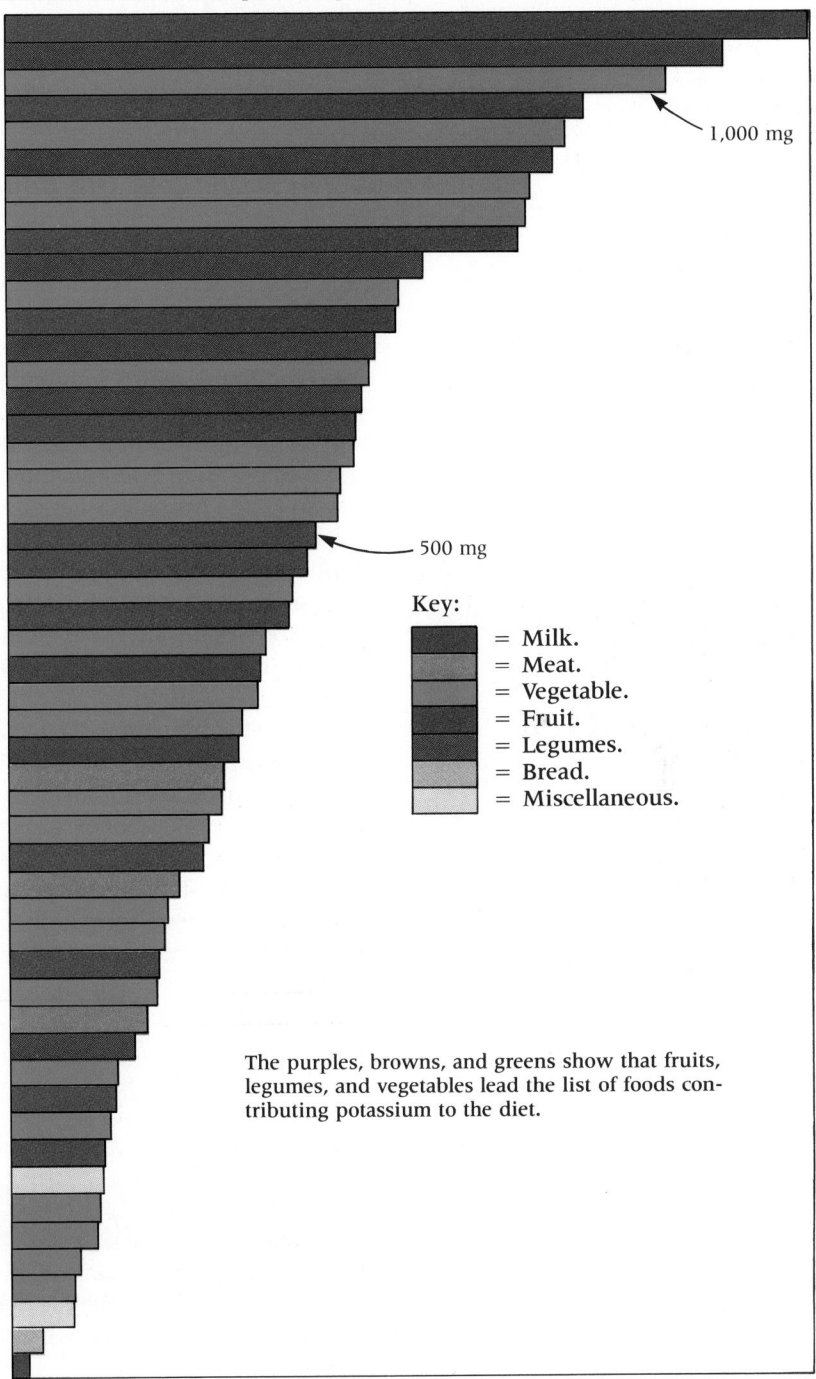

Estimated Safe and Adequate Daily Intake = 1,875 to 5,625 milligrams

1,000 mg

500 mg

Key:
= Milk.
= Meat.
= Vegetable.
= Fruit.
= Legumes.
= Bread.
= Miscellaneous.

The purples, browns, and greens show that fruits, legumes, and vegetables lead the list of foods contributing potassium to the diet.

Milligrams/Serving

person with heart disease; it does not result from foods. The body protects itself from toxicity as best it can. If you consume more potassium than you need, the kidneys accelerate their excretion and so maintain control. If you exceed your kidneys' limit (if you ingest too much potassium too fast), a vomiting reflex is triggered. However, if the GI tract is bypassed, and potassium is injected into a vein at a high rate, it can stop the heart.

Nutrients and the Bones

The previous chapter told of how vitamin A assists in remodeling bones as they grow larger; of how its deficiency alters the shape of bones and causes their growth to cease; and of how its toxicity accelerates bone dismantling and causes painful joints. It also told of how another member of the bone-building team, vitamin D, assists in mineralizing the bones. A lack of vitamin D causes legs to bow and ribs to bead; an excess promotes the withdrawal of calcium from the bones. Vitamins A and D cooperate with a number of other nutrients and compounds in building and maintaining the bones of the body, including vitamin C; the hormones parathormone and calcitonin; the protein collagen, which provides the underlying framework of bone; and the minerals calcium, phosphorus, magnesium, and fluoride, which compose the inorganic bone material built onto that framework. Calcium, phosphorus, and magnesium receive most of the attention for the remainder of this chapter; fluoride appears in both Highlight 10 and Chapter 11.

Figure 10–7 shows the three phases of bone development throughout life. From birth to approximately age 20, the bones are actively growing in length, width, and shape. This rapid growing phase overlaps with the next period of peak bone mass development that occurs between the ages of 12 and 40.[8] During this period, bones grow both thicker and denser by losing some existing bone and depositing more new bone. The final phase, which begins between 30 and 40 years of age and continues throughout life, finds bone loss exceeding new bone formation.

■ **FIGURE 10–7**
Phases of Bone Development throughout Life
The active growth phase occurs from birth to approximately age 20. The next phase of peak bone mass development occurs between the ages of 12 and 40. The final phase, when bone resorption exceeds formation, begins between ages 30 and 40 and continues throughout life.

Source: Adapted from L. K. DeBruyne and S. R. Rolfes, *Life Cycle Nutrition: Conception through Adolescence* (St. Paul, Minn.: West, 1989), p. 9.

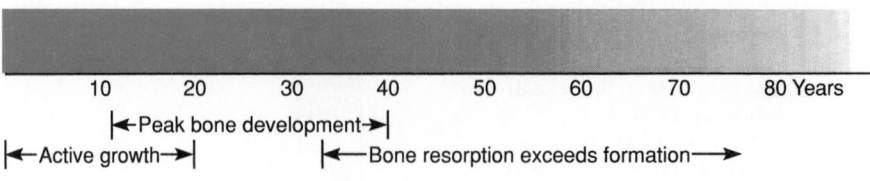

Nearly all people experience some bone loss as they grow older—especially women after menopause or hysterectomy, suggesting that hormonal changes are responsible. Because women's bones are less dense than men's and their hormonal changes accelerate losses, the extensive adult bone loss of osteoporosis is eight times more common in women than in men. Osteoporosis leads to crippling deformities, irreparable fractures, and even death.

While bone loss is a natural process that cannot be completely prevented, it can perhaps be minimized by starting early in life. The goal is to build maximally dense bones during the years of growth and development. Women whose bone mass does not reach its full potential in the younger years are likely to face osteoporosis earlier in life.[9] The amount and quality of bone laid down in those early years and maintained throughout midlife depends on many factors—most notably, genetics—and one of these factors may be the amount of calcium ingested. Prolonged inadequate calcium uptake during childhood and adulthood may result in less than optimal calcium deposition in bones.

The causes of osteoporosis seem to be multiple. In addition to calcium and vitamin D, the other previously mentioned minerals and vitamins required to form and stabilize the structure of bones may be essential for preventing osteoporosis. Weight-bearing exercise such as walking, dancing, or jogging is also necessary, for bones lay down minerals in response to the demands of bearing weight.

Nondietary factors, particularly age-related changes in female hormone activity, also affect the development of osteoporosis, probably even more than any dietary factor. No matter how high calcium intake is, it cannot override the acceleration of bone loss caused by hormonal changes. To prevent the further depletion of bone mineral, physicians often prescribe a combination of estrogen therapy and calcium (either dietary or supplementary). (Estrogen also helps to counter some of the other effects of menopause.)

Other factors that affect the likelihood of bone loss include both hereditary and lifestyle items. Among the hereditary ones are not only sex (women lose more bone), but also race (Scandinavians lose more; blacks resist bone loss) and probably other factors (blonds lose more bone than dark-haired people). Among lifestyle factors that promote bone loss are lack of exercise, excessive dieting, smoking, alcohol abuse, and abuse of many other drugs.

Nutrition-conscious people necessarily emphasize prevention, rather than attempts at remediation, in dealing with osteoporosis. Perhaps the best advice is to eat a well-balanced diet, to drink milk while you are young to build dense bones for later life, and to continue to drink milk throughout adulthood to minimize the losses from your bones. Also, exercise regularly to make your bones strong and to keep them that way. Regular exercise helps to maintain peak bone mass.[10]

osteoporosis (oss-tee-oh-pore-OH-sis): reduced density of the bones.
osteo = bones
porosis = porous

■ *Calcium*

Calcium holds the honor of being the most abundant mineral in the body. Its importance is gaining recognition, as evidenced by the many new calcium-fortified foods appearing on grocery shelves and magazine articles on osteoporosis.

Calcium in the Body

Ninety-nine percent of the body's calcium is stored in the bones. The other 1 percent is in the blood and body fluids. Blood calcium is very active metabolically. It has been estimated that about a fourth of the calcium in the blood is exchanged with bone calcium every minute. Calcium's blood concentration is tightly controlled by a system of hormones and vitamin D. Whenever the blood calcium concentration rises too high, these agents promote its deposit into bone. Whenever the blood concentration falls too low, the regulatory system acts in three locations to correct it:

- Intestine: increase calcium absorption.
- Bone: increase calcium release.
- Kidney: reduce calcium excretion.

Thus the blood calcium concentration returns to normal.

Food calcium never affects *blood* calcium, but this is not to say that blood calcium never changes. It does change, but in response to changed regulatory control, not to diet. When blood calcium rises above normal, the result is known as calcium rigor: the muscle fibers contract and cannot relax. Similarly, calcium levels may fall below normal in the blood, causing calcium tetany—also characterized by uncontrolled contraction of muscle tissue due to a change in the stimulation of nerve cells. These conditions do *not* (we repeat) reflect a *dietary* lack or excess of calcium; they are caused by a lack of vitamin D or by glandular malfunctions that result in abnormal amounts of the hormones that regulate blood calcium concentration.

On the other hand, a chronic *dietary* deficiency of calcium or a chronic deficiency due to poor absorption over the course of years can diminish the savings account in the bones. Because this is an important concept, we repeat once more: it is the *bones*, not the blood, that are depleted by calcium deficiency.

Many factors affect calcium absorption. The stomach's acidity favors it by helping to keep calcium soluble. Vitamin D aids in calcium absorption by helping to make the necessary calcium-binding protein. It is no accident that milk is chosen as the vehicle for fortification with vitamin D. The lactose in milk also seems to facilitate calcium absorption by a mechanism as yet unknown.[11]

As mentioned, calcium absorption depends on the help of a calcium-binding protein in the intestinal tract. The body is able to regulate calcium absorption by altering its production of the calcium-binding protein. More of this protein is made if more calcium is needed. Thus you will absorb more when you need more. This system is most obviously reflected in the increased absorption of calcium by a pregnant woman, who absorbs 50 percent of the calcium from the milk she drinks instead of only 30 percent, as she formerly did. Similarly, growing children absorb 50 to 60 percent of ingested calcium; when their growth slows or stops (and their bones no longer demand a net increase in calcium content each day), their absorption falls to the adult level of about 30 percent.[12]

Some foods contain binders that combine chemically with calcium and other minerals such as iron and zinc to prevent their absorption, carrying them out of the body with other wastes. For example, phytic acid renders the calcium (as well as iron and zinc) in certain foods less available than it might be otherwise; oxalic acid also binds calcium and iron. Phytic acid is found in

The regulators are hormones from the parathyroid and thyroid glands, as well as vitamin D. One, **parathormone**, raises blood calcium. The other, **calcitonin**, lowers it by inhibiting release of calcium from bone. The hormonelike **vitamin D** raises blood calcium by acting at the three sites listed.

calcium rigor: hardness or stiffness of the muscles caused by high blood calcium concentrations.

calcium tetany: intermittent spasms of the extremities due to nervous and muscular excitability caused by low blood calcium concentrations.

calcium-binding protein: a protein in the intestines, made with the help of vitamin D, that facilitates calcium absorption.

binders: chemical compounds occurring in foods, that can combine with nutrients (especially minerals) to form complexes the body cannot absorb. Examples of such binders include **phytic** (FIGHT-ic) and **oxalic** (ox-AL-ic) **acids.**

oatmeal and other whole-grain cereals, and oxalic acid is present in rhubarb and spinach, among other foods. Fiber in general seems to hinder calcium absorption, so it is especially important that a diet high in fiber be adequate in calcium. This doesn't affect the overall value of high-fiber foods; they are nutritious for many reasons, but they are not useful as calcium sources.

Dietary phosphorus has been thought to affect calcium balance, favoring calcium retention when ingested in a 1-to-1 ratio and inducing calcium losses when phosphorus intakes greatly exceed calcium intakes. However, most researchers now agree that as long as calcium intake is adequate, its absorption will not be inhibited by phosphorus.

Protein also affects calcium status, but not by affecting absorption. Excess protein in the diet increases the amount of calcium excreted.[13] This is why calcium recommendations in the United States and Canada (where protein intakes are often double those recommended) are greater than for people in countries where protein intakes are lower. Another recommendation is to maintain protein intake at moderate levels.

To sum up, positive calcium balance is favored by the hormonal team that promotes growth (as in pregnancy), stomach acid, vitamin D, lactose, and phosphorus (in up to a 1:1 ratio). It is opposed by high-fiber foods and diets excessively high in protein. Calcium absorption also varies between individuals and within the same individual. Average calcium absorption in adults is 30 percent.[14]

The calcium that circulates in the body fluids plays many roles. Some calcium is found in close association with cell membranes, where it helps to regulate the transport of other ions in and out. It is essential for muscle action and so helps maintain the heartbeat. Calcium must be present between nerve and nerve, and between nerve and muscle, for the reception and interpretation of nerve impulses; and when it enters cells, it delivers important messages to intracellular receptors. The protein within cells that relays calcium's messages is calmodulin.

Several of the messages calcium delivers have to do with blood pressure. Calcium's role in maintaining blood pressure is discussed in Chapter 28.

Calcium must also be present if blood clotting is to occur, because it is one of the 14 factors directly involved in this process. (The other 13 are proteins; vitamin K is needed, too, for the synthesis of some of these proteins.) Calcium also acts as a cofactor for several enzymes. These roles, as well as deficiency symptoms and food sources, appear in Table 10–9.

As for the calcium in bone, it plays two important roles. One, as already mentioned, is to serve as a bank to prevent alteration of the all-important blood calcium concentration. The other is structural. The bones provide a rigid frame to hold the body upright and serve as attachment points for muscles, making motion possible.

Calcium Deficiency

Calcium is not abundant in the diet, and low intakes are widespread in human societies. As you know, deficient calcium uptake threatens the integrity of the bones. The bone disease rickets was mentioned in Chapter 9, for vitamin D deficiency is the most common cause of rickets. In vitamin D

Table H29–2 in Highlight 29 lists foods containing considerable amounts of oxalate.

Factors that enhance calcium balance:
- Hormones that promote growth.
- Stomach acid.
- Vitamin D.
- Lactose.

Factors that impair calcium balance:
- High-fiber diet.
- High-protein diet.
- Phytic and olaxic acids.

calmodulin (cal-MOD-you-lin): an inactive protein concentrated within cells that becomes active when bound to calcium; then it becomes a messenger that tells other proteins what to do. The system serves as interpreter for hormone- and nerve-mediated messages arriving at cells.

cofactor: a mineral element that, like a coenzyme, works with an enzyme to facilitate a chemical reaction. The cofactor occurs at the active site, maintains the structural integrity of the enzyme, and may also facilitate the enzyme's catalytic activity.

Altered composition of the bones is reflected in **osteomalacia**, the condition in which the bones become soft (see p. 254). Osteomalacia is sometimes called **adult rickets**.

■ TABLE 10–9
Calcium—A Summary

Chief Functions in the Body	Deficiency Symptoms	Toxicity Symptoms	Significant Sources
The principal mineral of bones and teeth; also involved in normal muscle (including heart muscle) contraction and relaxation, proper nerve functioning, blood clotting, blood pressure, and immune defenses	Stunted growth in children; bone loss (osteoporosis) in adults	Excess calcium is excreted except in hormonal imbalance states (not caused by nutritional deficiency)	Milk and milk products, small fish (with bones), tofu (bean curd), greens (broccoli, chard), legumes

deficiency, the production of the calcium-binding protein slows. Even when the amount of calcium in the diet is adequate, the calcium passes through the intestinal tract without being absorbed into the body, leaving the bones undersupplied. In children, the failure to deposit sufficient calcium in bone causes growth retardation, bowed legs, and other skeletal abnormalities. In adults, the same disease may set in after a normal childhood during which calcium intake and absorption were adequate, and after the skeleton has become fully calcified. In later adult life, osteoporosis occurs, as already mentioned.

The urgency of obtaining enough calcium has to be learned through education, because the body sends no signals saying it is deficient. Most nutrient deficiencies make themselves known by way of symptoms that can be felt or seen, such as pain, skin lesions, tiredness, and the like. But a developing calcium deficiency is utterly silent; it becomes apparent only when a hip or pelvic bone suddenly breaks and will not heal. No evidence of a developing calcium deficiency can be found in a blood sample, because blood calcium remains normal no matter what the bone content may be. Nor does depletion of bone calcium show up in an x-ray examination until it is so far advanced as to be virtually irreversible.

The first photograph in Figure 10–8 shows a hipbone sliced lengthwise so that you can see the lacy network of calcium-containing crystals inside the bone. These are the deposits in the body's calcium bank, which are drawn on whenever the supply from the day's diet runs short. Invested in savings during the milk-drinking years of childhood and young adulthood, these calcium deposits provide a nearly inexhaustible fund of calcium. The other parts of Figure 10–8 show the effects of bone loss on the spine and on a person's height. The skeleton literally sags and shrinks when it loses bone material.

Calcium Requirements and Intakes

Calcium RDA: 800 mg/day.
Canadian RNI: 700 mg/day (women).
800 mg/day (men).

The recommended intake of calcium, arrived at by way of balance studies, is 700 to 800 milligrams (0.7 to 0.8 grams) per day for adults in both the United States and Canada. Adults can stay in balance on intakes lower than this if they adapt over a long period of time to lower intakes, and the World Health

A. Cross section of bone. The lacy structural elements are **trabeculae** (tra-BECK-you-lee), which can be drawn on to replenish blood calcium.

6 inches lost

50-year-old

80-year-old

C. Effects of osteoporosis on a woman's height. On the left is a woman at menopause and on the right, the same woman 30 years later. Notice that collapse of her vertebrae has shortened her back; the length of her legs has not changed.

B. A healthy spine (*left*) and one that has deteriorated from adult bone loss, or osteoporosis (*right*). Notice how the vertebrae are being compressed by the weight of the head and shoulders.

■ **FIGURE 10–8**
Normal and Osteoporotic Bone

■ **FIGURE 10–9**
Daily Dietary Calcium Intake

Source: Calcium: A summary of current research for the health professional (Rosemont, Ill.: National Dairy Council, 1984), p.15. Courtesy of National Dairy Council.

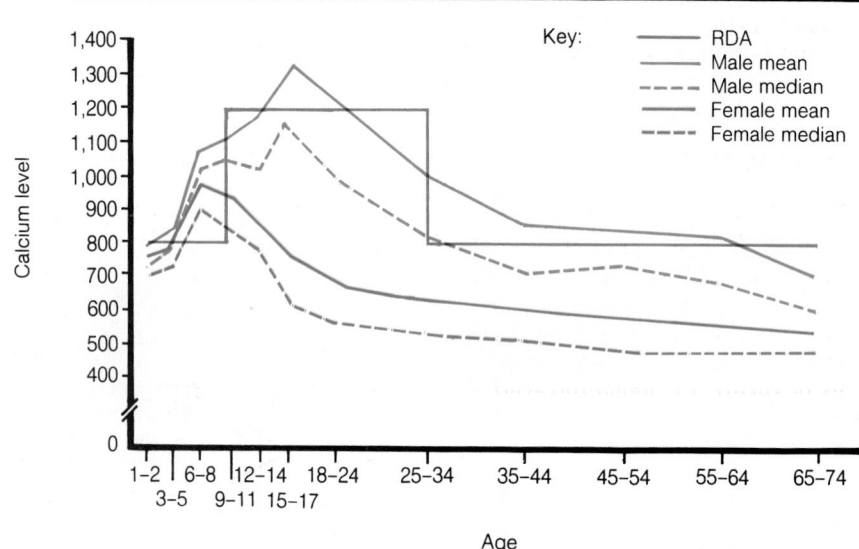

The Four Food Group Plan recommends daily milk servings (1 c):
- Children under 9: 2 to 3
- Children 9 to 12: 3 or more
- Teenagers: 4 or more
- Adults: 2
- Pregnant women: 3 or more
- Lactating women: 4 or more
- Older women: 3

Milk and milk products are rightly famous for their calcium contents.

Organization recommends only 400 to 500 milligrams per day for adults. However, as mentioned earlier, high protein intakes increase calcium excretion, and in the United States and Canada, where diets are rich in protein, 700 to 800 milligrams for adults and 1,200 milligrams for pregnant and lactating women seems to be a protective recommendation. Many authorities advocate even more—1,200 to 1,500 milligrams a day—for women over 50. Figure 10–9 shows that many people, particularly women, have dietary calcium intakes below the RDA.

The predominance of blue bars in Table 10–10 shows that calcium is found almost exclusively in a single class of foods—milk and milk products. The abundant green bars point out the significant calcium content of certain vegetables as well, at a lower energy cost. Nonfat milk offers 300 milligrams of calcium in an 86-kcalorie cup, for example, while greens (depending on the variety chosen) offer 100 milligrams or more in a 20-kcalorie cup. The greens would seem to be the better choice per kcalorie, but a complication enters in—they contain binders that inhibit absorption. Calcium absorption from green vegetables is not always efficient, whereas calcium is known to be efficiently absorbed from milk. The *NRC Recommendations* advise daily consumption of low- or nonfat milk products to help maintain an adequate calcium intake.

The word *daily* should be stressed with respect to food sources of calcium. Because of the body's limited ability to absorb calcium, it cannot handle massive doses periodically, but instead needs frequent opportunities to take in small amounts. The word *milk* products should also be stressed, rather than *dairy* products. Butter and cream contain negligible calcium, because calcium is not soluble in fat.

One slice of cheese (1 ounce) contains about two-thirds as much calcium as a cup of milk—at a kcalorie cost of 80 to 120 kcalories. A cup of cottage cheese offers less calcium (135 milligrams) for more kcalories (235), and so it is a poor source by this standard; for the person with an unlimited kcalorie

■ TABLE 10–10
Calcium in Commonly Eaten Foods Ranked Richest to Poorest

Food, Serving Size (Energy)

Sardines, 3 oz canned with bones (175 kcal)
Kefir, 1 c (160 kcal)
Goat's milk, 1 c (168 kcal)
Shrimp, 3.5 oz boiled (109 kcal)
Milk plus solids, 1 c nonfat (91 kcal)
Milk plus solids, 1 c 1% low-fat (105 kcal)
Romano cheese, 1 oz (110 kcal)
Milk or yogurt, 1 c nonfat (86 kcal)
Milk, 1 c 1% low-fat (102 kcal)
Milk, 1 c whole (150 kcal)
Buttermilk, 1 c (99 kcal)
Milk, 1 c whole chocolate (210 kcal)
Swiss cheese, 1 oz (107 kcal)
Spinach, 1 c canned (50 kcal)
Spinach, 1 c fresh cooked (41 kcal)
Cheddar cheese, 1 oz (114 kcal)
Muenster cheese, 1 oz (104 kcal)
Oysters, 1 c raw (160 kcal)
Turnip greens, 1 c cooked (29 kcal)
Broccoli, 1 c cooked (46 kcal)
Salmon, 3 oz canned with bones (120 kcal)
Beet greens, 1 c cooked (40 kcal)
Bok choy, 1 c cooked (20 kcal)
Cottage cheese, 1 c 2% low-fat (205 kcal)
Dandelion greens, 1 c cooked (35 kcal)
Soybeans, 1 c cooked (235 kcal)
Collards, 1 c cooked (20 kcal)
Tofu (soybean curd), 1 block (86 kcal)
Mustard greens, 1 c cooked (21 kcal)
Parsley, 1 c chopped fresh (20 kcal)
Almonds, 1 oz whole dried (167 kcal)
Kidney beans, 1 c canned (230 kcal)
Parmesan cheese, 1 tbsp (23 kcal)
Green beans, 1 c cooked (44 kcal)
Spinach, 1 c fresh chopped (12 kcal)
Okra pods, 8 fresh cooked (27 kcal)
Orange, 1 fresh medium (60 kcal)
Summer squash, 1 c cooked (36 kcal)
Seaweed (kelp), 1 oz raw (12 kcal)
Loose-leaf lettuce, 1 c (10 kcal)
Cauliflower, 1 c cooked (30 kcal)
Cabbage, 1 c raw shredded (16 kcal)
Cantaloupe, ½ (94 kcal)
Whole-wheat bread, 1 slice (70 kcal)
Oatmeal, 1 c cooked (145 kcal)
Peanuts, 1 oz dried unsalted (161 kcal)
Celery, 1 large outer stalk (6 kcal)
Sole/flounder, 3 oz baked (120 kcal)
Chicken breast, ½ roasted (142 kcal)
Apple, 1 fresh medium (80 kcal)
Sirloin steak, 3 oz lean (180 kcal)

U.S. RDA = 1,000 milligrams

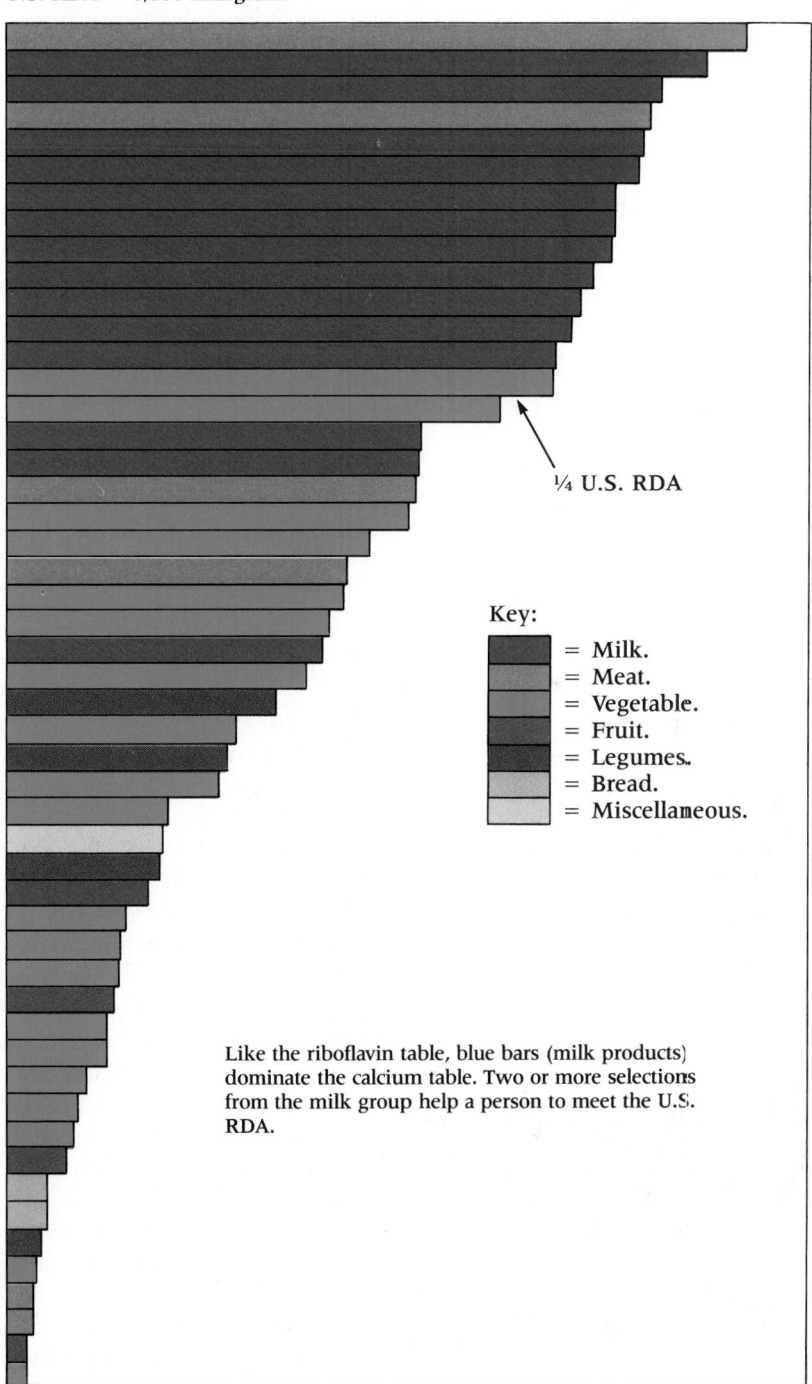

¼ U.S. RDA

Key:
= Milk.
= Meat.
= Vegetable.
= Fruit.
= Legumes.
= Bread.
= Miscellaneous.

Like the riboflavin table, blue bars (milk products) dominate the calcium table. Two or more selections from the milk group help a person to meet the U.S. RDA.

Milligrams/Serving

allowance, though, it can help meet the calcium need. Other high-kcalorie acceptable substitutes for regular milk include ice cream, ice milk, whole-milk yogurt, puddings, and custards.

Milk and milk products can be concealed in foods. Powdered nonfat milk, which is an excellent and inexpensive source of protein, calcium, and other nutrients, can be added to many foods (such as casseroles and meat loaf) in preparation; this is probably the best way for older women to obtain the calcium they need beyond the amount they can practicably get from liquid milk.

To make it easier for people to obtain the calcium they need from milk, the dairies are experimenting with a form of milk fortified so as to deliver twice as much calcium as regular milk; 1 cup would therefore do the job of two. Some brands of tofu, corn tortillas, some nuts (such as almonds), and some seeds (such as sesame seeds) supply calcium in reasonable quantities, for the person who is avoiding milk products.

A generalization that has been gaining strength throughout this book is supported by the information given here about calcium. A balanced diet that supplies a variety of foods is the best guarantee of adequacy for all essential nutrients. All food groups should be included, and none should be overused. In our culture, calcium is usually lacking wherever milk is underemphasized in the diet—whether through ignorance, simple dislike, fad dieting, lactose intolerance, or allergy. By contrast, iron is usually lacking whenever milk is overemphasized, as Chapter 11 will show.

Calcium Supplements

Calcium supplements are recommended only as a last resort. The reason is simply that they are not foods. They do not offer the variety of nutrients foods do, and their calcium is not, for the most part, absorbed as well as that from milk.

Calcium supplements have become popular among people who wish to prevent adult bone loss and who cannot or will not drink milk. Evidence that these supplements will prevent bone loss is inconclusive—it *may* slow the rate of bone loss in postmenopausal women who are not receiving an adequate calcium intake.[15] But the final word on calcium supplements has not been spoken—until then, all we know with any certainty is that low calcium intakes from food, early in life, correlate with osteoporosis late in life. Supplements are woefully inferior to milk for many reasons, but for the person who uses them, here are some facts about them.

First, regular vitamin-mineral pills contain little calcium, as you can tell from the labels. Don't be fooled; the label may list some number of milligrams of calcium that sounds like a lot, but the U.S. RDA for calcium is 1 gram—1,000 milligrams. So let's start with a list of the possible candidates that will offer 1,000 milligrams or so a day. (The 1984 Consensus Conference on Osteoporosis recommended that women consume 1,000 to 1,500 milligrams a day, and intakes of up to 2,500 milligrams a day are known to be safe for healthy people.[16])

Calcium supplements are available in three forms. Simplest are the purified calcium compounds—such as calcium carbonate, citrate, gluconate, lactate, malate, phosphate, and compounds of calcium with amino acids (called amino acid chelates). Then there are mixtures of calcium with other compounds—such as mixtures of calcium carbonate with magnesium carbonate, with aluminum salts (as in some antacids), or with vitamin D. Then there are powdered forms of calcium-rich materials—such as bonemeal, powdered bone, oyster shells, or dolomite (limestone). If you wanted a calcium supplement, which of these should you choose? In comparing them, you should address several questions.

Before comparing calcium supplements on any other basis, you should eliminate some right away as potentially unsafe. Some preparations of bonemeal and dolomite, for example, have been found to be contaminated with amounts of arsenic, cadmium, mercury, and lead high enough to cause a hazard to the health of the person who takes them routinely.[17] Antacids that contain aluminum and magnesium hydroxides can accelerate calcium loss (Rolaids is an example; Tums is not).[18] Supplements that contain vitamin D present a toxicity risk; the user must be careful to take an amount that will provide enough, but not too much, vitamin D, and to eliminate any other concentrated vitamin D sources. The risk of kidney stone formation may also be a problem with some supplements: when rats were fed calcium phosphate dibasic as their sole calcium source, they deposited abnormal amounts of calcium in their kidneys.[19] Some people are genetically susceptible to stone formation; they need to know who they are and to avoid calcium supplements.

The next question to ask is how well the body absorbs and uses the calcium from various supplements. Based on limited research to date, it seems that most healthy people absorb calcium equally well—and as well as from milk—from any of the following supplements: amino acids chelated with calcium, calcium acetate, calcium carbonate, calcium citrate, calcium gluconate, calcium lactate, calcium phosphate dibasic, and oyster shells. People absorb calcium less well from a mixture of calcium carbonate and magnesium carbonate, from oyster shell calcium fortified with inorganic magnesium, from a chelated calcium-magnesium combination, or from calcium carbonate fortified with vitamins and iron.[20] This raises the specter of interactions, and with it, another question: Do calcium supplements, themselves, interfere with the absorption of other nutrients?

The answer, unfortunately, is yes. Calcium phosphate dibasic inhibits magnesium absorption. The same amount of calcium in milk does not. If the calcium phosphate dibasic is fortified with magnesium, then it interferes with iron absorption. Calcium carbonate also interferes with iron absorption; so does calcium hydroxyapatite. A way to get around this may be to take calcium supplements between, not with, meals—but this is not a satisfactory solution, for only a meal enhances the absorption of the calcium.[21]

Supposing that you can absorb the supplement taken between meals, and that your body will use it well, then the next question to ask is, Which contains the most calcium per pill? The more calcium in a single pill, the fewer pills you have to take. Read the label to find out. Calcium carbonate is 40 percent calcium; calcium gluconate, only 9 percent; so they vary a lot. Then consider that when manufacturers compress large quantities of calcium into small pills, the stomach acid has difficulty breaking up the compound. To test a supplement's absorbability, drop it into a 6-ounce cup of vinegar, and stir occasionally. A high-quality formulation will be 75 percent dissolved within a half hour.[22]

Finally, consider the cost, and choose a supplement. Establish a routine so that you will not forget to take it. Take it with snacks or meals and take it several times a day in divided doses rather than all at once; divided doses can increase absorption by up to 20 percent.[23]

But think one more time before you commit yourself to this course of action. You may need as much as 1,000 milligrams or more of calcium every day for the rest of your life. Are you absolutely sure you cannot get it from milk, milk products, or other foods? Everyone seems to prefer that you use foods. The Consensus Conference on Osteoporosis recommended milk. The American Society for Bone and Mineral Research recommends foods as a source of calcium in preference to supplements.[24] Nutrition authorities Jean Mayer and Jeanne Goldberg, whose syndicated column on nutrition reaches newspaper readers nationwide, state, "We stand firmly in favor of dietary measures to meet the RDA . . . of calcium."[25] Seldom is such a consensus seen among nutritionists.

Supplements contain only calcium; they don't offer the other nutrients that accompany it as fringe benefits in a food such as milk—thiamin, riboflavin, niacin, potassium, phosphorus, vitamin A, and all the rest. Therefore, the person who omits milk and attempts to make up for it by taking supplements still is left with the task of obtaining all the other nutrients, and for some of these, milk is an excellent source. Milk's other essential nutrients are present in appropriate amounts; imbalances are not likely, and overdoses are impossible. Milk's long-term safety is assured. The habit of drinking milk is easy to sustain, once established, because it fits with meals, provides energy, and can be served in delicious forms. It is low in cost, and fits well into a food budget. Milk drinking squares with the philosophy that using whole foods is preferable to taking supplements.

■ *Phosphorus*

Phosphorus is the mineral in the second largest quantity in the body. About 85 percent of it is found combined with calcium in the crystals of the bones and teeth. There it occurs as any of several salts of calcium phosphate, including hydroxyapatite, one of the compounds in the crystals that give strength and rigidity to these structures.*

hydroxyapatite (high-drox-ee-APP-ah-tite):the major calcium-containing crystal of bones and teeth.

The concentration of phosphorus in blood plasma is less than half that of calcium: 3.5 milligrams per 100 milliliters of plasma. But as part of one of the body's major buffers (phosphoric acid and its salts), phosphorus is found in all body cells. It is a part of DNA and RNA, the genetic code material present in every cell. Thus phosphorus is necessary for all growth, because new DNA and RNA have to be made to provide the building instructions whenever new cells are formed.

Phosphorus also plays many key roles in energy transfers occurring during cellular metabolism. Many enzymes and the B vitamins become active only when a phosphate group is attached. (The B vitamins, you will recall, play major roles in energy metabolism.) ATP itself, the energy carrier of the cells,

---

*The suffix *ate* in *calcium phosphate* indicates that the phosphorus has undergone a chemical reaction with oxygen and is bonded to calcium through oxygen atoms. Phosphate is the salt form of phosphoric acid.

■ **TABLE 10–11**
Phosphorus—A Summary

Chief Functions in the Body	Deficiency Symptoms	Toxicity Symptoms	Significant Sources
A principal mineral of bones and teeth; part of every cell; important in the genetic material, as part of phospholipids, in energy transfer, and as buffer systems that maintain acid-base balance	Deficiency unknown	Excess phosphorus may draw calcium out of the body in being excreted	All animal tissues

contains three phosphate groups and uses these groups to do its work (see Figure 7–3 in Chapter 7).

Some lipids contain phosphorus as part of their structure. These phospholipids help to transport other lipids in the blood; they also reside in cell membranes, where they affect transport of nutrients into and out of the cells. (Table 10–11 lists functions and food sources of phosphorus.)

Animal protein is the best source of phosphorus, because phosphorus is so abundant in the energetic cells of animals. In addition to foods from the milk and milk products group and the meats and meat alternates group, processed foods (including soft drinks) are usually high in phosphorus. The recommended intakes for phosphorus are the same as those for calcium. Few people would have trouble meeting that intake; deficiencies are unknown.

Phosphorus RDA: 800 mg/day.
Canadian RNI: 850 mg/day (women).
1,000 mg/day (men).

■ *Magnesium*

Magnesium barely qualifies as a major mineral. Only about 1¾ ounces of magnesium is present in the body of a 130-pound person, most of it in the bones. Bone magnesium seems to be a reservoir to ensure that some will be on hand for vital reactions, regardless of recent dietary intake.

Magnesium also acts in all the cells of the soft tissues, where it forms part of the protein-making machinery, and where it is necessary for the release of energy. A major role seems to be as a catalyst in the reaction that adds the last phosphate to the high-energy compound ATP. Magnesium also helps relax muscles after contraction and promotes resistance to dental caries by holding calcium in tooth enamel. See Table 10–12 for a summary of magnesium.

Dietary intake of magnesium in the U.S. population is generally lower than the RDA, although the development of deficiency symptoms in the absence of disease is unlikely.[26] A magnesium deficiency may occur as a result of vomiting, diarrhea, alcohol abuse, protein malnutrition, or renal or endocrine disorders; in postsurgical clients who have been fed incomplete fluids into a vein for too long; or in people using diuretics. A severe deficiency causes

Magnesium RDA: 350 mg/day (men).
280 mg/day (women).
Canadian RNI: 3.4 mg/kg/day.

■ **TABLE 10–12**
Magnesium—A Summary

Chief Functions in the Body	Deficiency Symptoms	Toxicity Symptoms	Significant Sources
Involved in bone mineralization, the building of protein, enzyme action, normal muscular contraction, transmission of nerve impulses, and maintenance of teeth	Weakness; confusion; depressed pancreatic hormone secretion; if extreme, convulsions, bizarre muscle movements (especially of the eye and facial muscles), hallucinations, and difficulty in swallowing; in children, growth failure[a]	Not known; large doses have been taken in the form of the laxative Epsom salts, without ill effects except diarrhea	Nuts, legumes, whole grains, dark green vegetables, seafood, chocolate, cocoa

[a]A still more severe dificiency causes tetany, an extreme, prolonged contraction of the muscles similar to that caused by low blood calcium.

neuromuscular symptoms such as tetany, an extreme and prolonged contraction of the muscles very much like the reaction of the muscles when calcium levels fall. Magnesium deficit also impairs the central nervous system activity; it is thought to cause the hallucinations experienced by people withdrawing from alcohol overdoses. Symptoms of a marginal deficiency are less clear.

Food sources are shown in Table 10–13. Like all the other nutrients discussed so far, magnesium has its own pattern of distribution in foods. The colored bars at the top of the table indicate that legumes, seeds, and nuts make significant magnesium contributions; vegetables are also noteworthy.

■ *Sulfur*

The body does not use sulfur by itself as a nutrient (see Table 10–14); the reason sulfur is mentioned here is that it occurs in nutrients that the body does use, such as thiamin and certain amino acids. Sulfur is present in all proteins and plays its most important role in determining the contour of protein molecules. Sulfur helps the strands of protein to assume a particular shape and hold it—and so to do their specific jobs, such as enzyme work. Some of the amino acids contain sulfur in their side chains, and once built into a protein strand, one of these amino acids can link to another by way of sulfur-sulfur bridges. The bridges stabilize the protein structure. Skin, hair, and nails contain some of the body's more rigid proteins, and these have a high sulfur content.

There is no recommended intake for sulfur, and no deficiencies are known. Only when people lack protein to the point of severe deficiency will they lack the sulfur-containing amino acids.

Amino acids containing sulfur are methionine and cysteine. Cysteine in one part of a protein chain can bind to cysteine in another part of the chain by way of a sulfur-sulfur bridge (see the drawing of insulin with its disulfide bridge on p. 136). Two cysteine molecules linked this way are called cystine (see Appendix C).

■ TABLE 10–13
Magnesium in Commonly Eaten Foods Ranked Richest to Poorest

Food, Serving Size (Energy)

Spinach, 1 c cooked (41 kcal)
Tofu (soybean curd), 1 block (86 kcal)
Sesame seeds, ¼ c dry (221 kcal)
Sunflower seeds, ¼ c dry (205 kcal)
Black-eyed peas, 1 c cooked (190 kcal)
Garbanzo beans, 1 c cooked (270 kcal)
Shrimp, 3.5 oz boiled (109 kcal)
Beet greens, 1 c cooked (40 kcal)
Broccoli, 1 c cooked (46 kcal)
Navy beans, 1 c cooked dry (225 kcal)
Lima beans, 1 c cooked (260 kcal)
Kidney beans, 1 c canned (230 kcal)
Cashew nuts, 1 oz roasted (163 kcal)
Wheat germ, ¼ c raw (68 kcal)
Beets, 1 c cooked (52 kcal)
Figs, 5 dried (239 kcal)
Baked potato, 1 whole (220 kcal)
Peach halves, 10 dried (311 kcal)
Oysters, 1 c raw (160 kcal)
Peanuts, 1 oz dried unsalted (161 kcal)
Wheat bran, ¼ c (19 kcal)
Summer squash, 1 c cooked (36 kcal)
Zucchini, 1 c cooked (29 kcal)
Asparagus, 1 c cooked (44 kcal)
Seaweed (kelp), 1 oz raw (12 kcal)
Milk, 1 c whole (150 kcal)
Turnip greens, 1 c cooked (29 kcal)
Green beans, 1 c cooked (44 kcal)
Clams, 3 oz raw meat (65 kcal)
Milk or yogurt, 1 c nonfat (86 kcal)
Whole-wheat bread, 1 slice (70 kcal)
Parsley, 1 c chopped fresh (20 kcal)
Popcorn, 1 c popped in oil salted (55 kcal)
Chicken breast, ½ roasted (142 kcal)
Sirloin steak, 3 oz lean (180 kcal)
Popcorn, 1 c air popped (30 kcal)
Bean sprouts, 1 c fresh (32 kcal)
Mustards greens, 1 c cooked (21 kcal)
Sole/flounder, 3 oz baked (120 kcal)
Cantaloupe, ½ (94 kcal)
Brewer's yeast, 1 tbsp (25 kcal)
Bok choy, 1 c cooked (20 kcal)
Mushroom pieces, 1 c cooked (42 kcal)
Tomato, 1 whole raw (24 kcal)
Orange, 1 fresh medium (60 kcal)
Green pepper, 1 whole (18 kcal)
Cabbage, 1 c raw shredded (16 kcal)
Cheddar cheese, 1 oz (114 kcal)
Loose-leaf lettuce, 1 c (10 kcal)
Apple, 1 fresh medium (80 kcal)
Celery, 1 large outer stalk (6 kcal)

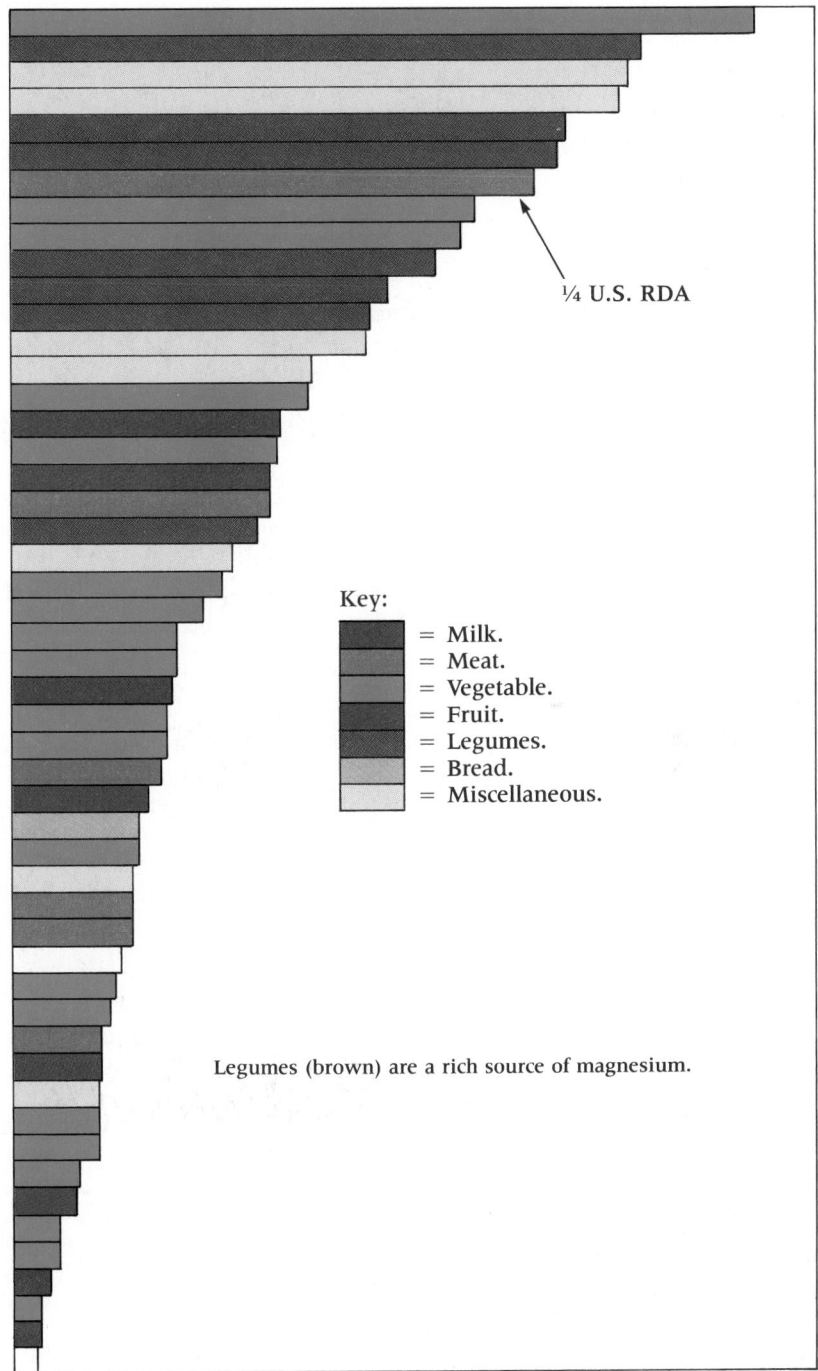

U.S. RDA = 400 milligrams

¼ U.S. RDA

Key:
= Milk.
= Meat.
= Vegetable.
= Fruit.
= Legumes.
= Bread.
= Miscellaneous.

Legumes (brown) are a rich source of magnesium.

Milligrams/Serving

■ TABLE 10–14
Sulfur—A Summary

Chief Functions in the Body	Deficiency Symptoms	Toxicity Symptoms	Significant Sources
As part of proteins, stabilizes their shape by forming sulfur-sulfur bridges; part of the vitamins biotin and thiamin and the hormone insulin; involved in the body's detoxification processes (combines with toxic substances to form harmless compounds)	None known; protein deficiency would occur first	Toxicity would occur only if sulfur amino acids were eaten in excess; this (in animals) depresses growth	All protein-containing foods

The major minerals, especially sodium, chloride, and potassium, influence the body's fluid balance and acid-base balance. Each of the major minerals also plays a variety of specific other roles in the body. Calcium, phosphorus, and magnesium, in particular, contribute to the structure of the bones. When you consider the tasks these minerals perform, you can appreciate their great importance to life.

SELF STUDY *Evaluate Your Intakes of Major Minerals*

1. Look up and record your recommended intake of calcium. Also record your actual intake, from the average derived on Form 2. What percentage of your recommended intake did you consume? Was this enough? What foods contribute the greatest amount of calcium to your diet? If you consumed more than the recommendation, was this too much? Why or why not? In what ways would you change your diet to improve it in this respect?

2. To estimate sodium intake, it is necessary either to add no salt at the table or to measure the amount you do add. The easiest way to measure salt used is to weigh the saltshaker on a gram balance at the start of the day, use only that salt-shaker all day and only for yourself, and weigh it again at the end of the day. The number of grams of salt used, times 0.40, is the number of grams of sodium used.

Estimate your sodium intake by totaling the sodium in the foods you consumed with that added at the table. Be careful to note whether the foods were home-prepared, with or without added salt, or whether they were preprepared. Read labels if you use processed foods. Be aware that sodium contents of foods are more difficult to estimate, because they are more variable, than other nutrient contents of foods.

Now compare your estimated intake with recommendations described in the chapter—not more than 6 grams (6,000 milligrams) of added salt per day. This means 2.4 grams (2,400 milligrams) of sodium in the added salt. (By "added salt," we mean salt added in processing or by you in cooking or at the table. It is assumed that foods you eat already contain about 3 grams of naturally occurring salt. So in comparing with recommendations, count only the sodium you find in processed foods and in the saltshaker.) If your typical intake is below this amount, congratulations.

3. Calculate your intakes of magnesium and potassium, and compare them with the recommended intakes. If you need to improve your diet with respect to these minerals, how will you go about doing so?

Study Questions

1. Name the organs, hormones, and major minerals responsible for regulating the constancy of body salts and water balance.
2. How does the body adjust its acid-base balance?
3. What is the major function of sodium in the body? Describe the role of the kidney in regulating blood sodium.
4. Describe bone development through the life cycle. Which nutrients and compounds are involved in building and maintaining bone?
5. List the roles of calcium in the body. How does the body maintain a constant blood level of calcium regardless of dietary intake? When would a calcium supplement be recommended? How would you go about choosing one?
6. List the roles of phosphorus in the body. Discuss the relationships between calcium and phosphorus.
7. State the major functions of chloride, potassium, magnesium, and sulfur in the body. Are deficiencies of these nutrients likely to occur in your own diet? Why?

Notes

1. Nutrition Committee, American Heart Association, *Dietary Guidelines for Healthy American Adults: A Statement for Physicians and Health Professionals* (Dallas, Tx.: American Heart Association, 1988).
2. M. Biertino, G. K. Beauchamp, and K. Engelman, Long-term reduction in dietary sodium alters the taste of salt, *American Journal of Clinical Nutrition* 36 (1982): 1134–1144.
3. M. J. Fregly, Sodium and potassium, in *Present Knowledge in Nutrition*, 5th ed. (New York: Nutrition Foundation, 1984), pp. 439–458.
4. N. Akaike, Sodium pump in skeletal muscle: Central nervous system-induced suppression by alpha-adrenoreceptors, *Science* 213 (1981): 1252–1254.
5. Fregly, 1984.
6. D. L. Costill, R. Cote, and W. J. Fink, Dietary potassium and heavy exercise: Effects on muscle water and electrolytes, *American Journal of Clinical Nutrition* 36 (1982): 266–271.
7. P. G. Lindner, Caution: All potassium supplements are not the same! *Obesity and Bariatric Medicine* 10 (1981): 87, 89, 92.
8. R. P. Heaney and coauthors, Calcium nutrition and bone health in the elderly, *American Journal of Clinical Nutrition* 36 (1982): 986–1013.
9. L. V. Avioli, Calcium and osteoporosis, *Annual Review of Nutrition* 4 (1984): 471–491.
10. L. Halioua and J. J. B. Anderson, Lifetime calcium intake and physical activity habits: Independent and combined effects on the radial bone of healthy premenopausal Caucasian women, *American Journal of Clinical Nutrition* 49 (1989): 534–541.
11. L. H. Allen, Calcium bioavailability and absorption: A review, *American Journal of Clinical Nutrition* 35 (1982): 783–808.
12. R. P. Heaney, R. R. Recker, and S. M. Hinders, Variability of calcium absorption, *American Journal of Clinical Nutrition* 47 (1988): 262–264.
13. Allen, 1982.
14. Heaney, 1988.
15. K. J. Polley, Effect of calcium supplementation on forearm bone mineral content in postmenopausal women: A prospective, sequential controlled trial, *Journal of Nutrition* 117 (1987): 1929–1935.
16. L. D. McBean, Food versus pills versus fortified foods, *Dairy Council Digest* 58 (March–April 1987), pp. 7–12.
17. McBean, 1987.
18. B. G. Shah, Calcium supplementation with antacids, *Journal of the American Medical Association* 257 (1987): 541.
19. J. L. Greger, Food, supplements, and fortified foods: Scientific evaluations in regard to toxicology and nutrient bioavailability, *Journal of the American Dietetic Association* 87 (1987): 1369–1373.
20. Greger, 1987; M. S. Sheikh and coauthors, Gastrointestinal absorption of calcium from milk and calcium salts, *New England Journal of Medicine* 317 (1987): 532–536.
21. R. P. Heaney and coauthors, Meal effects on calcium absorption, *American Journal of Clinical Nutrition* 49 (1989): 372–376.
22. Not all calcium pills provide calcium, *Tufts University Diet and Nutrition Letter* 6 (April 1988): 1.
23. More on supplementation: Calcium redux, *Nutrition Action*, December 1984, pp. 12–13.
24. McBean, 1987.
25. J. Mayer and J. Goldberg, Sufficient calcium intake still a major problem, *Tallahassee Democrat*, 5 November 1987.
26. P. O. Wester, Magnesium, *American Journal of Clinical Nutrition* 45 (1987): 1305–1312; Food and Nutrition Board, *Recommended Dietary Allowances*, 10th ed. (Washington, D.C.: National Academy Press, 1989), pp. 190–191.

Dental Health

People generally take their teeth for granted, as long as they are working well. They fail to appreciate the major contributions dental health makes to overall health. When things go wrong with a person's ability to chew, however, the whole body suffers. Dentists and periodontists know this, and they make strenuous efforts to inform their clients of the importance of attending to their dental health.

Nutrition plays several roles in supporting dental health. Nutrients influence the development of the teeth and food and eating habits affect the development of dental caries. Each of these is discussed in turn in the sections that follow.

Tooth Development

Primary tooth development in human beings begins during the first trimester of pregnancy. By the last trimester,

Good dental health shows itself in an attractive smile.

permanent teeth are forming in the fetus. Of the ultimate 52 primary and permanent teeth that human beings form, 32 have begun to develop during pregnancy.[1] Maternal nutrition during pregnancy therefore profoundly influences the development of the teeth. Maternal nutrients must supply the preeruptive teeth with the building materials needed to develop in the proper sequence.

To a great extent, heredity determines the potential arrangement of teeth, their eruption time, the tooth pattern and bite, the pits and fissures on the tooth surfaces, and the teeth's resistance to decay. Nutrition is one of several factors that help to determine the extent to which these potentials are realized. Chronic malnutrition during tooth development can interfere with tooth formation, delay the time of tooth eruption, and increase susceptibility of the teeth to caries.[2]

Figure H10–1 shows the anatomy of a tooth. The cells responsible for creating a tooth are odontoblasts (dentin-forming cells) and ameloblasts (enamel-forming cells). The dentin interior and the outer enamel shell of the tooth are built on protein matrices that are subsequently mineralized—primarily with calcium, magnesium, and phosphorus. For dentin, the protein foundation is a collagen matrix, which requires a variety of substances, including vitamin C, for proper formation. The protein matrix for enamel is keratin, which depends in part on vitamin A for its synthesis. If protein or either vitamin is deficient during tooth development, then an imperfect matrix is laid down, and even with successful mineralization, the final structure will be imperfect. Likewise, if the protein matrix is normal but mineralization is not, then the tooth will be poorly formed. Table

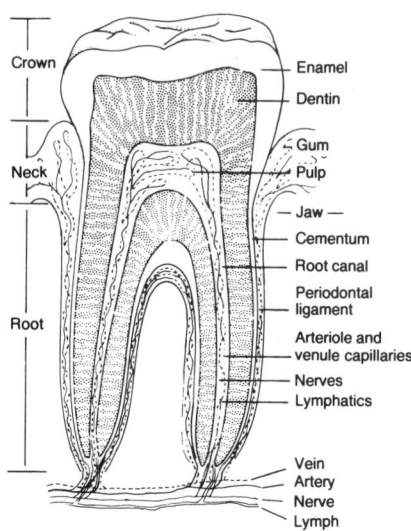

■ FIGURE H10–1
The Anatomy of a Tooth

H10–1 summarizes some of the effects of nutrient deficiencies on dental development.

The table shows the effects of deficiencies of all of the nutrients just mentioned—protein, the minerals that serve as building materials, and the vitamins that assist in the building of the tooth. In most instances, the effects are easily explained. As would be expected, protein deficiency makes teeth smaller, slower to erupt, and more irregularly shaped than normal.[3] The way in which it makes them susceptible to caries appears to be by reducing salivary flow.[4] Even when protein deficiency during pregnancy and early infancy is later corrected with an adequate diet, reduced salivary flow persists, reflecting an irreversible effect of early protein deficiency on gland function.

Iron deficiency appears to act in the same way. Prenatal iron deficiency, even if marginal, decreases salivary flow and salivary protein content in rats.[5] These salivary factors correlate with a high incidence of caries. Suboptimal zinc status prior to tooth eruption is also associated with an increase in dental caries.[6] The last nutrient mentioned in Table H10–1 is fluoride, known to be important in converting the basic tooth crystal, hydroxyapatite, to the more decay-resistant crystal, fluorapatite. Altogether, nutrition during tooth development clearly has a major influence on future dental health.

The 20 primary teeth (sometimes referred to as baby teeth) begin to erupt at around four months of age and continue erupting through the third year of life. Tooth development continues to depend on *systemic* nutrition—that is, nutrients supplied to the body by way of the vascular system—until the final tooth erupts at around age 13. The formation and mineralization of teeth continues to depend on all of the nutrients named in Table H10–1.

At the same time, as childhood progresses, the effect of nutrition on the teeth becomes increasingly more *environmental* than systemic; that is, the presence of food in the mouth increasingly affects the health of the teeth.

Dental Caries

Dental caries is an infectious oral disease that attacks the structure of the teeth. It is a pervasive health problem affecting 95 percent of the population.

The relationship between teeth, food, and caries development is complex and is complicated further by individual factors, such as the hormones and immunity, that affect susceptibility to caries. Additional considerations are the behaviors and lifestyles that influence food selection, eating habits, and oral hygiene.

Caries develops as the result of the metabolism of fuels by microorganisms that reside in plaque on the surface of the teeth. These microorganisms consume carbohydrates, producing organic acids such as lactic acid and

■ **TABLE H10–1**
Nutrient Deficiencies Affecting Tooth Development

Nutrient Deficiency	Effect on Tooth Development
Protein	Small, irregularly shaped teeth; delayed eruption; high caries susceptibility
Vitamin C	Disturbance of collagen matrix of dentin
Vitamin A	Disturbance of keratin matrix of enamel, delayed eruption, poor formation
Vitamin D	Poor mineralization, pitting, striations
Calcium	Poor mineralization
Phosphorus	Poor mineralization
Magnesium	Enamel underdeveloped
Iron	High caries susceptibility
Zinc	High caries susceptibility
Fluoride	High caries susceptibility

Source: Adapted from H. M. Leicester, Nutrition and the tooth, *Journal of the American Dental Association* 52 (1956): 284–289; A. E. Nizel, Preventing dental caries: The nutritional factors, *Pediatric Clinics of North America* 24 (1977): 141–155; J. H. Shaw and E. A. Sweeney, Oral health, in *Nutritional Support of Medical Practice*, eds. H. A. Schneider, C. E. Anderson, and D. B. Coursin (Philadelphia: Harper & Row, 1983) pp. 517–540.

pyruvic acid as wastes. These acids cause the pH in the plaque and saliva to fall, and this leads to demineralization of the basic crystal of the enamel, hydroxyapatite. Calcium and phosphorus dissociate from the hydroxyapatite crystals and diffuse into the plaque. Fortunately, salivary fluids dilute the contents of the mouth and salivary proteins buffer it, returning the pH to neutral. This results in plaque that is at neutral pH and supersaturated with calcium and phosphorus. A reverse flow of the calcium and phosphorus back into the enamel—that is, a remineralization of the enamel—can now occur. Until recently, caries development was considered to be a continuing demineralization process. Now it is viewed more as a dynamic process—one of alternating phases of demineralization and remineralization. When the net result is demineralization, caries develops.

Research conducted using animals reveals that at least two main ingredients are required to make dental caries: microorganisms and carbohydrates. Without microorganisms, there is no caries; that is, decay does not develop in a germ-free mouth, even with a cariogenic diet. Likewise, without a carbohydrate source, caries does not develop. Teeth remain caries-free when carbohydrate is fed via a tube into the GI tract, even when the mouth is infected with microorganisms.

This discussion of caries development begins with the microorganisms that inhabit the mouth, the saliva that influences the mouth, and the protective role of fluoride. The focus later shifts to the diet, the cariogenicity of foods, and the person's eating habits.

Microorganisms

The principal dental plaque–forming, caries–producing microorganism is *Streptococcus mutans*, although other microorganisms have been shown to cause caries. *S. mutans* is found in caries, adheres readily to tooth surfaces, and uses carbohydrate from food to produce acid. Research to develop a vaccine or oral antibiotics against dental caries is focusing on this organism.

In addition to acids, *S. mutans* produces sticky polysaccharides from sucrose and other carbohydrates. These polysaccharides allow the microorganisms to adhere to the smooth enamel surfaces, creating the clusters of plaque. As the bacteria continue to metabolize carbohydrates, the acids become concentrated at the site, and a carious lesion begins.

Saliva

Most people fail to fully appreciate the complexities and contributions of saliva to their oral health. Fluids secreted by the salivary glands vary according to stimulation, age, sex, time of day, diet, diseases, and drug intake. Approximately 1 liter of saliva is secreted in a day in response to the chewing of food. Salivary flow during other times of the day is small, and during sleep, it is minimal. One of the major actions of salivary fluids is protection against dental caries. Saliva dilutes acid and normalizes pH as mentioned earlier; rinses the mouth; provides minerals; and exerts antibacterial activity.[7] The power to elicit secretion of saliva is one of the factors that determines the cariogenicity of foods discussed later. When salivary flow is reduced, the mouth is less able to defend against caries.

Fluoride

The importance of fluoride to tooth protection has long been known. Numerous studies have shown that when fluoride is added to the water supply, the children in the community have fewer dental caries than children who drink nonfluoridated water. Children provided with optimally fluoridated water from birth have 50 to 70 percent fewer caries than otherwise expected.

Water fluoridation is the most effective, least expensive way to provide dental care to everyone. It protects the poor, the uninformed, and people who simply do not practice regular preventive measures or seek professional care. However, one-third of the U.S. population is not receiving fluoride because water fluoridation has not been adopted by their local communities or the private water companies that serve them.

The National Research Council of the National Academy of Sciences recommends fluoridation of drinking water to reach concentrations of approximately 1 part fluoride per 1 million parts water (1 ppm, which is the same as 1 milligram per liter). Water with 1 part per million fluoride offers the greatest caries protection at virtually no risk of fluorosis. Liquid fluoride supplements are available by prescription, and supplementation is recommended when the natural fluoride concentration in water is below 0.7 parts per million. Table H10–2 lists the American Dental Association's recommended supplement dosages by age.

All food and water supplies naturally contain variable amounts of fluoride in trace quantities.[8] About half of the U.S. population has access to water with an optimal fluoride concentration. Foods are not a major source of fluoride. The fluoride content of foods that are processed with fluoridated water, however, is higher than that of the same foods processed with fluoride-free water. The effect of water fluoridation on the food supply is becoming evident.

■ TABLE H10–2
American Dental Association's Recommended Fluoride Supplement Dosages for Low-Fluoride Areas

Age	Dosage
0 to 2 yr	0.25 mg/day
2 to 3 yr	0.50 mg/day
3 to 10+ yr	1.00 mg/day

Source: Adapted from Effect of fluoride on dental health, *Nutrition and the M.D.,* December 1980, pp. 3–4.

As would be expected, the fluoride content of beverages is also higher when they are processed with fluoridated water. The Food and Drug Administration has set limits on the natural and added fluoride content for domestic and imported bottled water. Most teas contain appreciable natural fluoride (contributing about 0.1 milligram fluoride per cup), even when brewed in fluoride-free water. An exception is herbal tea, popularly accepted as a caffeine-free alternative, which has negligible fluoride.

Excess fluoride causes dental fluorosis, a developmental imperfection of the tooth surface. At doses of 2 parts per million, the teeth appear extremely white; at doses greater than 4 parts per million, brown stains appear. (Stains on the teeth are also produced by other factors. For example, when taken prenatally or during the first eight years of life, tetracycline stains teeth. Like the fluoride stains, tetracycline stains are permanent but do not weaken the tooth structure.) Although the brown stains of fluorosis are cosmetically unattractive, dental fluorosis does not threaten health. Studies confirm that drinking water fluoridated to recommended levels poses no adverse health effects.[9]

The *preeruptive* maturation stage of tooth development is the critical time for *systemic* fluoride to offer its benefits in making the teeth resistant to caries throughout life.[10] This stage begins before birth and ends when the last molar erupts. It is during this time that the calcium and phosphate in the enamel are combining into hydroxyapatite, and systemic fluoride can convert it into fluorapatite—a combination of calcium fluoride and calcium phosphate. The benefit of this conversion is, as mentioned, that fluorapatite is more resistant than hydroxyapatite to the acid demineralization process that initiates dental caries.

The *posteruptive* maturation phase of tooth development is when *topical* fluoride makes the teeth resistant to caries.[11] Immediately after a tooth erupts, and for the following two to three years, the outer enamel surface is immature. This is an ideal time to expose the teeth to the protection of fluoride, because they can take up minerals. (They are also more prone to decay if exposed to harmful substances.) Topical fluoride produces calcium fluoride and fluorapatite compounds. Such fluoride application also disrupts the normal growth and activity of dental plaque bacteria.[12]

Fluoridated drinking water offers both systemic benefits to developing teeth and topical benefits to those teeth already present. Fluoride in the drinking water washes over the teeth during their development, enabling them to continuously incorporate fluoride into their crystals.

Topical fluoride can partially compensate for long periods of enamel formation without systemic fluoride, but the enamel thus produced is not as resistant to decay—it contains less fluorapatite. Even after teeth are formed, it is ideal to have fluoride continuously present in the mouth. Teeth continue to exchange materials with the surrounding fluid all the time. This is why fluoridation of water is preferable to topical fluoride. For children who do not drink fluoridated water, fluoride tablets or drops are an effective method of providing both topical and systemic benefits.

The rate of dental caries in the general population is declining, with major credit going to water fluoridation. Even in communities without fluoridated water, however, the prevalence of caries is declining.[13] This may be due to the increase of fluoride in the food supply, as already mentioned, because the use of fluoridated water in food processing is becoming increasingly common.[14]

Periodontal Disease

Although caries is declining, periodontal disease, or gum disease, still poses a large threat to most people, affecting over half of adults over age 45.[15] Periodontal disease is preventable with diligent oral hygiene, but if left untreated, it leads to bleeding gums, loosening of the teeth, and eventual loss of teeth.

Systemic nutrition may influence periodontal health by way of the immune system, bone metabolism, collagen formation, and epithelial tissue function. Consider, for example, that the oral epithelium has a rapid cell turnover rate, replacing cells every three to seven days. Any stress that compromises this ability to regenerate weakens the defense against microorganisms and, therefore, against gum disease.

The progress of gum disease can be slow and unnoticeable. It may first become evident when gums bleed while a person is brushing teeth. The same plaque that causes dental caries is the major initiating factor in gum disease. The plaque on tooth surfaces collects calcium salts, hardens, and turns into deposits of calculus, or tartar. The gums surrounding the tooth's root become inflamed and infected. If the infection progresses, resorption of the bone below the tooth begins, causing the tooth to lose its anchor.

Many factors contribute to gum disease. The primary cause, of course, is poor oral hygiene, but any irritation of the gums weakens their resistance to infection. Stresses such as bad tooth alignment, tooth loss, and tooth grinding can contribute to periodontal disease development.

Another nutrition connection, not often encountered but worth mentioning, is vitamin C, which has long been associated with the integrity of the gums. Gum deterioration is a classic clinical symptom of acute vitamin C deficiency. The effects of subclinical vitamin C deficiency are less well documented, but one study reports that subclinical vitamin C deficiency does influence the early stages of gingival inflammation, even under conditions of sustained good oral hygiene.[16] Gingival bleeding and inflammation varied directly with changes in vitamin C intake and serum concentrations. Vitamin C depletion did not affect other dental measurements observed, such as plaque accumulation.

Foods and Eating Habits to Foster Oral Health

Healthful eating habits from the nutrition standpoint are not necessarily healthful eating habits from the dental standpoint. A selection of foods may provide all the nutrients in adequate amounts to support overall health, but still may promote caries development. Of course, all meals should be followed by proper oral hygiene, but realistically, this does not always happen. The question of what foods are most and least cariogenic is therefore of interest.

The American Dental Association is trying to develop a rating system for the cariogenicity of foods. Most likely, it will be based on the key factor that results from all the characteristics of a food working together—namely, the amount of acid a food produces in plaque. Guidelines based on cariogenicity may eventually find their way to food labels. In Switzerland, foods that pass the acid-plaque test are labeled with a smiley-faced tooth to signify that the product is "safe for teeth." This positive labeling system encourages consumers to purchase such items for between-meal snacks.

Cariogenicity of Foods

The cariogenicity of a food depends on its chemical composition and physical form. The chemical composition of a food includes such things as the type of carbohydrate and the content of dietary acids, calcium, phosphorus, and fluoride. In addition, the food's ability to stimulate salivary flow is considered. The physical form of a food affects its retention in the mouth.

Prime among the relevant characteristics of foods is their

Miniglossary

ameloblasts (ah-MEL-oh-blasts): cells from which tooth enamel is formed.
   amel = enamel

buffer: a substance capable of neutralizing both acids and bases.

calculus: a general term for any abnormal concentration of mineral salts; also referred to as **tartar**.

caries (KARE-eez): the gradual decay and disintegration of a tooth.
   carius = rottenness

cariogenic: conducive to caries formation.

dentin: the main tissue of a tooth surrounding the pulp.
   dens = tooth

enamel: the hard, white, dense substance made up mainly of calcium and phosphorus that covers the crown of the teeth. Enamel is the hardest substance in the human body.

fluorapatite (floor-APP-ah-tite): the stabilized form of bone and tooth crystal (hydroxyapatite), in which fluoride replaces the hydroxy groups of the hydroxyapatite.

fluorosis (flur-OH-sis): mottling of tooth enamel caused by excess fluoride.

gingiva (jin-JYE-va, JIN-jih-va): the tissue surrounding the necks of the teeth and supporting bone; also called the **gums**. Gingival inflammation is known as **gingivitis** (jin-jih-VYE-tis).

hydroxyapatite (high-drox-ee-APP-ah-tite): the major calcium-containing crystal of bones and teeth. See also *fluorapatite*.

microorganisms: small living bodies, such as bacteria, not perceptible to the naked eye.

nursing bottle syndrome: extensive tooth decay due to prolonged tooth contact with formula, milk, fruit juice, or other carbohydrate-rich liquid offered to an infant in a bottle.

odontoblasts (oh-DON-toe-blasts): cells from which dentin is formed.

organic acid: any organic compound containing one or more acid (carboxyl) groups (for example, lactic and pyruvic acids).

periodontal: located around a tooth.

permanent teeth: the final set of 32 teeth that replace the primary teeth.

plaque (PLACK): a sticky, colorless cluster of microorganisms, protein, and polysaccharides that adheres to teeth and gums. Plaque contributes to dental caries and periodontal disease. When calcium combines with the plaque and hardens, it becomes **tartar**.

primary teeth: the first set of 20 teeth that are eventually replaced with permanent teeth; also called **deciduous teeth** or **baby teeth**.

tartar: calcium salts, mucin, and bacteria deposits found on the teeth and gums; also called **calculus**.

---

carbohydrate content. Carbohydrates are the fuel source for bacteria—carbohydrates of many kinds, not just refined table sugar (sucrose). Honey, molasses, brown sugar, glucose, fructose, and starches all have a strong cariogenic potential.

However, sugar alcohols, which are used as sugar substitutes, are either noncariogenic or have extremely low cariogenicity potential. Some may actually have anticariogenic effects. In experimental studies in rats, partial or total substitution of the sugar alcohol

xylitol for dietary sucrose results in caries reduction.[17] The effect is greater than just the displacement of sucrose—xylitol seems to have a therapeutic effect against caries. Rinsing with a xylitol solution after a sucrose-containing meal reduces the cariogenicity of the diet.

While xylitol solutions are not available to consumers, many sugar-free products containing xylitol are available. Children who chewed xylitol-sweetened gum three times a day for two years developed fewer dental cavities than did their classmates who chewed nonxylitol gum.[18] Xylitol stimulates salivary flow, increases pH, maintains a high pH, and resists microbial metabolism.

Other sugar substitutes, such as saccharin, aspartame, and cyclamate, are thought to be protective against caries simply because they are not metabolized to acids. However, one study concluded that saccharin actually inhibited caries in rats.[19] Rats fed a saccharin-supplemented diet developed fewer caries than rats fed the same diet without supplementation or with aspartame supplementation. Offsetting this effect of saccharin are other health risks, though, so its use should be moderate.

In addition to the presence of carbohydrate in foods, the retention of those foods in the mouth is critical.[20] Foods that stay in the mouth for a long time yield acid for a long time. Sticky foods are retained on tooth surfaces longer and present a greater risk than foods that are readily cleared from the mouth. For that reason, the sugar in a soft drink is less significant than that in caramels, pastries, or jelly. By the same token, the sugar in a sticky food such as dried fruit is more detrimental than its quantity alone would suggest.

Stickiness is not the only factor affecting food retention. Curiously, sugar speeds up the clearance rate of starchy foods from the mouth. Starchy foods with a high sugar content are removed more rapidly and lower the pH of the plaque for a shorter time than do starchy foods with less sugar.[21]

The sugar content of a food does not always parallel the amount of acid produced from that sugar or the amount of enamel dissolved.[22] Some foods, such as citrus fruits and carbonated beverages, contain acids of their own, and these acids can act directly on the tooth enamel. These dietary acids are strong enough to depress the pH below the point at which bacterial enzymes are active, so no new acid is formed, but the acid already present is strong enough to dissolve enamel significantly.[23]

Enamel erosion is also seen in people who chew vitamin C tablets for long times. Severe dental erosion was reported in a person who consumed one 12-ounce diet beverage and three chewable 500-milligram tablets of vitamin C daily for three years.[24] While the daily ingestion of carbonated beverages can damage the enamel, in this case the beverage was considered to be an additive, not a primary, factor. With a pH equivalent to that of stomach acid, vitamin C tablets are acidic enough to dissolve enamel. Researchers dissolved a chewable tablet in distilled water and observed the effects of this solution on a healthy tooth.[25] The first three days, the tooth surface was rough. During the fourth through eighth days of the experiment, the size of the tooth began to decrease, and the surface could be scraped away with a fingernail.

Interestingly, a high sugar concentration can also depress bacterial growth and activity. Foods with high concentrations of sugar (candies) rapidly leave the mouth and destroy less enamel than do foods with less sugar in combination with starch (breads and cookies).[26] This effect is not simply explained by the stickiness of the foods. A variety of other factors, including fat and salt content, also influence food clearance.[27] Thus, to predict which

foods will be cariogenic is not as easy as might be expected. Researchers often isolate one dietary factor to determine the extent of its effect on caries development, but when they do so, the usefulness of the findings is limited, because people eat meals that contain multiple dietary factors. Quite often, the findings of such research are variable and inconsistent. Researchers lack standardized reference foods and methods for assessing cariogenic potential. To establish a cariogenicity rating for a food is to rely on many questionable assumptions. Nevertheless, pieces are being collected and analyzed in the hope of assembling a puzzle in which, someday, they will all fit.

Some high-fiber carbohydrate foods are an example of anticariogenic foods. In particular, raw vegetables do not stick to the teeth, and they require vigorous, thorough chewing, which stimulates salivary flow. Increased saliva flow helps to clear the food from the mouth and buffer the plaque acid. The person wishing to minimize caries formation could munch on these types of foods at the end of any meal, if brushing was not feasible. Rinsing the mouth with water also helps, of course.

In contrast, although apples also stimulate salivary flow, they liberate sugar after they have been crushed by the teeth. The sugar contributes to acid formation, which soon offsets the buffering effect of the saliva. This example illustrates how foods may have both caries-promoting and caries-preventing effects.

The best foods to eat at the end of a meal are those that have a saliva-stimulating effect and do *not* depress pH. One example of such a food is cheese. Cheese is a powerful saliva stimulant, and its proteins also buffer pH in the mouth. Even when eaten immediately after sugary foods, cheese raises plaque pH.[28] A piece of cheese eaten at the end of a meal may therefore reduce the cariogenicity of the meal. A further contribution

cheese makes to dental health is its high calcium and phosphorus content.

Eating Habits

So far, these cariogenicity factors have been mentioned: the quantity of carbohydrate, the nature of the carbohydrate, its context (such as the stickiness of the food, or the acid or fiber present in it), and its saliva-stimulating effect. Another concern is the *frequency* of its consumption. Carbohydrate eaten between meals poses a greater risk of dental caries than does carbohydrate eaten with meals. Bacteria produce acid for 20 to 30 minutes after an exposure to sugar. So, if a person were to eat three pieces of candy at one time, the teeth would be exposed to approximately 30 minutes of acid demineralization. If that person were to eat three pieces of candy at half-hour intervals, the time of exposure to acid would increase to 90 minutes. Likewise, slowly sipping a sugar-sweetened soft drink between meals may be more harmful than drinking the entire soda at mealtime.

An extreme effect of prolonged tooth exposure to carbohydrate is seen in infants who are put to bed sucking on a bottle of formula, milk, or fruit juice, or who use such a bottle as a pacifier for extended periods of time. They experience extensive and rapid loss of tooth material. Prolonged sucking on such a bottle bathes the upper teeth for long periods in a carbohydrate-rich fluid. (The tongue covers and protects most of the lower teeth, although they, too, may be affected.) Salivary flow, which normally cleanses the mouth and neutralizes the acid, diminishes as the child falls asleep. The result is decayed teeth (nursing bottle syndrome). This syndrome has also been reported in breastfed infants offered the breast for extended times. To prevent it, children should not be given a bottle as a pacifier at bedtime. If a bottle is given, it should be filled with water. In fact, a mother would do well to offer her infant water after each feeding to rinse the mouth.

It makes sense to select foods with dental health, as well as nutrition, in mind. Of course, it is always best to brush and floss the teeth, or at least to rinse the mouth, after eating meals and snacks, but there is no harm in applying some knowledge of the relative cariogenicity of foods as well. For example, the person who likes raisins might be better advised to eat a carrot-raisin salad with meals after which toothbrushing will follow rather than to eat raisins between meals and let them stick to the teeth. Recommendations from the American Dental Association with respect to foods approved as snacks are provided in Table H10–3.

Teeth can last a lifetime with proper care. They do not have to loosen and fall out, even with old age. It is evident that diet and nutrition can promote dental health throughout life. The same balanced diet that promotes general health can also contribute to sound dental health, provided that, as the American Dental Association recommends, consumers control the frequency with which they eat cariogenic foods, especially when they cannot brush their teeth immediately afterwards. The following guidelines are offered to maximize protection against dental caries and gum disease:

- Do not allow infants to sleep with bottles of carbohydrate-rich liquids.
- Watch for hidden sugars in foods; use low-sugar or sugar-free products whenever possible.
- Restrict sweet treats to mealtimes.
- Practice oral hygiene after eating between-meal snacks.
- Limit the duration of time teeth are exposed to adhesive foods.
- Brush and floss daily, and visit a dentist for regular checkups.
- Rinse with water after eating if brushing and flossing are not possible.
- Drink fluoridated water; provide infants and children with fluoride supplements when such water is not available.
- Eat a balanced diet composed of a variety of foods that will maintain an adequate nutrition status.
- Eat foods rich in calcium and phosphorus.
- Eat a variety of firm, fibrous foods that will stimulate gum tissues, the jaw bones, and the salivary glands.

Other Habits

Dietary measures will serve personal dental health well. For the benefit of the younger generation, it is also important to make efforts to improve the social context so that it will better support their dental health. Unfortunately, much of the effort of the food industry is not directed toward this goal. Printed advertisements and television commercials compete to attract public attention to new items that delight the taste buds, but threaten the teeth. The average television-watching child sees over 21,000 commercials each year; approximately half of those commercials are for foods and beverages, most of which contain sugar.[29] Cereals, candy, and gum lead the list of kinds of foods advertised on the nation's airwaves. Cookies, crackers, desserts, and soft drinks follow close behind. At the bottom of the list are vegetables, citrus fruits and juices, and cheese. The tantalizing messages about high-sugar (and therefore low-nutrient) foods take unfair advantage of an impressionable, nutritionally naive audience.

Take a moment to consider this naive audience. Children spend about 70 hours a year learning about foods by way of television commercials— information that is almost invariably misleading. Compare that to the number of hours parents, teachers, and dentists spend each year providing children with sound nutrition and dental care information. Television commercials do not offer nutrition education, nor do they warn of

■ TABLE H10–3
Dietary Recommendations for Controlling Dental Caries

Food Group	Low Cariogenicity (use when teeth cannot be brushed immediately)	High Cariogenicity (do not use unless followed by prompt and thorough dental hygiene)
Dairy	Milk, cheese, plain yogurt	Chocolate milk, ice cream, ice milk, milk shakes, fruited yogurts, eggnog
Meats/meat alternates	Meat, fish, poultry, eggs, legumes	Peanut butter with added sugar, luncheon meats with added sugar, meats with sugared glazes
Fruits	Fresh, packed in water or juice	Dried, packed in syrup, jams, jellies, preserves, fruit juices and drinks
Vegetables	Most vegetables	Candied sweet potatoes, glazed carrots
Breads/cereals	Popcorn, soda crackers, toast, hard rolls, pretzels, corn chips, pizza	Cookies, sweet rolls, pies, cakes, cereals
Other	Sugarless gum, coffee or tea without sugar, nuts	Sugared soft drinks, candy, fudge, caramels, honey, sugars, syrups

problems certain foods pose to health. They could, however. The Netherlands require that commercials of sugary foods show an insignia of toothpaste being applied to a toothbrush during the last few seconds of the ad.

Consumers can influence television commercials. When the U.S. surgeon general warned of health problems associated with smoking, antismoking commercials were aired until cigarette advertising was eventually banned. Parents and health professionals need to continue making efforts to pressure the industry to respond to their concern for healthy teeth.

A poster in a dental office reminds clients, ''There is nothing the dentist can do that will overcome what the patient will not do.'' Professional dental care, in other words, augments, but does not replace, personal dental hygiene. Learning and practicing good dental hygiene habits, eating an adequate diet, and developing eating habits consistent with dental health will serve a person throughout life.

NOTES

1. F. B. Glenn, W. D. Glenn, and R. C. Duncan, Fluoride tablet supplementation during pregnancy for caries immunity: A study of the offspring produced, *American Journal of Obstetrics and Gynecology* 143 (1982): 560–564.

2. J. O. Alvarez and J. M. Navia, Nutrition status, tooth eruption, and dental caries: A review, *American Journal of Clinical Nutrition* 49 (1989): 417–426.

3. M. C. Alfano, Effect of diet and malnutrition during development on subsequent resistance to oral disease, in *National Symposium on Dental Nutrition*, ed. S. Wei (Iowa City: University of Iowa Press, 1979), p. 23, as cited by M. C. Alfano, Nutrition, sweeteners, and dental caries, *Food Technology* 34 (1980): 70–74.

4. L. Menaker and J. M. Navia, Effect of undernutrition during the perinatal period on caries development in the rat: V. Changes in whole saliva volume and protein content, *Journal of Dental Research* 53 (1974): 592, as cited by Alfano, 1980.

5. M. C. Alfano, J. Sintes, and D. P. DePaola, Effect of marginal dietary iron deficiency during development on caries susceptibility in rats, *Journal of Dental Research* 58 (Special Issue A, 1979): 422, as cited by Alfano, 1980.

6. Increased dental caries in young rats suckled by zinc-deficient rats, *Nutrition Reviews* 37 (1979): 232–233.

7. I. D. Mandel, Relation of saliva and plaque to caries, *Journal of Dental Research* 53: (1974): 246–266.

8. G. S. Rao, Dietary intake and bioavailability of fluoride, *Annual Review of Nutrition* 4 (1984): 115–136.

9. V. L. Richmond, Thirty years of fluoridation: A review, *American Journal of Clinical Nutrition* 41 (1985): 129–138.

10. A. E. Nizel, Preventing dental caries: The nutritional factors, *Pediatric Clinics of North America* 24 (1977): 141–155.

11. Nizel, 1977.

12. Nizel, 1977.

13. J. V. Kumar and coauthors, Trends in dental fluorosis and dental caries prevalences in Newburgh and Kingston, NY, *American Journal of Public Health* 79 (1989): 565–569.

14. D. H. Leverett, Fluorides in the changing prevalence of dental caries, *Science* 217 (1982): 26.

15. Dentistry at the crossroads: The future is uncertain, the challenges are many, *American Journal of Public Health* 72 (1982): 653–654.

16. P. J. Leggott and coauthors, The effect of controlled ascorbic acid depletion and supplementation on periodontal health, *Journal of Periodontology* 57 (1986): 480–485.

17. K. K. Makinen and A. Scheinin, Xylitol and dental caries, *Annual Review of Nutrition* 2 (1982): 133–150.

18. K. Makinen as cited in R. Weiss, Dentistry: A report from the American Dental Association/Federation Dentaire Internationale Joint World Congress, *Science News* 134 (1989): 270.

19. J. M. Tanzer and A. M. Slee, Saccharin inhibits tooth decay in laboratory models, *Journal of the American Dental Association* 106 (1983): 331–333.

20. B. G. Bibby and coauthors, Oral food clearance and the pH of plaque and saliva, *Journal of the American Dental Association* 112 (1986): 333–337.

21. Bibby and coauthors, 1986.

22. C. F. Schachtele and S. K. Harlander, Will the diets of the future be less cariogenic? *Journal of the Canadian Dental Association* 3 (1984): 213–219.

23. B. G. Bibby and S. A. Mundorff, Enamel demineralization by snack foods, *Journal of Dental Research* 54 (1975): 461–470.

24. J. L. Giunta, Dental erosion resulting from chewable vitamin C tablets, *Journal of the American Dental Association* 107 (1983): 253–256.

25. Giunta, 1983.

26. Bibby and Mundorff, 1975.

27. Bibby and Mundorff, 1975.

28. A. J. Rugg-Gunn and coauthors, The effect of different meal patterns upon plaque pH in human subjects, *British Dental Journal* 139 (1975): 351–356.

29. R. B. Choate, Selling cavities—U.S. style. Address presented at the American Dental Association Council on Dental Health Meeting, Miami Beach, Florida, 11 October 1977.

The Trace Minerals

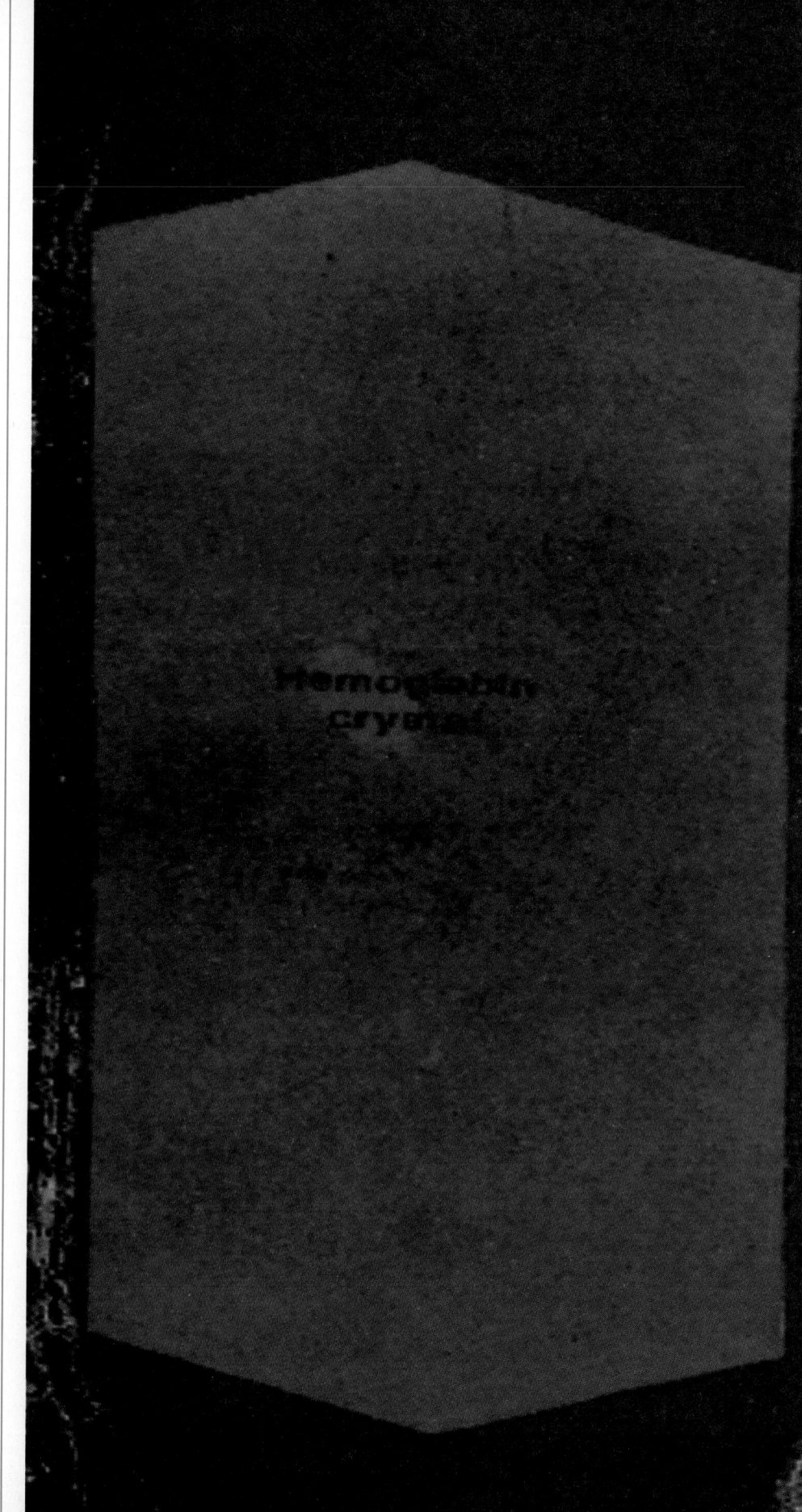

Hemoglobin
crystal

The red pigment of the blood cells is the protein hemoglobin, which contains iron. Hemoglobin is normally dispersed in the cell fluid, but here, due to an accident in preparation, the hemoglobin has crystallized, showing how abundant it is in the red blood cell. The cell is flanked by the walls of the capillary.

At the start of the last chapter, Figure 10–1 showed how tiny are the quantities of trace minerals in the human body. If you could collect them all, you would have only a bit of dust, hardly enough to fill a teaspoon. Yet each of the trace minerals performs some vital role for which no substitute will do. A deficiency of any of them may be fatal, and an excess of many is equally deadly. Remarkably, the way you eat and the way your body handles what you eat normally supplies you with just enough of these minerals to maintain your health.

The contributions of the best-known trace elements—iron, zinc, iodine, and selenium—to human nutrition have been extensively studied, and recommended dietary allowances have been established for them. For five others, the Committee on Dietary Allowances published tentative ranges for safe and adequate daily intakes. Still others are recognized as essential nutrients for some animals, but not proved to be required for human beings. Many other trace elements are presently under study to determine whether they, too, perform indispensable roles in the body.

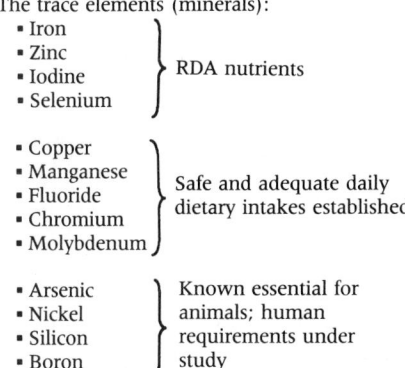

The trace elements (minerals):
- Iron
- Zinc
- Iodine
- Selenium

} RDA nutrients

- Copper
- Manganese
- Fluoride
- Chromium
- Molybdenum

} Safe and adequate daily dietary intakes established

- Arsenic
- Nickel
- Silicon
- Boron

} Known essential for animals; human requirements under study

▪ *Iron*

Iron is vital to cellular respiration—the processes by which cells generate energy. Every human cell, and in fact every living cell of every kind, contains iron. Iron is not rare in nature—but it has many hurdles to jump before assuming its duties in the body, and oftentimes, people simply don't maintain sufficient stores to support their health optimally. In fact, iron is a problem nutrient for millions of people, rich and poor, old and young, male and female, at home and abroad.

Iron in the Body

Iron has the knack of switching back and forth between two ionic states. In the reduced state, iron has lost two electrons, and so it carries two positive charges. Iron in the reduced state is known as ferrous iron. In the oxidized state, iron has lost three electrons, and so it carries three positive charges. Iron in the oxidized state is known as ferric iron. Thanks to this versatility, iron is the ideal mineral to work with proteins involved in oxidation-reduction reactions. In every cell, iron is found in several of the proteins at the end of the energy metabolic pathways. These proteins donate the hydrogens from energy nutrients to oxygen, completing the extraction of energy for the cell's use.

Since muscles use much of the body's energy, they contain much of its iron and use much of the oxygen delivered by the lungs. Oxygen keeps the energy-yielding pathway open so that the muscles can remain active. As the muscles use up and expel their oxygen (combined with carbons and hydrogens), the red blood cells shuttle between muscles and lungs to maintain fresh supplies.

Iron is also found in many enzymes that oxidize compounds, reactions so widespread in metabolism that they occur throughout the body. Iron is required for the making of new cells, of amino acids, of hormones, and of

Iron's two ionic states:
- **Ferrous iron** (reduced): Fe^{++}.
- **Ferric iron** (oxidized): Fe^{+++}.

For details about these ions, oxidation, and reduction, see Appendix B.

The iron-containing proteins at the end of the metabolic pathway include several TCA cycle enzymes and the electron carriers of the electron transport system—known as **cytochromes**. See Appendix C for these pathways.

hemoglobin: the oxygen-carrying protein of the red blood cells.

hemo = blood

globin = globular protein

myoglobin: the oxygen-holding protein of the muscle cells.

myo = muscle

The two proteins in the mucosal cells are (1) **mucosal transferrin** (trans-FERR-in), which passes the iron on to **blood transferrin**, and (2) **mucosal ferritin** (FERR-ih-tin), which holds it in the cell.

The storage proteins are **ferritin** (FERR-ih-tin) and **hemosiderin** (heem-oh-SID-er-in).

"Although erythrocytes occupy less than fifty percent of the volume of the blood fluid, they can absorb seventy-five times more oxygen than can possibly be dissolved in the plasma itself."

"Hemoglobin must be a tricky substance," said Mr. Tompkins thoughtfully.—George Gamow and Martynas Ycas, *Mr. Tompkins inside Himself*

■ **FIGURE 11–1**
Model of Hemoglobin
The hundred-odd stacked planes represent the contours of the coiled protein chains. The flat discs represent heme, nonprotein molecules containing iron that nestle inside of the hemoglobin protein. Oxygen binds to the iron in the heme portions of hemoglobin.

neurotransmitters. Iron also forms part of hemoglobin (the oxygen-carrying protein of the red blood cells) and myoglobin (the oxygen-holding protein in the muscle cells). Hemoglobin accounts for 80 percent of the iron in the body (see Figure 11–1 and Figure 6–5 in Chapter 6). Myoglobin contains smaller amounts, as do other iron-containing proteins.

Iron clearly is the body's gold, a precious mineral to hoard and guard closely. The number of special provisions for its handling, depicted in Figure 11–2, show how vital it is. To obtain iron, the body provides special proteins in the intestinal mucosal cells to help absorb it from food. Two proteins accomplish this. One transfers it to a carrier in the blood for transport; the other holds some iron in reserve in the mucosal cell. If that reserve iron is needed, it is released into the body; if it is not needed, it is shed from the body in the feces when the cell is shed. Intestinal mucosal cells are born, live, and die over about a three-day period, so this reserve provides a buffer against short-term changes in iron need or supply.

The blood protein transferrin captures the absorbed iron and carries it to the bone marrow and other blood-manufacturing sites. Each tissue takes up the amount of iron that it needs. The bone marrow takes large quantities, which are used to make new red blood cells; other tissues take less. In case a surplus accumulates, special storage proteins in the liver, bone marrow, and other organs store it. In a pregnant woman, the placenta avidly accepts iron, delivering large quantities to the fetus, even if this means depriving the mother's tissues of iron.

The average red blood cell lives about four months. When it has aged and is no longer useful, the spleen and liver cells remove it from the blood, take it apart, and prepare many of the degradation products for excretion. The liver saves the iron from broken-down blood cells. The liver can recycle the iron by attaching it to the blood carrier transferrin, which transports it back to the bone marrow. There, the iron is reused to make new red blood cells. Thus, although red blood cells are born, live, and die within a four-month cycle, the iron in the body recycles through each new generation. The body loses only tiny amounts of iron, principally in urine, sweat, shed skin, and blood (if bleeding occurs). The chief storage site for iron held in reserve is the liver.

Normally only about 10 to 15 percent of dietary iron is absorbed, although this amount varies widely from person to person and from time to time in the same person. The amount absorbed can be as low as 2 percent (in a person with GI disease) or as high as 35 percent (in a rapidly growing, healthy child), depending on circumstances. If the body's supply of iron is diminished, or if the need increases for any reason (such as pregnancy), absorption increases. More mucosal and blood transferrin is produced so as to pick up more iron from the intestines, and absorb more into the body.

Iron Deficiency

If stores are used up, or if absorption cannot compensate for losses or low dietary intakes, then iron deficiency sets in. Because so much of the body's iron is in the blood, iron losses are greatest whenever blood is lost. Women's menstrual losses make a woman's iron needs twice as great as a man's, but anyone who loses blood loses iron. Women are especially likely to experience

■ **FIGURE 11–2**
Iron Routes in the Body
Most iron is recycled. Some is lost with body tissues and must be replaced by eating iron-containing food.

Source: Adapted from L. Hallberg, Iron absorption and iron deficiency, *Human Nutrition: Clinical Nutrition* 36C (1982): 259–278.

Note: Ferritin is shown only in the intestinal mucosal cell, although it occurs in other body cells.

iron deficiency, because they not only lose more iron than men but they also eat less food, being smaller, on the average. Even though a woman may never have been diagnosed as iron deficient, she is likely to be deficiency-prone. Should she lose blood for any reason (even by giving a blood donation) or become pregnant (so that her blood volume would increase), she would need to pay special attention to her diet in an effort to maintain her iron stores. The information about iron in foods, which appears later in this chapter, is especially important for women.

The most common tests for iron deficiency are measures of the number and size of the red blood cells and of their hemoglobin contents. But before these levels fall, at the very beginning of an iron deficiency, the transferrin concentration *rises*. A sensitive test that will detect a developing iron deficiency, before it is full-blown, measures the amount of transferrin in the blood and the amount of iron it is carrying.*

When the hemoglobin concentration finally begins to fall, it is a sign that a long period of depletion of body stores has already occurred. In light of the debilitating effects of iron deficiency, it seems reasonable to try to achieve and maintain normal hemoglobin levels. The normal level for adult men is considered to be 14 to 18 grams per 100 milliliters (grams per deciliter); it is

Measurement of the red blood cell number is known as the **rbc count**. Measurement of the volume of the red blood cells packed by centrifuge in a given volume of blood is the **hematocrit**. The method of measuring blood transferrin and the iron bound to it is known as measuring the **transferrin saturation** and **total iron-binding capacity (TIBC)**. The direct test of stores measures **leukocyte ferritin**.

---

*Simultaneously with the rise in transferrin concentration, the concentration of a hemoglobin precursor rises, because without iron, it can't be converted into hemoglobin. The hemoglobin precursor is *erythrocyte protoporphyrin* which can be measured in the red blood cells. The determination of the blood cells' ferritin levels is also a sensitive measure of developing iron deficiency, because their ferritin contents parallel those of other body cells.

■ TABLE 11–1
Iron—A Summary

Chief Functions in the Body	Deficiency Symptoms		Toxicity Symptoms
Part of the protein hemoglobin, which carries oxygen from place to place in the body; part of the protein myoglobin in muscles, which makes oxygen available for muscle contraction; necessary for the utilization of energy as part of the cells' metabolic machinery	**Eyes** Blue sclerae **GI Tract** Lactose intolerance, and possibly intolerance to other sugars; increased risk of lead and cadmium poisoning **Immune System** Reduced resistance to infection (lowered immunity)		Infections
Significant Sources			
Red meats, fish, poultry, shellfish, eggs, legumes, dried fruits	**Nervous/Muscular Systems** Reduced work productivity, tolerance to work, and voluntary work; reduced physical fitness; weakness; fatigue; impaired cognitive function (children); reduced learning ability; increased distractibility (inability to pay attention); impaired visual discrimination; impaired reactivity and coordination (infants) **Skin** Itching; pale nailbeds, eye membranes, and palm creases; concave nails; impaired wound healing **General** Reduced resistance to cold, inability to regulate body temperature, pica (clay eating, ice eating)		

iron deficiency: the state of being without iron stores.

iron-deficiency anemia: the condition in which there are small, pale blood cells resulting from an iron deficiency.

12 to 16 for women.* Yet many people who have values lower than this have no obvious symptoms; apparently the hemoglobin level at which symptoms of deficiency begin to make themselves felt is an individual matter. Table 11–1 includes a list of the symptoms of iron deficiency.

About 20 percent of all women in the United States and Canada, and 3 percent of men, have no iron in their body stores (that is, they are iron deficient); some 8 percent of women and 1 percent of men have the outward symptoms of iron-deficiency anemia. This is an important distinction. Iron deficiency and anemia are not one and the same, though they often go hand in hand. People may be iron deficient without being anemic. The term *iron deficiency* refers to depleted body iron stores without regard to the degree of depletion or to the presence of anemia. The term *anemia* refers to the hematologic state resulting from a severe deficiency. In the case of iron-deficiency anemia, body iron stores are severely depleted, and hemoglobin concentration is low.

_____

*Standard international (SI) unit norms for hemoglobin are 140 to 180 grams per liter for men and 115 to 155 grams per liter for women.

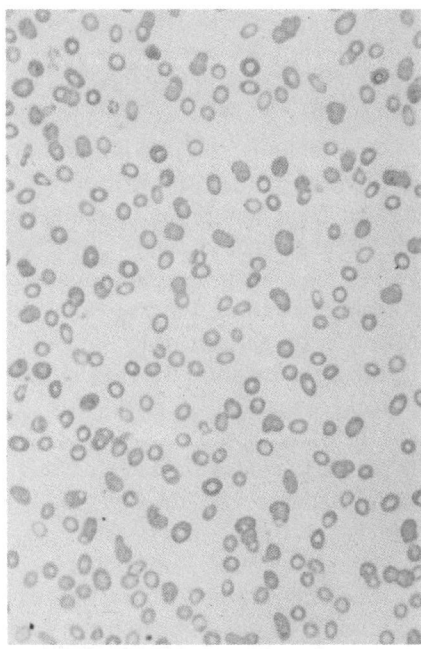

Normal blood cells. Both size and color are normal. The one large, purple cell is a normal white blood cell, stained purple.

Blood cells in microcytic hypochromic anemia such as that caused by iron deficiency. These cells are small and pale because they contain less hemoglobin.

When the body cannot make enough hemoglobin to fill its new red blood cells, the cells are small. Since hemoglobin is the bright red pigment of the blood, the skin of a fair person who is anemic may become noticeably pale. The blood of a person with iron-deficiency anemia contains smaller cells that are a lighter red than normal (Figure 11–3). The undersized cells can't carry enough oxygen from the lungs to the tissues, so energy release in the cells is hindered. Every cell of the body feels this effect; the result is fatigue, weakness, headaches, and apathy.

It is difficult to convey the extent and severity of iron deficiency among the world's people. The incidence of outright anemia can be stated, but people begin to feel the impact of iron deficiency, without knowing it, long before anemia is diagnosed. Iron deficiency occurs in as many as *half* of all persons in some settings, even in developed countries—most predictably in inner-city and rural poor. Long before the mass of the red blood cells is affected, a developing iron deficiency affects behavior. Even at slightly lowered iron levels, the complete oxidation of pyruvate is impaired, reducing physical work capacity and productivity. Children deprived of iron become irritable and restless, due to abnormal levels of the stress hormones in their systems. These symptoms are among the first to appear when the body's iron level begins to fall and among the first to disappear when iron intake is increased again.[1] With reduced energy available to work, plan, think, play, sing, or learn, people simply do these things less. They don't appear to have an obvious deficiency disease; they just appear unmotivated and apathetic. Because they work and play less, they are less physically fit. The incidence in developed countries of iron-deficiency

In a dark-skinned person, paleness can be observed by looking in the corner of the eye. The eye lining, normally pink, will be very pale, even white.

Iron-deficiency anemia is a **microcytic** (my-cro-SIT-ic) **hypochromic** (high-po-KROME-ic) **anemia**.
micro = small
cytic = cells
hypo = too little
chrom = color

There is more on the effects of iron deficiency on children's behavior in Chapter 15.

anemia ranges from 10 to 20 percent; it is higher in the developing countries. Therefore, the incidence of iron deficiency not severe enough to cause anemia must be higher still.[2] If this one worldwide malnutrition problem could be alleviated, the whole world's morale would improve. True, it is only one of many problems, but it is a major one.

The cause of iron deficiency is usually nutrition—that is, inadequate intake, from ignorance of what foods to choose, from sheer lack of food altogether, or from high consumption of iron-poor foods. In the Western world, high sugar and fat intakes are often responsible for low iron intakes. Among nonnutritional causes, blood loss is the primary one, caused in many countries by parasitic infections of the GI tract. In some countries, people go through their entire lives losing blood daily and do not know what it is like to feel energetic.

One of the more recently recognized symptoms of iron deficiency is poor tolerance to cold. You may have seen the headlines "Warm Up with Iron" and "Iron Deficiency Might Give You a Big Chill." While newspaper editors and television commentators were scrambling for the story, researchers were studying the connections between iron and body temperature regulation.[3] In its infinite wisdom, the body has several ways to increase heat production and to minimize heat loss when the environmental temperature drops below the internal body temperature. One of the ways to increase heat production involves the neurotransmitter norepinephrine and the thyroid gland, which releases its hormones to regulate both the metabolic rate and heat production. The body uses its fat stores for insulation to protect against heat losses. Iron deficiency impairs temperature regulation in both animals and human beings, most likely because a lack of iron interferes with normal production of norepinephrine and thyroid hormones. This is apparent even when researchers compare subjects with equal amounts of body fat.

A curious symptom seen in some iron-deficient people is an appetite for ice, clay, paste, and other unusual substances that do not contain iron and so do not remedy the deficiency. In fact, the clay actually inhibits iron absorption. This may explain the iron deficiency seen in people exhibiting such behavior.[4] This behavior has been observed for years, especially in women and children of low-income groups, and has been given the name *pica*.

Many of the symptoms associated with iron deficiency are easily mistaken for "mental" symptoms. A restless child who fails to pay attention in class might be thought contrary. An apathetic homemaker who has let housework pile up might be thought lazy. But the possibility is real that both these persons' problems are nutritional.

No responsible nutritionist would ever claim that all mental problems are caused by nutrient deficiencies. But poor nutrition is always a possible cause or contributor to problems like these. When you are seeking the solution to a behavioral problem, it makes sense to check the adequacy of the diet and to have the results of a routine physical examination before undertaking more expensive and involved diagnostic and treatment options.

pica (PIE-ka): a craving for nonfood substances. Also known as **geophagia** (gee-oh-FAY-gee-uh) when referring to clay eating and **pagophagia** (pag-oh-FAY-gee-uh) when referring to ice craving.

picus = woodpecker or magpie
geo = earth
phagein = to eat
pago = frost

Iron Overload

iron overload: toxicity from iron overdose.

The body absorbs less iron if its stores are full, but iron toxicity can occur; it is rare, but not unknown. Two kinds of iron overload are known. One is caused by a hereditary defect, the other by the ingestion of too much iron, usually in combination with excessive alcohol consumption.* Tissue damage, especially to the liver, occurs in both, and infections are likely, because bacteria thrive on iron-rich blood. The effects are most severe in those who also drink large quantities of alcohol, because alcohol not only damages the liver but also damages the intestine, breaking down its defenses against the absorption of excess iron. Certain wines (especially red wines) contain substantial amounts of iron, as well as sugars that enhance iron absorption; so the overconsumption of wine is particularly risky.

Iron overload is more common in men than in women. An argument against the fortification of foods with iron to protect women is that it might put more men at risk of overload. Indeed, some evidence from Sweden, where foods are generously fortified with iron, indicates that food fortification has increased the incidence of iron overload in men. Unfortunately, a measure meant to promote the health of one sex might put the other at risk.

The ingestion of massive amounts of iron can cause death within four hours after exposure. The second most common cause of accidental poisoning in small children (after aspirin) is ingestion of iron supplements or vitamins with iron. Symptoms of intoxication include nausea, vomiting, diarrhea, rapid heart beat, weak pulse, dizziness, shock, and confusion. As few as 6 to 12 iron tablets have caused death in a child. A child suspected of iron poisoning should be rushed to the hospital to have the stomach pumped; 30 minutes may make a crucial difference.

Iron in Foods

To obtain enough iron from foods, a person must not only select foods that are rich in iron, but must also eat so as to maximize iron *absorption*. This discussion begins by identifying iron-rich foods, then goes on to the problem of absorption.

The usual Western mixed diet provides only about 6 to 7 milligrams of iron in every 1,000 kcalories. The recommended daily intake for an adult man is 10 milligrams, and most men easily eat more than 2,000 kcalories; so a man can meet his iron needs without special effort. The recommendation for a woman during her childbearing years, however, is 15 milligrams.[5] To get 15 milligrams iron from the diet, a woman must emphasize the most iron-rich foods in every food group. On the average, women receive only 10 to 11 milligrams iron per day. The RDA committee attempted to define the dietary intake that would provide for 300 milligrams of iron stores, assuming that this level meets the nutritional needs of all healthy people.

Table 11–2 shows the amounts of iron in foods ranked by iron per serving. As you can see, meats, fish, and poultry rank highest, providing about one-third of the iron in the average diet. Eggs provide some iron, but an

Iron RDA: 15 mg (women during childbearing years).
   10 mg (women after menopause).
   10 mg (men).
Canadian RNI: 13 mg (women during childbearing years).
   8 mg (women after menopause).
   9 mg (men).

Hemochromatosis (heem-oh-crome-a-TOCE-iss) is a hereditary defect in iron metabolism characterized by deposits of iron-containing pigment in many tissues, with tissue damage. *Hemosiderosis* (heem-oh-sid-er-OH-sis) is iron overload characterized by excessive iron deposits in hemosiderin, the normal iron-storage protein.

■ TABLE 11–2
Iron in Commonly Eaten Foods Ranked Richest to Poorest

Food, Serving Size (Energy)

Oysters, 1 c raw (160 kcal)
Spinach, 1 c cooked (41 kcal)
Lima beans, 1 c cooked (260 kcal)
Braunschweiger sausage, 2 pieces (205 kcal)
Beef liver, 3 oz fried (185 kcal)
Peach halves, 10 dried (311 kcal)
Navy beans, 1 c cooked (225 kcal)
Soybeans, 1 c cooked (235 kcal)
Kidney beans, 1 c canned (230 kcal)
Parsley, 1 c chopped fresh (20 kcal)
Sauerkraut, 1 c canned (44 kcal)
Split peas, 1 c cooked (230 kcal)
Black-eyed peas, 1 c cooked (190 kcal)
Green peas, 1 c cooked (67 kcal)
Beef pot roast, 3 oz lean (232 kcal)
Prune juice, 1 c bottled (181 kcal)
Sirloin steak, 3 oz lean (180 kcal)
Baked potato, 1 whole (220 kcal)
Beet greens, 1 c cooked (40 kcal)
Sardines, 3 oz canned (175 kcal)
Clams, 3 oz raw meat (65 kcal)
Tofu (soybean curd), 1 block (86 kcal)
Shrimp, 3.5 oz boiled (109 kcal)
Dandelion greens, 1 c cooked (35 kcal)
Broccoli, 1 c cooked (46 kcal)
Bok choy, 1 c cooked (20 kcal)
Apricot halves, 10 dried (83 kcal)
Green beans, 1 c cooked (44 kcal)
Oatmeal, 1 c cooked (145 kcal)
Brewer's yeast, 1 tbsp (25 kcal)
Butternut squash, 1 c baked (83 kcal)
Asparagus, 1 c cooked (44 kcal)
Wheat germ, ¼ c (68 kcal)
Wheat bran, ¼ c (19 kcal)
Whole-wheat bread, 1 slice (70 kcal)
Peanuts, 1 oz dried unsalted (161 kcal)
Chicken breast, ½ roasted (142 kcal)
Mushrooms, 1 c raw sliced (18 kcal)
Seaweed (kelp), 1 oz raw (12 kcal)
Loose-leaf lettuce, 1 c (24 kcal)
Summer squash, 1 c cooked (36 kcal)
Tomato, 1 whole raw (24 kcal)
Cauliflower, 1 c raw (24 kcal)
Cantaloupe melon, ½ (94 kcal)
Cabbage, 1 c raw shredded (16 kcal)
Sole/flounder, 3 oz baked (120 kcal)
Apple, 1 fresh medium (80 kcal)
Cheddar cheese, 1 oz (114 kcal)
Orange, 1 fresh medium (80 kcal)
Milk or yogurt, 1 c nonfat (86 kcal)

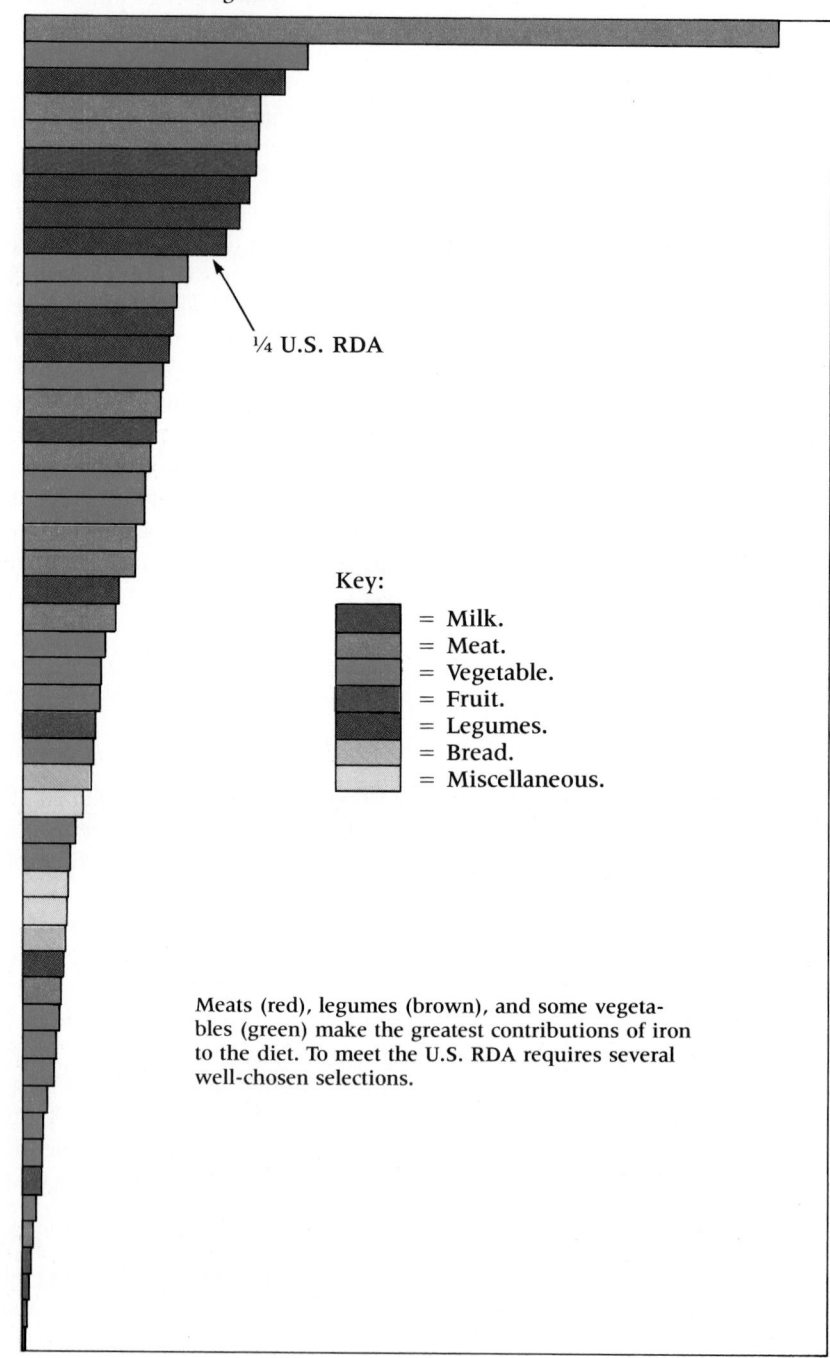

U.S. RDA = 18 milligrams

¼ U.S. RDA

Key:
= Milk.
= Meat.
= Vegetable.
= Fruit.
= Legumes.
= Bread.
= Miscellaneous.

Meats (red), legumes (brown), and some vegetables (green) make the greatest contributions of iron to the diet. To meet the U.S. RDA requires several well-chosen selections.

Milligrams/Serving

How the Recommended Daily Intake for Iron Is Calculated

To calculate the recommended daily iron intake, a number of factors need to be considered. For example, for an adult woman:

■ Losses from urine and shed skin: 1.0 mg.
■ Losses through menstruation (about 15 mg total averaged over 30 days): 0.5 mg.
■ Average daily need (total): 1.5 mg.
■ Average iron intake: 10 to 11 mg/day (provides adequate stores for most women).
■ Added margin of safety to cover the needs of essentially all adult women.

Assuming that an average of 10 to 15% of ingested iron is absorbed, the RDA is set at 15 mg.

---

absorption-inhibiting factor in eggs makes them a poor source. On a per-kcalorie basis, vegetables compare favorably with all other foods.

Foods in the milk group are notoriously poor iron sources, as poor in iron as they are rich in calcium. Although these foods are an indispensable part of the diet, they should not be overemphasized. In considering the grain foods, iron is one of the enrichment nutrients. Whole-grain or enriched breads and cereals—not refined, unenriched pastry products—are the best choices and provide about one-third of the iron in diets nationwide. Finally, among other plant foods, the legume family, the dark greens, and some fruits are the richest in iron.

Now, how can a person eat so as to maximize iron absorption? Iron occurs in two forms in foods: as heme iron, bound into the iron-carrying proteins hemoglobin and myoglobin in meats, poultry, and fish; and as nonheme iron. (Another form of iron that may occur in foods is contamination iron—inorganic salts, which are discussed in the next section.) Heme iron from meat, fish, and poultry contributes only 1 to 2 of the 10 to 20 milligrams of iron the average person consumes in a day; the majority of dietary iron is nonheme iron from vegetables, fruits, grains, eggs, meat, fish, and poultry. Healthy people who are not deficient in iron absorb heme iron at a relatively constant rate of about 23 percent over a wide range of meat intakes. People absorb nonheme iron at a lower rate (2 to 20 percent); its absorption depends on dietary factors and iron stores. People with severe iron deficiency absorb both heme and nonheme iron more efficiently and are more sensitive to dietary enhancing factors than people with better iron status.[6]

Dietary enhancing factors include MFP and vitamin C. Meat, fish, and poultry contain a factor ("MFP factor") other than heme that promotes the absorption of iron, even of the iron from other foods eaten at the same time as the meat. Vitamin C also helps you to absorb iron when it is consumed in the same meal. Vitamin C captures iron and keeps it in a soluble form ready for absorption. Its influence is greatest on nonheme iron absorption. For maximum iron absorption, use one or both of these enhancing factors at every meal. By manipulating the factors affecting nonheme iron absorption,

heme (HEEM): the iron-holding part of the hemoglobin and myoglobin proteins. About 40% of the iron in meat, fish, and poultry is bound into heme; the other 60% is nonheme iron.

MFP factor: a special factor found in meat, fish, and poultry that enhances iron absorption.

Factors that enhance iron absorption:
▪ MFP factor.
▪ Vitamin C.
▪ Other acids and organic acids.
▪ Sugars (including the sugars in wine).

consumers can double or triple the amount of iron their bodies actually derive from foods—an advantage for the person whose energy, and therefore iron, intakes are limited. A system of calculating the iron absorbed from a meal has been worked out by Dr. E. R. Monsen and her coworkers and reveals some of the factors worthy of attention (see box).[7]

This calculation does not predict perfectly the amounts of iron that will be absorbed from meals. One flaw is that it gives credit to vitamin C for enhancing nonheme iron absorption only up to a point. Actually, the absorption-enhancing effect of vitamin C continues to rise as the amount of vitamin C in the meal rises, up to a much higher vitamin C dose than 75 milligrams.[8] Still, the implications of the calculation of Monsen and coauthors are valid in a general way.

Some dietary factors inhibit iron absorption. These include phytates, fibers, soy, and tea.

The differences in iron absorption are so great that to present a table of the iron contents of foods without putting them in context would be misleading. (This is often the case when nutrition theory is compared with reality. The reality is more complex.) Table 11–2 permits you to select servings of foods that are high in iron, but the usefulness of these foods can only be fully realized if they are combined artfully into absorption-enhancing meals.

Factors that reduce iron absorption:
- Phytates; fibers.
- Soy, soy protein, and soy fiber.
- Other legumes.
- Tea (tannic acid); coffee.
- Nuts.

Contamination, Supplement, and Fortification Iron

contamination iron: iron found in foods as the result of contamination by inorganic iron salts from iron cookware, iron-containing soils, and the like.

Contamination iron may increase the diet's iron. In fact, in populations notable for unusually high iron stores, contamination iron from soil or cookware is usually responsible. The knowledge that iron salts can contribute to iron intakes has led people to recommend that consumers cook their foods in iron cookware. For example, the iron content of a half cup of spaghetti sauce simmered in a glass dish is 3 milligrams, but it's 87 milligrams when the sauce is cooked in an iron skillet. Even in the short time it takes to scramble eggs, you can triple their iron content by cooking them in an iron pan. Admittedly, the absorption of this iron may be poor (perhaps only 1 to 2 percent, depending on what else is in the meal), but every little bit helps.

Even after implementing all the strategies recommended so far, a woman may not accumulate enough storage iron to prepare her for the increased demands of pregnancy and childbirth. The Committee on Dietary Allowances and the Canadian RNI acknowledge that pregnant women may need supplemental iron. Iron from supplements is far less well absorbed than that from food, so the doses have to be high. The absorption of iron from iron sulfate, or when taken as an iron chelate, is better than that from other iron supplements. Absorption of iron from supplements also improves when they are taken with meat or with vitamin C-rich foods or juices. Look for the ferrous form, too; it is better absorbed than the ferric form.

The use of enriched or fortified foods, such as breads and cereals, is another option for obtaining an adequate iron intake. These food sources may not be "good" in the sense that single servings convey much iron into the body, but they may be "important," because people eat so much of them that they derive significant iron from the total. Iron added to foods is similar to contamination iron, though; it may boost apparent intakes, but its absorption may be so poor that it may do little or nothing to improve people's iron status.

An iron skillet adds a much-needed nutrient to foods.

This chili dinner provides iron from meat, iron from legumes, and vitamin C from tomatoes. The combination of heme iron, nonheme iron, MFP, and vitamin C helps to achieve maximum iron absorption.

Calculation of Iron Absorbed from Meals

Three factors go into the calculation of the amount of iron absorbed from a meal: first, how much of the iron in the meal was heme and how much was nonheme iron; second, how much vitamin C was in the meal; and third, how much total meat, fish, and poultry (MFP) was consumed. (It is assumed your iron stores are moderate; otherwise, you'd have to take this into consideration, too.) Write down the foods you eat at a typical meal, look up their iron content in Appendix H, and then answer these six questions:

1. How much iron was from animal tissues (MFP)? _____ mg.
2. 40% of (1), on the average, is heme iron: (1) _____ mg × 0.40 = _____ mg heme iron.
3. How much iron was from other sources? _____ mg.
4. This (3), plus 60% of (1), is nonheme iron: (3) _____ mg + 0.60 × (1) _____ mg = _____ mg nonheme iron.
5. How much vitamin C was in the meal? Less than 25 mg is low; 25 to 75 mg is medium; more than 75 mg is high. _____ mg.
6. How much MFP was in the meal? Less than 1 oz lean MFP is low; 1 to 3 oz is medium; more than 3 oz is high.* _____ oz.

Now calculate:
You absorbed 23% of the heme iron, or (2) _____ mg × 0.23 = _____ mg heme iron absorbed.

Now, take your best score from (5) and (6). If either vitamin C or MFP was high or if both were medium, the availability of your nonheme iron was high. If neither was high, but one was medium, the availability of your nonheme iron was medium. If both were low, your nonheme iron had poor availability. You absorbed:

- High availability: 8% of the nonheme iron.
- Medium availability: 5% of the nonheme iron.
- Poor availability: 3% of the nonheme iron.

Now calculate:
You absorbed _____ % of the nonheme iron, or (4) _____ mg × _____ = _____ mg nonheme iron absorbed.
Your total: _____ mg nonheme iron absorbed.
Add the two together:

- _____ mg heme iron absorbed.
- _____ mg nonheme iron absorbed.

Total = _____ mg iron absorbed.
The RDA assumes you will absorb 10% of the iron you ingest. Thus, if you are a man of any age or a woman over 50 years old (RDA 10 mg), you need to absorb 1 mg per day; if you are a woman 11 to 50 years old (RDA 15 mg), you need to absorb 1.5 mg per day. If you have higher menstrual losses than the average woman, you may need still more.

---

*Note on #6: We have adapted the calculation of Monsen and coauthors, stating it in ounces. Her actual numbers are less than 23 g cooked meat, low; 23 to 46 g, medium; and 69 g or more, high.

Source: E. R. Monsen and coauthors, Estimation of available dietary iron, *American Journal of Clinical Nutrition* 31 (1978): 134–141.

In the right food carrier, though, perhaps it can make a difference, and in some cases it may even contribute to iron overload, at least in men. At present, 25 percent of all the iron consumed in the United States derives from foods to which iron has been added, including enriched breads and cereals, and fortified breakfast cereals that boast that they contain 100 percent of the U.S. RDA for iron.

Whatever the iron in the food supply, it is clearly the responsibility of consumers themselves to see that they get enough. Of all the strategies suggested here, the most effective, least expensive one is not to take supplements, but to eat some meats, fish, and poultry frequently, and vegetables and legumes abundantly. The accompanying nutritional benefits would be great.

In case any reader should be left in doubt about whether foods are a better source of iron than fortification or supplements, this discussion of iron closes with two stories—one that took place in the United States, the other in West Java. The first was a study of over 200 adults in Boston who had hemoglobin levels below 13. Two-thirds were given iron-fortified foods for six to eight months; the others were given the same foods without added iron. At the end of the study, the hemoglobin levels of *all* had increased equally. In addition, three months of iron supplements given to those adults whose hemoglobin remained low had no effect. Unfortunately, iron intake prior to intervention was not determined; perhaps both groups increased their dietary iron intakes (one more so than the other). In any case, foods made the difference, with or without added iron.

The study in West Java involved rubber plantation workers with iron-deficiency anemia. The more anemic they were, the less work they could do, and the more often they got sick with infections. Half were given an iron supplement, the other half a placebo—and unexpectedly, both experienced recovery from their anemia and improved markedly in work output. At first glance, it would seem that all the improvement in both groups must have been due to the placebo effect—and clearly the placebo effect did improve both sets of workers' outputs at first. But placebo effects don't usually last beyond a few weeks, and this effect lasted longer. On close inspection, it turned out that the increased work output in both groups had led to increased pay, and they spent the added pay on food. The food supplied 3 to 5 extra milligrams of iron a day, together with vitamin C. Careful analysis of all the circumstances revealed that it was neither the placebo effect nor the iron supplement, but increased iron intakes from food, that accounted for relief of the anemia and its symptoms.[9]

A placebo is a dummy medication, used for its psychological effect, as described on p. 232.

Zinc

cofactor: a mineral element that works with an enzyme to facilitate a chemical reaction; see also p. 293.

Zinc is active everywhere in the body, as the cofactor for more than 70 enzymes that perform specific tasks in the eyes, liver, kidneys, muscles, skin, bones, and male reproductive organs. Much can be understood about its importance and uses by simply reflecting on its close ties to protein. Wherever protein is, there zinc is; and it helps with whatever jobs proteins do. It is so tightly tied up in the body's tissues that it can be made available, in the case of deficiency, only by breaking them down. A regular dietary supply is therefore important.

Zinc in the Body

Among the proteins zinc assists are many whose actions have been mentioned in earlier chapters: an enzyme that frees the vitamin folate so that it can move across cell membranes, an enzyme that helps make parts of the genetic materials DNA and RNA, an enzyme that manufactures heme, an enzyme involved in essential fatty acid metabolism, an enzyme that releases vitamin A from its storage place in the liver, and many others. Zinc is also important in the immune function of white blood cells, in amino acid metabolism, in lipid transport, and in growth and development. Zinc associates with the hormone insulin (although it does not appear necessary for insulin's action), interacts with platelets in blood clotting, affects thyroid hormone function, and affects behavior and learning performance. It is essential to normal salt-taste perception, wound healing, the making of sperm, and the development of the fetus. Zinc deficiency impairs all these and other functions, underlying the vast importance of proteins as the machines that do the body's work.

Zinc, like iron, helps protect the body from heavy metal poisoning—for example, poisoning by lead and cadmium. This is especially important during development of the fetus and during other times of growth. The following highlight reveals the damage these heavy metals can do, and shows the importance of dietary adequacy of zinc and iron in helping ward it off.

The body handles zinc somewhat differently from iron, but with interesting similarities. In the intestine, the mucosal cells provide a two-way passage for zinc from the intestine to the blood (like iron) and back again (unlike iron). Intestinal cells take zinc up for transfer into the blood, where it can travel to the pancreas. The pancreas uses zinc to make some of its digestive enzymes, which it then squirts into the intestine at mealtimes. The intestine thus receives two doses of zinc with each meal—one from ingested foods, and the other from the zinc-rich pancreatic secretions. The circulation of zinc in the body from the pancreas to the intestines and back to the pancreas is referred to as the enteropancreatic circulation of zinc.

After zinc has entered a cell lining the intestine, it may become involved in the metabolic functions of the cell itself or pass through the far side of the cell into the blood going to the liver. The absorbed zinc may also become retained within the cell by a special binding protein similar to the one described earlier for iron and be released at a later time. Thus even zinc that has already entered the body is rescreened periodically by the intestine and can be refused entry or tied up in intestinal cells on any of its times around (see Figure 11–4). Zinc also has its own intracellular storage protein, analogous to iron's ferritin, to hold it inside cells. Zinc exits the body in feces; urine; and shed tissues, including skin, mucosal cells, menstrual fluids, and semen.

A homeostatic mechanism seems to be at work to regulate the amount of zinc entering the body. Extra zinc (like iron) is held within the intestinal cell, and only the amount needed is released into the bloodstream. The zinc status of the individual influences the percentage of zinc absorbed from the diet; if

The binding protein for zinc is a sulfur-rich protein known as **metallothionein** (meh-TAL-oh-THIGH-oh-neen).

metallo = containing a metal
thio = containing sulfur
ein = a protein

The small molecule that assists in zinc absorption is known as the **zinc-binding ligand** (LYE-gand, LIG-and), or **ZBL**.

■ **FIGURE 11–4**
Zinc's Routes in the Body
The bold arrows show the enteropancreatic
circulation of zinc.

more is needed, more is absorbed. Cells are shed daily from the intestinal lining and excreted in the feces; if the zinc trapped in them hasn't been released into the blood by that time, it is shed with them. Figure 11–4 shows the probable body pathways for zinc.

Zinc's two main transport vehicles in the blood are the major blood proteins albumin and transferrin—the same transferrin that carries iron in the blood. This accounts for the observation that zinc absorption is impaired in several conditions. Pregnancy and malnutrition, which lower plasma albumin levels, lower plasma zinc levels as well. Anything that binds transferrin might also hinder zinc absorption. In normal individuals, transferrin is usually less than 50 percent saturated with iron, but in cases of iron overload, it is more saturated. Iron excess thus leaves too few binding sites available, thereby impairing zinc absorption. Dietary iron-to-zinc ratios of greater than 2:1 inhibit zinc absorption, which is another reason why iron supplements need to be used conservatively.

Zinc Deficiency

Data from a nationwide survey have been used to assess the extent of zinc deficiency in the United States. Zinc deficiencies occur in the most vulnerable groups of our population—pregnant women, young children, the elderly, and the poor.

A deficiency of zinc in human beings was first reported in the 1960s from studies with growing children and adolescent males in Egypt, Iran, and Turkey. The native diets were typically low in animal meats and high in whole grains and beans; consequently, they were low in zinc and high in fiber and phytates. Furthermore, the bread they ate was unleavened. In unleavened bread, the phytates are not broken down by yeast in the process of fermentation. Diets high in phytates can impair zinc absorption, and the ratio of phytate to zinc in the diet is used as an index of zinc bioavailability. The zinc deficiency was marked by severe growth retardation and arrested sexual maturation—symptoms that were responsive to zinc supplementation. The World Health Organization recommends an increased zinc intake for populations that use unleavened whole-grain bread as their staple grain product.

Since the 1960s, zinc deficiency has been recognized elsewhere, and it is known to affect much more than just growth. It alters digestive function profoundly by creating deficits in pancreas function, abnormalities in chylomicron formation, and defects in the GI tract lining. It causes diarrhea, which worsens the malnutrition already present, with respect to not only zinc, but all nutrients. It drastically impairs the immune response, making infections more likely—among them, infections of the intestinal tract, which worsen malnutrition, including zinc malnutrition (a classic evil cycle). Chronic zinc deficiency impairs central nervous system and brain functioning. Both older people with senile dementia and younger people with early senility have lower blood zinc concentrations than their lucid peers.[10] Zinc deficiency directly interferes with folate absorption, and it impairs vitamin A metabolism, so the symptoms of those vitamin deficiencies often appear. It disturbs thyroid function and metabolic rate. It alters taste, causes anorexia, slows wound healing—in fact, its symptoms are so all-pervasive that generalized malnutrition and sickness are more likely to be the diagnosis than simple zinc deficiency. Many of the symptoms are similar to those of aspirin toxicity, perhaps because zinc, like aspirin, interacts with the hormonelike prostaglandin system. Table 11–3 includes a list of the symptoms of zinc deficiency.

Generally, zinc deficiency is not widespread in developed countries, although cases have occurred in U.S. and Canadian schoolchildren.[11] A number of Denver children had low hair zinc levels, poor growth, poor appetite, and decreased taste sensitivity.* The children were described as ''picky eaters'' and ate less than an ounce of meat per day. When pediatricians or other health workers evaluating children's health note poor growth accompanied by poor appetite, they should think zinc.

The Egyptian boy in the picture is 17 years old but is only 4 feet tall, like a 7-year-old in the United States. His genitalia are like those of a 6-year-old. The retardation, known as **dwarfism**, is rightly ascribed to zinc deficiency, because it is partially reversible when zinc is restored to the diet.

Zinc Toxicity

Zinc can be toxic if consumed in large enough quantities. Zinc doses two to three times the RDA lower the body's copper content—an effect that, in animals, leads to degeneration of the heart muscle. Higher doses affect cholesterol metabolism, alter lipoprotein levels, and appear to accelerate the development of atherosclerosis. Accidental consumption of high doses of zinc

*Hair analysis used to assess zinc status provides valid information.

■ **TABLE 11–3**
Zinc—A Summary

Chief Functions in the Body	Deficiency Symptoms[a]	Toxicity Symptoms
Part of many enzymes; associated with the hormone insulin; involved in making genetic material and proteins, immune reactions, transport of vitamin A, taste perception, wound healing, the making of sperm, and the normal development of the fetus	**Blood**	
	Tendency to atherosclerosis, elevated ammonia levels, decreased alkaline phosphatase, decreased insulin concentration	Anemia: reduced hemoglobin production
	Bones	
	Growth retardation, abnormal collagen synthesis	Growth in length, but without normal zinc content
	Cells/Metabolism	
	Decreased DNA synthesis, impaired cell division and protein synthesis	Raised LDL, lowered HDL
Significant Sources	**Digestive System**	
Protein-containing foods: meats, fish, poultry, grains, vegetables	Reduced sense of smell, reduced sensitivity to the taste of salt, weight loss, delayed glucose absorption, diarrhea, nausea, impaired folate absorption	Diarrhea, vomiting, decreased calcium and copper absorption
	Eyes	
	Night blindness	
	Glandular System	
	Delayed onset of puberty, small gonads in males, decreased synthesis and release of testosterone, abnormal glucose tolerance, reduced synthesis of adrenocortical hormones, altered thyroid function	
	Immune System	
	Altered skin test responses, reduced numbers of white blood cells and antibody-forming cells, thymus atrophy, increased susceptibility to infection	Fever, elevated white blood cell count
	Kidney	
		Renal failure
	Liver/Spleen	
	Enlargement	
	Nervous/Muscular Systems	
	Anorexia (poor appetite), mental lethargy, irritability	Muscular pain and incoordination, heart muscle degeneration, exhaustion, dizziness, drowsiness
	Reproductive System	
	Impaired reproductive function (rats), low sperm counts	Reproductive failure
	Skin	
	Generalized hair loss; lesions; rough, dry appearance; slow healing of wounds and burns	

[a]A rare inherited disease, *acrodermatitis enteropathica*, causes additional and more severe symptoms.

may cause vomiting, diarrhea, fever, exhaustion, and many other symptoms (see Table 11–3). Large doses are even fatal in experimental animals.[12]

Overdoses of zinc supplements can be toxic. Also, acidic foods or drinks that have been stored in galvanized containers may contain toxic doses of zinc.

Zinc in Foods

In setting the RDA for zinc, the committee assumed that 20 percent of dietary zinc is available to the body. The RDA for all age groups are given inside the front cover, left. Requirements for infants and children are relatively high, due to the role of zinc in normal growth and development.

Zinc-rich foods include oysters, meat, and poultry; whole-grain breads; legumes and nuts; and milk.

Table 11–4 shows zinc amounts in foods per serving. Zinc is highest in foods of high protein content, such as shellfish (especially oysters), meats, and liver. As a rule of thumb, two ordinary servings a day of animal protein will provide most of the zinc a healthy person needs. Eggs and whole-grain products are good sources of zinc if large quantities are eaten; the phytate in grains does not inhibit the absorption of zinc in people consuming ordinary diets. Cow's milk protein (casein) binds zinc avidly and seems to prevent its absorption somewhat; infants absorb zinc better from human breast milk. However, in the adult diet, so long as adequate amounts of animal protein are included, milk does not inhibit zinc absorption.

Zinc RDA: 15 mg/day (men).
            12 mg/day (women).
Canadian RNI: 12 mg/day (men).
              9 mg/day (women).

Contamination zinc, like contamination iron, may add to people's intakes. Vegetables vary in zinc content depending on the soil in which they are grown. The zinc content of cooking water also varies from region to region. Galvanized cooking pots, in earlier times, contributed zinc to foods, especially to acid foods, but with the increased use of stainless steel and plastic utensils to prepare and store food, this source of zinc is no longer significant. Galvanized pipes, used in plumbing, may contribute zinc to people's intakes.

galvanized: term referring to metal containers that have been treated with a zinc-containing coating to prevent rust.

Zinc supplements are seldom appropriate. Much excitement surrounded the 1984 publication of a research study that showed that zinc lozenges shorten the duration of the common cold.[13] Unfortunately, results from many other studies attempting to confirm this finding have contradicted it.[14] Differences in formulation of the lozenges may account for the inconsistency.[15] Different zinc salts have been used in different studies, and some lozenges have zinc chelators to enhance flavor. Depending on the chelator, zinc absorption may be promoted or prevented; thus the studies cannot be compared. The question remains open whether zinc lozenges help prevent colds.

Zinc supplements are useful in two instances, though: one, when used to remedy an accurately diagnosed zinc deficiency; and the other, when used to displace other ions in unusual medical circumstances. Otherwise, it should be possible to obtain enough zinc from the diet without resorting to the use of supplements.

■ Iodide

Like chlorine gas, iodine gas is poisonous; however, the iodide ion, which occurs in foods, is far less toxic. and traces of it are indispensable to life.

■ TABLE 11–4
Zinc in Commonly Eaten Foods Ranked Richest to Poorest

Food, Serving Size (Energy)

Oysters, 1 c raw (160 kcal)
Crabmeat, 1 c canned (135 kcal)
Beef pot roast, 3 oz lean (231 kcal)
Sirloin steak, 3 oz lean (180 kcal)
Beef liver, 3 oz fried (185 kcal)
Lamb chop, 3 oz braised (238 kcal)
Ground beef, 3 oz 10% fat (230 kcal)
Corned beef, 3 oz canned (185 kcal)
Shrimp, 3.5 oz boiled (109 kcal)
Black-eyed peas, 1 c cooked (190 kcal)
Miso, 3 tbsp (88 kcal)
Wheat germ, ¼ c raw (68 kcal)
Turkey, 3 oz (145 kcal)
Pinto beans, 1 c cooked (265 kcal)
Sardines, 3 oz canned (175 kcal)
Kidney beans, 1 c canned (230 kcal)
Clams, 3 oz raw meat (65 kcal)
Spinach, 1 c cooked (41 kcal)
Wheat bran, ¼ c (19 kcal)
Swiss cheese, 1 oz (107 kcal)
Buttermilk, 1 c (99 kcal)
Milk, 1 c whole (150 kcal)
Collards, 1 c cooked (20 kcal)
Peanuts, 1 oz dried unsalted (161 kcal)
Milk or yogurt, 1 c nonfat (86 kcal)
Cheddar cheese, 1 oz (114 kcal)
Tofu (soybean curd), 1 block (86 kcal)
Asparagus, 1 c cooked (44 kcal)
Chicken breast, ½ roasted (142 kcal)
Dandelion greens, 1 c cooked (35 kcal)
Beet greens, 1 c cooked (40 kcal)
Sole/flounder, 3 oz baked (120 kcal)
Summer squash, 1 c cooked (36 kcal)
Brewer's yeast, 1 tbsp (25 kcal)
Green peas, 1 c cooked (67 kcal)
Mushrooms, 1 c raw sliced (18 kcal)
Whole-wheat bread, 1 slice (70 kcal)
Green beans, 1 c cooked (44 kcal)
Parsley, 1 c chopped fresh (20 kcal)
Bok choy, 1 c cooked (20 kcal)
Bean sprouts, 1 c fresh (32 kcal)
Cantaloupe, ½ (94 kcal)
Mustard greens, 1 c cooked (21 kcal)
Cauliflower, 1 c cooked (30 kcal)
Alfalfa seeds, 1 c sprouted (10 kcal)
Broccoli, 1 c cooked (46 kcal)
Romaine lettuce, 1 c chopped (9 kcal)
Loose-leaf lettuce, 1 c (10 kcal)
Orange, 1 fresh medium (60 kcal)
Apple, 1 fresh medium (80 kcal)

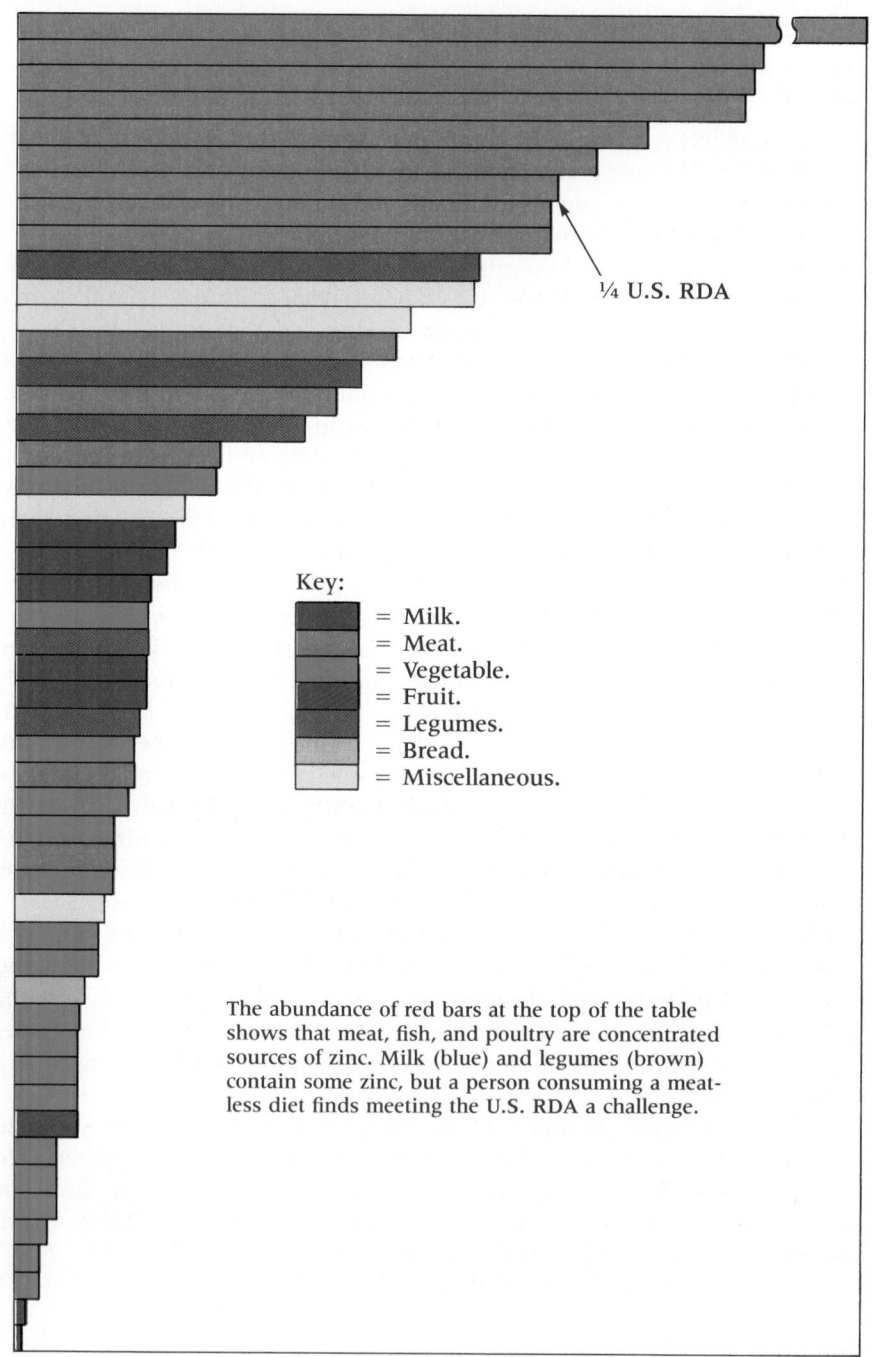

U.S. RDA = 15 milligrams

¼ U.S. RDA

Key:
■ = Milk.
■ = Meat.
■ = Vegetable.
■ = Fruit.
■ = Legumes.
■ = Bread.
□ = Miscellaneous.

The abundance of red bars at the top of the table shows that meat, fish, and poultry are concentrated sources of zinc. Milk (blue) and legumes (brown) contain some zinc, but a person consuming a meatless diet finds meeting the U.S. RDA a challenge.

Milligrams/Serving

Dietary iodine is converted to iodide in the GI tract. Iodide occurs in the body in an infinitesimally small quantity, but its principal role in human nutrition is well known, and the amount needed is well established. Iodide is part of the thyroid hormone, which regulates body temperature, metabolic rate, reproduction, growth, the making of blood cells, nerve and muscle function, and more.* This hormone enters every cell of the body to control the rate at which the cells use oxygen. This is the same as saying that thyroxin controls the rate at which energy is released.

Iodide must be available for thyroid hormones to be synthesized. The amount in the diet is variable and generally reflects the amount present in the soil in which plants are grown or on which animals graze. Iodide is plentiful in the ocean, so seafood is a dependable source. Land masses that have been under the ocean have soils rich in iodide; those that have not have iodide-poor soils. In the United States and Canada, the soil is iodide-poor in the area around the Great Lakes and the inland valleys of Oregon. The iodization of salt in these regions eliminated the widespread misery caused by iodide deficiency in the local people during the 1930s.

A specific hormone regulates thyroid gland activity by trapping iodide ions for the synthesis (and secretion) of thyroid hormones.** When the iodide level of the blood is low, the cells of the thyroid gland enlarge, so as to trap as many atoms of iodide as possible. If the gland enlarges until it is visible (Figure 11–5), the condition is called a simple goiter. Goiter afflicts about 200 million people the world over, many of them in Africa. In all but 4 percent of these cases, the cause is iodide deficiency. As for the 4 percent (8 million), who are mostly in Africa, they have goiter because they overconsume plants of the cabbage family and others that contain an antithyroid substance (goitrogen) whose effect is not counteracted by dietary iodide. The goitrogens present in plants serve notice that even natural components of foods can cause harm when eaten in excess, a topic described further in Chapter 16.

An iodide deficiency causes sluggishness and weight gain. During pregnancy, it may have serious effects on the development of the fetus in the uterus. Severe thyroid undersecretion during pregnancy causes the extreme and irreversible mental and physical retardation known as cretinism. An infant with cretinism has an IQ as low as 20 and a face and body with many abnormalities. Much of the mental retardation associated with cretinism can be averted by diagnosis of iodide deficiency and its treatment early in pregnancy.

The recommended intake of iodine for adults is a minuscule amount. The need for iodide is easy to meet by consuming seafood, vegetables grown in iodide-rich soil, and (in iodide-poor areas) iodized salt. In the United States, you have to read the label to find out whether salt is iodized; in Canada, all table salt is iodized.

Excessive intakes of iodide can also cause an enlargement of the thyroid gland, just as deficiency can. This goiterlike condition can be so severe as to block the airways in infants and cause suffocation. A dramatic increase in

■ **FIGURE 11–5**
Simple Goiter
In iodide deficiency, the thyroid gland enlarges.

thyroxin (thigh-ROX-in): a hormone secreted by the thyroid gland; it regulates the basal metabolic rate.

goiter (GOY-ter): an enlargement of the thyroid gland due to an iodide deficiency, malfunction of the gland, or over consumption of a goitrogen. Goiter caused by iodide deficiency is **simple goiter**.

goitrogen (GOY-troh-jen): a thyroid antagonist found in food; causes **toxic goiter**.

cretinism (CREE-tin-ism): an iodide-deficiency disease characterized by mental and physical retardation.

Iodine RDA: 150 μg/day.
Canadian RNI: 160 μg/day.

2 g iodized salt (less than ½ tsp) contains the RDA for iodine.

---

*The thyroid gland actually secretes two hormones, triiodothyronine (T_3) and tetraiodothyronine (T_4), more commonly known as *thyroxin*.

**The regulating hormone is thyrotropic hormone or thyroid stimulating hormone (TSH), a hormone secreted from the pituitary to act on the thyroid gland.

■ TABLE 11–5
Iodide—A Summary

Chief Functions in the Body	Deficiency Symptoms	Toxicity Symptoms	Significant Sources
A component of the thyroid hormone thyroxin, which helps to regulate growth, development, and metabolic rate	Enlargement of the thyroid gland, weight gain, mental and physical retardation of an infant	Enlargement of the thyroid gland, depressed thyroid activity	Iodized salt, seafood, plants grown in most parts of the country and animals fed those plants
Deficiency Disease Name			
Simple goiter, cretinism			

iodide intakes in the United States over the past several decades concerns some observers. Average consumption rose from 150 micrograms per day in 1960 to over 450 micrograms in 1970, and reached an all-time high of over 800 micrograms per day in 1974. It has since declined to about 200 to 500 micrograms with the recent emphasis on restricted salt intake to control high blood pressure. The toxic level at which detectable harm results is thought to be over 2,000 micrograms per day for an adult—several times higher than current average consumption levels.

Some of the excess iodide seems to be coming from fast foods, in which iodized salt is liberally used. Some comes from iodates—dough conditioners used in the baking industry—and from milk produced by cows exposed to iodide-containing medications and disinfectants. In some local areas, overuse of the seaweed kelp and powders made from it has caused iodide toxicity. Now that the problem has been identified, the food industries have reduced their use of these compounds, but the sudden emergence of this problem points to a need for continued surveillance of the food supply. Table 11–5 provides a summary of iodide.

■ *Copper*

The body contains about 75 to 100 milligrams of copper, which performs several vital roles. It is a part of several enzymes. As a catalyst in the formation of hemoglobin, it helps to make red blood cells. It is involved in the manufacture of collagen and the healing of wounds, and it helps to maintain the sheath around nerve fibers. Most of what is known about copper comes from animal research, which has provided clues to its possible roles in human beings. Copper's critical roles seem to have to do with helping iron shift back and forth between its ferrous and ferric states. This means that copper is needed in many of the reactions related to respiration and the release of energy.

Copper deficiency is rare, but not unknown. It has been seen in children with protein deficiency and iron-deficiency anemia and can severely disturb growth and metabolism. Excess zinc, as mentioned, interferes with copper absorption and can cause deficiency.

Estimated safe and adequate dietary intake for copper: 1.5 to 3.0 mg/day.

■ TABLE 11–6
Copper—A Summary

Chief Functions in the Body	Deficiency Symptoms	Toxicity Symptoms
Necessary for the absorption and use of iron in the formation of hemoglobin; part of several enzymes; a factor that helps to form the protective covering of nerves	Anemia, bone changes (rare in human beings)	Vomiting, diarrhea
Significant Sources		
Meat, drinking water		

Copper toxicity symptoms include vomiting and diarrhea at intakes of 10 to 15 milligrams.[16] Larger amounts can be fatal.

The best food sources of copper include grains, nuts, organ meats, and seeds. About a third of the copper taken in food is absorbed, and the rest is eliminated in the feces. Water also provides copper; its content varies with the type of plumbing pipe and hardness of the water. See Table 11–6 for a summary of copper.

■ Manganese

The human body contains a tiny 20 milligrams of manganese, mostly in the bones and glands. Still, this represents billions on billions of molecules. Animal studies suggest that manganese cooperates with many enzymes, helping to facilitate dozens of different metabolic processes. Manganese deficiency in animals deranges many systems, including the bones, reproduction, the nervous system, and fat metabolism.

Deficiencies of manganese have not been seen in human beings. Toxicity may be severe, but is more likely to occur when the environment is contaminated with manganese than from dietary intake. Miners who inhale large quantities of manganese dust on the job over prolonged periods show many of the symptoms of a brain disease, with frightening abnormalities of appearance and behavior. A summary of manganese is given in Table 11–7.

Estimated safe and adequate dietary intake for manganese: 2.5 to 5.0 mg/day.

■ TABLE 11–7
Manganese—A Summary

Chief Functions in the Body	Deficiency Symptoms	Toxicity Symptoms
Facilitator, with enzymes, of many cell processes	(In animals): poor growth, nervous system disorders, reproductive abnormalities	Nervous system disorders
Significant Sources		
Widely distributed in foods		

hydroxyapatite (high-drox-ee-APP-uh-tite): the major calcium- containing crystal of bones and teeth. The stabilized form of bone and tooth crystal, in which fluoride has replaced the hydroxy groups of hydroxyapatite, is **fluorapatite** (floor-APP-uh-tite).

Highlight 10 describes the contributions fluoride makes to tooth development and dental health.

Fluoride

Only a trace of fluoride occurs in the human body, but studies have demonstrated that wherever diets are high in fluoride, the crystalline deposits in bones and teeth are larger and more perfectly formed. When bones and teeth become mineralized, first a crystal called hydroxyapatite is formed from calcium and phosphorus. Then fluoride replaces the hydroxy (OH) portions of the crystal, rendering it more resistant to decay.

Dental caries ranks as the nation's greatest health problem in terms of persistence and the numbers of people affected. By fluoridating the drinking water, a community offers its people, particularly its children, a safe, economical (less than 40 cents per person per year), practical, and effective

 NUTRITION DETECTIVE WORK

The first water fluoridation program was implemented in 1945 and raised fluoride concentrations to 1 part fluoride per 1 million parts water (1 ppm). At this concentration, developing teeth receive the greatest protection against dental caries without health risk to children (Highlight 10 discusses the role of fluoride in dental health). While all food and water contain some fluoride naturally, controversy surrounds the addition of fluoride to water for the purpose of defending against dental caries.

Whenever the issue of water fluoridation arises, people in the community voice their opinions. Although most of the arguments sound logical, if you listen closely to them, you will hear a mixture of facts, fears, and faith. A nutrition detective entering the fluoridation controversy would point out errors, set value judgments aside, and stick to—as Sergeant Joe Friday would say—"Just the facts, ma'am." A look at some of the comments of a person reluctant to fluoridate the water supply and the responses of a nutrition detective might be enlightening.

"Fluorine is a poisonous gas, and I don't want my water poisoned." The thoughtful detective carefully provides the rest of the story. True, *fluorine* gas is poisonous, but the ionic form found in water is *fluoride*. While fluoride, like any substance, including water, can be toxic if consumed in excess (fluoride is fatal at 2,500 ppm), such doses far exceed the standard recommendation (1 ppm).

"Fluoride causes a number of side effects, including tooth discoloration." Once again, the partial story omits pertinent facts, and the detective must fill in the information gaps. High fluoride concentrations (2 to 10 ppm) can stain tooth enamel, and wherever the water supply naturally contains such high concentrations of fluoride, it can be treated to remove the excess. But again, programs add fluoride to reach a concentration of only 1 ppm.

way to prevent dental caries. Wherever the natural concentration falls short of optimal levels, fluoride should be added.

Fluoride is required for growth in animals and is an essential nutrient for human beings; in fact, the continuous presence of fluoride in body fluids is desirable. Drinking water is the usual source of fluoride, although fish and tea may supply substantial amounts.

Estimated safe and adequate dietary intake for fluoride: 1.5 to 4.0 mg/day.

The role of fluoride in protecting against adult bone loss (osteoporosis) is less clear than in protecting against tooth decay. Early studies reported that the incidence of osteoporosis was higher in areas where the fluoride content of the water was low compared with high-fluoride areas. A more recent study found no protective effect with high-fluoride water intake.[17] High fluoride in combination with adequate calcium and vitamin D increases bone mass and reduces the incidence of fractures. Side effects of fluoride therapy include GI distress and nausea.

"Fluoride, even at low concentrations, causes cancer." Few words capture the attention of an audience quicker than *cancer*. Fear takes a strong hold over facts. When rumors of cancer surface, the detective turns to the authorities and finds no scientific evidence to support a link between fluoride and cancer. The World Health Organization, the National Cancer Institute, the U.S. surgeon general, the Centers for Disease Control, and the National, Heart, Lung, and Blood Institute all confirm this conclusion.[18]

"I don't want the government interfering with my water and infringing on my freedom." Being a scientist and not an attorney, the detective seeks legal counsel on this argument and learns that fluoridation has not been considered by the U.S. Supreme Court, but that lower courts have upheld its legality. The courts find that the freedom to derive the well-known benefits from fluoride in drinking water outweighs the freedom from being coerced to drink fluoridated water.

"If fluoride is so safe and effective, why the controversy?" The controversy over the safety of fluoride is not among scientists. A small group of people who usually oppose a number of public health measures, such as polio vaccines and milk pasteurization, use misinformation and fear to convince uninformed people to oppose fluoridation. Scientists and health professionals fully endorse the fluoridation of public drinking water as an effective measure against dental disease.

"If we were meant to consume that much fluoride, the water supply would contain enough of it naturally." The detective realizes that this statement is based on faith alone and recognizes that each of us is entitled to our own beliefs. The role of a scientist is to present the facts, not to pass judgment. With that in mind, the nutrition detective just summarizes the facts, leaving it to the public to recognize the value of water fluoridation.

■ TABLE 11–8
Fluoride—A Summary

Chief Functions in the Body	Deficiency Symptoms	Toxicity Symptoms	Significant Sources
An element involved in the formation of bones and teeth; helps to make teeth resistant to decay	Susceptibility to tooth decay	Fluorosis (discoloration of teeth), nausea, diarrhea, chest pain, itching, vomiting	Drinking water (if naturally fluoride containing or fluoridated), tea, seafood

fluorosis: discoloration of tooth enamel caused by excess fluoride.

Fluoride is toxic in excess, but toxicity symptoms appear only with very high doses or after chronic intakes of 20 to 80 milligrams a day over many years. They include fluorosis, nausea, diarrhea, chest pain, itching, and vomiting. The amount consumed from fluoridated water is typically about 1 milligram a day. Table 11–8 summarizes fluoride's roles, sources, and symptoms of deficiency and toxicity.

■ *Chromium*

glucose tolerance factor (GTF): a small organic compound containing chromium that enhances insulin's action. (Because other nonchromium factors may also enhance insulin's action, "biologically active chromium" may better describe this molecule in the future.)

Like iron, chromium can have different charges. In the case of chromium, the Cr^{+++} ion seems to be the best absorbed and most effective in living systems. Chromium absorption increases with low dietary intake and decreases with high dietary intake. Chromium also occurs in association with several different complexes in foods. The one that is best absorbed and most active is a small organic compound named the glucose tolerance factor (GTF). This compound has been extracted from brewer's yeast, but its complete structure and function still elude researchers.

Chromium is an essential mineral that participates in carbohydrate and lipid metabolism. Experiments on animals have shown that chromium works closely with the hormone insulin, facilitating the uptake of glucose into cells and the release of energy. When chromium is lacking, the effectiveness of insulin is impaired, and a diabeteslike condition results (high blood glucose). Chromium deficiency in experimental animals raises serum cholesterol and LDL concentrations and lowers HDL concentrations; in human beings, it is associated with coronary artery disease.

Estimated safe and adequate dietary intake for chromium: 50 to 200 μg/day.

Chromium deficiency is unlikely given the small amount required and its presence in a variety of foods.[19] The more refined foods are eaten, the less chromium people obtain from their diets; unrefined foods are the best sources, particularly liver, brewer's yeast, whole grains, nuts, and cheeses. Older people are most susceptible to marginal chromium intakes, because many lack an appetite or the desire to prepare and eat meals.

In experimental studies, chromium supplements seem to correct glucose imbalances in both directions. The supplements lower high blood glucose concentrations in people with diabetes and raise low blood glucose concentrations in people with hypoglycemia.[20] Chromium supplements to treat adult-onset diabetes should only be used under medical supervision for

■ TABLE 11–9
Chromium—A Summary

Chief Functions in the Body	Deficiency Symptoms	Toxicity Symptoms	Significant Sources
Associated with insulin and required for the release of energy from glucose	Diabeteslike condition marked by an inability to use glucose normally; associated with coronary artery disease	Unknown as a nutrition disorder; occupational exposures damage skin and kidneys	Meat, unrefined foods, fats, vegetable oils

people with signs of a chromium deficiency. Table 11–9 provides a summary of chromium.

■ *Selenium*

Selenium is a trace element that functions as part of an enzyme. The enzyme acts as an antioxidant and, like vitamin E, can prevent oxidation of polyunsaturated fatty acids, providing an additional source of protection for them.* Selenium's role as an antioxidant is complementary to that of vitamin E; neither can replace the other.

In some parts of China, selenium deficiency has precipitated heart disease in hundreds of thousands of children; not until the 1970s, however, was the cause of their heart trouble confirmed and remedied with selenium supplements. The regions of China in which the selenium-deficiency heart disease is prevalent are regions where the soil and foods are selenium-poor.

Regions in the United States and Canada produce crops on selenium-poor soil, but the people are protected from deficiency because of wide food distribution patterns and high meat intakes. Meats and other animal products are reliable sources of selenium, because selenium is associated with the protein parts of foods.

In other parts of the world, selenium-poor soil has been found to correlate with certain kinds of cancer. The question of whether selenium protects against cancer has stimulated research with both animal and human subjects, and it seems possible that dietary selenium adequacy may be one of the many health factors that defend against cancer. Results of research to date have not been clear, however, and there is "no justification at this time for the use of selenium supplements by people living in a low selenium area."[21]

High doses of selenium are toxic, causing loss of hair and nails, lesions of the skin and nervous system, and possibly damage to the teeth. An outbreak of selenium poisoning arose in China in the 1960s, when a local rice crop failed and inhabitants of five villages consumed vegetables from a region where selenium-rich coal contaminated the soil in which the vegetables were

selenium (se-LEEN-ee-um): a trace element.

Selenium RDA: 55 μg/day (women). 70 μg/day (men).

The heart disease caused by selenium deficiency is named **Keshan disease**, for one of the provinces of China where it was studied.

---

*The enzyme of which selenium is a part is glutathione peroxidase, which destroys oxidative compounds that could otherwise oxidize other compounds in the cell.

■ TABLE 11–10
Selenium—A Summary

Chief Functions in the Body	Deficiency Symptoms	Toxicity Symptoms
Part of an enzyme that works with vitamin E to protect body compounds from oxidation	Anemia (rare); heart disease	Digestive system disorders, loss of hair and nails, skin lesions, nervous system disorders, tooth damage
Significant Sources		
Seafood, meat, grains		

grown. Some 50 percent of the villagers became seriously ill before the cause was discovered.[22] See Table 11–10 for a summary of selenium.

■ *Molybdenum*

molybdenum (mo-LIB-duh-num): a trace element.

metalloenzyme: an enzyme that contains one or more minerals as part of its structure.

Estimated safe and adequate dietary intake for molybdenum: 75 to 250 μg/day.

Molybdenum is an important mineral in human and animal physiology that functions as a working part of several metalloenzymes, some of which are giant proteins. One metalloenzyme, for example, contains two atoms of molybdenum and eight of iron. Deficiencies of molybdenum are unknown in animals and human beings, because the amounts needed are minuscule—as little as 0.1 part per million parts of body tissue. Excess molybdenum causes goutlike symptoms in human beings. For a summary of molybdenum, see Table 11–11.

■ *Other Trace Minerals*

The trace minerals have been known for decades, but their roles as essential nutrients make up a rapidly growing area of nutrition research. Nickel is now recognized as important for the health of many body tissues; deficiencies harm the liver and other organs. Silicon is known to be involved in bone calcification, at least in animals. Tin is necessary for growth in animals, and probably in human beings. Vanadium, too, is necessary for growth and bone development, and also for normal reproduction; human intakes of vanadium may be close to the minimum needed for health. Cobalt is recognized as the mineral in the large vitamin B_{12} molecule (see Figure 11–6); the alternative name for vitamin B_{12}, cobalamin, reflects the presence of cobalt (see Table

■ TABLE 11–11
Molybdenum—A Summary

Chief Functions in the Body	Deficiency Symptoms	Toxicity Symptoms
Facilitator, with enzymes, of many cell processes	Unknown	Enzyme inhibition, goutlike symptoms
Significant Sources		
Legumes, cereals, organ meats		

11–12). Boron may play a key role in bone development and minimize demineralization in osteoporosis.[23] In the future we may discover that many other trace minerals also play key roles: silver, mercury, lead, barium, and cadmium. Even arsenic—famous as the poisonous agent of death in many murder mysteries and known to be a carcinogen—may turn out to be an essential nutrient for human beings in tiny quantities.

■ *The Trace Minerals—In Summary*

After the discussion of each of the trace minerals presented in this chapter, it is appropriate to make a few general statements about them. The body requires trace minerals in minuscule quantities (hence, their name), and they function in similar ways, assisting the many enzymes that busily work all over the body. If you were to create a list of outstanding food sources for each of the trace minerals (and add that to the lists of outstanding foods for all the other nutrients mentioned in this book), you would be convinced that a variety of foods would serve you best. A well-balanced diet of whole foods provides adequate quantities to meet trace mineral requirements.

The trace mineral contents of foods often vary depending on the soil and water supply, as well as on processing. Even taking these variations into account, available data on the composition of foods reveal no information as to how well the body will absorb a trace mineral. Many dietary factors and homeostatic mechanisms affect absorption and availability.

Severe deficiencies of the better-known minerals are easy to recognize; deficiencies of the others and mild deficiencies of all of them are less readily diagnosed. In general, the most common result of a deficiency is failure to grow and thrive, for the minerals are evident in all the body systems—the GI tract, cardiovascular system, blood, muscles, bones, and central nervous system. These systems are also impaired when intake is excessive.

Toxicity of the trace elements occurs at a level not far above the estimated requirement. Thus it is as important not to overdose as it is to have an adequate intake. The RDA committee underscores this point by adding a special note to its trace mineral table to not habitually exceed the upper end of the range of recommended intakes. The National Nutrition Consortium, too, worries that now that more trace minerals are known, they will be added to vitamin-mineral pills, making toxic overdoses more likely. The FDA is not

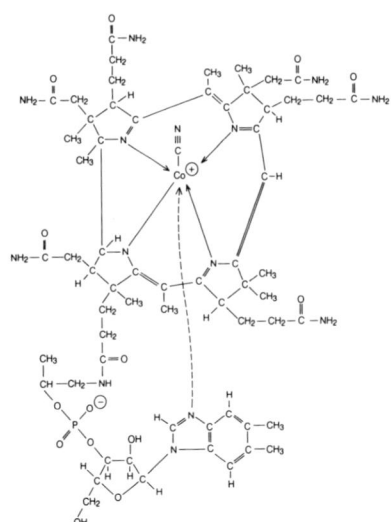

■ FIGURE 11–6
Cobalt with Vitamin B$_{12}$
The intricate vitamin B$_{12}$ molecule contains one atom of cobalt.

■ TABLE 11–12
Cobalt—A Summary

Chief Functions in the Body	Deficiency Symptoms	Toxicity Symptoms	Significant Sources
Part of vitamin B$_{12}$ and therefore involved in nerve cell function and in the process of blood formation	Unknown in human beings except in vitamin B$_{12}$ deficiency	Unknown as a nutrition disorder; occupational exposures damage skin and red blood cells	Vitamin B$_{12}$–containing foods (meat, milk and milk products)

permitted to enforce limits on the amounts of trace minerals added to supplements, because some consumers have insisted they must have the freedom to choose their own doses of nutrients; thus this is an area in which buyers must beware. In fact, it is best to avoid supplements that contain trace minerals in amounts larger than trace amounts (as reflected in the RDA tables). It is safer to consume a diet that provides foods from a variety of sources than to try to put together a combination of pills that will meet all needs without causing toxicity.

As research on the trace minerals continues, many interactions between them are also coming to light. An excess of one may cause a deficiency of another. (A slight manganese overload, for example, may aggravate an iron deficiency.) A deficiency of one may open the way for another to cause a toxic reaction. (Iron deficiency, for example, makes the body much more susceptible than normal to lead poisoning.) These examples point out the need to balance nutrient intakes and to steer clear of supplement use. Good food sources of one nutrient are poor food sources of another; and factors that cooperate with some trace elements oppose others. (Vitamin C, for example, enhances the absorption of iron and depresses that of copper.[24]) The continuous outpouring of new information about the trace minerals is a sign that we have much more to learn.

SELF STUDY *Evaluate Your Intakes of Trace Minerals*

1. Look up and record your recommended intake of iron. Also record your actual intake. What percentage of your recommended intake did you consume? Was this enough?
2. Which of the foods you eat supply the most iron? Rank your top five iron contributors. How many were meats? Legumes? Greens? Did any of them fall outside these classes? If so, what were they? How much of a contribution does enriched or whole-grain bread or cereal make to your iron intake? Are there refined bread/cereal products in your diet, such as pastries, that you could replace with enriched or whole-grain products to increase your iron intake?
3. Compute your iron absorption from a meal of your choosing, using the Monsen method (p. 325). The RDA assumes you will absorb 10 percent of the iron you ingest. What percentage did you absorb? If you are a man of any age or a woman over 50 years old, you need to absorb about 1 milligram per day; if you are a woman 11 to 50 years old, 1.5 milligrams. How could you eat differently to improve your iron absorption?
4. Are you in an area of the country where the soil is iodine-poor? If so, do you use iodized salt?
5. Record your recommended zinc intake and the amount you actually consumed. What percentage of your recommended intake did you obtain from your diet? Which were your best food sources? What guidelines do you need to follow to be sure of obtaining enough zinc from the foods you eat?
6. Repeat exercise 5, using magnesium as the subject.
7. Is the water in your county fluoridated? (Call the county health department.) If not, how do you and your family ensure that your intakes of fluoride are optimal?
8. Review your three-day food record (Self-Study 1), and separate the foods you ate into two categories: predominantly natural, unprocessed foods like those on the exchange lists; and highly processed foods, such as TV dinners, pastries, and instant gravies. Beside each food, record its kcalorie value. How many total kcalories did you consume in three days? Of these, what percentage came from highly processed foods? In light of the discussion of trace elements in this chapter, what implications do you suppose this estimate has for the nutritional adequacy of your diet?

Study Questions

1. Distinguish between iron deficiency and iron-deficiency anemia. What are the symptoms of iron-deficiency anemia?
2. Distinguish between heme and nonheme iron. Discuss the factors that enhance iron absorption.
3. Discuss possible reasons for a low intake of zinc. What factors affect the bioavailability of zinc?
4. Describe the principal functions of iodide, copper, fluoride, chromium, and selenium in the body.
5. What public health measure has been used in preventing simple goiter? What measure has been recommended for protection against tooth decay?
6. Discuss the importance of a balanced and varied diet in obtaining all the essential trace minerals and avoiding toxicities.

Notes

1. L. Hallberg, Iron, in *Present Knowledge in Nutrition*, 5th ed. (New York: Nutrition Foundation, 1984), pp. 459–478.
2. N. S. Scrimshaw, Functional consequences of iron deficiency in human populations, *Journal of Nutrition Science and Vitaminology* 30 (1984): 47–63.
3. J. Beard and M. Borel, Iron deficiency and thermoregulation, *Nutrition Today* 23 (1988): 41–45.
4. E. R. Monsen, Iron nutrition and absorption: Dietary factors which impact bioavailability, *Journal of the American Dietetic Association* 88 (1988): 786–790.
5. Food and Nutrition Board, *Recommended Dietary Allowances*, 10th ed. (Washington, D. C.: National Academy Press, 1989).
6. Monsen, 1980.
7. E. R. Monsen and coauthors, Estimation of available dietary iron, *American Journal of Clinical Nutrition* 31 (1978): 134–141.
8. Vitamin C increases iron absorption linearly up to a vitamin C dose of 1,000 milligrams. J. D. Cook and E. R. Monsen, Vitamin C, the common cold, and iron absorption, *American Journal of Clinical Nutrition* 30 (1977): 235–241.
9. Scrimshaw, 1984.
10. R. Hullin, Zinc deficiency: Can it cause dementia? *Therapaeia*, September 1983, pp. 26, 27.
11. R. S. Gibson and coauthors, A growth-limiting, mild zinc-deficiency syndrome in some Southern Ontario boys with low height percentiles, *American Journal of Clinical Nutrition* 49 (1989): 1266–1273.
12. T. Li and B. L. Vallee, The biochemical and nutritional roles of other trace elements, in *Modern Nutrition in Health and Disease*, eds. R. S. Goodhart and M. E. Shils (Philadelphia: Lea and Febiger, 1980), pp. 408–441.
13. G. A. Eby, D. R. David, and W. W. Halcomb, Reduction in duration of common colds by zinc gluconate lozenges in a double-blind study, *Antimicrobial Agents and Chemotherapy* 25 (1984): 20–24.
14. J. C. Godfrey, Zinc for the common cold, *Antimicrobial Agents and Chemotherapy* 32 (1988): 605–606; W. Al-Nakib, Prophylaxis and treatment of rhinovirus colds with zinc gluconate lozenges, *Journal of Antimicrobial Chemotherapy* 20 (1987): 893- 901; B. M. Farr and coauthors, Two randomized controlled trials of zinc gluconate lozenge therapy of experimentally induced rhinovirus colds, *Antimicrobial Agents and Chemotherapy* 31 (1987): 1183–1187.
15. Stability constants of zinc complexes affect common cold treatment results, *Antimicrobial Agents and Chemotherapy* 32 (1988): 606–607.
16. J. R. Turnlund, Copper nutriture, bioavailability, and the influence of dietary factors, *Journal of the American Dietetic Association* 88 (1988): 303–308.
17. M. R. Sowers, R. B. Wallace, and J. H. Lemke, The relationship of bone mass and fracture history to fluoride and calcium intake: A study of three communities, *American Journal of Clinical Nutrition* 44 (1986): 889–898.
18. Fluoridation (a report by the American Council on Science and Health, June 1983).
19. E. G. Offenbacher and F. X. Pi-Sunyer, Chromium in human nutrition, *Annual Review of Nutrition* 8 (1988): 543–563.
20. Effect of Cr on glucose tolerance, *Nutrition and the M.D.*, March 1988, p. 2.
21. T. D. Schultz and J. E. Leklem, Selenium status of vegetarians, nonvegetarians, and hormone-dependent cancer subjects, *American Journal of Clinical Nutrition* 37 (1983): 114-118.
22. G. Yang and coauthors, Endemic selenium intoxication of humans in China, *American Journal of Clinical Nutrition* 37 (1983): 872–881.
23. Dietary boron and osteoporosis, *Nutrition and the M.D.*, April 1988, p. 4.
24. W. Mertz, The essential trace elements, *Science* 213 (1981): 1332–1338.

Our Children's Daily Lead*

At nine months, Joey crawled about, exploring the world around him—touching and tasting everything, as all babies do. At two, his parents proudly watched as he began to toddle about. At four, he amused his parents when he'd chase after balls tossed his way. At five, he exhibited remarkable carefulness, holding tightly to the stair railings with both hands as he slowly climbed up or down.

Unfortunately, although his parents didn't notice it, Joey's health was gradually deteriorating throughout his young childhood. That Joey was late in walking, and that he rarely caught a ball or skipped and jumped at the playground like other kids his age were tiny clues. So was his small size, as was his clinging to the stair railings. The kindergarten teacher's report that Joey had some difficulty hearing and that his progress was slower than expected provided additional small clues, but each clue was easily dismissed with a comment that children progress at different paces. Nobody noticed that lead toxicity was inflicting its burden on young Joey.

The signs of mild lead poisoning include such nonspecific symptoms as diarrhea, irritability, and lethargy. With higher levels of lead, the symptoms become more pronounced, yet still difficult to pinpoint to a cause. Children lose their sense of balance and their general cognitive, verbal, and perceptual abilities, developing learning disabilities and behavior problems. Even more worrisome is that only one year of exposure can permanently impair the brain, nervous system, and psychological functioning.[1] Furthermore, recent experiments have shown that the

*Title borrowed from M. A. Wessel and A. Dominski, Our children's daily lead, *American Scientist* 65 (1977): 294–298.

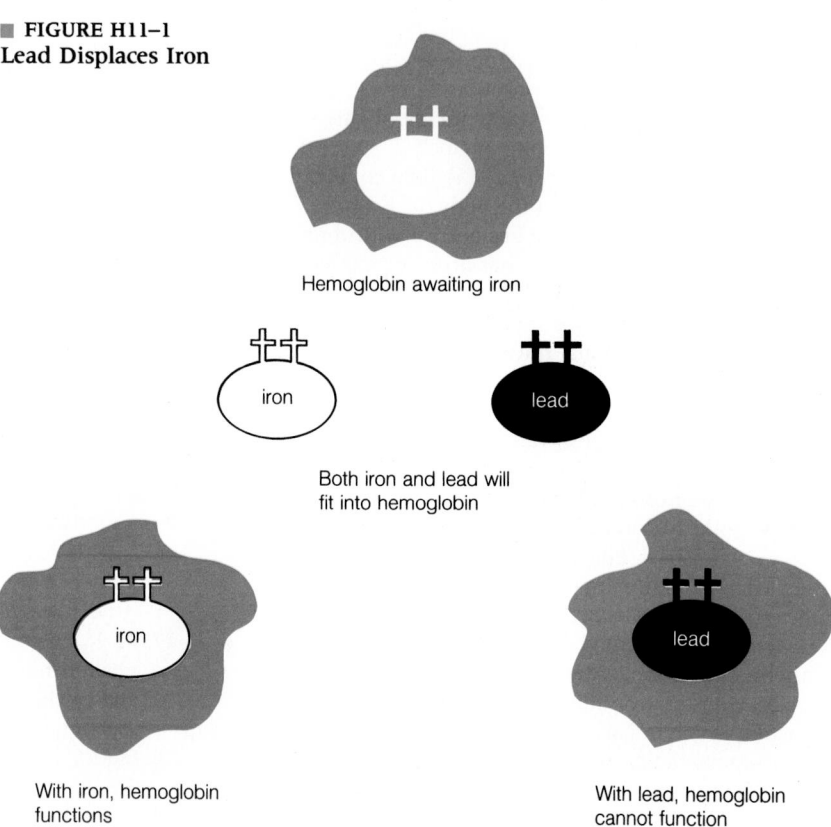

■ **FIGURE H11–1**
Lead Displaces Iron

Hemoglobin awaiting iron

iron

lead

Both iron and lead will fit into hemoglobin

iron

lead

With iron, hemoglobin functions

With lead, hemoglobin cannot function

effects occur with *lower* doses than has been thought in the past.[2] The Public Health Service has singled out lead poisoning as the worst environmental threat to children.[3]

This highlight begins with a discussion of the ways lead interacts with nutrients and disrupts the body's processes; it then looks for the sources of lead in our environment. Perhaps by learning about the problem, we can make changes that will safeguard the health of our children.

Lead in the Body

Chapters 10 and 11 told of the many ways minerals serve our bodies—maintaining fluid and electrolyte balance, providing structural support to the bones, transporting oxygen, and assisting enzymes. In contrast to those minerals that our bodies require, the mineral lead impairs the body's growth, work, and general health.

The indestructible element lead is a metal ion with two positive charges, similar in some ways to nutrient minerals like iron, calcium, and zinc. In fact, lead displaces them from some of the slots they normally occupy in the body, but then it is unable to fulfill their roles (see Figure H11–1). Consequently, lead interferes with many of the body's systems, particularly the vulnerable tissues of the nervous system, kidney, and bone marrow.[4]

■ FIGURE H11–2
Sources of Lead Exposure

Lead aggressively attacks fetuses, infants, and children, because the body absorbs lead most efficiently during times of rapid growth.[5] Lead readily transfers across the placenta, inflicting severe damage on the developing fetal nervous system. Infants and young children absorb five to ten times as much lead as adults do. One out of every six children between the ages of 6 months and 5 years and one out of every nine fetuses are exposed to threatening levels of lead.[6] Lead toxicity prevails primarily in children less than six years old and is associated with iron, calcium, or zinc deficiencies—the nutrient deficiencies most common in young children.

Blood concentrations of lead generally reach a peak in children at age two, the typical time of exploring the surroundings "hand to mouth" and ingesting lead-tainted dirt and debris (see Figure H11–2).[7] Tragically, a child's neuromuscular system is maturing at precisely the same time. No wonder children with high blood concentrations of lead show poor balance and delayed motor development. Lead interferes with the relay of nerve messages to and from the brain. Blood lead concentrations at two and three years inversely relate to the child's development at age four.[8]

Malnourished children are especially vulnerable to lead poisoning. They absorb more lead if their stomachs are empty; if they have low calcium or zinc intakes; and, of greatest concern because it is so common, if they have iron deficiencies. Excess lead in the blood also deranges the structure of red blood cell membranes, making them leaky and fragile. Lead interacts with white blood cells, too, impairing their ability to fight infection, and it binds to antibodies, thereby reducing the body's resistance to disease.

Iron deficiency contributes to lead toxicity. A child with adequate iron stores is not immune to an excess of blood lead, but a child with iron-deficiency anemia is three times as likely to have elevated blood lead concentrations.[9] This is especially unfortunate because the two conditions overlap considerably: the very same children who are most likely to be deficient in iron are also most likely to be exposed to environmental lead. The two problems are of equal magnitude in prevalence and severity, affecting 1 out of every 50 children in rural areas and more than 1 out of every 10 inner-city children.[10]

Iron deficiency impairs the body's defenses against absorption of lead. Conversely, lead toxicity contributes to iron deficiency. One of lead's actions is to interfere with iron's incorporation into heme, resulting in symptoms of anemia. Thus the combination of iron deficiency and lead toxicity is greater than the effect of either alone. Any study of the mental development of young children must consider the roles of these confounding variables.[11]

Similarly, a diet low in calcium enhances the risk of lead toxicity. A significant inverse relationship between dietary calcium and blood lead levels has been observed, leading researchers to speculate that an inadequate calcium intake enhances lead absorption and retention.[12]

Prevention of lead toxicity rests primarily on reduced exposure, but parents might also protect their children by making sure that the children receive an adequate calcium intake.[13]

Zinc status also appears to influence lead toxicity in that zinc deficiency enhances both tissue accumulation of lead and sensitivity to its effects.[14] Serum zinc concentrations are frequently low in children with elevated lead levels.[15]

The actions of lead typify the ways heavy metals behave in the body—they interfere with nutrients that are trying to do their jobs. The "good guys" in nutrition cannot help being shoved aside by the "bad guy" contaminants.

Lead in the Environment

All foods contain some lead. Much, perhaps all, of it is from industrial pollution. People are exposed to lead in gasoline, paint, newspaper ink, batteries, shotgun ammunition, and pesticides, as well as in industrial processes that release it into the air and water. Lead works its way through rainfall and soil and then into plants and animals that people use for food. Lead also enters food from food containers such as tin cans sealed with lead solder and old or imported pottery decorated with lead glazes.[16] Pipelines with lead solder joints also release lead into drinking water, in which it is the nation's most significant contaminant.[17]

A standard has been recommended for weekly acceptable intakes of lead,* but no monitoring system keeps track

---

*The World Health Organization suggests not more than 3 milligrams lead per individual for adults. Evaluation of mercury, lead, cadmium and the food additives amaranth, diethylpyrocarbonate and octyl gallate, *WHO Food Additives*, series no. 4, (Geneva: WHO), as cited by D. G. Lindsay and J. C. Sherlock, Environmental contaminants, in *Adverse Effects of Foods*, eds. E. F. P. Jelliffe and D. B. Jelliffe (New York: Plenum Press, 1982), pp. 85–110.

of the amounts to which people are actually exposed. Exposures are highest in urban and industrial areas, near highways, and in slums where old leaded paint peels from the buildings. People suffering the effects of lead exposure are most often black, male, and from low-income families.

Reductions in the use of leaded products, mandated by federal law in recent years, have helped to limit the amount of lead in the environment—and in the blood. The decline in blood lead concentrations in children during the late 1970s paralleled exactly the decline in the nation's use of leaded gasoline, leaded house paint, and lead-soldered food cans.[18] Even so, preschool children's blood lead concentrations are still unacceptably high in 4 to 6 percent of cases (when *acceptable* is defined at the 1988 Centers for Disease Control standard of 30 micrograms per deciliter). Leaded gas is still being sold at quantities greater than anticipated, and leaded paint is still being used on nonresidential structures, so there is still considerable lead appearing newly in the environment.

Ironically, even as people become more aware of the sources of accidental ingestion of lead, some parents are intentionally giving their children lead to remedy common ailments. Traditional folk medicine in the American Southwest uses lead to cure constipation (and it does!); the people of Southeast Asia use lead to soothe teething babies; and people in parts of Africa use lead to prevent umbilical cord infections.[19]

Defining the Limits

Based on evidence of neurotoxic effects at low blood lead concentrations, the Centers for Disease Control have revised *downward* their definition of "excessive blood lead" in children from 30, to 25, micrograms per deciliter of blood, and the Environmental Protection Agency (EPA) has advised that the level be reduced further, to as low as 10

micrograms per deciliter. To change the level so drastically would raise the percentage of U.S. children defined as carrying an excessive burden of lead to 88 percent, and would put 77 percent of adults in that category. Among the findings behind the EPA recommendation: blood pressure in men increases as blood lead increases from 10 to 20 micrograms per deciliter;[20] a linear relationship exists between elevated blood lead concentration and diminished height and IQ in children from 7 micrograms per deciliter on up;[21] low birthweight and slowed neuromotor development in children appear with blood lead concentrations from about 10 to 15 micrograms per deciliter on up.[22] Ideally, pediatricians would detect and treat children with low blood lead levels before overt clinical symptoms appeared. Unfortunately, in many parts of this country, such screening is not a reality.

The available evidence has not yet been deemed conclusive enough to justify lowering the definition of "excessive blood lead" below 25 micrograms per deciliter, but more studies continue to indicate that even lower lead exposures impair functioning. Of particular interest was a study specifically designed to determine whether children with moderately elevated blood lead concentrations would show significant cognitive deficits when their performance was compared with that of matched controls using a comprehensive neuropsychological battery of tests. They did show such deficits—in speed, dexterity, verbal memory, language functions, concentration, and reasoning. These were children who "had never attained markedly elevated blood levels, were generally treated early and aggressively, and had maintained levels of less than 30 μg/dl for at least a year prior to testing." The researchers noted that the test scores were consistently low across the children tested, rather than being pulled down by a few large-magnitude differences; and they concluded that "in the United States alone, perhaps more than 1 million children are at higher risk than our subjects."[23] They urged "great caution before disregarding" these seemingly small differences in functioning, citing the observation that "if the IQ scores of all children decreased by less than 0.5 standard deviation," twice as many children would be within the retarded range.[24]

With respect to drinking water, too, the tolerance levels are being lowered. Federal standards limit the amount of lead in drinking water to 50 parts per billion. As of June 1988, the EPA was considering lowering the line defining excess lead in water to 20 parts per billion. (In 1986, the EPA had reported that 42 million people were exposed to drinking water with lead concentrations of more than 20 parts per billion.) Even lower limits have been recommended; a panel of scientists participating in a 1987 Conference on Heavy Metals in the Environment recommended 10 parts per billion. The EPA requires suppliers to notify customers about *any* amount of lead in their water and to provide information on lead's health effects. Information must include what the source may be, what the supplier is doing about it, what the health effects may be, how to reduce the level, and related concerns.[25] The new regulation does not require any action if lead is less than 50 parts per billion. With Congress's ban on the use of lead-containing plumbing in new construction and water treatment methods that slow the leaching of lead from pipes, meeting lower standards is gradually becoming a feasible goal.

Strategies

Three major discoveries about lead toxicity have occurred simultaneously. Lead poisoning appears to have more *subtle* effects than have heretofore been appreciated; the effects are more *permanent* than known earlier; and

they occur at *lower levels of exposure* than realized before. Consumers would be wise to take ultraconservative measures to protect themselves, and especially their small and unborn children, from lead poisoning.

Practical implications of these findings include:

- In contaminated environments, prevent hand-to-mouth ingestion (keep small children from putting dirty or old painted objects in their mouths).
- Do not make baby formula from canned, evaporated milk.
- Once you have opened canned food, immediately remove it from the can and keep it in a storage container, to minimize lead migration into the food.
- Consume a diet adequate in calcium, iron, and zinc.

The EPA also publishes a booklet, *Lead and Your Drinking Water,* in which the following cautions appear:

- Have the water in your home tested by a competent laboratory.
- Use only cold water for drinking, cooking, and making baby formula (cold water absorbs less lead).
- When water has been standing in pipes, flush the cold-water pipes by running water through them until it is as cold as it can get (this may take as long as two minutes).

If lead contamination of your water supply seems probable, obtain additional information and advice from the EPA and your local public health agency.[26]

NOTES

1. Getting the lead out, *Science News* 132 (1987): 269.
2. D. Faust and J. Brown, Moderately elevated blood lead levels: Effect on neuropsychological functioning in children, *Pediatrics* 80 (1987): 623–629.
3. U.S. Department of Health and Human Services, Public Health Service, *Promoting Health, Preventing Disease: Objectives for the Nation* (Washington, D.C.: Government Printing Office, 1980), p. 34.

4. Y. H. Neggers and K. R. Stitt, Effects of high lead intake in children, *Journal of the American Dietetic Association* 86 (1986): 938–940.
5. Neggers and Stitt, 1986.
6. R. W. Miller, The metal in our mettle, *FDA Consumer,* December 1988-January 1989, pp. 24–27.
7. J. Raloff, Lead effects show in child's balance, *Science News* 135 (1989): 54.
8. A. J. McMichael and coauthors, Port Pirie Cohort study: Environmental exposure to lead and children's abilities at the age of four years, *New England Journal of Medicine* 319 (1988): 468–475.
9. M. Clark, J. Royal, and R. Seeler, Interaction of iron deficiency and lead and the hematologic findings in children with lead poisoning, *Pediatrics* 81 (1988): 247–254; W. S. Watson and coauthors, Food iron and lead absorption in humans, *American Journal of Clinical Nutrition* 44 (1986): 248–256.
10. Update: Childhood lead poisoning, *Journal of the American Dietetic Association* 80 (1982): 592, 594.
11. Environmental exposure to lead and cognitive deficits in children, *New England Journal of Medicine* 320 (1989): 595–596.
12. K. Mahaffey and coauthors, Blood lead levels and dietary calcium intake in 1- to 11-year-old children: The Second National Health and Nutrition Examination Survey, 1976–1980, *Pediatrics* 78 (1986): 257–262.
13. K. R. Mahaffey, P. S. Gartside, and C. J. Glueck, Inverse associations of dietary calcium and blood lead in 3513 one to eleven year old black and white children: The NHANES II study, *American Journal of Clinical Nutrition* 41 (1985): 836.
14. K. R. Mahaffey, Nutritional factors in lead poisoning, *Nutrition Reviews* 39 (1981): 353–362.
15. M. E. Markowitz and J. F. Rosen, Zinc and copper metabolism in CaNa$_2$EDTA–treated children with plumbism (abstract), *Pediatric Research* 15 (1981): 635.
16. Miller, 1989.
17. Getting the lead out, 1987.
18. E. Yetley, Nutritional applications of the Health and Nutrition Examination Surveys (HANES), *Annual Review of Nutrition* 7 (1987): 441–463.
19. A cure that's worse than the ailment, *Science News* 135 (1989): 135.
20. W. R. Harlan and coauthors, Blood lead and blood pressure, *Journal of the American Medical Association* 253 (1985): 530–534.
21. *Pediatrics,* March 1986, as cited by Faust and Brown, 1987.
22. Excess lead: Its evolving definition, *Science News,* 22 November 1986, p. 333.
23. Faust and Brown, 1987.
24. M. Rutter, Raised lead levels and impaired cognitive/behavioral functioning: A review of the evidence, *Development Medicine and Child Neurology* 22, supplement 42 (1980): 1–26, as cited by Faust and Brown, 1987.
25. Getting the lead out, 1987.
26. U.S. Environmental Protection Agency, Office of Water, *Lead and Your Drinking Water,* publication no. OPA 87-006, (Washington, D.C.: Government Printing Office, April 1987.)

12

Energy Balance and Weight Control

Contents

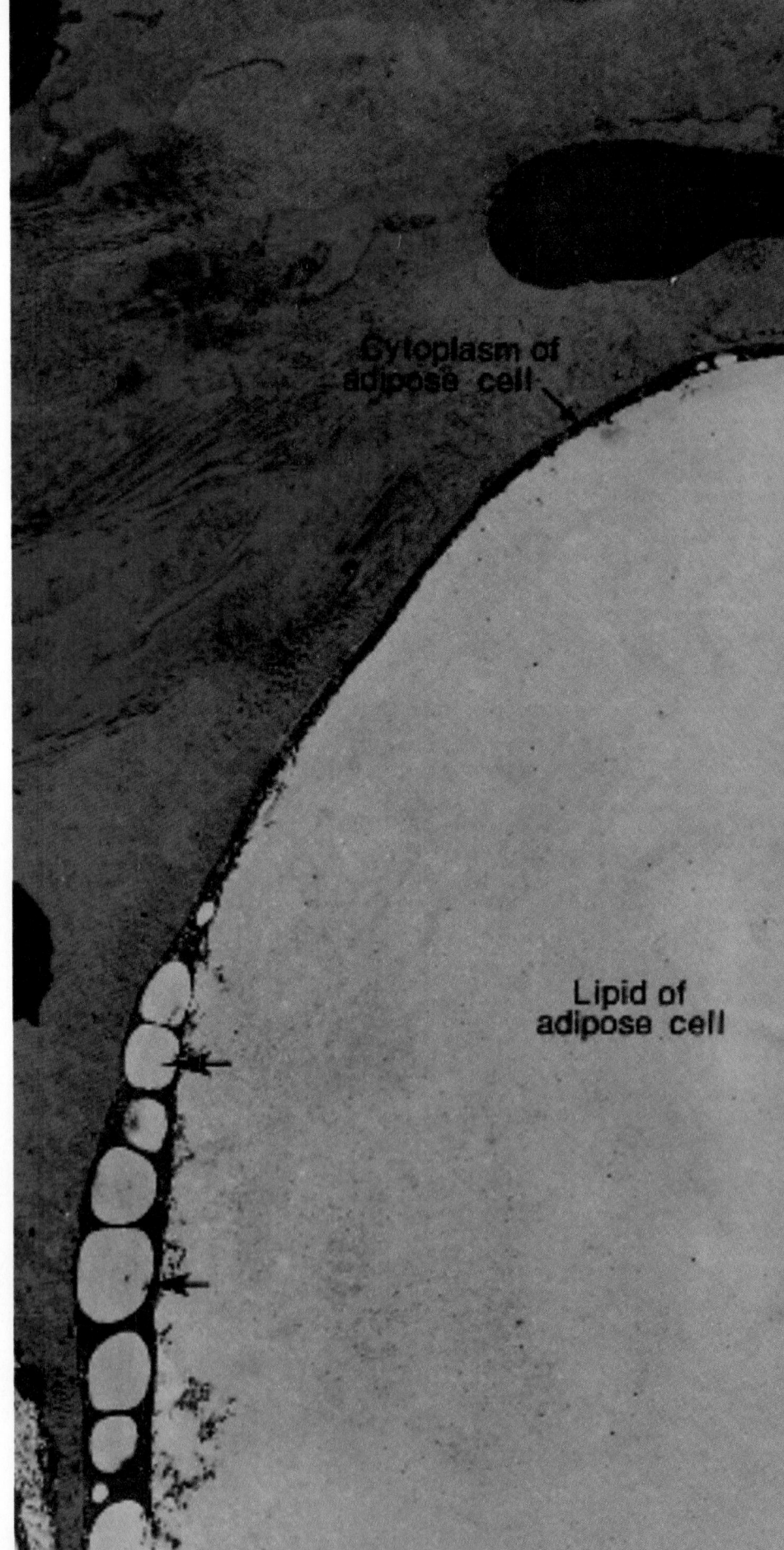

Cytoplasm of adipose cell

Lipid of adipose cell

Fat cells can expand immensely as their fat stores increase. The cell material (cytoplasm) is pushed to the very edge of the cell; the center is a giant fat reservoir. New fat being synthesized first forms small droplets near the edge of the cell (arrows); then the droplets merge into the central reservoir.

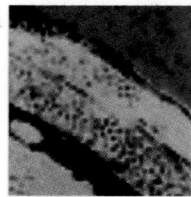

Obesity is a major malnutrition problem, largely unexplained. Much speculation, debate, and frustration surrounds the question of why and how obesity occurs and what can be done about it. For the obese person who has earnestly tried every known means of losing weight only to fail, frustration can turn to despair. Equally frustrating is the problem of the underweight person who finds it as hard to gain weight as the obese person does to lose it.

This chapter emphasizes the problems of overweight and obesity, partly because they have been more intensively studied, and partly because they are a more widespread health problem in the developed countries; information on underweight is presented whenever appropriate. The highlight that follows this chapter delves into the eating disorders anorexia nervosa and bulimia.

Overweight and underweight both result from unbalanced energy budgets. The overweight person has consumed food energy in excess of expenditures and has banked the surplus in body fat. The underweight person has not consumed enough food energy, and so has depleted body fat stores and possibly lean tissues as well. Energy itself doesn't weigh anything and can't be seen, but when it exists in the form of chemical bonds in nutrients or body fat, the material that it holds together is bulky, heavy, and visible.

The amount of body fat you might deposit in, or withdraw from, your "savings" on any given day depends on your energy balance for that day—the amount you consume (energy in) versus the amount you expend (energy out). You can reduce your fat deposits by withdrawing more energy from them than you put in.

■ **FIGURE 12–1**
Bomb Calorimeter
When an organic substance such as food is burned, the energy in the chemical bonds that held its carbons and hydrogens together is released in the form of heat. The amount of heat released can be measured; this direct measure of the amount of energy that was stored in the food's chemical bonds is termed **direct calorimetry**.

As the chemical bonds in food are broken, the carbons and hydrogens combine with oxygen to form carbon dioxide and water. Measuring the amount of oxygen consumed in the process gives an indirect measure of the amount of energy released, termed **indirect calorimetry**.

■ *Energy In: The kCalories in Food*

To find out how many kcalories a food provides, a laboratory scientist can burn the food in a bomb calorimeter (see Figure 12–1). This device can reveal food energy values in two ways—directly, by measuring the heat given off (kcalories are units of energy defined in terms of heat), or indirectly, by measuring the amount of oxygen consumed in the burning.

The number of food kcalories as determined by direct calorimetry exceeds the number of kcalories that same food gives to the human body. The body is less efficient; it does not metabolize all of the food all the way to carbon dioxide and water, as the calorimeter does. Researchers can correct mathematically for this discrepancy, and so can use calorimetry to make useful tables of the energy values of foods (such as Appendix H). Another way to arrive at the energy values of foods is to compute them from the amounts of protein, fat, and carbohydrate (and alcohol, if present) in the foods.*

You can also estimate the numbers of kcalories in foods roughly, using the exchange system described in Chapter 2. Take the foods depicted in Figure 12–2, for example. You could look them up one by one in Appendix H, but

calorimetry (cal-o-RIM-uh-tree): the measurement of energy as heat.
  calor = heat
  metron = measure

The number of kcalories that the human body derives from a food, as contrasted with the number of kcalories determined by calorimetery, is the **physiolgical fuel value**.

Remember:
  • 1 g carbohydrate = 4 kcal.
  • 1 g fat = 9 kcal.
  • 1 g protein = 4 kcal.
  • 1 g alcohol = 7 kcal.

---

*Some of the food energy values in the table of food composition in Appendix H were derived by bomb calorimetry, and many were derived by calculation from their energy-yielding nutrient contents.

■ FIGURE 12–2
kCalorie Quiz
Use the exchange system to estimate how
many kcalories are in the meal depicted here.
The answer is provided in Figure 12–3.

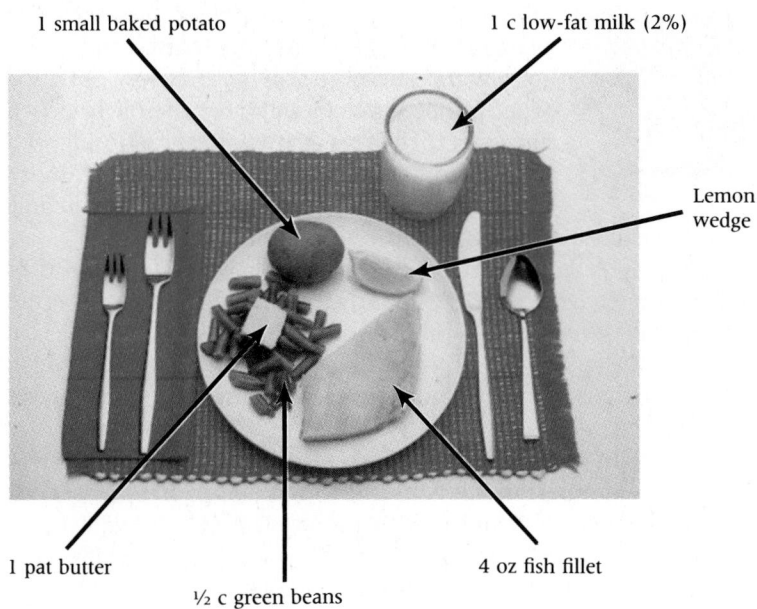

1 small baked potato

1 c low-fat milk (2%)

Lemon wedge

1 pat butter

½ c green beans

4 oz fish fillet

it is quicker to translate them into exchanges and add up the kcalorie values (see Figure 12–3). With some practice, you can look at any plate of food and "see" the number of kcalories on it. Only seven values need be learned as a start toward gaining this skill (see Table 12–1).

Perhaps even more important than "seeing" the kcalories in foods is seeing the fat (review Figure 12–3 and see Table 12–2 with an eye open for fat). It seems that not all kcalories are created equal, but that energy derived from fat is more fattening than energy from carbohydrate or protein.* Not only does fat

---

*Researchers have proposed that the physiological fuel value of fat be raised from 9 kcalories per gram to 11 kcalories per gram.

■ TABLE 12–1
Food Energy Values

Food	Energy
1 c nonfat milk	90 kcal
(1 c low-fat milk)	(120 kcal)
(1 c whole milk)	(150 kcal)
½ c vegetable[a]	25 kcal
1 portion[a] fruit (unsweetened)	60 kcal
1 portion grain or starchy vegetable	80 kcal
1 oz lean meat (1 exchange)	55 kcal/oz[b]
(1 oz medium-fat meat)	(75 kcal/oz)
(1 oz high-fat meat)	(100 kcal/oz)
1 tsp fat or oil	45 kcal
1 tsp sugar	20 kcal

[a]For the distinction between vegetables and starchy vegetables, the sizes of fruit portions, and other details, see the exchange lists in Appendix G. An introduction to the exchange system was given in Chapter 2.
[b]An ounce is not a typical serving of meat. Typical servings are 3, 4, or more ounces. A 4-oz portion of lean meat would be 220 kcal; of medium-fat meat, 300 kcal of high-fat meat, 400 kcal.

■ TABLE 12–2
Food Fat Values

Food	Fat kCalories	% kCalories Fat
1 c nonfat milk	Trace	Trace
(1 c low-fat milk)	45	38
(1 c whole milk)	72	48
½ c vegetable[a]	0	0
1 portion[a] fruit (unsweetened)	0	0
1 portion grain or starchy vegetable	Trace	Trace
1 oz lean meat (1 exchange)	27	49
(1 oz medium-fat meat)	45	60
(1 oz high-fat meat)	72	72
1 tsp fat or oil	45	100
1 tsp sugar	0	0

[a]For the distinction between vegetables and starchy vegetables, the sizes of fruit portions, and other details, see the exchange lists in Appendix G. An introduction to the exchange system was given in Chapter 2.
[b]An ounce is not a typical serving of meat. Typical servings are 3, 4, or more ounces. A 4-oz portion of lean meat would be 220 kcal; of medium-fat meat, 300 kcal of high-fat meat, 400 kcal.

provide over twice as many kcalories per gram (9 compared with 4), but when the total kcalories in two foods are equal, the food higher in fat contributes more to obesity. The body uses energy from dietary fat more efficiently than from carbohydrate; it loses less while metabolizing the dietary fat to body fat. Even when total energy intake is restricted, if dietary fat is high, it is more readily converted to body fat.[1] Immediately after a meal, when fat levels in the blood are high, fat stores eagerly take their fill. Once deposited in storage, fat becomes a less readily available energy source. In contrast, large intakes of carbohydrates encourage glycogen storage instead of fat deposition.[2] To store dietary fat in body fat tissues costs just 3 percent of the

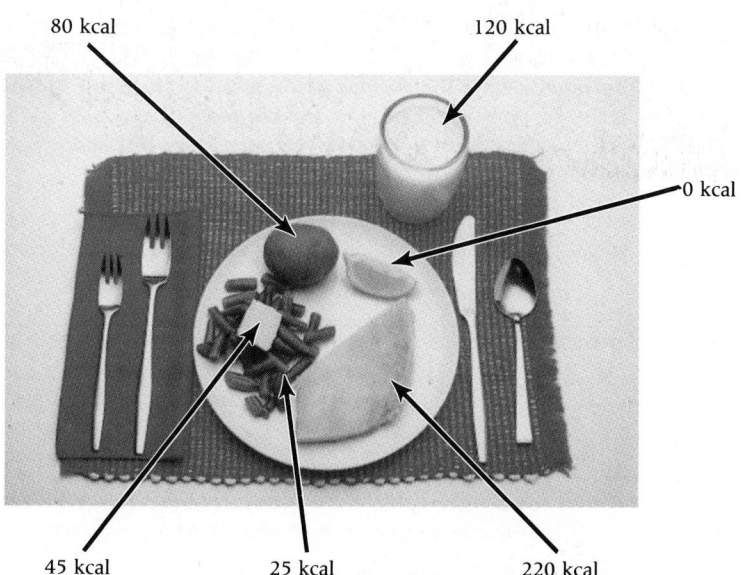

80 kcal   120 kcal

0 kcal

45 kcal   25 kcal   220 kcal

■ FIGURE 12–3
Quiz Answers
We figure about 490 kcal for the meal.

Note: Appendix H values yield a total of about 432 kcal, lower because these foods are low-kcalorie choices within the exchange groups. Any answer within about 50 to 100 kcal of this is a good estimate.

Food	kCalories
1 c low-fat milk (1 lowfat milk)	120
½ c green beans (1 vegetable)	25
1 small baked potato (1 starchy vegetable)	80
1 pat butter (1 fat)	45
4 oz fish (4 lean meat, assuming no fat is added), at 55 kcal/oz	220
Lemon wedge	0
	490

Fat Content Of Foods

Determining the percentage of kcalories from fat will help you to develop a sense of the "fattening" power of different types of food. To calculate the percentage of kcalories that fat contributes to a food, first multiply the number of grams of fat in a food by 9 to get the number of kcalories provided by fat. Then divide that number by the total number of kcalories in the food, and multiply the result by 100:

Fat (g) $\times$ 9 (kcal/g) = fat (kcal).
(Fat kcal $\div$ total kcal) $\times$ 100 = % kcal from fat.

For one example:
1 oz cheddar cheese provides 9.4 g fat and 114 kcal.

9.4 g $\times$ 9 kcal/g = 84.6 kcal from fat.
(84.6 kcal from fat $\div$ 114 total kcal) $\times$ 100 = 74% kcal from fat.

(Alternatively, estimating from the exchange system, 1 oz cheddar cheese provides 8 g fat and 100 kcal, for 72% kcal from fat.)
For another example:
1 c cooked egg noodles provides 2 g fat and 200 kcal.

2 g $\times$ 9 kcal/g = 18 kcal from fat.
(18 kcal from fat $\div$ 200 total kcal) $\times$ 100 = 9% kcal from fat.

(Using the exchange system, 1 c cooked egg noodles provides trace fat and 160 kcal, for essentially no kcalories from fat.)

This percentage reflects the fat content of the food for any amount of food; for example, 1 oz cheddar cheese derives 74% of its kcalories from fat, just as 1 lb cheddar cheese does. Such a calculation allows you to easily compare foods to recommendations; that is, you can easily see that cheddar cheese exceeds current recommendations to limit fat to 30% total kcalories. If you choose to eat cheddar cheese, you will need to balance it with other foods with a low percentage of kcalories from fat if you want your diet's average fat content to meet recommendations. Be careful, though: percentages cannot be added together or averaged to get a total percentage; that is, a dish composed of 1 c macaroni with 1 oz cheese does not have simply 9% kcal fat plus 74% kcal fat, nor does it have the average of 9% and 74% kcal fat. To determine its fat percentage, you would need to add the grams of fat from each and the kcalories from each and then calculate the percentage of kcalories of fat in the combination:

11.4 g fat $\times$ 9 kcal/g = 102.6 kcal from fat.
(102.6 kcal from fat $\div$ 314 total kcal) $\times$ 100 = 32.7% kcal from fat.

---

ingested energy intake; to store dietary carbohydrate in body fat requires an expenditure of 23 percent of ingested energy intake.[3]

As you might expect, when rats are allowed to eat as much as they want of a *high*-fat diet for a long time, they become obese (over 50 percent body fat).[4] What you might not expect is that when similar rats are allowed to eat as much as they want of a *low*-fat diet, they eat enough so that their total kcaloric intake is similar—but they deposit 20 percent less body fat. This

(Using the exchange system, this combination provides 28% kcal from fat, a slight underestimation. Some authorities suggest replacing 1 g fat for trace values to correct for this. Using such a correction makes the estimates more accurate.)

A second method of evaluating the fat content of a food is to note the actual gram weight of fat in a specified amount (usually a standard portion) of the food. This measure—grams per serving—is commonly used on food labels and in food composition tables such as the one in Appendix H.

One advantage of this measure is that it provides the actual quantity of fat, and so allows for easy comparison. You can see at a glance, without any mathematical calculations, that 1 c whole milk provides more grams of fat than 1 c 2% milk. This method also allows you to add and to average grams of fat from different foods consumed. For example, to find your total intake:

1 oz cheddar cheese provides	9.4 g fat
1 c cooked egg noodles provides	2.0 g fat
Total fat intake	11.4 g fat

Or, to determine your average intake:

Monday	75 g fat
Tuesday	100 g fat
Wednesday	65 g fat
3-day total	240 g fat
3-day average	80 g fat

A disadvantage is that because the measure depends on a specified portion, the portion size must be considered in making comparisons. This can be problematic when one food composition table lists a portion size for a food item as "1 c"; another, "100 g"; a food label, "½ c"; and a diet plan, "2 oz"—and your actual intake was "a small handful."

You can compare dietary recommendations given in percentages with food labels that give fat content in terms of grams. Use the rule of thumb that 3 g fat (27 kcal of fat) represents about 30% of the kcalories in 100 kcal food.

You can also calculate your recommended maximum daily fat intake in terms of grams as follows. Suppose you can afford 1,800 kcal/day and your goal is 30% kcal from fat:

1,800 total kcal × 0.30 from fat = 540 fat kcal.
540 fat kcal ÷ 9 kcal/g = 60 g fat.

With this number in mind, you can quickly evaluate the numbers of fat grams in foods you consider eating. One fast-food superburger alone could use up your entire fat allowance for a day.

Rule of thumb: 3 g fat ≈ 30% kcal fat in 100 kcal food.

suggests that obesity develops more readily from consuming a high-fat diet than from mere overeating.

Dietary guidelines state that total fat intake should not exceed 30 percent of dietary energy.[5] How well are we doing in meeting this goal? As long ago as 1910, fat provided 32 percent of energy consumed; it climbed to 43 percent in 1977, and then dipped slightly to 36 to 37 percent in 1985.[6]

■ *Energy Out: The kCalories the Body Spends*

Counting the kcalories provided by the food you eat tells you your food energy income, but to balance your energy budget, you also need to know your expenditure. How can you count the kcalories you expend in a day? One way is to assume you are a "typical citizen" of the United States or Canada, and to use the numbers your government uses as standards for its population studies.

Government Recommendations

The U.S. Committee on Dietary Allowances and the Canadian Ministry of Health and Welfare have published recommended energy intakes for various age-sex groups in their populations. These are useful for population studies, but the range of energy needs for any one group is so broad that it is impossible even to guess an individual's needs without knowing something about the person's lifestyle. The U.S. recommendations represent the energy allowances for adults engaged in light to moderate physical activity based on the median heights and weights of the population. For a 20-year-old woman, for example, the RDA assumes that she stands 5 feet 5 inches tall, weighs about 128 pounds, and needs about 2,200 kcalories a day to maintain her weight. The healthy 20-year-old man used as a reference figure stands 5 feet 10 inches tall, weighs 160 pounds, and needs about 2,900 kcalories a day. Taller people have a greater body surface area than shorter people, and therefore need proportionately more kcalories to balance their energy budgets. Older people generally need fewer kcalories, with the number diminishing by about 5 percent per decade beyond age 30. Appendix I provides the U.S. and Canadian energy allowances for various age groups.

Although few people fit these descriptions exactly, most fall close to the mean. For adults, it is believed that an 800-kcalorie range covers most individuals, but the total span of needs is broad, and some people have energy needs outside this range. In fact, in any group of 20 similar people with similar activity levels, one will expend twice as much energy per day as another. Clearly, it is impossible to pinpoint any one person's energy need within such a wide range without knowing more.

Light activity (for both women and men) is typically characterized by 10 hours a day at rest and 14 hours a day in light activity of the same intensity as ordinary walking.

Diet Record Method

To obtain an individualized estimate of your energy needs, monitor your food intake and body weight over a period of time in which your activities are typical. If you keep an accurate record of all the food and beverages you consume for a week or two, and if your weight does not change during that time, you can assume that your energy budget balances. Records have to be kept for at least a week, however, because intakes fluctuate from day to day. (On some days you eat less, and on others more, kcalories than the average.) This method identifies your personal *energy needs to maintain your current body weight* at your current intake and expenditure levels. In general, the more a person weighs, the more energy is required to maintain that weight.[7] The diet record method leaves you to identify any nutrient inadequacies or excesses and to make adjustments in energy intake and expenditure if you want to alter your body weight.

Laboratory Methods

Physiologists detect human energy expenditure as thermogenesis—the generation of heat. The body converts the energy of food to the energy of the temporary storage molecules, ATP (see p. 172), with about 50 percent efficiency. Then, when ATP energy is used to do work, about 50 percent is lost as heat. Thus the overall efficiency of the human body in converting food energy to work is 25 percent; the other 75 percent appears as heat.[8] The work itself, once done, generates heat as well, so a body's total heat production provides an index of the amount of energy it is spending.

Because energy expenditure always produces heat, a device that measures escaping heat gives a measure of the energy being spent. An alternative measure uses the principle that the amount of oxygen consumed and carbon dioxide expelled is in direct proportion to the heat released. Table 12–3 gives average energy expenditures for people engaged in different activities.

thermogenesis: the generation of heat; used in physiology and nutrition studies as an index of how much energy the body is spending. Four categories of thermogenesis account for the total energy a body spends:
- Basal thermogenesis—similar to basal metabolic rate, described in the next section.
- Exercise-induced thermogenesis—generation of heat by physical activity.
- Diet-induced thermogenesis—energy used while metabolizing food (normally 10% of energy input).
- Adaptive thermogenesis—adjustments in energy expenditure related to environment and physiological events such as cold, overfeeding, trauma, and changes in hormone status.

■ TABLE 12–3
Energy Spent on Various Activities

Activity	Intensity	Energy, Including BMR (kcal/kg/hr)	Energy, Excluding BMR (kcal/kg/hr)
Lying down	Asleep	0.9	0
	Awake	1.1	0.1
Sitting	Quiet/studying	1.2	0.2
	Eating/writing	1.5	0.5
	Driving car/typing rapidly	2.2	1.2
Standing	Relaxed	1.8	0.8
	Dressing	2.0	1.0
	Ironing/washing dishes	2.2	1.2
Walking	3 mph	3.3	2.3
	Vacuuming floor	4.2	3.2
Swimming (crawl)	20 yd/min	4.2	3.2
	45 yd/min	7.8	6.8
	50 yd/min	9.0	8.0
Bicycling	13 mph	6.0	5.0
	15 mph	6.6	5.6
	17 mph	7.8	6.8
	19 mph	10.2	9.2
	21 mph	12.0	11.0
	23 mph	14.4	13.4
	25 mph	18.6	17.6
Running	11.5 min/mi—5.2 mph	7.8	6.8
	9.0 min/mi—6.7 mph	11.4	10.4
	8.0 min/mi—7.5 mph	12.6	11.6
	7.0 min/mi—9.0 mph	13.8	12.8
	6.0 min/mi—10.0 mph	15.0	14.0
	5.5 min/mi—11.0 mph	17.4	16.4

Note: Skiing, squash, and handball require about the same energy as bicycling at 13 mph.

Source: Swimming, bicycling, and running data from G. P. Town and K. B. Wheeler, Nutritional concerns for the endurance athlete, *Dietetic Currents* 13 (1986): 7–12. Reprinted with the permission of Ross Laboratories, Columbus, OH 43216 from *Dietetic Currents*. Copyright 1986 Ross Laboratories.

Estimation from Metabolism and Activities

The two major contributors to human energy output under normal conditions are metabolic processes and voluntary activities. A way of estimating the total energy you spend is to estimate these components individually, then add them together.

Metabolic energy occupies the lion's share of most people's energy budgets—at least two-thirds of the energy spent in a day. It consists of the energy spent to keep the heart beating, the lungs inhaling and exhaling air, the cells conducting their metabolic activities, the nerves generating their continuous streams of electrical impulses—in short, the energy spent to keep all the processes going on that support life. People often do not realize that so much of their energy supports the basic work of their bodies' cells, because they are unaware of all the work these cells do to maintain life.

The basal metabolic rate (BMR) is the rate at which the body spends energy for these maintenance activities, usually expressed as kcalories per hour. This rate varies from one person to the next, and may vary for one individual with a change in circumstance or physical condition. The rate is lowest when a person is sleeping undisturbed, but since periodic tossing and turning increase it, it is usually measured with the subject lying down in a room with a comfortable temperature, and not digesting any food. (The difference from sleep can be discounted in all but the most precise laboratory measurements.)

Table 12–4 summarizes the factors that raise and lower BMR. In general, BMR is higher in people with greater lean body mass (growing children,

basal metabolism: the total energy output of a body at rest after a 12-hour fast. Also called **basal metabolic rate (BMR)**. The **resting metabolic rate (RMR)** is similar, but may be measured after less than 12 hours of fasting.

Weight: 8 units

Surface area
24 units   34 units

Both weigh the same, but the tall, thin structure will lose more heat to its surroundings.

■ TABLE 12–4
Factors that Affect BMR

Factor	Effect on BMR
Age	In youth, the BMR is higher; age brings less lean body mass and slows the BMR.[a]
Height	Tall, thin people have higher BMRs.[b]
Growth	Children and pregnant women have higher BMRs.
Body composition	The more lean tissue, the higher the BMR. The more fat tissue, the lower the BMR.[c]
Fever	Fever raises the BMR.[d]
Stress	Stress raises the BMR.
Environmental temperature	Both heat and cold raise the BMR.
Fasting/starvation	Fasting/starvation lowers the BMR.[e]
Malnutrition	Malnutrition lowers the BMR.
Thyroxin	The thyroid hormone thyroxin is a key BMR regulator; the more thyroxin produced, the higher the BMR.

[a]The BMR decreases by about 2%/decade after growth and development cease. A reduction in voluntary activity as well brings the total decline in energy expenditure to 5%/decade.
[b]Of two people who weigh the same, the taller, thinner person will have the faster metabolic rate, reflecting a greater skin surface, in proportion to the body's volume, through which heat is lost by radiation.
[c]In general, males tend to have higher BMRs than females due to their greater lean body mass.
[d]Fever raises BMR by 7% for each degree Fahrenheit.
[e]Prolonged starvation reduces the total amount of metabolically active lean tissue in the body, although the decline occurs sooner and to a greater extent than body losses alone can explain. More likely, the neural and hormonal changes that accompany fasting are responsible for changes in BMR.

pregnant women, and males), in people who are tall for their weight, in people with fever or under stress, and in people with high thyroid gland activity. It is lowered by loss of lean tissue and depression of thyroid hormone activity due to disease, inactivity, fasting, or malnutrition. The accompanying box shows how to estimate a person's basal metabolic energy.

The second component of energy output is physical activity voluntarily undertaken and achieved by use of the skeletal muscles. The amount of energy needed for any activity, whether it be playing tennis or studying for an

---

Estimation of Energy Output

Basal Metabolism. Use the factor 1.0 kcal/kg body weight/hour for men, or 0.9 for women (men's hormones induce them to develop more lean tissue than most women). Example (for a 150-lb man):

1. Change pounds to kilograms:

   150 lb ÷ 2.2 lb/kg = 68 kg.

2. Multiply weight in kilograms by the BMR factor:

   68 kg × 1 kcal/kg/hour = 68 kcal/hour.

3. Multiply kcalories used in one hour by hours in a day:

   68 kcal/hour × 24 hours/day = 1,632 kcal/day.

Energy for BMR equals 1,632 kcal/day.

Voluntary Muscular Activity. The following figures are crude approximations based on the amount of muscular work a person typically performs in a day. To select the one appropriate for you, remember to think in terms of the amount of *muscular* work performed; don't confuse being *busy* with being *active.* Rules of thumb to estimate the energy need for activities:

- For sedentary (mostly sitting) activity (a typist), add 40 to 50% of the BMR.
- For light activity (a teacher), add 55 to 65%.
- For moderate activity (a nurse), add 65 to 70%.
- For heavy work (a roofer), add 75 to 100% or more.

Suppose the man we are using as an example is a clerk. To estimate the energy he needs for physical activities (sedentary), multiply his BMR kcalories per day by 50%:

   1,632 kcal/day × 50% = 816 kcal/day.

Energy for activities equals 816 kcal/day.

Total. The man in our example spends, in a day:

   1,632 kcal/day + 816 kcal/day = 2,448 kcal/day.

Because the exact figure is based on several estimates, it's probably best to express the man's needs as falling within a 100-kcal range:

   Total energy needs equal about 2,400 to 2,500 kcal/day.

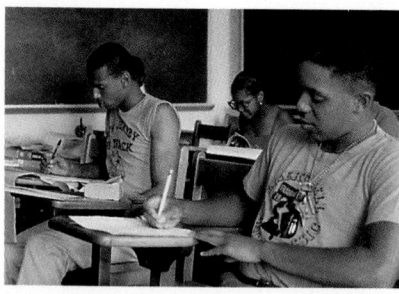

It feels like work, but studying requires only 0.2 kcalories per kilogram per hour more than resting.

Diet-induced thermogenesis is also sometimes called the **specific dynamic effect (SDE)** or **specific dynamic activity (SDA)** of food.

exam, depends on how many muscles are involved, and on how intensely and how long they have to work. Table 12–3 shows the amounts of energy spent on various activities by the average individual.

You may be disappointed to learn that intense mental activity such as studying requires only slightly more energy than resting, even though it may make you very tired. On the other hand, physical activity uses energy: the muscles must move the body, the heart must beat hard to send nutrients and oxygen to them, and the lungs must move fast to deliver oxygen and dispose of carbon dioxide.

A heavier person usually uses more energy to perform a task than does a lighter person, because it takes extra effort to move extra weight. Other factors may also alter the amount of energy spent, such as the person's skill or efficiency at performing the task. You can estimate the energy needed for activities by using the rules of thumb offered in the accompanying box.

The total energy a person spends in a day is derived by adding the two components together. The box shows that the man in our example spends about 2,400 to 2,500 kcalories per day on his BMR plus activities.

Some energy expenditure, not accounted for in this estimate, is that required for the body to manage food. When you eat food, many of your body's cells increase their activities. The GI tract muscles that move the food speed up their rhythmic contractions; the cells that manufacture and secrete digestive juices begin their tasks. These cells and others need extra energy as they come alive to participate in the digestion, absorption, and metabolism of food. This stimulation of cellular activity is diet-induced thermogenesis, which equals about 10 percent of the total food energy taken in. For purposes of rough estimates, diet-induced thermogenesis can be ignored; the 10 percent it might contribute to total energy output is smaller than the probable errors involved in estimating energy input from food or energy output for activities.

Finally, another category of energy expenditure is the energy required for adaptation to changed circumstances (adaptive thermogenesis, defined earlier). When the body has to adapt to physical conditioning, cold, overfeeding, starvation, trauma, or other types of stress, it has extra work to do, building the necessary tissues and secreting the necessary enzymes and hormones. Normally, this energy need not be taken into account in estimating a person's needs, but there are circumstances in which it makes a considerable difference. For example, a thin person who tries to gain weight may have to take in considerably more than 3,500 kcalories above normal energy expenditures to gain a pound. Another example: the person who undertakes a physical conditioning program may unexpectedly lose weight at first, even while increasing food intakes to cover apparent added energy expenditure.

■ Energy Balance: Weight Loss and Gain

Most of us maintain a steady energy balance over time. You may eat a little more or a little less on any given day, and your weight may go up or down a pound or two, but for the most part, you maintain a balance. When the balance shifts, your weight changes.

Hunger and Satiety Regulation

To manage its energy balance so as to meet its needs without storing too much or too little energy, the body must decide how often and how much to eat. Most researchers accept that the signals that regulate food intake—hunger and satiety—are responsible for this energy balance regulation. These signals seem to work well. Given the freedom to eat what they want, when they want, experimental animals regulate their energy balance with remarkable accuracy. This seems somewhat true for human beings, as well.[9]

Research devoted to discovering what stimulates and regulates eating behavior has been trying to answer the following questions: Why do we start to eat? Why do we eat as much as we do? Why do we stop?

Hunger and appetite both encourage eating—with a distinction. Hunger is physiological (an inborn instinct), whereas appetite is psychological (a learned response to food). We experience appetite without hunger when presented with an appealing food: "I'm not hungry, but I'd love to have a piece." We may experience the reverse, hunger without appetite, when faced with a stressful situation: "I know I must be hungry, but I just don't feel like eating."

After eating for a while, satiety signals feelings of fullness and satisfaction, and we stop eating. Satiety occurs when food accumulates in the stomach and passes into the intestine.[10] Most likely, the intestines signal satiety by releasing GI hormones and by firing intestinal nerves. Nerves of the intestine send messages to the brain—the cortex and the hypothalamus (see Figure 12–4). The hypothalamus integrates many signals received from the rest of the body, including information about the body's temperature, cell metabolism, and fuel availability (the concentrations of absorbed nutrients in the blood may also produce the ongoing sensation of satiety).* Damage to the hypothalamus alters eating behavior and body weight—in some cases causing severe weight loss; in others, vast overeating. In the person with a normal hypothalamus, however, eating behavior seems to be a response to a number of signals. Somehow these many inputs become integrated into a "final common path"—the act of eating. Figure 12–5 illustrates these and other factors thought to be involved in hunger and appetite.

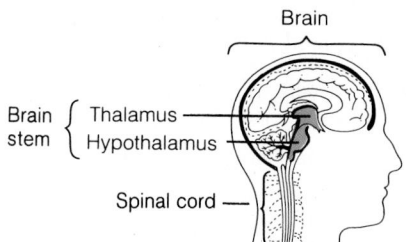

■ **FIGURE 12–4**
Hypothalamus
Researchers believe that the hypothalamus controls the sensations of hunger and satiety.

hunger: the physiological need to eat; a negative, unpleasant sensation.

satiety (sah-TIE-ah-tee): the feeling of fullness or satisfaction at the end of a meal, which prompts a person to stop eating.

appetite: the desire to eat, which normally accompanies hunger; by itself a pleasant sensation.

Shifting the Balance

A pound of body fat stores about 3,500 kcalories. To lose it, you must take in 3,500 kcalories less than you expend; to gain it, you must take in 3,500 kcalories more than you use. On the average, a deficit or excess of 500 kcalories a day brings about a weight loss or gain, respectively, at the rate of 1 pound a week; a deficit or excess of 1,000 kcalories a day, 2 pounds a week.

Extraordinarily active people, by virtue of their high energy expenditures, or extremely obese people, by virtue of their extra tissue and the energy cost of moving their bodies, can lose weight faster, but for most people, the maximum possible rate of *fat* loss is 1 to 2 pounds a week, which requires that

1 lb = 3,500 kcal. A pound of body fat (adipose tissue) is actually composed of a mixture of fat, protein, and water and yields 3,500 kcal on oxidation. (A pound of pure fat (454 g) would yield 4,086 kcal at 9 kcal/g.)

---

*In rats, the intestinal peptide hormone cholecystokinin (CCK) and the gastric peptide bombesin (BBS) both reduce food intake and elicit satiety. In human beings, both of these peptides hold promise for obesity treatment. In addition, the L-isomer of phenylalanine (which releases CCK) suppresses feeding in rats and rhesus monkeys.

■ **FIGURE 12–5**
Hunger and Appetite
This is a partial list of the factors thought
to be operating to control food intake.

Source: Adapted from T. W. Castonguay and coauthors,
Hunger and appetite: Old concepts/new distinctions,
Nutrition Reviews 41 (April 1983): 101–110.

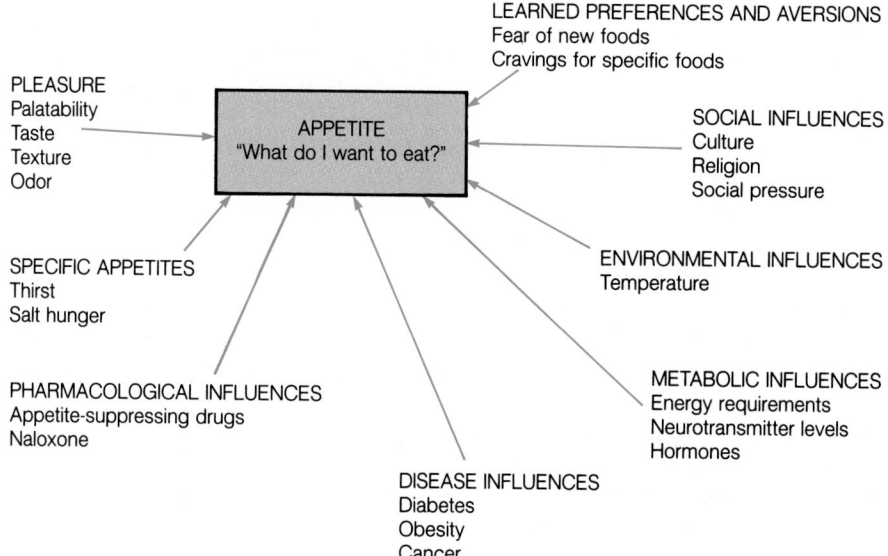

kcalories be restricted to about 1,000 to 1,500 a day. Below 1,200 kcalories, most dieters lose lean tissue and are hard pressed to achieve adequacy for all the vitamins and minerals.

A pound or two gained or lost does not necessarily indicate body *fat* gained or lost. Changes in body weight reflect shifts in many materials—fat, large amounts of fluid, some bone minerals, and lean tissues such as muscles. People concerned with weight control must realize that quick changes in weight are not changes in fat. Normally, the composition of weight gained or lost is approximately 75 percent fat and 25 percent lean.[11] This is not an unvarying rule; during starvation, losses are about equal. Before exploring the problems of overweight and underweight, the following section looks at body weight and body composition.

■ *Body Weight and Body Composition*

An average man or woman about 5 feet 10 inches tall who weighs 150 pounds carries about 90 of those pounds as water and 30 as fat. Most of the water is associated with the other 30 pounds—the lean tissues—muscles; organs such as the heart and liver; and, to a lesser degree, the bones of the skeleton. Stripped of water and fat, then, the person weighs only 30 pounds! This lean tissue with its associated water is vital to health. The person who seeks to lose weight wants, of course, to lose fat, not this precious lean tissue. And for someone who wants to gain weight, it is desirable to gain lean and fat in proportion, not just fat. As you can see, then, weight doesn't matter as much as body composition, especially body fat content.

Once upon a time, the definition of obesity was simple. A person's weight could be compared with that in the ideal weight tables. If the actual weight was 20 percent or more above the ideal weight, then the person was obese. Now (to tell a long story in a few words), the term *ideal weight* is subject to debate, and the definition of obesity is complex. A look at the measures and standards used in the assessment of body fatness will reveal some of the problems.

Body Weight

Body weight, by itself, says little about the body composition factor of interest: body fatness. A person who doesn't seem to weigh too much may be too fat; a person who seems to weigh too much may not be too fat. An athlete, whose muscles are well developed and whose bones have become well mineralized by responding to constant stress, may weigh the same as a sedentary person of the same height, yet the athlete may be at the right weight, and the sedentary person may be too fat. We can't look inside a person and see the bones, muscles, and fat.

Granted that weight poorly measures body fatness, it is still the measure people use as an index of body composition. Height-weight tables (such as Table 19–4 in Chapter 19) serve as the standards for comparison. These height-weight tables reflect the weight ranges that correlated some time ago with the greatest longevity in a population of people who had purchased life insurance, excluding those with major diseases such as heart disease, cancer, and diabetes. Some of them reported their weights verbally; others were weighed once. The weights were recorded at the time they applied for life insurance—not years later when, by dying, they provided the statistics the life insurance companies used to generate the weight tables.

A reevaluation of the statistics on which the 1959 weight tables were based showed that the weights should have been higher, and higher weights were published in 1983. These higher weights still fall below the average weights of the general population. Clearly, when a person's weight is compared with the table weight, it is not being measured against a standard, but simply compared with the average weight recorded years ago for a population of people who lived quite long after that until they died.

The 1983 Metropolitan Height and Weight tables appear in Table 19–4 on p. 618.

body mass index (BMI): an index of a person's weight in relation to height, determined by dividing the weight (in kilograms) by the square of the height (in meters):

$$BMI = \frac{weight\ (kg)}{height^2\ (m)}.$$

A BMI greater than 27.8 for men or 27.3 for women indicates overweight.

frame size: the size of a person's bones and musculature. A person with a large frame can weigh more than one the same height with a small frame before risk begins to increase.

A person whose weight is 10 to 20% above the weight on the life insurance tables is overweight; more than 20% above is obese.

The fatfold test provides an estimate of total body fat.

A standard derived from height and weight measures, which is useful for estimating the risk to health associated with obesity, is the body mass index (BMI). Appendix E presents a nomogram for determining BMI and the inside back covers provide BMI tables.

The extent to which weight reflects fatness depends partly on a person's frame size. The larger the frame, the heavier a person is expected to be, due to the density of bones and muscles. Only weight in excess of that appropriate for frame size should count towards excess body fat. However, frame size is hard to measure accurately. Researchers have determined that bone mass does correlate with muscle mass (that is, people with bigger bones do have greater muscle mass).[12] That means it should be possible to measure a bone to obtain an estimate of the body's fat-free mass.

The question of what bone to measure has been answered variously. Different measures have been suggested, including the breadth of the elbow bone, wrist bone, and ankle bone; the distance between the hip bones; a ratio of height to wrist circumference; and measures at the shoulder and knee. The wrist and ankle breadths seem to be associated *least* with total body fat; the insurance height-weight tables use the breadth of the elbow bone as an index of frame size (Appendix E describes how to measure elbow breadth to determine your body frame size). The compilers of these tables chose this particular measurement because a recent survey had provided extensive reference values for elbow breadth in U.S. adults.[13] Unfortunately, though, frame sizes based on elbow breadths tend to underestimate fat in lean people and overestimate it in obese people.

As a result of this uncertainty, height-weight tables have limited usefulness, but every bathroom and every doctor's office seems to have a scale, and the tables will doubtless continue to be used. If you choose to use them, be sure to add an inch to your barefoot height (you are assumed to be wearing shoes with 1-inch heels), and adjust for clothing (the tables assume 5 pounds for clothes for men and 3 pounds for women).

If the weight tables cause frustration in would-be users, perhaps that reaction brings with it a benefit—it leads them to ask deeper questions about the state of the body most compatible with good health and long life. Simple answers don't await the asker, but when answers do come, they will doubtless have to do with body composition.

Body Composition

Several laboratory techniques for directly estimating body composition have been developed. One way is to determine the body's density (weight compared with volume). Lean tissue is denser than fat tissue, so the more dense a person's body is, the more lean tissue it must contain. Weight is measured with a scale; volume measurement involves submerging the whole body in a large tank of water and measuring the amount of water displaced. From the density, an estimate of the percentage of body fat can be derived. This technique is not available in the typical home or doctor's office, for obvious reasons, but is in wide use on university campuses that pursue exercise physiology research. Underwater, or hydrostatic, weighing is the "gold standard" against which all other body composition measures are compared.

A simpler way to obtain an estimate of the amount of body fat is by taking a fatfold measure. The assessor lifts a fold of skin from the back of the arm, from the back, or from other body surfaces and measures its thickness with a caliper that applies a fixed amount of pressure. The fat under the skin in these regions represents about half of the body's total fat tissue, and on most people it is roughly proportional to total body fat. If the person gains body fat, the fatfold increases proportionately; if the person loses fat, it decreases. Measures taken from lower body sites (around the abdomen) better reflect changes in fatness than those taken from upper sites (arm and back). The fatfold test is a practical diagnostic procedure in the hands of trained people and is in increasingly wide use. Appendix E presents percentiles for fatfold measures for males and females.

The major limitation of the fatfold test is that fat may be thicker under the skin in one area than another. A pinch at the side of the waistline may not yield the same measurement as a pinch on the back of the arm. For this reason, an assessor may take measures at each of several different body sites. The measures at each site are then compared with standards; each site requires its own standard. The assessor can then average the results. For example, a person who has two fatfolds that indicate obesity and two that do not is moderately obese.

Another measure being tested for its usefulness in assessing body composition is bioelectrical impedance. The method is based on the principle that lean tissues are full of electrolyte-containing fluids—that is, fluids that readily conduct an electrical current. Fat, on the other hand, acts as an insulator and is a poor conductor. To obtain impedance data, electrodes are placed on a person's hand and foot on the same side of the body, and a small current is briefly transmitted. Values are then calculated according to mathematical formulas. Researchers are working on establishing the validity of bioelectrical impedance as a standard measure of body composition.

fatfold test: a clinical test of body fatness in which the thickness of a fold of skin on the back of the arm (on the triceps), below the shoulder blade (subscapular), or in other places is measured with a caliper. The older, less preferred, term for this is **skinfold test**.

What Is Ideal?

After you have a body fatness estimate, more questions arise. How do you interpret it? What is the "ideal" amount of fat for a body to have? The question "Ideal for what?" has to be answered first.

For competitive athletes, especially endurance athletes, the ideal is relatively easy to define. The amount of fat in the body should be as low as possible so as not to contribute excess weight for the muscles to carry but still above the minimum needed for essential functions such as providing fuel, insulation, and normal fat-soluble hormone activity. A man of normal weight may have, on the average, 10 to 20 percent fat; a woman, because of her greater quantity of essential fat, 20 to 30 percent. Endurance athletes consider it ideal to have lower fat percentages than these. Clinicians recommend an absolute *minimum* of 3 to 7 percent for men and 10 to 20 percent for women.[14]

For an Alaskan fisherman, the ideal percentage of body fat is probably higher than this. Fat provides an insulating blanket, and in cold climates, such a blanket confers an advantage. For a woman starting a pregnancy, the ideal percentage of body fat may be different again; the outcome of pregnancy is compromised if the woman begins it with too little body fat. Below a certain threshold body fat content, some individuals become infertile, develop depression, experience abnormal hunger regulation, or become unable to keep warm. These thresholds differ for each function and for each individual; much remains to be learned about them.

Just as there is a minimum percentage of body fat that is ideal for a given individual, there is also a maximum, and this, too, may differ from person to person. One major factor that determines where to draw the line is the blood pressure. Extra fat tissue requires the heart to work harder to pump blood through miles of extra capillaries that feed that fat tissue. Some people can tell you exactly at what weight their blood pressure begins to rise; when they lose weight to below that threshold, their blood pressure becomes normal again. Other risk indicators also rise and fall with body fatness—blood glucose and blood cholesterol, for example. For people with diabetes (Type II, or non-insulin-dependent type), hypertension, and high blood cholesterol, weight reduction is most critical.

The uncertainties surrounding the definition of ideal body composition reflect the newness of the branch of nutrition science that studies body weight and its regulation. The best definition of obesity would be body fatness significantly in excess of that consistent with optimal health, determined by a reliable measure—but the techniques to pinpoint it accurately are still to be worked out.

Besides having all the health implications that it does, body weight is also a social and personal matter. In some societies fatness is desired; it is equated with prosperity, comfort, and security. In others it is despised; it is considered undisciplined to be fat. In our society, social and economic disadvantages plague the fat person. Obese people are less often sought after for marriage, pay higher insurance premiums, meet discrimination when applying for college admissions and jobs, and are limited in their choice of sports. For many, guilt, depression, withdrawal, and self-blame are inevitable psychological accompaniments to obesity.

The person seeking a single, authoritative answer to the question "How much should I weigh?" is bound to be disappointed. No one can tell you *exactly* how much you should weigh—but with health as a value, at least you have a starting framework. Any of a wide range of weights is probably acceptable, and within that range, the exact weight to choose depends on your own preferences. The self-study exercise at the end of this chapter offers a procedure for selecting an appropriate weight for yourself. Outside the acceptable range, however, your athletic performance, fertility (in women), health, or longevity would be adversely affected. Within the range, the weight to pick is up to you; your own standards are important.

The branch of nutrition science concerned with weight control is **bariatrics** (barry-AT-ricks).

barys = weight

obesity: excessive body fatness, presently determined by comparing body weight with the life insurance tables. The person whose weight is more than 20% above the table weight is considered **obese**; 10% above the table weight is **overweight**; and 10% below the table weight is **underweight**.

◼ *Problems of Obesity*

However you define it, obesity does occur to an alarming extent and is increasing in the developed countries. In the United States, some 10 to 25 percent of all teenagers and some 25 to 50 percent of all adults are obese.

■ **TABLE 12–5**
Health Hazards Associated with Obesity

In General:
- Abdominal hernias
- Accidents
- Arthritis—especially in the knees, hips, and lower spine
- Complications after surgery
- Gout
- High blood cholesterol concentrations (a risk factor for coronary heart disease)
- Hypertension
- Respiratory problems
- Varicose veins

For Men:
- Risk of cancers of the colon, rectum, and prostate gland

For Women:
- Gynecological irregularities
- Pregnancy-induced hypertension
- Risk of cancers of the breast, uterus, ovaries, gallbladder, and bile ducts

Obesity brings many health hazards with it, as Table 12–5 demonstrates. Insurance companies report that fat people die younger from a host of causes, including heart attacks, strokes, and complications of (Type II) diabetes.* Even after the effects of diagnosed diseases are discounted, the risk of death remains twofold for obese people, especially for those with lifelong weight problems.

The location of fat on the body may be as critical as (or even more critical than) the total amount. Fat around the abdomen may represent a greater risk to health than fat elsewhere on the body. Abdominal fat (most common in males), even in the absence of obesity, is associated with heart disease, diabetes, and hypertension. In contrast, fat around the hips and thighs (most common in females) seems relatively harmless. If weight loss is to benefit health, then, it should reduce upper-body fat. Fatfold measurements do not take this fat distribution difference into account. A simple comparison of the waist to the hip measurement better assesses abdominal fat than other methods and is quickly becoming a standard part of the assessment of body fatness.

Beyond all these hazards is the risk incurred by millions of obese people throughout much of their lives—the risk of ill-advised, misguided dieting. Some fad diets are more hazardous to health than obesity itself. One survey of 29,000 claims, treatments, and theories for losing weight found fewer than 6 percent of them effective—and 13 percent dangerous![15]

Obesity is a severe physical handicap, but it is reversible. If it is corrected in time, some of its risks are, too. Mortality rates (from insurance data) are no higher for the formerly obese than for the never obese. Prevention is desirable, but where it has failed, treatment is needed.

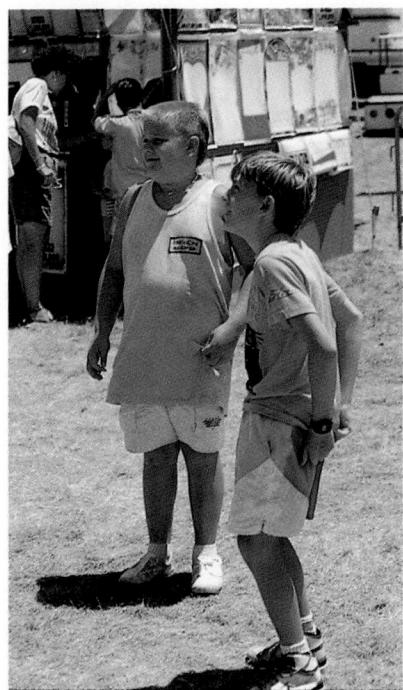

The overweight child who becomes obese invites a host of health risks and social disadvantages to follow in adult life.

---

*The greater the degree of overweight, the higher the excess death rate, especially in the young.

■ *Causes of Obesity*

Excess body fat accumulates when people take in more food energy than they need to provide for the day's metabolic, muscular, and digestive activities. Why do they do this? Is it genetic? Metabolic? Environmental? Psychological? Behavioral? Biological? All of these? Perhaps obesity has many causes; some experts in the field speak of many different *obesities*.

The next sections summarize current obesity research without coming to a final conclusion as to cause. Several lines of investigation seem promising, and the findings that are emerging suggest that no single answer will ever be found; obesity is multifactorial.

Genetics versus Environment

One way to approach the question of what causes obesity is to ask whether it is hereditary. In some animals, at least one kind of obesity is hereditary: strains of rats exist that are genetically fat, and they tend to be fat in any environment—that is, regardless of the kind or variety of food they eat. In human beings, family resemblance studies strongly support the impression that obesity runs in families. When one parent is obese, the chances of a child's becoming obese are greater (40 percent) than when neither parent is obese (7 percent); if both parents are obese, the chances become quite likely (80 percent).[16] While the weight-for-height measures of both parents correlate with their children's measures, mothers' measurements correlate more closely.[17]

Twin studies offer insights to help distinguish between genetic and environmental explanations for family resemblances. Results from twin studies suggest a genetic potential for obesity at least as strong as that seen in schizophrenia, alcoholism, and coronary heart disease.[18] Identical twins are twice as likely to be the same weight as fraternal twins.

Another approach is to study adopted children, to see whether they resemble their biological or adoptive parents. These studies also suggest that the tendency to obesity is inherited, but that the environment is influential in the sense that it can prevent or permit the development of obesity when the potential is there.

That obesity runs in families, though, does not support a hereditary cause alone, for clearly, learning plays a role. Habits learned in childhood tend to persist throughout life. Food-centered families encourage such behaviors as overeating at mealtimes, rapid eating, excessive snacking, and eating to meet needs other than hunger. Children readily imitate overeating parents, and their behavior at the table tends to persist outside the home. Obese children tend to take more bites of food per interval of time and to chew them less thoroughly than their nonobese schoolmates.

Fat-Cell Hypothesis

Still another approach to the question what causes obesity is to study people from childhood on, asking the question, Do fat babies become fat adults?

By setting an example, parents have the opportunity to influence their children's eating habits at every meal.

Several longitudinal studies have shown that most fat babies don't become fat adults; they grow out of their obesity in childhood. However, most overweight *children* (80 percent) remain overweight into adulthood. Something must therefore happen between infancy and childhood that contributes to adult obesity.

Research on fat cells suggests a possible reason why childhood-onset obesity is persistent. Simply stated, early overfeeding is thought by some researchers to stimulate fat cells so that they increase abnormally in *number*. The number of fat cells is thought to become fixed by adulthood; if it is, then a gain or loss in weight thereafter can take place only through an increase or decrease in the *size* of the fat cells.

Studies confirm that obese children have a greater number of fat cells than nonobese children. Their fat cells are also larger. The fat cells of obese children reach the size normal for nonobese adults even before the children enter their teen years.[19] It is most likely that an obese child whose *number* of fat cells already equals or exceeds that of the average adult will continue to be obese throughout life. Children with the greatest number of fat cells are least likely to lose weight successfully. However, a chubby child whose number of fat cells is within the normal range will more likely outgrow the baby fat.

The prognosis is different for a person who gains weight in adulthood. Such a person, according to the fat-cell theory, probably has a normal number of fat cells and therefore normal hunger regulation. The weight gain brought about only an increase in fat-cell *size*. Such a person needs only to reduce the size of the cells back to normal to return to normal weight.

The theory that the number of fat cells becomes fixed at a critical point in time, and thereafter sets a person's tendency to be normal weight or obese, has been debated without confirmation over the past 20 years. The theory has appeal because it agrees with other findings about critical periods. However, it has drawbacks because recent studies indicate that cell growth and development do not necessarily follow the simple pattern implied by this theory. Whatever the case, there are certain periods in life when body fat increases more rapidly than lean tissue: late infancy, early childhood (age six), and adolescence. The multiplication of fat cells that takes place at these times may be irreversible, so preventive efforts are most important then.

Fat is hard to lose, even if it is gained during adulthood. When fat cells enlarge, they become sluggish in their responses to insulin (the hormone that promotes the making and storage of fat), even though insulin concentrations are high.[20] One possible explanation is that excess glucose remains in the bloodstream longer than normal and stimulates the insulin-producing cells of the pancreas to secrete more insulin. When the fat cells finally respond, they store more fat than normal in response to the raised insulin level. As if this were not enough, enlarged fat cells tend also to be insensitive to hormones that promote fat breakdown. Weight loss restores insulin levels to normal, but it first has to be achieved against great odds.

A **longitudinal study** is one in which the subjects are studied over time—for example, in 1970 and again in 1980 and in 1990.

fat cell theory: the theory that during the growing years, fat cells respond to overfeeding by increasing in number; that the number of fat cells becomes fixed before adulthood; and that the number regulates hunger, so that an individual overfed during infancy or childhood will always overeat.

Obesity due to an increased *number* of fat cells is **hyperplastic obesity**. Obesity due to an increased *size* of fat cells is **hypertrophic obesity**.

critical period: a finite period during development in which certain events may occur that will have irreversible, determining effects on later development.

Set Point

Many internal physiological variables, such as blood glucose, blood pH, and body temperature, remain fairly stable under a variety of environmental conditions. Constant monitoring of the body's internal status and delicate changes maintain these variables within certain limits. The stability of such complex systems as the human body may depend on set-point regulators. These regulators maintain variables at specified values.

Research on the regulation of body weight has been influenced by this set-point concept. Researchers propose that each individual body has a set biological weight determined by genetic and environmental factors, a "set point." However, unlike body temperature, the range of body weight in human beings is large. For example, a reasonable weight for an adult woman, 5 feet 4 inches tall, is about 120 pounds. Yet it is easy to find women of that same height who weigh less than 100 pounds and others who weigh more than 200 pounds. Such large variation does not seem consistent with a tightly regulated set-point system. Such is the picture when we look at the population. A look at individuals, however, reveals another pattern. The range of one individual's body weight remains fairly narrow over long time spans.

It is thought that the body sends out signals to establish, regulate, and maintain the set point.[21] Yet these set-point regulators do more than maintain a constant body weight; they *defend* that body weight when it is challenged. People who have lost 25 percent of their body weight by restricting their dietary intake return to their normal weights when allowed to eat as they please. Similarly, people who increase their food energy intake and gain 15 to 25 percent of their body weight return to their normal weight when allowed to eat as usual. This tenacious defense of body weight deters obese people from losing weight and promotes the regain of any weight that is successfully lost.

The set-point theory is still controversial; even if it is valid, it is not yet possible to determine a person's set point independent of body weight—it can only be estimated from a person's weight over time. For example, a person who has weighed within a few pounds of 150 over the past several years is considered to have a set point of 150.

Metabolic theories such as the set-point theory have been advanced to explain how the body might be able to "choose" whether to store or spend energy, and may provide clues to the way the body maintains its weight. A person who eats more than usual on a given day may metabolize the food less efficiently (wasting more energy as heat) than usual, and gain less weight than expected. A person who eats less than usual might conserve more that day, and so lose less weight than expected. Such mechanisms might help to explain why gaining and losing weight are equally hard to do for a person at the set-point weight, and may also help to account for the mysterious plateaus at which both weight gainers and weight losers tend to get stuck.

Environment and Behavior

Earlier, we mentioned that some rats were genetically obese, no matter what they were fed; and the previous sections presented the possibility that some human beings might also be obese for genetic, biological, or metabolic reasons. Some direct evidence also suggests alternative possibilities for both animals and human beings. Experiments with "cafeteria rats" support the environmental obesity model. When ordinary rats eat regular rat feed they maintain normal weight (for rats). But, if those same rats are offered free

set point: the point at which controls are set (for example, on a thermostat). In the case of body weight, the set point is that point above which the body tends to lose weight and below which it tends to gain weight.

access to a wide variety of tempting, rich, highly palatable "cafeteria" foods, they greatly overeat and become obese. Evidently, the behavior of eating, which occurs appropriately in response to internal hunger signals, can also be triggered by external stimuli at times when it is not appropriate.

Some obese people, like cafeteria rats, tend to eat in response to external stimuli. Rather than responding only to internal, visceral hunger cues, they seem to respond helplessly to such external factors as the time of day ("It's time to eat") or the availability, sight, and taste of food ("That looks delicious!"). This is the basis of the external cue theory.

Experiments under controlled conditions confirm this. Lean and fat people respond differently to meals offered in monotonous liquid form from a feeding machine. The lean people eat enough to maintain their weight (responding to internal cues); the fat people drastically reduce their food intake and lose weight (responding to external cues). When kcalories are added to the formula, the lean people adjust their intakes to continue maintaining weight as if they had internal kcalorie counters, but the obese people continue drinking the same volume of formula as before, and stop losing weight.[22]

The implications for treatment of obesity are obvious. Such people need to learn several strategies—to avoid places where the "eat me" signals that foods send out are too overwhelming; to create environments for themselves where food stimuli are at a minimum; and to learn to say no in circumstances where tempting but unneeded foods are offered. This is difficult in an environment that is not conducive to weight control. The television offers delectable, technicolor food in its commercials. Fast-food places, complete with tempting aromas, line our main streets. Kitchen appliances such as the hamburger cooker and the doughnut maker make it all too easy to prepare and impulsively eat high-kcalorie foods.

external cue theory: the theory that some people eat in response to such external factors as the presence of food or the time of day rather than to such internal factors as hunger.

Psychological Factors

If the behavior of eating is appropriate as a response only to internal hunger sensations, and is inappropriate when triggered by chance offerings of food, it is even more inappropriate when triggered by psychological stimuli. Yet eating behavior easily becomes conditioned to occur automatically in response to a wide variety of inappropriate stimuli, because food itself rewards the eater with its good taste and calming effects. The routine is built in, in the brain's response to stressors such as pain, anxiety, arousal, excitement, and even the presence of food. On experiencing these stimuli, the brain responds by producing endogenous opiates. They soothe pain and lessen arousal, and they have two effects on energy balance. They enhance appetite for palatable foods, and they reduce activity.[23] Combine these effects with a tendency to be supersensitive to particular stressors anyway, and one is likely to overeat and gain weight in response to any kind of stress, positive or negative. (What do I do when I'm depressed? Eat. What do I do when I'm excited? Eat!) Some people do respond to anxiety, or in fact to any kind of arousal short of severe stress, by eating. (Highlight 1 described the reaction to severe stress, which is to stop eating.) Significantly, however, if stress eaters are able to give a name to their aroused condition, thereby gaining a feeling that they have some control over it, they are not as likely to overeat.[24]

endogenous opiates: morphinelike compounds produced in the brain in response to pain, stress, certain drugs, and other circumstances. They act as internal tranquilizers, reducing arousal level.

The term **arousal** has been used several times. The general meaning is self-evident, but in the sense in which it is used here, it refers to heightened activity of certain brain centers associated with excitement and anxiety.

Food behavior is also intimately connected to deep emotional needs such as the primitive fear of starvation and the infant's association of food with mother love. Yearnings, cravings, and addictions with profound psychological significance can express themselves in people's food behavior. An emotionally insecure person might eat rather than call a friend and risk rejection. Another might use eating to relieve boredom or to ward off depression.

Lack of physical activity fosters obesity.

Inactivity

The many possible causes of obesity mentioned so far all relate to the input side of the energy equation. What about output? People may be obese because they eat too much, but another possibility is that they spend too little energy. The control of hunger/appetite actually works quite well in active people and only fails when activity falls below a certain minimum level. Obese people under close observation are often seen to eat less than lean people, but they are sometimes so extraordinarily inactive or efficient in their way of moving that they still manage to have an energy surplus.

Despite evidence of the benefits of physical activity, fewer than half of all adults in the United States exercise regularly, although the number who exercise may be increasing. Underactivity is probably the most important single contributor to the obesity problem in our country. In turn, television may contribute most to physical inactivity.

Several effects of watching television could contribute to obesity. First, television viewing requires no energy beyond the resting metabolic rate. Second, it replaces time spent in more vigorous activities. Third, watching television correlates with between-meal snacking; eating the high-kcalorie, high-fat foods most heavily advertised on programs; and influencing family food purchases. The foods advertised on television tend not to be nutrient-dense foods, but rather foods that tend to be high in fat, sugar, and kcalories, and low in nutrients. Nonnutritious foods and beverages appear not only in commercials, but also within the television programs themselves. People may miss the message that eating and drinking high-kcalorie foods will bring about weight gain when they see television stars indulging in such behavior and remaining thin.

The question whether obesity was associated with increased television watching has been researched.[25] Two cross-sectional samples and one longitudinal sample of children and adolescents in the United States were used. The findings reflect that children who watched more television had a greater prevalence of obesity (they had a triceps fatfold measurement at or above the 85th percentile) and superobesity (triceps fatfold at or above the 95th percentile) than children watching less television. In addition, evidence supported a dose-response relationship between obesity and time spent watching television (see the Nutrition Detective Work box). The prevalence of obesity increased by 2 percent for each additional hour of television viewed per day. This relationship between television and obesity held strong when control variables such as prior obesity and socioeconomic class were considered.

Like all the other "causes" of obesity, inactivity alone fails to explain it fully. One study strapped mechanical devices to the arms and legs of overweight and normal weight people and found them to be equally active.[26]

NUTRITION DETECTIVE WORK

A dose-response relationship is a specific relationship between a substance or procedure and the response to it such that the greater the dose, the greater the response—persuasive evidence that the substance causes the response. In the case of children watching television, as the dose of the television-watching variable increased, the response (in this case, obesity) increased. The conclusion was drawn that the more time kids spend watching television, the more obese they become. A dose-response relationship provides stronger evidence that the one variable causes the other than a simple yes-no response (one group watches television and is obese; the other does not and is thin), because the correlation appears at all points along a continuum.

No two people are alike either physically or psychologically, and the causes of obesity may be as varied as the people who are obese. Many causes may contribute to the problem of obesity in a single person. Given this complexity, it is obvious that there is no panacea. The top priority should be prevention, but where prevention has failed, the treatment of obesity must involve a simultaneous attack on many fronts.

Before embarking on the discussion of healthful treatments for obesity, however, a word of advice might be beneficial. As mentioned later, repeated cycles of weight losses and gains make each attempt at weight loss more difficult. Consider your motivation seriously, and evaluate your weight-loss plan carefully, before embarking on a program. A modest weight loss is more likely to improve your health and minimize rebound weight gain than a dramatic weight loss undertaken impulsively.

Magical alternatives to this systematic, hard-work approach have been offered time and again over the centuries—ways to "shrink the stomach," to eat "negative kcalories," to "eat all you want and lose weight"—but they are born of wishful thinking. They are effective only when they directly affect the kcalorie balance. If they can be said to be successful in any sense, it is only because they are popular, not because they work.

▪ *Treatments of Obesity: Poor Choices*

Many people—those who are of normal weight as well as those who are obese—would like to lose weight. Anyone who could devise a quick and easy weight-loss plan would be highly praised and financially rewarded. Consequently, a number of alternative strategies for losing weight have been set forth. As you will see, some have limited usefulness, some are not useful at all, and some are actually harmful.

diuretic (dye-you-RET-ic): a drug that promotes water excretion; popularly, a "water pill."
> *dia* = through
> *ure* = urine

No matter how much you huff and puff, you can't just shake it off, rock it off, roll it off, knock it off or bake it off . . . The only way is to eat less and exercise more.—American Medical Association

Pills, Procedures, and Other Possibilities

When searching for ways to lose weight quickly, people sometimes take "water pills." The idea that excess weight is due to water accumulation is appealingly simple. Indeed, temporary water retention, seen in many women around the time of the menstrual period, may make a difference of several pounds on the scale.* If water retention is a medical problem, a physician can prescribe a diuretic. But obese—that is, overfat—people have a *smaller* percentage of body water than people of normal weight. If they take diuretics, the weight they lose will be water, not fat; the weight loss will last only half a day or so; and the price will be dehydration.

Some doctors prescribe amphetamines ("speed") to help with weight loss, such as Dexedrine and Benzedrine. These reduce appetite—but only temporarily. Typically, the appetite returns to normal after a week or two, the lost weight (and often more) is regained, and the user then has the problem of trying to get off the drug without gaining more weight. It is generally agreed that these drugs cause a dangerous dependency and are of little or no usefulness in treating obesity.[27]

People also buy over-the-counter medications to help with weight loss. The FDA has given approval to only two over-the-counter weight control aids. Most nonprescription weight control products contain phenylpropanolamine hydrochloride (as in Dexatrim and Appedrine), which is an amphetamine and carries the risk of stroke. The other approved drug is benzocaine (in a candy form), which anesthetizes the tongue, reducing taste sensations.

Bulk producers or fillers are products that swell when taken with water and produce a feeling of fullness in the stomach. The FDA considers them safe, but questions their effectiveness. It has withheld approval for "grapefruit diet pills" and states, as this book does, that the only demonstrated way to lose weight is to take in fewer kcalories than your body uses.[28]

A multitude of other drugs are presently under investigation: hormones and hormonelike compounds, inhibitors of nutrient absorption, inhibitors of fat synthesis, promoters of fat breakdown, other modifiers of metabolism—in short, every kind of agent that researchers can imagine might be effective in any way against obesity. Tests in human beings of any of these would be premature at present, and results in animals are not encouraging. Side effects, in many cases, are severe. In short, at present, no known drug is both safe and effective, and many are hazardous.

Perhaps the most promising antiobesity agents presently being tested are the synthetic fats described in Highlight 5. It remains to be seen, however, whether their long-term use will facilitate permanent weight loss or whether, like artificial sweeteners, they will become mere additions to the diet.

Other gimmicks that don't help with weight loss are found in salons and spas. Hot baths do not speed up the basal metabolic rate so that pounds can be lost in hours. Steam and sauna baths do not melt the fat off the body, although they may dehydrate people so that their weights on the scales change dramatically. Machines intended to jiggle parts of the body while

---

*Oral contraceptives may have the same water-retention effect. They may also promote actual fat gain in some women. A woman who has this problem should consult her physician about switching brands.

people lean passively on them provide pleasant stimulation, but no exercise, and so no expenditure of energy. Brushes, sponges, and massages intended to break down "cellulite" do nothing of the kind, because there is no such thing as cellulite.[29] Being passively moved provides no expenditure of energy.

Still another approach to weight control is surgery, which some obese people request out of sheer desperation. The use of surgery in some specific cases is justified, but potentially hazardous. Guidelines for client evaluation, selection, care, and follow-up have been published.[30] The person contemplating surgery for weight loss should think long and hard before submitting to it.

The most common operations for obesity alter the stomach's shape and size, sometimes by stapling the stomach. Gastric stapling forces the person to eat less. The theory may seem pleasingly simple, but stapling involves hazards in practice; stomach tissue is damaged, scars are formed, and staples pull loose.

Another surgical procedure is used not to treat obesity but to remove the evidence. Plastic surgeons can extract fat deposits by suction lipectomy, or "liposuction." This technique carries some risks and complications; most weight-control experts regard it as unsafe and ineffective.

Physicians can position and inflate a balloon inside the stomach to treat obesity without surgery, thus making a person feel uncomfortable when too much food is eaten. To minimize the risks of gastric ulcer, internal bruising, and intestinal blockage that commonly occur during the fourth month of use, the FDA requires removal of these balloons after three months.

Desperation of the same kind leads some clients to request that their jaws be wired shut so that they will be forced to consume a liquid diet. This does bring about weight loss, but when the wires are removed, there is "relentless weight gain . . . until the prewiring weight has been reached."[31]

Last, but not least, among poor choices in obesity treatment are the fad diets. Most of them are low-carbohydrate diets, whose hazards have already been described in Chapter 7. Table 12–6 lists questions you can ask to determine if a diet is safe.

cellulite (SELL-you-leet): supposedly a lumpy form of fat; actually a fraud. The skin sometimes appears lumpy in fatty areas of the body because strands of connective tissue attach the skin to underlying structures. These points of attachment may pull tight where the fat is thick, making lumps appear between them. The fat itself is not different from fat anywhere else in the body. So, if you lose the fat there, you lose the lumpy appearance.

Very-Low-kCalorie Diets

An important class of weight-loss diets is the very-low-kcalorie diets (VLCD) offered by medical centers with the claim that they are balanced and safe. These may be appropriate for some people, at certain times, under close medical supervision, but they require inspection with an eye to their consequences and the specific conditions that warrant their use.

For many obese people, compliance with a well-balanced, nutritionally adequate, kcalorie-restricted diet plan offers slow results compared with the number of pounds they have to lose. Quite often, frustration and a loss of hope take over before significant changes become apparent. For these people, a VLCD plan offers a short-term solution. It allows them to escape the necessity of having to deal with foods—no decisions about what to buy, how to prepare it, or how much of it to eat. They only need to drink a formula as prescribed.

This break from food is important to people who have a compulsive-addictive relationship with food. Unlike a recovering alcoholic, who can abstain from alcohol altogether, or a smoker, who can throw away all

■ TABLE 12–6
How to Evaluate Weight-Loss Diets

With a balanced perspective on foods and a sense of what is important in diet planning and what is not, you can evaluate the many different diets people consume. Here's a summary of the questions you might ask. Start with 100 points, and subtract if any of these criteria are not met:

1.   Does the diet provide a reasonable number of kcalories (about 10 kcalories per pound of current weight and not fewer than 1,200 kcal for the average-sized person)? If not, give it a **minus 10.**

2.   Does it provide enough, but not too much, protein (at least the recommended intake of RDA, but not more than twice that much)? If not, **minus 10.**

3.   Does it provide enough fat for balance and satiety, but not so much fat as to go against current recommendations (say, between 20 and 30% of the kcalories from fat)? If not, **minus 10.**

4.   Does it provide enough carbohydrate to spare protein and prevent ketosis (100 g of carbohydrate for the average-sized person or at least 55 percent of total kcalories)? Is it mostly complex carbohydrate (not more than 10% of the kcalories as concentrated sugar)? If no to either, or both, **minus 10.**

5.   Does it offer a balanced assortment of vitamins and minerals from meats, vegetables (especially dark green and yellow ones), fruits (especially citrus fruits), breads, cereals, legumes, and low-fat milk products? If a food group is omitted (for example, meats), is a suitable substitute provided? For *each* food group omitted and not adequately substituted for, **minus 10.**

6.   Does it offer variety, in the sense that different foods can be selected each day? If you'd class it as "monotonous," give it a **minus 10.**

7.   Does it consist of ordinary foods that are available locally (for example, in the main grocery stores) at the prices people normally pay? Or does the dieter have to buy special, expensive, or unusual foods to adhere to the diet? If you'd class it as "bizarre" or "requiring unusual foods," **minus 10.**

cigarettes, a person cannot go "cold turkey" with food. All people must eat, and to eat the appropriate quantities of the appropriate foods is to challenge obese people to a battle that they have lost before (usually many times). Compliance with a VLCD allows for a break in the pattern of poor eating habits; rapid weight loss (sort of a "jump start" on the journey); and an opportunity to begin good eating habits when the VLCD ends.

VLCDs provide significantly fewer kcalories than the kcalorie-restricted diets described in the following section. VLCD diets contain:

■ Between 400 and 800 kcalories.
■ A protein intake about twice the RDA.
■ Little or no fat.
■ Little carbohydrate (not enough to spare protein).
■ An assortment of vitamins and minerals from supplements.
■ A limited number of foods (primarily lean meats, fish, and poultry) each day or, more commonly, a powdered formula available by prescription only.

Formulas are designed to be nutritionally adequate, even when used as a sole source of nourishment over several weeks.[32] However, the body's response to these severe dietary restrictions is to adapt to a state of

■ TABLE 12–7
Signs and Symptoms Associated with Very-Low-kCalorie Diets

Cardiovascular/Respiratory
- Pulse rate declines.
- Respiratory rate declines.
- Blood pressure declines.
- Oxygen consumption declines.
- Carbon dioxide production declines.
- Cardiac output declines.

Digestive
- GI tract motility declines.
- Constipation develops.

Metabolic
- Cold intolerance occurs.
- Ketosis develops.
- Lean body tissues are lost.
- Basal metabolism declines.
- Dehydration may occur.

Blood
- Blood carotene concentrations increase.
- Blood cholesterol concentrations increase.
- Blood urea concentrations increase.

Physical
- Skin dries out.
- Hair dries out.
- Fatigue sets in.
- Sleeplessness may occur.

semistarvation. It does whatever it needs to do in order to survive, and that generally means it tries to conserve energy. As Chapter 7 describes, several changes occur in hormone concentrations, metabolic activities, fluid and electrolyte balances, and organ functions in an effort to meet the challenge of living on a much-less-than adequate kcalorie intake. For these reasons, a VLCD is appropriate only for short-term use and under close medical supervision. Table 12–7 lists common side effects of a VLCD.

One of the first responses a person on a VLCD notices is a rapid loss of weight; perhaps less noticeable is the frequent urination common in the first weeks. Much of the initial weight loss reflects water losses. On the return to eating a mixed diet, the person may notice a dramatic retention of fluids, swelling, and accompanying weight gain. Such shifts in water balance falsely encourage and distress a person looking for a loss of fat.

■ *Treatments of Obesity: Good Choices*

Dietary recommendations state that a person should maintain appropriate body weight. The only realistic and sensible way for the obese person to achieve and maintain a healthy body weight is to cut kcalories, to increase activity, and to maintain this changed lifestyle for life. This is a tall order. Only

5 to 20 percent of people who try meet with any success. To succeed means modifying all the attitudes and behaviors that have contributed to the problem in the first place, sometimes against factors that can't be changed. Still, it can be, and has been, done successfully. A multiple approach works best, involving changes in diet, exercise, behavior, and attitude.

The way a person loses weight is a highly individual matter. Two weight-loss plans may both be successful and yet have little or nothing in common. To heighten the sense of individuality, the following sections are written in terms of advice to "you." This is not intended to put "you" under pressure to take it personally, but to give you the illusion of listening in on a conversation in which an obese person (with, say, 50 pounds to lose) is being competently counseled by someone familiar with the techniques known to be effective. Margin notes at intervals highlight the principles involved.

Diet

No particular diet is magical, and no particular food must either be included or avoided. You are the one who will have to live with the diet, so you had better be involved in its planning. Don't think of it as a diet you are going "on"—because then you may be tempted to go "off." The diet can be called successful only if the pounds do not return. Think of it as an eating plan that you will adopt for life. It must consist of foods that you like, that are available to you, and that are within your means.

- Be involved in planning your own program.

To be successful, people have to first lose weight; then, maintain the weight loss. If you adopt an "eating plan" rather than "a diet," you can be practicing maintenance behaviors all the time you are losing weight. You will be ready to succeed for the rest of your life, once you arrive at your goal weight.

- Keep in mind that you will want to maintain your lost weight. Practice the needed behaviors as you go.

Choose an energy level you can live with. A deficit of 500 kcalories a day for seven days (3,500 kcalories a week) is enough to lose a pound of body fat. It is best to do this by increasing activity and reducing food intake. A rule of thumb is that you need at least 10 kcalories per pound of current weight.

Nutritional adequacy is difficult for most people to achieve on fewer than 1,200 kcalories a day—1,000 at the very least. You will experience a healthier and more successful weight loss with a small kcalorie deficit that provides an adequate intake than with a larger kcalorie deficit that creates feelings of starvation and deprivation, which can lead to an irresistible urge to binge. Table 12–8 presents a sample balanced 1,225-kcalorie weight-loss diet using the exchange system (introduced in Chapter 2).

- Adopt a realistic plan.

Put diet adequacy high on your list of priorities. This is a way of putting yourself first. "I like me, and I'm going to take good care of me" is the attitude to adopt. This means including low-kcalorie foods that are rich in valuable nutrients; tasty vegetables and fruits; whole-grain breads and cereals; modest portions of lean protein-rich foods like poultry, fish, and eggs; nutritious meat alternates like dried beans and peas; and low-fat milk products such as nonfat milk and yogurt. Within these categories, learn what foods you like, and use them often. If you plan resolutely to include a certain number of servings of food from each of these categories each day, you may be so busy making sure you get what you need that you will have little time or appetite left for high-kcalorie or empty-kcalorie foods.

- Make the diet adequate by emphasizing high-nutrient-density foods that you like.

- Make tasty vegetables and fruits central to your weight-control plan.

■ TABLE 12–8
A Sample Balanced Weight-Loss Diet[a]

Exchange Item	Number of Exchanges	Carbohydrate (g)	Protein (g)	Fat (g)
Starch/bread	6	90	18	Trace
Meat (lean)	4	0	28	12
Vegetables	4	20	8	0
Fruit	2	30	0	0
Milk (nonfat)	2	24	16	Trace
Fat	4	0	0	20
Total		164 g	70 g	32 g

[a]This 1,225-kcal diet typifies the balance recommended for a weight-loss diet: approximately 50% carbohydrate, 25% protein, and 25% fat. (Carbohydrate supplies 656 kcal; protein, 280 kcal; and fat, 288 kcal.) When the dieter returns to a maintenance plan by adding mostly carbohydrate foods, the ratio will resemble the 15% protein, 30% fat, and 55% carbohydrate recommended for a maintenance diet.

The carbohydrate-containing foods you eat should be largely unrefined, complex-carbohydrate foods of low energy density. People who eat these foods in abundance have been observed to spontaneously eat for longer times and to eat 22 to 33 percent fewer kcalories than when eating foods of high energy density.[33] The satiety signal indicating that you are full is sent after a 20- minute lag, so unless you slow down, you can eat a great deal more than you need before the signal reaches your brain.

- Select complex carbohydrate-rich foods high in bulk.

Confirming these statements, one research study reported that the eating of soup at either lunch or dinner reduces people's rate of eating. People who eat fewer than 20 kcalories per minute tend to lose more weight. The single suggestion that the subjects include soup in their meals helped them lose a pound a week.[34]

- Use low-fat soups often.

Measure your dietary fat with extra caution. A slip of the butter knife adds even more kcalories than a slip of the sugar spoon. Even given the same number of kcalories, less fat in the diet means less fat in the body. Dietary fat correlates positively with body fat, whereas, dietary carbohydrate and fiber correlate negatively with body fat.[35]

Less fat in the diet also means fewer kcalories. By lowering the kcaloric density of the diet, you will lower your total kcalorie intake. When women were given diets of foods similar in appearance and palatability, but varying in the percentages of kcalories from fat, they did not adjust their food intakes to compensate for kcalories.[36] The women who ate low-fat foods did not increase their food intakes, but instead, consumed fewer kcalories. If you can make low-fat food selections habitually, you need not limit the amount of food you eat. A low-fat diet has multiple health benefits. And speaking of empty kcalories, omit not only fat, but sugar and alcohol, too, if you are willing.

- Select low-fat foods regularly.

Learn to satisfy your thirst with water. Overeaters often use food to satisfy thirst; don't do that anymore. Drink plenty of water. A generous water intake will do several things for you. It will help to fill your stomach between meals, keep your mouth happy, and keep you busy. It will dilute the metabolic wastes you generate from breaking down fat so that you can excrete them easily. It will meet the water need that you formerly met by eating extra food

- Drink plenty of water.

- Anticipate a plateau (have realistic expectations from the start).

- Learn, practice, and eat right for the rest of your life.

weight cycling: the effect that repeated cycles of weight loss and gain, without exercise, have on body composition, in which the body fat content increases and kcaloric needs fall after each round, making the next round of weight loss harder; popularly called the **ratchet** or **yo-yo effect**.

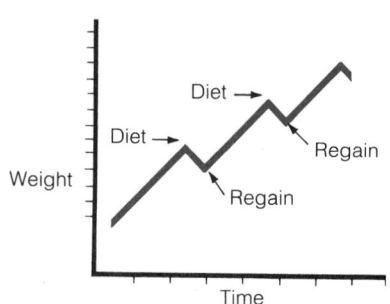

■ **FIGURE 12–6**
The Weight Cycling Effect of Repeated Dieting
Each round of dieting, without exercise, is followed by a rebound of weight to a higher level than before.

- Pave the way for later changes.

Benefits of exercise:
- Short-term increased energy output.
- Appetite control.
- Stress reduction.
- Control of stress-induced eating.
- Increased self-esteem.
- Physical well-being.

(food provides water, as you may recall). It is a kcalorie-free oral pleasure; cultivate it enthusiastically.

Take well-spaced weighings so you can see your progress. If you see a weight gain and you know you have strictly followed your diet, this probably represents a shift in water weight. Many dieters experience a temporary plateau after about three weeks—not because they are slipping, but because they have gained water weight temporarily while they are still losing body fat. If you faithfully follow your diet plan, one day the plateau will break. You can tell from your frequent urination.

A dieter who undertakes an exercise program may arrive at a plateau for another reason: gain in muscle mass at the expense of body fat. An upcoming section discusses the role of exercise in a weight-control program.

The focus of this section has been on "kcalorie-restricted" diets—those that provide fewer kcalories than you expend. By following such a diet you will experience a gradual weight loss and maintain the loss as long as you abide by the appropriate food selections and eating habits. People can live healthfully and happily on such diets for a *lifetime*.

Finally, plan to put as much effort into maintenance of goal weight as you did into achieving it. No doubt you've heard someone say as a joke, "I've lost 200 pounds, but I was never more than 20 pounds overweight." What this person means is that frequent dieting alternating with weight gain is an expected pattern of life. With each bout of dieting, this person is trading a small amount of healthy lean body tissue for a slightly higher body fat content. This weight cycling pattern, known as the ratchet or "yo-yo" effect of dieting, is illustrated in Figure 12–6.

Researchers studying this repeated pattern of weight loss and weight gain propose that the body adapts by increasing its food efficiency, thus creating a "dieting induced obesity."[37] This increased efficiency shows itself in a way familiar to dieters who have lost and gained—and lost and gained again. With each attempt, it becomes harder and takes longer to lose weight and easier and quicker to gain it back. The body's metabolic rate has declined so that the same body weight can be maintained on a lower food energy intake than was required prior to the dieting cycle. Don't let this happen to you.

Exercise

Some people who want to lose weight hate the very idea of exercise. Obese people often—understandably—do not enjoy moving their bodies. They feel heavy, clumsy, even ridiculous. A word to reassure them: weight loss is possible without exercise. In fact, obese women on a kcalorie-restricted diet who did not exercise lost the same amount of weight as obese women who exercised and dieted—with a notable difference. The exercise group lost more *fat*.[38] Even if you choose not to alter your habits at first, let your mind be open to the possibility that you will want to take up some activity later on. As the pounds come off, moving your body becomes a pleasure.

Exercise makes several contributions to a weight-control program. Exercise alters body composition in a desirable direction, thereby altering metabolism and making daily energy expenditures slightly higher, even during rest. It spends energy directly, too, of course. Exercise also offers the psychological benefits of looking and feeling healthy, and it reduces stress and stress-induced eating. Increased self-esteem accompanies these benefits, and this tends to support a person's resolve to persist in a weight-control effort—rounding out a beneficial cycle.

Exercise has two other beneficial effects. First, the conditioned body is "trained" to use fatty acids, rather than glucose, as fuel; therefore, after you've become conditioned, you'll tend to burn more body fat during exercise than you did when you were out of condition. The best kind of exercise for building up your fat-burning equipment is not severely strenuous, but easy-paced to moderate exercise of long duration (30 minutes or more). Second, regular vigorous exercise will speed the metabolism slightly for a day or so. The metabolism is stimulated by about 5 percent for as long as two days later.

Table 12–9 shows the energy in foods and how far you must run or how long you must walk to "work them off." People can take such charts out of context and say, "A sandwich and a glass of milk will cost me an hour of running . . . hmm, I think I'll skip lunch." Don't let the table fool you into thinking only in terms of kcalories. First, such charts refer only to kcalories eaten in *excess* of your daily maintenance level or the lower kcaloric level chosen for a weight-loss diet. Second, your body needs nutritious foods during weight loss as much as ever. So eat the sandwich, drink the milk, go do your workout, and know that you've found the best of both worlds.

Keep in mind that if exercise is to help with weight loss, it must be *active exercise*—voluntary moving of muscles. Being moved passively, as by a machine at a health spa or by a massage, does not increase kcalorie expenditure. The more muscles you move, the more kcalories you spend.

People sometimes ask about "spot reducing." Can you lose fat in particular locations? Unfortunately, muscles don't "own" the fat that surrounds them. All body fat is shared by all the muscles and organs, so "spot-reducing" exercises that work only the flabby parts won't help reduce the fat located there. There is some good news, though: tightening muscles in trouble spots

Moderate exercise of long duration, such as bicycling or walking, help to burn fat.

Two more benefits of regular exercise:
- Burning of more body fat during exercise by a conditioned body than by an unconditioned one.
- Long-term increase (slight) in BMR, with increased lean tissue.

■ TABLE 12–9
Activity Cost of Eating Foods beyond kCalorie Need[a]

To work off the kcalories from this food eaten beyond your energy need:	To have to walk:	Or jog:
Cookie, chocolate chip (50 kcal)	20 min	5 min
Ice cream, ⅔ c (200 kcal)	76 min	22 min
T-bone steak, 8 oz (800 kcal)	5 hr	1½ hr
Pizza, gooey, 1 slice (300 kcal)	2 hr	33 min
Beer or cola beverage, 12 oz (150 kcal)	58 min	16 min
Caramel candy, 1 oz, or potato chips, 10 chips (115 kcal)	44 min	13 min
Chocolate-coated peanuts, 8 (160 kcal)	1 hr	17 min

[a]For a 150-lb person, the energy cost of walking at 3.0 mph, exclusive of BMR, is 2.6 kcal/min; of running at 5.2 mph is 9.2 kcal/min.

by way of a balanced, all-over exercise program will help the appearance of the fatty areas.

Another thing to keep in mind is that the number of kcalories spent in an activity depends more upon your weight than on how fast you can do the exercise. For example, a person who weighs 120 pounds and runs a six-minute mile burns off 83 kcalories. That same person, ambling along for a mile in ten minutes, burns almost the same amount—76 kcalories. Similarly, a 220-pound person spends 148 kcalories on the six-minute mile, and only a little less—136 kcalories—on the ten-minute amble. The rule seems to be that you don't have to work fast to use up energy effectively. If you choose to walk the distance instead of run, you'll use up about the same energy; it'll just take you longer.

Behavior and Attitude

Diet and exercise are not the only prerequisites to achieving and maintaining appropriate body weight. Behavior and attitude are important supporting factors.

Behavior Modification   As an earlier section described, some people eat in response to external cues. Behavioral psychologists view human behavior as regulated by environmental conditions, those that precede a behavior and those that follow it—the antecedents and the consequences:

A (antecedents) $\longrightarrow$ B (behavior) $\longleftrightarrow$ C (consequences)

A behavior occurs in response to antecedents (cues or stimuli); the more intense they are, the more likely the behavior is to occur. The behavior leads to consequences, and the more intense these are, the more or less likely the behavior is to occur again. Behavior modification involves manipulating these environmental conditions so as to favor the repeated occurrence of desired behaviors and extinguish the occurrence of unwanted behaviors.

Behavior modification can be used to change the behaviors of overeating and underexercising that lead to and perpetuate obesity. Table 12–10 presents behaviors commonly used for weight loss.

First, set about controlling the stimuli that prompt you to eat inappropriately. This involves purchasing the appropriate foods, planning meals and exercise times, and altering food-related activities. Try to strengthen the cues to appropriate eating and exercise. For example, keep good foods in the front of the refrigerator, and make exercise equipment easily available. Resolve to respond only to one set of cues designed by you: one particular place in one particular room.

Second, alter the eating behavior itself. By chewing food thoroughly and putting the fork down between bites, you will eat more slowly (overeaters eat faster than others).

Third, make sure that positive consequences, including material rewards, follow your display of the desired behaviors. Friends and family may provide praise to reward you.

Fourth, monitor yourself. Keep a record of your present eating and activity behaviors against which to measure future progress. Keep a diary, like that

■ TABLE 12–10
Behavioral Principles of Weight Loss

1. Stimulus Control.

A. Shopping.
   1. Shop for food after eating.
   2. Shop from a list.
   3. Avoid ready-to-eat foods.
   4. Don't carry more cash than needed for shopping list.

B. Plans.
   1. Plan to limit food intake.
   2. Substitute exercise for snacking.
   3. Eat meals and snacks at scheduled times.
   4. Don't accept food offered by others.

C. Activities.
   1. Store foods out of sight.
   2. Eat all food in the same place.
   3. Remove food from inappropriate storage areas in the house.
   4. Keep serving dishes off the table.
   5. Use smaller dishes and utensils.
   6. Avoid being the food server.
   7. Leave the table immediately after eating.
   8. Don't save leftovers.

D. Holidays and parties.
   1. Drink fewer alcoholic beverages.
   2. Plan eating habits before parties.
   3. Eat a low-kcalorie snack before parties.
   4. Practice polite ways to decline food.
   5. Don't get discouraged by an occasional setback.

2. Eating Behavior.
   1. Put the fork down between mouthfuls.
   2. Chew thoroughly before swallowing.
   3. Prepare foods one portion at a time.
   4. Leave some food on the plate.
   5. Pause in the middle of the meal.
   6. Do nothing else while eating (e.g., read, watch television).

3. Reward.
   1. Solicit help from family and friends.
   2. Help family and friends provide this help in the form of praise and material rewards.
   3. Utilize self-monitoring records as a basis for rewards.
   4. Plan specific rewards for specific behaviors (behavioral contracts).

4. Self-Monitoring.
   Keep a diet diary that includes:
   1. Time and place of eating.
   2. Type and amount of food.
   3. Who is present/How you feel.

5. Nutrition Education.
   1. Use a diet diary to identify problem areas.
   2. Make small changes that you can continue.
   3. Learn nutritional values of foods.
   4. Decrease fat intake; increase complex carbohydrates.

6. Physical Activity.
   A. Routine activity.
      1. Increase routine activity.
      2. Increase use of stairs.
      3. Keep a record of distance walked each day.

   B. Exercise.
      1. Begin a very mild exercise program.
      2. Keep a record of daily exercise.
      3. Increase the exercise very gradually.

7. Cognitive Restructuring.
   1. Avoid setting unreasonable goals.
   2. Think about progress, not shortcomings.
   3. Avoid imperatives like *always* and *never*.
   4. Counter negative thoughts with rational restatements.
   5. Set weight goals.

Source: A. J. Stunkard and H. C. Berthold, What is behavioral therapy? A very short description of behavioral weight control, *American Journal of Clinical Nutrition* 41 (1985): 821–823. Copyright *American Journal of Clinical Nutrition*, American Society for Clinical Nutrition.

shown in Figure 12–7, to learn what your particular eating stimuli, or cues, are. Such a practice will give you an honest look at your kcalorie intake. It is not unusual for people to underestimate their kcalorie intakes.

Fifth, learn about nutrition. Be able to identify problem foods in your diet and make appropriate substitutions.

Sixth, increase your physical activity. Park the car at the far end of the parking lot; use the stairs instead of the elevator; do a deep knee bend each time you get up from your chair. These strategies don't add up to many kcalories each, but over a year's time they become significant. If you also

■ FIGURE 12–7
Food Diary
The record reveals problem areas, the first
step towards solving problems.

incorporate regular aerobic exercise into your schedule (see Chapter 13), your heart and lungs, as well as your muscles, will be fit.

The seventh principle involves cognitive restructuring. Set realistic goals and think positively about your progress toward reaching them.

From all the behavior changes available to you, you can choose the ones to begin with. Don't try to master them all at once. No one who attempts too many changes at one time is successful. Set your own priorities. Pick one trouble area that you think you can handle, start with that, and practice your strategy until it is habitual and automatic. Then you can select another trouble area to work on. Throughout the process, enjoy your new, emerging self.

Finally, be aware that it can be harder to maintain weight loss than to lose weight. On arriving at the goal weight after months of self-discipline and new habit formation, the victorious weight loser must at all cost avoid "celebrating" by resuming old eating habits. They are gone forever—remember? Membership in an ongoing weight-control organization and continued physical activity can provide indispensable support for the formerly fat person who wants to remain trim.

Personal Attitude   When behavior therapists view overeating and under-exercising as maladaptive behaviors that people can change, they ignore the positive contribution that overeating plays in a person's life. They also miss that being overweight may have become a part of a person's identity. For many people, overeating and being overweight have become integral parts of their lives, involving social, marital, and family relationships; community activities; work; health; self-concept; and emotional states.[39] To change diet and exercise behaviors without attention to the person's self-concept is to meet failure.

Sometimes habitual behaviors that are hazardous to health, such as smoking or drinking alcohol, contribute positively by becoming ways for people to adapt to stressful situations. Similarly, many people overeat to cope with the stresses of life. To break out of that pattern, they must first identify the particular stressors that trigger their urges to overeat. Then, when faced with these situations, they must learn to practice problem-solving skills. These skills will help them to learn appropriate responses to a variety of difficult situations.

All this is not to imply that psychological therapy holds the magic answer to a weight problem. Still, efforts to improve one's general well-being can result in weight loss even when weight control is not the goal. That is, when the problems that trigger the urge to overeat are dealt with in alternative ways, people may find they eat less and that their eating behavior begins to occur appropriately in response to internal cues of hunger rather than inappropriately to external signals of stress. The message is that sound emotional health supports your ability to take care of your health in all ways—including nutrition, weight control, and fitness.

Self-esteem underlies emotional health and facilitates personal growth. You can enhance your self-esteem by fostering a positive view of your inner self and by developing a healthy relationship with your outer self, your body. A technique for viewing your inner self positively is to practice positive thinking. By making affirmative statements about yourself and visualizing yourself succeeding at whatever task you choose, you can improve your self-esteem and enhance your chances for success. People who believe they can lose weight are more successful in losing weight than those who expect to fail; people who view themselves as "thin" are more successful in maintaining weight loss than those who view themselves as "fat" or even as "formerly fat."

You may find it helpful to join a group such as Take Off Pounds Sensibly (TOPS), Weight Watchers (WW), or Overeaters Anonymous (OA). A modest expenditure for your own health is well worthwhile (but avoid rip-offs, of course). Many dieters find it helpful to form their own self-help groups.

A surefire remedy for obesity has yet to be found, although most people find a combination of the approaches just described to be most effective. Diet and exercise shift energy balance so that more kcalories are being spent than taken in; the exercise maintains or even builds the lean body so that fat is preferentially lost and metabolic energy needs remain high; the behavior modification retrains habits so that once the weight is lost, it will not return; and the improvement in inner self helps a person to manage life without a dependency on food. This treatment package requires time, individualization, and skilled health care providers.

■ Underweight

Much of what has been said about obesity applies to underweight as well. No serious hazards accompany *mild* degrees of underweight. In fact, the only causes of death seen more often in thin people than in normal-weight people are wasting diseases such as tuberculosis and cancer. (Suicide is more common among underweight people, but the underweight is not thought to be a cause. The severe depression probably came first and caused anorexia, or lack of appetite.)

Underweight does pose hazards, however, when it is accompanied by undernutrition. An inadequate supply of vitamins, minerals, and energy leaves the body unprepared to handle its many metabolic and physical tasks.

The causes of underweight may be as diverse as those of overeating—hunger, appetite, and satiety irregularities; psychological factors; metabolic ones; hereditary tendencies. Habits learned early in childhood, especially food aversions, may perpetuate themselves.

The demand for energy to support physical activity and growth often contributes to underweight; an extremely active boy during his adolescent growth spurt may need more than 4,000 kcalories a day to maintain his weight. He may be too busy to take time to eat. Underweight people state with justification that it is as hard for them to gain weight as for overweight people to lose it. So much energy may be spent adapting to a higher food intake that at first, as many as 750 to 800 extra kcalories a day may be needed to gain a pound a week.[40] Like the weight loser, the person who wants to gain must learn new habits and learn to like new foods.

Weight-gain strategies center mostly on increasing food intake and eating foods that provide as many kcalories in as small a volume as possible. You won't gain much weight eating raw carrots, because they'll fill you up before they offer you enough energy. kCalorie-dense foods hold the key to weight gain (the ones the successful weight-loss dieter avoids). Pick the highest-

anorexia (an-o-REX-ee-uh): lack of appetite; commonly seen in illnesses such as cancer and GI disorders and in conditions such as depression and alcohol and drug abuse; in contrast, anorexia nervosa (the subject of Highlight 12) is not explainable by such circumstances.

an = not
orexis = appetite

kcalorie items from each food group. Consume milk shakes instead of milk, peanut butter instead of lean meat, avocados instead of cucumbers, and whole-wheat muffins instead of whole-wheat bread. Eat butter on cooked vegetables; add cream and sugar to coffee; use creamy dressings on salads, whipped cream on fruit, sour cream on potatoes, and so forth. (Because fat contains more than twice as many kcalories per teaspoon as sugar does, fat adds kcalories without adding much bulk.)

Be aware that a low-fat diet plan is recommended for the general U.S. population, because the general population is overweight and at risk for heart disease. These dietary recommendations may not apply to you; consult your physician. Consumption of high-fat foods is not healthy for most people, of course, but may be essential for an underweight individual who needs to gain weight.

Since you need substantially more kcalories per day, in addition to eating more kcalories per meal, you will need to eat more frequently. Between-meal snacking offers a solution. Make three sandwiches in the morning and eat them between classes in addition to the day's three regular meals. Most people who are underweight have simply been too busy (sometimes for months) to eat enough to gain or maintain weight. Therefore, preplan your meals. Spend more time eating each meal; learn to eat more food within the first 20 minutes of a meal. Don't start with soup or salad; eat meaty appetizers or the main course first.

Expect to feel full. Most underweight individuals are accustomed to small quantities of food. When they begin eating significantly more, they feel uncomfortable. This is normal, and it passes over time.

For people who are underweight due to illness, however, concentrated liquid formulas are often recommended, because a weak person can swallow them with a minimum of effort. A physician or registered dietitian can recommend high-protein, high-kcalorie formulas to help the underweight person maintain or gain. Used in addition to regular meals, these can help considerably.

No known pill, shot, hormone, or surgical procedure will increase weight safely, and although physical activity costs kcalories, it is essential for health, unless an underweight condition has become life threatening. The healthy way to gain weight is to build up muscle tissue by patient and consistent training and, at the same time, to take in enough energy to support the weight gain. If you are not dangerously underweight, you can adopt an exercise program designed to increase lean body tissue (for more details on exercise, see Chapter 13).

As with weight loss, the person attempting a weight gain must anticipate a plateau. At that time a further increase in food intake will be necessary to continue the gain.

An extreme underweight condition known as anorexia nervosa is sometimes seen in young people, usually young women, who exercise heroic self-denial in order to control their weight. They actually go to such extremes that they become severely undernourished, finally achieving a body weight of 70 pounds or even less. The distinguishing feature of this type of anorexic, as opposed to other thin people, is that the starvation is intentional.

Anorexia nervosa is one of two eating disorders that are becoming widespread in our society today. The other is bulimia— compulsive overeating. These two disorders are the subject of the highlight that follows this chapter.

Choose a Goal Weight and Plan a Diet

What is an appropriate weight for you? When physical health alone is considered, a wide range of weights is acceptable for a person of a given height. Within the safe range, the definition of appropriate weight is up to the individual, depending on factors such as family history, occupation, physical and recreational activities, and personal preferences.

1. Determine the safe range for a person your height and sex.

- Record your height: _____ ft _____ inches.
- Look up the acceptable weight range for a person your height and sex in the tables on the inside back cover. Record the entire range: _____ to _____ lb.

2. If your weight is below the bottom end of this safe range, you need to gain weight for your health's sake. If your weight is above the top end of the range, check your health history for further confirmation. A family or personal medical history of diabetes (non-insulin-dependent type), hypertension, or high blood cholesterol indicates the need for weight loss.

3. Choose a goal weight within the acceptable range. Answering the following questions should help you to determine where, within the safe range, your personal appropriate weight may be:

- Does your occupation demand that you have a certain body shape? Record the weight, within the safe range, that would most nearly approximate this body shape: _____ lb.
- Do you engage in a sport or other physical activity that requires a particular body weight for optimal performance? Consult your instructor or other expert in that sport or activity, and record the weight recommended on that basis: _____ lb.
- Do you hope to start a pregnancy soon? If so, consult your health care provider about the ideal weight with which to begin a pregnancy: _____ lb.
- Undress and stand before a mirror. Do you think you need to gain or lose weight? Add or subtract pounds to arrive at a personal goal weight (but be sure to stay within the safe range): _____ lb.

Based on all of these considerations, choose a final goal weight. No formula exists for this estimate, but don't choose a weight outside the acceptable range without a professional assessment.

Your goal weight: _____ lb.

Diets can be planned using the exchange system to gain weight, lose weight, or stay the same. For practice in the use of this convenient system, try planning two diets, one for weight maintenance or gain, the other for weight loss.

Diet for Weight Maintenance or Gain

1. Set your daily energy level. If you choose to maintain weight, this energy level should be equal to your daily energy expenditure (see p. 357). If you wish to gain weight, it should be at least 500 kcalories above that.

2. Decide on the proportions in which protein, fat, and carbohydrate kcalories will be represented in the diet. A suggested ratio is about 10 to 15 percent of the energy from protein, not more than 30 percent from fat, and the rest from carbohydrate. Given the daily kcalorie level you choose, how many kcalories will you allot to each nutrient?

3. Translate these kcalorie amounts into grams. (Remember, 1 gram protein or carbohydrate = 4 kcalories; 1 gram fat = 9 kcalories.) Enter these gram amounts and your intended kcalorie total at the top of Form 6 (Appendix K).

4. Now decide how many exchanges of milk, vegetables, and fruit you'd like to have each day; enter these numbers in the form; and compute the number of grams of carbohydrate, protein, and fat they will deliver (don't compute kcalories yet). See p. 28 or Appendix G for the exchange system values. (Caution: Use pencil. You'll want to change these numbers several times before you finalize your plan.)

Only one more set of foods—the bread exchanges—contributes any carbohydrate to the diet. Select the number of bread exchanges that will bring your total carbohydrate intake close to the amount you want. Adjust the numbers of these four exchanges until they seem reasonable to you.

Suggestions: Diets for adults should include 2 to 3 milk exchanges daily, 2 or more vegetable exchanges, and at least 2, and preferably more, fruit exchanges. The number of bread exchanges is variable, but the bread list includes many nutritious foods containing complex carbohydrates. It is not unusual for women's diets to include 4 to 6 bread exchanges and for men's to include twice as many or even more. High-kcalorie diets can have many more of all of these carbohydrate-containing exchanges.

If you have a special fondness for sugar or sugar-containing foods, add a line to Form 6 under "Bread," and allow yourself some

(continued)

"sugar exchanges" (see pp. 96–97). At the end of this step, you should have a carbohydrate gram total within about 10 percent of the number you planned in step 3.

5. Subtotal the protein grams delivered by these four types of foods. Only one more list of foods—the meat exchanges—will contribute any protein to the diet. Select the number of meat exchanges you need to bring your total protein intake close to what you planned in step 3.

   Note: The recommended intake of carbohydrate is high compared with what many people are used to. Planners often find that once they have completed step 4 of this procedure, they have almost used up their protein allowance and must therefore drastically limit their consumption of meat exchanges. If it works out this way for you, you have two choices. You can accept the dictates of this pattern and resolve to limit your intake of meats and meat substitutes accordingly. Or you can increase the number of protein grams you will allow yourself (step 3) and reduce carbohydrate and/or fat to keep the kcalorie level within bounds. At the end of this step, you should have a protein gram total that agrees (within 10 percent) with your plan of step 3, and falls between your protein RDA and twice the RDA.

6. Subtotal the fat grams delivered by these five categories of foods. Now use the fat exchanges to bring your total fat intake up to the level planned in step 3.

7. Fill in the kcalorie amounts contributed by the exchanges you have selected, and check to see that the total agrees (within 10 percent) with the kcalorie level you set in step 1. The completed form now indicates the total exchanges of each type that you will consume on each day of your diet.

8. Distribute the exchanges you have selected into a meal pattern like that on Form 7 (see Appendix K). You may want to plan four to six meals a day or to have only one snack; if so, or if you have other preferences, make your own form.

9. Finally, to see how your diet plan might work out on an actual day, make a sample menu. Look over the exchange lists, and choose foods you would like to eat that fit the pattern you worked out in step 8.

For example:

My meal pattern for breakfast specifies:

- 1 fruit exchange.
- 2 grain/starchy vegetable exchanges.
- 1 milk exchange.
- 1 sugar exchange.
- 1 fat exchange.

So I might choose:

- ½ cup orange juice.
- ¾ ounce dry cereal and 1 slice bread, toasted.
- ½ cup milk on the cereal and ½ cup milk in a glass.
- 1 teaspoon sugar on the cereal.
- 1 pat margarine on the toast.

Diet for Weight Loss

1. Set your daily kcalorie level. If you wish to lose a pound a week, set it 500 kcalories per day below your energy need (p. 357). You could set it higher or lower than this, but on no account should you set it below 1,000 kcalories per day unless your height is below average.

2. Decide on the proportions in which protein, fat, and carbohydrate kcalories will be represented in the diet. A suggested ratio is about 50 percent of the kcalories from carbohydrate, and 25 percent each from protein and fat.

3. Translate these kcalorie amounts into grams, as in the previous diet plan, and enter them and your kcalorie level into Form 6.

4. Now, using pencil on Form 6 (Appendix K), decide on the number of carbohydrate-containing exchanges you'll have, as in step 4 of the first plan. Try to include 2 milk, 2 vegetable, and at least 2 fruit exchanges, and make up the rest of your carbohydrate intake with bread exchanges. Allow no sugar unless you really can't do without it. At the end of this step you should have a carbohydrate gram total within about 10 percent of the number you planned in step 3.

5. Now subtotal the protein grams you have so far, and bring your total protein intake up to the level of your plan by adding meat exchanges. At the end of this step, you should have a protein gram total that agrees (within 10 percent) with your plan of step 3.

6. Now subtotal the fat grams you have so far, and add fat exchanges to bring your total fat intake up to the level planned in step 3.

7. Fill in the kcalorie amounts contributed by the exchanges you have selected, and check to see that the total agrees (within 10 percent) with the kcalorie level you set in step 1.

8. Distribute the exchanges into a meal pattern, using Form 7 (Appendix K) or your own form based on your own preferences.

9. Make a day's sample menus, as in step 9 of the first plan.

Study Questions

1. Discuss the limitations for the definition of ideal or desirable weight.
2. List the factors that affect the basal metabolic rate (BMR), and discuss the effect on the BMR that these factors have.
3. How do you calculate the total energy that a person spends in a day?
4. List the factors that tend to increase the risk of obesity. What are the dangers of excess weight?
5. What considerations are essential to any successful weight-loss program?
6. Discuss strategies suitable for achieving weight gain.
7. What are the benefits of increased physical activity in a weight-loss program?
8. Describe the behavior modification techniques recommended for changing an individual's dietary habits.

Notes

1. K. Donato and D. M. Hegsted, Efficiency of utilization of various sources of energy for growth, *Proceedings of the National Academy of Sciences* 82 (1985): 4866–4870.
2. K. J. Acheson and coauthors, Glycogen storage capacity and de novo lipogenesis during massive carbohydrate overfeeding in man, *American Journal of Clinical Nutrition* 48 (1988): 240–247; J. P. Flatt, Effect of carbohydrate and fat intake on postprandial substrate oxidation and storage, *Topics in Clinical Nutrition*, April 1987, pp. 15–27.
3. D. M. Dreon and coauthors, Dietary fat: Carbohydrate ratio and obesity in middle-aged men, *American Journal of Clinical Nutrition* 47 (1988): 995–1000.
4. L. B. Oscai, M. M. Brown, and W. C. Miller, Effect of dietary fat on food intake, growth and body composition in rats, *Growth* 48 (1984): 415–424.
5. National Academy of Sciences report on diet and health, *Nutrition Reviews* 47 (1989): 142–149.
6. L. S. Sims, Contributions of the US Department of Agriculture, *American Journal of Clinical Nutrition* 47 (1988): 329–332.
7. G. B. Forbes and M. R. Brown, Energy need for weight maintenance in human beings: Effect of body size and composition, *Journal of the American Dietetic Association* 89 (1989): 499–502.
8. Refractory obesity and energy homeostasis, *Nutrition Reviews*, November 1983, pp. 349–351.
9. G. H. Anderson, N. Hrboticky, and L. A. Leiter, Macronutrient-specific appetites: Their importance in obesity, in *Dietary Treatment and Prevention of Obesity*, eds. R. T. Frankle and coeditors (London: Libbey, 1985), pp. 21–31.
10. J. Gibbs, Gut peptides in obesity: Can we use them to learn and to treat? in *Dietary Treatment and Prevention of Obesity*, eds. R. T. Frankle and coeditors (London: Libbey, 1985), pp. 97–103.
11. J. S. Garrow, Energy balance in man—An overview, *American Journal of Clinical Nutrition* 45 (1987): 1114–1119.
12. T. B. Van Itallie, When the frame is part of the picture (editorial), *American Journal of Public Health* 75 (1985): 1054–1055.
13. First National Health and Nutrition Examination Survey (NHANES I), as cited by Van Itallie, 1985.
14. T. G. Lohman, Body composition methodology in sports medicine, *The Physician and Sports Medicine* 10 (1982): 47–58.
15. M. Simonton, An overview: Advances in research and treatment of obesity, *Food and Nutrition News*, March–April 1982.
16. M. Winick, Childhood obesity, *Nutrition Today*, May–June 1974, pp. 6–12.
17. R. E. Patterson and coauthors, Factors related to obesity in preschool children, *Journal of the American Dietetic Association* 86 (1986): 1376–1381.
18. A. J. Stunkard, T. T. Foch, and Z. Hrubec, A twin study of human obesity, *Journal of the American Medical Association* 256 (1986): 51–54.
19. J. L. Knittle, Obesity in childhood: A problem in adipose tissue cellular development, *Journal of Pediatrics* 81 (1972): 1048–1059.
20. D. R. Krieger and L. Landsberg, Role of hormones in the etiology and pathogenesis of obesity, in *Obesity and Weight Control: The Health Professional's Guide to Understanding and Treatment*, eds. R. T. Frankle and M. Yang, (Rockville, Md.: Apsen Publishers, 1988) pp. 35–54.
21. R. E. Keesey, A set-point analysis of the regulation of body weight, in *Obesity*, ed. A. J. Stunkard (Philadelphia: W. B. Saunders, 1980), pp. 144–165.
22. T. B. Van Itallie and R. G. Campbell, Multidisciplinary approach to the problem of obesity, *Journal of the American Dietetic Association* 61 (1972): 385–390.
23. A. Mandenoff, F. Fumeron, and M. Apfelbaum, Endogenous opiates and energy balance, *Science* 215 (1982): 1536–1538.
24. J. Slochower and S. P. Kaplan, Anxiety, perceived control, and eating in obese and normal weight persons, *Appetite* 1 (1980): 75–83.
25. W. H. Dietz, Jr., and S. L. Gortmaker, Do we fatten our children at the television set? Obesity and television viewing in children and adolescents, *Pediatrics* 75 (1985): 807–812.
26. W. W. Tryon, Activity as a function of body weight, *American Journal of Clinical Nutrition* 46 (1987): 451–455.
27. A. C. Sullivan, C. Nauss-Karol, and L. Cheng, Pharmacological treatment, in *Obesity*, ed. M. R. C. Greenwood (New York: Churchill Livingstone, 1983), pp. 123–158.

28. Diet plans, *Consumer News,* February 1976.

29. D. C. Fletcher, What is cellulite? (letter to the editor), *Journal of the American Medical Association* 235 (1976): 2773. The FDA concurs that cellulite is a fraud, in a leaflet: L. Fenner, *Cellulite: Hard to Budge Pudge,* HHS publication no. FDA 80–1078 (Washington, D.C.: Government Printing Office, 1982), reprinted from *FDA Consumer,* May 1980.

30. Task Force of the American Society for Clinical Nutrition, Guidelines for surgery for morbid obesity, *American Journal of Clinical Nutrition* 42 (1985): 904–905.

31. A. E. Kark, Jaw wiring, *American Journal of Clinical Nutrition* 33, supplement 2 (February 1980): 420–424.

32. J. S. Garrow, Are liquid diets safe or necessary? *Recent Advances in Obesity Research,* vol. 5 (Westport, Conn.: Food and Nutrition Press, 1987), pp. 327–331.

33. R. L. Hammer and coauthors, Calorie-restricted low-fat diet and exercise in obese women, *American Journal of Clinical Nutrition* 49 (1989): 77–85; K. H. Duncan, J. A. Bacon, and R. L. Weinsier, The effects of high and low energy density diets on satiety, energy intake, and eating time of obese and nonobese subjects, *American Journal of Clinical Nutrition* 37 (1983): 763–767.

34. H. A. Jordan, L. S. Levitz, K. L. Utgoff, and H. L. Lee, Role of food characteristics in behavioral change and weight loss, *Journal of the American Dietetic Association* 79 (1981): 24–29.

35. Dreon and coauthors, 1988.

36. L. Lissner and coauthors, Dietary fat and the regulation of energy intake in human subjects, *American Journal of Clinical Nutrition* 46 (1987): 886–892.

37. L. Buckmaster and K. D. Brownell, Behavior modification: The state of the art, in *Obesity and Weight Control: The Health Professional's Guide to Understanding and Treatment,* eds. R. T. Frankle and M. U. Yang (Rockville, Md.: Aspen, 1988), pp. 225–240.

38. J. O. Hill and coauthors, Effects of exercise and food restriction on body composition and metabolic rate in obese women, *American Journal of Clinical Nutrition* 46 (1987): 622–630; S. B. Heymsfield and coauthors, Kinetics of weight loss during underfeeding: Relation to level of physical activity (abstract) *American Journal of Clinical Nutrition* 45 (1987): 868.

39. R. B. Stuart and C. Mitchell, Indirection in the management of obesity: A new treatment rationale, in *Dietary Treatment and Prevention of Obesity,* eds. R. T. Frankle and coeditors (London: Libbey, 1985), pp. 31–45.

40. Questions doctors ask, *Nutrition and the M.D.,* June 1978.

Eating Disorders

Anorexia nervosa and bulimia affect an estimated 1 million teenagers.[1] Specific causes of these eating disorders still baffle clinicians. Some speculate that society's excessive pressure to be thin is to blame, others point to neurological links with depression and impulsive behaviors or other biological malfunctions, and still others believe the cause to be an inability to cope. Their point of agreement is that the disorders are most likely multifactorial—sociocultural, neurochemical, and psychological—and that treatment requires a multidisciplinary approach. The nutrition component of treatment requires both intervention and education.[2]

Anorexia Nervosa

Julie is 18 years old. She has always been a beautiful girl, and a superachiever in school. She prides herself on her fine figure and watches her diet with great care. She exercises daily, maintaining a heroic schedule of self-discipline. She is thin, but she is not satisfied with her weight and is determined to lose more. She is 5 feet 6 inches tall and weighs 85 pounds. She has anorexia nervosa.

Julie is unaware that she is undernourished, and she sees no need to obtain treatment, but her friends and family have become concerned about her. She stopped menstruating (developed amenorrhea) several months ago and has become moody. She insists that she is too fat, although her eyes lie in deep hollows in her face. She denies that she is ever tired, although she is obviously close to physical exhaustion. Her family is reluctant to push her, but has insisted that she see a psychiatrist. The psychiatrist has evaluated her case and

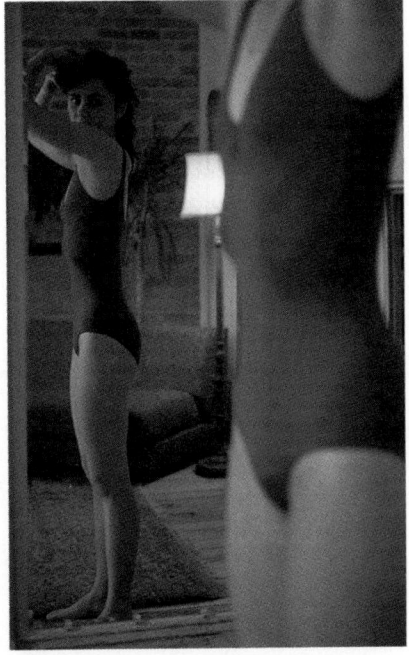

Women with anorexia nervosa see themselves as fat, even when they are dangerously underweight.

has decided to begin group therapy immediately with a warning that if she does not begin to gain weight she will need to be hospitalized.

Most people with anorexia nervosa are white females from middle- or upper-class families; males account for less than 10 percent of the cases.[3] A typical psychological profile includes depression, early developmental failure, and a characteristic cluster of family circumstances. Such families are usually mother dominated, with absentee or distant fathers. They value achievement and outward appearances more than an inner sense of self-worth and self-actualization. Julie works hard to please her parents and shows a high degree of perfectionism. The parents cherish and indulge the

child, so the intermeshing of needs is tight.

Julie identifies so strongly with her parents' ideals and goals for her that she sometimes feels she has no identity of her own. She can't get in touch with her own feelings, and she sometimes feels like a robot. She earnestly desires to control her own destiny, but she feels controlled by others. When she does not eat, she gains control.

Anorexia resembles an addiction. The characteristic behavior is obsessive and compulsive, and often there are other addictions in the family. Biological links between addictions and eating abnormalities are mushrooming in scientific literature.[4]

As almost always happens, Julie began to develop anorexia nervosa within half a year after her menstrual periods started. She was distressed by the signs that she was turning into a woman and afraid of the changes that were taking place in her body. If she remained thin, she felt, she might escape being enveloped in a woman's body with hips, belly, and breasts—which frightened and revolted her. Julie's anorexia has tightened the bonds between herself and her mother, stabilizing her in a juvenile state and making it unnecessary for either of them to deal with the other problems that they face in their lives.

You may wonder how a person as thin as Julie could possibly continue to diet. Julie controls her food intake with tremendous discipline. She avoids carbohydrates and fats as if they were poison and eats strictly limited amounts of lean meat and low-kcalorie vegetables. She knows the number of kcalories per serving of dozens of different foods, and thinks and talks about food constantly. She

---

Miniglossary

anorexia nervosa: a disorder seen (usually) in teenage girls, involving self-starvation to the extreme.

an = without
orex = appetite
nervos = of nervous origin

bulimia, alternative spelling **bulemia** (byoo-LEEM-ee-uh): recurring binge eating combined with a morbid fear of becoming fat, sometimes followed by self-induced vomiting or purging; other terms used to describe this eating behavior include **compulsive eating**, **bulimarexia** (byoo-lee-ma-REX-ee-uh), and **bulimia nervosa**.

buli = ox

cathartic: a strong laxative.

emetic (em-ETT-ic): an agent that causes vomiting.

---

cooks elaborate meals for her mother and her mother's friends, but she never partakes of them herself. If she feels that she has gained an ounce of weight, she runs or jumps rope until she is sure she has exercised it off. Her favorite sports are solitary; she doesn't participate in team sports. Once in a while she slips and eats more than she intends to, and when she has done that, she takes laxatives to hasten the exit of the food from her system. She is unaware that this doesn't work, because her other ways of staying thin are so effective. Her preoccupation with foods reveals that she is starving and is desperately hungry; the reason she doesn't eat is because of her fierce determination to achieve self-control, not because she isn't hungry.

When Julie looks at herself in the mirror, she sees herself as fat. The psychiatrist who tested her gave her a visual self-image test, and she drew a picture of herself that was grossly distorted. The psychiatrist took this as an index of the severity of her illness, knowing that the more she overestimated her body size, the more resistant she would be to the treatment, and the more unwilling to examine her faulty values and misconceptions.[5] When asked to draw her best friend, Julie rendered an accurate image.

The physical consequences of anorexia nervosa are similar to those of starvation. They include many hormonal aberrations. The heart pumps less efficiently, the heart muscle becomes weak and thin, the chambers diminish in size, and the blood pressure falls. Sudden stopping of the heart, perhaps due to lean tissue loss and mineral deficiencies, accounts for many cases of sudden death among severely emaciated subjects.

The person with anorexia nervosa also has many abnormalities of immune function. There may be anemia. As the person becomes thinner and thinner, abnormalities of the GI system also occur. Peristalsis becomes sluggish, and if the person eats too fast, the stomach becomes overfull, because it empties abnormally slowly. The lining of the digestive tract atrophies, and on eating food again the person may have diarrhea, because the system can't absorb nutrients well. The pancreas becomes unable to secrete many enzymes, as does the lining of the intestinal tract.

Other starvation effects include altered serum lipid levels, high concentrations of vitamin A and carotene in the blood, reduced blood proteins, an increased amount of fine body hair, skin dryness, and decreased skin and core temperatures. The electrical activity of the brain becomes abnormal, sleep is disturbed, and bad dreams are common. The person with anorexia nervosa may complain of never feeling rested.

Women with the disorder always have amenorrhea, and in 25 percent of cases, that symptom precedes the weight loss.[6] Young men with the disorder lose their sex drive and become impotent. To resume normal cycling, a female must gain body fat to at least 17 percent of her body weight. Sometimes it requires 22 percent fat content before periods may resume, and some never restart even after they have gained the weight. It isn't clear whether the hormonal change is first or whether stress precedes the hormonal change. (Stress induces amenorrhea in up to three out of every four women in concentration camps and virtually all women on death row.) The likely sequence in the development of anorexia nervosa is stress; then hormonal abnormalities; then food restriction, amenorrhea, and weight loss.[7]

Anorexia nervosa is hard to diagnose, because nearly everyone in our society is engaged in the "pursuit of thinness." Some women *without* weight loss meet all the criteria for the diagnosis of anorexia nervosa based on their eating attitudes and behaviors, as if they had a subclinical or premorbid disorder. Anorexialike thought patterns are common among fashion models, long-distance runners, and dancers. Many young women, on learning of the disorder, state that they wish they had "a touch" of it, in order to get thin.

It takes a skilled clinician to make a diagnosis. Denial runs high among people with anorexia, and they deceive their families effectively. Table H12–1 shows the diagnostic criteria for anorexia nervosa.

Treatment artfully combines medical and dietary information to initiate and sustain weight gain, as well as psychological techniques to resolve personal and family problems. Teams of physicians, nurses, psychiatrists, family psychologists, and dietitians work together to treat clients with anorexia nervosa.

Treatment programs of recent date have been more successful than in the past, and residential treatment centers specializing in eating disorders are often especially successful. The person who works most closely with the client should aim at four goals:

- To support her own feeling of autonomy—her feeling that she can control her own life, feel her own feelings, and choose her own behaviors.
- To earn her trust by being honest, acknowledging that the treatment for anorexia nervosa may be uncomfortable at first and that for a while things may seem worse before they begin to get better; to acknowledge the client's feelings about this, too.
- To involve the family, so that they will not continue to reinforce maladaptive behavior, but will help the client gain weight by providing positive reinforcement.
- To make connections with other health care agencies, depending on individual needs.

The malnutrition of anorexia nervosa can be so severe as to throw a person into severe electrolyte imbalance, create tremendous metabolic stress by way of infection, cause depression to the point of suicide, and even stop the heart. Appropriate nutritional treatment is crucial and needs to be tailored to the client's needs. Table H12–2 lists principles of nutrition intervention in anorexia nervosa. People with anorexia nervosa are usually younger than people with other medical conditions and are usually not ill with other diseases, so they are under less physical stress. Seldom are they willing to feed themselves, but if they are, chances are they can recover without other interventions.

■ TABLE H12–1
Diagnostic Criteria for Anorexia Nervosa

- Refusal to maintain body weight over a minimal normal weight for age and height, e.g., weight loss leading to maintenance of body weight 15% below that expected; or failure to make expected weight gain during period of growth, leading to body weight 15% below that expected.
- Intense fear of gaining weight or becoming fat, even though underweight.
- Disturbance in the way in which one's body weight, size, or shape is experienced; e.g., the person claims to "feel fat" even when emaciated, or believes that one area of the body is "too fat" even when obviously underweight.
- In females, absence of at least three consecutive menstrual cycles when otherwise expected to occur (primary or secondary amenorrhea). (A women is considered to have amenorrhea if her periods occur only following hormone, e.g., estrogen, administration.)

Source: American Psychiatric Association, *Diagnostic and Statistical Manual of Mental Disorders*, 3rd edition, revised 1987 (Washington, D.C.: American Psychiatric Association, 1987), p. 67, with permission.

It is suggested that clients be classed as being at low, intermediate, or high risk, depending on how they score on several indicators of protein-energy malnutrition.* Low-risk people need nutrition counseling by a dietitian and psychological counseling simultaneously. Intermediate-risk

*Indicators of protein-energy malnutrition: the percentage of body fat, serum albumin, serum transferrin, and immune reactions.

people may need nutritional supplements such as high-kcalorie, high-protein formulas besides regular meals but may not have to be hospitalized. The initial goal is to provide 250 to 500 kcalories above the daily energy requirement—about the maximum that most people are willing and able to accept. Drugs may be used to improve gastric motility and help people become able to tolerate larger meals. If the risk is

■ TABLE H12–2
Principles of Nutrition Intervention in Anorexia Nervosa

- Increase kcalorie intake slowly, beginning with 800 to 1,200 kcal/day.
- Prescribe well-balanced diets, with *some* individual variations according to client preferences (e.g., vegetarian).
- Give multiple vitamin-mineral supplements at RDA levels.
- Enhance elimination with dietary fiber from grain sources.
- Reduce sensations of bloating with small, frequent feedings.
- In behavioral programs, link rewards to kcalorie intake, not weight gain.
- Use liquid supplements when the client cannot achieve desired intake with solid food.
- Reduce satiety sensations with cold or room-temperature foods and with finger foods (e.g., snacks).
- Provide interactive nutrition counseling as an ongoing process.
- Reduce excessive caffeine intake.
- Provide parenteral nutritional support only in severe states of ill health, malnutrition, and wasting.

Source: Adapted from C. L. Rock and J. Yager, Nutrition and eating disorders: A primer for clinicians, *International Journal of Eating Disorders* 6 (1987): 276, as cited in *Nutrition and the M.D.*, July 1988, with permission. Reprinted with permission of John Wiley & Sons, Inc., copyright 1987.

high, then hospitalization is indicated, daily kcalorie supplementation may be greater, and tube feeding may have to be instituted. The hope is that the person will gain about 1 to 2 kilograms (2 to 4 pounds) a month. For a person who refuses to eat, forcible methods may be necessary to forestall death. These are in the hands of the physician and will not be described here. Drug therapies may be used as accompaniment.

Three-quarters of those in treatment may regain weight up to within 25 percent of the desired weight. Half to three-quarters may resume normal menstrual cycles. About two-thirds fail to eat normally on follow-up, but they may eat better than they did before. About 6 percent die, 1 percent by suicide.* Social and family relationships may remain impaired. It seems that anorexia nervosa can adversely affect a person's social, psychological, and family functioning for life.

Bulimia

Sophie is a charming, intelligent woman of normal weight who thinks constantly about food. She alternately starves herself and binges, and when she has eaten too much, she vomits. Probably few people would fail to recognize these characteristics as the description of bulimia, for although the disease was recognized and named only in 1980, it has received much media attention.

Bulimia is a distinct eating disorder that shares some characteristics with anorexia nervosa. It is more common than anorexia nervosa. Like anorexia

*This is from a review of 19 studies on about 1,000 clients over a five-year period. Other deaths are from infection; heart disease; lung disease; and iatrogenic causes including aspiration, electrolyte imbalance from intravenous therapy, and vitamin D poisoning. M. A. Balaa and D. A. Drossman, *Anorexia Nervosa and Bulimia: The Eating Disorders*, Disease-a-Month (Chicago: Year Book Medical Publishers, June 1985), p. 34.

For many people with bulimia, guilt, depression, and self condemnation follow a binge-eating episode.

nervosa, bulimia is more common in females than in males, although the proportion of males with bulimia outnumbers that of males with anorexia nervosa. The possibility exists that only the reporting of bulimia is increasing, but the incidence seems to be rising, ranging anywhere from 5 to 20 percent of women.

Like the person with anorexia nervosa, the person with bulimia spends much time thinking about her body weight and food. Her preoccupation with food manifests itself in secretive binge-eating episodes followed by self-induced vomiting, fasting, or the use of laxatives and diuretics.[8] Such behaviors typically begin in late adolescence after a long series of various unsuccessful weight-reduction diets. People with bulimia commonly follow a pattern of restrictive dieting interspersed with

bulimic behaviors and experience weight fluctuations of more than 10 pounds up and down over short periods of time. The secretiveness of bulimic behaviors makes recognition of the problem difficult, even though actual diagnosis is not difficult when symptoms present themselves, because no other diseases present similar symptoms (see Table H12–3).

Like the "typical" person with bulimia, Sophie is single, Caucasian, and in her early 20s. She is well educated and close to her ideal body weight. She binges periodically, and when she does so, it is in secret, usually at night, and lasts an hour or more. Sophie seldom lets binging interfere with her work or social activities, although a third of all bingers do; she is like most people with bulimia (60 percent) in that she starts the binge after having gone through a period of rigid dieting, so that her eating is accelerated by her hunger. Each time, she eats anywhere from one thousand to many thousands of kcalories of food containing little fiber or water, smooth in texture, and high in sugar and fat, so that it is easy to consume vast amounts rapidly, with little chewing. Typically, she chooses cookies, cake, ice cream, or bread, although sometimes she binges on atypical foods—for example, vegetables—when she is dieting. After the binge, she pays the price of having swollen hands and feet, bloating, fatigue, headache, nausea, and pain.

■ TABLE H12–3
Diagnostic Criteria for Bulimia

- Recurrent episodes of binge eating (rapid consumption of a large amount of food in a discrete period of time).
- A feeling of lack of control over eating behavior during the eating binges.
- Regular practice of either self-induced vomiting, use of laxatives or diuretics, strict dieting or fasting, or vigorous exercise in order to prevent weight gain.
- A minimum average of two binge eating episodes a week for at least three months.
- Persistant overconcern with body shape and weight.

Source: American Psychiatric Association, *Diagnostic and Statistical Manual of Mental Disorders*, 3rd edition, revised 1987 (Washington, D.C.: American Psychiatric Association, 1987), pp. 68–69, with permission.

The binge itself is not like normal eating. It is not primarily a response to hunger, apparently, and the food is not consumed for its nutritional value. It is a compulsion and usually occurs in several stages: "anticipation and planning, anxiety, urgency to begin, rapid and uncontrollable consumption of food, relief and relaxation, disappointment, and finally shame or disgust."[9]

As Sophie repeats and repeats this behavior, she faces more and more serious consequences, including medical ones. Fluid and electrolyte imbalance caused by vomiting can lead to abnormal heart rhythms and injury to the kidneys, which have to cope with the altered balance. Infections of the bladder and kidneys can lead to kidney failure. Vomiting causes irritation and infection of the pharynx, esophagus, and salivary glands; erosion of the teeth; and dental caries. The esophagus may rupture or tear, as may the stomach. Sometimes the eyes become red from pressure on vomiting. The hands may be bruised and lacerated from scraping on the teeth while inducing vomiting.

Some people use cathartics—violent laxatives that can injure the lower intestinal tract. Others use emetics to induce vomiting. Repeated use can lead to heart failure due to poisoning; it was emetic abuse that caused the death of popular singer Karen Carpenter in 1983.

What makes a person become bulimic? Again, Sophie is typical. From early in her childhood, she has been a high achiever, with a strong feeling of dependence on her parents. Her mother is a bright, well-educated woman who abandoned a promising career in order to stay home and raise the family; she has taught her children a high degree of respect for their father, who is a powerful but distant figure. Sophie experiences considerable social anxiety and has difficulty in establishing personal relationships. She is sometimes depressed and often exhibits impulsive behavior. Some people with bulimia exhibit antisocial behavior, including drug abuse, kleptomania, and sexual promiscuity.

Unlike Julie, Sophie is aware of the consequences of her behavior, feels that it is abnormal, and is deeply ashamed of it. She feels inadequate, unable even to control her eating, and so she tends to be passive and to look to men for confirmation of her sense of worth. When rejected, either in reality or in her imagination, her bulimia becomes worse. If Sophie gets carried away by bulimia, she may not only experience a deepening of her depression, but may move on to drug or alcohol abuse.

A food-centered society that favors thinness in women puts a woman in a bind. Bulimia has been described as socially sanctioned and almost required among upper-class women who must attend many dinners and cocktail parties. Typically, they have been raised in families that encouraged hearty eating, and there is much socializing around the dinner table. Food is always involved in celebrations and also is used to console the family during periods of mourning. When a child raised in such a setting is also made socially conscious and is told she must become thin, she may perceive that she has little alternative but to celebrate or mourn with the family; indulge in vast quantities of food; and then vomit, crash diet, or fast to "undo" her possible weight gain.

Bulimia is in many respects easier to treat than anorexia nervosa, because it seems to be more of a chosen behavior. People with bulimia know that their behavior is abnormal, and many are willing to try to cooperate.

The goal of a dietary plan to treat bulimia is to help clients gain control and establish regular eating patterns.[10] Initial dietary management requires a structured eating plan with little flexibility. The person needs to learn to eat a quantity of nutritious food sufficient to nourish her body and leave her satisfied without bringing on the feared and detested weight gain. Such an approach has been used successfully in the treatment of many people with severe bulimia; it requires that they eat no less than 1,500 kcalories a day.[11] Table H12–4 lists diet recommendations for the person with bulimia.

■ TABLE H12–4
Diet Recommendations for Bulimia

- Avoid finger foods; plan meals with foods that require the use of utensils.
- Increase meal satiety by including warm foods, rather than cold or room-temperature foods.
- Include vegetables, salad, and/or fruit at a meal, to prolong the meal duration; choose whole-grain and high-fiber breads and cereals.
- Prescribe a well-balanced diet and meals, both to increase satiety and to increase the variety of foods eaten.
- Use foods that are naturally divided into portions, such as potatoes (rather than rice or pasta); 4- and 8-oz containers of yogurt, ice cream, or cottage cheese; precut steak or chicken parts; and frozen dinners and entrées.
- Include foods containing adequate amounts of complex carbohydrates (which promote meal satiety) and fat (which slow gastric emptying and further enhance the feeling of fullness).
- Make sure meals and snacks are eaten sitting down.
- Plan meals and snacks, and keep a food diary by recording food prior to eating.

Source: Adapted from C. L. Rock and J. Yager, Nutrition and eating disorders: A primer for clinicians, *International Journal of Eating Disorders* 6 (1987): 276, as cited in *Nutrition and the M.D.*, July 1988, with permission. Reprinted with permission of John Wiley & Sons, Inc., copyright 1987.

A mental health professional should be on the treatment team. Almost 90 percent of people with bulimia are clinically depressed, and the rates of alcohol, marijuana, and cigarette abuse are high.[12]

Long-term follow-up studies remain to be undertaken. It isn't clear what becomes of people with bulimia in later life. Possibly, there are roughly three categories: college students who engage in the disorder briefly and then recover; bingers/vomiters who also begin during college and who require more intensive therapy and hospitalization; and older people who have chronic and stable bulimia and whose binge-eating and self-starving or vomiting patterns are regular and established. These people might be said to be socially adjusted, in a way, because their behavior fits in with their other activities.

Eating Disorders in Our Society

Anorexia nervosa, bulimia, and their combination (bulimarexia or bulimia nervosa) are relatively new eating disorders. Anorexia nervosa was first described 100 years ago; bulimia was first defined as a medical disorder only in 1980. Both are known only in developed nations and become more prevalent as wealth increases. Some people point to the vomitoriums of ancient peoples and claim that bulimia is nothing new, but the two are actually quite distinct. The ancient people were eating for pleasure, without guilt, and in the company of others; they vomited so that they could rejoin the feast. Bulimia is a disease of isolation and is always accompanied by self-hate and low self-esteem.

If asked today, Julie might describe herself as proud of her achievements in dieting and eager to achieve more. She has, after all, made significant progress toward achieving her goal—to be thin. Sophie, on the other hand, would describe herself as unhappy, because she has failed to control her eating. She is longing for the time when she'll be happy—that is, when she's thin. It's not uncommon in our society for some women to develop a kind of Cinderella complex—to hide behind obstacles, real or imaginary, waiting and hoping for some event or some person to "bring them happiness."

At so tender an age as 12 years, beautifully growing, normal-weight female youngsters are already worried that they are too fat. Most are "on diets." Magazines, newspapers, and television all present the message that to be beautiful and happy is to be thin. Anorexia nervosa and bulimia are not a form of rebellion against these unreasonable expectations, but rather the exaggerated acceptance of them. Perhaps a person's best defense against these disorders is to learn to appreciate her own uniquenesses. The author Eda LeShan beautifully described her recovery from overeating: "Deep inside there had always been a small child begging for my attention. . . . All I gave her was food. Now I give her love."[13] To respect and value oneself may be lifesaving.

NOTES

1. D. Farley, Eating disorders: When thinness becomes an obsession, *FDA Consumer*, May 1986, pp. 20–23.

2. Position of the American Dietetic Association: Nutrition intervention in the treatment of anorexia nervosa and bulimia, *Journal of the American Dietetic Association* 88 (1988): 68.

3. Farley, 1986.

4. F. S. Sizer, *Addiction, Brain Chemistry, and Eating Disorders*, a monograph (1989) available from J. B. Lipincott Co., East Washington Sq., Philadelphia, PA 19105.

5. H. Bruch, Anorexia nervosa, *Nutrition Today,* September–October 1978, pp. 14–18.

6. M. A. Balaa and D. A. Drossman, *Anorexia Nervosa and Bulimia: The Eating Disorders,* Disease a Month, (Chicago: Year Book Medical Publishers, June 1985), pp. 1–52.

7. Balaa and Drossman, 1985.

8. Balaa and Drossman, 1985.

9. Balaa and Drossman, 1985.

10. M. Story, Nutrition management and dietary treatment of bulimia, *Journal of the American Dietetic Association* 86 (1986): 517–519.

11. S. Dalvit-McPhillips, A dietary approach to bulimia treatment, *Physiology and Behavior* 33 (1984): 769–775.

12. J. D. Killen and coauthors, Depressive symptoms and substance use among adolescent binge eaters and purgers: A defined population study, *American Journal of Public Health* 77 (1987): 1539–1541; Health and Public Policy Committee, American College of Physicians, Eating disorders: Anorexia nervosa and bulimia, *Annals of Internal Medicine* 105 (1986): 790–794.

13. E. LeShan, *Winning the Losing Battle: Why I Will Never Be Fat Again* (New York: Crowell, 1979).

13

Exercise, Nutrients, and Body Adaptations

Muscle cells can work without oxygen, using glycogen for fuel. This strand of muscle is peppered with glycogen (dark spots). Nearby are two mitochondria to oxidize both glycogen and fat breakdown products when oxygen is available.

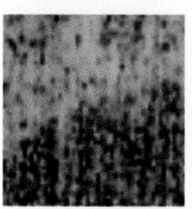

In the body, nutrition and exercise go hand in hand. The working body demands that the energy-yielding nutrients provide fuel for the increased metabolism of exercise. One of these fuels is the body's stored fat, and using body fat in exercise pushes body composition toward the lean.

Exercise contributes to the output side of the energy balance equation. The *NRC Recommendations* encourage all healthy people to maintain physical activity at a moderately active level and to improve physical fitness. Most health professionals accept that health depends on a certain minimum daily or weekly amount of exercise. In fact, an RDA for exercise would be useful, although no such specific recommendation has yet been made. Stretching the point, we can even think of the need for exercise as analogous with the need for nutrients, and speak of "exercise deficiency," just as we speak of nutrient deficiencies. Such a deficiency would lead to accelerated development of the diseases associated with sedentary life—cardiovascular disease, obesity, intestinal disorders, apathy, insomnia, accelerated bone losses, and many more.

Exercise, or its lack, affects everyone's nutrition and overall health, so this chapter is written for "you"—the athlete, the health seeker, the sports player, the weight-loss seeker, and you who have yet to begin exercising. To understand the interactions between exercise and nutrition, you must first know a few things about exercise.

■ *The Essentials of Exercise*

For the person seeking health, exercise is as important as nutrition or sleep.[1] It promotes fitness and enhances appearance, for a fit body looks healthy and attractive. Fitness doesn't require that you develop a Ms. Olympia or Mr. Universe body; rather, you need to develop to your own potential along several lines. You need to achieve enough of the four components of fitness— flexibility, strength, muscle endurance, and cardiovascular endurance—to allow you to meet the everyday demands of life, plus some to spare. Nutrition alone cannot endow you with fitness or athletic ability, but it can augment the effort you put forth to obtain them. Conversely, unwise food selections can stand in your way.

Researchers have yet to discover how little exercise is too little and how much might be too much. Some authorities believe that a minimum of 20 minutes of the kind of exercise that produces cardiovascular endurance three times or more each week is necessary for a strong heart. Others argue that the amount of energy (number of kcalories) spent in exercise is the key to heart health. Exercises that improve cardiovascular endurance raise the heart rate for more than 20 minutes, and use most of the large muscle groups of the body (legs, buttocks, and abdomen). Such exercises are aerobic and include swimming, cross-country skiing, rowing, fast walking, jogging, fast bicycling, soccer, hockey, basketball, water polo, lacrosse, and rugby. Activities equally difficult to perform, but that do not improve cardiovascular endurance, include ballet dancing, tennis (doubles), and golf (riding instead of walking).

aerobic (air-ROE-bic): requiring oxygen.

Miniglossary of Fitness Terms

fitness: the body's ability to meet physical demands, composed of four components:
- Flexibility.
- Strength.
- Muscle endurance.
- Cardiovascular endurance.

flexibility: the ability to bend without injury; flexibility depends on the elasticity of muscles, tendons, and ligaments and on the condition of the joints.

strength: the ability of muscles to work against resistance.

endurance: the ability to sustain an effort for a long time. One type, **muscle endurance**, is the ability of a muscle to contract repeatedly within a given time without becoming exhausted. Another type, **cardiovascular endurance**, is the ability of the cardiovascular system to sustain effort over a period of time.

Regular aerobic exercise improves the cardiovascular system. In cardiovascular conditioning, the total blood volume and number of red blood cells increase, so that the blood can carry more oxygen. The heart muscle becomes stronger and larger, and each beat empties the heart's chambers more completely, so that the heart pumps more blood per beat. This makes fewer beats necessary, so the pulse rate falls. The muscles that inflate and deflate the lungs gain strength and endurance, allowing breathing to become more efficient. Blood moves easily through the body's blood vessels because the muscles of the arteries contract powerfully, and movement of the skeletal muscles pushes the blood through the veins. This facilitates normal blood pressure, because vessel resistance diminishes. Figure 13–1 shows the major relationships between the heart, lungs, and muscles.

In contrast, anaerobic exercise generally does not bring about cardiovascular conditioning, but develops strength and bulk of muscles. It involves sudden, all-out exertions of muscles that last less than 90 seconds and thus

cardiovascular conditioning: the effect of regular exercise on the cardiovascular system—including improvements in heart, artery, and lung function and increased blood volume.

anaerobic (AN-air-ROE-bic): not requiring oxygen.

How to Check Your Pulse

An informal pulse check can give you some indication of how conditioned your heart is. As a rule of thumb, the average resting pulse rate for adults is around 70 beats per minute, but the rate can be higher or lower. Active people can have resting pulse rates of 50 or even lower. To take your pulse, place your finger over a pulse point (the side of the throat, for instance), and count the number of beats in 15 seconds; multiply by 4 to get beats per minute.

Cardiovascular conditioning is characterized by:
- Increased blood volume and oxygen delivery.
- Increased heart strength and stroke volume (amount of oxygenated blood ejected by the heart with each beat).
- Slowed resting pulse.
- Increased breathing efficiency.
- Improved circulation.
- Reduced blood pressure.

■ **FIGURE 13–1**

Delivery of Oxygen by the Heart and Lungs to the Muscles

The more fit a muscle is, the more oxygen it draws from the blood. That oxygen is drawn from the lungs, so the person with more fit muscles extracts from the inhaled air more oxygen than a person with less fit muscles. The cardiovascular system responds to the demand for oxygen by building up its capacity to deliver oxygen. Researchers can measure cardiovascular fitness by measuring the amount of oxygen a person consumes per minute while working out, a measure called **VO_2 max.**

VO_2 max: the maximum volume of oxygen consumed per minute.

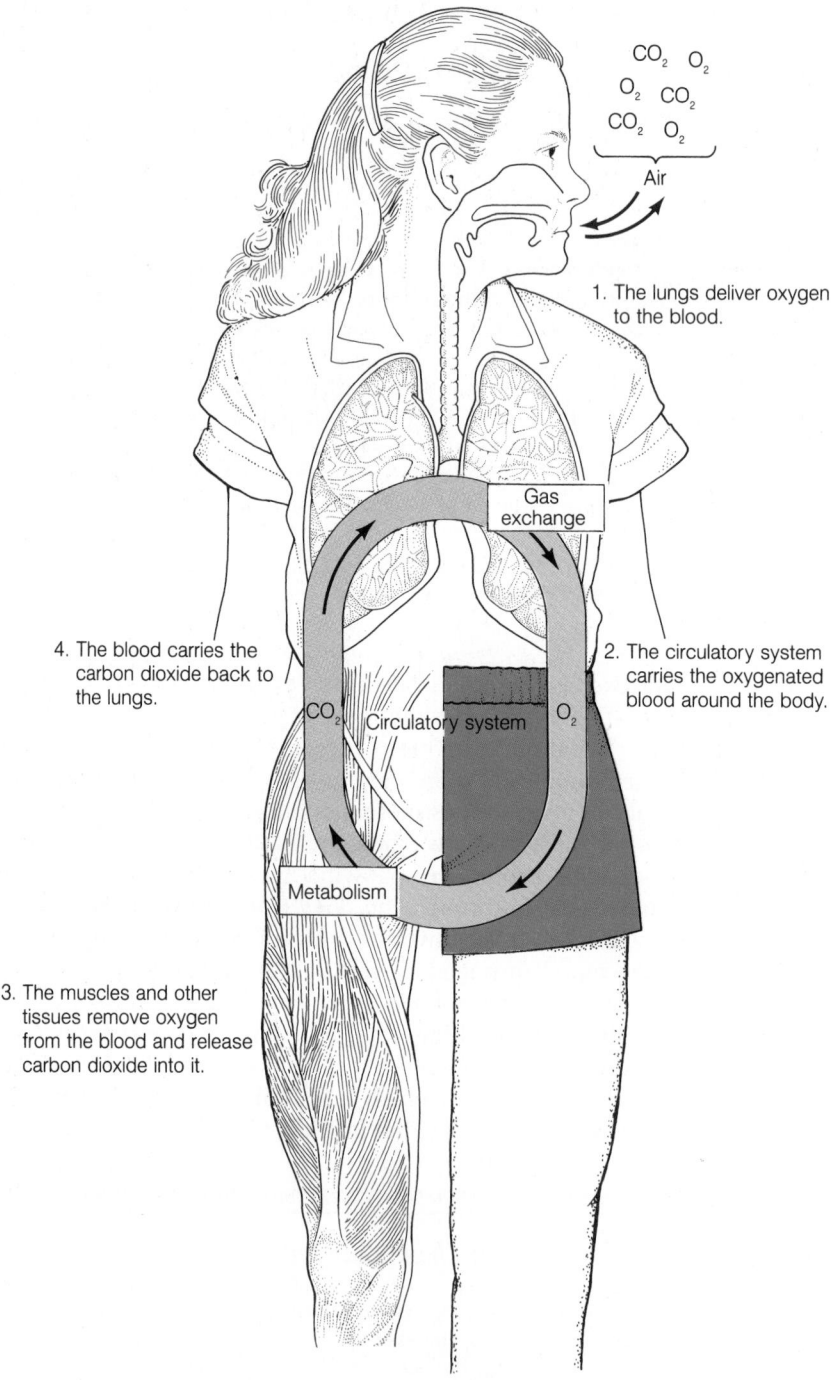

CO_2 O_2
O_2 CO_2
CO_2 O_2
Air

1. The lungs deliver oxygen to the blood.

Gas exchange

4. The blood carries the carbon dioxide back to the lungs.

CO_2 Circulatory system O_2

2. The circulatory system carries the oxygenated blood around the body.

Metabolism

3. The muscles and other tissues remove oxygen from the blood and release carbon dioxide into it.

require almost no fresh oxygen. Examples include sprinting (100-meter dash), serving a tennis ball, jumping a fence, or lifting a weight.

As important as cardiovascular conditioning is, it is only one facet of fitness. All fitness components are important to health and appearance. For balanced fitness, stretching exercises can enhance flexibility, while weight work or calisthenics can develop strength and muscle endurance.

People shape their bodies by what they do and by what they choose not to do. The use-disuse principle governs this fact: muscle cells and tissues respond to the overload of exercise by gaining strength and size, a response called hypertrophy. The converse is also true: if not called on to perform, muscles atrophy. Thus cyclists often have well-developed legs but little arm or chest strength; a tennis player may have one superbly strong arm, while the other is just average. A swimmer usually develops in a balanced way—arms, legs, back, and chest all perform and so develop uniformly. This doesn't mean that everyone should give up tennis and cycling for swimming, but only that a variety of kinds of exercise will produce the most uniform overall fitness. This is one of the reasons why people are told to work different muscle groups from day to day. Another reason is that it takes a day or two to restore muscle fuel supplies, and to repair any slight damage incurred through exercise.

Less obvious than muscle development are the multitude of specific adaptations the body makes to facilitate the type of exercise performed. The muscle cells of a superbly trained weight lifter have equipped themselves with extra glycogen and have built up their strong, quick muscle fibers, thereby increasing their work capacity. This athlete's muscle cells, although superbly suited for work that requires strength and quickness, could not do well in endurance competition. In the same way, the muscle cells of a distance swimmer equip themselves for prolonged exertion, but would soon give up in power competition. This means that people who wish to play a sport should train mainly by playing that sport, to develop the specific metabolic equipment most needed in the game. However, each person is born with a set number of each type of muscle fiber and genetic potential that cannot be changed, even through hard work. In sports, only those born with the right fibers and who work with devotion to develop their potential can join the ranks of elite athletes.

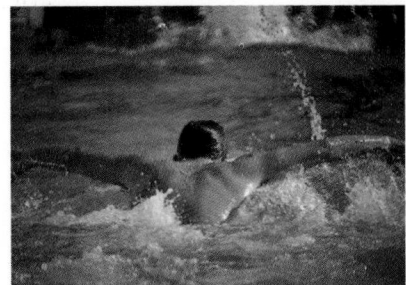

People's bodies are shaped by the activities they perform.

use-disuse principle: the principle that fitness develops in response to demand and diminishes in response to a lack of demand. Related terms are **hypertrophy** (high-PURR-tro-fee), an increase in size in response to use, and **atrophy** (AT-tro-fee), a decrease in size because of disuse.

overload: an extra physical demand placed on the body; an increase in the frequency, duration, or intensity of an exercise. A principle of training is that for a body system to improve, it must be worked at frequencies, durations, or intensities that increase by increments over time.

▪ Exercise and the Body's Use of Fuels

As a person exercises, the body adapts to the exercise by adjusting its fuel metabolism. In addition, the body's composition begins to change, and this also changes metabolism.

When you begin to exercise, hormones, including epinephrine and norepinephrine, are released into the bloodstream and signal the liver and fat cells to liberate their stored energy nutrients, glucose and fatty acids. Thus hormones set the table for the muscles' energy feast, and the muscles help themselves to the fuels passing by in the blood.

During rest, the body uses slightly more fat than carbohydrate for its fuel, along with a small percentage of protein. How much of which fuels the muscles actually use during exercise depends on an interplay between the fuels available, the intensity of the exercise, and the availability of oxygen. Later sections of this chapter explain these relationships. First, take a look at how metabolism supports body movement when a person decides to get up and go.

The First Fuels of Exercise—ATP and PC

Have you noticed how fast muscles can contract? When called upon, a muscle responds instantaneously, without taking time to metabolize fat or carbohydrate for energy. In the first fractions of seconds of exercise, muscles depend on pools of free quick-energy molecules they maintain for this purpose.

The first of these molecules is the high-energy compound adenosine triphosphate (ATP), introduced in Chapter 7.[2] ATP provides the chemical driving force for muscle contraction. Ultimately, the energy of all the energy-yielding nutrients is transferred to ATP, the final product in a series of reactions that transform chemical into mechanical energy. A tiny, but essential, ATP pool stands ready to meet sudden demands for movement. When ATP is split, its energy is released, and the muscle cells channel most of this energy into mechanical movement. The conversion is imperfect, however. Some ATP energy escapes as heat—heat you can feel building up during exercise.

Unlike a single reflexive muscle jerk, exercise involves sustained or repeated muscle contractions that demand a continuous supply of ATP. The muscles' use of ATP reserves signal that ATP is in demand, and more must be made. Before muscle ATP pools dwindle, a muscle enzyme is signaled to break down another high-energy compound, phosphocreatine (PC). Phosphocreatine yields more ATP to drive the muscles' work. Still, PC supplies last only a little while—perhaps only about 20 seconds. Fortunately, if the demand for fuel continues beyond this time, other systems respond quickly to generate ATP from the body's more abundant fuel reserves—carbohydrate (glucose), fat, and protein. The following sections look at each of these fuels and their roles in exercise, how the body adapts to exercise, and how diet affects exercise performance.

Glucose Use in Exercise

Glucose, stored in the liver and muscles as glycogen, is vital to exercise. During exercise, the liver releases its glucose into the bloodstream. The muscles pick up this glucose and use it in addition to their own private glycogen stores. Compared with ATP or PC, glycogen supplies are abundant; compared with fat, though, the glycogen stores are limited. A person with 30 pounds of body fat to spare may have only a pound or so of glycogen to draw on.

The body constantly uses and replenishes its glycogen stores. The size of glycogen stores depends partly on the carbohydrate content of the diet—how much carbohydrate you eat affects how much glycogen you can store. In muscles, exercise also affects the size of glycogen stores—the more that muscles deplete their glycogen through work, the more they develop their capacity to store glycogen to support that work. The size of your glycogen stores influences the rate at which you will use glycogen in any given exercise.[3] Thus dietary carbohydrate bears on performance, because the more glycogen you store, the longer the stores will last during exercise.

A classic study compared fuel use during exercise among three groups of runners, each on a different diet. For several days before testing, one of the groups consumed a normal mixed diet (55 percent kcalories from carbohy-

ATP is the fuel that provides the chemical energy that drives muscle contraction.

phosphocreatine (PC): a high-energy compound in muscle cells that acts as a reservoir of energy for the maintenance of a steady supply of ATP; it provides the energy for short bursts of activity.

Fat-and-protein diet

Normal mixed diet

High-carbohydrate diet

Maximum endurance time:

57 min

114 min

167 min

■ **FIGURE 13–2**
The Effect of Diet on Physical Endurance
A high-carbohydrate diet can triple an athlete's endurance.

Source: Data from P. Astrand, Something old and something new . . . very new, *Nutrition Today*, June 1968, pp. 9–11.

drate), a second group consumed a high-carbohydrate diet (83 percent kcalories from carbohydrate), and the third group consumed a no-carbohydrate diet (94 percent kcalories from fat, 6 percent from protein). Figure 13–2 shows the results of the study. The high-carbohydrate diet increased the athletes' glycogen stores, thereby allowing them to work longer before exhaustion. This study and many others that followed suggest that a high-carbohydrate diet enhances an athlete's endurance by ensuring ample glycogen stores. The last section of this chapter describes how to choose a performance diet with special attention paid to carbohydrate.

How long an exercising person's glycogen will last depends not only on diet, but also partly on the intensity of the exercise. The most intense activities, such as sprinting, quickly use up glycogen.[4] Other, less intense activities, such as jogging, are more conservative of glycogen, but joggers still use it, and eventually they will run out of it. Glycogen depletion usually occurs in less than two hours of vigorous exercise.

The relationship between the intensity of exercise and the amount of glucose used as fuel depends on oxygen availability. Oxygen plays a key role in the workings of the muscles' metabolic engines. With ample oxygen, muscles can extract all available energy from glucose, and during *moderate* exercise, the lungs and circulatory system have no trouble keeping up with the muscles' need for oxygen. The exerciser breathes deeply and easily, and the heart beats steadily—the exercise is aerobic. You may recognize Figure 13–3 from Chapter 7; it is repeated here to emphasize that oxygen is necessary for aerobic metabolism. Because aerobic metabolism extracts all of the usable energy from each glucose molecule, moderate aerobic exercise

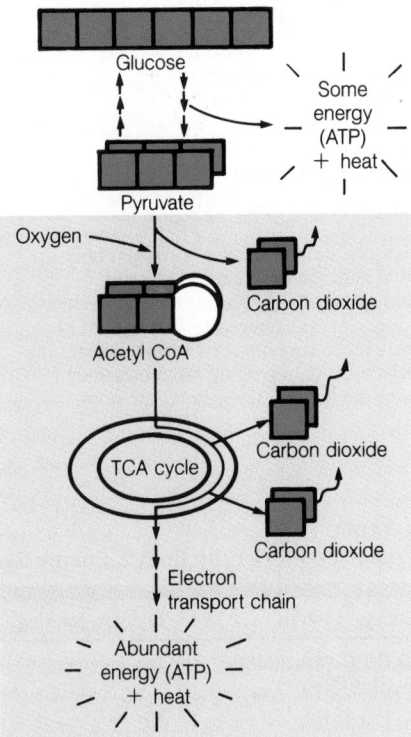

Glucose

Some energy (ATP) + heat

Pyruvate

Oxygen

Carbon dioxide

Acetyl CoA

TCA cycle

Carbon dioxide

Carbon dioxide

Electron transport chain

Abundant energy (ATP) + heat

■ **FIGURE 13–3**
Glucose in Aerobic Metabolism
The trained body uses its glucose most efficiently in aerobic metabolism, extracting from each molecule the maximum energy (ATP). The body can conserve its glucose because the trained heart and lungs provide abundant oxygen to the exercising muscles, and so permit them to use carbohydrate aerobically. The shaded area represents aerobic metabolism.

conserves glycogen, and uses mostly fat. Table 13–1 shows how the use of fuels changes according to the intensity of the exercise.

Intense exercise presents a different picture. The heart and lungs can provide only so much oxygen, only so fast. When muscle exertion is so great that the demand for energy outstrips the oxygen supply, aerobic metabolism cannot sufficiently meet energy needs. Muscles must instead draw more heavily on their limited supply of glucose, because glucose can be metabolized *anaerobically*, part of the way to its end products. Figure 13–4 shows that glucose metabolism cannot go to completion without ample oxygen in the muscles, but it can proceed partway anaerobically during oxygen deficit. The anaerobic part ends when glucose reaches pyruvate, and pyruvate is shunted on to a metabolic sidetrack and held as lactic acid until oxygen becomes available to complete its breakdown.

At this point, the exerciser's body is said to be building up an oxygen debt. During oxygen debt, pyruvate molecules accumulate, and oxygen is needed faster than it can be delivered to break them down completely. If you are exercising this intensely, you may have to slow down or even stop to "catch your breath" (replenish your oxygen supply). When you do, your body begins producing energy aerobically once more. (That's why this physiological state is called a *debt;* oxygen can be "repaid" later.) The nervous and hormonal systems respond to these pyruvate molecules by speeding up the heart and lungs, but a point comes at which they can't keep up with the pyruvate load. At this point, the pyruvate molecules are converted to lactic acid.

Lactic acid buildup can cause burning pain, especially in untrained muscles. Lactic acid accumulation can lead to muscle exhaustion within seconds if the blood cannot clear it away. A strategy for dealing with lactic acid buildup is to relax the muscles at every opportunity, so that the circulating blood can carry the lactic acid away and bring oxygen to support aerobic metabolism. This is what mountaineers are doing when they relax their leg muscles at each step (the "mountain rest step").

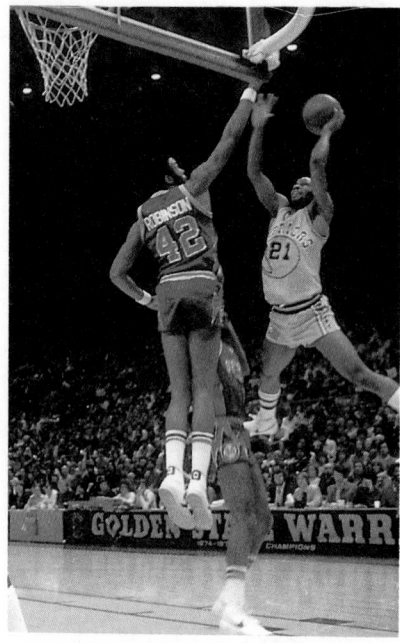

The jump of a basketball player requires anaerobic metabolism.

lactic acid: an acid produced from pyruvate during anaerobic metabolism.

oxygen debt: a deficit of oxygen built up by a body performing exercise so demanding that the cardiovascular system cannot deliver oxygen fast enough to the muscles to support aerobic metabolism; the debt must be repaid by rapid breathing after the activity slows down or stops.

■ **TABLE 13–1**
Characteristics of the Body's Energy Systems

Energy System	Oxygen Needed?	Exercise Duration	Exercise Intensity	Activity Example
ATP-PC (immediate availability)	No	Less than 30 sec	All initially; extreme thereafter	100-yd dash, shot put
ATP from carbohydrate (lactic acid)	No (anaerobic)	30 sec to 3 min	Very high	¼-mi run at maximal speed
ATP from carbohydrate	Yes (aerobic)	3 min to 20 min	High	Cross-country skiing, distance swimming or running
ATP from fat	Yes (aerobic)	More than 20 min	Moderate	Distance running or jogging

Source: Adapted from M. H. Williams, Human energy, in *Nutritional Aspects of Human Physical and Athletic Performance*, 2nd ed. (Springfield, Ill.: Charles C. Thomas, 1985), pp. 21-57; E. L. Fox, Sports activities and the energy continuum, in *Sports Physiology*, 2nd ed. (New York: W. B. Saunders Company, 1984), pp. 26–39.

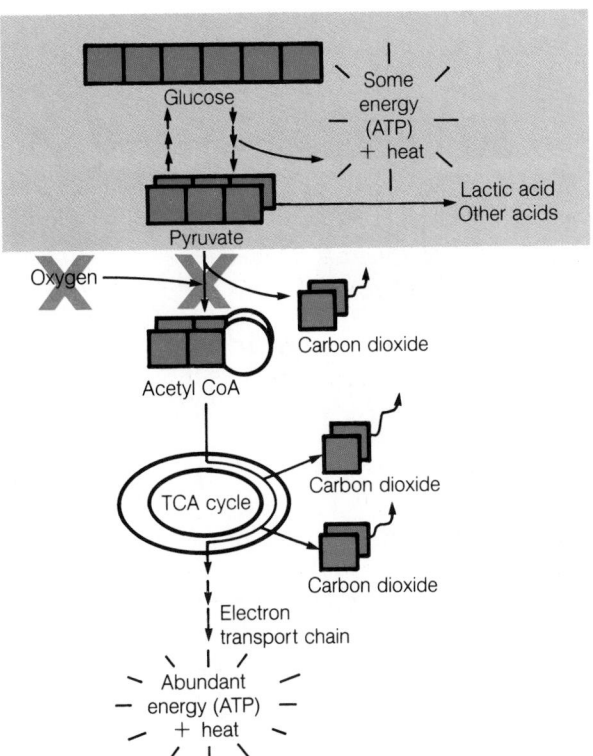

Glucose in Anaerobic Metabolism
The untrained body delivers less oxygen to its working muscles, so they extract just a little energy from glucose. Even the trained body may be unable to meet oxygen needs during intense exercise. Without ample oxygen, working muscles resort to breaking down most of their glucose molecules anaerobically until pyruvate has been produced. Anaerobic metabolism is shown in the shaded area.

Figure 13–5 shows that when oxygen is restored, much of the lactic acid is routed to the liver, where it is converted to glucose. A little lactic acid remains in muscle tissue, where it is completely oxidized when the oxygen supply is once again sufficient.

Glycogen use during exercise depends not only on the *intensity,* but also on the *duration,* of the exercise—how long it continues. Within the first 20 minutes or so of moderate exercise, a person uses up about one-fifth of the available glycogen.[5] As the muscles devour their own glycogen, they become ravenous for more glucose and increase their uptake of blood glucose 20-fold or more.[6] If you tested a person's blood glucose during this period, you would see it rise for a while, signaling that the liver is pouring out its stored carbohydrate for use by muscles. The muscles' accelerated use of blood glucose keeps the blood glucose concentration from rising too high, and indeed, it will soon begin to decline.

A person who continues exercising moderately (mostly aerobically) for longer than 20 minutes begins to use less and less glycogen, and more and more fat, for fuel (review Table 13-1). Still, glycogen use continues, and if the exercise goes on for long enough and at high enough intensity, muscle and liver glycogen stores will run out almost completely. Exercise can continue for a short time thereafter, only because the liver scrambles to produce from available lactic acid and certain amino acids the minimum amount of glucose needed to forestall hypoglycemia briefly.

When hypoglycemia hits, it brings nervous system function almost to a halt, making exercise difficult, if not impossible. This is "hitting the wall" in a marathon, and different from the sudden fatigue that a weight trainer feels

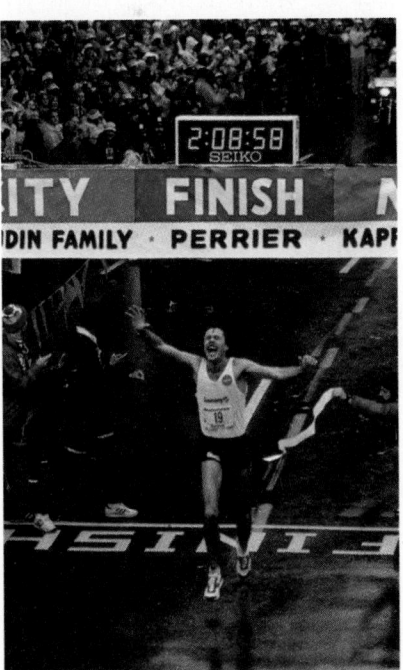

Running a marathon requires aerobic metabolism.

■ **FIGURE 13–5**
The Liver Recycles Glucose from Lactic Acid
Energy release is completed when oxygen is again available. The muscles are not forced to use glucose anaerobically. Lactic acid travels to the liver, where it is converted back to glucose and freed into the bloodstream to be used by the muscles.

after only a few seconds of lifting heavy weights. The weight lifter works at such a high intensity that the muscles' energy needs outstrip their quick-energy supply. The muscles' fatigue is the result of the depletion of PC within each muscle cell. The weight trainer may also feel pain from buildup of wastes, but a few minutes of relaxation will relieve this and permit another lift of the weights.

Since hypoglycemia brings on fatigue, people who compete try to maintain their blood glucose concentrations. It used to be thought that sugar taken during exercise might bring on hypoglycemia due to the insulin reaction to glucose, which normally stimulates all tissues of the body to take up glucose from the blood and stow it away. Exercise is a special case, though; during exercise, the body wisely releases the hormone epinephrine, which keeps the insulin level from rising too high in response to glucose in the blood. Exercise also increases muscle sensitivity to insulin so that muscle tissue is singled out as the main recipient of blood glucose. The enhancing effect of exercise on insulin activity lasts beyond the exercise period, and makes exercise helpful in the defense against the disease diabetes. People with diabetes who begin to exercise regularly can often reduce their daily requirements of insulin or insulin-eliciting drugs. (Another benefit to those with diabetes: exercise helps in weight loss, and excess body fatness is a key risk factor for Type II diabetes.)

The effect of exercise on insulin is important to endurance athletes, who often run short of glucose at the end of a competitive event. At such times, glucose can make its way slowly from the digestive tract to the muscles. The glucose from dilute sugared drinks can augment the body's supply of glucose just enough to forestall exhaustion.[7]

Before concluding that sugar might be good for your own performance, consider first whether you engage in *endurance* activity—that is, do you run, swim, bike, or ski nonstop at a rapid pace for more than 1½ hours at a time? If not, the sugar picture changes. For an everyday jog or swim, sugar won't help performance, and unless the timing is right, it may actually be a hindrance. If an exerciser makes the mistake of taking sugar within the three hours *before* exercise, before insulin secretion is suppressed, it will stimulate insulin to pour forth, and hypoglycemia then becomes likely. Research on runners shows that a sugar drink taken directly before exercise can reduce athletic performance by 25 percent.

One more factor affects carbohydrate use during exercise—the degree of training of the muscles doing the exercise at hand. A well-trained body can exercise at high intensities somewhat longer than a less-trained body; trained muscles can burn more fat and thus require less glucose, even during strenuous exercise. When you first attempt an activity, you use much more glucose than an athlete who is trained to perform it. Oxygen delivery to the muscles by the heart and lungs plays a role in this effect; but equally important, untrained muscles are less well equipped to *use* their oxygen, and so depend heavily on the anaerobic breakdown of glucose, even when the exercise is just moderate.

Trained muscles also store more glycogen within each cell than untrained muscles, especially if they have trained at high-intensity work. This is one of the microscopic adaptations that cells make during conditioning. Hard work depletes cellular glycogen stores, but within a day or two, the muscle cells replenish their supply from the carbohydrate in the diet. A later section explains how, by carbohydrate loading and exercise, some athletes stimulate their muscles to store larger-than-normal amounts of glycogen for competition.

Fat Use in Exercise

If a person should eat nothing but fat and protein, with no measurable carbohydrate, that person would burn more fat than normal during exercise. However, that person would also sacrifice athletic performance, as Figure 13–2 showed, and would also suffer needless protein degradation as the body struggled to provide the glucose it needed from amino acids. When you add to these facts that a high-fat diet is a major risk factor for cardiovascular disease, and that even those who exercise are not immune to heart attacks and strokes, it is no wonder that every reliable source speaks out against high-fat diets for athletes.

In contrast to fat in the diet, *body* fat stores are of tremendous importance in exercise. Unlike glycogen stores, which are limited, body fat stores can fuel hours of exercise without running out; fat is a virtually unlimited source of energy. Early in exercise, the blood fatty acid concentration falls as the muscles begin to draw on the available fatty acids. If exercise continues for more than a few minutes, the hormone epinephrine is released and signals the fat cells to break apart their stored triglycerides and liberate fatty acids into the blood. After about 20 minutes of exercise, the blood fatty acid concentration rises and surpasses the normal resting concentration. It is during this phase of sustained, submaximal exercise—beyond the first 20 minutes—that the fat cells begin to shrink in size as they empty out their lipid stores.

Intensity and duration of exercise affect fat use. In general, the contribution fat makes to the total fuel required diminishes as the *intensity* of exercise increases. Fat can be broken down for energy in only one way—by aerobic metabolism; fat cannot supply energy without oxygen's simultaneously being consumed. In fact, the use of fatty acids for energy requires *more* oxygen per kcalorie delivered than does that of glucose. This is because the carbon chain of each fatty acid molecule must be cleaved into many two-carbon fragments before it can enter the TCA cycle, and each cleavage requires oxygen. Thus, for fat to fuel exercise, oxygen is indispensable, as Figure 13–6 shows.

Aerobic exercise draws heavily on fat for fuel, and the body's adaptations to exercise reflect that. For example, repeated aerobic exercise stimulates the muscle cells to manufacture more mitochondria, the intracellular organelles that perform aerobic metabolism. Another adaptation: the heart and lungs improve in their capacity to deliver oxygen to muscles. Thus the body that

mitochondria (my-toe-KON-dree-ah): the cellular organelles responsible for producing ATP aerobically, made of membranes (lipid and protein) with enzymes associated with them; **mitochondrion** is the singular.
mitos = thread (referring to their slender shape)
chondros = cartilage (referring to their external appearance)

organelles: subcellular structures such as chromosomes, mitochondria, and ribosomes.
organelle = little organ

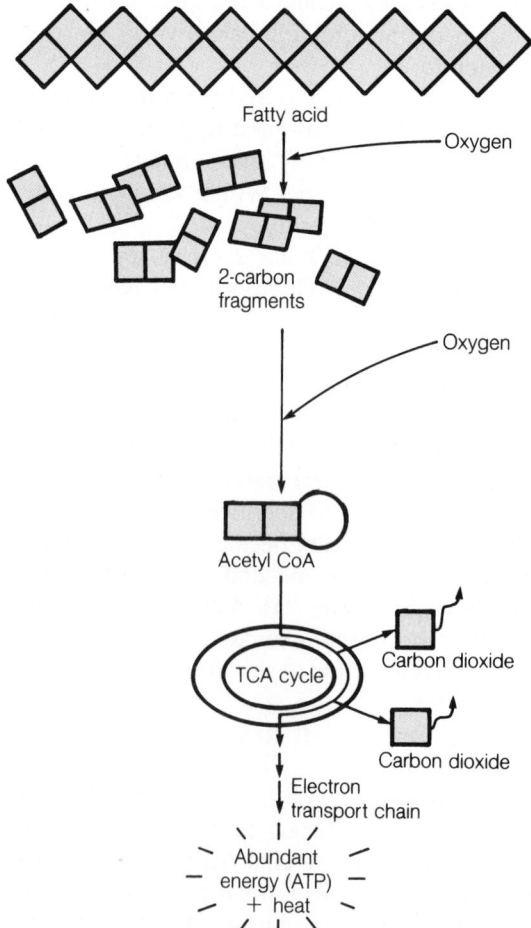

■ **FIGURE 13–6**
Fat Is an Aerobic Fuel
Abundant energy from fat breakdown can be obtained only through aerobic metabolism.

exercises aerobically becomes well-suited to the task; its muscle fibers contain more aerobic metabolic equipment, and the body has a greater heart and lung capacity. These adaptations are not reserved for trained athletes only. The first section of this chapter recommended aerobic exercise to develop cardiovascular endurance. Just 20 minutes of aerobic exercise, three times each week, stimulates even the untrained body to adapt by packing its cells with more fat-burning enzymes and by improving the ability of the heart and lungs to deliver oxygen.

The key to burning fat is slow, steady, long-duration exercise.

The body's adaptations to aerobic exercise benefit people who want to lose weight. For example, insulin levels during exercise decline in the trained person, slowing glucose release from the liver while encouraging fat use. The person who wishes to burn fat by exercising should know that patient, persistent, consistent low-intensity training, such as fast walking, is the road to maximum use of fat and conservation of carbohydrate. In general, the longer the *duration* of exercise, the greater the contribution fat makes to the total fuel required.

After exercise has ceased, fat use may continue at an accelerated rate for about a day. At least some evidence suggests that metabolism is stimulated by about 25 percent for as long as three hours after intensive exercise and may still be running 10 percent faster two days later. It takes energy to link glucose molecules back into glycogen and to build new muscle tissue; fat supplies some of this energy. Exercise favors the continued liberation of stored fat, too.[8] The body adapted to strenuous and prolonged aerobic exercise burns more fat all day long, not just during the exercise. In other words, intense exercise of more than an hour's duration probably raises a person's basal metabolic rate (BMR).

The fat used in exercise is liberated as fatty acids from the internal fat pads and from the fat under the skin. Areas that have the most fat to spare donate the greatest amounts of fatty acids to the blood (although they may not be the areas that appear most fatty). This is why "spot reducing" doesn't work—muscles do not own the fat that surrounds them. Fat cells release fatty acids not into the underlying muscles, but into the blood, and all the muscles share these fatty acids. Proof of this is found in a tennis player's arms—the fatfolds measure the same in both arms, even though the muscles of one arm are much better developed than those of the other. A balanced exercise program will, however, tighten muscles underneath the fat in trouble spots to improve the overall appearance.

Chapter 19 and Appendix E provide the details of fatfold measure.

Table 13–1 provides a summary of fuel use in exercise, as discussed so far. The next section describes the roles of protein in exercise. Protein is not a major source of energy for exercise, but it still provides some; more important, it provides the structural material of muscle tissue.

Protein Use in Exercise

If a high-fat diet is ill-advised for athletes, what about a high-protein diet? Science is just beginning to understand how exercise and training affect protein metabolism. With respect to exercise, the body uses protein primarily to build cell structures and secondarily as a fuel source. The body handles protein differently during exercise than at rest. Athletes' needs for protein may be just slightly higher than the needs of others, but are still well within the amount provided by a typical U.S. diet and the margin of safety in the RDA.

Synthesis of body proteins is suppressed during exercise, and for several hours afterwards. In the hours following this inactive period, though, protein synthesis rebounds beyond normal resting levels.[9] This may be the time in which the body adapts and builds the tissues and molecules it needs for the next time of exercise. Whenever the body remodels a part of itself, it must tear down the old structures to make way for the new ones. Repeated exercise, with just a slight overload, triggers the protein-dismantling and protein-synthesizing equipment of each muscle cell to make needed changes.

The physical work of each muscle cell acts as a signal to its DNA and RNA to begin producing the kinds of proteins that will best support that work.[10] Take jogging, for example. In the first difficult sessions, the body is not yet equipped to perform—for example, the muscle fibers have limited mitochondria for aerobic metabolism. But in those first sessions, the cells' genetic material gets the message that an overhaul is needed. In the hours that follow exercise, muscle cells start breaking down any unneeded protein structures. At the same time, the genes and protein-building equipment receive molecular messages that tell them what new structures are needed; and within the limits of their genetic potential, they build more. Among the new structures are more mitochondria to facilitate efficient aerobic metabolism. The muscles don't change appreciably in just one or two occasions of exercise, but within a few weeks, remodeling occurs and jogging becomes easier.[11]

Studies show that during active muscle-building phases of training, a weight lifter might add to existing muscle mass between ¼ ounce and 1 ounce (between 7 and 28 grams) of protein each day.[12] This only happens during periods of *building*, by exercising at high intensities, and not during maintenance exercise.

Not only do athletes retain more protein, but they also burn more protein as fuel, too. Studies of nitrogen balance show that muscles speed up their use of amino acids for energy during exercise, just as they speed up their use of fat and carbohydrate.[13] Protein is not a major source of energy—it is estimated to contribute an average of about 10 percent of the total fuel used, both during exercise and during rest.[14] Endurance athletes use up enormous amounts of total energy fuels during performance, though, and so they break down a proportionately larger amount of protein than do people who exercise moderately.

The factors that modify how much protein is used during activity seem to be the same three that modify the use of fat and carbohydrate—for one, diet. Athletes who consume diets rich in carbohydrate burn less protein than those who eat protein- and fat-rich diets.[15] This could be related to the protein-sparing effect of carbohydrate first discussed in Chapter 4. Some amino acids can, unlike fat, be converted into glucose. Fat can never provide glucose, and thus a high-fat diet necessitates the conversion of amino acids to glucose. Exercise requires glucose, and combined with a high-fat, low-carbohydrate diet, hastens the use of protein for fuel.

A second factor, the intensity and duration of the exercise, also modifies protein use.[16] Low- to moderate-intensity exercise of long duration demands large quantities of fuel, including protein. Short-duration, high-intensity anaerobic exercise demands less total protein fuel.[17]

A third factor also modifies the use of protein—the degree of training. The better trained the athlete, the less protein used during exercise.

As mentioned earlier, all athletes probably need just a little more protein than do sedentary people. Endurance athletes burn greater quantities of protein for fuel than power athletes do, and they retain some, especially in the muscles used for their sport. Power athletes use less protein for fuel than do endurance athletes, but still spend some, and they retain much more. Therefore, *all* athletes in training should attend to protein needs, but should not neglect carbohydrate needs in the process. Otherwise, they will burn off as fuel the very protein that they wish to retain as muscle.

How much protein should an athlete consume? The American Dietetic Association (ADA) recommends 1 gram protein per kilogram of body weight each day, an amount somewhat higher than the 0.8 gram per kilogram body weight per day recommended for sedentary people.[18] The association acknowledges a study showing that young men who ate diets containing 1 gram protein per kilogram body weight per day and then began training developed negative nitrogen balance—the men lost body protein, at least at first. Later in the study, as training progressed, the men's nitrogen balance gradually became positive—they built up body protein while still eating the diet containing 1 gram protein per kilogram body weight per day.[19] This shift from negative to positive nitrogen balance with no change in diet supports the ADA protein recommendation. The initial protein losses in the study could have been caused by something other than insufficient dietary protein, such as the training itself.

Other experts disagree with the ADA and recommend higher protein intakes. For example, one group of researchers found that 2 grams protein per kilogram body weight per day during the early stages of training effectively maintained positive nitrogen balance during that time and prevented a drop in the levels of certain blood proteins, including hemoglobin, observed at lower protein intakes.[20] Still another authority suggests different protein levels for different sports: endurance athletes in hard training for an hour each day should consume between 1.0 and 1.2 grams protein per kilogram body weight per day, and power athletes who are increasing muscle bulk should take in between 1.3 and 1.6 grams protein per kilogram body weight per day. Thus an athlete weighing 70 kilograms might choose any level of intake from among those shown in Table 13–2. After considering these

■ TABLE 13–2
Total Daily Protein Needs of a 70-Kilogram Athlete

Authority	Recommendation (g/kg/day)	Protein/Day (g)
Food and Nutrition Board (RDA)	0.8	56
American Dietetic Association	1.0	70
Brotherhood (endurance athletes)	1.0 to 1.2	70 to 84
Brotherhood (power athletes)	1.3 to 1.6	91 to 112
Yoshimura (early training)	2.0	140

Source: Data from Food and Nutrition Board, *Recommended Dietary Allowances*, 10th ed. (Washington, D.C.: National Academy of Sciences, 1989); Position of the American Dietetic Association: Nutrition for physical fitness and athletic performance for adults, *Journal of the American Dietetic Association* 87 (1987): 933–939; J. R. Brotherhood, Nutrition and sports performance, *Sports Medicine* 1 (1984): 350–389; H. Yoshimura and coauthors, Anaemia during hard physical training (sports anaemia) and its causal mechanism with special reference to protein nutrition, *World Review of Nutrition and Dietetics* 35 (1980): 1–86.

recommendations, an athlete might well wonder what level is best and how the recommendations translate into diet. Before drawing conclusions about what foods to eat, read the later section about choosing a diet, where these questions are answered.

■ Vitamins, Minerals, and Performance

Vitamins and minerals assist in releasing energy from fuels and in transporting oxygen. Table 13–3 lists some vitamins and minerals and their functions crucial to physical performance.

Vitamins and Performance

Popular belief has it that vitamin supplements offer athletes both health benefits and improved athletic performance. (Highlight 13 explores the many nutrition, and other, tricks athletes use in the hope of enhancing performance.) According to one survey, 84 percent of world-class athletes use vitamin supplements.[21] It goes without saying that athletes need adequate

■ TABLE 13–3
Roles of Vitamins and Minerals Important in Exercise

Vitamin or Mineral	Function
Thiamin, riboflavin, niacin	Energy-releasing reactions
Vitamin B_6, zinc	Building of muscle protein
Folate, vitamin B_{12}	Building of red blood cells to carry oxygen
Vitamin C	Collagen formation for joint and other tissue integrity; hormone synthesis
Iron	Transport of oxygen in blood and in muscle tissue; energy transformation reactions
Calcium, vitamin D, vitamin A, phosphorus	Building of bone structure; muscle contractions; nerve transmissions; component of high-energy molecules
Sodium, potassium, chloride	Maintenance of fluid balance; transmission of nerve impulses for muscle contraction
Chromium	Assistance in insulin's energy-storage function
Magnesium	Cardiac and other muscle contraction; energy-releasing reactions

Note: This is just a sampling. Other vitamins and minerals play equally indispensable roles in exercise.

vitamins and minerals to do what they do, as Table 13–3 showed. But are the amounts that are adequate for sedentary people also adequate for active people? If not, which nutrients do active people need more of? The answers remain uncertain, but science is searching for them in the metabolic workings of the muscles, and in the roles that vitamins play there.

If asked to guess which vitamins an athlete might need more of, a logical reply might be that, since athletes use more energy in a day, they might need more of the vitamins involved in the breakdown of energy-yielding nutrients—the B vitamins. The RDA for several of the B vitamins, remember, is expressed in amounts per 1,000 kcalories of food energy required to support energy needs.[22]

Scientists have studied the effects of thiamin supplements on athletes. They gave supplements to one group of athletes, and compared the physical performance of that group to that of athletes eating only a regular adequate diet.[23] They found that extra thiamin did not benefit performance. They concluded that the thiamin in an *adequate* diet supplies all the thiamin a person needs, even an athlete doing heavy work. This is because almost any kind of unprocessed food supplies thiamin. Most diets are adequate in thiamin, and even athletes do not need more than the RDA.

This does not mean that thiamin or any of the other vitamins are not important. The words *adequate diet* are weighty in this regard. To be adequately nourished, most of the athletes' extra energy needs must be met with nutrient-dense foods, not fats and sweets. Even sedentary people who consume a diet of foods relatively empty of nutrients can become thiamin deficient. This effect is magnified for the exerciser who spends many more kcalories of energy each day than do others.

Riboflavin, another B vitamin, also plays a role in energy release. The link between riboflavin and physical performance arises from its role as part of the coenzyme flavin adenine dinucleotide (FAD), which is central to the mitochondrial oxygen-requiring reactions that generate ATP from energy-yielding nutrients. To try to answer the question of whether riboflavin, at levels beyond the RDA, assists in athletic performance, researchers studied groups of overweight, sedentary women who began an exercise regimen in addition to weight-loss dieting.[24] One group of women consumed the RDA of riboflavin, while the other group consumed slightly more (an additional 0.2 milligrams). Blood tests to evaluate riboflavin activity seemed to indicate a deficiency in the group that consumed only the RDA amounts. However, the aerobic capacity of both groups increased similarly. Extra riboflavin did not improve this aspect of physical performance over the RDA amount, but other indexes of physical performance were not studied. To answer questions about riboflavin requirements during exercise will require more research. Riboflavin is abundant in the diets of developed countries, so outward symptoms of deficiency are rarely seen.

Unlike the two other B vitamins just discussed, niacin may affect performance more directly, especially when taken as a supplement. Niacin taken before exercise suppresses the release of fatty acids, forcing muscles to use extra glycogen. Whether this impairs performance is unknown, but it probably shortens the time to glycogen depletion and makes the work seem more difficult to the exerciser.[25] Exercisers need no more niacin than that supplied by a nutrient-dense diet, and people who take niacin supplements before exercise probably impair their workouts.

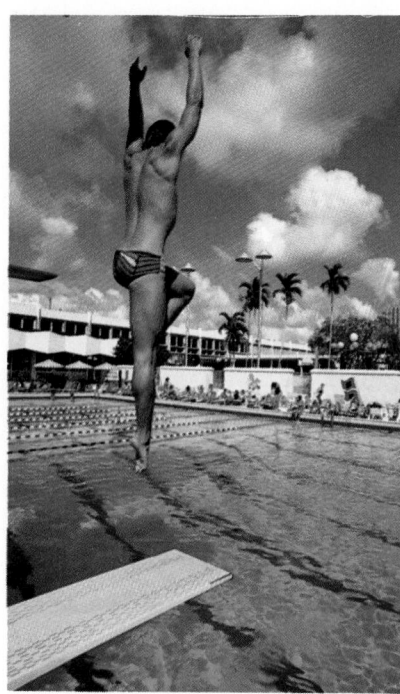

For perfect functioning, every nutrient is needed.

You may recall that vitamin B_6 participates in numerous enzyme systems involved with the metabolism of protein and the other energy-yielding nutrients. It functions in the breakdown of glycogen and in the formation of hemoglobin. Such roles are the basis for claims that vitamin B_6 in amounts greater than the RDA promotes aerobic endurance. Thus far, research does not support these theories. Experimentally, supplementation with vitamin B_6 does not improve aerobic performance.[26] To ensure that the diet is adequate in vitamin B_6, a person need only include some leafy green vegetables, meats, fish, legumes, fruits, and whole grains. Pills, even those containing megadoses of vitamin B_6, can't compete with an optimal diet.

The belief that vitamin B_{12} supplementation will enhance performance stems from its role in the production of red blood cells. In anemia, a diminished number of circulating red blood cells robs the blood of its oxygen-carrying capacity, starving the cells and restricting aerobic energy metabolism. Vitamin B_{12} deficiency is only one cause of anemia. Iron and folate deficiencies are equally destructive to performance, as are medical anemias.

Some athletes take vitamin B_{12} prior to competition because they believe that they can enhance endurance and oxygen delivery in this way. The limited research thus far does not support this concept. In fact, taking *any* vitamin directly before competition runs contrary to science. Vitamins function only as small parts of larger working units, coenzymes, inserted into enzymes. A molecule of a vitamin floating around in the blood is simply waiting for the tissues to combine it with its appropriate other parts so that it can do its work. This takes time—hours or days. Vitamins taken right before competition are still waiting in the blood during exercise and are useless for improving performance during that event, even if the person actually is deficient in that vitamin. Vitamin B_{12} supplements are the appropriate treatment for a vitamin B_{12} deficiency. For a well-nourished athlete, any perceived benefits from their use are based on psychology, not physiology.[27]

Years ago, evidence that excretion of vitamin C was increased after exercise seemed to indicate that vitamin C in amounts two to three times the RDA might best serve the needs of the athlete. Since that time, the great bulk of work designed to explore this theory has disproved it. Most experiments show that athletes perform no better when taking vitamin C supplements than when they receive the RDA amount from food.

Even so, athletes are often told by "advisors" in health food stores to ingest huge quantities of vitamin C, measured in multiples of a gram. These amounts are clearly beyond those indicated as potentially useful, and they could be harmful. Besides, if an athlete eats mostly unprocessed foods, it is almost impossible *not* to receive two to three times the RDA for vitamin C. A person who drinks a small glass of orange juice and eats a baked potato and a serving of broccoli in a day will receive about five times the RDA for vitamin C from these foods alone. When shown the full array of values for vitamins and minerals, including vitamin C, in foods such as these, athletes have been known to throw away their pills and learn to cook broccoli.

Of the fat-soluble vitamins, supplemental A and D have been shown not to benefit athletic performance, and they are toxic in excess. One other fat-soluble vitamin, vitamin E, has been promoted for athletes. In its role as an antioxidant of polyunsaturated fatty acids, it is as important to athletes as to anyone else. Vitamin E protects lipids of cell and mitochondrial membranes against destruction by oxygen. In the mitochondria, vitamin E may similarly protect a part of the metabolic equipment that transforms energy fuels into ATP, obviously important to athletes.*

The effect of training on vitamin E is only just beginning to be explored by research. In one recent study, researchers found that even though trained muscles contain many mitochondria, and even though mitochondria need vitamin E to prevent their own destruction by oxygen, trained muscles contain no more vitamin E than do untrained muscles.[28] It is too early to say how this can be applied to the diets of athletes. Many facts are still unknown, but the evidence indicates that extra vitamin E as supplements does not enhance athletic performance.

As the oxygen carriers for the body, red blood cells need the protection that vitamin E has to offer. If there is too little vitamin E, red blood cell membranes weaken and break open, spilling out their hemoglobin. The result is anemia. Without a doubt, the anemia of vitamin E deficiency would hinder athletic performance, should it occur in people, but that is unlikely. As Chapter 9 described, vitamin E is widespread in foods, and its deficiency is practically unheard of. Still, vitamin E is one of the many nutrients sold to athletes under the guise of promoting performance, as Highlight 13 describes.

Minerals and Performance

Like the vitamins, minerals are essential to exercise. Calcium and iron stand out among minerals of importance because deficiencies of them are likely. Nutrition counselors may find athletes particularly motivated to dietary change, and with respect to calcium and iron, such change is oftentimes needed.

Osteoporosis, the condition of reduced bone mass, increases susceptibility to fractures, including stress fractures and bone breaks that are due to exercise. Chapter 10 pointed out that moderate exercise protects against bone loss, but extremes in exercise may be detrimental to the bone health of some young women.[29] A side effect of endurance training for some women is athletic amenorrhea, characterized by low estrogen concentrations and possibly increased calcium requirements. A recent study of ballet dancers found that those with extremely low body fat content and who suffered from amenorrhea incurred more bone injuries than did those with more normal body fatness.[30] Considering that the food energy intakes of some amenorrheic athletes are abnormally low, and that the calcium intakes of women in the United States are also low, amenorrheic athletes with low body fatness may be at much greater risk for osteoporosis than other women.[31]

In one survey, one-third of female athletes questioned practiced some sort of pathological eating behavior, many of the type that characterizes anorexia nervosa and bulimia (discussed in Highlight 12).[32] These behaviors are harmful to bone health and general health, and they impair physical performance. It goes without saying that such women are in need of treatment for their eating behaviors before they can hope to compete with

stress fracture: bone damage or breakage caused by stress on bone surfaces during exercise.

athletic amenorrhea: the cessation of menstruation associated with strenuous athletic training.

---

*The molecule believed to be protected is coenzyme Q.

well-nourished athletes in sports. Some authorities have suggested that at least part of the reason so many athletic women engage in self-destructive behaviors related to their body weights is because they have adopted weight standards that are invalid for athletes. Women athletes are taller and are heavier for their heights (they have more healthy muscle and bone tissue) than other women. When the athletes consult weight standards designed for sedentary women, they can easily be misled into believing, wrongly, that they are too fat. Many resort to bulimic techniques in an attempt to lose weight and solve the imaginary problem.[33] Standard height and weight charts should not be applied to athletes. Underwater weighing and other body composition measures are more appropriate for them.

Endurance athletes, and especially women athletes, are prone to iron deficiency. Vegetarian women athletes may be especially at risk for low iron status.[34] A recent nutrition survey found that more than one-third of the women runners had diminished iron stores.[35] Habitually low intakes of iron-rich foods and increased iron losses may cause iron deficiency in young women athletes. In addition, exercise may cause small blood losses through the GI tract, at least in some athletes. A little iron is also lost in sweat.

Iron-deficiency anemia reduces the oxygen-carrying capacity of the blood and inhibits mitochondrial enzyme function, thereby dramatically impairing physical performance. Even marginal iron deficiency without clinical signs of anemia impairs physical performance to some extent. On the other hand, low iron indicators in the blood do not always accompany decreases in performance. In a study of male marathon runners, blood iron measures indicated that the men suffered from marginal anemia. Even so, their running speeds remained unchanged.[36] The below-normal blood iron measures observed in these men are not unusual for distance runners and may indicate a particular type of iron-deficiency anemia, runner's anemia.

runner's anemia: a true iron-deficiency anemia that develops in many high-mileage runners.

Iron status might be affected by exercise in any of several ways. One possibility is that iron lost in sweat creates the deficiency, although the sweat of trained athletes contains less iron than the sweat of others (another adaptation of conditioning). Another possible route to iron loss is red blood cell destruction; blood cells are squashed when body tissues (such as the soles of the feet) make contact with an unyielding surface (such as the ground). Perhaps more significant than these losses is reduced iron absorption in some athletes, as well as increased iron uptake from blood for use by muscles to make the iron-containing molecules of the mitochondria and the iron-containing muscle protein, myoglobin.

sports anemia: a transient condition of low hemoglobin in the blood, associated with the early stages of sports training or other strenuous activity.

The condition known as sports anemia is distinct from the true iron-deficiency condition runner's anemia. Sports anemia is characterized by a temporary decrease in hemoglobin concentration after a sudden increase in aerobic exercise. Its exact cause remains controversial, but marginal iron intakes may contribute to it. In addition, strenuous aerobic exercise promotes destruction of fragile, older red blood cells, and increases the plasma volume of the blood. Sports anemia appears to be an adaptive, temporary response to endurance training. Iron-deficiency anemia requires iron-supplementation therapy; sports anemia goes away by itself.

The best strategy concerning iron may be to try to determine your individual needs. Many young menstruating women probably border on iron deficiency even without the additional iron losses incurred through exercise.

Especially for teen and adult women, then, prescribed supplements may be needed to correct a deficiency of iron as determined by medical testing.

Other minerals are affected by athletic training, too. Three trace minerals—chromium, zinc, and copper—are of current scientific interest. These minerals have been found to be excreted in larger amounts when people exercise than when they are sedentary.[37] So far, it is too early to say whether the excretion is meaningful in terms of people's nutrition, but studies of runners have shown that even with low zinc levels in their blood, running performance is not hindered.[38]

For the most part, studies indicate that athletes who take supplements gain no competitive advantage.[39] What the studies consistently find, however, is that compromised nutrition status impedes performance. Not all, or even most, athletes are well nourished, for even a prodigy on the playing field can be a dunce in the dining room. A human body, even one in superb condition, cannot wring from high-fat, empty-kcalorie foods the nutrients it needs. For the most part, active people who choose foods with care can be sure of meeting their vitamin and mineral needs without supplements. After all, they eat more food; it stands to reason that with the right choices, they'll get more nutrients.

■ *Fluids and Electrolytes*

As Chapter 10 described, the human body relies on watery fluids as the medium for all of its life-supporting chemistry, and its need for water far surpasses that for any other nutrient. Should the body lose too much water, as in dehydration, its chemistry becomes compromised. The first symptom of dehydration is fatigue. A rapid water loss equal to 5 percent of the body weight can reduce muscular work capacity by 20 to 30 percent.[40]

Most obviously, the body loses water via sweat; second to that, breathing costs water, exhaled as vapor. In exercise, both routes can be significant, but sweat is the greater. Earlier, it was said that working muscles produce heat as a by-product of ATP breakdown. One of the adjustments the body makes to rid itself of excessive heat is to route its blood supply, which carries heat, through the capillaries just under the skin. At the same time, sweat is secreted and cools the skin by evaporation. The heated blood flows under the cooled skin, and it is cooled for its return trip to the deeper body chambers.

In humid, hot weather, sweat doesn't evaporate well because the surrounding air is already laden with water. Body heat builds up and triggers maximum sweating—the body's only defense against excess heat. Still, without much evaporation, little cooling takes place. In such conditions, active people must take precautions to prevent heat stroke, the dangerous accumulation of body heat with accompanying loss of body fluid. The only way to prevent heat stroke is to drink enough fluid before and during the activity, to rest in the shade when tired, and to wear lightweight clothing that allows evaporation. (Hence the danger of rubber or heavy suits sold supposedly to promote weight loss during exercise—they promote profuse sweating, prevent sweat evaporation, and invite heat stroke.) If you ever experience any of the symptoms of heat stroke, stop your activity, sip fluids, seek shade, and ask for help—the condition can be fatal and demands medical attention.

heat stroke: an acute and dangerous reaction to heat buildup in the body. Symptoms include headache, nausea, dizziness, clumsiness, stumbling, changes in normal sweating (more or less), and confusion or other mental changes.

Athletes can lose 2 to 4 quarts of fluid in *every hour* of heavy exercise. The digestive system can absorb only about a quart an hour. Hence the athlete must hydrate before, and rehydrate during and after, exercise to replace it all. Even then, in hot weather, the GI tract may not be able to absorb enough water fast enough to keep up with an athlete's sweating losses, and some degree of dehydration becomes inevitable. Athletes who are preparing for competition are often advised to drink extra fluids in the few days before the event, especially if they are in training. The extra water is not stored in the body, but drinking extra water ensures maximum levels of hydration at the start of the event. A caution is in order—some coaches and athletes withhold water during practice because they believe the body can adapt to use less water. This false and dangerous idea has extracted a toll on the health of athletes, and some have even died. Full hydration is imperative for every athlete in training, as well as in competition. The athlete who arrives even slightly dehydrated from chronic underconsumption of fluid arrives with a disadvantage. Drinking a few extra glasses of water a day causes no harm, and it may be protective.

Even casual exercisers must attend conscientiously to their fluid needs. Exercise blunts the thirst mechanism, especially in cold weather. During heavy exercise, thirst signals too late, after fluid stores are depleted. Don't wait to feel thirsty before drinking. Table 13–4 presents one schedule of hydration for exercise. To find out how much water is needed to replenish losses after a workout, weigh yourself before and after—the difference is all water. One pound equals roughly 2 cups fluid (a quart equals 2 pounds).

What is the best fluid for an exercising body? Surprisingly, cool water, especially in warm weather. It is best for two reasons—because it rapidly leaves the digestive tract to enter the tissues where it is needed, and because it cools the body.

hypothermia: a below-normal body temperature.

In cold weather, *hypo*thermia, or loss of body heat, can pose as serious a threat as heat stroke. During exercise in cold weather, the body still sweats and needs fluids, but the fluids should be warm or at room temperature, not cold. Under these conditions, the absorption advantage conferred by drinking cool water is overshadowed by the threat of hypothermia.

When you sweat, electrolytes—the charged minerals sodium, potassium, chloride, and magnesium—are lost from the body along with water. People who are just beginning an exercise regimen lose electrolytes to a much greater extent than do trained people; as the body adapts to exercise, it becomes

■ TABLE 13–4
Schedule of Hydration Before and During Exercise

When to Drink	Amount of Fluid
2 hr before exercise	About 3 c
10 to 15 min before exercise	About 2 c
Every 60 to 90 min during exercise	About 1 qt (or 1 liter)
After exercise	Replace each pound of body weight lost with 2 c (½ liter) fluid

Source: Adapted from J. B. Marcus, ed., *Sports Nutrition* (Chicago: American Dietetic Association, 1986), p. 57; American College of Sports Medicine position stand on the prevention of thermal injuries during distance running, *Medicine and Science in Sports and Exercise* 19 (1987): 529–533.

better at conserving electrolytes. An exception is magnesium; its losses in sweat are about the same for trained and untrained individuals. One study found magnesium levels in the blood serum to be lower in exercising people than in others; the effect remained even three months after the exercise

---

Sports Drinks

Most fitness authorities agree that water best meets the body's fluid needs, yet manufacturers market many good-tasting drinks for active people. Manufacturers reason that if a drink tastes good, people will drink more, thereby ensuring adequate hydration. In addition, they claim the drinks attempt to duplicate the fluid lost in sweat (most fall short with respect to magnesium), and so can facilitate performance. Furthermore, the drinks supply energy from carbohydrate—another proposed edge over plain water. Exercise physiologists counter most of these claims.

For one thing, immediate replacement of the minerals lost in sweat isn't necessary; within hours of competition is soon enough. Further, a major ingredient in the drinks is salt, and most people already ingest so much salt as to aggravate hypertension in salt-sensitive people—and hypertension is a major health problem in this country. Salt-containing drinks could counteract the blood pressure-normalizing effects of exercise. In rare cases of the most strenuous competition at the world-class level, heavy sweating for many days in a row has been reported to dilute the blood concentration of sodium, and in these few cases, sodium repletion was needed. For the average exerciser, though, salt in drinks is excessive—it causes loss of potassium and places an extra burden on the kidneys to excrete both sodium and potassium.

On one aspect of the needs of the athlete, researchers agree with the beverage companies: a beverage that supplies glucose in some form might be desirable during endurance activity lasting longer than two hours. It used to be thought that the sugar in the drinks slowed fluid absorption, but recent research indicates that fluid transport to the tissues is equally rapid from beverages containing up to 6% glucose as from plain water.[42] Some manufacturers of the commercial drinks claim that formulas that replace glucose with starchlike glucose polymers are more rapidly absorbed, but this question is still open.

While carbohydrate is known to enhance the performance of an endurance athlete in grueling competitive events, it is of no value to the average exerciser, and is counterproductive if weight loss is a goal. Glucose is sugar, and like candy, it provides only empty kcalories—no nutrients. Sports drinks contain about half the sugar of ordinary soft drinks; that is, about 5 tsp in each 12 oz.

In choosing a sports drink or formula, be aware. Some drinks contain the sugar fructose, because fructose does not elicit as high an insulin response as does glucose and so does not drive energy-yielding nutrients into storage. Fructose causes other problems, though, at least for some people, such as gas, bloating, pain, and diarrhea—deterrents to performance.

Commercial products for athletes provide a psychological edge for some people who equate the drinks with athletes and sports. The need to belong is valid, and if the drinks are used with care, they may do no harm and might provide a needed boost to morale.

glucose polymers: compounds that supply glucose, not as single molecules, but linked in chains somewhat like starch. The object is to attract less water from the body into the digestive tract (osmotic attraction depends not on the size, but on the number, of particles).

program began.[41] This could mean that a magnesium deficiency was coming on, or it could mean that the magnesium had moved out of the blood and into the tissues in response to training.

As for potassium, it usually remains safely inside the cells, where it does its work. However, in prolonged dehydration from profuse sweating, it may migrate outside of cells and be lost by excretion in the urine. Even so, it is easily replaced with just a few servings of fresh fruits and vegetables. Avoid potassium supplements unless prescribed by a physician, because, while they better some conditions, they worsen others.

As the previous box on sports drinks states, most times, athletes need make no special effort to replenish lost electrolytes; a regular diet that meets their energy and nutrient needs also supplies all the electrolytes they need. There is also no need to replace electrolytes during exercise, unless the athlete works up a drenching sweat exceeding 5 to 10 pounds a day (3 percent of body weight) for several consecutive days. Under such exertion, a commercial "sweat replacer" beverage, diluted by half with water, may be drunk for fluid replacement; a homemade mixture of ⅓ teaspoon salt (sodium chloride) and 1 cup fruit juice (to provide potassium and carbohydrate) added to each quart of water will also serve the purpose. Avoid electrolyte or salt tablets; they increase potassium losses, can irritate the stomach, can cause vomiting, and always cause water to flow into the GI tract from the tissues at first, thereby temporarily worsening dehydration and impairing performance.

■ *Diets for Athletes*

No particular diet supports an athlete's performance perfectly; many different diets can be excellent for athletes. However, food choices must be made within the framework of rules for diet adequacy first presented in Chapter 2.

Choosing a Performance Diet

First, athletes need a nutrient-dense diet composed mostly of unprocessed foods—foods that supply maximum vitamins and minerals for the energy they provide. When athletes rely heavily on processed foods that have suffered nutrient losses and contain added sugar and fat, nutrition status suffers. Even if these foods are fortified or enriched, manufacturers cannot replace the whole range of nutrients and nonnutrients lost in processing. Consider, for example, that manufacturers mill and process the trace minerals magnesium and chromium out of foods but do not replace them, and that they are essential to optimal performance. This doesn't mean that athletes can *never* choose a white bread, bologna, and mayonnaise sandwich for lunch, but only that later, to compensate, they should drink a glass of milk and eat a large, fresh salad or big portions of vegetables and whole-grain breads. That way, the nutrient-dense foods provide most of the needed nutrients, including magnesium and chromium; the bologna sandwich, high in fat and salt, and of low nutrient density, simply added extra kcalories.

Beyond eating for adequacy, athletes must eat for energy, and energy needs may be immense. The athlete may want full glycogen stores as well. Too,

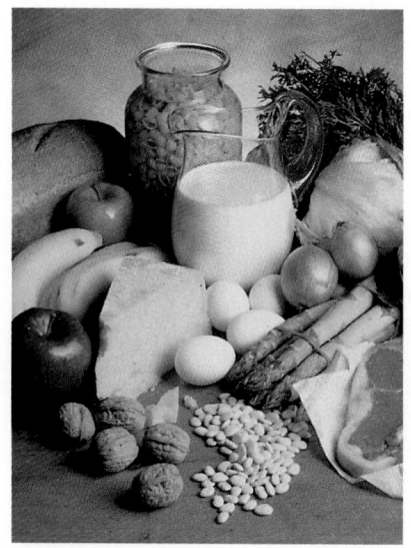

A variety of foods is the best source of nutrients for athletes.

athletes are not immune to heart disease or cancer, and so must limit fats while still trying to eat enough food to provide all the needed energy. Simply stated, a diet that is high in carbohydrate (65 percent of total kcalories or more), low in fat (20 percent or less), and adequate in protein (12 to 15 percent) while meeting the athlete's energy needs works best to ensure full glycogen and other nutrient stores. Even if the athlete does not compete in glycogen-depleting events, such a diet will help to control weight (thus reducing diabetes and other disease risks) and to provide adequate fiber while supplying abundant nutrients. For the athlete who competes in glycogen-depleting events, the accompanying box describes carbohydrate loading.

Adding more carbohydrate-rich foods is a sound and reasonable option for increasing energy intake, up to a point. The point at which it becomes unreasonable is when the person's energy needs outstrip the capacity to eat enough food to provide them. At that point, the person must find ways of adding food energy to the diet, mostly through the addition of refined sugars and even some fat. Still, this energy-rich diet must be superimposed on the nutrient-rich choices for adequacy. Energy alone is not enough.

In addition to carbohydrate, athletes need protein. How much of what kinds of foods can supply enough protein to meet the needs of athletes? The

---

Carbohydrate Loading

When the facts about glycogen stores and endurance performance first became known, athletes naturally wanted to make sure they had glycogen to spare. Some used a technique called carbohydrate loading to trick their muscles into storing extra glycogen before a competition. In the early days, athletes were taught to restrict carbohydrates and exercise heavily to empty their muscles of glycogen. Before the event, they cut back on exercise and switched abruptly to an extremely high-carbohydrate diet. Muscle glycogen rebounded to as high as three to four times the normal amount.

Carbohydrate loading practiced this way can have side effects that outweigh any performance advantage, including abnormal heartbeat, swollen and painful muscles (glycogen attracts and holds water), and weight gain immediately before competition. Exercise physiologists now recommend a modified plan that confers similar benefits without the side effects. First, the athlete increases exercise intensity *without* restricting carbohydrates. Next, during the week before competition, the athlete gradually cuts back on exercise, rests completely the day before, and eats a very-high-carbohydrate diet for a few days before competition. In the modified plan, athletes never restrict carbohydrate intake; they only manipulate exercise levels and pack extra carbohydrate in at the end. Endurance athletes who follow this plan can keep going longer than their competitors without ill effects. In a hot climate, extra glycogen confers an additional advantage; as glycogen breaks down, it releases water, which helps to meet the athlete's fluid needs.

Extra glycogen benefits only those who exercise long enough (at least 90 minutes) and hard enough to deplete their stores; the regular, everyday exerciser won't benefit from having larger stores. What that person does need, though, is *adequate* glycogen from eating a diet high in complex carbohydrates.

carbohydrate loading: a regimen of exhaustive exercise followed by consuming a high-carbohydrate diet, which enables muscles to store glycogen beyond their normal capacity; also called **glycogen loading** or **glycogen supercompensation**.

To make glycogen, muscles need carbohydrate, but they also need rest, so vary daily exercise routines to work different muscles on different days.

exchange lists, of course, point out rich protein sources, and meats and milk head the list. To recommend that athletes eat plenty of meat would be narrow advice for many reasons. For one thing, athletes must protect themselves from heart disease, and even lean meats contain fat, much of it saturated fat. For another, athletes need a diet high in carbohydrates to support performance, and of course, meats have none to offer.

Earlier in this chapter, Table 13–2 showed some possible protein intakes for a 70-kilogram athlete based on recommendations of various authorities. It is likely that an athlete weighing 70 kilograms who exercised vigorously on a daily basis could require more than 3,000 kcalories per day. To meet such an energy requirement, the athlete could select from a variety of nutrient-dense foods. Figure 13–7 provides one example; it itemizes the foods added to the original meal selections pictured in Chapter 2 to attain a 3,000-kcalorie diet. In addition to the items listed, low-fat (2 percent) milk replaced the nonfat milk. These meals supply 124 grams protein, an amount greater than all but the highest recommended level of 2 grams per kilogram body weight per day (140 grams per day) for such a person. Obviously, the more energy an athlete requires, the more protein that athlete will receive, assuming wise food choices. This relationship between energy and protein intakes breaks down when athletes meet their energy needs with high-fat, high-sugar confections. The meals shown in Figure 13–7 provide 61 percent of their kcalories from carbohydrate. Athletes who train exhaustively and who train for endurance events may want to aim for somewhat higher carbohydrate levels—from 65 to 70 percent. Beyond these specific concerns of total energy, protein, and carbohydrate, the diet most beneficial to athletic performance is remarkably similar to the diet of most people.

Table 13–5 shows some sample diet plans for athletes who wish to increase their energy and carbohydrate intakes. These plans are effective only if the user chooses foods to provide nutrients as well as energy—extra milk for calcium and riboflavin; many fruits and vegetables for folate, vitamin A, and vitamin C; meat or alternates for iron and other vitamins and minerals; and whole grains for B vitamins, magnesium, zinc, and chromium. In addition, these foods provide plenty of sodium, potassium, and chloride.

■ TABLE 13–5
Diet Plans for High-kCalorie, High-Carbohydrate Intakes

Use the number of exchanges indicated to arrive at the specified energy levels.

	Energy (kCal)		
Exchange	3,100	3,900	4,600
Milk	3	5	6
Vegetables	9	11	13
Fruits	9	11	15
Starch/bread	15	19	20
Meat	6	7	10
Fat	9	11	11

These plans supply 55 to 60% of kcalories as carbohydrate and less than 30% as fat. To increase the carbohydrate content to over 60%, substitute ⅓-c servings of legumes for the meats.

The original breakfast *plus:*
  2 pieces whole-wheat toast
  4 tsp jelly
  ½ c orange juice
  2 tsp brown sugar on the oatmeal

■ **FIGURE 13–7**
Meal Choices of an Athlete
Figure 2–7 in Chapter 2 introduced a set of meals (see p. 36). This figure presents them again with the addition of the foods listed and the substitution of 2% low-fat milk for nonfat milk. These changes help to meet an athlete's greater need for energy and appropriate amounts of protein and carbohydrate.

> **Total kcal: 3,119**
>   61% kcal from carbohydrate
>   24% kcal from fat
>   15% kcal from protein

The original morning snack

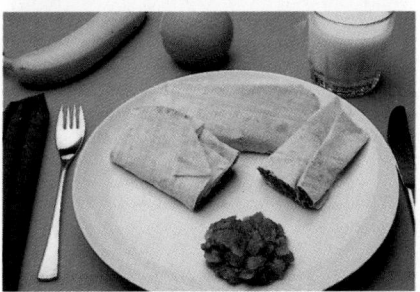

The original lunch *plus:*
  1 bean burrito
  1 banana

Plus an afternoon snack:
  1 c 2% low-fat milk
  1 piece angel food cake

The original dinner *plus:*
  1 dinner roll
  2 tsp butter
  ¼ c noodles
  ½ c sherbet

Caffeine and Alcohol

Athletes, like others, sometimes drink beverages that contain caffeine or alcohol. Both substances are diuretics, and both promote the excretion of water; of vitamins such as thiamin, riboflavin, and folate; and of minerals such as calcium, magnesium, and potassium—exactly the wrong effect for fluid balance and nutrition. It is hard to overstate alcohol's detrimental effects on physical activity. In addition, drinking alcohol is equivalent to taking a diuretic (water pill) as far as its effects on the body's fluid balance are concerned, and both practices make heat stroke much more likely.

Caffeine is a stimulant, and athletes sometimes use it to enhance performance. Highlight 13 includes a discussion of how athletes use caffeine to mobilize fat from stores and reduce early glycogen use.

Unlike caffeine, alcohol has no redeeming benefits in exercise metabolism, and in fact impairs athletic performance. Alcohol not only causes excess excretion of fluid, vitamins, and minerals, as mentioned earlier, but also alters perceptions, slows reaction time, and deprives people of their judgment, compromising their safety in sports. Many sports-related fatalities and injuries each year involve alcohol or other drugs. (Read about alcohol's effects on the brain in Highlight 7.)

The Pregame Meal

No single food is known to confer specific physical benefits to athletic performance, although some kinds of foods are preferable to others. The individual athlete may eat particular foods or practice pregame rituals that convey psychological advantages. As long as these foods or rituals remain harmless, they should be respected.

The recommended pregame meal is light, easy to digest, and eaten three to four hours before competition to allow time for the stomach to empty before the event. The meal or snack should contain between 300 and 1,000 kcalories, although the lighter the better.[43] Breads, potatoes, pasta, and fruit juices—carbohydrate-rich foods low in fat, protein, and fiber—are the basis of the pregame meal. Fiber-rich carbohydrate foods such as raw vegetables or whole grains, while usually desirable, are best avoided at the pregame meal. Fiber in the digestive tract attracts water out of the blood and can cause stomach discomfort during performance. Some athletes prefer liquid meals, which are commercially available and easily digested.

The person who wants to excel physically will apply the most accurate possible knowledge, along with dedication to rigorous training. A diet that provides ample fluid and consists of a variety of nutrient-dense foods in quantities to meet energy needs will not only enhance athletic performance, but overall health as well. Training and genetics being equal, you can easily guess who would win a competition—the person who habitually consumes half or less of the needed nutrients, or the one who arrives at the event with a long history of full nutrient stores and well-met metabolic needs.

Some athletes learn of the ways that nutrition can support their physical performance and turn to pills and powders instead of foods. In case you need further convincing that a healthful diet surpasses such potions, the following highlight addresses this issue.

Study Questions

1. List the diseases associated with a sedentary lifestyle.
2. Define fitness, and list and define the four components of fitness.
3. Define aerobic and anaerobic exercise, and list corresponding exercises.
4. Describe the body's use of fuel during moderate exercise.
5. List the roles of vitamins and minerals in exercise.
6. Define runner's anemia and sports anemia.
7. Discuss the importance of hydration during training, and list recommendations to maintain proper hydration.
8. Describe a healthy diet for athletic performance.

Notes

1. Much of the discussion about fitness is derived from F. S. Sizer and E. N. Whitney, *Life Choices: Health Concepts and Strategies* (St. Paul, Minn.: West, 1988), chap. 7.
2. The ideas presented here were inspired by F. S. Sizer and L. K. DeBruyne, *Nutrition for Sport*, a monograph (1988) available from J. B. Lipponcott, Route 3, Box 20B, Hagerstown, IN 21740.
3. J. P. Flatt, Dietary fat, carbohydrate balance, weight maintenance: Effects of exercise, *American Journal of Clinical Nutrition* 45 (1987): 296–306.
4. E. H. Christensen and O. Hansen, Arbeitsfahigkeit und ehrnahrung, *Skandinavisches Archiv fuer Physiologie* 8 (1939): 160–175, as cited by E. L. Fox, *Sports Physiology*, 2nd ed. (New York: Saunders, 1984): 40–57.
5. E. Jequier, Carbohydrates: Energetics and performance, *Nutrition Reviews* 44 (1986): 55–59.
6. R. C. Hickson, Carbohydrate metabolism in exercise, in *Report of the Ross Symposium on Nutrient Utilization during Exercise*, ed. E. L. Fox (Columbus, Ohio: Ross Laboratories, 1983), pp. 1–8.
7. J. M. Davis and coauthors, Carbohydrate-electrolyte drinks: Effects on endurance cycling in the heat, *American Journal of Clinical Nutrition* 48 (1988): 1023–1030.
8. R. Bielinski, Y. Schutz, and E. Jequier, Energy metabolism during the postexercise recovery in man, *American Journal of Clinical Nutrition* 42 (1985): 69–82.
9. P. W. R. Lemon, K. E. Yarasheski, and D. Dolny, The importance of protein for athletes, *Sports Medicine* 1 (1984): 474–484.
10. P. Babij and F. W. Booth, Biochemistry of exercise: Advances in molecular biology relevant to adaptation of muscle to exercise, *Sports Medicine* 5 (1988): 137–143.
11. J. F. Hickson and coauthors, Failure of weight training to affect urinary indices of protein metabolism in men, *Medicine and Science in Sports and Exercise* 18 (1986): 563–567.
12. J. R. Brotherhood, Nutrition and sports performance, *Sports Medicine* 1 (1984): 350–389.
13. Lemon, Yarasheski, and Dolny, 1984.
14. Brotherhood, 1984.
15. P. W. R. Lemon, Protein and exercise: Update 1987, *Medicine and Science in Sports and Exercise* 19 (1987): S179–S188.
16. Lemon, 1987.
17. G. J. Kasperek and R. D. Snider, Effect of exercise intensity and starvation on activation of branched-chain keto acid dehydrogenase by exercise, *American Journal of Physiology* 252 (1987): E33–E37, as cited by Lemon, 1987.
18. Position of the American Dietetic Association: Nutrition for physical fitness and athletic performance for adults, *Journal of the American Dietetic Association* 87 (1987): 933–939; Food and Nutrition Board, *Recommended Dietary Allowances*, 10th ed. (Washington, D.C.: National Academy of Sciences, 1989).
19. I. Gontzea, R. Sutzescu, and S. Dumitrache, The influence of adaptation to physical effort on nitrogen balance in man, *Nutrition Reports International* 11 (1975): 231–236.
20. H. Yoshimura and coauthors, Anaemia during hard physical training (sports anaemia) and its causal mechanism with special reference to protein nutrition, *World Review of Nutrition and Dietetics* 35 (1980): 1–86.
21. Use of nutritional supplements by athletes, in *Nutrition and Athletic Performance*, eds. W. Haskell, J. Scala, and J. Whitman (Palo Alto, Calif.: Bull Publishing, 1982): 106–155.
22. Food and Nutrition Board, *Recommended Dietary Allowances*, 10th ed. (Washington, D.C.: National Academy of Sciences, 1989).
23. M. H. Williams, *Nutritional Aspects of Human Physical and Athletic Performance*, 2nd ed. (Springfield, Ill.: Charles C. Thomas, 1985), 147–185.
24. A. Belko and coauthors, Effects of exercise on riboflavin requirements: Biological validation in weight reducing women, *American Journal of Clinical Nutrition* 41 (1985): 270–277.
25. Williams, 1985.
26. Williams, 1985.
27. V. Herbert, N. Colman, and E. Jacob, Folic acid and vitamin B_{12}, in *Modern Nutrition in Health and Disease*, 6th ed., eds. R. S. Goodhart and M. E. Shils (Philadelphia: Lea and Febiger, 1980): 229–259.
28. K. Gohil and coauthors, Effect of exercise training on tissue vitamin E and ubiquinone content, *Journal of Applied Physiology* 63 (1987): 1638–1641.
29. M. E. Nelson and coauthors, Diet and bone status in amenorrheic runners, *American Journal of Clinical Nutrition* 43 (1986): 910–916.

30. J. E. Benson and coauthors, Relationship between nutrient intake, body mass index, menstrual function, and ballet injury, *Journal of the American Dietetic Association* 89 (1989): 58–63.

31. B. B. Peterkin, Women's diets: 1977 and 1985, *Journal of Nutrition Education* 18 (1986): 251–257.

32. L. W. Rosen, Pathogenic weight-control behavior in female athletes, *Physician and Sports Medicine* 14 (1986): 79–86.

33. P. K. Welch and coauthors, Nutrition education, body composition, and dietary intake of female college athletes, *The Physician and Sports Medicine* 15 (1987): 63–64, 67–69, 73–74.

34. A. C. Snyder, L. L. Dvorak, and J. B. Roepke, Influence of dietary iron source on measures of iron status among female runners, *Medicine and Science in Sports and Exercise* 21 (1989): 7–10.

35. P. A. Deuster and coauthors, Nutritional survey of highly trained women runners, *American Journal of Clinical Nutrition* 44 (1986): 954–962.

36. R. H. Dressendorfer, C. E. Wade, and E. A. Amsterdam, Development of pseudoanemia in marathon runners during a 20-day road race, *Journal of the American Medical Association* 246 (1981): 1215–1218.

37. W. W. Campbell and R. A. Anderson, Effects of aerobic exercise and training on the trace minerals chromium, zinc, and copper, *Sports Medicine* 4 (1987): 9–18.

38. Williams, 1985, p. 213.

39. M. H. Williams, Vitamin supplementation and physical performance, in *Report of the Ross Symposium on Nutrient Utilization during Exercise*, ed. E. L. Fox (Columbus, Ohio: Ross Laboratories, 1983), pp. 26–30.

40. J. E. Greenleaf and coauthors, Drinking and water balance during exercise and heat acclimation, *Journal of Applied Physiology: Respiratory, Environmental and Exercise Physiology* 54 (1983): 414–419.

41. G. Stendig-Lindberg, Changes in serum magnesium concentration after strenuous exercise, *Journal of the American College of Nutrition* 6 (1987): 35–40.

42. J. M. Davis and coauthors, Carbohydrate-electrolyte drinks: Effects on endurance cycling in the heat, *American Journal of Clinical Nutrition* 48 (1988): 1023–1030.

43. Position of the American Dietetic Association, 1987.

Athletic Hocus-Pocus—Supplements and Ergogenic Aids Athletes Use

Many people advise athletes to eat a variety of concoctions to enhance endurance and strengthen muscles. Some say to take protein supplements, carbohydrate drinks, and muscle-building powders, while others recommend electrolyte pills, vitamin pills, and "ergogenic" foods. This highlight looks at some of the magical potions that promise to improve physical performance.

Many supplements that claim to benefit athletes boast of being *ergogenic*, implying that they generate energy. Except for providing kcalories, as any food does, supplements offer no energy-boosting magic. At best, they may provide a psychological boost; at worst, they may bring on a host of side effects and actually impair performance. When you hear a claim that a product is ergogenic, remember to consider the source of the claim and to ask who may gain from the sale.

Athletes generally make easy targets for quacks because they have invested much time and effort in training, and they are open to regimens that might improve their performances. If a salesperson or advertisement can convince athletes that a product might provide their competitors a winning edge in their field, they may fear that by not using it, they would deny themselves equal advantage. Of course, simply purchasing and swallowing a product cannot provide competitors a winning edge, but the *fear* that it could is powerful. Casual exercisers are also susceptible to unfounded product claims; they, too, are lured by promises of better performance through pills.

Nutrient Supplements

A variety of supplements base their claims on misunderstood nutrition

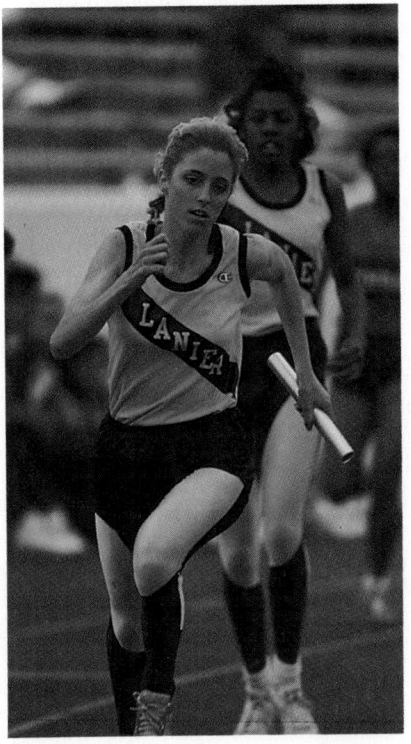

Training serves an athlete better than any pills or powders.

principles. The claims tend to sound good, but the rationale for their use has no factual basis. Among the pills and powders hawked to athletes are amino acid supplements. As Chapter 6 pointed out, amino acid supplements have no value, and they may even be dangerous.

Drinks that manufacturers claim provide "complete" nutrition offer mixtures of carbohydrate, protein (usually amino acids), and certain vitamins and minerals. They usually taste good and provide additional food energy for those who need it. In providing "complete" nutrition, they fall short. As for boosting performance or building muscle, they

are useless when taken in addition to a balanced diet.

Such a nutritionally "complete" drink could be of use in one case, however: that of the nervous athlete who cannot tolerate solid food the day of an event. A liquid meal three or four hours before competition can supply the needed fluid and carbohydrate to replace the pregame meal. Just as effective, a milk shake of nonfat milk and ice milk blended with flavorings could do the same thing, and less expensively than the commercial drink.

Some athletes take vitamin and mineral supplements in the last hours before competition with the expectation that the pills will benefit performance. Chapter 13 explained that taking niacin before exercise could actually have negative results by suppressing fatty acid release. Other vitamins and minerals simply have no effect, because they have not been assembled into their working molecules. The body's enzymes can ensure successful performance only when they are fully supplied daily with all the vitamins and minerals they require, including the ones not present in supplements, but only in unprocessed foods.

Most nutrition experts and exercise physiologists agree that supplements do not help the performance of a well-nourished person. If a diet lacks nutrients, it should be modified to provide the needed nutrients. In the case of a clinical nutrient deficiency identified by a health professional, the appropriate nutrient supplements may be prescribed—in addition to dietary modification.

An ordinary multivitamin and mineral supplement might be prudent when an athlete's need for energy outstrips the ability to eat the quantity

Miniglossary

This miniglossary lists and describes some of the products used by athletes in the hope of improving performance.

bee pollen: a product consisting of bee saliva, plant nectar, and pollen that confers no benefit to athletes and may cause an allergic reaction in individuals sensitive to it.

brewer's yeast: a preparation of yeast cells, containing a concentrated amount of B vitamins and some minerals; often mistakenly used by athletes as an energy supplement.

caffeine: a natural stimulant found in many plants, including coffee, tea, and the cocoa bean (from which chocolate is made).

DNA (deoxyribonucleic acid): a necessary chemical in protein synthesis, falsely promoted as an ergogenic aid.

ergogenic aids: the term *ergogenic* implies "energy giving," but in fact, no products impart such a quality.

ergo = work
genic = gives rise to

gelatin: a soluble form of the protein collagen, used to thicken foods, and sometimes falsely promoted as an ergogenic aid.

ginseng: a plant whose extract has been inappropriately promoted as an ergogenic aid; side effects of chronic use include nervousness, confusion, and depression.

glycine: a nonessential amino acid, promoted as an ergogenic aid because it is a precursor of the high-energy compound phosphocreatine.

growth hormone releasers: a product supposedly composed of hormone-regulating factors falsely promoted for enhancing athletic performance.

octacosanol: an alcohol isolate extracted from wheat germ, often falsely promoted to enhance athletic performance.

phosphate pills: a product demonstrated to increase the levels in red blood cells of a metabolically important phosphate compound (diphosphoglycerate) and the potential of the cells to deliver oxygen to the body's muscle cells, but that does not improve the ability to perform endurance exercise nor increase the efficiency of aerobic metabolism.

RNA (ribonucleic acid): a necessary chemical in protein synthesis, falsely promoted to enhance athletic performance.

royal jelly: the substance produced by worker bees and fed to the queen bee; there is no evidence of its enhancing athletic performance.

spirulina: a microscopic blue-green alga inappropriately used by athletes; potentially toxic.

superoxide dismutase (SOD): an enzyme that protects cells from oxidative damage. When taken orally, the body digests and inactivates this protein enzyme; it is useless to athletes.

wheat germ oil: the oil from the wheat kernel, often falsely promoted as an ergogenic aid.

they supply, though, requires processing by vitamin- and mineral-containing enzymes. Consequently, the need for these nutrients is greater in proportion to that energy. Thus, for a short time during the heaviest training, a supplement might be appropriate. Choose one on the basis of the information in Highlight 9, and do not be led astray by the words *athlete* or *fitness* on a label.

One other instance justifies supplementation: the need for iron. Long-distance runners (especially women) may lose iron through red blood cell destruction, reduced absorption, and increased excretion so that their reserves become dangerously low and their performance in sports impaired. In these cases, treatment with iron reverses the condition, but the dosage should be individualized and prescribed by a physician.

Caffeine

Athletes can improve their endurance and make their work seem easier with moderate caffeine consumption (2 milligrams per pound of body weight or 2 to 3 cups of coffee) one hour prior to exercise.[1] Caffeine is a stimulant that elicits a number of physiological and psychological effects in the body. One of its effects is to stimulate the release of fatty acids. As a result, caffeine facilitates the utilization of the body's free fatty acids as an energy source during exercise, thus helping to spare the use of muscle glycogen for the later stages of prolonged aerobic endurance events. (In Chapter 15, Table 15−3 provides a list of common caffeine-containing beverages, foods, and medicines and the doses they deliver.) Of course, athletes and exercisers can make their work seem easier without consuming caffeine, by warming up with light activity. Activity warms the muscles and connective tissues, making them more flexible and less easily injured; caffeine does not.

of food required to supply it. In this case, many athletes must turn to concentrated energy sources, such as

candies and fats. While such foods supply abundant energy, they lack vitamins and minerals. The energy

The possible benefits of caffeine use must be weighed against its adverse effects—stomach upset, nervousness, irritability, headaches, and diarrhea. Caffeine is potentially hazardous, particularly to individuals who are sensitive to it or who perform endurance exercises in a hot environment. Caffeine-containing beverages should be used in moderation, and *in addition* to other fluids, not as a substitute for them.[2] College, national, and international athletic competitions forbid the use of caffeine in amounts greater than the equivalent of 5 or 6 cups of coffee consumed within a short period of time.

Anabolic Steroids

Some athletes, both men and women, take anabolic steroids in the attempt to accelerate muscular development. (Men produce larger amounts of certain steroid hormones in their bodies than do women, and this induces them to develop bulkier muscles in response to exercise.) The results of these practices show that anabolic steroids can increase body weight (especially lean body weight) and, in combination with high-intensity weight training, can increase muscular strength in some highly conditioned athletes.[3] However, no extra aerobic capacity can be gained by steroid drug use.[4]

To athletes struggling to excel, the promise of bigger, stronger muscles, beyond those that training alone can produce, has been tempting. Athletes who lack superstar genetic material and who normally would not be able to break into the elite ranks can suddenly compete with true champions with the help of steroids. This leaves other athletes faced with an unfair challenge, and many feel compelled to use the drugs themselves. Especially in professional circles, where monetary rewards for excellence are sky-high, steroid use is common, despite its illegality.

The medical community has voiced its concerns about the safety of athletes' use of anabolic steroids. For one thing, all steroid users experience a sharp change in their blood lipid profile to that associated with a high risk of heart disease.[5] For another, steroids damage the liver, creating cancerous tumors, impairing its function, and causing it to rupture and hemorrhage.[6] In addition, they permanently alter the reproductive system and facial appearance. Testicular shrinkage in men and masculinization of women are inevitable.[7] Psychological changes attributed to steroids include mood swings, aggressive behavior, and changes in libido.[8] Further, athletes who take human growth hormone develop symptoms of the disease acromegaly—huge body size, widened jawline, widened nose, protruding brow and teeth, and an increased likelihood of death before age 50.[9]

Serious athletes must make a hard choice—to use no steroids and face a large field of artificially endowed opponents, or to use the drugs and risk their side effects. Judging from athletes' extensive use of steroids, they must consider the drug risks less severe than the disadvantages in competitive events.

The American Academy of Pediatrics and the American College of Sports Medicine condemn the use of anabolic steroids by athletes. They cite the known toxic side effects, state the belief that taking these drugs is a form of cheating, and say that competitors who use them put other athletes in the difficult position of either conceding an unfair advantage to the abusing competitors or ''taking them and accepting the risk of untoward side effects.''[10] Young athletes should not be placed in the situation of having to make such a choice.

Some manufacturers promote the use of specific herbs as legal substitutes for steroid drugs. They make false claims that these special herbs contain hormones, enhance the body's natural hormonal activity, or both. In some cases, the herb does contain a steroid, but not of the type that functions anabolically. Nor does the body convert any of the herbal compounds to anabolic steroids. In short, none of these products has any proven anabolic steroid activity, nor can any increase muscle strength.[11]

Blood Doping

Nutrition supplements and drugs are not alone in the collection of things athletes use to improve athletic performance. One of the most popular physiological ergogenic aids is blood doping: injecting red blood cells to enhance aerobic capacity.[12] The athlete donates blood a week or two prior to the event and banks it while his body makes more blood to replace it. Then, at the time of competition, he receives it back again, thus bringing his total red blood cell count above normal.

Blood doping has been accepted by some and rejected by others in various studies as a viable way to improve athletic performance. Admissions by world-class athletes—including members of the victorious U.S. bicycling team in the l984 Olympics—that they used blood doping to reduce race times continue to stimulate questions about both sports ethics and whether the procedure actually works. Several studies confirm an aerobic benefit to the athlete as a result of blood doping, but the possible negative health consequences remain to be determined.[13]

The search for a single food, nutrient, drug, or technique that will safely and effectively enhance athletic performance will no doubt continue for as long as people strive to achieve excellence in sports. So far it seems that when athletic performance does improve after use of an ergogenic aid, it can probably be attributed to the placebo effect. The placebo effect is strongly at work in athletes, so even if a reliable source reports a performance boost from a newly tried product, give it time to fade away. Chances are excellent that the effect simply reflects the power of the mind over the body.

The overwhelming majority of potions sold for athletes are frauds. Wishful thinking will not substitute for talent, hard training, adequate diet, and mental preparedness in competition. But don't discount the power of mind over body for a minute—it is formidable, and sports psychologists dedicate their work to harnessing it. You can use it by imagining yourself as a winner and visualizing yourself as excelling in your sport. You don't have to buy magic to obtain a winning edge; you already possess it—your mind.

NOTES

1. D. L. Costill, G. P. Dalsky, and W. J. Fink, Effects of caffeine ingestion on metabolism and exercise performance, *Medicine and Science in Sports* 10 (1978): 155–158.
2. F. T. O'Neil, M. T. Hynak-Hankinson, and J. Gorman, Research and application of current topics in sports nutrition, *Journal of the American Dietetic Association* 86 (1986): 1007–1015.
3. P. G. Dyment and B. Goldberg, Anabolic steroids and the adolescent athletes, *Pediatrics* 83 (1989): 127–128.
4. H. Haupt and G. D. Rovere, Anabolic steroids: A review of the literature, *American Journal of Sports Medicine* 12 (1984): 469–484.
5. M. Alen and P. Rahkila, Reduced high-density lipoprotein-cholesterol in power athletes: Use of male sex hormone derivatives, an atherogenic factor, *International Journal of Sports Medicine* 5 (1984): 341–342; O. L. Webb, P. M. Laskarzewski, and C. J. Glueck, Severe depression of high-density lipoprotein cholesterol levels in weight lifters and body builders by self-administered exogenous testosterone and anabolic-androgenic steroids, *Metabolism* 33 (1984): 971–975.
6. Haupt and Rovere, 1984.
7. Haupt and Rovere, 1984.
8. Dyment and Goldberg, 1989.
9. D. R. Lamb, Anabolic steroids in athletics: How well do they work and how dangerous are they? *American Journal of Sports Medicine* 12 (1984): 31–38.
10. Dyment and Goldberg, 1989.
11. V. E. Tyler, "Bodybuilding" herbs, *Nutrition Forum*, March 1988, p. 23.
12. M. H. Williams, Introduction, in *Nutritional Aspects of Human Physical and Athletic Performance* (Springfield, Ill.: Charles C. Thomas, 1985), pp. 3–19.
13. Controversial blood doping revisited, *Science News* 131 (1987): 344.

14

Life Cycle Nutrition: Pregnancy and Infancy

Contents

All that is needed to form a new human being is a single, fertilized egg cell containing instructions (in DNA) to make proteins. The rest will follow. This is a human embryo, three days old; the single egg cell has divided five times, producing 32 cells.

A person's diet can have a great effect on that person's life, and even on the life of another human being. A woman's nutrition prior to and throughout pregnancy is crucial to her health and to the growth, development, and health of the infant she conceives. Sound nutrition during infancy promotes the rapid growth that characterizes this stage of life. This chapter focuses on the special importance of nutrition during pregnancy and infancy.

■ *Pregnancy: The Impact of Nutrition on the Future*

Pregnancy has such a major impact on an infant's development that it is best if a woman can enter pregnancy prepared. Nutrition preparation involves filling nutrient stores, establishing sound eating habits, and achieving a healthy body weight.

Preparing for Pregnancy

In the early weeks of pregnancy, before many women are even aware that they are pregnant, significant developmental changes occur that depend on a woman's nutrient intake and nutrient stores. A woman who eats a variety of nutrient-dense foods prior to pregnancy establishes eating habits that will optimally nourish the growing fetus and herself. If dietary changes do not correct deficiencies, nutrient supplementation may be warranted.

Appropriate weight for height prior to pregnancy also benefits pregnancy outcome. Women who enter pregnancy 10 percent or more below or 20 percent or more above standard weight for height and age face a greater risk than normal-weight women of impaired pregnancy outcome.[1] Underweight women are therefore advised to try to gain weight before becoming pregnant, and overweight women are wise to lose excess weight, to maximize the chances of having healthy babies, as well to maintain their own good health.

A strong correlation exists between prepregnancy weight and infant birthweight. In turn, infant birthweight is the most potent single indicator of the infant's future health status. A low-birthweight baby, defined as one who weighs less than 5½ pounds (2,500 grams), has a statistically greater chance than a normal-weight baby of contracting diseases and of dying early in life. About 1 in every 15 infants born in the United States is a low-birthweight infant, and about one-fourth of these die within the first month of life.[2]

A major reason why the mother's prepregnancy nutrition is so crucial to a healthy pregnancy is that it determines whether she will be able to grow a healthy placenta during the first month of gestation. The only way nutrients can reach the developing fetus in the uterus is through the placenta (see accompanying miniglossary for definitions of fetal development terms). The placenta is shown in Figure 14–1; it is a sort of cushion in which the mother's and baby's blood vessels intertwine and exchange materials. The fetus receives nutrients and oxygen across the placenta; the mother's blood picks up carbon dioxide and other waste materials to be excreted via her lungs and

low birthweight (LBW): a birthweight of 5½ lb (2,500 g) or less; indicates probable poor health in the newborn and poor nutrition status of the mother during and/or before pregnancy. Some low-birthweight infants are **premature**; they are born early and are the right size for their gestational age. Others have suffered growth failure in the uterus; they may or may not be born early, but they are **small for gestational age (small for date).**

gestation: the period from conception to birth; for human beings, the normal length of gestation is from 38 to 42 weeks.

uterus (YOO-ter-us): the womb, the muscular organ within which the infant develops before birth.

placenta (pla-SEN-tuh): an organ that develops inside the uterus early in pregnancy in which the mother's and fetus's circulatory systems intertwine, and in which exchange of materials between maternal and fetal blood takes place.

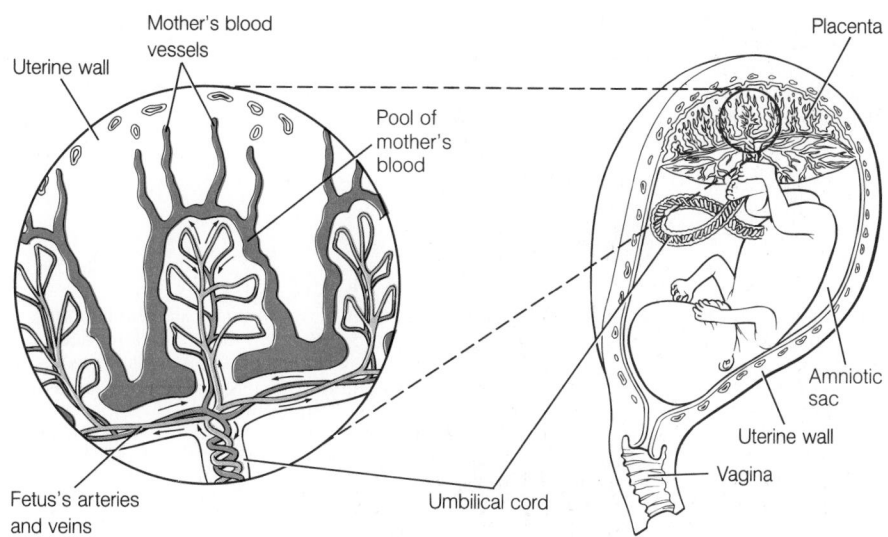

■ **FIGURE 14–1**
The Placenta
The placenta is the tissue in which maternal blood vessels lie side by side with fetal blood vessels entering through the umbilical cord. This close association between the two circulatory systems permits the mother's bloodstream to deliver nutrients and oxygen to the fetus and carry fetal waste products away.

kidneys. The placenta must develop normally if the developing fetus is to attain full genetic potential.

If the mother's nutrient stores are inadequate during placental development, then no matter how well she eats later, the fetus will not receive optimum nourishment. The infant will be a low-birthweight baby, with all of the attendant health consequences. If the infant is a female, she too may be unable to store sufficient nutrients as a young adult, and so she may also be unable to grow an adequate placenta. In her turn, she may bear an infant who is unable to reach full developmental potential. Thus the poor nutrition of a woman during her early pregnancy can theoretically have an impact on the health of her *grandchild*, even after that child has become an *adult*.[3]

Implantation and Embryonic Development

The implantation of a newly fertilized ovum, or zygote, in the uterine wall induces placental growth. This event, too, depends on conditions in the uterus at the time of conception. During the two weeks following fertilization, the zygote divides into many cells, and these cells sort themselves into three

implantation: the stage of development in which the fertilized egg embeds itself in the wall of the uterus and begins to develop, during the first two weeks after conception.

ovum: the egg, produced by the mother, which unites with a sperm from the father to produce a zygote.

Miniglossary of Fetal Development Terms

zygote (ZYE-goat): the product of the union of ovum and sperm during the first two weeks after fertilization.
embryo (EM-bree-oh): the developing infant during its third to eighth week after conception.
fetus (FEET-us): the developing infant from eight weeks after conception until its birth.

1. A newly fertilized ovum is about the size of the period at the end of this sentence. This zygote, less than one week after fertilization, is not much bigger and is ready for implantation.

3. A fetus after 11 weeks of development is just over an inch long; notice the umbilical cord and blood vessels connecting the fetus with the placenta.

2. An embryo 5 weeks after fertilization is about the size of the capital A that began this sentence; after implantation, the placenta develops and begins to provide nourishment to the developing embryo.

4. A newborn infant after nine months of development measures close to 20 inches in length. From eight weeks to term, this infant grew 20 times longer and 50 times heavier.

■ **FIGURE 14–2**
Stages of Embryonic and Fetal Development

Source: Adapted from L. K. DeBruyne and S. R. Rolfes, *Life Cycle Nutrition: Conception through Adolescence*, ed. E. N. Whitney (St. Paul, Minn.: West, 1989), p. 63.

critical period: see p. 367. A critical period is usually a period of cell division in a body organ.

layers. Minimal growth in size takes place at this time, but it is a critical period developmentally. Adverse influences at this time lead to failure to implant or to other disturbances so severe as to cause loss of the zygote, possibly even before the woman knows she is pregnant. A prudent course of action for a potential mother is to avoid all drugs, even familiar over-the-counter drugs. Both mother and child will benefit most from an optimal supply of nutrients uncontaminated by other materials.

The next six weeks, the period of embryonic development, register astonishing physical changes (see Figure 14–2). Beginning at eight weeks, the embryo is called a fetus and has a complete central nervous system, a beating heart, a fully formed digestive system, and the beginnings of facial features.

The growth of each organ and tissue type has its own characteristic pattern and timing. Each organ is most dependent on an adequate supply of nutrients during its own intensive growth period. In the fetus, for example, the heart and brain are well developed at 14 weeks, even though the lungs are still nonfunctional 10 weeks later. Therefore, early malnutrition affects the heart and brain; later malnutrition affects the lungs.

Events during a critical period can occur at only that time, and at no other. Whatever nutrients and other environmental conditions are necessary during this period must be supplied on time if the organ is to reach its full potential. If the development of an organ is limited during a critical period, recovery is impossible. Thus early malnutrition can have irreversible effects, although they may not become fully apparent until maturity. Table 14–1 provides a list of nutrient deficiency effects during pregnancy.

The effect of malnutrition during critical periods is seen in the shorter height of people who were undernourished in their early years and in the poor dental health of children whose mothers were malnourished during pregnancy, to give but two examples. The irreversibility of these effects is

■ TABLE 14–1
Effects of Nutrient Deficiencies during Pregnancy

Nutrient	Deficiency Effect
Energy	Low infant birthweight
Protein	Reduced infant head circumference
Folate	Miscarriage and neural tube defect
Vitamin D	Low infant birthweight
Calcium	Decreased infant bone density
Iron	Low infant birthweight and premature birth
Iodide	Cretinism (varying degrees of mental and physical retardation in the infant)
Zinc	Congenital malformations

Source: Adapted from L. K. DeBruyne and S. R. Rolfes, *Life Cycle Nutrition: Conception through Adolescence*, ed. E. N. Whitney (St. Paul, Minn.: West, 1989), p. 68.

obvious when abundant, nourishing food fed after the critical time fails to remedy the growth deficit.

The last seven months of pregnancy, the fetal period, bring about a tremendous increase in the size of the fetus. Critical periods of cell division and development occur in organ after organ. The amniotic sac fills with fluid to cushion the infant. The mother's uterus and its supporting muscles increase greatly in size, her breasts change and grow in preparation for lactation, and her blood volume increases by half to accommodate the added load of materials it must carry. The gestation period, which lasts approximately 40 weeks, ends with the birth of the infant.

amniotic (am-nee-OTT-ic) **sac**: the "bag of waters" in the uterus, in which the fetus floats.

Nutrient Needs

A woman's nutrient needs during pregnancy and lactation are higher than at any other time in her adult life and are greater for certain nutrients than for others, as Figure 14–3 shows. A study of the figure reveals some of the key needs.

Energy   One of the smallest increases apparent is in energy: a daily increase of 300 kcalories (during the second and third trimesters) above the allowance for nonpregnant women is recommended. Pregnant teenagers, underweight women, or physically active women may require more. In each case, enough energy is needed to spare the protein needed for growth.

Recommended energy intake during pregnancy: 40 kcal/kg (18 kcal/lb). Minimum energy intake: 36 kcal/kg (17 kcal/lb).
For a 120-lb woman, this represents at least 2,000 kcal/day, and preferably 2,200 kcal/day.

Protein   The recommendation for protein allows an additional 10 grams per day throughout pregnancy. The results of food consumption surveys indicate that many women in the United States exceed the recommended protein intake each day.[4] Thus some women may already receive the 10 grams of additional daily protein recommended during pregnancy. Adequate protein consumption during pregnancy is important, but excessive protein may have adverse effects, as Chapter 6 described.

Chapter 15 provides a discussion of the nutrient needs of pregnant teenagers.

Recommended protein intake: 60 g/day.

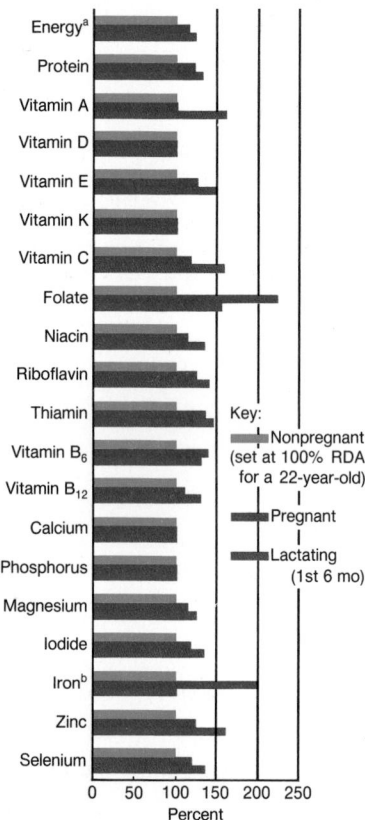

■ FIGURE 14-3
Comparison of Nutrient Needs of Nonpregnant, Pregnant, and Lactating Women

[a]Energy allowance during pregnancy is for 2nd and 3rd trimesters; no additional allowance is provided during the 1st trimester.
[b]The increased needs of pregnancy cannot be met by diet or by existing iron stores. Therefore, pregnant women need to take an iron supplement.

Recommended carbohydrate intake: more than 50% of energy intake. In a 2,000 kcal/day intake, this represents at least 1,000 kcal of carbohydrate, or about 250 g. Four cups of milk a day will contribute about 50 g carbohydrate. An apple provides 15 g carbohydrate, and a slice of bread provides 15 g, so generous intakes of fruit and bread exchanges are clearly beneficial.

The RDA for folate more than doubles during pregnancy, increasing from 180 µg to 400 µg per day.

Some people choose to exclude all foods of animal origin from their diets. For these individuals, the selection of protein-rich foods is limited, and the need for abundant high-quality protein during pregnancy demands careful attention. The inclusion of adequate food energy each day and several servings of plant-protein foods such as legumes, whole grains, nuts, and seeds in generous quantities is imperative.

Carbohydrate   Pregnant women need generous amounts of carbohydrate to spare the protein they eat. If added energy is needed, it is best obtained from carbohydrate.

Vitamins   The nutrients required for blood production and rapid cell proliferation are required in large amounts during pregnancy. The pregnant woman's extraordinary need for folate is due to the great increase in her blood volume and the rapid growth of the fetus. It is possible to obtain the recommended folate amounts from foods, but some diets may be inadequate in this respect. Table 8-11 in Chapter 8 shows that vegetables and legumes lead the list of folate-rich foods. Inadequate folate intake is common during pregnancy, and folate supplements are often prescribed for pregnant women. The determination of folate status by way of a diet history and possibly laboratory tests may be more important than previously thought. Folate supplements taken unnecessarily, especially in combination with iron supplements (as occurs in most prenatal supplements), can compromise the zinc status of women with marginal zinc stores.[5]

Because many vitamin recommendations are based on food energy and protein intakes (which increase during pregnancy), and because tissue synthesis is so rapid, the recommendations for the water-soluble vitamins are slightly higher during pregnancy. The RDA for the fat-soluble vitamins change slightly, or not at all.

Minerals   Among the minerals, those involved in building the skeleton—calcium, phosphorus, and magnesium—are in great demand during pregnancy. Intestinal absorption of calcium doubles early in pregnancy; the mother's bones store the mineral. Later, as the fetal bones begin to calcify, there is a dramatic shift of calcium across the placenta, and the mother's bone stores are drawn upon. Recommendations for calcium and phosphorus are 1,200 milligrams per day. The recommendation for magnesium during pregnancy is slightly higher than for nonpregnant women based on its role in maternal and fetal tissue growth.

The body conserves iron even more than usual during pregnancy: menstruation ceases, and absorption of iron increases up to threefold due to a rise in the blood concentration of the blood's iron-absorbing and iron-carrying protein, transferrin. However, iron stores dwindle during pregnancy and iron losses occur with the blood losses inevitable at the time of birth. The developing fetus draws on maternal iron stores to create stores of its own to last through the first three to six months of life. These drains on the mother's supply may precipitate a deficiency. Fetal deaths, prematurity, and low birthweight occur more frequently when maternal iron status (by tests of hemoglobin or hematocrit) is poor.[6]

Few women enter pregnancy with adequate iron stores, so the RDA committee recommends an iron supplement throughout pregnancy.[7] The physician administering prenatal care determines the exact amount of the iron supplement. Table 11–2 in Chapter 11 shows that meats and legumes top the list of iron-rich foods.

Zinc is another nutrient of vital importance in pregnancy; it is required for DNA and RNA synthesis and thus for protein synthesis. Zinc is most abundant in foods of high protein content, such as shellfish, meat, and nuts, but the presence of other trace elements and fiber in foods may adversely affect zinc absorption. One study of pregnant women found that their dietary zinc intake averaged less than two-thirds of the RDA.[8] Zinc nutrition is the focus of intense study at the present time, and many questions remain to be answered regarding zinc metabolism and availability from foods. In the meantime, however, daily consumption of zinc-rich foods is no doubt beneficial to the pregnant woman and her fetus. Table 11–4 in Chapter 11 shows that meats and legumes are rich in zinc.

Mineralization of the primary teeth begins in the fifth month after conception. For this and for the bones, fluoride may be needed. Fluoride does cross the placenta, but whether the placenta can defend against excess intakes is questionable. Therefore, fluoride supplements are not recommended for pregnant women who drink fluoridated water. However, in one study, children of mothers who took 1 milligram fluoride supplements when pregnant in addition to using fluoridated water have been observed to have teeth that are more decay-free at the ages of five and six than children whose mothers had only used fluoridated water.[9] For women who live in communities without fluoridated water, a fluoride supplement may protect fetal teeth.

Food Choices   Because energy needs increase less than nutrient needs, the pregnant woman must select foods of high nutrient density. For most women, appropriate choices include foods like nonfat milk, cottage cheese, lean meats, legumes, eggs, liver, dark green vegetables, vitamin C–rich fruits, and whole-grain breads and cereals. Table 14–2 provides a suggested food pattern.

Does a pregnant woman have the right to nudge the baby's father out of bed at 2 AM to make her a dish of pickles with chocolate sauce? Perhaps

In pregnancy, hemoglobin values of 12 g/100 ml are not unusual, and 11 g is where the line defining "too low" is often drawn. It is usually desirable to use more sensitive measures than hemoglobin tests if questions about the woman's iron status arise.

■ TABLE 14–2
Four Food Group Plan for Pregnant and Lactating Women[a]

| | Number of Servings | |
Food Group	Adult	Pregnant or Lactating Women
Meat and meat alternates	2	3
Milk and milk products	2	4
Vegetables and fruits	4	4
Breads and cereals	4	4

[a] See Figure 2–4 in Chapter 2 and Appendix G for a more detailed summary of serving sizes and food sources.

Craving of nonfood items such as clay, ice, and cornstarch is known as **pica**.

not—although he may choose to humor her anyway if he is generous. Individual food cravings during pregnancy do not seem to reflect real physiological needs.[10] In other words, a woman who craves pickles does not necessarily need salt, nor does a chocolate craving indicate a need for caffeine or fat. The craving for ice cream is the most common craving in pregnancy, but does not signify a calcium deficiency. Food aversions and cravings may arise during pregnancy, but are probably due to changes in taste and smell sensitivities.

Weight Gain and Exercise

The pregnant woman must gain weight. A pregnancy weight gain of 22 to 28 pounds is recommended for most women (see Table 14–3). Ideally, weight gain follows a pattern of about 2 to 4 pounds during the first three months, and about a pound per week thereafter. Underweight women and teenagers need to gain more. Women who are 10 percent or more above the standard weight for height at the start of pregnancy need to gain between 16 and 24 pounds (depending on prepregnancy weight).[11] Women lose some of the weight gained during pregnancy at delivery, and most of the remainder within a few weeks or months, as blood volume returns to normal and accumulated fluids are lost.

Some researchers have recommended the use of new weight-gain standards for pregnancy, based on larger, more diverse groups of women. They suggest that studies to develop new pregnancy weight-gain charts include adolescents, obese and underweight women, and women who are carrying more than one fetus.[12]

If a woman has gained more than the expected amount of weight early in pregnancy, dieting in the last weeks does not compensate, nor is it recommended. Women have been known to gain up to 60 pounds in pregnancy without ill effects. (A *sudden* large weight gain, however, is a danger signal that may indicate the onset of pregnancy-induced hypertension (see the later section, ''Medical Complications and Other Problems of Pregnancy'').

Weight gain during pregnancy, like prepregnancy weight, directly relates to infant birthweight.[13] If the mother does not gain the full amount of weight recommended, she may give birth to a low-birthweight baby.

Pregnant women can enjoy the benefits of exercise.

■ TABLE 14–3
Ideal Components of Weight Gain during Pregnancy

Development	Weight Gain (lb)
Infant at birth	7½
Placenta	1
Increase in mother's blood volume to supply placenta	4
Increase in size of mother's uterus and muscles to support it	2½
Increase in size of mother's breasts	3
Fluid to surround infant in amniotic sac	2
Mother's fat stores	2 to 8
Total	22 to 28

Another lifestyle component that promotes health and well-being is exercise. The active, physically fit woman experiencing a normal pregnancy can continue to enjoy the benefits of exercise throughout the pregnancy, adjusting the duration and intensity as needed. One study found that women who participated in a balanced, 45-minute exercise session, 3 days per week, had fewer surgical births, shorter hospital stays, and their infants were in stronger physical condition at birth than those who did not.[14] Common sense and consultation with physician are recommended.

Some general rules for exercise during pregnancy:
- Stop exercising if you feel overheated.
- Drink plenty of fluids before you exercise.
- Avoid exercising in hot, humid weather.
- Protect the abdomen from injury, especially in games like baseball or basketball in which accidents are likely.
- Discontinue any exercise that causes discomfort.
- Do not exercise while lying on your back after about the fourth month.
- Do not allow your heart rate to exceed 140 beats per minute.

Potential Hazards of Pregnancy

A general guideline can be offered to the pregnant woman: eat a normal, healthy diet, and practice moderation. Factors associated with malnutrition in pregnancy are listed in the margin. Some truly harmful substances and their potential impact receive attention in the following paragraphs.

One member of this group of substances to limit is caffeine. The equivalent of 1 cup of coffee or tea a day probably falls within safe limits, but caffeine is a potentially harmful drug, and it does cross the placenta.[15] The developing fetus has a limited ability to metabolize caffeine. One study links the daily use of 2 cups or more of coffee (or the equivalent in caffeine) to an increased risk of spontaneous abortion in women.[16] Caffeine consumption during pregnancy should be minimal (less than 150 milligrams per day, the amount contained in 1 cup of coffee or two 12-ounce cola drinks). Table 15-3 in Chapter 15 lists the caffeine contents of beverages, foods, and over-the-counter drugs.

Another clearly harmful practice is smoking. Smoking restricts the blood supply to the growing fetus and so limits the delivery of oxygen and nutrients and the removal of wastes. It stunts growth, thus increasing the risk of retarded development, low birthweight, and complications at birth. Alarming facts about the effects of smoking during pregnancy continue to be revealed. One study has found that the incidence of cancer and leukemia in children of women who smoke while pregnant is twice as high as in nonsmokers.[17] The surgeon general warns that smoking can be a direct cause of fetal or neonatal death in an otherwise normal infant.[18]

Drugs taken during pregnancy can cause serious birth defects. We live in a society in which the use of over-the-counter drugs is routine for many people, and drugs of abuse are a major problem. Research shows that the use of marijuana or cocaine during pregnancy adversely affects fetal growth and development.[19] Without prior physician consultation, the use of any drugs or even vitamin supplements is contraindicated.

Dieting, even for short periods, is hazardous during pregnancy. Low-carbohydrate diets or fasts that cause ketosis deprive the growing brain of needed glucose and may impair its development.[20] Such diets are also likely to be deficient in other nutrients vital to fetal growth. Energy restriction during pregnancy is dangerous for all women, regardless of their prepregnancy weight.

Most important, alcohol consumption during pregnancy can cause irreversible brain damage and mental and physical retardation in the fetus (fetal alcohol

Most severe risk factors for malnutrition in pregnancy:
- Age 15 or under.
- Alcohol abuse.
- Chronic disease requiring special diet.
- Drug addiction.
- Food faddism.
- Heavy smoking.
- History of poor outcome of pregnancy.
- Many pregnancies close together.
- More than 10% underweight.
- More than 20% overweight.
- Poverty.
- Unwanted pregnancy.

These factors at the start of pregnancy indicate that poor nutrition is very likely to be present and to affect the pregnancy adversely.

syndrome is the topic of Highlight 14). Another hazard of alcohol abuse is malnutrition, which, as discussed, is potentially damaging to mother and fetus. The surgeon general warns that pregnant women should avoid alcohol.

Medical Complications and Other Problems of Pregnancy

To alleviate the most common problems encountered during pregnancy, some additional measures are helpful. Pregnancy precipitates the onset of diabetes in some women. This condition is known as gestational diabetes. Without proper management, gestational diabetes can lead to infant sickness and death. Health care professionals screen all pregnant women for diabetes at or before the sixth month.

A certain degree of edema is to be expected in late pregnancy. This is due to the raised secretion of the hormone estrogen, which promotes water retention and helps to ready the uterus for delivery, toward the end of pregnancy. For some women, however, edema may be a part of a larger problem known as pregnancy-induced hypertension (PIH). Preexisting hypertension and PIH are the most common medical complications of pregnancy. They can cause maternal death, infant death, retarded growth, lung problems, and other birth defects. Prenatal care includes keeping track of maternal blood pressure throughout pregnancy, and if PIH is diagnosed, initiating treatment promptly.* Treatment requires medical attention; salt restriction is not a part of treatment until and unless the kidneys prove unable to handle a normal sodium load. A normal salt intake is necessary for health.[21]

The nausea of "morning" (actually, anytime) sickness seems unavoidable, because it arises from the hormonal changes taking place early in pregnancy, but it can often be alleviated. A strategy some expectant mothers have found effective in quelling nausea is to start the day with a few sips of water and a few nibbles of a soda cracker or other bland carbohydrate food, to get something in their stomachs before getting out of bed. Carbonated beverages also may help.

Later, as the hormones of pregnancy alter her muscle tone and the thriving infant crowds her intestinal organs, an expectant mother may complain of constipation. A high-fiber diet and a plentiful water intake will help to relieve this condition. Daily exercise, if the physician approves, may also be beneficial. The woman should use laxatives only if the physician prescribes them, and the physician should determine the type to take.

Pregnancy is a time of adjustment to major changes. The woman who is expecting a baby senses that her lifestyle will have to change as she takes on the responsibility of caring for a child. Ideally, she will be encouraged to develop this sense of responsibility by caring for herself during pregnancy. The expectant mother needs support in thinking of herself as a worthwhile and important person with a new and challenging task that she can and will perform well.

---

gestational diabetes: the appearance of abnormal glucose tolerance during pregnancy, with subsequent return to normal postpartum.

The normal edema of pregnancy responds to gravity; blood pools in the ankles. The edema of PIH is a generalized edema. The distinction helps with diagnosis.

pregnancy-induced hypertension (PIH), formerly known as **toxemia** (tox-EEM-ee-uh): a cluster of symptoms seen in pregnancy, including edema, hypertension, and kidney complications. A variety of terms are associated with PIH. Most common is **eclampsia**; its symptoms include convulsions and coma, associated with hypertension, edema, and protein in the urine. Eclampsia may be preceded by **preeclampsia**, an abnormal condition of pregnancy characterized by edema, increasing hypertension, and protein in the urine.

---

*Blood pressure of 140/90 mm mercury during the second half of pregnancy in a woman who has not previously exhibited hypertension indicates PIH. So does a rise in systolic blood pressure of 30 mm or in diastolic blood pressure of 15 mm on at least two occasions more than six hours apart. R. J. Worley, Pathophysiology of pregnancy-induced hypertension, *Clinical Obstetrics and Gynecology* 27 (1984): 821–835.

■ *Breastfeeding: The Mother's Nutrient Needs*

Adequate nutrition of the mother makes a highly significant contribution to successful lactation; without it, lactation is likely to falter or fail. An inadequate diet does not support the stamina, patience, and self-confidence that nursing an infant demands. By continuing to eat high-quality foods, not restricting weight gain unduly, and enjoying ample food and fluid at frequent intervals throughout lactation, the mother who chooses to breastfeed her infant will be nutritionally prepared to do so.

A nursing mother produces approximately 23 ounces of milk a day, with wide variations possible. At 23 kcalories per ounce, this milk output amounts to about 530 kcalories per day. In addition, her body requires extra energy to produce this milk. The energy allowance for a lactating woman is a generous 640 kcalories a day above her ordinary need during the first six months of lactation. The Committee on Dietary Allowances suggests that 500 kcalories come from added food, and the rest from the body stores of fat accumulated during pregnancy for that purpose.[22] Severe energy restriction hinders milk production.

The period of lactation is the natural time for a woman to lose that extra body fat, which was accumulated to support lactation. If she chooses nutrient-dense foods, she will gradually lose weight, even though her energy intake may be greater than normal.[23] Fat can only be mobilized slowly, however, and too large an energy deficit, especially early on, will inhibit lactation.

In addition to providing energy, the foods consumed by the nursing mother should offer abundant nutrients—especially those needed to make milk, such as vitamin A, protein, riboflavin, zinc, and plenty of fluid. Figure 14–3 shows the differences between a lactating woman's nutrient needs and those of a nonpregnant woman, and Table 14–2 shows a food pattern that meets them.

Despite previous misconceptions, increasing maternal fluid intake does not increase breast milk volume.[24] Nevertheless, a lactating woman will want to drink at least 2 quarts of liquids each day to protect herself from dehydration. A convenient way to ensure adequate fluid consumption is to drink a glass of milk, juice, or water each time the baby nurses, as well as at mealtimes.

The question is often raised whether a mother's milk may lack a nutrient if she fails to get enough in her diet. The answer differs from one nutrient to the next, but in general, the effect of nutritional deprivation of the mother is to reduce the *quantity,* not the *quality,* of her milk. For protein, carbohydrate, and most minerals, the milk of a healthy mother has a fairly constant composition. The taking of a vitamin-mineral supplement that contains nutrient levels close to 100 percent of the RDA seems not to raise nutrient concentrations in the breast milk of an otherwise well-nourished mother. The concentrations of some of the water-soluble vitamins reach saturation levels in well-nourished women; excesses are excreted. The levels of fat-soluble vitamins in human milk can be altered by excessive or deficient intakes of the mother. For example, large doses of vitamin A correspondingly raise the concentration of this vitamin in breast milk. Vitamin supplementation of

Nutritious foods support successful lactation.

undernourished women, however, appears to raise the vitamin concentration of their milk, and may be beneficial.[25]

Some substances impair maternal milk production or enter the breast milk and interfere with infant development. Alcohol enters breast milk and large amounts consumed over a short time easily reach the nursing infant. Large amounts of alcohol also reduce milk production. An occasional glass of wine or beer is within safe limits. Excessive caffeine consumption during lactation may cause irritability and wakefulness in the breastfed infant. The use of illegal drugs is incompatible with breastfeeding, and prescription medications should be taken only after physician consultation.

Foods with strong or spicy flavors may alter the taste of breast milk. A sudden change in the taste of the milk may annoy some infants. Infants who are sensitive to particular foods such as cow's milk protein may become uncomfortable when the mother's diet includes these foods. While this may be true of a few infants, it is not basis for all nursing mothers to avoid cow's milk. The nutrients provided by milk products make a significant contribution to both the infant's and the mother's health. A nursing mother can eat whatever nutritious foods she chooses; then, if she suspects a particular food of causing the infant discomfort, she can try eliminating that food from her diet and see if the problem goes away.

■ *Nutrition of the Infant*

For a while, the infant drinks only breast milk or formula, but later it becomes appropriate to introduce other foods. All those involved in caring for an infant need to understand the nutrient needs and proper feeding of infants. Early nutrition affects later development and early feeding sets the stage for eating habits that will influence nutrition status for a lifetime.

Trends change and experts argue about the fine points, but properly nourishing a baby is relatively simple, overall. Common sense in the selection of infant foods and a nurturing, relaxed environment go far to promote an infant's health and well-being.

Nutrient Needs

An infant grows faster during the first year than ever again, as Figure 14–4 shows. The growth of infants and children directly reflects their nutritional well-being and is an important parameter in assessing their nutrition status. The birthweight doubles around four months of age, and it triples by the age of one year. (Consider that if an adult, starting at 150 pounds, were to do this, the person's weight would increase to 450 pounds in a single year.) By the end of the first year, the growth rate slows considerably, so that between the first and second birthdays, the weight gained amounts to less than 10 pounds.

The rapid growth and metabolism of the infant demands an ample supply of *all* the nutrients. However, the energy nutrients and those vitamins and minerals critical to the growth process, such as vitamin A, vitamin D, calcium, and iron, have special importance during infancy.

Infant's metabolism
- Heart rate: 120 to 140 beats per minute.
- Respiration rate: 20 per minute.

Adult's metabolism
- Heart rate: 70 to 80 beats per minute.
- Respiration rate: 12 to 14 per minute.

■ **FIGURE 14–4**
Weight Gain of Human Infants in Their First Five Years of Life
The colored vertical bars show how the yearly increase in weight gain diminishes over the years.

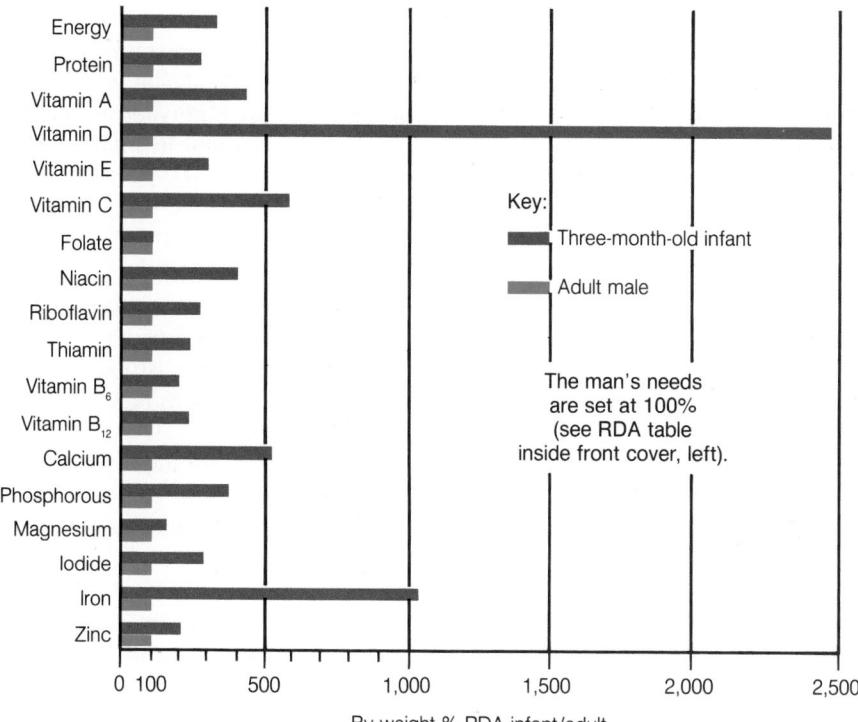

■ **FIGURE 14–5**
Nutrient Needs of a Three-Month-Old Infant and
an Adult Male Compared on the Basis of Body Weight

Infants, because of their small size, need smaller total amounts of the nutrients than adults do; but as a percentage of body weight, infants need over twice as much of most nutrients. Figure 14–5 compares a three-month-old infant's needs per kilogram body weight with those of an adult man; as you can see, some of the differences are extraordinary. After six months, energy needs increase less rapidly as the growth rate begins to slow down, but some of the energy saved by slower growth is spent in increased activity.

Observers note wide variations in actual energy intakes of infants. Current recommendations reduce energy intakes per kilogram body weight at six months of age, but a study of breastfed infants in the United States and Canada found that a spontaneous decline may occur actually earlier than six months.[26]

The most important nutrient of all, for infants as for everyone, is the one easiest to forget: water. The younger the infant, the greater the percentage of body weight is water. Proportionately more of the infant's body water than the adult's is between the cells and in the vascular space, so this water is easy to lose. Conditions that cause fluid loss, such as vomiting, diarrhea, sweating, or obligatory urinary loss without replacement, can rapidly propel an infant into life-threatening dehydration. In early infancy, breast milk or infant formula normally provides enough water for a healthy infant to replace water losses from the skin, lungs, feces, and urine.[27] An infant who is exposed to hot weather, has diarrhea, or vomits repeatedly needs supplemental water to prevent dehydration. Infants cannot tell you what they are crying for; remember that they may need water, and let them drink it until they quench their thirst.

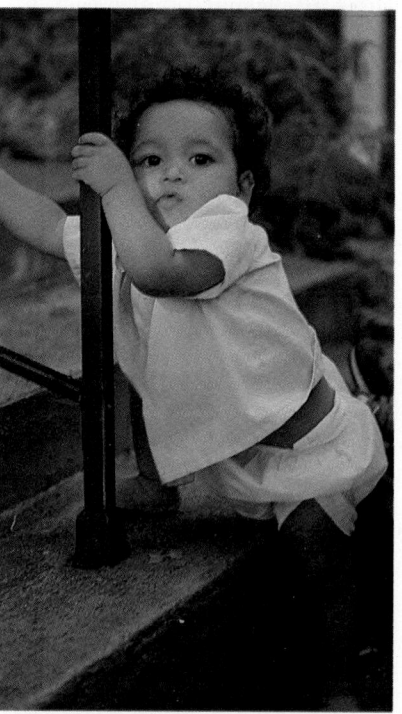

After six months, energy saved by slower growth is spent in increased activity.

Breastfeeding is a natural extension of pregnancy—of the mother's body nourishing the infant.

alpha-lactalbumin (lact-AL-byoo-min): the chief protein in human breast milk, as opposed to **casein** (CAY-seen), the chief protein in cow's milk.

lactoferrin (lak-toe-FERR-in): a factor in breast milk that binds iron and keeps it from supporting the growth of the infant's intestinal bacteria.

In developed, well-nourished countries, such as the United States and Canada, the dietary practices that influence infants' nutrition status the most center upon which type of milk the infant receives and the age at which solid foods are introduced. The remainder of this discussion is devoted to feeding the infant and identifying the nutrients most often deficient in infant diets.

Breast Milk

Breast milk excels as the most desirable source of nutrients for the young infant. The Committee on Nutrition of the American Academy of Pediatrics (AAP) and the Nutrition Committee of the Canadian Pediatric Society have issued this joint statement: "Breastfeeding is strongly recommended for full-term infants, except in the few instances where specific contraindications exist."[28]

With the possible exceptions of vitamin D and fluoride, breast milk provides all the nutrients needed by the healthy infant for the first four to six months of life. But the attributes of breast milk go beyond its nutrient content, as the later section on immunological protection describes.

Energy-Yielding Nutrients   Tailor-made to meet the nutrient needs of the human infant, breast milk offers its carbohydrate as lactose and its fat as a mixture with a generous proportion of the essential fatty acids. The unique composition of the fat in breast milk, in combination with the fat-digesting enzymes present, contributes to highly efficient fat absorption by the breast-fed infant.

The protein in breast milk is largely alpha-lactalbumin, a protein the human infant can easily digest. Another protein component of breast milk, lactoferrin, indirectly benefits the baby's iron nutrition and at the same time, acts as an antibacterial agent. Lactoferrin is an iron-grabbing compound that keeps bacteria from getting the iron they need to grow on, helps absorb iron into the infant's bloodstream, and also works directly to kill some bacteria.[29]

Vitamins   The vitamin content of breast milk is ample. Even vitamin C, for which cow's milk is a poor source, is supplied generously by breast milk from a well-nourished mother. The concentration of vitamin D in breast milk, however, is low.[30] Vitamin D deficiency causes impaired bone mineralization in children. Manufacturers fortify cow's milk and infant formulas with vitamin D, but the concentration in breast milk falls short of adequacy. The vitamin is formed by the action of sunlight on the skin; the amount formed depends on skin color, exposure time, atmospheric pollution, time of year (summer versus winter), and latitude (how far from the sun). Lack of daily sunlight exposure; prolonged, unsupplemented breastfeeding; and pigmented skin are risk factors for vitamin D deficiency in infants. For this reason, vitamin D supplements are routinely prescribed for breastfed infants in the United States and Canada.

Minerals   As for minerals, calcium, phosphorus, and magnesium are present in amounts appropriate for the rate of growth expected in a human infant. Breast milk is low in sodium. The iron in breast milk is highly absorbable, and its zinc, too, is absorbed better than from cow's milk, thanks

■ TABLE 14–4
Supplements for Full-Term Infants

	Vitamin D[a]	Iron[b]	Fluoride[c]
Breastfed infants:			
Birth to six months of age	√		√
Six months to one year	√	√	√
Formula-fed infants:			
Birth to six months of age			√
Six months to one year		√	√

[a]Vitamin D supplements are recommended for breastfed infants for as long as breast milk is the major milk the infant consumes. Once infant formula or vitamin D–fortified cow's milk replaces breast milk in the infant's diet, vitamin D supplements are no longer needed.

[b]Iron-fortified infant cereal is a reliable source of iron for both breastfed and formula-fed infants during the second half of the first year. The Committee on Nutrition of the American Academy of Pediatrics recommends the use of iron-fortified infant formula by four months of age for formula-fed infants. Most pediatricians recommend the use of iron-fortified formula from birth for formula-fed infants, although some infants are fed noniron-fortified formula for the first few months.

[c]The use of fluoride supplements for infants less than six months of age is controversial. The Committee on Nutrition of the American Academy of Pediatrics recommends initiating fluoride supplements for breastfed infants, formula-fed infants who receive ready-to-use formulas (these are prepared with water low in fluoride), or those who receive formula mixed with water that contains little or no fluoride (less than 0.3 ppm) shortly after birth. The committee acknowledges that fluoride supplementation could be initiated at six months of age, however.

Source: Adapted from Committee on Nutrition, American Academy of Pediatrics, Vitamin and mineral supplement needs of normal children in the United States, in *Pediatric Nutrition Handbook*, 2nd ed., eds. G. B. Forbes and C. W. Woodruff (Elk Grove Village, Ill.: American Academy of Pediatrics, 1985), pp. 37–48.

to the presence of a zinc-binding protein.[31] Normally, given the nutrient composition of breast milk, infants do not require nutrient supplements, with the possible exceptions of vitamin D and fluoride. After age four to six months, depending on food intake, infants may also require iron supplements, as Table 14–4 shows.

Immunological Protection Breast milk offers the infant unsurpassed protection against infection. This barrier of protection includes antiviral agents such as immunoglobulins, antibacterial agents such as lactoferrin, and other infection inhibitors.

During the first two or three days of lactation, the breasts produce colostrum, a premilk substance containing antibodies and white cells from the mother's blood. Colostrum is sterile as it leaves the breast, and the baby cannot contract a bacterial infection from it even if the mother has one. Because it contains maternal immune factors, colostrum helps protect the newborn infant from those infections against which the mother has developed immunity. These diseases are the ones in her environment, and precisely those against which the infant needs protection. Entering the infant's body with the milk, maternal antibodies inactivate harmful bacteria within the digestive tract, where they would otherwise cause harm. Later, breast milk also delivers antibodies, although not as many as colostrum.

Other powerful agents against bacterial infection also are found in colostrum and breast milk. Certain factors known as bifidus factors favor the growth of the "friendly" bacteria *Lactobacillus bifidus* in the infant's digestive tract, so that other, harmful bacteria cannot grow there. Another factor present in colostrum and breast milk stimulates the development of the

colostrum (co-LAHS-trum): a milklike secretion from the breast, rich in protective factors, present during the first day or so after delivery, before milk appears.

bifidus (BIFF-id-us, by-FEED-us) **factors**: factors in colostrum and breast milk that favor the growth, in the infant's intestinal tract, of the "friendly" bacteria *Lactobacillus* (lack-toh-ba-SILL-us) *bifidus*, so that other, less desirable intestinal inhabitants will not flourish.

infant's digestive tract.[32] Worn cells in the infant's digestive tract are promptly replaced, and the protective factors within the tract remain intact.

Other factors in breast milk include several enzymes, several hormones (including thyroid hormone and prostaglandins), and lipids, all of which protect the infant against infection.[33] Prolonged breastfeeding (six months or more) has been shown to reduce the incidence of allergic disease in babies with a family history of allergies.[34] Much remains to be learned about the composition and characteristics of human milk, but clearly it is a very special substance.

Contraindications to Breastfeeding   If a woman has an ordinary cold, she can go on nursing without worry. If susceptible, the infant will catch it from her anyway, and thanks to immunological protection, a breastfed baby may be less susceptible than a formula-fed baby would be. If a woman has a communicable disease such as tuberculosis or hepatitis that could threaten the infant's health, then mother and baby have to be separated. Breastfeeding would be possible only by pumping the mother's breasts several times a day.

Similarly, if a nursing mother must take medication that is secreted in breast milk and that is known to affect the infant, then breastfeeding is contraindicated. Drug addicts, including alcohol abusers, are capable of taking such high doses that their infants can become intoxicated and addicted by way of breast milk; in these cases, too, breastfeeding is contraindicated. Many prescription drugs do not reach nursing infants in sufficient quantities to affect them adversely. Some, however, do. As a precaution, a nursing mother should consult with the prescribing physician prior to ingesting any drugs.

A lactating woman is wise to avoid oral contraceptives until after she has weaned her infant, and to use another method of contraception in the meantime. Standard oral contraceptives contain estrogen, which reduces milk volume and the protein content of breast milk.[35]

A woman sometimes hesitates to breastfeed because she has heard that environmental contaminants may enter breast milk and harm her infant. The decision whether to breastfeed on this basis might best be made after consultation with a physician or dietitian familiar with the local circumstances.

For more about contaminants and nutrition, turn to Chapter 16.

Infant Formula

The substitution of formula feeding for breastfeeding involves copying nature as closely as possible. Human and cow's milk differ; cow's milk contains significantly higher concentrations of protein, calcium, and phosphorus, for example, to support the calf's fast growth rate. But a formula can be prepared from cow's milk that closely approximates human milk; the manufacturers dilute the milk and then add carbohydrate and nutrients to make it nutritionally comparable to human milk.

Like the breastfeeding mother, the mother who feeds infant formula deserves support in her choice. Bearing and nurturing an infant involves much more than merely providing nutrients. The mother who offers formula to her infant may have valid reasons for making her choice, and her feelings should be honored. She and the infant can benefit in many ways from the supportive approval of those around them.

Formula preparation:
- Liquid concentrate (inexpensive, relatively easy)—mix with equal part water.
- Powdered formula (cheapest, lightest for travel)—read label directions.
- Ready-to-feed (easiest, most expensive)—pour directly into clean bottles.
- Whole milk—do not use before six months.

Formula feeding offers a major advantage to the mother whose attempts at breastfeeding have met with frustration. If a woman truly doesn't want to breastfeed, or worse, if she earnestly does want to and can't, continuing to try is an agonizing course, as hard on the infant as on the mother. When the mother finally accepts the necessity of formula feeding and weans the infant to the bottle, a period of anguish for both may be followed by the onset of peace and the first real opportunity to develop the all-important mother-child love. Formula feeding also allows other family members to enjoy feeding the infant.

Health care professionals who advise on breastfeeding versus formula feeding must remember the advantages of both methods. In fact, when addressing any audience, keep in mind that some members of that audience will be women who feed their babies each way. To praise breastfeeding out of proportion or without qualification can only make some mothers feel guilty or angry.

Many mothers choose to breastfeed at first but wean within the first one to six months. Prior to six months of age, mothers must wean their infants onto *infant formula*, not onto plain milk of any kind—whole, low-fat, or nonfat.

The American Academy of Pediatrics recommends the use of iron-fortified infant formula by four months of age for formula-fed infants. Most pediatricians are more cautious and practical, recommending iron-fortified formula from birth for these infants. Only formula, not plain milk, contains enough iron (to name but one of many, many factors) to support normal development in the infant's first months of life.

Standards National and international standards have been set for the nutrient contents of infant formulas. The Infant Formula Act of 1980 requires that formulas meet nutrient standards based on the American Academy of Pediatrics recommendations, and in 1982 the FDA adopted quality control procedures to ensure that they do. Formulas that meet the standard are nutritionally similar; small differences in nutrient content are sometimes confusing, but not usually important.

Table 14–5 shows the AAP standard for the bulk ingredients of infant formulas and permits comparison with human milk and with typical formulas. As you can see, the AAP standard recommends higher protein than human milk contains; this is because the cow's milk protein offers a less-than-perfect balance of amino acids for the human infant. You can also see that the formulas meet the AAP standard for the nutrients listed.

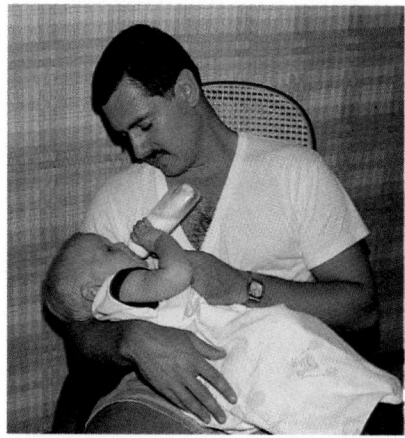

The infant thrives on infant formula offered with affection.

wean: to gradually replace breast milk with infant formula or other foods appropriate to an infant's diet.

■ TABLE 14–5
AAP Standard Compared with Human Milk and Infant Formula

Content	Mature Human Milk	AAP Standard	Infant Formula[a]
Energy (kcal/100 ml)	67 to 75	60 to 80	67
Protein (% of kcal)	5.2	7 to 18	9
Fat (% of kcal)	35 to 58	30 to 55	47 to 50
Carbohydrate (% of kcal)	35 to 44	35 to 50	41 to 43

[a]Five formulas were used to generate these data: Similac (Ross), Similac 60/40 (Ross), Enfamil (Mead Johnson), SMA (Wyeth), and Nan (Nestlé).

Source: Adapted from K. Brostrøm, Human milk and infant formulas: Nutritional and immunological characteristics, in *Textbook of Pediatric Nutrition,* ed. R. M. Suskind (New York: Raven Press, 1981), p. 43.

Special Formulas   Standard formulas are inappropriate for some infants. For example, premature babies require special formulas. Special formulas based on soy protein are available for infants allergic to milk protein, and formulas with the lactose replaced can be used for infants with lactose intolerance. For infants with other special needs, many other variations have been formulated.

In an infant's first six months, the choice of formula is important, because whatever is chosen must supply the nutrients of human milk in similar forms and proportions. After the first year, the exact formulation of the milk selected is less critical, but the choice remains important—milk or its substitute occupies a place in the diet that no other type of food can fill. If an infant requires supplements in addition, the type of formula determines what the supplements should contain (review Table 14–4).

Introducing Cow's Milk   As long as formula is the baby's major food, ordinary milk is an inappropriate replacement—primarily because cow's milk provides insufficient vitamin C and iron. Once the baby is obtaining at least a third of the total daily food energy from a balanced mixture of cereals, vegetables, fruits, and other foods (usually after six months of age), then whole cow's milk in any form, fortified with vitamins A and D, is acceptable as an accompanying beverage.[36] The AAP recommends the introduction of cow's milk at six months, but many pediatricians advise continued use of infant formula throughout the first year because of the iron it provides. (Don't offer plain, unmodified cow's milk before six months; the infant's digestive tract may be sensitive to the protein content, and if so, may bleed.) Infants under a year old should not drink low-fat or nonfat milk routinely; they need the fat of whole milk. Powdered milk is usually skimmed, but fat-containing varieties are available. Parents are advised to use vitamin A– and vitamin D–fortified whole milk.

Introducing First Foods

Changes in body organs during the first year affect the baby's readiness to accept solid foods. The immature stomach and intestines can digest milk sugar (lactose), but they don't develop the ability to digest starch until they are several months old. This is one of the many reasons why breast milk and formula are such good foods for babies; they provide simple, easily digested carbohydrate, supplying energy for the baby's growth and activity.

The infant's kidneys are unable to concentrate waste efficiently, so an infant must excrete relatively more water than an adult to carry off a comparable amount of waste. This means that the risk of dehydration is even greater once solid foods are introduced. Because infants can communicate their needs only by crying, it is important to remember that they may be crying for fluid. All infants require supplemental water once they receive solid foods in the diet. Foods with a high protein or electrolyte content, such as meat and eggs, in the absence of adequate water, can promote water loss to the point of dehydration. Water also provides fluid without additional food energy. Many adults would no doubt be healthier had they learned early to quench their thirst with water.

The timing for adding solid foods (beikost) to an infant's diet depends on several factors. As long as the infant receives formula or breast milk from a healthy, well-nourished mother, additions to the diet are not needed until the infant is four to six months old, but infants who do not receive solid foods before the end of the first year may suffer delayed growth.[37] Foods may be started gradually beginning sometime between four and six months, depending on readiness. Indications of readiness include:

beikost (BYE-cost): supplemental or weaning foods.

- When the infant has doubled the birth weight, or
- When the infant can consume 8 ounces of formula and still is hungry in less than four hours, or
- When the infant can sit up, or
- When the infant is consuming 32 ounces a day and wanting more, or
- At six months.

Solids should not be introduced too early, because infants are most likely to develop allergies to them in the early months. But infants differ, and the program of additions depends on the individual baby's developmental readiness, not on any rigid schedule. Table 14–6 presents a suggested sequence for introducing new foods.

The addition of foods to an infant's diet should be governed by three considerations: the infant's nutrient needs, the infant's physical readiness to handle different forms of foods, and the need to detect and control allergic reactions. With respect to nutrient needs, the nutrient needed earliest is iron, then vitamin C.

Iron deficiency is a common nutrition problem, especially in young children, throughout the world. Iron deficiency is most prevalent in children between the ages of six months and three years due to their rapid growth rate and the significant place that milk, which is a poor source of iron, has in their

■ TABLE 14–6
First Foods for the Infant

Age (months)	Addition
4 to 6	Iron-fortified rice cereal, followed by other cereals (for iron; baby can swallow and can digest starch now)[a]
5 to 7	Strained vegetables and/or fruits and their juices,[b] one by one (perhaps vegetables before fruits, so the baby will learn to like their less sweet flavors)
6 to 8	Protein foods (cheese, yogurt, tofu, cooked beans, meat, fish, chicken, egg yolk)
9	Finely chopped meat (baby can chew now), toast, teething crackers (for emerging teeth)
10 to 12	Whole egg (allergies are less likely now), whole milk

[a]Later you can change cereals, but don't forget to keep on using the iron-fortified varieties. According to *Nutrition and the M.D.*, April 1981, the iron in cereal specially prepared for babies is so bioavailable that three level tablespoons a day is all they need.
[b]All baby juices are fortified with vitamin C. Orange juice causes allergies in some babies; apple juice is often recommended as the first juice to feed. Juices should be offered in a cup, not a bottle, to prevent nursing bottle syndrome.

Source: Adapted from the 1979 *Recommendations for Infant Feeding Practices of the California Department of Health Services*, as presented in Current infant feeding practices, *Nutrition and the M.D.*, January 1980.

diets. An infant's stored iron supply from before birth runs out after the birthweight doubles thus setting the stage for iron deficiency by the end of the first year. Therefore the infant's iron recommendations increase to 10 milligrams per day at 6 months of age. One study showed that infants who were started on whole milk at six months of age had 33 percent lower serum ferritin concentrations than those who continued to drink iron-fortified formula until one year of age.[38] Iron ranks highest on the list of nutrients most needing attention in infant nutrition.[39] Formula with iron, iron-fortified cereals, and later, meat or meat alternates such as legumes, are recommended to deliver iron to infants.

Vitamin C's best vehicles are fruits and vegetables. Some authorities suggest that the early introduction of sweet fruits to infants' diets might favor the development of a preference for sweets and lessen the liking for vegetables introduced later. To prevent this, the order can be reversed: vegetables first, fruits later. This practice now has a wide following. As for sweets of any other kind (including baby food "desserts"), they have no place in a baby's life. The added food energy they contribute can promote obesity, and they convey no nutrients to support growth.

Physical readiness for food handling develops in many small steps. For example, the ability to swallow solid food develops at around four to six months, and experience with the spoon and solid food at that time helps to develop swallowing ability by desensitizing the gag reflex. Later still, a baby can sit up, can handle finger foods, and begins to teethe. At that time, hard crackers and other hard finger foods may be introduced to promote the development of manual dexterity and control of the jaw muscles. These feedings must occur under the watchful eye of an adult, because the infant can also choke on such foods.

Some parents want to feed solids at an earlier age, on the theory that "stuffing the baby" at bedtime promotes sleeping through the night. There is no proof for this theory. On the average, babies start to sleep through the night at about the same age, regardless of when solid foods are introduced, and by three months, 75 percent of infants sleep through the night regardless of whether they are receiving any solid foods.[40]

New foods should be introduced singly and slowly, so that allergies can be detected. For example, when cereals are introduced, rice cereal is offered first for several days; it causes allergy least often. Wheat cereal is offered last; it is the most common offender. If a cereal causes an allergic reaction (irritability due to skin rash, digestive upset, or respiratory discomfort), its use should be discontinued before going on to the next food.

As for the choice of foods, baby foods commercially prepared in the United States and Canada are generally safe, nutritious, and of high quality. In response to consumer demand, baby food companies have removed all of the added salt and much of the sugar their products contained in the past, and baby foods also contain few or no additives. They generally have high nutrient density, except for mixed dinners and heavily sweetened desserts. An alternative for the parent who wants the baby to have family foods is to "blenderize" a small portion of the table food at each meal. This necessitates cooking without salt, though; foods adults prepare for themselves often contain much more salt than commercial baby foods.

Some foods are best omitted from a baby's diet. Canned vegetables are inappropriate for infants; they often contain too much sodium. Honey should

■ **TABLE 14–7**
Meal Plan for a One-Year-Old

Breakfast	**Snack**
1 c milk	½ c milk
3 tbsp cereal	Teething crackers
2 to 3 tbsp fruit	1 tbsp peanut butter
Teething crackers	
Lunch	**Supper**
1 c milk	1 c milk
2 to 3 tbsp vegetables	1 egg
2 tbsp chopped meat or well-cooked, mashed legumes	2 tbsp cereal or potato
	2 to 3 tbsp vegetables
	2 to 3 tbsp fruit

never be fed to infants because of the risk of botulism. Babies and even young children have difficulty swallowing foods such as popcorn, whole grapes, whole beans, hot dog slices, and nuts, and they can easily choke on these foods. It's not worth the risk. Also an infant's caretaker must be on guard against food poisoning and take the precautions against it as described in Chapter 16.

At a year of age, milk remains the obvious food to supply most of the nutrients the infant needs; 2 to 3½ cups a day meets those needs sufficiently. More milk than this displaces foods necessary to provide iron and can cause the iron-deficiency anemia known as milk anemia. Other foods—meat, iron-fortified cereal, enriched or whole-grain bread, fruits, and vegetables— should be supplied in variety and in amounts sufficient to round out total energy needs. Ideally, a one-year-old will sit at the table, eat many of the same foods everyone else eats, and drink liquids from a cup—not a bottle. Table 14–7 shows a meal plan that meets the requirements for the one-year-old.

milk anemia: iron-deficiency anemia caused by drinking so much milk that iron-rich foods are displaced from the diet.

Looking Ahead

The first year of life lays the foundation for future health. From the nutrition standpoint, the relevant problems most common in later years are obesity and dental disease. Prevention of obesity can also help prevent the development of the obesity-related diseases such as atherosclerosis and diabetes.

Infant obesity should be avoided. Probably the most important single measure to undertake during the first year is to encourage eating habits that will support continued normal weight as the child grows. Primarily, this means introducing a variety of nutritious foods in an inviting way; not forcing the baby to finish the bottle or the baby food jar; avoiding concentrated sweets and empty-kcalorie foods; and encouraging physical activity.

To discourage development of the behaviors and attitudes that plague obese people, parents should avoid teaching infants to seek food as a reward, to expect food as comfort for unhappiness, or to associate food deprivation with punishment. If infants cry for thirst, give them water, not milk or juice. Infants seem to have no internal "kcalorie counter," and they stop eating when their stomachs feel full. Nutrient-dense, low-kcalorie foods will satisfy as long as they provide bulk.

A "prudent diet," like that recommended for heart clients (restrict fat, increase the ratio of polyunsaturated to saturated fat, and reduce cholesterol intake), is inappropriate for infants. The AAP recommends against a fat-modified diet during infancy, stating that the evidence so far is insufficient and does not warrant dietary manipulation to lower serum cholesterol.[41]

Normal dental development is promoted by the same strategies outlined above: supplying nutritious foods, avoiding sweets, and discouraging the association of food with reward or comfort. Dental health is the subject of Highlight 10.

Mealtimes

The wise parent of a one-year-old offers nutrition and love together. Both promote growth. "Feeding with love" produces better growth in both weight and height of children than feeding the same food in an emotionally negative climate.[42] It also promotes better brain development. The formation of nerve-to-nerve connections in the brain depends both on nutrients and on environmental stimulation.[43]

The person feeding a one-year-old has to be aware that this is a period in the child's life when exploring and experimenting are normal and desirable behaviors. The child is developing a sense of autonomy that, if allowed to flower, will provide the foundation for later confidence and effectiveness as an individual. The child's impulses, if consistently denied, can turn to shame and self-doubt. In light of the developmental and nutrient needs of one-year-olds, and in the face of their often contrary and willful behavior, a few feeding guidelines may be helpful:

- Firmly discourage unacceptable behavior (such as standing at the table or throwing food) by removing the child from the table to wait until later to eat. Be consistent and firm, not punitive. The child will soon learn to sit and eat.
- Do let the child explore and enjoy food, though, even if this means eating with fingers for a while. Use of the spoon will come in time.
- Don't force food on children. Provide children with nutritious foods, and let them choose which ones and how much they will eat. Gradually they will acquire a taste for different foods. If children refuse milk, provide it in the form of cheese, cream soups, and yogurt.
- Limit sweets strictly. Infants have no room in their 1,000-kcalorie allowance each day for empty-kcalorie sweets, except occasionally.

These recommendations reflect a spirit of tolerance that serves the best interest of the child emotionally as well as physically. The next chapter continues with the special nutrient needs of people throughout life.

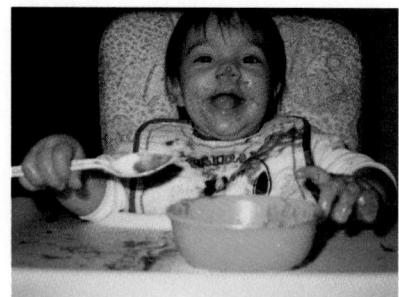

This child's first encounter with black beans and rice was a delightful and delicious, albeit messy, experience.

Study Questions

1. Discuss the special problems and energy needs of pregnancy. Describe the currently recommended pattern and extent of weight gain during pregnancy.
2. What substances should be avoided during pregnancy?
3. What are the advantages of breastfeeding? How does the recommended diet for a lactating woman differ from that of a pregnant woman?
4. What are the advantages of formula feeding? What criteria would you use in selecting an infant formula?
5. Why are solid foods not recommended for an infant during the first few months of life? Name the indicators of readiness for adding solid foods to an infant's diet.

Notes

1. M. C. Mitchell and E. Lerner, Weight gain and pregnancy outcome in underweight and normal weight women, *Journal of the American Dietetic Association* 89 (1989): 634–638, 641; R. M. Pitkin, Assessment of nutritional status of mother, fetus, and newborn, *American Journal of Clinical Nutrition* 34 (1981): 658–668.
2. National Institute of Child Health and Human Development, *Facts about Premature Birth*, publication no. 461–338–814/25324 (Washington, D.C.: Government Printing Office, 1985).
3. E. Hackman and coauthors, Maternal birth weight and subsequent pregnancy outcome, *Journal of the American Medical Association* 250 (1983): 2016–2019.
4. B. H. Dennis and coauthors, Nutrient intakes among selected North American populations in the Lipid Research Clinics prevalence study: Composition of energy intake, *American Journal of Clinical Nutrition* 41 (1985): 312–329.
5. K. Simmer and coauthors, Are iron-folate supplements harmful? *American Journal of Clinical Nutrition* 45 (1987): 122–125.
6. S. M. Garn, M. T. Keating, and F. Falkner, Hematological status and pregnancy outcomes, *American Journal of Clinical Nutrition* 34 (1981): 115–117.
7. Food and Nutrition Board, *Recommended Dietary Allowances*, 10th ed. (Washington, D.C.: National Academy of Sciences, 1989).
8. K. M. Hambidge and coauthors, Zinc nutritional status during pregnancy: A longitudinal study, *American Journal of Clinical Nutrition* 37 (1983): 429–442.
9. F. B. Glenn, W. D. Glenn, and R. C. Duncan, Fluoride tablet supplementation during pregnancy for caries immunity: A study of the offspring produced, *American Journal of Obstetrics and Gynecology* 143 (1982): 560–564.
10. B. Worthington-Roberts and coauthors, Dietary cravings and aversions in the postpartum period, *Journal of the American Dietetic Association* 89 (1989): 647–651.
11. R. L. Naeye, Weight gain and the outcome of pregnancy, *American Journal of Obstetrics and Gynecology* 135 (1979): 3–9; J. E. Brown and coauthors, Prenatal weight gains related to the birth of healthy-sized infants to low-income women, *Journal of the American Dietetic Association* 86 (1986): 1679–1683.
12. A. L. Pederson, B. Worthington-Roberts, and D. E. Hickok, Weight gain patterns during twin gestation, *Journal of the American Dietetic Association* 89 (1989): 642–646; P. Rosso, A new chart to monitor weight gain during pregnancy, *American Journal of Clinical Nutrition* 41 (1985): 644–652.
13. B. Luke, M. A. Jonaitis, and R. H. Petrie, A consideration of height as a function of prepregnancy nutritional background and its potential influence on birth weight, *Journal of the American Dietetic Association* 84 (1984): 176–181.
14. D. Hall and D. Kaufmann, Effects of aerobic and strength conditioning on pregnancy outcomes, *American Journal of Obstetrics and Gynecology* 157 (1987): 1199–1203.
15. National Institute of Nutrition in Canada, Caffeine: A perspective on current concerns, *Nutrition Today*, July–August 1987, pp. 36–38.
16. W. Srisuphon and M. B. Bracken, Caffeine consumption during pregnancy and association with late spontaneous abortion, *American Journal of Obstetrics and Gynecology* 154 (1986): 14–20.
17. M. Stjernfeldt and coauthors, Maternal smoking during pregnancy and risk of childhood cancer, *Lancet* 1 (1986): 1350–1352.
18. Pregnancy and infant health, in *Smoking and Health*, a report of the surgeon general, January 1979, available from Superintendent of Documents, U.S. Government Printing Office, Washington, D.C. 20402.
19. B. Zuckerman and coauthors, Effects of maternal marijuana and cocaine use on fetal growth, *New England Journal of Medicine* 320 (1989): 762–768.
20. National Dairy Council, Nutrition and pregnancy outcome, *Dairy Council Digest*, May–June 1983, pp. 13–18.
21. F. P. Zuspan, Chronic hypertension in pregnancy, *Clinical Obstetrics and Gynecology* 27 (1984): 854–873.
22. Food and Nutrition Board, 1989.
23. M. Brewer, M. R. Bates, and L. P. Vannoy, Postpartum changes in maternal weight and body fat depots in lactating vs nonlactating women, *American Journal of Clinical Nutrition* 49 (1989): 259–265.

24. Maternal nutrition during lactation, *Nutrition and the M.D.*, February 1987.

25. Maternal nutrition, 1987.

26. R. G. Whitehead and coauthors, A critical analysis of measured food energy intakes during infancy and early childhood in comparison with current international recommendations, *Journal of Human Nutrition* 35 (1981): 339–348.

27. Committee on Nutrition, American Academy of Pediatrics, *Pediatric Nutrition Handbook*, 2nd ed., eds. G. B. Forbes and C. W. Woodruff (Elk Grove Village, Ill.: American Academy of Pediatrics, 1985), p. 31.

28. Committee on Nutrition, American Academy of Pediatrics, and Nutrition Committee of the Canadian Pediatric Society, Breast-feeding: A commentary in celebration of the international year of the child, 1979, *Pediatrics* 62 (1978): 591–601.

29. B. Lonnerdal, Biochemistry and physiological function of human milk proteins, *American Journal of Clinical Nutrition* 42 (1985): 1299–1317.

30. Committee on Nutrition, American Academy of Pediatrics, 1985, pp. 37–48.

31. C. Eckhert, Isolation of a protein from human milk that enhances zinc absorption in humans, *Biochemical and Biophysical Research Communications* 130 (1985): 264–269.

32. G. Carpenter, Epidermal growth factor is a major growth-promoting agent in human milk, *Science* 210 (1980): 198–199.

33. K. M. Shahani, A. J. Kwan, and B. A. Friend, Role and significance of enzymes in human milk, *American Journal of Clinical Nutrition* 33 (1980): 1861–1868; Thyroid hormones in human milk, *Nutrition Reviews* 37 (1979): 140–141; Prostaglandins in human milk, *Nutrition Reviews* 39 (1981): 302–303; J. J. Kabara, Lipids as host-resistance factors of human milk, *Nutrition Reviews* 38 (1980): 65–73.

34. C. Briggs, Recent developments in infant feeding and nutrition, in *Nutrition Update*, vol. 1, eds. J. Weininger and G. M. Briggs (New York: Wiley, 1983), pp. 227–261.

35. Committee on Drugs, American Academy of Pediatrics, The transfer of drugs and other chemicals into human breast milk, *Pediatrics* 72 (1983): 375–381; Task Force on Oral Contraceptives of the WHO Special Programme of Research, Effects of hormonal contraceptives on milk volume and infant growth, *Development and Research Training in Human Reproduction*, December 1984, pp. 505–522.

36. Committee on Nutrition, American Academy of Pediatrics, The use of whole cow's milk in infancy, *Pediatrics* 72 (1983): 253–255.

37. M. Winick, Infant nutrition: Formula or breast feeding? *Professional Nutritionist*, Spring 1980, pp. 1–3.

38. Ross Laboratories, Perspectives on nutrition in latter infancy, *Public Health Currents* 28 (1988): 17–20.

39. G. H. Johnson, G. A. Purvis, and R. D. Wallace, What nutrients do our infants really get? *Nutrition Today*, July–August 1981, pp. 4–10, 23–26.

40. L. L. Clark and V. A. Beal, Age at introduction of solid foods to infants in Manitoba, *Journal of the Canadian Dietetic Association* 42 (1981): 72–78.

41. A "prudent diet" for infants? *Nutrition and the M.D.*, May 1983.

42. E. M. Widdowson, Mental contentment and physical growth, *Lancet* 1 (1951): 1316–1318.

43. J. Cravioto, Nutrition, stimulation, mental development and learning, *Nutrition Today*, September–October 1981, pp. 4–8. ·

Fetal Alcohol Syndrome

As Chapter 14 mentioned, drinking excess alcohol during pregnancy endangers the fetus. Alcohol crosses the placenta freely and enters the fetal brain, causing both glucose and oxygen deficits, to which developing nervous tissue is extremely vulnerable. The result may be fetal alcohol syndrome (FAS), a combination of growth retardation, mental retardation, and physical defects. At its most severe, FAS involves:

- Prenatal and postnatal growth retardation.
- Impairment of the brain and nerves, with consequent mental retardation, poor coordination, and hyperactivity.
- Abnormalities of the face and skull (see Figure H14–1).
- Increased frequency of major birth defects (cleft palate and defects in major organ systems—heart, ears, genitals, urinary system).

About 1 in every 750 children born in the United States is a victim of this preventable damage.[1] For every baby born with the symptoms of classic FAS, ten more are born with subtle symptoms. These symptoms have been seen often enough to be given the name subclinical FAS, or fetal alcohol effects. The mothers of these children drank, but not enough to cause visible, obvious effects. The subtle abnormalities associated with subclinical FAS hide under a normal-looking exterior. Without the clue from the classic facial abnormalities to alert them to the condition's presence, parents, as well as physicians, may not suspect the presence of defects. Yet they can be substantial: learning disabilities, behavioral abnormalities, motor impairments, and more.

This highlight asks several questions. How much alcohol causes FAS? When during pregnancy is the damage done? Can a pregnant woman safely drink

any alcohol at all? The precise answers to all of these questions remain elusive. Yet because alcohol consumption during pregnancy has severe consequences, and because this birth defect can only be prevented—it cannot be treated—this highlight offers conservative answers based on the available evidence.

When alcohol crosses the placenta to the fetus, fetal blood-alcohol concentrations rise until they reach an equilibrium with maternal blood-alcohol concentrations.[2] This might not seem to be a problem if the

■ FIGURE H14–1
Fetal Alcohol Syndrome (FAS)
These facial traits are typical of fetal alcohol syndrome, caused by drinking during pregnancy—low nasal bridge, short eyelid opening, underdeveloped groove in center of the upper lip below the nose, thin reddish upper lip, small midface, short nose, and small head circumference. Irreversible abnormalities of the brain and internal organs accompany these surface features.

mother is functioning well (is not drunk), but while blood levels are the same for the mother and fetus, the fetus's body is significantly smaller and its detoxification system is less developed. Blood-alcohol concentrations tend to fall more slowly in the fetus than in the mother, and alcohol can be detected in fetal blood after it has totally disappeared from maternal blood.

How much alcohol is too much? The surgeon general has issued a statement that pregnant women should drink absolutely no alcohol, and the editors of the *Journal of the American Medical Association* have taken the position that women should stop drinking as soon as they *plan* to become pregnant.[3] The responsibility of caring for another life requires that women abstain from alcohol during pregnancy. So far, no "safe" level of alcohol consumption during pregnancy has been established, and there is no evidence of benefits to mother or fetus. Thus, such advice is in the best interest of both mother and fetus.

Not everyone agrees that women need to abstain totally from alcohol use during pregnancy. Some authorities recommend that women be cautious about alcohol use during pregnancy, and advise a daily limit of two 12-ounce beers, two 4-ounce glasses of wine, or two drinks with 1½ ounces of 80-proof liquor.[4] They maintain that the health risks associated with this level of alcohol consumption are fairly insignificant in comparison with most others. The mother's socioeconomic status, age, emotional stability, diet, drug use, smoking habits, genetic makeup, and prenatal care all play at least as great a role as an alcoholic beverage or two.

The difference between a "no-drinks" position and an "occasional-drinks" position is one of

---

Miniglossary

fetal alcohol syndrome (FAS): the cluster of symptoms seen in an infant or child whose mother consumed excess alcohol during pregnancy, including retarded growth, impaired development of the central nervous system, and facial malformations.

subclinical FAS or **fetal alcohol effects**: a subtle version of FAS, with hidden defects including learning disabilities, behavioral abnormalities, and motor impairments.

---

philosophy. No one contests that excessive alcohol consumption is hazardous to the fetus, though. It is therefore important to distinguish between heavy drinking, which almost invariably affects the unborn child, and moderate drinking, which in some cases does not. There is undeniably a risk associated with *any* drinking during pregnancy; the moderate alcohol intake position simply states that at some level, that risk is small enough to be negligible.

Now it remains to define moderate drinking. A pregnant woman need not be an alcoholic in order to give birth to a baby with FAS characteristics. She only needs to drink in excess of the liver's capacity to detoxify alcohol. Reports from mothers of FAS children reveal they consumed an average of five or more drinks daily throughout their pregnancies. Does this mean that four drinks or less per day are safe? Probably not, for researchers cannot be sure they are obtaining accurate measures of alcohol consumption, nor do they agree on the criteria used to define safety. The extent of damage varies with intake.

Most FAS studies speak only of average intake. Little is known about the effects of periodic binge drinking. How does a drinking binge at a critical time compare with the same amount of alcohol consumed over a longer period of time? Most likely it depends on the frequency of binges, the quantity consumed, and the stage of fetal development at the time of each drinking episode.

In conclusion, it is impossible to say whether small amounts of alcohol are safe during pregnancy. The risk associated with occasional drinking is less than that associated with heavy drinking, but why take any risk? The mother who chooses to drink during pregnancy, even moderately, is at greater risk than the mother who abstains completely.

When during the pregnancy is the damage done? There is no time when drinking excessively is safe. The type and extent of abnormality observed in a FAS infant seems to depend on the developmental events that are occurring at the time the fetus is exposed to alcohol.

Different dangers are associated with each trimester of the pregnancy.[5] In the first trimester, developing organs such as the brain, heart, and kidneys may be malformed. During the second trimester, the risk of spontaneous abortion increases. During the third trimester, when the fetus is fully formed and rapidly growing, body and brain growth may be retarded.

In experiments on laboratory animals, the effects of alcohol on fetal development are most marked when the female takes alcohol during the earliest period—that of organ formation. Effects also appear when a dose of alcohol elevates the female's blood-alcohol level immediately prior to conception; the amount of alcohol in the female's blood is critical.

Male alcohol ingestion may also affect fertility and fetal development. Animal studies have found decreased litter size, birthweight, survival, and learning ability in the offspring of males consuming alcohol prior to conception.[6] One human study found an association between paternal alcohol intake one month prior to conception (defined as an average of two or more drinks daily or at least five drinks on one occasion) and low infant birthweight.[7] This relationship was independent of parents' smoking or maternal use of alcohol, caffeine, or other drugs.

In view of these findings, it is important to advise women not to drink, or to be *extremely* conservative if they choose to drink, during pregnancy. Everyone should be aware that the pregnant woman who drinks is more likely to give birth to a baby with FAS defects. The woman who is addicted to alcohol should be advised to avoid pregnancy at all costs.[8] The U.S. Government has taken steps to ensure that everyone gets the message about alcohol consumption causing birth defects. A federal law requires warning labels on all containers of beer, wine, and liquor.

Of the leading causes of mental retardation, FAS is the only one that is totally preventable. Every female, indeed every person, should know the potential dangers of alcohol use during pregnancy. Proper health care education begins *before* conception. The message is clear: FAS can be prevented by maternal avoidance of alcohol.

NOTES

1. K. K. Sulik, M. C. Johnston, and M. A. Webb, Fetal alcohol syndrome: Embryogenesis in a mouse model, *Science* 214 (1981): 936–938.
2. C. F. Enloe, How alcohol affects the developing fetus, *Nutrition Today*, September/October 1980, pp. 12–15.
3. Even moderate drinking may be hazardous to maturing fetus (Medical News), *Journal of the American Medical Association* 237 (1977): 2535.
4. A Report by the American Council on Science and Health, *Alcohol Use during Pregnancy*, 1981.
5. H. L. Rosett and L. Weiner, Alcohol and pregnancy: A clinical perspective, *Annual Review of Medicine* 36 (1985): 73–80.
6. L. F. Soyka and J. M. Joffe, Male mediated drug effects on offspring, *Progress in Clinical and Biological Research* 36 (1980): 49–66.
7. R. E. Little and C. F. Sing, Father's drinking and infant birth weight: Report of an association, *Teratology* 36 (1987): 59–65.
8. *Nutrition Today* (letter), 8 April 1981.

15

Life Cycle Nutrition: Children, Teenagers, and Adults

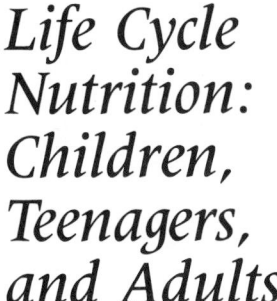

Contents

Early and Middle Childhood

The Teen Years

Adulthood and the Later Years

Highlight: Nutrition and the Aging Brain

Growth requires that cells duplicate all their materials and copy their DNA instructions so each daughter will have a set; and then portion out the two sets to the two daughters. This dividing cell is sorting out its genetic material so that one complete copy will be delivered to each daughter cell. Much energy and many nutrients are needed to support cell division.

Nutrient needs change steadily throughout life, depending on the rate of growth, gender, and many other factors. Nutrient needs also vary from individual to individual, but generalizations are possible and useful. This chapter brackets the adult years, beginning with children's and teenager's needs and ending with the special concerns of older adults.

■ *Early and Middle Childhood*

After the age of one, a child's growth rate slows, but the body continues to change dramatically. At one, infants have just learned to stand and toddle; by two, they can take long strides with solid confidence and are learning to run, jump, and climb. One of the internal changes that makes these new accomplishments possible is the accumulation of a larger mass and greater density of bone and muscle tissue. Thereafter, the same trend—a lengthening of the long bones and an increase in musculature—continues, unevenly and more slowly, until adolescence.

Growth and Nutrient Needs

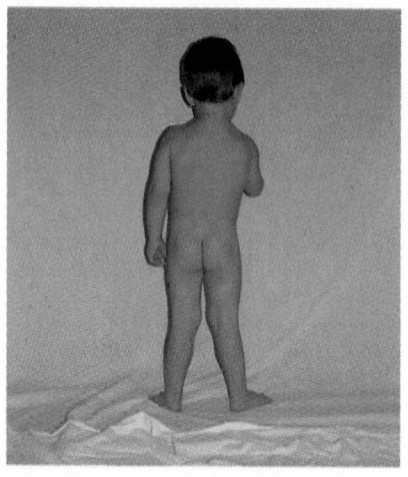

The body shape of a one-year-old (above) changes dramatically by age two (below). The two-year-old has lost much of the baby fat; the muscles (especially in the back, buttocks, and legs) have firmed and strengthened; and the leg bones have lengthened.

An infant's appetite decreases markedly near the first birthday, in line with the great reduction in growth rate. Thereafter, the appetite fluctuates; at times children seem to be insatiable, and at other times they seem to live on air and water. Parents need not worry about this—a child will need and demand more food during periods of rapid growth than during slow periods. The perfection of appetite regulation in children of normal weight guarantees that their food energy intakes will be right for each stage of growth.

People are mistaken in believing that it is necessary to control children's portion sizes; an innovative study has proven otherwise.[1] Children ate puddings that contained either 40 kcalories or 150 kcalories. The children were then given lunch. They compensated for the kcaloric difference: those who had eaten the high-kcalorie pudding ate less lunch than those who had eaten the low-kcalorie pudding. (Overweight children, however, may eat in response to external cues, disregarding appetite-regulation signals.)

A one-year-old child needs perhaps 1,000 kcalories a day; a three-year-old needs only 300 kcalories more. At age ten a child needs about 2,000 kcalories a day. The total energy needs increase slightly with age, but when the child's size is considered, the energy needs are actually declining gradually. Individual children's energy needs vary widely, depending on their physical activity, and an inactive child can become obese even when consuming a diet that is below average in kcalories.

Steady growth during childhood is reflected in gradually increasing needs for all nutrients. The RDA table and the RNI for Canadians list average nutrient intakes recommended for each span of three years. Before adolescence, children accumulate stores of nutrients. Then, when they take off on the adolescent growth spurt, there comes a time during which their nutrient intakes cannot meet the demands of rapid growth, and they draw on the nutrient stores accumulated earlier. This is especially true of calcium; the denser the bones are in childhood, the better prepared they will be to support teen growth and still withstand the inevitable bone losses of later life.

As in infancy, iron-deficiency anemia is the most prevalent nutrient deficiency of condition U.S. children and adolescents.[2] To avert it, children's foods must deliver 10 milligrams iron or more per day. To achieve this goal, milk intakes must be limited after infancy, because milk is a poor iron source; children should receive enough milk products to ensure adequate calcium and riboflavin intakes, but no more. That means 2 to 3 cups of milk per day up to age three, grading on up to 3 to 4 cups per day from ages six to twelve (see Table 15–1). After age two, if low-fat milk is used instead of whole milk, saved kcalories can be invested in such iron-rich foods as lean meats, fish, poultry, eggs, and legumes. Whole-grain or enriched products also contribute iron.

To provide all the needed nutrients, a variety of foods from each of the food groups is recommended. Table 15–1 offers a daily food pattern for children. The portion sizes increase with the child's age. For the person who needs to estimate portion sizes of meat, fruits, and vegetables for children, a portion is loosely defined as 1 tablespoon per year. Thus at four years of age, a serving of meat, fruit, or vegetable would be 4 tablespoons (¼ cup); at eight years it would be ½ cup. Because the portion sizes adjust as the child grows older, this rule of thumb is appropriate from age two to the teen years.

Careful food selection is essential to ensure adequate nutrition. When a child skips breakfast, or when more-sugary foods take the place of some of the nourishing ones, it is virtually assured that the child will fail to get enough of several nutrients. The nutrients missed from a skipped breakfast won't be "made up" at lunch and dinner, but will be completely left out, that day. A child can't be trusted to choose nutritious foods on the basis of taste alone; the preference for sweets is innate.

Experimentation with children's diets shows that children must practically exclude candy, cola, and other concentrated sweets if their diets are to supply

■ TABLE 15–1
Children's Daily Food Patterns for Good Nutrition

Food Group	Servings per Day	Average Size of Serving		
		1 to 3 Years	4 to 6 Years	7 to 12 Years
Milk and milk products[a]	4	½–¾ c	¾ c	¾–1 c
Meat and meat alternates[b]	2 or more	1–2 oz	1–2 oz	2–3 oz
Fruits and vegetables[c]	4 or more	2–4 tbsp or ½ c juice	¼–½ c or ½ c juice	½–¾ c or ½ c juice
Bread and cereals (whole grain or enriched)[d]	4 or more	½ slice	1 slice	1 to 2 slices

[a]½ c milk = ½ c cottage cheese, pudding, yogurt; ¾ oz cheese; 2 tbsp dried milk.
[b]1 oz meat, fish, poultry = 1 egg, 1 frankfurter, 2 tbsp peanut butter, ½ c legumes.
[c]Vitamin C source (citrus fruits, berries, tomatoes, broccoli, cabbage, cantaloupe) daily; Vitamin A source (spinach, carrots, squash, tomato, cantaloupe) 3 to 4 times weekly.
[d]1 slice bread = ¾ c dry cereal, ½ c cooked cereal, ½ c potato, rice or noodles.

Source: Adapted from P. M. Queen and R. R. Henry, Growth and nutrient requirements of children, in *Pediatric Nutrition*, eds. R. J. Grand, Jr. L. Sutphen, and W. H. Dietz, Jr. (Boston: Butterworths, 1987), p. 347.

The energy from ice cream can fuel the play of a well-fed child.

the needed nutrients. Only if a child is of normal weight and active is it appropriate to offer sweets, and even then the treats should be nutritious foods: ice cream or pudding from the milk group, whole-grain or enriched cake and cookies from the bread group. These foods are made from milk and grain, they carry valuable nutrients, and they encourage a child to learn, appropriately, that eating is fun. If nonnutritious foods are permitted in large quantities, however, the only possible outcomes are nutrient deficiencies, obesity, or both. The following section discusses the effects of nutrient deficiencies on behavior in children.

The Effects of Nutrient Deficiencies on Behavior

Nutrient deficiencies bring a host of physical symptoms, many of which are described in earlier chapters. Of particular interest to people concerned with caring for children is that nutrient deficiencies might also have behavioral symptoms.

Most people are familiar with the role of iron in carrying oxygen in the blood. Another extremely important function of iron is transporting that oxygen within cells, where it is used to help produce energy. A lack of iron not only causes an energy crisis but also directly affects behavior, mood, attention span, and learning ability. Iron is involved in the functioning of many molecules in the brain and nervous system. Deficiencies of iron produced experimentally in animals have caused abnormal synthesis and degradation of neurotransmitters, and notably those that regulate the ability to pay attention, crucial to learning.[3]

Iron deficiency, as already emphasized, is the most common nutrient deficiency in U.S. children. It is usually diagnosed from a deficit of iron indicators in the *blood,* after the deficiency has progressed all the way to overt anemia. A child's *brain,* however, is sensitive to slightly lowered iron levels long before the blood effects appear. Iron's effects are hard to distinguish from the effects of other factors in children's lives, but it is likely that iron deficiency manifests itself in a lowering of the ''motivation to persist in intellectually challenging tasks,'' a shortening of the attention span, and a reduction of overall intellectual performance. Anemic children perform less well on tests and have more conduct disturbances than their nonanemic classmates.[4]

Iron is not the only nutrient that can be displaced from a diet high in nutrient-poor foods. Any of several dozen nutrients may be lacking as well, and the deficiencies of those nutrients may also cause behavioral, as well as physical, symptoms.

A child with the behavioral symptoms of nutrient deficiencies might be irritable, aggressive, disagreeable, or sad and withdrawn. One might label such a child ''hyperactive,'' ''depressed,'' or ''unlikable,'' when in fact these traits might arise from simple, albeit marginal, malnutrition. In any such case, inspection of the child's diet by someone knowledgeable about children's nutrient needs is clearly in order. Should suspicion of dietary inadequacies be raised, *no matter what other causes may be implicated,* the people responsible for feeding the child should take steps to correct those inadequacies promptly.

Malnutrition is quite often a complex condition involving multiple nutrients and other factors. Highlight 11 described one example of a possible complicating factor: lead poisoning can cause iron-deficiency anemia, and iron deficiency impairs the body's defenses against absorption of lead. The anemia brought on by lead poisoning may be mistaken for a simple iron deficiency. Lead toxicity symptoms are widespread among children—one out of every six children between the ages of 6 months and 5 years are affected with lead poisoning.[5] Such problems are important to investigate, but even before they have been identified, the child should be fed properly.

Parents and medical practitioners often overlook the possibility that malnutrition may account for abnormalities of appearance and behavior. Consider the behavior of a well-nourished child: alert, energetic, responsive to external stimuli; in other words, healthy. Any departure from normal, healthy appearance and behavior is a possible sign of poor nutrition.

Food Allergies

Food allergies are frequently blamed for physical and behavioral abnormalities in children. A true food allergy—appropriately called a food-hypersensitivity reaction—occurs when a whole food protein or other large molecule enters the system and elicits an immunologic response. (Recall that large molecules of food are normally dismantled in the digestive tract to smaller ones that are absorbed without problem.) The body's immune system reacts to a food protein or other large molecule as it does to an antigen—by producing antibodies, histamines, or other defensive agents.

Allergies may have one or two components. They always involve antibodies; they may or may not involve symptoms. A person may produce antibodies *without* having any symptoms (known as asymptomatic allergy) or may produce antibodies *and* have symptoms (known as symptomatic allergy). Symptoms without antibody production are food intolerances and are *not* due to allergy. This means that allergies cannot be diagnosed from symptoms alone; they have to be diagnosed by testing for antibodies. Even if a child's symptoms are exactly like those of an allergy, they may not be caused by one.

Depending on the location of the allergic reaction in the body, a symptomatic allergy will exhibit different symptoms. In the digestive tract, it may cause nausea or vomiting; in the skin, it may cause rashes; and in the nasal passages and lungs, it can cause inflammation or asthma. A generalized, all-systems reaction is anaphylactic shock.

Allergic reactions to food can occur with different timings, simply classified as immediate and delayed. In both, the interaction of the antigen with the immune system is immediate, but the appearance of symptoms may come within minutes or after several (up to 24) hours.[6] Identifying the food that causes an immediate allergic reaction is easy, because symptoms correlate closely with the time of eating the food. Identifying the food that may cause a delayed reaction is more difficult, because the symptoms may not appear until a day after the offending food is eaten; by this time, many other foods will have been eaten, too, complicating the picture.

The foods that most often cause immediate allergic reactions are listed in Table 15–2. According to one investigator, 91 percent of adverse reactions are caused by only four major foods—nuts (43 percent), eggs (21 percent), milk (18 percent), and soy (9 percent).[7] Allergic reactions to single foods are common. Reactions to multiple foods are the exception, not the rule.

■ TABLE 15–2
Foods That Most Often Cause Allergies

Nuts	Peanuts
Eggs	Chicken
Milk	Fish
Soybeans	Shellfish
Wheat	Mollusks

Source: Adapted from D. D. Metcalfe, Diseases of food hypersensitivity, *New England Journal of Medicine* 321 (1989): 255–257; C. D. May, Food allergy: Perspective, principles, practical management, *Nutrition Today*, November-December 1980, pp. 28–31.

Miniglossary of Food Allergy Terms

anaphylactic (an-AFF-ill-LAC-tic) **shock**: a whole-body allergic reaction to an offending substance that may result in death. Symptoms: abdominal pain, nausea, vomiting, diarrhea, inflamed nasal membranes, chest pain, hives, swelling, low blood pressure.

antibody: a large protein that is produced in response to an antigen, and that inactivates the antigen.

antigen: a substance foreign to the body that elicits the formation of antibodies or an inflammation reaction from immune system cells. Food antigens are usually glycoproteins (large proteins with glucose molecules attached).

food allergy: a term generally synonymous with food hypersensitivity although often used to denote any unusual response to food. Allergies may be **symptomatic** or **asymptomatic**.

food-hypersensitivity reaction: an adverse reaction to foods that involves an immune response.

food intolerance: an adverse reaction to foods that does not involve an immune response.

histamine: a substance produced by cells of the immune system as part of a local immune reaction to an antigen; participates in causing inflammation.

A number of tests and food challenges are required to identify a true food allergy. Allergies are not always diagnosed by these time-consuming, laborious methods, however. In fact, the term *food allergy* is used loosely, even by many physicians, as a catch-all term for any unexplained adverse reaction to foods. Among reactions to foods that are confused with true food allergies are:

■ Allergic reactions to molds, antibiotics, and other contaminants of foods.

■ Chinese restaurant syndrome, a reaction specific to the flavor enhancer monosodium glutamate, or MSG (trade name, Accent). Incidence: one in several hundred.

■ Reactions to bacterial toxins, such as botulinal toxin, and other food poisoning.

■ Reactions to chemicals in foods, such as the natural laxative in prunes.

■ Symptoms of digestive diseases such as hernias and ulcers, aggravated by eating any food.

■ Enzyme deficiencies, such as lactose intolerance, which cause symptoms superficially indistinguishable from those of food allergy.

■ Psychological reactions based on the belief that certain foods cause certain symptoms.[8]

These reactions should be called *food intolerances*, not *allergies*.[9]

A parent whose child has any kind of discomfort after eating—stomachache, headache, pain, rapid pulse rate, nausea, wheezing, hives, bronchial irritation, cough, or any other—may decide that an allergy is responsible, when in fact the cause is something else entirely. Only careful, skilled testing can distinguish the many possibilities, and such testing is seldom done.

Parents are advised to watch for signs of food dislikes and take them seriously. Children's food aversions may be the result of nature's efforts to protect them from allergic or other adverse reactions. Although many cases of suspected allergies turn out to be something else, real allergies do exist, as do other valid reasons to avoid certain foods. Don't prejudge, in any case. Test, and then apply nutrition knowledge conscientiously in deciding how to alter the diet. Don't risk feeding the child an unbalanced diet, which could lead to nutrient deficiencies. Whenever a food is excluded from the diet, care must be taken to include other foods that offer the same nutrients as the omitted food contains. Remember that children with allergies need all their nutrients, just as other children do.

Hyperactivity and Diet

In searching for explanations for a child's misbehavior, many people have looked to the kitchen. One such attempt is to blame food for hyperactivity. Hyperactivity, one kind of learning disability, occurs in 5 to 10 percent of young school-age children—that is, in 1 or 2 in every classroom of 20 children.[10] It can lead to academic failure and major behavior problems. Parents and teachers need to deal effectively with it wherever it appears, to avert the grief that can otherwise result.

Physicians often diagnose hyperactivity by conducting a trial with stimulant drugs. Stimulants normally speed up people's activity, but they have a paradoxical effect with hyperactivity; they normalize it. (Perhaps they stimulate control centers in the brain.) If a child responds to stimulant drugs by calming down, that indicates that the drugs may be correcting a biochemical imbalance in the nervous system, and can be used to help control the behavior. *In children who are responsive,* prescription medication should at least be considered as the treatment of choice.

Many parents fail to appreciate the utility of drug treatment for hyperactivity, and resist its use, especially when they believe a solution may lie in manipulating the diet. Diet is one aspect of a child's life over which parents feel they can have some control. If problems can be solved by adding carrots or deleting cookies, then parents are eager to give diet advice a try. While it is true that nutrition should be considered whenever a person's physical or mental health is less than optimal, caution is advised not to jump at appealing solutions that are unfounded.

No behavior problems originate with diet other than the general misery caused by malnutrition. Food allergies do not cause hyperactivity. Misbehavior is seldom, if ever, attributable or even linked to dietary causes, although poor diet may be part of a cluster of factors seen in an unmanageable child's life.

One dietary excess that can irritate children is that of caffeine, a matter of some concern to pediatricians. A 12-ounce cola beverage may contain as much as 50 milligrams caffeine; two or more such beverages are equivalent in the body of a 60-pound child to the caffeine in 8 cups of coffee for a 175-pound man. Chocolate bars also contribute caffeine. Children can be troubled by sleeplessness, restlessness, and irregular heartbeats due to excess caffeine consumption. A survey of over 1,000 children between the ages of 1 and 17 years found that 77 percent of them were caffeine consumers.[11] (The accompanying box describes caffeine's effects in more detail and Table 15–3 lists the caffeine

hyperactivity syndrome in children: a cluster of symptoms in which the essential features are signs of developmentally inappropriate inattention, impulsivity, and high levels of motor activity. Other important features are onset before age seven, duration of six months or more, and proven absence of mental illness or mental retardation. Other names associated with hyperactivity: attention deficit disorder, hyperkinesis, minimal brain damage, minimal brain dysfunction, minor cerebral dysfunction.

learning disability: a defect in the ability to learn basic cognitive skills such as reading, writing, and mathematics; causes vary.

contents of commonly used beverages, foods, and drugs.) As long as such undeniably attractive temptations as cola beverages and chocolate bars surround children, barriers against their abuse have to be provided by concerned adults until the children learn to control consumption themselves.

■ TABLE 15–3
Caffeine Content of Beverages, Foods, and OTC Drugs

	Average (mg)	Range (mg)
Beverages and Food		
Coffee (5-oz cup)		
Brewed, drip method	130	110–150
Brewed, percolator	94	64–124
Instant	74	40–108
Decaffeinated, brewed or instant	3	1–5
Tea (5-oz cup)		
Brewed, major U.S. brands	40	20–90
Brewed, imported brands	60	25–110
Instant	30	25–50
Iced (12-oz glass)	70	67–76
Soft drinks (12-oz can)		
Dr. Pepper		40
Colas and cherry cola		
Regular		30–46
Diet		2–58
Caffeine-free		0–trace
Jolt		72
Mountain Dew, Mello Yello		52
Fresca, Hires Root Beer, 7-Up,		
Sprite, Squirt, Sunkist Orange		0
Cocoa beverage (5-oz cup)	4	2–20
Chocolate milk beverage (8 oz)	5	2–7
Milk chocolate candy (1 oz)	6	1–15
Dark chocolate, semisweet (1 oz)	20	5–35
Baker's chocolate (1 oz)	26	26
Chocolate flavored syrup (1 oz)	4	4
Drugs[a]		
Cold remedies (standard dose)		
Dristan		0
Coryban-D, Triaminicin		30
Diuretics (standard dose)		
Aqua-ban, Permathene H₂Off		200
Pre-Mens Forte		100
Pain relievers (standard dose)		
Excedrin		130
Midol, Anacin		65
Aspirin, plain (any brand)		0
Stimulants		
Caffedrin, NoDoz, Vivarin		200
Weight-control aids (daily dose)		
Prolamine		280
		200
Dexatrim, Dietac		

[a]Because products change, contact the manufacturer for an update on products you use regularly.

Source: Data from C. Lecos, The latest caffeine scoreboard, *FDA Consumer,* March 1984, p. 14; Measuring your life with coffee spoons, *Tufts University Diet and Nutrition Letter,* April 1984, pp. 3–6; Institute of Food Technologists, Expert Panel on Food Safety and Nutrition, *Evaluation of Caffeine Safety,* a publication (1986) available from the Institute of Food Technologists, 221 N. LaSalle St., Chicago, IL. 60601.

See pg. 426 Highlight

Without any magical answers, parents still have to deal with excitable, rambunctious, and unruly children; all children at times get wild and "hyper." There are many normal, everyday causes of such behavior:

- Desire for attention.
- Lack of sleep.
- Overstimulation.
- Too much TV.
- Lack of exercise.

Together, these produce the tension-fatigue syndrome, which can be relieved by giving more consistent care to the child's welfare. It helps especially to insist on regular hours of sleep, regular mealtimes, and regular outdoor exercise.

tension-fatigue syndrome: apparent hyperactivity produced in a child by the combination of lack of sleep and overstimulation with anxiety.

A Comment on Caffeine

Caffeine occurs in several plants, including the familiar coffee bean and tea leaf—and the cocoa bean, from which chocolate is made. Nearly every human society uses one or another plant to deliver caffeine.

The effects of this stimulant drug differ for each individual depending on a variety of factors, including the quantity of caffeine consumed, whether that quantity was taken all at once or over time, and to what extent the user has developed a tolerance to caffeine. Most people develop a tolerance to caffeine rather quickly. For those who are unaccustomed to caffeine use, caffeine may increase blood pressure, raise blood cholesterol concentrations, and cause irregular heartbeats.[12] Caffeine stimulates the digestive tract, promoting efficient elimination, and its "wake-up" effect is also well known. Curiously, the wakefulness of caffeine may actually be moderated by its ability to increase brain serotonin concentrations, which are generally associated with drowsiness.[13]

Caffeine, at doses equivalent to 1 c coffee, raises the metabolic rate slightly for a couple of hours. If a person wanting to lose weight could refrain from making up this energy deficit with food, these small changes in the metabolic rate (75 to 100 kcal/day) could lead to substantial weight loss.[14]

Caffeine seems to be relatively harmless when used by healthy (nonpregnant) adults in moderate doses (the equivalent of, say, two average-sized cups of coffee a day). In larger amounts, caffeine can produce reactions that are indistinguishable from those caused by anxiety. People who drink between 8 and 15 c coffee a day, for example, have been known to seek help from health care providers for complaints such as dizziness, agitation, restlessness, recurring headaches, intestinal discomfort, and sleep difficulties. Before prescribing a tranquilizer, the physician would do well to inquire about the caffeine consumption of such clients.

Like some other drugs, caffeine is addictive, in that the body adapts to its presence. Sudden abstinence after long use (even if use has been moderate), cutting back from a high to a low dose, or switching to a decaffeinated product causes a characteristic withdrawal headache. This kind of headache is so common that many pain relievers include caffeine in their formulas, even though caffeine is ineffective for relieving other types of pain. As is true of many other substances, moderation in the use of caffeine-containing foods and beverages is advisable.

See pg 426 highlight

Regularity of Meals

Children who eat no breakfast perform poorly in tasks of concentration, their attention spans are shorter, and they even show lower IQs on testing than their well-fed peers; malnourished children are particularly vulnerable.[15] Common sense tells us that it is unreasonable to expect anyone to learn and perform work when no fuel has been provided. By the late morning, discomfort from hunger may become distracting even if a child has eaten breakfast.

The problem that arises for children who attempt morning schoolwork on an empty stomach appears to be at least partly due to hypoglycemia. The average child up to the age of ten or so needs to eat every four to six hours to maintain a blood glucose concentration high enough to support the activity of the brain and nervous system. A child's brain is as big as an adult's, and the brain is the body's chief glucose consumer. A child's liver is considerably smaller—and the liver is the organ responsible for storing glucose (as glycogen) and releasing it into the blood as needed. A child's liver can't store more than about four hours' worth of glycogen; hence the need to eat fairly often. Teachers aware of the late-morning slump in their classrooms wisely request that a midmorning snack be provided; it improves classroom performance all the way to lunchtime. But for the child who hasn't had breakfast, the morning is lost altogether.

Nutrition at School

While parents are doing what they can to establish favorable eating behaviors during the transition from infancy to childhood, other factors are entering the picture. During preschool or grade school, the child encounters foods prepared and served by outsiders. The U.S. government funds several programs to provide nutritious, high-quality meals for children at school. (School lunches in Canada are administered locally and therefore vary from area to area.) School lunches are designed to meet certain requirements. They must include specified servings of milk, protein-rich foods (meat, poultry, fish, cheese, eggs, legumes, or peanut butter), vegetables, fruits, and breads or other grain foods. The design is intended to provide at least a third of the RDA for each of the nutrients. Table 15–4 shows school lunch patterns for different ages.

Parents rely on the school lunch program to meet a significant part of their children's nutrient needs on school days. Indeed, students participating in the school lunch program have higher intakes of energy and nutrients than students who do not. Children don't always like what they are served, and school lunch programs attempt to feed them both what they want and what will nourish them. In response to children's differing needs and tastes, the trend is:

■ To increase the variety of offerings and allow children to choose what they are served.
■ To vary portion sizes, so that little children may take little servings.
■ To involve students (in secondary schools) in the planning of menus.
■ To improve the scheduling of lunches so that children can eat when they are hungry and can have enough time to eat well.

■ TABLE 15–4
School Lunch Patterns for Different Ages

Food Group	Preschool (age)		Grade School through High School (grade)		
	1 to 2	3 to 4	K to 3	4 to 6	7 to 12
Meat or Meat Alternate					
1 serving:					
Lean meat, poultry, or fish	1 oz	1½ oz	1½ oz	2 oz	3 oz
Cheese	1 oz	1½ oz	1½ oz	2 oz	3 oz
Large egg(s)	1	1½	1½	2	3
Cooked dry beans or peas	½ c	¾ c	¾ c	1 c	1½ c
Peanut butter	2 tbsp	3 tbsp	3 tbsp	4 tbsp	6 tbsp
Vegetable and/or Fruit					
2 or more servings, both to total	½ c	½ c	½ c	¾ c	¾ c
Bread or Bread Alternate					
Servings[a]	5 per week	8 per week	8 per week	8 per week	10 per week
Milk					
1 serving of fluid milk	¾ c	¾ c	1 c	1 c	1 c

[a]A serving is 1 slice of whole-grain or enriched bread; a whole-grain or enriched biscuit, roll, muffin, and so on; or ½ c cooked pasta or other cereal grain such as bulgur or grits.

Source: School lunch patterns: Ready, set, go! *School Food Service Journal,* August 1980, p. 31.

Many schools are attempting to meet today's ideals of healthful food. They offer low-fat or nonfat milk instead of whole milk. To economize, they do not require that children be served every item, but permit them to select what they will eat, so that little food will be wasted. Many schools offer salad bars, potato bars, and taco bars, providing students an opportunity to create their own meals from a selection of nutritious foods.

Whether to eat the school's lunch is not the only choice facing children in the school. Some children bring lunch from home, whereas others rely on vending machines. The American Dental Association (ADA) would like to eliminate the sale of confections as snacks in schools, but so far has met with little success. Most progress has been made by way of individual, voluntary initiatives. Experiments have shown that children choose more nutritious snacks if they are offered side by side with the sugary foods. When apples are made available in vending machines, children choose chocolate bars less often. When milk is made available, soft drink use drops considerably. Coincident with the school lunch program is a program of nutrition education and training (NET program) in all the public schools. This program is minimally funded, but program administrators are ingenious and creative in accomplishing its highest-priority objectives. Children need not only to be fed well, but to learn enough about nutrition to become able to make healthy food choices when the choices become theirs to make.

Television's Influence on Nutrition

On the average, children in the United States spend as much time watching television as they do attending school. Little wonder that television viewing

Television watching influences children's eating habits and activity patterns.

The *NRC Recommendations* are presented in Chapter 2.

has become associated with a variety of child and teen behaviors. Television's influence is evident in childhood obesity as Chapter 12 explained (see p. 370). Television may also influence dental health as decribed in Highlight 10 (see pp. 312–313).

Mealtimes

The childhood years are a parent's last chance to influence food choices. By fostering the development of healthy eating habits, parents help determine whether development will take place in a positive or negative direction for the rest of life. Food choices can not only promote healthy growth, but can also help prevent the degenerative diseases of later life—cardiovascular disease, cancer, diabetes, and osteoporosis. Many experts seem to agree that early childhood is the time to put practices into effect that, until recently, were recommended only for adults.

Most important is to avoid obesity. Train preschool children to "eat thin." Teach children to eat slowly, to pause and enjoy their table companions, and to stop eating when they are full. Serve small portions of food that can be followed by additional servings, if needed. Discourage snacking on high-fat, high-sugar foods. Encourage frequent adequate milk consumption. Follow recommendations like those of the *NRC Recommendations,* emphasizing foods with high nutrient density. Encourage physical activity on a daily basis. Later chapters offer many more pointers on nutrition for disease prevention.

It is desirable for children to learn to like nutritious foods in all the food groups. With one exception, this liking usually develops naturally. The exception is vegetables, which young children frequently dislike and refuse. Even a tiny serving of spinach, cooked carrots, or squash may elicit an expression that registers the utmost in negative feelings. Since most young-sters need to eat more vegetables, the next few paragraphs are addressed to this problem.

Try to remember how you felt when first offered a cup of vegetable soup, a serving of runny spinach, or a pile of peas and carrots. If the soup burned your tongue, it may have been years before you were willing to try it again. As for the spinach, it was suspiciously murky looking. (Who could tell what might be lurking in that dark, stringy stuff?) The peas and carrots troubled your sense of order. Before you could eat them, you felt compelled to sort the peas onto one side of the plate and the carrots onto the other. Then you had to separate, into a reject pile, all those that got mashed in the process or contaminated with gravy from the mashed potatoes. Only then might you be willing to eat the intact, clean peas and carrots one by one—perhaps with your fingers, since the peas, especially, kept rolling off the fork.

Researchers attempting to explain children's food preferences are met with contradictions. Children describe liking colorful foods, yet vegetables are most often rejected, and brown peanut butter and white potatoes, apple wedges, and bread are among their favorites. Raw vegetables are better accepted than cooked ones, so it is wise to offer vegetables that are raw or slightly undercooked and crunchy, bright in color, served separately, and easy to eat. They should be warm, not hot, because a child's mouth is much more sensitive than an adult's. The flavor should be mild (a child has more taste buds), and smooth foods such as mashed potatoes or pea soup should have no lumps in them (a child wonders, with some disgust, what the lumps might be). Children prefer foods that are familiar to them, so offer foods regularly.

When feeding children, parents must always be alert to the dangers of choking. A choking child is a silent child—an adult should be present whenever a child is eating. Encouraging the child to sit when eating is also a good practice; choking is more likely when a child is running or falling. Round foods such as grapes, nuts, hard candies, and hotdog pieces are difficult to control in a mouth with few teeth and can easily become lodged in the small opening of a child's trachea. Other potentially dangerous foods include tough meat, popcorn, and chips. (Highlight 3 provides a description of the Heimlich maneuver in Figure H3–2.)

Wise parents allow children to help make the family's choices, including the right to say no at times. At the same time, of course, parents are sensible to prevent children from dominating the family. Allowing children to help plan and prepare the family's meals provides enjoyable learning experiences that encourage children to eat the foods they have prepared.

Little children like to eat at little tables and to be served little portions of food. Teaching children how to serve themselves the quantity they will eat minimizes waste. Never force children to clean their plates. This practice can lead to behaviors that encourage obesity. Instead, allowing children to stop eating when they are full encourages them to listen to their bodies.

Children like to eat with other children and have been observed to stay at the table longer and eat much more when in the company of their peers. Children are also more likely to overcome their prejudices against foods their peers are eating.

When introducing new foods at the table, parents are advised to offer them one at a time—and only a small amount at first. The more often a food is presented to a young child, the more likely the child will like that food. Whenever possible, the new food should be presented at the beginning of the meal, when the child is hungry. Offer the new food, and allow the child to make the decision; whether the child accepts or rejects the new food is okay. Never make an issue of food acceptance, not even to reward acceptance. When children are pushed to try new foods, even by way of rewards, they are less likely to try those foods again than children who are left to decide for themselves.[16] One authority on childrens' eating behaviors makes a point relevant to the research just discussed: the parent is responsible for *what* the child is offered to eat, but the child is responsible for *how much* and even *whether* to eat.[17]

Parents may find that their children often snack so much that they aren't very hungry at mealtimes. Instead of teaching children *not* to snack, parents might be wise to teach them *how* to snack. Provide snacks that are as nutritious as the foods served at mealtime. Snacks can even be mealtime foods that are served individually over time, instead of all at once on one plate. When providing snacks to children, a smart parent thinks of the four food groups and offers pieces of cheese, tangerine slices, carrot sticks, and peanut butter on whole-wheat crackers. Snacks need to be easy to prepare and readily available to children. This is particularly important to children who return home after school without parental supervision.

A bright, unhurried atmosphere free of conflict is conducive to good appetite. Parents who serve meals in a relaxed and casual manner, without anxiety, provide the climate in which a child's negative emotions will be

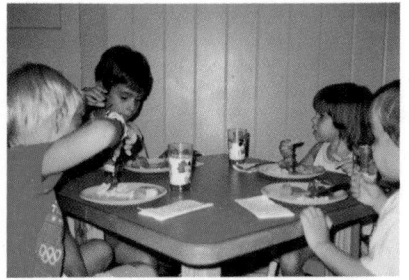

Eating is more fun when the fork fits your hand and your friends are there.

minimized. Conflicts can be promoted by unaware parents, even if they have the best of intentions. Parents who beg, cajole, and demand that their child eat deny the child an opportunity to develop self-control. Instead, the child enters a battle that takes on more importance than hunger. The power struggle almost invariably results in a confirmed pattern of resistance and a permanently closed mind on the child's part. Mealtimes can be nightmarish for the child who is struggling with personal and parental problems. If, as a child sits down to the table, a barrage of accusations is shouted—"Your hands are filthy . . . your report card . . . and clean your plate! Your mother cooked that food!"—mealtimes may be unbearable. The stomach may recoil, because the body, as well as the mind, reacts to stress of this kind.

In an effort to practice these many tips, parents may overlook perhaps the single most important influence on their child's food habits—themselves. Parents who don't eat carrots shouldn't be surprised when their child refuses to eat carrots. Likewise, parents who dislike the smell of brussels sprouts may not be able to persuade a child to like them. A child learns much through imitation. Parents set an irresistable example by enjoying nutritious foods.

While serving and enjoying food, caretakers can promote not only physical, but also emotional, growth at every stage of a child's life. If the beginnings are right, children will grow without the kind of conflict and confusion over food that can lead to nutrition problems. In the interest of promoting both a positive self-concept and a positive attitude toward good food, it is important for parents to help their children remember that they are good kids. What they *do* may sometimes be unacceptable; but what they *are*, on the inside, are normal, healthy, growing, fine human beings.

The Teen Years

Few teenagers become interested in nutrition for its contribution to growth and health. Lessons (and misinformation) in nutrition come to them by way of personal experiences—related to how diet can improve their lives now—crash dieting in order to buy a new bathing suit, avoiding greasy foods in an effort to clear acne, or eating a large plate of spaghetti in preparation for a big sporting event. The next few sections examine the nutrient needs of adolescents and how this unique time of life influences their food intakes.

Chapter 12 discusses fad diets. Chapter 13 provides tips for the pregame meal.

Growth and Nutrient Needs

The fairly steady rate of growth throughout childhood rises rather abruptly and dramatically with the onset of adolescence. Prior to adolescence, female and male growth patterns differ little; with the onset of puberty, they become distinct. A female's adolescent growth spurt begins at age 10 or 11 and reaches its peak at 12. A male's growth spurt begins at 12 or 13 and peaks at 14. Gender differences also become apparent in the skeletal system, lean body mass, and fat stores. In females, fat becomes a larger percentage of the total body weight, and in males, the lean body mass—muscle and bone—becomes much greater. This intensive growth period brings not only a dramatic

adolescence: the period from the beginning of puberty until maturity.

puberty: the period in life in which a person becomes physically capable of reproduction.

increase in height and weight, but also hormonal changes that profoundly affect every organ of the body (including the brain) and that culminate in the emergence of physically mature adults within two or three years.

Tremendous individual variations occur in teenagers' rates and patterns of growth. Growth charts used for children must be abandoned when the signs of puberty begin to appear. Age in years signifies little about development; the only way to be sure a teenager is growing normally is to compare his or her height and weight with previous measures taken at intervals. If reasonably smooth progress is being made, all is well.

There is also tremendous variation in the energy needs of adolescents. The rapid growth of adolescence, especially if coupled with high activity, incurs high energy needs. An active male of 15 may need 4,000 kcalories or more a day just to maintain his weight. On the other hand, when growth and activity are minimal, energy needs may be minimal. An inactive female of 15 whose growth is nearly at a standstill may need fewer than 2,000 kcalories if she is to avoid becoming obese.

Total nutrient needs are greater during adolescence than at any other time of life, with the exception of pregnancy and lactation. Again, iron stands out as a nutrient deserving of special mention. Iron needs increase during adolescence due to the onset of menstruation in females and to the greater development of lean body mass in males. Other nutrients are also required in greater quantities during adolescence than in childhood. These nutrient requirements either level off or diminish slightly as the adolescent passes into adulthood.

Many teenagers are well nourished, but some have nutritional problems. One study of adolescent nutrient intake found that males met the RDA for all nutrients; the females in this study failed to meet the RDA for iron, calcium, and vitamin A.[18] Other studies have reported dietary inadequacies of vitamin B_6, zinc, folate, iodide, vitamin D, and magnesium prevalent among adolescent women.[19] The gender difference in diet adequacy primarily reflects the males' consuming larger quantities of food.

The insidious problem of obesity becomes more apparent in adolescence and often continues into adulthood, mostly in females, and especially in black females. Young women who become interested in nutrition may make choices that will benefit their health, may become obsessed with weight control (see Highlight 12), or may be persuaded to take supplements they do not need.

Drugs, Alcohol, and Tobacco

The teen years are a critical time in the development of problem behaviors such as drug, alcohol, and tobacco use. Three of every five high school seniors report that they have at least tried an illicit drug, most commonly marijuana.[20] Like all substances entering the body, marijuana must be processed. The active ingredients are rapidly and almost completely (90 percent) absorbed from the lungs.[21*] Then, being fat soluble, these substances

---

*The active ingredient of marijuana primarily responsible for its intoxicating effects is delta-9-tetrahydrocannabinol, or THC.

are packaged (most likely in lipoproteins) before being transported by the blood to the various body tissues.[22] They are processed by many tissues (not just by the liver), and they persist for several days in the body, being excreted over a period of a week or more after the smoking of a single marijuana cigarette.[23] With repeated exposure, these substances accumulate and become concentrated in body fat, the lungs, the liver, the reproductive organs, and the brain.[24]

Smoking a marijuana cigarette has several characteristic effects on the body, altering, among other things, the sense of taste. Among the apparent taste changes induced by marijuana is an enhanced enjoyment of eating, especially of sweets, commonly known as "the munchies." Why or how this effect occurs is not known.[25] Some investigators speculate that the hunger induced by marijuana is actually a social effect caused by the suggestibility of the group in which it is smoked.[26] Prolonged use of the drug does not seem to bring about a weight gain.

Cocaine elicits such effects as intense euphoria, restlessness, heightened self-confidence, irritability, insomnia, and loss of appetite. Weight loss is a common side effect, and cocaine abusers often meet the criteria for eating disorders.[27] Repeated use can cause rapid heart rate, irregular heartbeats, heart attacks, and even death.

Drug abusers face multiple nutrition problems:

- They spend money for drugs that could be spent on food.
- They lose interest in food during "high" times.
- Some drugs induce at least a temporary depression of appetite.
- Their lifestyle often lacks the regularity and routine that promote good eating habits.
- They may contract hepatitis, a liver disease common in drug abusers, which causes taste changes and loss of appetite.
- Their nutrient status may be altered by treatments and medicines.
- They often become ill with infectious diseases, which increases their need for nutrients.

During withdrawal from drugs, an important aspect of treatment is the identification and correction of nutrition problems.

At some point during adolescence, teenagers face the decision whether or not to drink alcohol. Even though the law forbids the sale of alcohol to people under a specific age, alcohol is still available to many teenagers who seek it.

Many teenagers find that alcohol and marijuana serve similar purposes, and the pattern of substance use indicates parallel consumption, not a displacement of one by the other.[28] Some teenagers use alcohol as an escape or for support—an ineffective way to cope with problems that leads to greater problems. Dependency on alcohol or any drug has major adverse effects on the growth and development of adolescents and deserves attention, but is beyond the scope of this text.

People use alcohol to help them relax or to relieve anxiety. They think that alcohol is a stimulant, because it seems to make them lively and uninhibited at first. Actually, though, the way it does this is by sedating inhibitory nerves, which are more numerous than excitatory nerves. Ultimately, alcohol acts as a depressant and sedates all the nerve cells.

Alcohol is an empty-kcalorie beverage and can displace needed nutrients from the diet while simultaneously altering metabolism so that even good nutrition cannot normalize it. Highlight 7 provides a basis for understanding the effects of alcohol on a person's body and nutrition status.

Cigarette smoking is a pervasive health problem causing thousands of people to suffer from cancer and diseases of the cardiovascular, digestive, and respiratory systems. These effects are beyond the scope of this text, but there are a few nutrition connections to be explored. Smoking cigarettes does influence hunger, body weight, and nutrient status. There are also links between nutrients and lung cancer.

Smoking a cigarette eases feelings of hunger. When smokers receive a hunger signal, they can quiet it with a cigarette instead of food. Such behavior ignores body signals and postpones energy and nutrient intake.

Indeed, smokers tend to weigh less than nonsmokers and to gain weight upon cessation of smoking.[29] Weight gain is often a concern for people contemplating giving up cigarettes. The decision to quit weighs unhealthy smoking against unattractive (and potentially unhealthy) weight gain. The message to smokers wanting to quit is to adjust diet and exercise habits in order to maintain weight during and after cessation.

Nutrient intakes of smokers and nonsmokers differ. Smokers have lower intakes of dietary fiber, vitamins, and minerals, even when their energy intakes are quite similar.[30] The association between smoking and low vitamin intake may be noteworthy, considering the altered metabolism of vitamin C in smokers and the protective effect of vitamin A against lung cancer.

Results of one research study indicate that the vitamin C requirement of smokers may exceed that of nonsmokers. Smokers break down vitamin C faster, thus requiring more vitamin C to achieve steady body pools comparable to those of nonsmokers.[31] Beta-carotene, a precursor to vitamin A found in vegetables, has anticancer activity.[32] Specifically, the risk of lung cancer is greatest for smokers who have the lowest intake of carotene. Of course, conclusions from such evidence cannot be made in haste. Teenagers cannot be led to believe that as long as they eat their carrots they can safely smoke their cigarettes. However, it is important to encourage teenagers to eat foods rich in carotene, a nutrient many of them lack in their diets.

The vitamin C RDA for people who regularly smoke cigarettes is 100 mg/day.

Teenage Pregnancy

Teenage pregnancy presents a special case of nutrient needs. Even when not pregnant, a teenage female is hard put to meet her own nutrient needs at this time of maximal growth. Nourishing a growing fetus adds to her burden. Her own high nutrient requirements can compete with those of her fetus, especially if she is going through her most rapid growth phase. Adequate nutrition can substantially improve the course of events and the health of the mother and infant; it is an essential component of prenatal care.[33] To support the needs of both mother and fetus, young teenagers (13 to 16 years old) are encouraged to gain approximately 35 pounds during pregnancy. Young teenagers who gain less, even if they gain the 24 to 27 pounds recommended for older pregnant women, have smaller newborns.[34] As discussed in Chapter 14, small newborns have a high risk of disease and death.

Little information is available on the specific nutrient needs of pregnant adolescents. For some nutrients, estimates of nutrient needs are made by adding the increments of recommended nutrients for the pregnant adult woman to the RDA for nonpregnant females 15 to 18 years of age; for other nutrients, the RDA during pregnancy is set for all ages. Figure 15–1 shows that a pregnant teenager's needs for many nutrients increase more than does her energy allowance. If a young woman starts pregnancy already malnourished or lacks education, resources, and support, she may encounter serious medical problems. Table 15–5 provides a daily food guide for pregnant and lactating teenagers based on the Four Food Group Plan.

The complications of pregnancy and the acute and long-lasting consequences of poor nutrition at this time were discussed in Chapter 14. Complications are common in pregnant teenagers. The greatest risk of a teenage pregnancy is death of the infant. The infant mortality rate for mothers under age 20 is high, with mothers under 15 having the highest rate of all age groups.

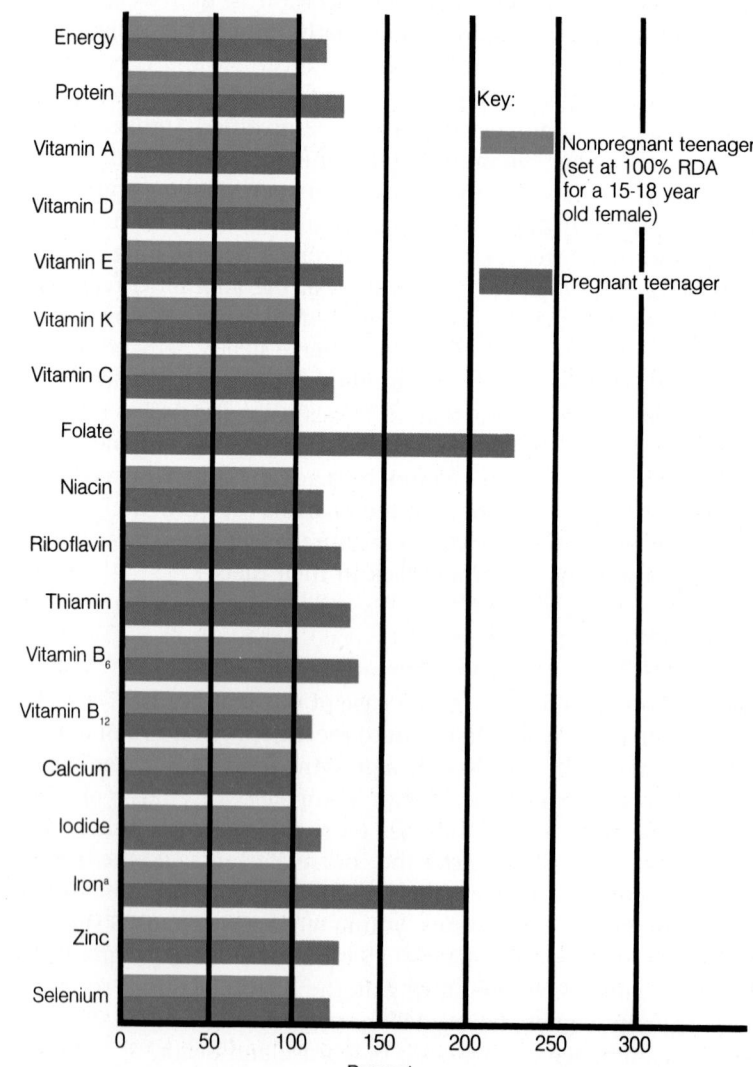

Key:

▬ Nonpregnant teenager (set at 100% RDA for a 15-18 year old female)

▬ Pregnant teenager

■ FIGURE 15–1
Comparison of the Nutrient Needs of a Nonpregnant Teenager with Those of a Pregnant Teenager
These values derive from adding the increment of recommended nutrients for the pregnant adult woman to the RDA for females 15 to 18 years of age.

[a]The pregnant teenager may need to take an iron supplement.

■ TABLE 15–5
Four Food Group Plan for Pregnant and Lactating Teenagers[a]

| | Number of Servings | |
Food Group	Teenagers	Pregnant or Lactating Teenagers
Meat and meat alternates	2	3
Milk and milk products	4	5
Vegetables and fruits	4	4
Breads and cereals	4	4

[a]See Figure 2–4 in Chapter 2 for a more detailed summary of serving sizes and food sources.

Teenage pregnancy is common. About one out of every five babies is born to a teenager, and more than a tenth of these mothers are 15 or younger. Emphasis on preparing adolescents for future pregnancy is needed in public schools and public health programs. A model program for giving nutrition help to teenage mothers is the WIC (Women's, Infants' and Children's) program. WIC is described in Chapter 17.

Food Choices and Eating Habits of Teenagers

Teenagers are not fed; they eat. For the first time in their lives, they assume primary responsibility for their own food intakes. Teenagers come and go as they choose and eat what they want when they have time. With a multitude of after-school, social, and job activities, they almost inevitably fall into irregular eating habits. The adult becomes a gatekeeper, controlling the availability, but not the consumption, of food in the teenager's environment. The adult can't nag, scold, or pressure teenagers into eating, because teens typically turn a deaf ear to coercion, and often to persuasion. The gatekeeper who wants to promote the desired choices effectively provides access to nutritious and economical energy foods that are low in sugar and fat at home and limits access to nonnutritious foods. The teenage snacker who finds only nutritious foods around the house is well provided for. Table 15–5 provides a daily food guide for teenagers based on the Four Food Group Plan.

Snacks provide about a fourth of the average teenager's total daily food energy intake. Teens receive substantial amounts of protein, thiamin, riboflavin, vitamin B$_6$, magnesium, and zinc from snacks, and even calcium (if they snack on dairy products). The nutrients they most often fail to obtain are iron, vitamin A, and folate. Protein usually need not be stressed, but many teenagers need to be encouraged to recognize and consume more dairy products (for calcium) and more vegetables (for vitamin A and folate). (Wherever vitamin A is lacking, folate generally is, too, because both are found in green vegetables.) Iron-rich snacks include hard-boiled eggs, bran muffins, and peanut butter and crackers.

Inevitably, teenagers do a lot of eating away from home. There, as well as at home, their nutritional welfare is favored or hindered by the choices they make. A lunch of a hamburger, a chocolate shake, and french fries supplies

gatekeeper: with respect to nutrition, a key person who controls other people's access to foods and thereby has a profound impact on their nutrition; examples are the spouse who buys and cooks the food, the parent who feeds the children, and the caretaker in a day-care center.

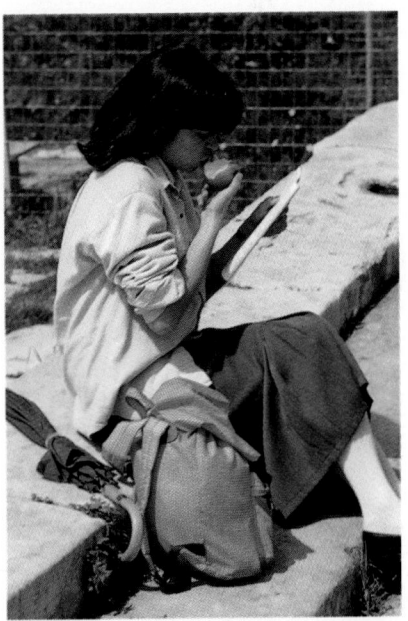

Nutritious snacks play an important role in an active teen's diet.

■ **TABLE 15—6**
Selected Nutrients in a Hamburger, Chocolate Shake, and Fries (Percentage of RDA)

Nutrient	Male[a]	Female[a]
Energy	27	37
Protein	41	55
Calcium	32	32
Iron	30	24
Zinc	23	28
Vitamin A	8	10
Thiamin	34	47
Riboflavin	53	73
Niacin	32	43
Folate	23	26
Vitamin C	16	16

[a]RDA for an 18-year-old, moderately active, person of average height and weight.

The nutritive value of selected fast foods is presented in Appendix H.

nutrients in the amounts shown in Table 15—6, at a kcalorie cost of 820. For the most part, these are substantial percentages of recommended intakes at an energy cost many teenagers can afford. Depending on how they adjust their breakfast and dinner choices, teenagers may meet their nutrient needs more than adequately with this sort of lunch. They need only select fruits and vegetables (for vitamins A and C), good fiber sources, and more good folate, iron, and zinc sources at their other meals.

Calcium is sometimes a problem nutrient for teenagers. The requirement for calcium reaches its peak during these years. Unfortunately, many teens reject milk as a "child's drink" and opt instead for soft drinks with their lunches, dinners, and snacks. As might be expected, the more soft drinks teenagers drink, the less likely they are to meet their RDA for calcium.[35]

Teenagers are intensely involved in day-to-day life with their peers and in preparation for their future lives as adults. Adults need to remember that teenagers have the right to make their own decisions—even if they are in opposition to the adults' own views. The gatekeeper can set up the environment so that nutritious foods are available, and can stand by with reliable nutrition information and advice, but the rest is up to the teenagers. Ultimately, they make the choices.

The nutrition choices people make as teenagers and young adults have immediate, as well as long-term, effects on their health. The rest of this chapter is devoted to how people's nutrition throughout their lives influences their health later on, and to the nutrition concerns of older adults.

▓ Adulthood and the Later Years

Most of this book has been about adult nutrition. This chapter and the previous one focus on other specific stages of the life cycle that require special nutrition attention. To this point, pregnancy, lactation, infancy, childhood, and adolescence have been addressed. To discuss the needs of adults would be to review this text; accordingly, the remainder of this chapter describes aging and the later adult years.

As people age, a lifetime of nutrition choices incur consequences for the better or for the worse. While each day's intakes of nutrients may have only a minute effect on body organs and their functions, over years and decades their repeated effects accumulate to have major impacts. One writer has put it this way: "By age 65, the average American will have consumed 100,000 pounds of food, give or take a few tons. . . . Neglect will almost certainly be reflected in the state of his or her health by age 65, if not long before."[36] This being the case, it is of great importance for everyone to pay close attention now to nutrition.

The majority of the U.S. population is now middle-aged. As that group ages, the ratio of old people to young is growing larger, as Figure 15—2 shows. The fastest-growing age group is people over 85.

In 1983 in the United States, the life expectancy for women was 78 years and for men was 71 years, up from about 45 years in 1900. Advances in medical science—antibiotics and other treatments—are largely responsible for almost doubling the life expectancy in this century. Still, a biological schedule

life expectancy: the average number of years lived by people in a given society.

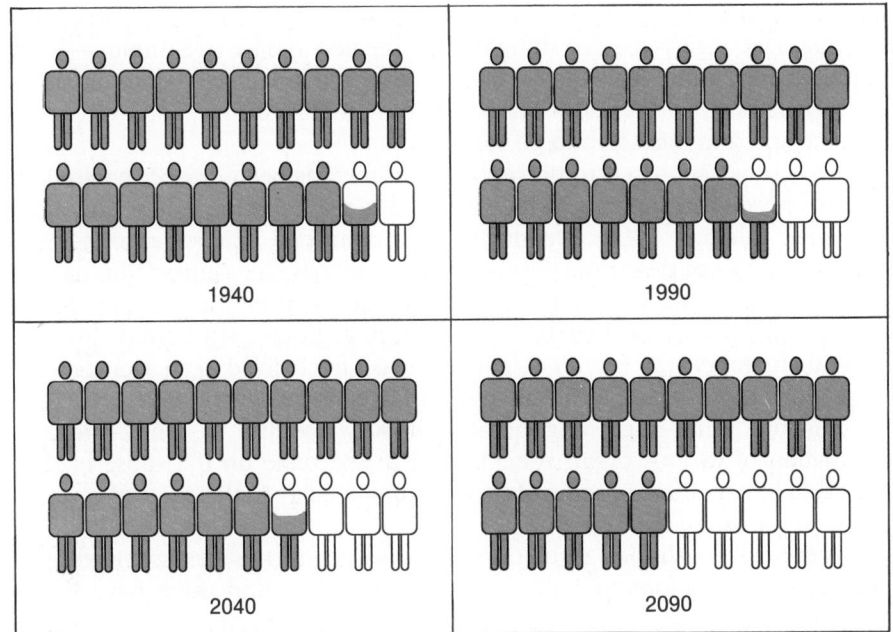

1940   1990   2040   2090

■ **FIGURE 15–2**

The Aging of the U.S. Population
(👤 = 65 years or older)

In 1940, 6.8 percent of the population was 65 or older. Today, 12.7 percent of us have reached age 65; by 2040, 21.7 percent will have reached age 65; and a century from now, nearly one out of four Americans will be 65 and older. An estimated 25,000 Americans now living are 100 years old or older.

Source: K. Flieger, Why do we age? *FDA Consumer,* October 1988, pp. 20–25.

is built into the human organism (we call it aging) that cuts off life at a genetically fixed point in time. The life span (the maximum length of life possible for a species) of human beings—115 years—has not changed over the years and is probably the upper limit of human longevity.

The study of the aging process in human beings is among the youngest of the scientific disciplines. It is only in this century that human beings have achieved a life expectancy worthy of a science devoted to studying it.[37] What has been learned so far about the effects of nutrition and environment on longevity provides incentive for researchers to keep asking questions about how and why human beings age. Among the questions they are asking are:

■ To what extent is aging inevitable? Can we retard it through changes in lifestyle and environment?

■ What roles does nutrition play in aging, and what roles can it play in retarding aging?

With respect to the first question, it seems that aging is an inevitable, natural process, programmed into the genes at conception, but that people can adopt lifestyle habits such as exercising and attention to work and recreational environments that will slow the process within the natural limits set by heredity. With respect to the second question, clearly, good nutrition can retard and ease the aging process in many significant ways.

One approach to the prevention of aging has been to study other cultures in the hope of finding an extremely long-lived race of people and then learning from them the secrets of long life. Scientists have found people who claimed to have lived over 100 years in two different geographical areas. Further study revealed, however, that some of these people only claimed to be 100 or older, because in their societies age was venerated. Still, some did prove not only to be remarkably old, but also remarkably healthy. The credit

life span: the maximum number of years of life attainable by a member of a species.

longevity: long duration of life.

did not go to nutrition: these people did not eat according to any particular formula. The secret—the one thing they all seemed to have in common—was that they lived a physically active life, and they remained active into old age. A recent study on longevity bears this out in this society, too; vigorous exercise and long life seem to go together.[38]

Still another approach to prevention of aging has been drastic manipulation of the diet in animals, which has given rise to some interesting and suggestive findings.[39] Rats live longer when their food intake is restricted in the early weeks of their lives, or even when it is restricted during adulthood. The life spans of rats also were lengthened by drastic restrictions of their food intakes, and especially their fat intakes, during the growth period. In one experiment, for example, animals allowed to eat freely lived to an average 656 days, while those whose feed was restricted lived to an average 949 days. The experiments were interesting because it was possible to study growth retardation of various organ systems, and to speculate on the cause of the increased length of life of some of the animals—a delay in the onset of certain diseases, for example.

Experiments with food restriction and longevity in rats has *not* suggested any direct applications to human nutrition, though, and there have been distinct disadvantages to the animals given restricted feedings. For example, half of the restricted animals died *very* early (before 300 days). The average length of life for the restricted rats was long because the few survivors lived a long time. Also, the restriction was severe: "even the shortest period of food restriction in this study was comparable to restriction of the food intake of a human infant kept in an isolated environment for 20 to 25 years to an amount that would permit the infant during that time to grow to about the size of a one-year-old child."[40] Furthermore, the restricted animals that survived were retarded and malformed in a number of ways. Extreme starvation to extend life, like any extreme, is not worth the price.

The views of the experts on food restriction can best be summed up by saying that disease can shorten people's lives, and that poor nutrition practices make diseases more likely or worse. Adequate nutrition, then, by postponing and slowing disease processes, can help an individual reach the maximum life span—but cannot extend it further.

The idea that nutrition can influence the way human bodies age is particularly appealing, since it is one factor that people can control and change. One of the ways that nutrition affects aging and longevity is by way of its role in disease prevention. (Nutrition and disease prevention is the topic of the next chapter.) Nutrition alone cannot ensure a long and robust life. However, many diseases are nutrition sensitive, even if also responsive to other factors.

Among the better-known relationships between nutrition and disease are the following:

- Appropriate energy intake helps prevent *obesity, diabetes,* and related *cardiovascular diseases* such as atherosclerosis and hypertension (Chapters 12, 27, and 28), and may influence the development of some forms of *cancer* (Chapter 30).
- Adequate intakes of essential nutrients prevent *deficiency diseases* such as scurvy, goiter, anemia, and the like (Chapters 8, 9, 10, and 11).

- Variety in foods, as well as certain vegetables, may be protective against certain types of *cancer* (Chapter 30).
- Moderation in sugar intake helps prevent *dental caries* (Highlight 10).
- Appropriate fiber intakes help prevent malfunctions of the digestive tract such as *constipation, diverticulosis,* and possibly *colon cancer* (Highlight 3 and Chapters 4, 24, and 25).
- Moderate sodium and adequate intakes of potassium, calcium, and other minerals help prevent *hypertension,* at least in people who are genetically predisposed to it (Chapters 10 and 28).

Other, less well established links between nutrition and disease are being discovered each day. Highlight 15, discusses the relationship between nutrition and brain degeneration.

Another age-related change is seen in the lens of the eye: cataracts, thickenings of the lenses that impair vision and ultimately lead to blindness. Cataracts occur even in well-nourished individuals due to injury, viral infections, toxic substances, and genetic disorders, but most cataracts are vaguely called senile cataracts—meaning "caused by aging." Scientists have searched for a possible role of nutrient deficiencies, excesses, and imbalances in cataract causation. They have observed several possible (and, it should be emphasized, highly tentative) links: to protein, fat, or sugar (fructose derived from sucrose) excess; to excess food energy intake (in people with diabetes); to deficiencies of the vitamins riboflavin or vitamin E; and to deficiencies of the minerals selenium or zinc. A link between lactose intolerance and cataracts is gaining strength, and researchers are trying to determine whether the presence of the milk sugar itself, or the dehydration caused by diarrhea in lactose-intolerant people, is the associated factor.[41]

cataract: clouding of the eye lens that diminishes vision.

Another major disease that disables the elderly is arthritis, a painful swelling of the joints that troubles many people as they grow older. During movement, the normal ends of bones are protected from wear by cartilage and by small sacs of fluid that act as a lubricant; but with age, bones sometimes disintegrate, and the joints become malformed and painful to move. The cause of arthritis is unknown, but it afflicts millions around the world and is a major problem of the elderly.

arthritis: a usually painful inflammation of a joint caused by many conditions, including infections, metabolic disturbances, or injury; joint structure is usually altered, with loss of function.

Arthritis has for centuries been ascribed to poor diet, many times to promote quack remedies, including many bizarre diets advertised as arthritis cures. Two or three new popular books on diet for arthritis come out every year, urging people to eat no meat, or drink no milk, or eat all their food raw, or eat only "natural" food, or avoid all additives, or—who knows what will be next? Actually no known diet prevents, relieves, or cures arthritis, but as long as people keep buying the books that make these claims, the law of supply and demand dictates that such books will keep coming out.[42]

One possible true link between arthritis and diet is through the immune system. It could be that in some cases of arthritis, the immune system has become defective and attacks the tissues of the bone coverings as it normally would an invader. The integrity of the immune system depends on adequate nutrition, and a poor diet probably worsens the condition. It is also possible that foods may stimulate the immune system to attack.[43] Another nutrient link to arthritis is the now-famous fatty acid found in fish oil, EPA. Chapter 5 introduced EPA and Chapter 28 will tell more about EPA and heart health;

Not effective against arthritis:
- Watercress.
- Burdock root.
- Vitamin D.
- Celery juice.
- Calcium.
- Megadoses of vitamins.
- Fasting.
- Fresh fruit.
- Honey.
- Lecithin.
- Yeast.
- Kelp.
- Raw liver.
- Alfalfa tea.
- *Aloe vera* liquid.
- Superoxide dismutase (SOD).
- 100 other substances.

research shows that the same diet recommended there—one low in saturated fat from red meats and dairy products and high in the fish oil EPA—can reduce the suffering of people with arthritis after three months of use.[44] The seemingly all-purpose low-fat diet with EPA added may prevent the inflammation in the joints that makes arthritis so painful. Researchers theorize that EPA probably interferes with the action of prostaglandins, chemicals involved in the inflammatory response of body tissues.

Weight loss is important for overweight persons with arthritis, because the joints affected are often weight-bearing joints that are stressed and irritated by having to carry excess poundage. Weight-loss diets alone often relieve the worst of the pain in arthritis clients, even that of arthritis in the hands (not weight bearing). Perhaps the drastic reduction in fat intake that accompanies the adoption of a kcalorie-restricted diet is beneficial for arthritis relief, with or without EPA added. Important to note: jogging and other weight-bearing exercise is not related to the development of arthritis—even in marathon runners.[45] Drugs are commonly used to relieve arthritis. Some drugs may affect nutrient availability and require attention to nutrition status when used over a prolonged time, as a later section of this chapter describes.

These brief discussions of cataracts and arthritis could be multiplied manyfold, both to provide further details and to add other diseases (as other chapters and highlights have), but they have sufficed to show that nutrition can provide at least some protection against certain diseases commonly associated with aging. In fact, in general, it is beginning to look as if nutrition through the prime years may play a greater role than has been realized in preventing many changes once thought to be inevitable consequences of growing older.

Nutrient Needs and Nutrition Status of Older Adults

As mentioned earlier, old age is a relatively new phenomenon—only recently have the ranks of senior citizens been growing larger. Scientists are working to find out how nutrient needs change as advancing age changes the body. So far, there are no RDA for older age groups—everyone over 50 is grouped together, even though needs change as aging progresses. Clearly, the need for such standards is urgent and will become more so as the bulk of the population ages. As people age, their individual histories determine their nutrient needs, depending on diseases they have suffered and on their genetic predispositions to faulty nutrient absorption. Until an improved version of the RDA exists, the present RDA for adults will have to serve. The next sections give special attention to a few nutrients of concern.

Water recommendation for adults: 1 to 1½ oz/kg actual body weight.

Water   Chapter 10 described the importance of water. Older people need to be reminded to drink water and other fluids. Dehydration is a risk for older adults, who may not notice or pay attention to their thirst, or who are unable to obtain water because of immobility. An intake of six to eight glasses of water a day is recommended, enough to bring urine output to about 6 cups per day. A large percentage of nursing home operators note that one of the biggest problems with their elderly clients is getting them to drink more water and fruit juices.

Energy and Energy-Yielding Nutrients Energy needs decrease with advancing age. For one thing, the number of active cells in each organ decreases, bringing about a reduction in the body's overall metabolic rate, although this is not inevitable. For another, older people usually reduce their physical activity (although they need not do so). The recommended food energy intakes for older people reflect an estimated reduction of about 5 percent per decade in energy output. The recommended energy intake for men over the age of 50 is 2,300 kcalories per day; for women, 1,900 kcalories per day. For people 75 and older the requirements are somewhat less.

On such a limited energy allowance, all foods must be nutrient dense. There is little leeway for such low-nutrient-density foods as sugars, fats, oils, or alcohol. Because overweight is well recognized as a shortener of the life span, these seem to be life-sustaining recommendations.

Activities of all kinds are recommended for maintenance of good health. Ideally, exercise should be part of each day's schedule, intense enough to increase the heartbeat and respiration rate for at least 20 minutes, and to prevent muscle atrophy. Many older persons believe that they can't participate in strenuous exercise, but studies have shown that they can do more than they think they can. Any exercise—even a ten-minute walk a day—is better than none, and with persistence, great improvement can be achieved at any age. Training not only improves muscles but also increases the blood flow to the brain. Another reason to exercise: a person spending energy in physical activity can afford to eat more food, and with it, more nutrients.

Energy like this requires continued physical activity and all the nutrients to support it.

The protein needs of older adults appear to be about the same as, or even greater than, those of younger people. Energy needs decrease, however, so the protein has to be obtained from low-kcalorie sources of high-quality protein.

Abundant carbohydrate is needed to protect protein from being used as energy. Complex carbohydrate foods such as vegetables, whole grains, and fruits are also rich in fiber and essential vitamins and minerals.

High-fiber foods can alleviate constipation—a condition prevalent among older adults, and especially among nursing home residents.[46] One group of researchers found that fiber intakes of older adults are not as low as might be expected.[47] The researchers compared the dietary fiber intakes of independent-living older adults and nursing home residents. The researchers discovered that the fiber intakes of the two groups were similar (18 grams per day), and were comparable to the fiber content of typical diets, although still lower than current recommendations (20 to 35 grams).[48] Constipation was more prevalent among the nursing home residents, however. Physical inactivity and greater medication use among the nursing home residents probably contributed to a higher incidence of constipation.

Fiber is discussed in more detail in Chapter 4.

As is true for people of all ages, fat needs to be limited in the diet of older adults, for many reasons. Cutting fat helps cut kcalories and may also help retard the development of atherosclerosis, cancer, and other degenerative diseases (as Chapters 28 and 30 describe). The challenge for older adults is to restrict fat intake to less than 30 percent of total energy while on a limited energy intake.

Vitamins The roles of specific vitamins in disease prevention and development and the age-related physiological changes that affect vitamin metabolism remain unclear. In the meantime, vitamin recommendations for older adults are no different than those for younger adults. Vitamins A and D illustrate why research focusing on the vitamin needs of older adults deserves attention.

Vitamin A stands alone in that there is an apparent *increase* in absorption with aging. When the vitamin A intake and plasma retinol concentrations of healthy older adults and young adults were compared, the older people had higher mean plasma vitamin A concentrations despite little difference in dietary intake between the two groups.[49] This research supports the position to lower the RDA for vitamin A but research into the role of the vitamin A precursor beta carotene in preventing cancer must also be considered in establishing dietary recommendations.

Older adults face a greater risk of vitamin D deficiency than younger people do. Many older adults drink little or no milk.[50] Only vitamin D-fortified milk provides significant amounts of vitamin D. As many as one-third of older adults have vitamin D intakes of less than half of the RDA.[51] Further compromising the vitamin D status of many older people is their limited exposure to sunlight, especially among those in nursing homes.[52] Finally, the potential for vitamin D deficiency in older people is favored by age-related changes in vitamin D synthesis and metabolism.[53] Some authorities suggest that the RDA for vitamin D for older people should be set at 15 to 20 micrograms per day, rather than the 5 micrograms suggested for all adults over age 25.[54]

Adequate vitamin intakes can be ensured by including foods from all food groups. Studies have shown that the one food group omitted most often by the elderly is the vegetable group.[55] About 18 percent of older people are reported to eat no vegetables at all. Fruit is lacking in many diets, and up to one of every three older people reports never eating fruit. Some older adults do not eat whole-grain breads and cereals, a significant source of many B vitamins. Highlight 15 discusses the relationship between some of the B vitamins and the aging brain.

Minerals Among the minerals, iron deserves first mention. Iron-deficiency anemia is not as common in older adults as it is in younger people, but it still occurs in some, especially in those with low food energy intakes.[56] Aside from diet, other factors in many older people's lives increase the likelihood of iron deficiency:

- Chronic blood loss from ulcers, hemorrhoids, or other disease conditions.
- Poor iron absorption due to reduced stomach acid secretion.
- Antacid use, which interferes with iron absorption.
- Use of medicines that cause blood loss, including anticoagulants, aspirin, and other arthritis medicines.

Anyone concerned with the nutrition status of an older person should not forget these possibilities.

Older adults commonly consume diets low in zinc, but this does not appear to jeopardize their zinc status.[57] It is possible that improved absorption compensates for low zinc intakes, but this has not been confirmed; indeed, some research suggests that older adults absorb zinc less efficiently than younger people do.[58] The bright side of the zinc story is that intakes below the RDA may be adequate for some healthy older adults.[59]

The importance of abundant dietary calcium throughout life, especially for women after menopause, to protect against osteoporosis was discussed in Chapter 10. Controversy surrounds the question of what the appropriate calcium intake for older adults is. Some researchers argue that current recommendations are too low for postmenopausal women.[60] Others contend that people adapt to lower calcium intakes by way of increased absorption, so higher intakes are not needed.[61]

While researchers attempt to reach agreement about the calcium requirements of older adults, especially those of women, one aspect of calcium nutriture is not controversial—calcium intakes of many people, especially women, in the United States are well below the RDA. If fresh milk causes stomach discomfort, as some older people report, then cheese should be included in the diet. Dry nonfat milk can be incorporated into many foods.

The determination of mineral requirements for older adults poses many challenges for researchers. Food composition tables are inadequate with respect to some of the minerals. The accuracy of dietary intake studies is thereby hindered when it is not known how much of a certain nutrient is present in foods. Interactions of minerals with other nutrients and drugs affect the bioavailability of the minerals, complicating the process still further. When age-related metabolic changes and disease conditions are superimposed, the task of determining mineral requirements for older people becomes increasingly difficult, but not impossible. The ever-growing number of older people in the world creates an urgency to know more about how their nutrient needs differ from those of younger people, and how such knowledge can enhance their health. In the meantime, people judge for themselves how to manage their nutrition, and some turn to supplements.

Supplements for Older Adults

Advertisers target older people for supplements and "health foods" by claiming that their products prevent disease and promote longevity, claims that attract older people. Despite this, and much to their credit, older adults are, for the most part, reasonable in their approach to so-called health foods—most avoid health food stores, or they buy less there than others do.[62]

Older adults are not always so reasonable in their approach to supplement use. A study in a California retirement community showed that 72 percent of those surveyed were taking supplements—mostly vitamins C and E—but that these choices were not related to the users' dietary intakes.[63] The vitamins they were taking were not the ones they may have needed. Furthermore, some of the older people in this study consumed toxic levels of vitamin A (more than 25,000 IU per day) and more than ten times the RDA of vitamins C and E. One study found that supplement use correlated with medical problems and living alone.[64] Certain diseases or health problems may require supplements, but in this study the vitamins taken were often inappropriate and not prescribed by a health care professional.

Can supplements meet the needs of older people? The answer is sometimes, depending on the nutrient being supplemented. For instance, calcium supplements for osteoporosis or iron for anemia, when recommended by a health care professional, may be beneficial. In most cases, though, the money people spend on supplements would be better spent on nutritious foods. The National Institute on Aging (NIA) states that a well-balanced diet will provide most healthy older people with the nutrients they need.[65] The NIA advises that a well-balanced diet consist of two servings of milk or milk products; two servings of protein-rich foods such as lean meat, fish, and legumes; four servings of fruits and vegetables; and four servings of whole-grain breads and cereals. The chosen foods should be low in fat and high in fiber.

Older adults with food energy intakes less than about 1,500 kcalories should probably take a vitamin-mineral supplement—not a megavitamin, but just a once-daily type of supplement. Many older adults fall into this category and might benefit from a supplement; physically active older adults whose energy needs remain high are an exception. They need to keep in mind that food is the best source of nutrients for everybody and that supplements are just that—supplements to foods, not substitutions for it. For anyone who is motivated to obtain the best possible health, it is never too late to learn to eat well, exercise regularly, and adopt other lifestyle changes to achieve that goal. Inactive adults, rather than taking supplements, would do well to become active and earn the right to eat more food.

The Effects of Drugs on Nutrients

As people get older, illnesses tend to set in, and the use of medicines—from over-the-counter (OTC) types such as aspirins and laxatives to prescription drugs of all kinds—becomes commonplace. Most drugs interact with one or more nutrients in several ways, usually resulting in greater-than-normal needs for these nutrients (see Chapter 18 for more details).

The most common drug that can affect nutrition in older people is alcohol. A recent estimate sets the incidence of alcoholism in people over 60 in our society at 2 to 10 percent. The effects of alcohol on a person of any age are explained in Highlight 7.

OTC drugs are readily available and can be harmful to nutrition. These drugs are useful aids in the self-treatment of minor conditions, but they can easily be misused. For example, a person who uses laxatives daily for a long time may find that the intestines can no longer function without them. This dependence can lead to malnutrition. Laxatives cause a rapid transit time through the intestine, so many vitamins do not have time to be absorbed. The use of mineral oil as a laxative robs the person of the fat-soluble vitamins, including vitamin D. The vitamins dissolve in the indigestible oil and are excreted; calcium, too, is excreted. Antacids also have nutrition effects. A person who takes Alka-Seltzer may not realize it, but it is loaded with sodium—a single 2-tablet dose exceeds some people's safe sodium intake for a whole day. Another antacid (Tums) makes claims to supplement calcium to the diet, but its action as a drug makes it unsuitable for this purpose. It neutralizes stomach acid, on which the absorption of many nutrients (possibly including calcium itself) depends. Taking Tums or any other antacid regularly will cause the body to excrete many nutrients as wastes, rather than absorb them.

Older people use more medications than any other age group. They often take multiple drugs simultaneously, and need to be particularly aware of the nutrition consequences.

Drugs change food intake by:
- Altering the appetite.
- Interfering with taste.
- Inducing nausea or vomiting.
- Causing sores in the mouth.

Drugs change nutrient absorption by:
- Changing GI tract acidity.
- Altering digestive juices.
- Altering GI motility.
- Inactivating enzymes.
- Damaging intestinal cells.

Drugs change nutrient metabolism by:
- Interfering with enzymes.
- Binding to nutrients.

Drugs change nutrient excretion by:
- Altering kidney reabsorption.
- Displacing nutrients from their carriers.

Food Choices and Eating Habits of Older Adults

Research and knowledge about the nutrient requirements of older people are of little use if what is learned cannot be practically applied to benefit those being studied. If nutrition strategies and intervention are to be effective in improving the nutrition status of older adults, then the food likes and dislikes, as well as the living conditions, economic status, and medical conditions, of this diverse group of people must also be considered. It is essential to know what foods older adults prefer, in what settings they like to eat these foods, and whether they can buy and prepare meals, if nutrition intervention is to be successful.

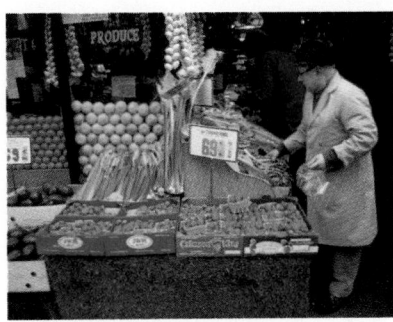

Taking time to nourish your body well is a gift you give yourself.

Many factors affect food choices, eating habits, and the nutrition status of older adults. Information about specific subgroups of older people is lacking, making it difficult to interpret existing research. For instance, nutrition surveys seldom differentiate among older people living alone, those living with others, and those in institutions.[66] Evidence shows that these factors play a significant role in food practices of older adults.[67] One study found higher nutrition scores for diets of older people who lived independently and could maintain traditional eating habits.[68] In a different study, work experience, education, housing (federally funded versus privately owned), and gender influenced food intake.[69] The results indicated that older adults most likely to be at risk of malnutrition were women, those with the least education, those living alone in federally funded housing, and those who had recently experienced a change in lifestyle.

Information about older persons' food consumption and nutrition status is inconsistent, primarily because of differences in socioeconomic status, race, and living conditions of those studied. Overall, it appears that the nutrition status of older adults as a group, in the United States, is better than previously thought. Subgroups of this population may need programs designed to meet specific nutrient deficiencies. Despite the diversity in living conditions and economic status among older adults, some consistency in food choices emerges. For one thing, older people eat limited amounts of fresh plant foods—fruits and especially vegetables. When almost 500 participants in a meal program were surveyed about their food likes and dislikes, nine of the top ten most-disliked foods were vegetables, which are often overcooked or canned in such programs.[70] In a study designed to determine eating habits of older adults, a list of core foods was developed based on how frequently specific foods were eaten.[71] Few fruits and vegetables were among the common core foods. Women eat more fruits and vegetables than men do. In both of these studies and in another one, potatoes were well liked and eaten frequently.[72] Orange juice and bananas were the favorite fruits. Nonfat milk is not well-liked by older adults, probably because they are not accustomed to its taste.

Breakfast appears to be the favorite meal of older adults, and many of them eat a nutritious breakfast daily.[73] In the study of core foods mentioned previously, a large percentage of the foods on the list were breakfast foods such as cereals, eggs, orange juice, and whole-wheat bread.[74] Cheese and meat are also favorite foods.

Taste and health beliefs exert greater influence on food selection by older adults than convenience or price do, although these are influential as well.[75] The importance of diet and health beliefs in food selection is evidenced by surveys indicating that older adults are heavy users of bran cereal, egg substitutes, and decaffeinated coffee.[76] Older people are less likely to diet to lose weight than younger people are, and more likely to diet for medical reasons such as blood sugar control, cholesterol control, and sodium control.

Knowledge about the kinds of foods older people prefer and the reasons why they select or reject foods should be used for developing nutrition intervention programs and acceptable food products. Most older people are independent, productive, health-conscious consumers who know what they want from the foods they purchase. Older people spend more money per person on food they eat at home than other age groups and less money on food away from home.[77] Manufacturers would be wise to cater to the preferences of older adults by providing good-tasting, nutritious foods in easy-to-open, single-serving packages with labels that are easy to read.

Researchers studying nutrition and aging are challenged by the physiological and psychosocial diversity of older adults. Many of the health problems older adults experience are presently attributed to normal, age-related processes, perhaps to the point of overexaggeration.[78] Research that focuses on how nutrition and other life factors affect aging and disease processes is vital to ensuring that more and more people can look forward to long, healthy lives.

Study Questions

1. What is the most prevalent nutrient deficiency among children and adolescents in the United States? What dietary strategies can help prevent this deficiency?
2. Present a daily food pattern to provide good nutrition for children.
3. How do children learn about nutrition outside the home? Discuss the impact of the School Lunch Program, television, and vending machines on the nutrition status of children. How would you encourage children to be more involved in their own nutrition?
4. Discuss the potential benefits and disadvantages of snacking during the teen years. What nutrition problems are common among teenagers?
5. What are some of the physiological changes that occur in the body's systems with aging? Can aging be prevented?
6. What roles does nutrition play in aging, and what roles can it play in retarding aging?
7. Discuss the nutrient needs of the elderly. Which nutrients need special consideration? Explain why.
8. What are some physical, psychological, and financial conditions that may contribute to malnutrition in older people?

Notes

1. L. L. Birch and M. Deysher, Caloric compensation and sensory specific satiety: Evidence for self-regulation of food intake by young children, *Appetite* 7 (1986): 323–331.
2. *Iron Nutrition Revisited—Infancy, Childhood, Adolescence,* The 82nd Ross Conference on Pediatric Research (Columbus, Oh.: Ross Laboratories, 1981), p. 1.
3. D. M. Tucker and H. H. Sandstead, Body iron stores and cortical arousal, in *Iron Deficiency: Brain Biochemistry and Behavior,* eds. E. Pollitt and R. L. Leibel (New York: Raven Press, 1982), pp. 161–182.
4. J. D. Haas and M. W. Fairchild, Summary and conclusions of the International Conference on Iron Deficiency and Behavioral Development, October 10–12, 1988, *American Journal of Clinical Nutrition* 50 (1989): 703–705.
5. R. W. Miller, The metal in our mettle, *FDA Consumer,* December 1988-January 1989, pp. 24–27.
6. S. L. Taylor, Food allergy—The enigma and some potential solutions, *Journal of Food Protection* 43 (1980): 300–306.
7. C. D. May, Food allergy: Perspective, principles, practical management, *Nutrition Today,* November-December 1980, pp. 28–31.
8. R. H. Buckley and D. Metcalfe, Food allergy, *Journal of the American Medical Association* 248 (1982): 2627–2631.
9. D. D. Metcalfe, Diseases of food hypersensitivity, *New England Journal of Medicine* 321 (1989): 255–257.
10. *Diagnostic and Statistical Manual (DSM III),* 3rd ed. (Washington, D.C.: American Psychiatric Association, 1980), p. 41.

11. M. L. Arbeit and coauthors, Caffeine intakes of children from a biracial population: The Bogalusa Heart Study, *Journal of the American Dietetic Association* 88 (1988): 466–471.

12. T. K. Leonard, R. R. Watson, and M. E. Mohs, The effects of caffeine on various body systems: A review, *Journal of the American Dietetic Association* 87 (1987): 1048–1053.

13. Caffeine can increase brain serotonin levels, *Nutrition Today* 46 (1988): 366–367.

14. A. G. Dulloo and coauthors, Normal caffeine consumption: Influence on thermogenesis and daily energy expenditure in lean and postobese human volunteers, *American Journal of Clinical Nutrition* 49 (1989): 44–50.

15. E. Pollitt, R. Leibel, and D. Greenfield, Brief fasting, stress and cognition in children, *American Journal of Clinical Nutrition* 34 (1981): 1526–1533; D. T. Simeon and S. Grantham-McGregor, Effects of missing breakfast on the cognitive functions of school children of differing nutritional status, *American Journal of Clinical Nutrition* 49 (1989): 646–653.

16. L. L. Birch, D. W. Marlin, and J. Rotter, Eating as the "means" activity in a contingency: Effects on young children's food preference, *Child Development* 55 (1984): 431–439.

17. E. M. Satter, *Child of Mine: Feeding with Love and Good Sense* (Palo Alto, Calif.: Bull Publishing, 1986).

18. J. D. Skinner and coauthors, Appalachian adolescents' eating patterns and nutrient intakes, *Journal of the American Dietetic Association* 85 (1985): 1093–1099.

19. J. A. Driskell, A. J. Clark, and S. W. Moak, Longitudinal assessment of vitamin B₆ status in southern adolescent girls, *Journal of the American Dietetic Association* 87 (1987): 307–310; P. Thompson and coauthors, Zinc status and sexual development in adolescent girls, *Journal of the American Dietetic Association* 86 (1986): 892–897; H. McCoy and coauthors, Nutrient intakes of female adolescents from eight southern states, *Journal of the American Dietetic Association* 84 (1984): 1453–1460; A. J. Clark, S. Mossholder, and R. Gates, Folacin status in adolescent females, *American Journal of Clinical Nutrition* 46 (1987): 302–306.

20. L. D. Johnston, P. M. O'Malley, and J. G. Bachman, Psychotherapeutic, licit, and illicit use of drugs among adolescents, *Journal of Adolescent Health Care* 8 (1987): 36–51.

21. L. J. King, J. D. Teale, and V. Marks, Biochemical aspects of cannabis, in *Cannabis and Health,* ed. J. D. Graham (New York: Academic Press, 1976).

22. L. E. Hollister, Marihuana in man: Three years later, *Science* 172 (1971): 21–29.

23. King, Teale, and Marks, 1976; Hollister, 1971.

24. N. C. Doyle, Marihuana and the lungs, a bulletin (November 1979) distributed by the American Lung Association.

25. E. L. Abel, Effects of marihuana on the solution of anagrams, memory and appetite, *Nature* 231 (1971): 260–261; C. T. Tart, Marihuana intoxication: Common experiences, *Nature* 226 (1970): 701–704.

26. L. E. Hollister, Hunger and appetite after single doses of marihuana, alcohol, and dextroamphetamine, *Clinical Pharmacology and Therapeutics* 12 (1971): 44–49; J. D. P. Graham and D. M. F. Li, The pharmacology of cannabis and cannabinoids, in *Cannabis and Health,* 1976.

27. J. M. Jonas and M. S. Gold, Cocaine abuse and eating disorders, *Lancet* 1 (1986): 390–391.

28. Johnston, O'Malley, and Bachman, 1987.

29. R. M. Carney and A. P. Goldberg, Weight gain after cessation of cigarette smoking: A possible role for adipose-tissue lipoprotein lipase, *New England Journal of Medicine* 310 (1984): 614–616.

30. A. M. Fehily, K. M. Phillips, and J. W. G. Yarnell, diet, smoking, social class, and body mass index in the Caerphilly Heart Disease Study, *American Journal of Clinical Nutrition* 40 (1984): 827–833.

31. A. B. Kallner, D. Hartmann, and D. H. Hornig, On the requirements of ascorbic acid in man: Steady-state turnover and body pool in smokers, *American Journal of Clinical Nutrition* 34 (1981): 1347–1355.

32. Dietary carotene and the risk of lung cancer, *Nutrition Reviews* 40 (1982): 265–268.

33. Position of the American Dietetic Association: Nutrition management of adolescent pregnancy, *Journal of the American Dietetic Association* 89 (1989): 104.

34. A. R. Frishancho, J. Matos, and L. A. Bollettino, Influence of growth status and placental function on birth weight of infants born to young still-growing teenagers, *American Journal of Clinical Nutrition* 40 (1984): 801–807.

35. P. M. Guenther, Beverages in the diets of American teenagers, *Journal of the American Dietetic Association* 86 (1986): 493–499.

36. L. Hofmann, ed., *The Great American Nutrition Hassle* (Palo Alto, Calif.: Mayfield Publishing, 1978), p. 89.

37. E. L. Schneider and J. D. Reed, Life extension, *New England Journal of Medicine* 312 (1985): 1159–1168.

38. R. S. Paffenbarger and coauthors, Physical activity, all-cause mortality, and longevity of college alumni, *New England Journal of Medicine* 314 (1986): 605–613.

39. Curtailing calories may lengthen life, *FDA Consumer,* February 1989, pp. 3–4; E. J. Masoro, Food restriction in rodents: An evaluation of its role in the study of aging, *Journal of Gerontology* 43 (1988): B59–64.

40. A. E. Harper, Nutrition, aging, and longevity, *American Journal of Clinical Nutrition* (supplement) 36 (1982): 737–749.

41. The nutritional origin of cataracts, *Nutrition Reviews* 42 (1984): 377–379; F. Rosales and coauthors, Lactose digestion and milk consumption pattern in Guatemalan

cataract patients (abstract), *American Journal of Clinical Nutrition* 43 (1986): 700.

42. The items shown in the margin were listed by K. A. Meister, Can diet cure arthritis? *ACSH News and Views,* September-October 1980, p. 10; and in Morsels and tidbits, *Nutrition and the M.D.,* January 1982.

43. L. G. Darlington, N. W. Ramsey, and J. R. Mansfield, Placebo-controlled, blind study of dietary manipulation therapy in rheumatoid arthritis, *Lancet* 1 (1986): 236–238.

44. J. M. Kremer and coauthors, Fish-oil fatty acid supplementation in active rheumatoid arthritis: A double-blind, controlled crossover study, *Annals of Internal Medicine* 106 (1987): 497–503.

45. N. E. Lane, D. A. Block, and H. H. Jones, Long distance running, bone density, and osteoarthritis, *Journal of the American Medical Association* 255 (1986): 1147–1151.

46. H. Kallman, Constipation in the elderly, *American Family Physician* 27 (1983): 179–184, as cited by E. J. Johnson and coauthors, Dietary fiber intakes of nursing home residents and independent-living older adults, *American Journal of Clinical Nutrition* 48 (1988): 159–164.

47. Johnson and coauthors, 1988; P. M. Suter and R. M. Russell, Vitamin requirements of the elderly, *American Journal of Clinical Nutrition* 45 (1987): 501–512.

48. Position of the American Dietetic Association: Health implications of dietary fiber, *Journal of the American Dietetic Association* 88 (1988): 216.

49. P. J. Garry and coauthors, Vitamin A intake and plasma retinol levels in healthy elderly men and women, *American Journal of Clinical Nutrition* 46 (1987): 989–994.

50. A. M. Parfitt and coauthors, Vitamin D and bone health in the elderly, *American Journal of Clinical Nutrition* (supplement) 36 (1982): 1014–1031.

51. P. J. Garry and coauthors, Nutritional status in a healthy elderly population: Dietary and supplemental intakes, *American Journal of Clinical Nutrition* 36 (1982): 319–331.

52. Vitamin D status of the elderly: Contributions of sunlight exposure and diet, *Nutrition Reviews* 43 (1985):78–80.

53. D. M. Slovik and coauthors, Deficient production of 1,25-dihydroxyvitamin D in elderly osteoporotic patients, *New England Journal of Medicine* 305 (1981): 372–374.

54. Parfitt and coauthors, 1982.

55. V. Holt, J. Nordstrom, and M. B. Kohrs, Food preferences of older adults (abstract), *Journal of the American Dietetic Association* 87 (1987): 1597.

56. S. R. Lynch and coauthors, Iron status of elderly Americans, *American Journal of Clinical Nutrition* (supplement) 36 (1982): 1032–1045.

57. C. A. Swanson and coauthors, Zinc status of elderly adults: Response to supplement, *American Journal of Clinical Nutrition* 48 (1988): 343–349.

58. J. R. Turnlund and coauthors, Stable isotope studies of zinc absorption and retention in young and elderly men

59. Turnlund and coauthors, 1986.

60. H. Spencer, Minerals and mineral interactions in human nutrition, *Journal of the American Dietetic Association* 86 (1986): 864–867.

61. L. H. Allen, The role of nutrition in the onset and treatment of metabolic bone disease, *Nutrition Update* 1 (1983): 263–282.

62. L. Yung, I. Contento, and J. D. Gussow, Use of health foods by the elderly, *Journal of Nutrition Education* 3 (1984): 127–131.

63. G. E. Gray and coauthors, Vitamin supplement use in a Southern California retirement community, *Journal of the American Dietetic Association* 86 (1986): 800–802.

64. B. S. Ranno, G. M. Wardlaw, and C. J. Geiger, What characterizes elderly women who overuse vitamin and mineral supplements? *Journal of the American Dietetic Association* 88 (1988): 347–348.

65. C. Lecos, Diet and the elderly, *FDA Consumer,* November 1984, p. 7.

66. Food and nutrient intakes of individuals in one day in the United States: Spring 1977, USDA/SEA Nationwide Food Consumption Survey, 1977–78, preliminary report no. 2, September 1980, as cited by M. Krondl and coauthors, Food use and perceived food meanings of the elderly, *Journal of the American Dietetic Association* 80 (1982): 523–529.

67. J. S. Atkins and coauthors, Cluster analysis of food consumption patterns of older Americans, *Journal of the American Dietetic Association* 86 (1986): 616–624.

68. M. Clark and L. M. Wakefield, Food choices of institutionalized vs. independent-living elderly, *Journal of the American Dietetic Association* 66 (1975): 600–604.

69. P. O'Hanlon and coauthors, Socioeconomic factors and dietary intake of elderly Missourians, *Journal of the American Dietetic Association* 82 (1983): 646–653.

70. Holt, Nordstrom, and Kohrs, 1987.

71. Krondl and coauthors, 1982.

72. M. Fanelli and K. J. Stevenhagen, Characterizing consumption patterns by food frequency methods: Core foods and variety of foods in diets of older Americans, *Journal of the American Dietetic Association* 85 (1985): 1570–1575.

73. M. Chou, Selling to older Americans (abstract), *Journal of the American Dietetic Association* 80 (1982): 277.

74. Krondl and coauthors, 1982.

75. Krondl and coauthors, 1982; Fanelli and Stevenhagen, 1985.

76. S. B. Sellery, New product opportunities: Diet food for older Americans (abstract), *Journal of the American Dietetic Association* 85 (1985): 128.

77. Chou, 1982.

78. J. W. Rowe and R. L. Kahn, Human aging: Usual and successful, *Science* 237 (1987): 143–149.

(abstract), *Journal of the American Dietetic Association* 86 (1986): 1762.

Nutrition and the Aging Brain

This highlight is dedicated to a topic of great interest to researchers today—the interactions between nutrition and the aging brain. Because the area of inquiry is new and difficult, this discussion comes to no specific conclusions or practical applications. It asks more questions than it can find answers to—and the occasional answers don't always provide an understanding of the relationships between nutrient deficiencies, cognition, and the aging brain. While many of the research implications are only speculative, however, they are fascinating enough to be worth reporting and thinking about.

First, it is necessary to lay groundwork in three areas: the brain, the aging brain, and some of the nutrients essential to brain function. The final section then presents research about nutrient deficiencies, cognition, and the aging brain.

The Brain

The old adage "You can't tell a book by its cover" seems especially apropos of the brain. To look at it, the brain seems an unimpressive lump of convoluted matter, rather like a large sea sponge. Microscopically, though, the brain takes on intrigue as a fantastic communications network more intricate than any man-made computer, possessing billions of connections between its cells. Functionally, it is the body's awesome master, coordinating muscular movement, life-support functions, sensory integrations, thought and memory, and human emotions. Though it accounts for only about 2 percent of an adult's body weight, and though it expends no energy in physical movement, the brain receives 20 percent of the body's blood flow

Cerebral cortex
Cerebrum

■ **FIGURE H15–1**
A Section of the Human Brain

and uses one-quarter of the available oxygen.

Figure H15–1 shows a midsection of a human brain and the accompanying miniglossary defines related terms. The outermost layer, the cerebral cortex, confers the ability to think, remember, and reason. Underlying the cortex is the site of motor coordination (the cerebrum). The centermost structures of the brain make up the limbic system, the seat of the emotions and learning. Although structurally distinct, the various brain parts communicate with one another through numerous physical connections much like telephone wires. Each part acts on information it receives from a variety of sources: from the other brain parts, from the outside world, from stored memory. The brain, of course, dictates the actions of the body at large, everything from orchestrating the many subtle muscular movements needed to play a flute to instructing

the blood vessels to expand or contract.

The cells of the brain are of two types: the neurons, which specialize in transmitting information; and the glial cells, which play a supporting role. Like benevolent caretakers, the glial cells embrace each neuron and sustain its life by providing nutrients and removing wastes via their own internal metabolism.

The structure of a neuron reveals its function (see Figure H15–2). Each neuron possesses thousands of short, spidery projections, the dendrites, through which it receives messages from other neurons. Each neuron also has a long, fiberlike structure, an axon, through which it sends messages to other nerve cells or to target organs. The axons of some neurons in the brain are so long that they run all the way down the spinal cord, where they terminate in thousands more projections, disseminating information to as many

---

Miniglossary

axon: a major fiber emanating from the cell body of a neuron. The axon transports signals away from the cell body.

cerebral cortex: the outer surface of the cerebrum.

cerebrum: the largest part of the brain; it controls voluntary muscle function and higher mental functions.

dendrites: fibrous branches emanating from the cell body of a neuron. Dendrites receive incoming signals.

glial (GLY-al) **cell**: a cell that surrounds, supports, and nourishes a neuron.

limbic system: a group of brain structures whose primary responsibility is the regulation of emotional behavior.

neuron: a nerve cell; the structural and functional unit of the nervous system. Neurons initiate and conduct nerve transmissions.

neurotransmitter: a chemical agent released by one neuron that acts upon a second neuron or upon a muscle or gland cell and alters its electrical state or activity.

senile dementia (SEE-nile dee-MEN-she-ah): the loss of brain function beyond the normal loss of physical adeptness and memory that occurs with aging.

senile dementia of the Alzheimer's type (SDAT): a degenerative disease of the brain involving memory loss and major structural changes in neuron networks; also known as **primary degenerative dementia of senile onset** or **chronic brain syndrome**, and often simply called **Alzheimer's disease**.

synapse: an anatomically specialized junction between two neurons where the activity in one neuron influences the excitability of the second.

---

receiving cells. The brain contains 100 *billion* neurons, each with thousands of sending sites and thousands of receiving sites.

A neuron functions somewhat as a gun does—that is, it either fires a transmission or remains silent. Neurons do not partially fire. Subtle shadings of human experience—for example, how hard a pianist strikes a key—are determined by how many neurons fire and how rapidly. A strong reaction is the result of many neurons' firing in rapid succession. For a lesser reaction, fewer fire in less rapid succession. A neuron fires whenever it receives instructions to do so. When the signals received at the dendrites add up to a threshold level that can make the neuron fire, a chemical chain reaction involving the transfer of electrically charged ions (sodium and potassium) across the axon's

membrane generates an electrochemical signal. That signal travels down the length of the axon along the cell membrane, somewhat as an electrical current travels down a wire.

When a nerve impulse reaches the end of an axon, it transfers the signal to the next neuron through the fluid that separates their membranes. To do this, the neuron releases chemicals, called neurotransmitters, into the fluid-filled space. Neurotransmitters send and receive messages from cell to cell. Figure H15–3 demonstrates how a nerve impulse crosses from one neuron to the next.

Neurons make their own neurotransmitters from the nutrient supplies in the blood that reaches the brain. For a nutrient, or any substance, to reach the brain, it must

have received special clearance, for the body protects the brain from harmful influences more completely than any other organ.

Three barriers offer the brain protection. First, the GI tract cells selectively allow absorption of specific substances. Second, the substances absorbed circulate through the liver, which selectively removes toxins, drugs, and excess quantities of nutrients before allowing the blood to reach other parts of the body. Third, the brain presents its own barrier: a molecular sieve. Called the blood-brain barrier, this protective device normally lets in only those substances the brain cells particularly need: glucose (or ketones), oxygen, amino acids, and other nutrients.

The brain cells make complex molecules for themselves out of the simple building blocks they accept from the passing blood supply. If there is a *deficiency* of an essential nutrient in the blood supply, the brain's supply falls short; if there is an *excess*, or if substances are circulating in the body that the brain doesn't need, the contents of brain cells do not usually reflect these fluctuations. Thus, in general, substances in the brain don't necessarily reflect blood concentrations, but the neurotransmitters are an exception.

At least some of the neurotransmitters are unusual in being subject to precursor control; that is, the neurons respond to a larger or smaller supply of building blocks (precursors) by making larger or smaller amounts of neurotransmitters. Furthermore, these building blocks (nutrients derived from food) are able to penetrate the blood-brain barrier. Thus the food you eat can influence your brain chemistry, to the extent that it produces high concentrations of the precursor nutrients in an available form. These facts link nutrition to brain activity in some intriguing ways.

The neurons store their neurotransmitters in saclike vesicles at the terminal ends of their axons. When the time comes to transmit a message, a neuron opens its vesicles and releases the contents into the space (the synapse) between the two cell membranes. The neurotransmitters traverse the synapse and come to rest on specialized membranes of the receiving cell's dendrites (see Figure H15–3). The receiving cell, recognizing the chemical message, becomes either excited or inhibited, and as mentioned, will fire a signal of its own when excitatory messages have built up to the needed threshold.

The neurotransmitters' life in the synapse is short. After transmission of an impulse, the neuron that released the neurotransmitters whisks them back in or enzymes in the synaptic space destroy them. This wipes clean the synaptic slate for the next rapid-fire message. All of this synaptic activity occurs at lightning speed.

The brain is thought to contain dozens of different types of neurotransmitters, each conveying a unique message. Which message the neighboring cell receives depends upon which type of neurotransmitter is released, and whether that cell's membrane is equipped to recognize it. Some neurotransmitters excite the receiving neurons to fire, and some inhibit such excitation. The sum of many such messages simultaneously arriving at a single receiving cell determines whether that cell will fire or remain silent.

The human nervous system is a communications system of almost unlimited capacity and has many ways to compensate for injury and disease. Yet it is also vulnerable to injury, disease, and aging, just as the rest of the body is—and in some ways, even more so. The next section focuses on the aging brain.

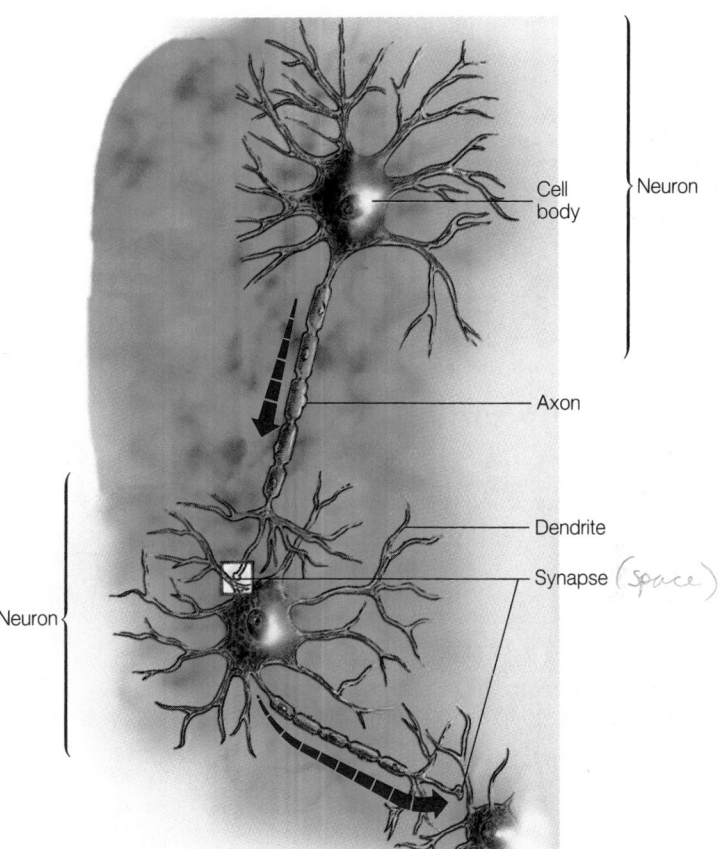

■ FIGURE H15–2
The Structure of a Neuron
The mature human brain is composed of about 100 billion nerve cells, or neurons, which communicate with one another using a combination of electrical and chemical signals. Each neuron is a long, slim cell with receiving structures (dendrites) at one end; a transmitting structure (the axon) at the other; and a bulge, the cell body, between. Electrical impulses arise in the dendrites, pass through the cell body, and continue down the axon to its terminal. When an impulse arrives at the axon terminal, neurotransmitter molecules are released, thus transferring the signal to the next neuron through the fluid that separates their membranes.

The Aging Brain

The choices people make throughout their lives about diet, alcohol and drug use, smoking, and exercise either improve or harm their health, including the health of their brains. Over time, the health effects of these choices accumulate, affecting each organ and in turn, the whole body. The brain, like all of the body's organs, is influenced by both genetic and environmental factors that can enhance or diminish its amazing capacities. One of the challenges researchers face when studying the aging process in human beings is to distinguish among disease processes, normal age-related physiological changes, and changes that are the result of cumulative, extrinsic factors such as diet.

Alzheimer's disease falls in the first of these categories; it is a nonreversible, probably hereditary, dementia. The accompanying box describes its course and its few relationships to nutrition.

The brain ages in some characteristic ways. The number of neurons decreases as people age, and so does blood flow to the brain. When nerve cells in one part of the cerebral cortex

■ **FIGURE H15–3 Nerve Impulse Transmission**

A. The impulse arrives at the end of the first nerve cell. Clustered just inside the nerve cell ending are a multitude of little sacs (vesicles) filled with neurotransmitters.

B. The vesicles fuse with the nerve cell membrane, releasing the neurotransmitters into the gap between cells (synapse).

C. The neurotransmitters arrive at the receiver cell and (in this instance) stimulate it to generate an impulse that will travel along its length. Simultaneously, the receiver cell destroys the molecules of neurotransmitter at its membrane, or the transmitter cell takes them up again to reuse them. Total elapsed time: a fraction of a second.

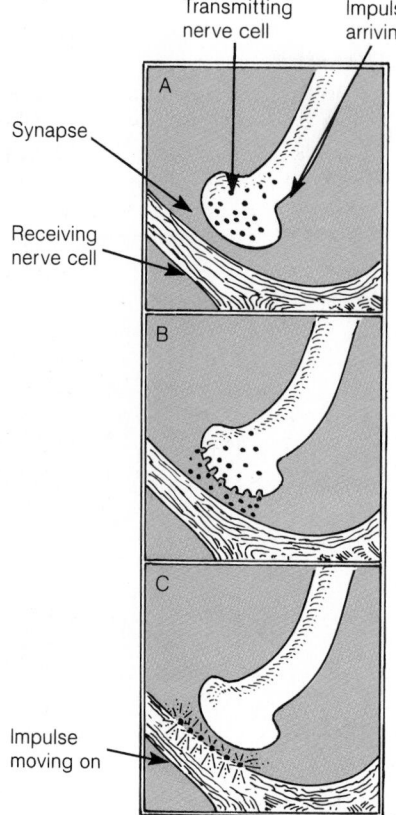

Transmitting nerve cell

Impulse arriving

Synapse

Receiving nerve cell

Impulse moving on

Tryptophan

5-hydroxytryptophan (5-HT)

5-hydroxytryptamine, or serotonin

5-hydroxyindole acetic acid (5-HIAA)

■ **FIGURE H15–4**
The Making of a Neurotransmitter
In the brain, tryptophan is converted to the neurotransmitter serotonin in two steps. Serotonin is then converted to the inactive product 5-HIAA, and 5-HIAA leaves the brain to be excreted. The chemical drawings shown here are simplified by omission of the Cs and Hs in the ring structures.

diminish in number, hearing and speech are affected. Losses of neurons in other parts of the cortex can impair memory and cognitive function. When the number of neurons in the hindbrain diminishes, balance and posture are affected. Losses of neurons in other parts of the brain affect still other functions.

Clinicians now recognize that much of the cognitive loss and forgetfulness generally attributed to aging is due in part to extrinsic, and therefore controllable, factors. In some instances, the degree of cognitive loss is extensive and attributable to a specific disorder that may respond to treatment; many dementias are treatable.

The rest of this discussion explores the concept that moderate, long-term nutrient deficiencies may contribute to the loss of memory and cognition that some older adults may experience. The exploration begins with a brief description of the roles of certain nutrients in brain metabolism. It then goes on to discuss the nutrition status of older adults, along with research that examines the relationship between moderate nutrient deficiencies and cognition.

Nutrition and the Aging Brain

The normal development of the brain depends on an adequate supply of nutrients. For example, severe malnutrition in early childhood curtails the normal increase in brain cell number.[3] The importance of adequate nutrition to the brain continues long after its development, however. As mentioned earlier, the ability of neurons to synthesize specific neurotransmitters depends in part on the availability of precursor nutrients that are obtained from the diet. For example, the neurotransmitter serotonin derives from the amino acid tryptophan (see Figure H15–4).

The enzymes involved in neurotransmitter synthesis require vitamins and minerals for activity.[4] For example, the vitamin B_6 coenzyme, pyridoxal phosphate, is needed for the synthesis of the compound gamma-aminobutyric acid (GABA), which acts as the neurotransmitter at the synapses of inhibitory cells in the nervous system. Vitamin B_6 deficiency interferes with GABA synthesis in the brain. Low concentrations of GABA are associated with convulsions, a symptom common to vitamin B_6 deficiency.

Research on animals and human beings clearly shows that severe dietary deficiencies of thiamin, niacin, vitamin B_6, vitamin B_{12}, folate, and vitamin C impair mental ability, including memory.[5] Trace elements such as iodine, iron, copper and zinc also support normal brain function.[6] For example, many of the enzymes that participate in the synthesis and catabolism of neurotransmitters depend on iron. Iron deficiency may thus interfere with the ability of the neurons to transmit signals to other neurons by way of impaired neurotransmitter synthesis or degradation. Zinc is also essential to many enzymatic systems, including those involved in DNA synthesis, repair, replication, and transcription. One researcher speculates that zinc deficiency impairs enzyme synthesis, causing a cascade of effects in the central nervous system.[7]

Researchers have begun exploring the possibility that the memory impairments observed in people and animals with severe nutrient deficiencies could develop in older adults who have experienced moderate (subclinical) deficiencies for long times. Diet is one of the more controllable components of people's lives. If research reveals significant links between moderate nutrient deficiencies and loss of cognitive function with aging, then through diet, the loss may be preventable, or at least diminished or delayed.

Nutrition and Cognition
Research on both animals and human beings has contributed to present knowledge about nutrition and cognitive function. Caution is necessary when applying the results of animal research to human beings, but animal research enables scientists to conduct studies on the brain that would otherwise be impossible, and to determine directions for future

Alzheimer's Disease

Lately, much attention has focused on the *abnormal* aging of the brain called senile dementia of the Alzheimer's type (SDAT). SDAT may be the most common acquired progressive brain syndrome, afflicting 5 percent of the population by the age of 65 and 20 percent of those over 80.[1]

Physicians can conduct preliminary tests to rule out other possible disorders, but they can only diagnose SDAT with certainty upon autopsy. Its characteristic symptoms make its presence known: gradual loss of memory; loss of the ability to communicate; loss of physical capabilities; and eventually, death.

The cause of SDAT continues to elude researchers, although it appears that there are genetic factors involved. Consequently, researchers have yet to find a cure for this devastating degenerative disease. Treatment involves providing relief and support to both the clients and their families.

Some SDAT characteristics may be relevant to nutrition. For example, normally, as blood flow to the brain diminishes with age, the brain compensates by absorbing more glucose and oxygen. In SDAT, no such compensation occurs, and glucose and oxygen concentrations decline. Whether the brain's diminished capacity to get glucose and oxygen causes or results from SDAT remains unclear. Another abnormality of interest involves the extremely low concentrations of the enzyme that makes the neurotransmitter acetylcholine from choline and acetyl CoA.

You may have heard that aluminum contributes to the development of SDAT, although its role, if any, has not yet been defined. Brain concentrations of aluminum in SDAT people do exceed normal brain concentrations by some 10 to 30 times—but blood and hair levels remain normal, indicating that the accumulation is caused by something in the brain itself, not by something in the environment. However, an epidemiological survey found that the risk of SDAT was 1½ times greater in areas where water aluminum concentrations were high compared with areas where concentrations were low, indicating that environmental aluminum may have a role.[2] Current research is investigating the relationship between dietary aluminum and SDAT in individuals; aluminum cookware can increase the aluminum content of foods slightly, but whether this significantly affects the progress of SDAT is unknown.

Maintaining appropriate body weight may be the most important nutrition concern for the person with SDAT. Depression and forgetfulness can lead to a poor dietary intake, and restlessness may increase energy needs. Perhaps the best that a caretaker can do nutritionally for an SDAT client is to supervise food planning and mealtimes. Providing well-balanced meals and snacks in a cheerful atmosphere encourages food consumption. To minimize confusion, offer a few ready-to-eat foods (in bite-size pieces, with seasonings and sauces) appropriate to the person's likes. To avoid mealtime disruptions, control distractions such as television, children, and the telephone.

research. Further research is needed to determine whether mild, long-term nutrient deficiencies result in brain cell changes similar to those observed in, for example, rats with severe deficiency, but the studies reported here represent a start in that direction. In human beings, multiple nutrient deficiencies are more likely than individual deficiencies, because nutrients occur in foods in combination. A lifetime of multiple nutrient deficiencies could conceivably contribute to mental impairment in later life by way of brain cell degeneration.

The studies that follow each take a different tack. None alone provides direct evidence of the effect nutrition has on brain activity, but together, they show that nutrient deficits do hasten the onset of impaired cognitive functioning, and they give the impression that adequate nutrition would forestall, if not reverse, the observed degeneration.

Water-Soluble Vitamins
One group of researchers studied the relationship between nutrition status and cognitive functioning in more than 200 healthy, independent-living men and women over 60 years of age.[8] The researchers evaluated nutrient intakes by way of diet records, and nutrition status by way of biochemical tests. Participants in the study were given two tests of cognitive function. One was a test of short-term memory (Wechsler Memory Test) and the other, a test of problem-solving ability (Halstead-Reitan Categories Test). Participants with low blood concentrations of vitamin C or vitamin B_{12} scored worse than better-nourished participants on both tests. Those with low blood concentrations of riboflavin or folate scored worse on the problem-solving test.

It is important to note that even the lowest scores in this study were still within the normal range for men and women of the same age. The researchers point out that the relationship between poor cognition

and poor nutrition might be compared with the question of whether the chicken or the egg came first. It is possible that poor cognition is, itself, a risk factor for poor nutrition. People with impaired cognition might be less adept at meal preparation. However, the participants in this study had no history of dementia or impaired mental status, and so the researchers concluded that poor nutrition status might contribute to poor cognitive functioning in healthy elderly people. Studies of older populations at greater risk of malnutrition than this population might provide more insight into the relationship between nutrition and the aging brain.

Vitamin B_{12}
Memory impairment due to vitamin B_{12} deficiency can precede the blood symptoms of deficiency by years.[9] Dietary deficiency of vitamin B_{12} is rare, but inadequate absorption is common, accounting for more than 95 percent of deficiencies seen.[10] As many as 50 percent of people over the age of 60 are affected by atrophic gastritis, a condition that can impair vitamin B_{12} absorption.[11]

Evidence that vitamin B_{12} deficiency accounts for some cognitive deficits in older people comes from a study that revealed abnormal short-term memory in more than two-thirds of clients with pernicious anemia.[12] Treatment with vitamin B_{12} restored memory within one month in three-fourths of the clients. The researchers recommend that a diagnosis of senile dementia should not be made, even in the absence of anemia, until vitamin B_{12} status is determined biochemically.

Thiamin
It is estimated that as many as 3 million people over the age of 60 abuse alcohol.[13] As Highlight 7 describes, alcohol displaces food from the diet and alters normal nutrient metabolism, causing multiple nutrient deficiencies. Thiamin deficiency is common in alcoholics and is at least partially responsible for the mental

symptoms that can accompany alcoholism.[14]

Surveys indicate that 5 percent of people over the age of 60 have impaired thiamin status.[15] Small amounts of thiamin are present in nearly all whole foods, but people with low food energy intakes or those who do not eat foods from all four food groups risk thiamin deficiency. As Chapter 15 mentioned, energy intake declines with age, and older people frequently fail to eat foods from all four groups.[16]

It is clear that mental impairment occurs with severe thiamin deficiency, but it is unclear whether mental impairment accompanies moderate deficiency. Limited research suggests that older people may be more susceptible to the effects of subclinical thiamin deficiency than younger people.[17] When thiamin was restricted in the diets of ten women between the ages of 52 and 72, irritability, fatigue, and headaches occurred after 12 days. Women between the ages of 18 and 21 did not experience these symptoms with the same level of thiamin restriction.

Copper and Vitamin B_6
One study showed that changes in the brains of young rats subjected to dietary deficiencies of copper and vitamin B_6 resembled the degenerative changes that occur in the brains of human beings as they age.[18] The rats in this study ate diets extremely deficient in vitamin B_6, an unlikely situation for human beings, but vitamin B_6 intakes of many older adults vary, and many people are ingesting amounts well below recommendations.[19]

Iron
Iron deficiency is prevalent worldwide, especially among infants, children, and young women. Research on children shows a relationship between iron deficiency and cognitive function.[20] Researchers examining iron status and cognition in college students found a relationship between body iron stores

and cognition.[21] The exact relationship is unclear, but iron status appeared to influence tasks dominated by the left side of the brain differently from tasks dominated by the right side. For example, higher iron status was associated with better word fluency performance (a left brain–dominated task), but with poorer performance of right brain–dominated tasks. (All of the students in this study were right-handed.) Animal research further supports a relationship between iron deficiency and cognition.[22] The offspring of rats fed an iron-deficient diet were less responsive (they reared on their hind legs and stood immobile less frequently) to adverse, novel stimuli than were the offspring of iron-sufficient mice.

Iron deficiency is not as widespread among older adults as it is among other groups, but it does occur. Perhaps more significant with respect to iron and cognitive function in later life are the effects of long-term moderate deficiency so common in women prior to menopause—especially women with either repeated pregnancies or limited food energy intakes. In view of the widespread occurrence of iron deficiency, its role in mental function deserves further research.

Zinc

Surveys indicate that zinc intakes in the United States are below recommended levels.[23] As many as one-fourth of older women have zinc intakes less than one-half of the recommended allowance.[24] A study in England showed that people with senile dementia had much lower levels of zinc than those without dementia.[25] As the number of people over age 65 continues to grow, the urgent need for solutions to the problems that this major portion of the population faces becomes apparent. Senile dementia and other losses of brain function afflict millions of older adults. Some may be inevitable, but some are preventable. The search for ways to prevent or delay brain dysfunction

should be a high priority for researchers investigating nutrition for older people. The findings reported here on possible relationships between dementia and nutrition offer promise as a reasonable approach to a devastating problem.

It is clear that severe nutrient deficiencies impair cognition, but the effects of moderate deficiencies are less clear. It is also clear that a person's nutrition status affects the health and functioning of the whole body. Eating a nutritious, balanced diet throughout life seems a minimal effort to make in support of continued health and the enjoyment of later life.

In addition, there is much people can do, besides obtaining adequate nutrition, to support a high quality of life into old age. By practicing stress-management skills, maintaining physical fitness, participating in activities of interest, and cultivating spiritual health, a person can grow old gracefully.

NOTES

1. Much of the discussion on Alzheimer's disease came from M. S. Claggett, Nutritional factors relevant to Alzheimer's disease, *Journal of the American Dietetic Association* 89 (1989): 392–396.
2. C. N. Martyn and coauthors, Geographical relation between Alzheimer's disease and aluminum drinking water, *Lancet* 1 (1989): 59–62.
3. M. Winick and P. Rosso, The effect of severe early malnutrition on cellular growth of human brain, *Pediatric Research* 10 (1976): 57–61.
4. W. M. Lovenberg, Biochemical regulation of brain function, *Nutrition Reviews* (supplement), May 1986, pp. 6–11.
5. K. Yoshimura and coauthors, Animal experiments on thiamine avitaminosis and cerebral function, *Journal of Nutritional Science and Vitaminology* 22 (1976): 429–437, as cited by A. Cherkin, Effects of nutritional factors on memory function, in *Nutritional Intervention in the Aging Process*, eds. H. J. Armbrecht, J. M. Prendergast, and R. M. Coe (New York: Springer-Verlag, 1984), pp. 229–249; M. K. Horwitt, Niacin, in *Modern Nutrition in Health and Disease*, 6th ed., eds. R. S. Goodhart and M. S. Shils (Philadelphia: Lea and Febiger, 1980), pp. 204–208; C. S. Russ and coauthors, Vitamin B_6 status of depressed and obsessive-compulsive patients, *Nutrition Reports International* 27 (1983): 867–873; J. S. Goodwin, J. M. Goodwin, and P. J. Garry, Association between nutritional status and cognitive functioning in a healthy elderly population, *Journal of the American Medical Association* 249 (1983): 2917–2921.
6. H. Sandstead, A brief history of the influence of trace elements on brain function, *American*

Journal of Clinical Nutrition 43 (1986): 293–298.
7. F. M. Burnet, A possible role of zinc in the pathology of dementia, *Lancet* 1 (1981): 186–188.
8. Goodwin, Goodwin, and Garry, 1983.
9. Cherkin, 1984.
10. V. Herbert, Recommended dietary intakes (RDI) of vitamin B_{12} in humans, *American Journal of Clinical Nutrition* 45 (1987): 671- 678.
11. M. Siurala and coauthors, Prevalence of gastritis in a rural population, *Scandinavian Journal of Gastroenterology* 3 (1968): 211–223, as cited by P. Suter and R. M. Russell, Vitamin requirements of the elderly, *American Journal of Clinical Nutrition* 45 (1987): 501–512.
12. R. W. Strachan and J. G. Henderson, Psychiatric syndromes due to avitaminosis B_{12} with normal blood and marrow, *Journal of Medicine* 34 (1965): 303–317, as cited by Cherkin, 1984.
13. P. J. Bloom, Alcoholism after sixty, *American Family Physician* 28 (1983): 111–113.
14. M. Victor, Alcohol and nutritional diseases of the nervous system, *Journal of the American Medical Association* 167 (1958): 65–71.
15. F. L. Iber and coauthors, Thiamin in the elderly—Relation to alcoholism and to neurological degenerative disease, *American Journal of Clinical Nutrition* 36 (1982): 1067–1082.
16. V. Holt, J. Nordstrom, and M. B. Kohrs, Food preferences of older adults (abstract), *Journal of the American Dietetic Association* 87 (1987): 1597.
17. H. G. Oldham, Thiamin requirements of women, *Annals of the New York Academy of Sciences* 378 (1982): 542–549, as cited by R. H. Haas, Thiamin and the brain, in *Annual Review of Nutrition*, eds. R. E. Olson, E. Beutler, and H. P. Broquist (Palo Alto, Calif.: Annual Reviews, 1988), pp. 483–515.
18. E. J. Root and J. B. Longenecker, Brain cell alterations suggesting premature aging induced by dietary deficiency of vitamin B_6 and/or copper, *American Journal of Clinical Nutrition* 37 (1983): 540–552.
19. P. J. Garry and coauthors, Nutritional status in a healthy elderly population: Dietary and supplemental intakes, *American Journal of Clinical Nutrition* 36 (1982): 319–331; J. R. Turnlund, Copper nutriture, bioavailability, and the influence of dietary factors, *Journal of the American Dietetic Association* 88 (1988): 303–308.
20. E. Pollitt and coauthors, Iron deficiency and behavioral development in infants and preschool children, *American Journal of Clinical Nutrition* 43 (1986): 555–565.
21. D. M. Tucker and coauthors, Iron status and brain function: Serum ferritin levels associated with asymmetries of cortical electrophysiology and cognitive performance, *American Journal of Clinical Nutrition* 39 (1984): 105–113.
22. J. Weinberg, Behavioral and physiological effects of early iron deficiency in the rat, in *Iron Deficiency: Brain Biochemistry and Behavior*, eds. E. Pollitt and R. L. Leibel (New York: Raven Press, 1982), pp. 93–123.
23. K. Patterson and coauthors, Zinc, copper, and manganese intake and balance for adults consuming self-selected diets, *American Journal of Clinical Nutrition* 40 (1984): 1397–1403.
24. Garry and coauthors, 1982.
25. R. Hullin, Zinc deficiency: Can it cause dementia? *Therapaeica*, September 1983, pp. 26, 27, 30.

16

Consumer Concerns about Foods

Contents

People seldom realize that the foods they eat often have a complex microstructure, as do their own bodies' tissues. Shown here is a sample of dough; the large spheres are starch granules, and the coating is a film of gluten (protein).

494

To this point, this book has focused primarily on the nutrients and how your body handles them. Along the way, it has offered some practical pointers about foods—but no chapter has focused on foods themselves. What do they contain, besides nutrients? What are the contaminants, pesticides, and additives in foods, and what are their effects? What does public water contain, and is it safe to drink?

This chapter provides answers to some of these consumer questions. The chapter takes up the following concerns in the order in which the FDA has prioritized them:

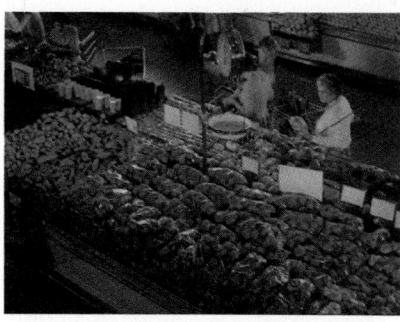

Consumers can select from an abundant supply of a large variety of safe foods.

1. Food-borne illnesses.
2. Nutritional adequacy of foods (reserved for the end of this chapter and Highlight 16, "Nutrition Labeling").
3. Environmental contaminants.
4. Naturally occurring toxicants in foods.
5. Pesticide residues.
6. Food additives.

The chapter closes with a look at public drinking water. The miniglossary here identifies the various food regulatory agencies by their abbreviations.

Before beginning the following sections on each of these areas of concern, take a moment to consider the vastness of the task at hand—supplying food to over 250 million people in the United States. To feed this nation requires farmers to grow and harvest crops; dairy producers to supply milk products and eggs; ranchers to raise livestock; shippers by land, sea, and air to deliver food products to manufacturers and markets; manufacturers to prepare, process, preserve, and package the products for the refrigerated food cases and

---

Miniglossary of Agencies That Monitor the Food Supply

CDC (Centers for Disease Control): a branch of the Department of Health and Human Services, responsible for, among other things, monitoring food-borne diseases.

EPA (Environmental Protection Agency): a federal agency responsible for, among other things, regulating pesticides and establishing water quality standards.

FAO (Food and Agriculture Organization): an international agency that has adopted standards to regulate pesticide use, among other responsibilities.

FDA (Food and Drug Administration): a part of the Department of Health and Human Services' Public Health Service responsible for ensuring the safety and wholesomeness of all foods sold in interstate commerce except for meat, poultry, and eggs (which are under the jurisdiction of the USDA).

USDA (U.S. Department of Agriculture): the federal agency responsible for enforcing standards for the wholesomeness and quality of meat, poultry, and eggs produced in the United States; conducting nutrition research; and educating the public about nutrition.

WHO (World Health Organization): an international agency that has adopted standards to regulate pesticide use, among other responsibilities.

grocery store shelves; and grocers to store the food and supply it to the consumers. After much time, many people, and extensive transport, an abundant supply of a large variety of safe foods finally reaches the consumers at reasonable market prices.

Monitoring any system as large as this requires a nationwide network of people and sophisticated equipment. In addition, government monitoring agencies must stay within their budgets. While consumers can rely on sound standards set by these agencies, individual infractions of those standards occasionally escape enforcement, at least temporarily. Often, consumers can protect themselves by knowing of the risks and learning how to avoid them. This chapter presents some of the knowledge that can help you avoid becoming ill.

■ Food-Borne Illnesses

food-borne illness: illness transmitted to human beings through food, caused by either a poisonous substance *(food intoxication)* or an infectious agent *(food-borne infection)*.

Food-borne illnesses top the FDA's list of food hazard priorities; over 40 percent of the FDA's budget and close to half of its personnel are dedicated to food-borne illnesses. Just about everyone experiences a food-borne illness (whether they realize it or not) at least once a year.[1] For some people—the very young, the very old, the sick, and the malnourished—the symptoms can be so severe as to cause death. If you take the proper precautions, however, you can reduce your chances of ever having it again.

The term *food-borne illness* refers to both food-borne infections and food intoxications. Table 16–1 summarizes some of the more common food-borne illnesses, their most frequent food sources, and general symptoms. Food-borne infections are caused by eating foods contaminated by infectious microbes. The most common infectious microbe is *Salmonella*, which enters the GI tract within contaminated foods such as poultry and eggs. Symptoms generally include abdominal cramps, headache, vomiting, and diarrhea. If you experience these symptoms as the major or only symptoms of your next bout of "flu," chances are excellent that what you really have is a food-borne illness.*

Food intoxications are caused by eating foods containing natural toxins or, more likely, microbes that produce toxins. The most infamous, but not common, example is *Clostridium botulinum*, the organism that can grow in improperly canned foods and that produces the deadly botulinum toxin. Botulism danger signs include double vision, weakening muscles, and difficulty swallowing or breathing. Botulism requires immediate medical attention, and even then, survivors suffer the effects for months or years. An amount of botulinum toxin as tiny as a single crystal of salt can kill several people within an hour.

botulism (BOTT-you-lism): an often-fatal food-borne illness caused by the ingestion of foods containing **botulinum** (bot-you-LINE-um) **toxin**, a toxin produced by bacteria that grow in improperly canned foods.

Between 21 million and 81 million cases of diarrhea related to food-borne illness are treated in the United States each year; infection from one major food supplier can cause many thousands of cases of illness. For example, when a major dairy experienced a flaw in its pasteurization system, over 16,000 confirmed, and as many as 200,000 suspected, cases of food poisoning resulted; in another episode, 100 people died of infection.[2] Consumers have little protection against such large-scale calamities; they must trust federal

*Some viruses do cause intestinal distress, and those that do are usually transmitted via food; true influenza viruses cause symptoms primarily in the upper respiratory tract.

■ TABLE 16–1
Food-Borne Illnesses

Disease and Organism That Causes It	Most Frequent Food Source	General Symptoms
Botulism Botulinum toxin (produced by *Clostridium botulinum* bacteria)	Anaerobic (no oxygen) environment of little acidity, such as canned corn, peppers, green beans, soups, beets, asparagus, mushrooms, ripe olives, spinach, tuna, chicken, chicken liver, liver pâté, luncheon meats, ham, sausage, stuffed eggplant, lobster, and smoked and salted fish.	Onset: 4 to 36 hr after eating. Nervous system symptoms, including double vision, inability to swallow, speech difficulty, and progressive paralysis of the respiratory system; often fatal; leaves prolonged symptoms in survivors.
Campylobacteriosis *Campylobacter jejuni* bacteria	Poultry, beef, lamb, milk.	Onset: 2 to 5 days after eating. Diarrhea, abdominal cramping, fever and sometimes bloody stools; lasts 7 to 10 days.
Giardiasis *Giardia lamblia* protozoa	Contaminated water; uncooked foods.	Diarrhea (but occasionally constipation), abdominal pain, gas, abdominal distention, digestive disturbances, anorexia, nausea, and vomiting.
Perfringens food poisoning *Clostridium perfringens* bacteria	Meats and meat products stored at between 120 and 130° F.	Onset: 8 to 12 hr (usually 12) after eating. Abdominal pain and diarrhea, sometimes nausea and vomiting; symptoms last a day or less and are usually mild; can be more serious in old or weak people.
Salmonellosis *Salmonella* bacteria (more than 2,000 kinds)	Raw meats, poultry, milk and other dairy products, shrimp, frog legs, yeast, coconut, pasta, and chocolate.	Onset: 6 to 48 hr after eating. Nausea, vomiting, abdominal cramps, diarrhea, fever, and headache; can be fatal.
Staphylococcal food poisoning Staphylococcal toxin (produced by *Staphylococcus aureus* bacteria)	Toxin produced in meats, poultry, egg products, tuna, potato and macaroni salads, and cream-filled pastries.	Onset: ½ to 8 hr after eating. Diarrhea, vomiting, nausea, abdominal cramps, and prostration; mimics flu; lasts 24 to 48 hr; rarely fatal.

Source: Adapted from F. E. Young and K. J. Skinner, Summer food safety tips, *FDA Consumer,* June 1987, pp. 17–19.

agencies to enforce strict standards to prevent all but truly unavoidable accidents. Fortunately, large-scale incidents, while dramatic, make up only a fraction of the total food poisoning cases each year. Most arise from one person's error in a small setting, and affect just a few victims. Some people have come to accept a yearly bout or two of intestinal illness as inevitable, but in truth, most of these illnesses can be prevented.

In general, commercially prepared food is usually safe. Batch numbering makes it possible for suppliers to recall contaminated foods through public announcements via newspapers, television, and radio. In the grocery store, carefully inspect the seals, safety "buttons," and wrappers of packages. A broken seal or mangled package fails to protect the product against microbes, insects, and spoilage. Raw foods from the grocery store, especially meats and poultry, contain microbes. Whether microbes multiply and cause illness depends, in part, on what you do or fail to do in the grocery store and in your own kitchen.

The "2–40–140" rule will help you to remember the time and temperature danger zone for foods—no more than 2 hr between 40° F and 140° F.

Safety in the Kitchen

Almost one-third of all food-borne illnesses arises from home kitchens.[3] For the most part, illness episodes can be prevented by doing three simple things: keeping hot food hot; keeping cold food cold; and keeping hands, utensils, and the kitchen clean.

Keeping hot food hot includes allowing sufficient cooking time for food to reach safe internal temperatures during cooking, and holding the food at a high enough temperature to prevent bacterial growth until it is served. Keeping cold food cold begins when you go directly home upon leaving the grocery store and immediately unpack foods into the refrigerator or freezer upon your arrival. Keeping a clean kitchen requires that you wash the countertops, your hands, and utensils in warm, soapy water before and after each step of food preparation. (See Table 16–2 for specific food safety tips.)

■ TABLE 16–2
How to Prevent Food-Borne Illnesses

To Keep Hot Foods Hot
- When cooking meats or poultry, use a thermometer to test the internal temperature. Insert the thermometer between the thigh and the body of the turkey, or in the thickest part of other meats, making sure the tip of the thermometer is not in contact with bone or the pan. Cook to the temperature indicated for that particular meat; cook hamburgers to at least medium well-done.
- Cook stuffing separately, or stuff poultry just prior to cooking.
- Do not cook large cuts of meats or turkeys in a microwave oven.
- Cook eggs before eating them (boiled for 7 min, poached for 5 min, and fried for 3 min on each side).
- When serving foods, maintain temperatures above 140° F.
- Heat leftovers thoroughly.

To Keep Cold Foods Cold
- When running errands, stop at the grocery store last. When you get home, refrigerate the perishable groceries (such as meats and dairy products) immediately. Do not leave perishables in the car any longer than it takes for ice cream to melt.
- Buy only those foods that are solidly frozen and stored below the frost line in store freezers.
- Keep cold foods at 40° F or less.
- Refrigerate leftovers promptly; use shallow containers to help foods cool faster.
- Thaw meats or poultry in the refrigerator, not at room temperature. If you must hasten thawing, use cool running water or a microwave oven.

To Keep a Clean Kitchen
- Use hot, soapy water to wash hands, utensils, dishes, nonporous cutting boards, and countertops. Use a bleach solution to clean wooden cutting boards.
- Avoid cross-contamination by washing all surfaces that have been in contact with raw meats, poultry, or eggs.
- Mix foods with utensils, not hands; keep hands and utensils away from mouth, nose, and hair.
- Anyone may be a carrier of bacteria and should avoid coughing or sneezing over food. A person with a skin infection or infectious disease should not prepare food.

Meat requires special handling. It may contain bacteria, and its moist, nutrient-rich environment favors microbial growth. (Ground meat is especially susceptible, because it receives more handling than other kinds of meat, and has more surface exposed to bacterial contamination.) Consumers have no way to detect the presence of harmful bacteria in or on meat. A USDA seal on raw meat or poultry indicates that it has been inspected for quality, but does not guarantee that it is free of potentially harmful bacteria. When buying meat, consumers take on the responsibility of handling it in such a way that the bacteria present won't cause a food-borne illness. Wash any surfaces (such as cutting boards or platters) that have been in contact with raw meat with hot, soapy water before using them again for the cooked meat or raw produce; otherwise, the bacteria inevitably left on the surfaces from the raw

■ **TABLE 16–2** (continued)

- Wash or replace sponges and towels regularly. (Cook wet sponges and cloths on "high" in a microwave oven until they are steamy and hot, or launder them with bleach; sponge a bleach solution over the cutting board, to sterilize two kitchen items at once.)
- Clean up food spills and crumb-filled crevices.

In General
- Throw out foods with danger-signaling odors. Be aware, though, that most food poisoning bacteria are odorless, colorless, and tasteless.
- Do not even taste food that is suspect.
- Do not buy or use items that appear to have been opened.
- Follow label instructions for storing and preparing packaged and frozen foods.

For Specific Food Items
- *Canned goods.* Discard food from cans that leak or bulge in a manner that will protect other people and animals from its accidental ingestion; before canning, seek professional advice from the USDA Extension Service (check your phone book under United States government listings, or ask directory assistance).
- *Cheeses.* Aged cheeses, such as Cheddar and Swiss, do well for an hour or two without refrigeration, but should be refrigerated or stored in an ice chest for longer periods.
- *Eggs.* Use clean eggs with intact shells.
- *Honey.* Honey may contain dormant bacterial spores, which can awaken in the human body to produce botulism. In adults, this poses little hazard, but infants under one year of age should never be fed honey. Honey can accumulate enough toxin to kill an infant; it has been implicated in several cases of sudden infant death. (Honey can also be contaminated with environmental pollutants picked up by the bees.)
- *Mayonnaise.* Commercially prepared mayonnaise may actually help a food to resist spoilage because of its acid content. Still, keep mayonnaise cold after opening.
- *Mixed salads.* Mixed salads of chopped ingredients spoil easily because they have extensive surface area for bacteria to invade, and they have been in contact with cutting boards, hands, and kitchen utensils that easily transmit bacteria to food (regardless of their mayonnaise content). Chill them well before, during, and after serving.
- *Picnic foods.* Choose foods that last without refrigeration such as fresh fruits and vegetables, breads and crackers, and canned spreads and cheeses that can be opened and used immediately.

meat can recontaminate the cooked meat or start to grow in the other foods. (This is called *cross-contamination*.)

Eating raw or lightly steamed seafood is a risky proposition, even if it is eaten in sushi prepared by a master Japanese chef.[4] The microorganisms that lurk in seafood are undetectable without a microscope. As population density increases along the shores of seafood-harvesting waters, pollution of those waters inevitably invades the creatures living there. Watchdog agencies that monitor the commercial fishing waters to keep harvesters out of contaminated areas catch some cheaters, but they cannot catch them all, and unwholesome foods can reach the market.[5] In one season alone, black-market dealers sold millions of dollars worth of clams and oysters taken illegally from closed harvesting areas.[6]

The food-borne infections that lurk in normal-appearing seafood can cause severe illnesses—hepatitis, worms, parasites, viral intestinal disorders, and other diseases. People who love raw seafood and have eaten it for years may try to brush off these threats because they have never experienced serious illness. Now, though, experts say that the risks of consuming raw or lightly cooked seafood are unacceptably high.

Finally, keep in mind that fresh food generally smells fresh. You cannot detect all types of food poisoning by odor, but some bacterial wastes produce off odors. These odors can serve as a signal that the numbers of bacteria in the food exceed safety limits. If an abnormal odor exists, consider the food spoiled, and throw it out or return it to the grocery store. Do not even taste it.

Local health departments and the USDA Extension Service can give further information about food safety, especially about issues in your particular area. Should precautions fail and mild food-borne illness develop, drink clear liquids to replace fluids lost through vomiting and diarrhea. If serious food-borne illness is suspected:

1. Call your physician.
2. Wrap and label the remainder of the suspected food, along with its container, so that it cannot be mistakenly used; place it in the refrigerator; and hold it for possible inspection by health authorities.
3. Notify the Health Hazard Evaluation Board of the FDA's Bureau of Foods, a panel of scientists and health experts who assess how serious a threat to health a food may be (see Appendix F for the FDA's address).

Food Safety while Traveling

If you travel to distant lands, you have a 50–50 chance of contracting traveler's diarrhea, a sometimes serious, always annoying, bacterial infection of the digestive tract. The risk is high because, for one thing, other countries' cleanliness standards are often lower than those at home. For another, every region's microbes are different, and while you are immune to those in your own neighborhood, you have had no chance to develop immunity to the pathogens in a place you are visiting for the first time. You can take some steps to protect your health against disease-causing organisms not found at home.

To avoid illness:

- Wash your hands often with soap and water, especially before handling food or eating.
- Eat only cooked food and commercially canned items. Eat raw fruit or vegetables only if you have washed them in sterile water and peeled them yourself. Skip salads and salad dressings.
- Drink only boiled, canned, or bottled beverages, and drink them without ice, even if they are not chilled to your liking.
- Sterilize or boil the local water before using it, even if you are just brushing your teeth.
- Check with your physician before you leave on the trip for recommendations on which medicines to take along in case your efforts to avoid illness fail.

Chances are excellent, if you follow the rules above, that you will avoid food-borne illness.

The FDA maintains food-borne illness as the number 1 food safety concern, because episodes of food poisoning far outnumber episodes of any other kind of food contamination, affecting millions of people every year. The second concern, environmental contaminants in foods, grows in importance as the world grows more populated and more industrialized.

■ *Environmental Contaminants*

A contaminant of a food is anything that does not belong there. The term used broadly includes the microbes already discussed, harmful substances from industry, pesticide residues, bits of packaging, and ordinary dirt. The term as used here applies to harmful substances from industry; it includes pesticides only when they are accidentally spilled in large quantities into food. A later section deals with pesticides as ordinarily used, and bits of packaging are classed as incidental additives, discussed still later.

contaminant: a substance that does not normally occur in a food.

The potential harmfulness of a contaminant depends in part on its persistence—the extent to which it lingers in the environment or in the human body. If the environment can break the contaminant down before it enters the food chain, then there may be no cause for concern; but when a substance resists breakdown, and furthermore accumulates from one species to the next, it builds up in the food chain. Figure 16–1 shows how this happens. Similarly, if the body can rapidly excrete the contaminant or metabolize it to a harmless compound, then its ingestion may not give cause for concern; the body may be able to survive a brief exposure time. But if the contaminant enters and interacts with the body's systems, without being metabolized or excreted, then it presents a danger. Additional doses may accumulate and cause significant harm. Figure 16–2 shows how contaminants find their way into our food.

persistence: stubborn or enduring continuance; with respect to food contaminants, the quality of persisting in the bodies of animals and human beings.

Contaminants can be difficult to regulate. Many of them have been around for only a short time. Sometimes they are hard to identify, and sometimes their presence is not even known. We have yet to learn of the effects of prolonged

■ **FIGURE 16–1**

How a Food Chain Works

A person whose principal animal-protein source is fish may consume about 100 lb of fish in a year. These fish will, in turn, have consumed a few tons of plant-eating fish in the course of their lifetimes. The plant eaters, in their lifetimes, will have consumed several tons of photosynthetic producer organisms.

The concern about persistent contaminants is implicit in this pyramid. Assuming 100% retention of the contaminant at each level (an oversimplification), a person, being at the top of the food chain, could ingest in a year the amount of contaminant that had accumulated in several tons of producer organisms.

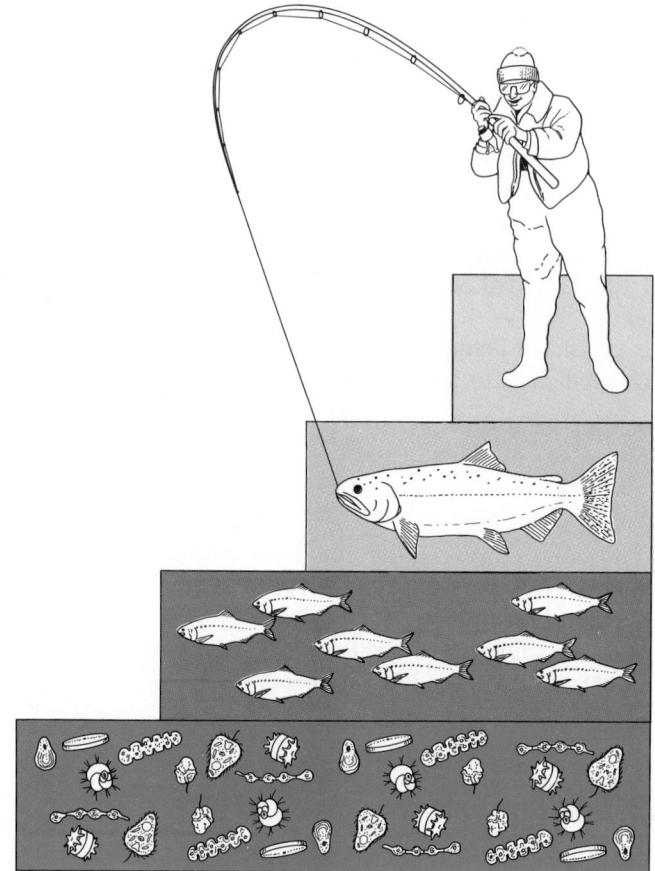

Level 4
A 150-pound person

Level 3
A hundred pounds of fish

Level 2
A few tons of plant-eating fish

Level 1
Several tons of producer organisms

exposure to them. Many cause delayed reactions, especially those that poison the nerves or cause cancer. Many toxins collect in fatty tissues, sequestered away from the rest of the body—harmless until that fat becomes mobilized.

How threatening are environmental contaminants to the food supply? For the most part, the hazards appear to be small, because the FDA regulates the presence of contaminants in foods and removes foods with unsafe contamination.[7] But in the event of an accidental spill, the risk of toxicity can suddenly become great.

Much of our knowledge derives from episodes of acute contamination of limited populations. For example, in 1953, a number of people in Minamata, Japan, became ill with a disease no one had seen before. By 1960, 121 cases had been reported, including 23 in infants. Mortality was high; 46 died, and in the survivors the symptoms were "progressive blindness, deafness, inco-ordination, and intellectual deterioration."[8] The cause was ultimately revealed to be methylmercury contamination of fish from the bay these people lived on. The infants who contracted the disease had not eaten any fish, but their mothers had, and even though the mothers exhibited no symptoms during their pregnancies, the poison had been affecting their unborn babies. Manufacturing plants in the region were discharging mercury into the waters

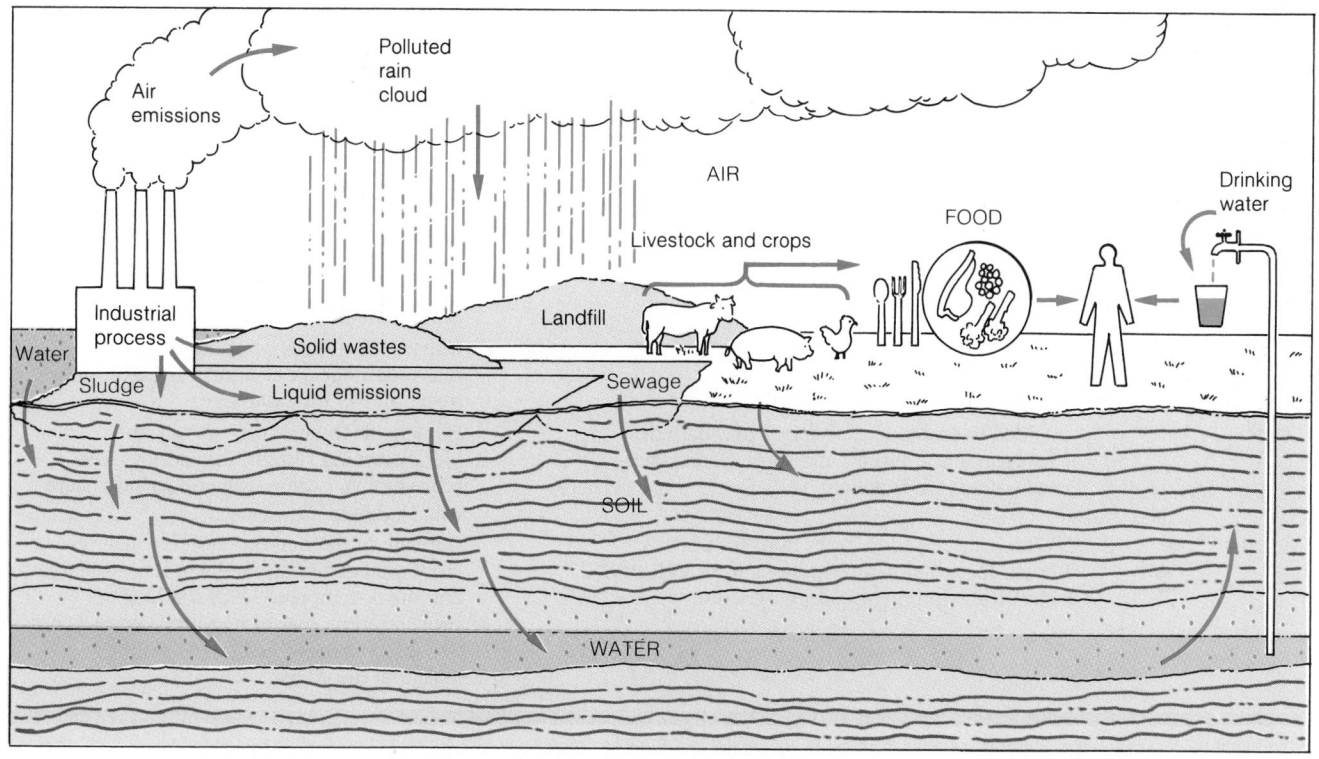

of the bay, the mercury was turning to methylmercury on leaving the factories, and the fish in the bay were accumulating this poison in their bodies. Some of the families who were affected had been eating fish from the bay every day.

In 1973, in Michigan, half a ton of polybrominated biphenyl (PBB), a toxic chemical, was accidentally mixed into some livestock feed that was distributed throughout the state. The chemical found its way into millions of animals and then into people who ate their meat. The seriousness of the accident began to come to light when dairy farmers reported their cows' going dry, aborting their calves, and developing abnormal growths on their hooves. Although more than 30,000 cattle, sheep, and swine and more than a million chickens were destroyed, effects on people were not prevented. By 1982, it was estimated that 97 percent of Michigan's residents had become contaminated with PBB. Nervous system aberrations and alterations in the liver and immune systems were among the effects in exposed farm residents.[9]

Mercury is a heavy metal, and PBB is an organic halogen. These two classes of chemicals are among the most toxic and are still being liberated into our environment daily, although at lower levels than those that caused the tragedies reported in the previous paragraphs. The number of contaminants we could discuss here, and the amount of information available about them, is far beyond our scope. Table 16–3 selects a few metal contaminants of great concern in foods to show how pervasively a contaminant can affect the body, and Highlight 11 focuses on the heavy metal lead and its toxic effects.

■ **FIGURE 16–2**
How Contaminants Find Their Way into Foods

heavy metal: any of a number of mineral ions such as mercury and lead, so called because they are of relatively high atomic weight. Many heavy metals are poisonous.

organic halogen: an organic compound containing one or more atoms of a **halogen**—fluorine, chlorine, iodine, or bromine.

■ **TABLE 16–3**
Examples of Metal Contaminants

Metal	Common Sources	Toxic Effects
Aluminum	Used to manufacture or process foods, cosmetics, and medicines; to purify water.	Spinal cord and brain disease, skeletal pain.
Cadmium[a]	Used in industrial processes, including electroplating, plastics, batteries, vapor lamps, alloys, pigments, and as a substitute for tin in solder; present in cigarette smoke.	Emphysema, fatigue, headache, vomiting, anemia, loss of smell, kidney failure.
Chromium	Used in car manufacturing.	Lung cancer, kidney damage.
Cobalt	Used as a superalloy for jet engines.	Nausea, vomiting, anorexia, ear ringing, nerve damage, respiratory diseases, goiter, heart and kidney damage.
Lead[b]	Added to gasoline, newspaper ink, batteries, shotgun ammunition, and some nonresidential paints (see Highlight 11).	Damage to the nervous system, the blood-forming system, the kidneys, the reproductive system, the endocrine system (see Highlight 11).
Mercury[c]	Widely dispersed in gases from the earth's crust; local high concentrations from industry, electrical equipment, paints, agriculture.	Damage to the nervous system causing emotional disturbances, including excitability and quick-tempered behavior, lack of concentration, loss of memory, depression, fatigue, weakness, headache, stomach and intestinal disorders.

[a]The World Health Organization suggests not more than 400 to 500 μg per individual per week.
[b]The World Health Organization suggests not more than 3 mg per individual for adults.
[c]The World Health Organization notes adverse health effects at 200 μg/L blood.
Source: Adapted from R. W. Miller, The metal in our mettle, *FDA Consumer*, December 1988–January 1989, pp. 24–27.

■ *Natural Toxicants in Foods*

Contamination of foods is not alone in presenting hazards to consumers. Many commonly used plants and plant products contain naturally occurring toxic substances. Mushrooms are a familiar example, but a number of other common foods have been observed to cause toxic effects. For example, cabbage, mustard, and other plants contain goitrogens; if these plants are consumed as a steady diet, they can enlarge the thyroid gland. Similarly, spinach and rhubarb contain oxalates; these are tolerable as usually consumed, but one normal serving of rhubarb contains one-fifth the toxic dose for humans. Honey can be a host to the botulinum organism and can accumulate enough toxin to kill an infant.[10]

Even the humble potato can present a hazard if improperly stored: green potato skins contain solanine, a powerful inhibitor of nerve impulses. Ordinary consumption of potatoes delivers one-tenth the dose of solanine that would be toxic. When potatoes are exposed to light, they develop more solanine; it is in the green layer that develops just beneath the skin. (Throw such potatoes away; don't eat them.)

Some 700 other plants have caused serious illnesses or deaths in the Western Hemisphere.[11] Some fish are also naturally toxic, presenting hazards from mild illness to instant death. A well-known environmental scientist has said, "One can predict that if the standards used to test manmade chemicals were applied to 'natural' foods, fully half of the human food supply would have to be banned."[12]

This brief look at naturally occurring toxicants should serve as a reminder of two principles. First, anything can be toxic when consumed in excess; use moderation in the use of all foods. Second, poisons are poisons whether made by people or nature. Thus consumers who fear only "chemicals" that come from laboratories are slightly off the mark. It is not the source of a chemical that makes it hazardous; it is its chemical formula.

■ Pesticides

Pesticides differ from the other contaminants of foods in that they are used on purpose. Because pesticides leave residues in foods, their use is regulated so as not to present a significant hazard to consumers. They are necessary, for pests destroy about one-third of the world's food crops every year, even with extensive pesticide use.[13] The use of pesticides ensures an adequate food supply at a reasonable cost, but high doses of some pesticides have caused birth defects, sterility, tumors, organ damage, and central nervous system impairment in animals.[14] Little wonder that fear of pesticides in the food supply is the American public's number 1 food safety concern.

residues: that which remains after the pesticide has been broken down, washed away, or evaporated.

Ideally, man-made pesticides destroy the pest, and then quickly degenerate to nontoxic products so that by the time consumers eat the food, no harmful residues remain. Unfortunately, no such perfect pesticide exists. (Pesticides also occur in nature—the nicotine in tobacco is an example—but they are less damaging to other living things and less persistent in the environment than the man-made ones.) Development of new pesticides and monitoring of their use is an ongoing activity that requires continued vigilance on the part of government agencies.

Consumers cannot usually see or taste pesticides in their foods; they depend on agencies such as the EPA to keep the levels within safe limits. The EPA oversees pesticide use in several ways. It regulates the manufacture, use, and labeling of pesticides. It monitors their presence in fish, birds, and mammals; in water, air, and food; and in human beings.[15] Also, the EPA sets tolerances for pesticide residues in foods, which are enforced by the FDA and the USDA. The EPA establishes these tolerance levels by weighing the risks and benefits of pesticide use and applying a judgment factor to protect public health as well as provide an adequate, wholesome, and economical food supply. Tolerance levels are generally 100 to 1,000 times lower than the level that caused "no effect" in laboratory animals.[16] (EPA tolerances reflect the quantities needed to get the job done, and not necessarily the maximum safe levels of pesticides in foods. Actual residues may be lower than maximum legal residues.)

tolerance level: the maximum level of a substance allowed.

Over 10,000 tolerance regulations state the maximum levels for over 300 pesticide ingredients used on various specific crops. The FDA samples thousands of food shipments, both domestic and imported, for illegal use of pesticides—including residues above tolerances, use of unapproved pesticides, or uses of particular pesticides on crops for which they have not been approved. The agency reports compliance with the law in 96 to 98 percent of the samples tested; over 50 percent of the samples have no detectable levels of pesticides.[17] Regulations in foreign countries are more lenient than in this country; consequently, imported foods contain both higher concentrations of pesticides than domestic foods and also contain pesticides that have been banned in this country.

In addition to sampling the food supply in the field, the FDA conducts the Total Diet Study four times a year. The FDA purchases and prepares over 200 foods typical of the U.S. diet to analyze them for pesticides and other chemicals. This provides an estimate of the amount of pesticide residues that remain in foods as they are usually eaten—after they have been washed, peeled, and cooked. Reports state that while some samples contain residues, they are well below EPA tolerances and below WHO's "acceptable daily intake—one that appears to present no appreciable risk to health if consumed every day over a lifetime."[18]

Consumer groups are not completely reassured by this information; they still have concerns about pesticides. They point out that the FDA does not sample all food shipments, and test for all pesticides in each sample. True, the agency staffs fewer than 700 inspectors and scientists to test food samples from the multitude of farms, groves, docks, airports, warehouses, and processing plants it oversees. It is a *monitoring* agency, and as such, it cannot (nor can it be expected to) guarantee 100 percent safety in the food supply. What it can do is set conditions so that injuries are unlikely, and act promptly when problems or suspicions arise.

safety: the practical certainty that injury will not result from the use of a substance.

Whether you are ingesting significant pesticide residues depends on a number of factors, including:

- The food (what kind it is and how much of it you eat).
- The pesticide (what kind it is and how much was used).
- The weather conditions (whether they promoted pest growth and thereby necessitated additional pesticide use, or they washed away pesticides before harvest).
- The time (how long since the food was last sprayed).
- The preparation (how well you washed the fresh produce and whether you peeled or cooked it).

With this many factors, and so many of them out of your control, it is difficult to know whether, or to what extent, you are ingesting pesticide residues. Table 16–4 offers a few guidelines for minimizing your risks.

To feed a nation with fewer pesticides requires employing creative farming methods. Organic farming, without the use of inorganic fertilizers and pesticides, can provide produce for only a small percentage of the population. Other alternatives to heavy pesticide use include such efforts as releasing predators into fields to destroy pests and nearby planting of nonfood crops that attract pests away from the food crops.

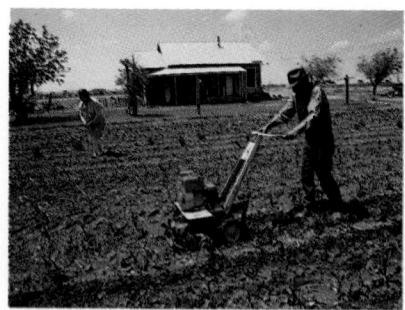

People can avoid the use of inorganic pesticides and fertilizers when their garden or farm is relatively small.

■ **TABLE 16–4**
Food Selection and Preparation to Minimize Risks Associated with Pesticides

- Trim the fat from meat, and remove the skin from poultry and fish; discard fats and oils in broths and pan drippings. (Pesticide residues concentrate in the animals' fat.)
- Wash fresh produce in water. Use a scrub brush, and rinse thoroughly.
- Use a knife to peel an orange or grapefruit; do not bite into the peel.
- Discard the outer leaves of leafy vegetables such as cabbage and lettuce.
- Peel waxed cucumbers; waxes don't wash off and can seal in pesticide residues.
- Peel vegetables such as carrots and fruits such as apples when appropriate. (Peeling offers a trade between removing pesticides that remain in or on the peel and removing fibers, vitamins, and minerals.)

■ *Food Additives*

Additives confer on foods a number of benefits. In some cases, they reduce the risk of food-borne illness (for example, nitrites used in curing meat to prevent poisoning from the botulinum toxin). In others, they enhance the nutrient quality of a product (as in vitamin D-fortified milk). Most additives make a larger variety of foods available at a reasonable market price by preventing spoilage. Some additives simply make foods look and taste good.

Intentional additives are substances put into foods on purpose, while incidental additives are those that may get in by accident before or during processing. This discussion begins with the regulations that govern additives, then discusses intentional additives class by class, and finally goes on to say a word about the incidental additives.

additives: substances not normally consumed as foods but added to food either intentionally or by accident.

intentional additives: additives intentionally added to foods, such as nutrients or colors.

incidental additives: substances that can get into food as a result of contact with foods during growing, processing, packaging, storing, or some other stage before the foods are consumed; also called **indirect** or **accidental additives**.

Regulations Governing Additives

The FDA's authority over additives hinges primarily on their safety. To receive permission to use a new additive in food products, a manufacturer must satisfy the FDA that the additive is:

- ■ Effective (it does what it is supposed to do).
- ■ Detectable and measurable in the final food product.
- ■ Safe when fed in large doses to animals under strictly controlled conditions (it causes no cancer, birth defects, or other injury).

On approving an additive's use, the FDA writes a regulation stating in what amounts, and in what foods, the additive may be used. No additive receives permanent approval; all receive periodic review.

Many substances in common use were exempted from complying with this procedure when the law on additives came into being, because no hazards

GRAS (generally recognized as safe) list: a list, established by the FDA in 1958, of food additives that had long been in use and were believed safe. The list is subject to revision as new facts become known.

Delaney Clause: a clause in the Food Additive Amendment to the Food, Drug, and Cosmetic Act that states that no substance that is known to cause cancer in animals or human beings at any dose level shall be added to foods.

toxicity: the ability of a substance to harm living organisms. All substances are toxic if high enough concentrations are used.

hazard: a state of danger; used to refer to any circumstance in which toxicity is possible under normal conditions of use.

were known to attend their use at that time. Some 700 substances were put on the GRAS (generally recognized as safe) list, including such items as salt, sugar, and herbs. However, any time substantial scientific evidence or public outcry has questioned the safety of any substance on the GRAS list, it has been reevaluated. Substances about which any legitimate question is raised are usually removed or reclassified (for the exceptions, see the accompanying Nutrition Detective Work box). Meanwhile, the entire GRAS list is subject to ongoing review.

To remain on the GRAS list, an additive must not have been found to be a carcinogen in any test on animals or human beings. The Delaney Clause (the part of the law that states this criterion) is uncompromising in addressing carcinogens in foods and drugs; in fact, it has been under fire in recent years for being too strict and inflexible.

An important distinction that governs determinations of additives' safety is the one between *toxicity* as a property of substances and the *hazard* associated

---

▶▶ NUTRITION DETECTIVE WORK

The Delaney Clause states that "no additive shall be deemed to be safe if it is found to induce cancer when ingested by man or animal." That sounds simple and clear enough, yet you may be aware of additives in products on the market that don't meet that criteria. Saccharin paved the way for exceptions to the rule. In the 1970s, when the FDA tried to ban saccharin because tests had revealed that it caused cancer in animals, Congress made a special exception that allowed saccharin to remain on the market as long as products containing it carried a warning. This was their best effort in trying to balance the Delaney Clause with current food safety and cancer knowledge. A little historical background may provide some insight.

When the Delaney Clause was adopted over 30 years ago, scientists knew that radiation, tobacco smoke, a chemical used to make dyes, and soot caused cancer. Since then, researchers have identified more than three dozen human carcinogens and several hundred animal carcinogens. In addition, technology has advanced so that substances once detectable only in parts per thousand can now be measured in parts per billion, or even per trillion. (One part per trillion is equivalent to about one grain of sugar in an Olympic-sized swimming pool or one hair on 10 million heads, assuming none are bald.) An FDA official states, "Given the extraordinarily low levels at which analytical chemists could measure chemical contaminants in food or anything else, all substances, no matter how pure, could be shown to be contaminated with one carcinogen or another."[19] In other words, we cannot provide absolute protection from all carcinogens in foods, as Congressman Delaney once thought we could. In fact, such a practice could actually be detrimental to the primary goals of the FDA in protecting the public health.[20] Instead, the FDA deems additives safe if they present no more than a one-in-a-million risk of cancer to human beings from lifetime use.

with substances. "Toxicity—the capacity of a chemical substance to harm living organisms—is a general property of matter; hazard is the capacity of a chemical to produce injury under conditions of use. All substances are potentially toxic, but are hazardous only if consumed in sufficiently large quantities."[21] An additive is not considered to be a hazard if it becomes toxic only when people consume some impossibly immense amount. The additive is a hazard only if it is toxic under the conditions of its actual use. However, food additives are supposed to have wide margins of safety.

Additives are allowed in foods at levels 100 times or more below those at which the risk is still known to be zero; their margin of safety is less than or equal to 1/100. Experiments to determine the extent of risk involve feeding test animals the substance at different concentrations throughout their lifetimes. The additive is then permitted in foods at 1/100 the level that can be fed under these conditions without causing any harmful effect whatever. In many foods, naturally occurring substances appear at levels that bring their margin of safety closer to 1/10. Even nutrients, as you have seen, involve risks at high dose levels. The margin of safety for vitamins A and D is 1/25 to 1/40; it may be less than 1/10 in infants. For some trace elements, it is about 1/5. People consume common table salt daily in amounts only three to five times less than those that cause serious toxicity.

Additives are in foods because they offer benefits that outweigh the risks they present or that make the risks worth taking. When the benefit to be gained from an additive is small, as in the case of color additives that only enhance the appearance of foods but do not improve their health value or safety, then the risks may be deemed not worth taking. In contrast, the FDA finds that it is worth taking the minimal risks associated with the use of nitrites on meat products to inhibit the formation of the deadly botulinum toxin.

It is the manufacturers' responsibility to use no more of an additive than is necessary to get the needed effect. The FDA also requires that additives *not* be used:

- To disguise faulty or inferior products.
- To deceive the consumer.
- Where they significantly destroy nutrients.
- Where their effects can be achieved by economical, sound manufacturing processes.

The regulations governing the use of intentional additives are well conceived and have been effective. The following sections focus on those additives that have received the most negative publicity, because people ask questions about them most often.

Intentional Food Additives

Intentional food additives are substances put into foods to give them some desirable characteristic: color, flavor, texture, stability, nutritional value, or resistance to spoilage. The accompanying miniglossary defines the categories of additives.

Artificial Colors Only 33 color additives remain on the GRAS list, a highly select group that has survived intense investigations. In fact, coloring agents

margin of safety: as used when speaking of food additives, a zone between the concentration normally used and that at which a hazard exists. For common table salt, for example, the margin of safety is 1/5 (five times the concentration normally used would be hazardous).

Miniglossary of Intentional Food Additives

antimicrobial agents: preservatives that prevent microorganisms from growing.

antioxidants: chemicals that prevent rancidity of fats and other damage to food caused by oxygen.

artificial colors: certified food colors, added to enhance appearance. (*Certified* means approved by the FDA.)

artificial flavors, flavor enhancers: chemicals that mimic natural flavors and those that enhance flavor.

nutrient additives: vitamins and minerals added to improve nutritive value

radiation: radioactivity used to sterilize and protect food.

---

are much better known than the *natural* pigments of plants, and we can state the limits on the safety of their use with greater certainty.[22] One natural pigment (and its synthetic counterparts) commonly used by the food industry is the vitamin A precursor beta-carotene.[23] Carotenoids add the colors yellow, red, and orange to products such as margarine, cheese, and macaroni.

Still, the food colors have been heavily criticized because they are dispensable. Simply stated, they only make foods pretty, whereas other additives, such as preservatives, make foods safe. Hence with food colors we can afford to require that their use entail no risk.[24] With other additives, we may have to compromise between the risks of using them and the risks of *not* using them.

Artificial Flavors and Flavor Enhancers Numbering close to 2,000, flavoring agents are the largest single group of food additives. One of the best-known members of this group is monosodium glutamate, or MSG (trade name, Accent)—the monosodium salt of the amino acid glutamic acid. MSG is used widely in restaurants, especially Asian restaurants, as a flavor enhancer. In addition to enhancing flavor, MSG may itself possess a basic taste independent of the well-known sweet, salty, bitter, and sour perceptions. MSG has received publicity because it may produce an adverse reaction in some individuals—the so-called Chinese restaurant syndrome—involving burning sensations, chest and facial flushing or pain, and throbbing headaches. MSG has been investigated extensively enough to be deemed safe for adults to use (except people who react adversely to it).

Antimicrobial Agents Foods can go bad in two ways: by becoming hazardous to health and by merely losing their flavor and attractiveness. An example of the former: microbes growing in foods can cause food-borne illnesses (as described earlier). Preservatives known as antimicrobial agents protect foods from these microbes.

The best known, most widely used antimicrobial agents are the two common substances salt and sugar. Salt has been used since before recorded history to preserve meat and fish; sugar serves the same purpose in canned and frozen fruits, as well as in jams and jellies. (Any jam or jelly that toots its "no preservatives" horn is exaggerating. The sugar makes it needless to add

Chinese restaurant syndrome: an intolerance reaction that may occur in one out of several hundred people, 20 min after the ingestion of the additive MSG (monosodium glutamate, or Accent). Symptoms include burning sensations, chest and facial flushing and pain, and throbbing headaches.

NUTRITION DETECTIVE WORK

The case of Chinese restaurant syndrome illustrates human suggestibility. No one really knows how common it is, or why it might occur. First reported less than 20 years ago, it was at that time thought to be quite rare, but as more and more people have learned of it, more and more people have developed the impression that they suffer from it. Meanwhile, some research demonstrates that MSG is not the only cause of the syndrome, and that if people don't know they are eating MSG, they may not have the symptoms.[25] This indicates a strong placebo effect at work. Some skepticism is in order as to just how extensive the syndrome is, what causes it, and who has it or what else they might have.

other preservatives.) Other additives, such as potassium sorbate and sodium propionate, are also used to extend the shelf lives of baked goods, cheese, beverages, mayonnaise, margarine, and many other products.

Another group of antimicrobial agents is the nitrites, added to foods for three main purposes: to preserve their color (especially the pink color of hot dogs and other cured meats), to enhance their flavor by inhibiting rancidity (especially in cured meats), and to protect against bacterial growth. In amounts smaller than those needed to confer color, nitrites prevent the growth of the bacteria that produce the deadly botulinum toxin, the most potent biological poison known.

Nitrites clearly serve a useful purpose, but they have been the object of much controversy. In the human body, nitrites can be converted to nitrosamines (see Figure 16–3). At nitrite levels higher than those used in food products, nitrosamine formation causes cancer in animals. The food industry uses the minimal amount of nitrites necessary to receive the protection they offer, and nitrosamines have not been known to cause cancer in human beings. Nitrosamines are the subject of continuing research.

nitrites: salts added to food to prevent botulism; one example is sodium nitrite, used to preserve meats.

nitrosamines (nigh-TROHS-uh-meens): derivatives of nitrites that may be formed in the stomach when nitrites combine with amines; nitrosamines are carcinogenic in animals.

Antioxidants The other way in which food can go bad is by undergoing changes in color and flavor caused by exposure to air (oxidation). Oftentimes, these changes involve no hazard to health, but they damage the food's

$$H^+ + NO_2^- \longrightarrow HNO_2$$

From acid · Nitrite salt · Nitrous acid

In an acid environment such as the stomach, nitrite salts form nitrous acid.

$$O=N-O-H \; + \; H-\overset{|}{N}- \longrightarrow O=N-\overset{|}{N}-$$

Nitrous acid · Amine · Nitrosamine

Nitrous acid reacts with amines to form nitrosamines. Amines are numerous in foods. (Water, H — O — H, is a by-product.)

■ FIGURE 16–3
Nitrosamine Formation

appearance, flavor, and nutritional quality. Familiar examples of these changes are the ways sliced apples or potatoes turn brown, or oil goes rancid. Preservatives known as antioxidants protect food from this kind of spoilage.

The FDA approves a total of 27 antioxidants for use in foods, including vitamin C (ascorbate) and vitamin E (tocopherol). Vitamin E is added to bacon to prevent nitrosamine formation while assisting nitrite's antioxidant activity. When the vitamin E additive is present in bacon along with the regular amount of nitrite preservative, nitrosamine formation is inhibited by more than half.*

sulfites: salts containing sulfur, added to fresh and frozen fruits and vegetables to prevent spoilage.

Another, less expensive group of preservatives, the sulfites, also prevents oxidation in many processed foods, alcoholic beverages, and drugs. The use of sulfites on salad bars to keep raw fruits and vegetables looking fresh has been banned. The ban came after sulfites caused adverse reactions in some people who have asthma—reactions that were sometimes serious, and for a few, deadly.[26] The FDA has taken a number of steps to protect people who are allergic to sulfites. It prohibits sulfite use on food intended to be consumed raw (except grapes) and requires that foods declare sulfites in their ingredient lists. For most people, sulfites do not pose a hazard in the amounts used in products,[27] but there is one more consideration: sulfiting agents destroy an appreciable amount of the vitamin thiamin in foods. A person choosing a food that contains sulfites should not count on that food to provide a share of the daily need for thiamin.

The ban on sulfites has stimulated research to look for alternatives. For example, some producers use honey to clarify browned apple juice, and agriculturists have created a hybrid apple that doesn't brown.[28] One manufacturer has combined four GRAS additives to create a product that can substitute for sulfites.[29]**

Two other antioxidants in wide use are the well-known BHA and BHT, which prevent rancidity in baked goods and snack foods. BHT provides a refreshing change from the tales of woe and cancer scares associated with many of the other additives. Among the many tests that were performed on BHT were several showing that animals fed large amounts of this substance developed *less* cancer when exposed to carcinogens and lived *longer* than controls. BHT apparently protects against cancer through its antioxidant effect, which is similar to that of vitamin E. To obtain this effect from BHT, though, a large amount of the substance must be present in the diet—larger by far than the amount in the U.S. diet. (A caution: at levels of intake even higher than this, the substance has experimentally produced cancer.) Vitamin E and vitamin C remain the most important dietary antioxidants to strengthen defenses against cancer.[30]

Upon learning of studies that show BHA and BHT to inhibit cancer in rats, some people came to a wrong conclusion—that what works for rats must work for people, too. Manufacturers have begun marketing capsules of the preservatives as anticancer pills, and recommend taking amounts far beyond the FDA's limit of safety. In fact, the daily dose recommended by the makers

---

*The additive is Cure-trol, created by the Diamond Salt Company of St. Claire, Michigan.
**Monsanto Company has developed a sulfite alternative, called Snow Fresh, from citric acid, ascorbic acid, sodium acid pyrophosphate, and calcium chloride.

of these pills is almost lethal. Ironically, health food stores sell the capsules of BHT and BHA right alongside the packages of ''no additives'' foods.

Nutrient Additives   As mentioned earlier in the chapter and in Highlight 16, manufacturers sometimes add nutrients to improve or maintain the nutritional value of foods. Included among these are the four nutrients added to refined grains to enrich them; the iodine added to salt; the vitamins A and D added to dairy products; and the nutrients added to fortified breakfast cereals. When nutrients are added to a nutrient-poor food, it may appear to the consumer to be nutrient-rich. It is, but only in those nutrients chosen for addition—and the absorption of these nutrients may be poor. The appropriate use of nutrient additives is to:[31]

Grain products are enriched with iron, thiamin, riboflavin, and niacin.

- Correct an existing dietary insufficiency known to result in a deficiency disease.
- Restore nutrients to levels found in the food before storage, handling, and processing.
- Balance the vitamin, mineral, and protein content of a food in proportion to the kcalorie content.
- Avoid nutritional inferiority in a food that replaces a traditional (more nutritious) food.

Nutrients are sometimes also added for other purposes. Vitamins C and E were already mentioned for their antioxidant properties and beta-carotene (a vitamin A precursor), for its color.

Radiation   The food-processing industry is using ionizing radiation as an alternative to chemical additives for certain FDA-approved foods.* Radiation kills microorganisms and insect pests, inhibits the growth of sprouts on potatoes and onions, extends refrigerated shelf life, and delays ripening in some fruits. The radiation doses required to achieve these different effects vary. Ideally, a food receives no more than the dose sufficient for the desired effect. For many foods, treatment with radiation does not alter flavor, texture, or color. The nutrient quality of irradiated foods is equal to foods processed by other commercial processing methods.[32]

Irradiation never makes foods radioactive. It does, however, create small chemical changes. These result from radiation's striking the atoms in the molecules of the food, causing them to lose electrons and form ions or free radicals. How these charged and uncharged particles react with one another and other food constituents is the focus of much research.[33] Compounds produced as a result of the irradiation process are unique radiolytic products, or simply, radiolytic products. The long-term safety of their consumption is being investigated.

radiolytic (RAY-dee-oh-LIT-ic) **products** (**RP**): products formed during the irradiation of food; also called **unique radiolytic products (URP).**

Many consumers react negatively to the use of radiation on foods, associating radiation with cancer. Some may confuse it with food contamination by radioactive particles, such as occurs in the aftermath of a nuclear accident. For this reason, some proponents of irradiation suggest using the

*The food-processing industry uses gamma radiation, a high-energy form of light with greater penetrating power than X rays, primarily generated from cobalt 60 or cesium 137.

This symbol identifies foods that have been irradiated.

ultrahigh temperature treatment: short-time exposure of a food to temperatures above those normally used, in order to sterilize it.

pasteurization: the treatment of milk with heat sufficient to kill certain pathogens (disease-causing microbes) commonly transmitted through milk, not a sterilization process. Pasteurized milk retains bacteria that cause milk spoilage. Unpasteurized ("certified" raw) milk transmits many food-borne diseases to people each year and should be avoided.

term *pico wave*, believing consumers will accept that term as readily as they did microwave. (Speaking of microwaves, like irradiation, microwaves sterilize foods.* Unlike irradiation, though, microwaves cook the food as they pass through it.)

The FDA considers irradiation an additive and permits its use at low concentrations to perform those functions mentioned earlier; to replace postharvest pesticide fumigation of certain foods; and to kill *Trichinella*, the dangerous parasitic worms that are sometimes found in pork. The FDA has also approved high-dose treatment of teas, dried spices, and other seasonings to sterilize them. Milk products change flavor when irradiated and so are not candidates for the treatment. (Incidentally, those boxes of milk kept at room temperature on the shelves of the grocery store are not irradiated, but processed with an ultrahigh temperature treatment; the milk is exposed to temperatures above those of milk pasteurization for a short time—just long enough to sterilize it.)

Irradiation cuts down on food wastage and can replace some costly pesticides. Unfortunately, poor countries that have many hungry people and little food for them lack irradiation technology, and much of their food rots or is eaten by insects. Where irradiation technology is available, its use must be carefully scrutinized. The likelihood of environmental contamination by the radioactive material used in the process exists, but there is no possibility of a meltdown or nuclear disaster, because food irradiation plants are not nuclear reactors. Strict controls on the transport of radioactive materials, adequate safety operations at facilities, and proper disposal of the wastes generated are indispensable to prevent hazards to workers and the environment.

The FDA requires that each food treated with radiation bear a label indicating that it was "treated with radiation" or "treated by irradiation." This requirement informs consumers of this method of preservation. Unfortunately, the FDA does not require label statements for other treatments that perform similar functions, such as postharvest fumigation with pesticides. If all treatment methods were declared, consumers could make fully informed choices.

On the whole, the benefits of food additives seem to justify the risks associated with their use. The FDA closely regulates and monitors all intentional additives. Still, some people wish to avoid them, and one way to do this is to eat a diet of mostly whole foods—fresh fruits, vegetables, whole grains, meats, and milk products.

Incidental Food Additives

Incidental, accidental, or indirect additives are all substances that find their way into food as the result of some phase of harvesting, production, processing, storage, or packaging. For example, among incidental additives are tiny bits of plastic, glass, paper, tin, and other substances from packages, as well as chemicals from processing, such as the solvent used in some processes for decaffeinating coffee. Since packaging and processing materials,

---

*Gamma waves used in irradiation have a wavelength of 10^{-12} m; microwaves have a wavelength of 10^{-2} m. As a point of reference, light bulbs emit wavelengths in the range of 10^{-7} m.

unlike pesticides or environmental contaminants, are required to be safe as used, their occasional migration into foods presents considerably less of a hazard to consumers.

Incidental additives are well regulated, just as intentional additives are. All food packagers are required to perform specific tests to discover whether materials are migrating into foods; if they are, the safety of these materials must be confirmed by strict procedures similar to those governing intentional additives. Incidental additives sometimes find their way into foods, but adverse effects are rare.

■ *The Water Supply*

The foregoing discussions of food have omitted water, but water, of course, can contain the same nonnutrients that food does. Water from the tap may contain naturally occurring minerals, toxic heavy metals, live microorganisms, and a miscellany of organic compounds. In addition, chlorine may have been added to it to kill disease-conveying microorganisms, and fluoride may have been added to it to protect against dental caries. A glass of "water" from the tap may be more than just H_2O.

Natural groundwaters contain all the major and trace mineral nutrients in varying concentrations. In some cases, the concentrations can be significant enough to affect a person's health. For example, in some communities, fluoride occurs naturally at a concentration that meets the human need for protection from dental caries.

Three minerals determine the "hardness" or "softness" of water, a distinction that has practical and health implications. Hard water contains high concentrations of calcium and magnesium; soft water contains mostly sodium. In terms of practical experience, soft water makes more bubbles with less soap; hard water leaves a bathtub ring, forms a residue of rocklike crystals in the tea kettle, and turns laundry gray.

hard water: water with a high calcium and magnesium concentration.

soft water: water with a high sodium concentration.

Consumers tend to prefer soft water and may even purchase water-softening equipment, which replaces magnesium and calcium with sodium. Consequently, soft water adds sodium to people's diets, and it appears to contribute to a higher incidence of hypertension and heart disease in areas where it is used. About half of the U.S. population drinks water containing more than 20 milligrams sodium per liter—an amount small enough for healthy people, but too much for persons who must restrict their sodium intakes severely. (Chapter 28 discusses nutrition and hypertension.)

Soft water also can dissolve certain toxic heavy metals, such as cadmium and lead, from pipes. Groundwater does not normally contain these metals, because in the wilderness, water usually undergoes a natural purifying process each time it cycles through living systems. The soil filters out animal waste excreted onto the earth, preventing it from reaching the underground water. (Plants use it as fertilizer, instead.) Soil holds pollutants, too—not beneficial to the soil, of course, but at least beneficial to the water. Pollutants entering rivers quickly disappear back into the earth as the rivers flow along, leaving the water pure. But neither the soil nor the rivers can purify completely the heavily polluted water expelled as city sewage or industrial

An abundant supply of fresh water is vital to life.

waste. Water leaving a factory may contain higher and higher concentrations of toxic metals as time goes on, especially if the water cycles through the same factory over and over again.

The metals of greatest concern are mercury, cadmium, and lead, whose toxic effects were already summarized in Table 16–3. These metals may be absorbed into the body, where they change cell membrane structure; alter enzyme or coenzyme functions; or even change the structure of the genetic material DNA, causing cancer or birth defects. If these metals happen to alter the DNA in the germ cells (eggs or sperm), the changes (mutations) will become hereditary. When combined with organic compounds, these metals may be absorbed especially rapidly and may damage body tissue even more.

Human technology bears the burden of purifying water contaminated by human technology. The Public Health Service sets drinking water standards (upper limits for the amounts of toxic substances permitted in water), and public law distributes the responsibility for adhering to these standards among the industries and the water-processing plants.

While the water supply naturally contains few, if any, heavy metals, it does naturally contain bacteria from the soil and from contamination with human sewage. The human digestive tract harbors many harmless, even beneficial, bacteria, and these are excreted into sewage; if they were its only inhabitants, there would be no concern about their presence in drinking water. Unfortunately, human pathogens are also excreted into sewage, and others are introduced into it by flies and other carriers. Before a sewage treatment plant releases water into the public water supply, it must reduce the bacterial count enough so that the further dilution that follows will make recycled water safe for drinking.

High standards for sewage treatment in the developed countries ensure safe drinking water for most people. For the rest of the world, however, microbial contamination remains the primary cause of human diseases and epidemics. Two of the most basic public health needs of the world's people are safe drinking water and an acceptable standard of waste disposal.

Organic compounds from sewage, insecticides, petroleum-based industries, highway runoff, and other sources may also occur in water. Researchers have identified some of these compounds and have found many of them to be toxic. Some cause birth defects; some cause cancer; some cause genetic mutations. Many contain chlorine, and some may be formed during the chlorination of water. The risks they present remain unknown; standards are being established, and if public water exceeds them, new filtering systems may be needed.

Many people use bottled water in order to control the quality of the water they drink. In contrast to Europeans, who drink bottled water for its mineral contents, people here drink it for its *lack* of specific contents, trying to choose beverages that are sugar-free, caffeine-free, sodium-free, preservative-free, kcalorie-free, or contamination-free. Whether to drink bottled water, and which brand to select, are individual choices; but in buying water, as in buying any product, consumers need to read labels carefully and be alert to fraudulent claims. Some waters contain minerals; others have been distilled. Mineral waters from famous springs offer no known health advantages and may be undesirably high in some minerals, such as sodium. Producers of bottled water sold in the United States must conduct yearly tests to confirm that the water at least equals the purity required of all public water supplies.

Water that is suitable for drinking is **potable** (POTE-ah-bul).

■ *Nutritional Adequacy of Foods and Diets*

The nutritional adequacy of foods and diets ranks high among the FDA's issues, second only to food-borne illness as a problem affecting consumers. The FDA's reason for concern is that many new foods have appeared on the market in recent decades—foods that are designed to appeal to people's tastes, but that may not deliver balanced assortments of the needed nutrients. Unlike the foods our ancestors used to eat, which were composed of the whole tissues of plants and animals, altered little or not at all before being eaten, many of the new foods have been formulated by manufacturers from *parts* of plant and animal tissues such as fat, sugar, and refined flour, or even constructed from entirely synthetic ingredients. Since the FDA is responsible for the wholesomeness, as well as the safety, of the U.S. food supply, it has become increasingly involved in attempting to ensure that these new foods are properly labeled and accurately advertised, so as to enable consumers to construct nutritionally adequate diets from them.

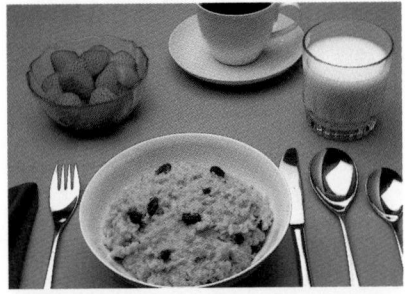

The highlight that follows this chapter deals with the nutrition labeling of foods, and it answers the questions consumers most often ask about the meanings of terms used to describe foods. This section focuses on you, the individual who makes food choices. What personal strategies can you use to enhance your nutrition status? Chapter 2 introduced two days' meal selections (see Figure 2–7). This discussion takes a closer look at some of the similarities and differences in the nutritional value of the meals. Remember that on Monday, the person chose an oatmeal breakfast, a burrito lunch, and a shrimp dinner; on Tuesday, the person selected an egg breakfast, a hamburger lunch, and a steak dinner.

Both Monday's and Tuesday's food choices provided fewer than 2,000 kcalories. This represents somewhat less than the RDA energy needs for young adults. An active man of average size or a large, active woman would require a larger energy intake; only a small man or woman wanting to lose weight might require a smaller one. The energy intakes of these two days were set at similar levels to illustrate the differences in what you can get for your "kcalorie dollar."

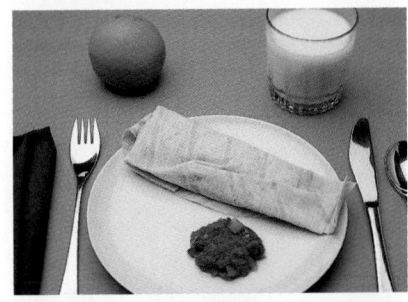

For the same number of kcalories, both sets of meals provided more than adequate protein. The Monday meals delivered a larger percentage of the kcalories from complex carbohydrates and naturally occurring simple carbohydrates; the Tuesday meals contributed a larger percentage of the kcalories from fat.

The abundance of plant foods in Monday's meals provided over 40 grams of fiber—too much, according to the American Dietetic Association (ADA). The bean burrito, oatmeal, strawberries, and orange together supplied a full half of the day's fiber intake. The ADA states that between 20 and 35 grams of dietary fiber daily is desirable and recognizes that the consumption of a diet too high in fiber on a regular basis can be as harmful as a diet too low in fiber.[34] To lower the fiber content without lowering the carbohydrate intake requires careful substitutions. A smart choice would be to replace the orange with orange juice; this would lower the day's fiber total by 10 percent without altering the overall nutrient profile.

Protein: 19% kcal.
Carbohydrate: 57% kcal.
Fat: 24% kcal.

Tuesday's meals

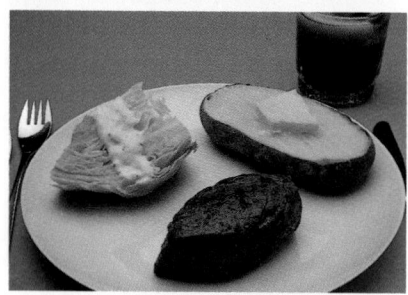

Protein: 23% kcal.
Carbohydrate: 33% kcal.
Fat: 44% kcal.

Just as Monday's fiber intake was too high, Tuesday's was too low. Tuesday's meals provided less than 10 grams of fiber. The dietary guidelines recommend high-fiber foods to promote GI tract and heart health; Tuesday's meals would benefit from *more* foods like the ones eaten on Monday.

Speaking of heart health, consider that Tuesday's meals provided almost twice as much fat as Monday's meals and violated dietary recommendations to limit fat intake to 30 percent. Furthermore, much of the fat was saturated (40 percent). In contrast, Monday's meals met recommendations to limit total fat and provided approximately equal amounts of saturated, monounsaturated, and polyunsaturated fats.

Figure 16–4 shows how the days' selections compared with one another and with the U.S. RDA for selected vitamins and minerals. As you might guess, Monday's meals fell short in the nutrients found more abundantly in foods derived from animals than from plants—niacin, vitamin B_{12}, and zinc. You also might guess, correctly, that the nutrients most notably lacking from Tuesday's meals are those that the vegetables and milk are famous for (folate, vitamin A, and calcium). Tuesday's meals also fell short in vitamin E, magnesium, and copper.

This meal comparison is informative. Clearly, neither set of meals is perfect. Monday's meals were too high in bulk for many people to eat; Tuesday's were too high in fat. Modifications in both could improve their health value. Monday's meals might be improved by adding a little meat or meat alternate. How could Tuesday's meals be improved?

People have tended to seek single servings of foods that would deliver large amounts of single nutrients—for example, a cup of milk for calcium. This approach works as far as obtaining the specific nutrients is concerned, but it fails to control fat and energy intake—you can't just keep adding a single food to the diet for each single nutrient until all nutrient needs are met. It's harder to visualize, but much more practical, to do this: select foods that provide many nutrients each and large quantities of nutrients per kcalorie.

If Tuesday's meals could get rid of some of their fat, there would be space to add the vegetables and milk they need in order to obtain the missing nutrients. Frankly, some effort had already been made to keep fat within reason—after all, the breakfast lacked bacon, the hamburger bore no cheese, and the baked potato went without its sour cream. Where's the fat? A full fourth of it is hidden in the hamburger. The french fries make a big contribution, too—almost 15 percent of the day's fat intake. By replacing this fast-food lunch with a visit to the salad bar, a person could lower fat intake significantly and pick up some fiber, vitamin A, and folate—all needed to improve the day's nutrient intakes.

Other ways the Tuesday choices might be improved have less dramatic effects, but every little change would help. Replacing the butter on the morning toast with jelly would save close to 8 grams of fat. Many such small changes could make Tuesday's meals, which exhibit the flaws of the typical American diet, higher in fiber and nutrients and lower in fat while still pleasing the eater.

Dramatic changes in lifestyle can be overwhelming, and often meet with failure. Even the smallest of dietary changes can make a difference, though. Small changes add up and set the momentum for other changes to follow in the right direction. By making minimal changes in their diets, most people

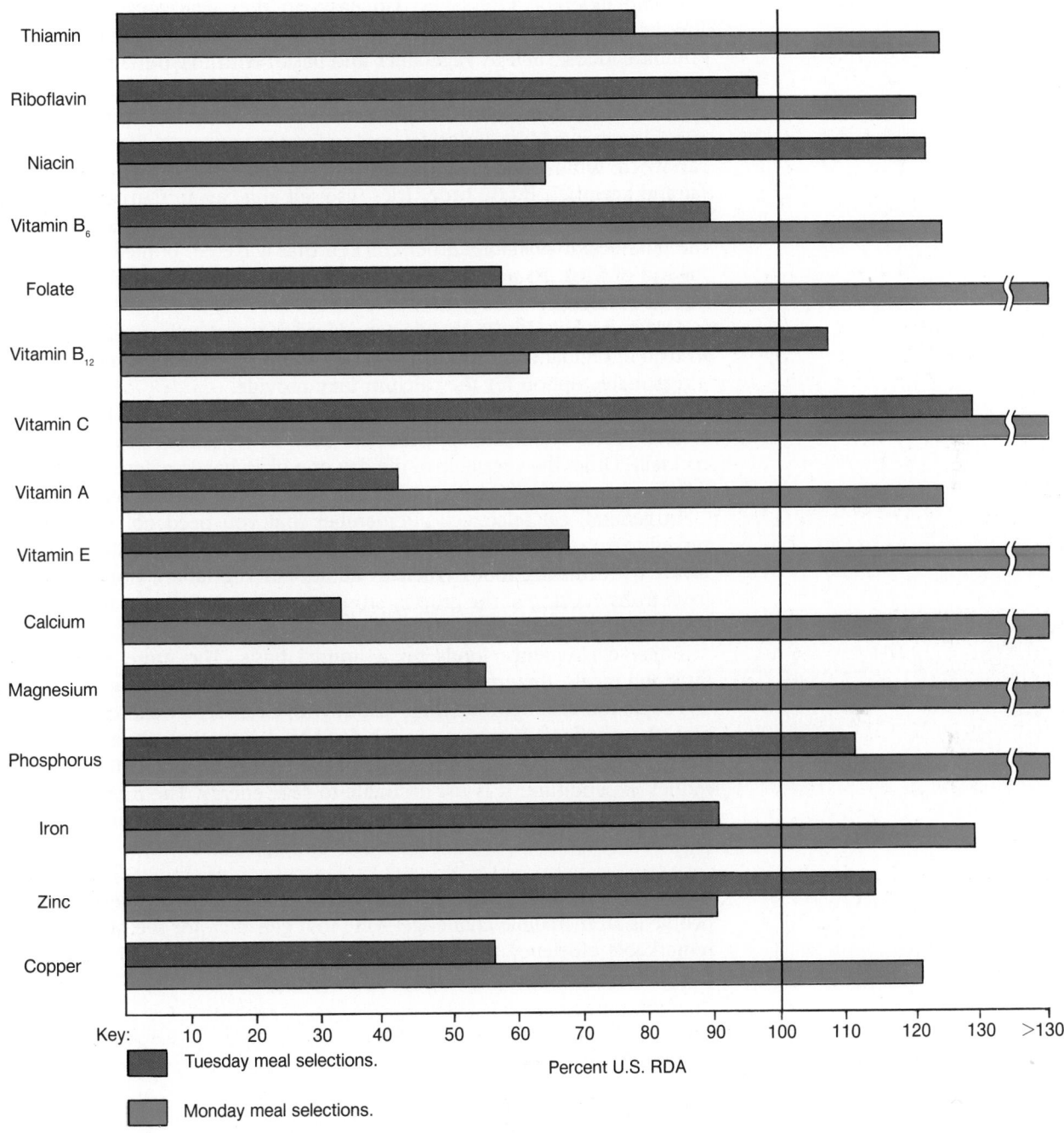

Key:

■ Tuesday meal selections.

■ Monday meal selections.

Percent U.S. RDA

can meet most dietary recommendations and improve their health.[35] Because quick meals and meals prepared by others play a major part in many people's lives, the following paragraphs suggest pointers for people who eat convenience foods, fast foods, airline meals, and the like from time to time—that is, most of us.

Many restaurants offer salad bars. Include plenty of fresh vegetables and fruits with your meal (or as your meal) to compensate for the nutrients that

■ **FIGURE 16–4**
Meal Selections Compared
Remember that the U.S. RDA are as high as, or higher than, the RDA and that comparisons with standards such as these are best done with several days' intakes averaged.

standard fast-food fare lacks. Go easy on the salad dressing, and select low-kcalorie dressings whenever possible. Steer clear of salad bar items that combine foods, such as vegetables and pasta, with mayonnaise.

At a fast-food hamburger place, if you don't want a salad, select a small regular hamburger; giant hamburgers with all the extras (like cheese and special sauces) add kcalories, fat, and sodium to your meal. If you prefer a fish sandwich, remove the breading. Avoid fries and desserts if you want to limit fat and kcalories. If you order fries, use salt and catsup sparingly, if at all.

At a fast-food chicken place, hold the butter on the roll and the gravy on the potatoes. If available, order chicken that is baked, broiled, or barbecued instead of fried. At a pizza restaurant, hold the ham, sausage, extra cheese, and anchovies.

Order diet soft drinks, unsweetened iced tea, orange juice, or low-fat milk instead of regular soft drinks. If you can afford the kcalories, milk shakes are a reasonable option for the calcium they provide.

At a regular restaurant, order a salad and share a meal with a friend, or order a small "meal" from the appetizer list (such as vegetable soup and a seafood cocktail). Order the vegetable of the day or a plain baked potato with butter on the side instead of fries. Select foods that have been broiled or baked, not fried.

In general, eat selectively. Remember that you need not eat everything served to you. Take leftovers home with you for another meal. Supplement meals with missing foods (such as additional vegetables, nonfat milk, and fresh fruits). A stop at the grocery store for such specific items may serve you better than a restaurant.

Enjoy convenience foods on a limited basis. The more often you eat fast-food meals, the greater their impact on your nutrition status.

People can also improve their health with exercise. By exercising, you can earn the privilege of eating enough food to deliver the nutrients you need. Energy expenditure, the output side of the energy budget, is the opposite of money expenditure: it is *not* desirable to save energy. The more energy you spend (within reason, of course), the more food you can afford to eat—both food delivering nutrients and food delivering pleasure.

As this chapter said at the start, supplying food safely to over 250 million people is an incredible challenge—one that gets met, for the most part, with remarkable efficiency. The next chapter describes a contrasting situation— that of the food supply not reaching the people.

■ Study Questions

1. Describe several measures that help prevent food-borne illness. In whom are these conditions most likely to be severe?
2. Describe how contaminants find their way into foods and how a contaminant buildup occurs in the food chain.
3. How do pesticides become a hazard to the food supply, and how are they monitored?
4. What is the difference between a GRAS substance and a regulated food additive? Give examples of each.

■ Notes

1. S. A. Miller, as quoted by C. Lecos, Worrying about the *right* issues in food safety, *FDA Consumer*, November 1986, pp. 24–27.
2. Lecos, 1986.
3. F. E. Young and K. J. Skinner, Summer food safety tips, *FDA Consumer*, June 1987, pp. 17–19.
4. P. M. Schantz, The dangers of eating raw fish, *New England Journal of Medicine* 320 (1989): 1143–1145.
5. D. L. Morse and coauthors, Widespread outbreaks of

SELF STUDY *Study Your Own Diet*

Now that you have analyzed the entire array of nutrients in your diet, it's time to reach some conclusions.

1. Review your findings and summarize the strong points and weak points of the way you eat at present. How is your diet presently successful in delivering the nutrients you need within an appropriate number of kcalories? In what respects does it have room for improvement? Describe specific steps you might take to set about improving it with respect to:

- Balance of meals.
- Number and regularity of meals.
- Specific food choices.

2. Having completed all the exercises to this point you are in a position to decide whether you really need a vitamin-mineral supplement or other supplements. For each nutrient you've studied, compare your RDA or RNI, the amount you consume, and the amount contributed by your supplement. Does the supplement make up for a deficit in your intake, or is it an unnecessary extra? Perhaps, with the appropriate food choices, you can dispense with it.

clam- and oyster-associated gastroenteritis: Role of Norwalk virus, *New England Journal of Medicine* 314 (1986): 678–681; H. L. Dupont, Consumption of raw shellfish—Is the risk now unacceptable? (editorial), *New England Journal of Medicine* 314 (1986): 707–708; Sushi lovers: Beware of parasites, *Science News*, 2 March 1985, p. 141.

6. V. Modeland, Fishing for facts on fish safety, *FDA Consumer*, February 1989, pp. 16–24.

7. D. Farley, Chemicals we'd rather dine without, *FDA Consumer*, September 1988, pp. 10–15.

8. W. A. Krehl, Mercury, the slippery metal, *Nutrition Today*, November–December 1972, pp. 4–15.

9. 97% of Michigan population contaminated by 1973 spills, *Tallahassee Democrat*, 16 April 1982.

10. R. W. Miller, Honey: Making sure it's pure, *FDA Consumer*, September 1979, pp. 12–13; I. B. Vyhmeister, What about honey? *Life and Health*, August 1980, pp. 5–7.

11. A. Brynjolfsson, Food irradiation and nutrition, *Professional Nutritionist*, Fall 1979, pp. 7–10.

12. R. Dubos, The intellectual basis of nutrition science and practice. Paper presented at the NIH Conference on the Biomedical and Behavioral Basis of Clinical Nutrition, 19 June 1978, in Bethesda, Md., and reprinted in *Nutrition Today*, July–August 1979, pp. 31–34.

13. D. Farley, Setting safe limits on pesticide residues, *FDA Consumer*, October 1988, pp. 8–11.

14. Farley, 1988.

15. M. G. Mustafa, Agricultural chemicals, in *Adverse Effects of Foods*, eds. E. F. P. Jelliffe and D. B. Jelliffe (New York: Plenum Press, 1982), pp. 111–128.

16. Farley, 1988.

17. Farley, 1988.

18. Farley, 1988.

19. Dr. W. Gary Flamm of the FDA's Center for Food Safety and Applied Nutrition, as cited by K. Flieger, The Delaney dilemma, *FDA Consumer*, September 1988, pp. 18–19.

20. W. J. Curran, The *de Minimus* rule versus the Delaney Clause, *New England Journal of Medicine* 319 (1988): 1262–1264.

21. F. M. Strong, Toxicants occurring naturally in foods, in *Present Knowledge in Nutrition*, 4th ed. (Washington, D. C.: Nutrition Foundation, 1976), pp. 516–527.

22. T. M. Parkinson and J. P. Brown, Metabolic fate of food colorants, *Annual Review of Nutrition* 1 (1981): 175–205.

23. Use of vitamins as additives in processed foods, *Food Technology*, September 1987, pp. 163–168.

24. Cancer-causing substances in food, drugs, and cosmetics, *New England Journal of Medicine* 320 (1989): 934–936.

25. M. Gore, The Chinese restaurant syndrome, in *Adverse Effects of Foods*, eds. E. F. P. Jelliffe and D. B. Jelliffe (New York: Plenum Press, 1982), pp. 211–223.

26. C. W. Lecos, Sulfites: FDA limits uses, broadens labeling, *FDA Consumer*, October 1986, pp. 10–13.

27. S. L. Taylor and R. K. Bush, Sulfites as food ingredients, *Contemporary Nutrition*, a publication (1986) available from the Nutrition Department, General Mills Inc., P.O. Box 1172, Minneapolis, MN 55440.

28. One honey of an alternative to sulfites, *Science News* 134 (1988): 218.

29. New "food freshener," *Nutrition Forum* 5 (1988): 49.

30. W. F. Wilkens and J. I. Gray, Reduce N-nitrosamine formation in bacon, *Food Engineering* 58 (1986): 68–69; E. N. Frankel, Lipid oxidation: Mechanisms, products and biological significance, *Journal of American Oil Chemists' Society* 61 (1984): 1908–1917.

31. F. R. Shank and V. L. Wilkening, Considerations for food fortification policy, *Cereal Foods World* 31 (1986): 728–740.

32. *Irradiated Foods*, a report (December 1988) available from the American Council on Science and Health, 1995 Broadway, New York, NY 10023–5860.

33. A. Rogan and G. Glaros, Food irradiation: The process and implications for dietitians, *Journal of the American Dietetic Association* 88 (1988): 833–838.

34. Position of the American Dietetic Association: Health implications of dietary fiber, *Journal of the American Dietetic Association* 88 (1988): 216.

35. J. Hallfrisch and coauthors, Acceptability of a 7-day higher-carbohydrate, lower-fat menu: The Beltsville Diet study, *Journal of the American Dietetic Association* 88 (1988): 163–168.

People often ask what information a food label provides, and which kinds of foods are most and least nutritious. The person who wants to read food labels intelligently needs to know, first, what information they present. According to law, every food label must prominently display and express in ordinary words:

- The common name of the product.
- The name and address of the manufacturer, packer, or distributor.
- The net contents in terms of weight, measure, or count.

Then, unless the food has a standard of identity (explained later), the label must list:

- The ingredients, in descending order of predominance by weight.

All labels must state at least this much. Even if they say no more, you can learn a lot about the nutritional value of a product from the ingredient list. Consider the following products:

- An orange powder that contains "sugar, citric acid, orange flavor . . ." versus a juice can that contains "water; tomato concentrate; concentrated juices of carrots, celery. . ."
- A cereal that contains "puffed milled corn, sugar, corn syrup, molasses, salt . . ." versus one that contains "100 percent rolled oats."
- A canned fruit that contains "apples, water."

By knowing that the first ingredient named is the one that predominates by weight, you can tell what you are getting in the largest quantity.

A label that provides any nutrition information or makes any nutrition claim must meet additional labeling requirements. For example, if manufacturers add a nutrient to a food

(such as vitamin C to a breakfast drink), or if they make a specific advertising claim (such as "This food is a good source of vitamin A"), then the package must provide an information panel that conforms *fully* with the following format under the heading "Nutrition Information":

- Serving or portion size.
- Servings or portions per container.
- Food energy (in kcalories) per serving.
- Protein (grams) per serving.
- Carbohydrate (grams) per serving.
- Fat (grams) per serving.
- Sodium (milligrams) per serving.
- Protein, vitamins, and minerals as percentages of the U.S. RDA. (No claim may be made that a food is a significant source of a nutrient unless it provides at least 10 percent of the U.S. RDA of that nutrient in a serving.)

Furthermore, labels must list any additives used and their functions. Figure H16–1 demonstrates the reading of a label.

Labeling laws also specify just what words labels may use and what specific terms mean (see Figure H16–1 and the Miniglossary of Terms on Food Labels). With an understanding of the U.S. RDA (see Chapter 2 and the accompanying box), consumers can extract a lot of information from a nutrition label.

Even with a complete information panel, nutrition claims can still deceive consumers. Therefore, food labels may not claim:

- That a food is effective as a treatment for disease.
- That a balanced diet of ordinary foods cannot supply adequate amounts of nutrients (excepting the iron requirements of infants, children, and pregnant or lactating women).

- That the soil on which food is grown may be responsible for deficiencies in quality.
- That storage, transportation, processing, or cooking of a food may be responsible for deficiencies in its quality.
- That a food has particular dietary qualities when such qualities have not been shown to be significant in human nutrition.
- That a natural vitamin is superior to a synthetic vitamin.

The FDA permits some scientifically based health statements on labels, subject to approval.[1] The label information must emphasize the importance of the total diet without undue emphasis on the role of diet in disease prevention. It is permissible to state on the label of a high-fiber cereal, for example, that "a high-fiber diet may reduce your risk of some kinds of cancer." The statement is true, and it is phrased in terms of total diet, not in terms of the particular cereal in the box. The cereal, after all, may indeed provide abundant fiber, but it may also provide large quantities of fat, and yet this information does not receive equal billing on the label. Labels are permitted to deliver responsible nutrition education to the public, providing they include only truthful, nonmisleading claims based on scientific evidence.[2]

Some convenience foods have no information panels, and simply say "TV dinner" or "macaroni and cheese." FDA nutritional quality guidelines have been established for products such as frozen dinners, breakfast cereals, vitamin C-fortified beverages, and main dishes such as pizza or macaroni and cheese. If a product complies with these guidelines, it may carry on its label the statement that it "provides nutrients in

■ **FIGURE H16–1**
How to Read a Food Label

The ingredient list on the front or side panel names the ingredients in order of predominance by weight. Significance to you, the consumer: what appears first is present in the largest quantity. Only products with standards of identity (recipes defined by law) have no ingredient list.

The front of the package must always tell you the product name, the name and address of the company, and the weight or measure; and it may list the ingredients.

The label may also state information about sodium and kcalories.

Nutrition Information (per serving)[a]
Serving Size = ½ c
Servings per Container = 10

	Cereal	With ½ c nonfat milk (Vitamins A– and D–fortified)[b]
Calories	140	180
Protein (g)[c]	4	8
Total carbohydrates (g)[d]	32	38
Simple sugars (g)	11	17
Complex carbohydrates (g)	17	17
Fiber (g)	4	4
Fat (g)[e]	1	1
Cholesterol (mg)	0	0
Sodium (mg)[f]	55	120

Currently optional, dietary fiber and cholesterol will be required under new labeling laws. In addition to the information presented here, labels will provide the saturated fat content, and the number of kcalories from fat.

Percentage of U.S. Recommended Daily Allowances (U.S. RDA)[g]

Protein	6	15
Vitamin A	4	10
Vitamin C	*	2
Thiamin	25	30
Riboflavin	25	35
Niacin	25	25
Calcium	2	15
Iron	25	25

Some currently required information will become optional; for example, the U.S. RDA for protein and most vitamins and minerals. Vitamins A and C, and the minerals iron and calcium will remain.

* Contains less than 2% of the U.S. RDA of this nutrient.

[a]The nutrition information panel tells you the nutrients in a serving. The serving size may or may not be the same as the amount you eat. Check the servings per container to get an idea if it is.
[b]The nutrient contents are listed in the food and as served (after adding milk, in this example).
[c]The energy-yielding nutrients are given in grams (units of weight). This is especially meaningful with respect to protein, because you need 40 to 80 g/day, depending on your size and other factors. Protein is also given in percentage of U.S. RDA in the list below.
[d]The carbohydrate breakdown tells you how much simple sugar, starch, and dietary fiber is in the product.
[e]A fat breakdown may also be listed, including saturated fat, unsaturated fat, and cholesterol.
[f]Sodium is listed in milligrams. A safe minimum intake is 500 mg sodium/day; recommendations limit salt intake to 6,000 mg salt/day (2,400 mg sodium/day). A teaspoon of salt contains just over 2,000 mg sodium.
[g]Protein, vitamins, and minerals are given in percentages of U.S. RDA (see inside front cover, right). Significance to you, the consumer: if it meets 10% of the U.S. RDA, it almost undoubtedly meets at least 10% of your daily needs.

Miniglossary of Terms on Food Labels

Cholesterol
cholesterol-free: less than 2 mg/serving.
low-cholesterol: less than 20 mg/serving.
reduced cholesterol: processed to reduce the cholesterol content by at least 75%, compared with the original.

Energy
diet or dietetic: must meet criteria of either low-kcalorie or reduced-kcalorie food, or state otherwise.
low-kcalorie: no more than 40 kcal/serving or 0.4 kcal/g.
reduced kcalorie: at least one-third lower in kcalories than the food it most closely resembles.

Fat
extra lean: 95% fat-free by weight.
lean or **low-fat:** 90% fat-free by weight. (The word *lean* as part of the brand name—as in "Lean Supreme"—indicates that the product is 25% lower in fat than the regular variety of the same food.)
leaner or lower-fat: made with less fat than the regular variety of the same food.

Sodium
sodium-free: less than 5 mg/serving.
very-low-sodium: 35 mg or less per serving.
low-sodium: 140 mg or less per serving.
reduced sodium: processed to reduce the usual level of sodium by 75%.
unsalted, no added salt, salt-free: processed without the normally used salt (may still contain the sodium present in the food originally).
low-salt: made with less salt than the regular variety of the same food.

Sugar
sugar-free, sugarless, no sugar: no sugar, but may contain kcaloric sweeteners; must meet criteria of low-kcalorie or reduced-kcalorie food, or state otherwise.

Calculating Nutrient Amounts from the U.S. RDA Amounts on Labels

The "percentage of U.S. RDA" on a label describes the amount of each nutrient in a serving as compared with the U.S. RDA. To determine exactly how many *units* of a nutrient a serving provides, do a simple calculation. Find out from the U.S. RDA table on the inside front cover of this book how many units the U.S. RDA is. Multiply that number by the percentage on the label, and you have the answer.

Suppose a label says that a serving provides "25% of the U.S. RDA" for vitamin A, for example. Turn to the U.S. RDA table (inside front cover, right). It states that the U.S. RDA is 1,000 RE, so you can deduce that each serving must therefore offer 250 RE.

amounts appropriate for this class of food as determined by the U.S. government."*

Standards of Identity
Some labels offer nothing more than a name, such as *mayonnaise*. For this and other products, the law provides standards of identity and excuses manufacturers from the requirement of listing ingredients. Standards of identity exist for many common foods that at one time were often prepared at home, so that the basic recipe was understood by almost everyone. (Bread is another example.) To use the standard names, the foods must contain certain ingredients in specific percentages defined by law.** The FDA does not have the authority to require that ingredients be listed for these foods, but it urges manufacturers to give the consumer more detailed information, and many manufacturers do so voluntarily.

Imitation Foods
Foods developed in imitation of, and as substitutes for, familiar foods often concern consumers. With advancing food technology, many imitation food products may benefit consumers. For example, egg replacers may be superior to eggs for people who wish to reduce their cholesterol intakes. Highlight 5 gives other examples. In cases like this, to imply that imitations are inferior to traditional foods is to

---

*For example, frozen dinners must contain one or more sources of protein from meat, poultry, fish, cheese, or eggs, and these must make up at least 70 percent of the total protein; these products must include one or more vegetables or vegetable mixtures other than potatoes, rice, or cereal-based products; and they must have a certain minimum nutrient level for each 100 kcalories.

**Mayonnaise, for example, may use that name on the label only if it contains 65 percent by weight of vegetable oil, either vinegar or lemon juice, and egg yolk.

mislead the consumer. For this reason, the law requires that the word *imitation* be used on the label only if the product is "a substitute for and resembles another food but is *nutritionally inferior* to the food imitated. . . . Nutritional inferiority is defined as a reduction in the content of an essential vitamin or mineral or of protein that amounts to 10 percent or more of the U.S. RDA."

Enriched Foods

Terms commonly used to describe grain foods such as *refined, enriched,* and *whole grain* reflect the nutrient losses incurred during the milling of grains and the replacement of some nutrients in the making of products (see the Miniglossary of Grain Food Terms and Figure H16–2). When milling wheat and baking bread became a common and automated process, bread eaters suffered a tragic loss of many nutrients that they had formerly received from bread. As a consequence, the Enrichment Act of 1942 required that all grain products that cross state lines must be enriched with iron, thiamin, riboflavin, and niacin. Manufacturers restore iron and niacin to the levels found in whole wheat; and thiamin, and especially riboflavin, to higher levels. You can almost take it for granted that all breads, grains like rice, wheat products like macaroni and spaghetti, and cereals (both cooked and ready-to-eat types) have been enriched.

Enrichment doesn't make a single slice of bread "rich" in these added nutrients, but people who eat several servings of grain products a day obtain significantly more of these nutrients than they would from unenriched white bread. To a great extent, the enrichment of white flour helps to prevent deficiencies of these four nutrients, but it fails to compensate for other losses incurred during the refining of the grain—losses of many other nutrients and fiber. As Figure H16–3 shows, enrichment makes

---

> ### Miniglossary of Grain Food Terms
>
> **bran**: the chief fiber donator of a grain.
> **endosperm**: the bulk of the edible part of a grain, the starchy part.
> **enriched food**: a processed food to which nutrients have been added; specifically, in the case of refined bread or cereal, four nutrients have been added: thiamin, niacin, and riboflavin in amounts approximately equivalent to, or higher than, those originally present and iron in amounts to alleviate the prevalence of iron-deficiency anemia. The term *enriched* is also used with the meaning of *fortified,* described later.
> **germ**: the nutrient-rich inner part of a grain.
> **gluten**: an elastic protein formed in certain grain products by the mechanical action of kneading that confers structure and cohesiveness on them.
> **husk**: the outer, inedible part of a grain.
> **refined food**: a food from which the coarse parts have been removed; specifically, with respect to grains, a product from which the bran, germ, and chaff have been removed, leaving only the endosperm.
> **whole grain**: a grain milled in its entirety (all but the husk), not refined.

---

refined bread comparable to whole-grain bread only with respect to the four nutrients added back, and not with respect to others. Enrichment of wheat and other cereal products, in other words, doesn't improve them enough—whole-grain items still outshine them. If bread is a staple food in your diet—that is, if you eat it every day—you would be well advised to learn to like the hearty flavor of whole-grain bread.

Fortified Foods

Like an enriched food, a *fortified* food has had nutrients added to it, but in a fortified food, the added nutrients may or may not have been in the original product. Examples are:

- Milk, to which vitamins A and D are added.
- Soy milk, to which calcium and vitamin B_{12} are added.
- Salt, to which iodine is added.

> ### Miniglossary
>
> **fortified**: a term referring to the addition of nutrients to a food to correct or prevent a widespread nutrient deficiency; to balance the total nutrient profile of a food; or to restore nutrients lost in processing. Often, the added nutrients were not originally present and have been added in amounts greater than might be found there naturally.
> **standards of identity**: standards for the recipes manufacturers must use if they are to be permitted to use certain common names on labels.
> **supplement**: as used on food labels, a term that means that nutrients have been added in amounts greater than 50% above the U.S. RDA.

■ **FIGURE H16–2**
A Wheat Plant

To make flour and then bread, kernels are first separated from the stem of the wheat plant and then further broken apart by the milling process. A wheat kernel (a whole grain) has four main parts: the germ, the endosperm, the bran, and the husk. The germ is the seed that grows into a wheat plant, and so it is especially rich in vitamins and minerals to support new life. The endosperm is the soft, white inside portion of the kernel containing starch and proteins. The bran, a protective coating around the kernel similar in function to the shell of a nut, is also rich in nutrients and fiber. The husk, commonly called chaff, is unusable for most purposes except for animal feed. When made into white flour and mixed with liquid, the endosperm forms a stretchy protein called gluten. Gluten allows a lacy network of air bubbles to be baked in, making bread appealingly light and soft.

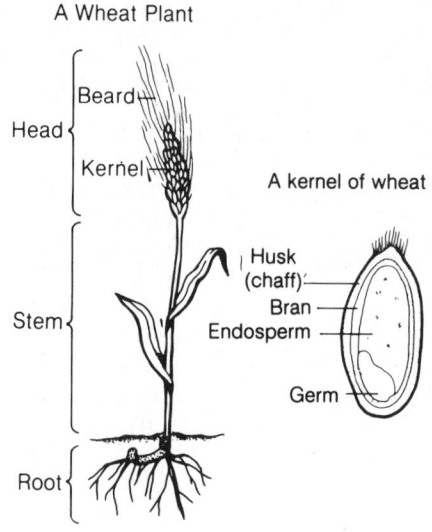

A Wheat Plant

Head — Beard, Kernel

Stem

Root

A kernel of wheat

Husk (chaff)
Bran
Endosperm
Germ

- A sweetened drink, to which vitamin C is added.
- A breakfast cereal, to which 100 percent of the U.S. RDA of several vitamins have been added.

The FDA has standards for the amounts of nutrients added to food products but does not require fortification of any products. Some fortified foods may *appear* to be nutritious because of the list of nutrients on their labels, but they may have lost many nutrients not listed, and which the original fresh foods naturally contained. To know whether a food is really nutritious for you, you have to view it in the context of your total diet. If it provides nutrients you need, then it is doing its job in your diet. Most nutritious foods do not come with labels (for example, oranges, broccoli, eggs, and chicken). You have to know more about foods than just what's on the label.

Breakfast cereals lead the list of the most highly fortified foods on the market; some of them have every vitamin and mineral of the U.S. RDA tables added. When a food has nutrients added in amounts greater than 50 percent above the U.S. RDA, it must be labeled as a "supplement," the same term that is used to describe a vitamin-mineral pill. This is an accurate term, for breakfast cereals made from refined flour and fortified with high doses of nutrients are actually more like pills in a cereal disguise than like whole grains. They may be nutritious—with respect to the nutrients added—but they still may fail to convey the full spectrum of nutrients that an unrefined food (or better, a mixture of such foods) might provide. Keep in mind that not all nutrients have assigned U.S. RDA values for labels.

Descriptive Terms

Some terms on labels, such as *health food* and *organic food,* have no legal definitions. The term *health food* is often used misleadingly on labels to imply unusual power to promote health. The term *organic* as used by a chemist denotes the presence of molecules with carbon atoms in them, but it also has a popular definition that is legal in some states: a food or nutrient produced without the use of chemical fertilizers, pesticides, or additives. Again, this term may be misleading, and it has not been legally defined by the FDA.

When used on meat and poultry labels, the word *natural* means that the product contains no artificial ingredients or chemical preservatives and that it has been minimally processed. When used on other foods, however, it can mean anything at all. The National Advertising Division of the Council of Better Business Bureaus has voluntarily adopted some guidelines. While these guidelines appear logical, they permit use of the word under conditions that might surprise consumers. Foods that can be labeled "natural" include ice cream, carbonated beverages, chewing gum, syrup, flavored drink mixes, pan spray coating, and purified fructose—even though they contain added refined sugar, added salt, added fat, or no nutrients at all.[3]

The meat and poultry industry uses the terms *light* or *lite* to describe

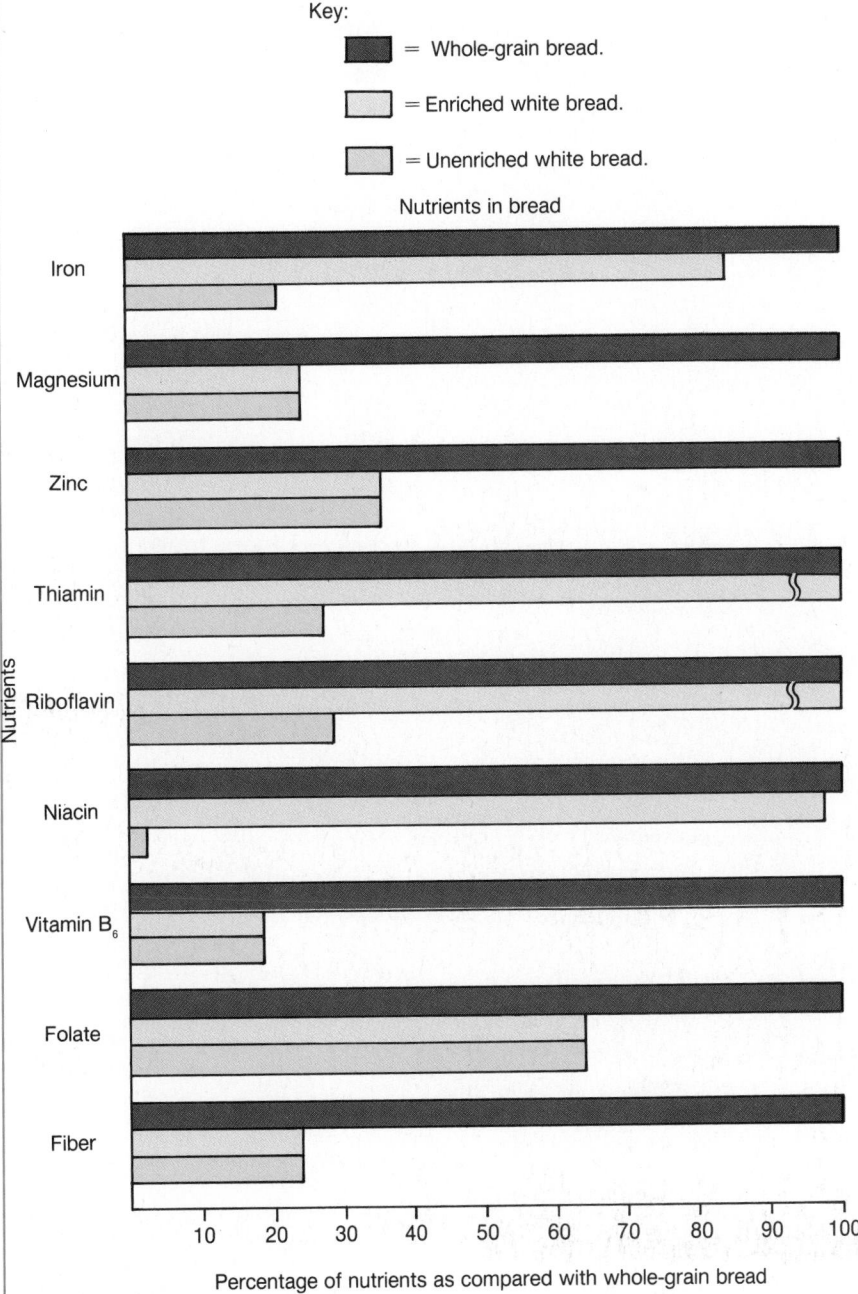

Key:
█ = Whole-grain bread.
▫ = Enriched white bread.
▪ = Unenriched white bread.

Nutrients in bread

Percentage of nutrients as compared with whole-grain bread

■ **FIGURE H16–3**
Nutrients in Bread
For iron, thiamin, riboflavin, and niacin, enriched bread provides about the same quantities as in whole-grain bread, and significantly more than unenriched bread. For fiber and the other nutrients (both those shown here and those not shown), enriched bread provides less than whole-grain bread.

products that contain 25 percent less of a stated ingredient (such as fat) than was originally present. Manufacturers of other products use these terms without legal guidelines. People hope these words mean that foods have been made with less fat, less cholesterol, less salt, fewer kcalories, less alcohol, or less sugar. Some products may be just what these consumers wanted, like thinly sliced whole-grain breads; others, such as light potato chips, may contain fewer kcalories per serving than the originals, but still provide plenty of fat and salt. As a national beer advertisement reminds us, we each have our own definition of light.

In 1990, legislation to extensively revise federal nutrition labeling laws was enacted and is scheduled to take effect by May 1992. Expect to see nutrition information for most grocery store items, including unpackaged foods such as produce and seafood. Serving sizes will be standardized and the U.S. RDA will reflect the latest RDA. In addition, FDA will define descriptive terms such as "high-fiber," and place conditions on the use of terms such as "cholesterol-free." For example, in addition to having minimal cholesterol, a "cholesterol-free" product must also contain less than 5 grams of fat with no more than 2 grams of saturated fat per serving.

Food labels contain a wealth of information. Armed with the knowledge of how to read a food label, consumers can make their selections with confidence.

NOTES
1. T. P. Labuza, A perspective on health claims in food labeling, *Cereal Foods World* 32 (1987): 256–267.
2. Nutrition information on food labels—ADA timely statement, *Journal of the American Dietetic Association* 89 (1989): 266–268.
3. Food cases involving "natural" claims, *NAD Case Report* (a newsletter from the Council of Better Business Bureaus, 845 Third Ave., New York, NY 10022), October 1984.

17

Domestic and World Hunger

These are microvilli on the surfaces of five neighboring cells of the cornea of the eye, viewed from the top (the opening art of Chapter 3 shows the microvilli on the surface of the GI tract lining viewed from the side). These intricate structures depend on vitamin A. Vitamin A malnutrition is the leading cause of childhood blindness in the world—and it is preventable.

Throughout this book, the problems of overnutrition—obesity, heart disease, cancer, and others—have guided recommendations, for these are the diseases of our society, of the economically developed nations. Not everyone shares these problems, though. People in developing nations, as well as people in the less-privileged parts of developed nations, suffer the problems of undernutrition, which is characterized by chronic debilitating hunger and malnutrition.* These conditions are most visible in times of famine, but they are widespread and persistent even when famine does not occur. They have been with us throughout history, and despite numerous development programs, they are not disappearing; the number of hungry and malnourished people continues to grow.

Everyone has known the uncomfortable feeling of hunger that signals "time to eat" and passes with the eating of the next meal. But many people know hunger more intimately, as a constant companion because a meal does not follow to quiet the signal. For them, hunger is ceaseless discomfort, weakness, and pain—the continuous lack of food and nutrients. People who live with chronic hunger either have too little food to eat or do not receive an adequate intake of the essential nutrients from the foods available to them—either way, malnutrition ensues.

To discuss hunger like this, though, is to fail to describe the depth of the experience of living without food. The following excerpt from a writer in Boston describes hunger in more personal terms:

> I've had no income and I've paid no rent for many months. My landlord let me stay. He felt sorry for me because I had no money. The Friday before Christmas he gave me ten dollars. For days I had had nothing but water. I knew I needed food; I tried to go out but I was too weak to walk to the store. I felt as if I were dying. I saw the mailman and told him I thought I was starving. He brought me food and then he made some phone calls and that's when they began delivering these lunches. But I had already lost so much weight that five meals a week are not enough to keep me going.
>
> I just pray to God I can survive. I keep praying I can have the will to save some of my food so I can divide it up and make it last. It's hard to save because I am so hungry that I want to eat it right away. On Friday, I held over two peas from the lunch. I ate one pea on Saturday morning. Then I got into bed with the taste of food in my mouth and I waited as long as I could. Later on in the day I ate the other pea.
>
> Today I saved the container that the mashed potatoes were in and tonight, before bed, I'll lick the sides of the container.
>
> When there are bones I keep them. I know this is going to be hard for you to believe and I am almost ashamed to tell you, but these days I boil the bones till they're soft and then I eat them. Today there were no bones.[1]

undernutrition (also called **hunger**): as used in this chapter, a term that describes the domestic and world food problem of a continuous lack of the food energy and nutrients necessary to achieve and maintain health and protection from disease.

malnutrition: the impairment of health resulting from a relative deficiency or excess of food energy and specific nutrients necessary for health.

famine: widespread lack of access to food due to natural disasters, political factors, or war; characterized by a large number of deaths due to starvation and malnutrition.

---

*A way of delineating developed versus developing countries is by the terms **First World, Second World,** and **Third World**. *First World* refers to the developed market economy nations (Western Europe, North America, Japan, Australia, and New Zealand). *Second World* refers to developed nations within centrally planned economies (Eastern Europe and the U.S.S.R.). *Third World* is used for the developing countries. (The term *Fourth World* is sometimes used to refer to the poorest of the Third World countries.)

Feeding the hungry—in the United States.

Feeding the hungry—in Nepal.

In this excerpt, a person in the Third World describes hunger in another way:

For hunger is a curious thing: at first it is with you all the time, waking and sleeping and in your dreams, and your belly cries out insistently, and there is a gnawing and a pain as if your very vitals were being devoured, and you must stop it at any cost, and you buy a moment's respite even while you know and fear the sequel. Then the pain is no longer sharp but dull, and this too is with you always, so that you think of food many times a day and each time a terrible sickness assails you, and because you know this you try to avoid the thought, but you cannot, it is with you. Then that too is gone, all pain, all desire, only a great emptiness is left, like the sky, like a well in drought, and it is now that the strength drains from your limbs, and you try to rise and you cannot, or to swallow and your throat is powerless, and both the swallow and the effort of retaining the liquid tax you to the uttermost.[2]

This chapter examines the extent of hunger and malnutrition in the United States and around the world; it offers suggestions for personal involvement with the issues presented. The highlight that follows this chapter describes the profound relationships between people, their food, and the planet's well-being through a discussion of the world's environment. As you read, challenge yourself with the answers to the following questions: What problems would you attack first in solving the problem of hunger and malnutrition? To what extent should the First World get involved in tackling problems related to Third or Fourth World hunger? Should we solve our own hunger problems first? These issues are complex and often overwhelming from an individual's standpoint. Remember, however, as you read, that it is better to light one small candle than to curse the darkness.

■ *Hunger and Undernutrition*

All people need food. Regardless of race, religion, sex, or nationality, our bodies experience similarly the effects of hunger and its companion malnutrition—listlessness, weakness, failure to thrive, stunted growth, mental retardation, muscle wastage, scurvy, pellagra, beriberi, anemia, rickets, osteoporosis, goiter, tooth decay, blindness, and a host of other effects, including death. Apathy and shortened attention span are two of a number of behavioral symptoms that are often mistaken for laziness, lack of intelligence, or mental illness in undernourished people.

The Food and Agriculture Organization (FAO) estimates that of the more than 5 billion people in the world, at least half a billion suffer some form of undernutrition. About 250 million are children of preschool age, and 10 million of these weigh less than 60 percent of the standard weight for their age. You may recall from Chapter 9 that an estimated 250,000 children are blinded every year by xerophthalmia (see p. 245), the leading cause of preventable blindness in children, as a result of an insufficiency of vitamin A in the diet. Vitamin A deficiency is also associated with other forms of malnutrition, infection, diarrhea, and a high rate of mortality.

Hunger was once viewed as a problem of overpopulation and inadequate food production, but now many people recognize it as a problem of poverty (see Figure 17–1). Poverty exists for many reasons, including overpopula-

poverty: the state of having too little money to meet minimum needs for food, clothing, and shelter. As of the late-1980s, the U.S. Department of Health and Human Services defined a poverty-level income as $10,650 annually for a family of four.

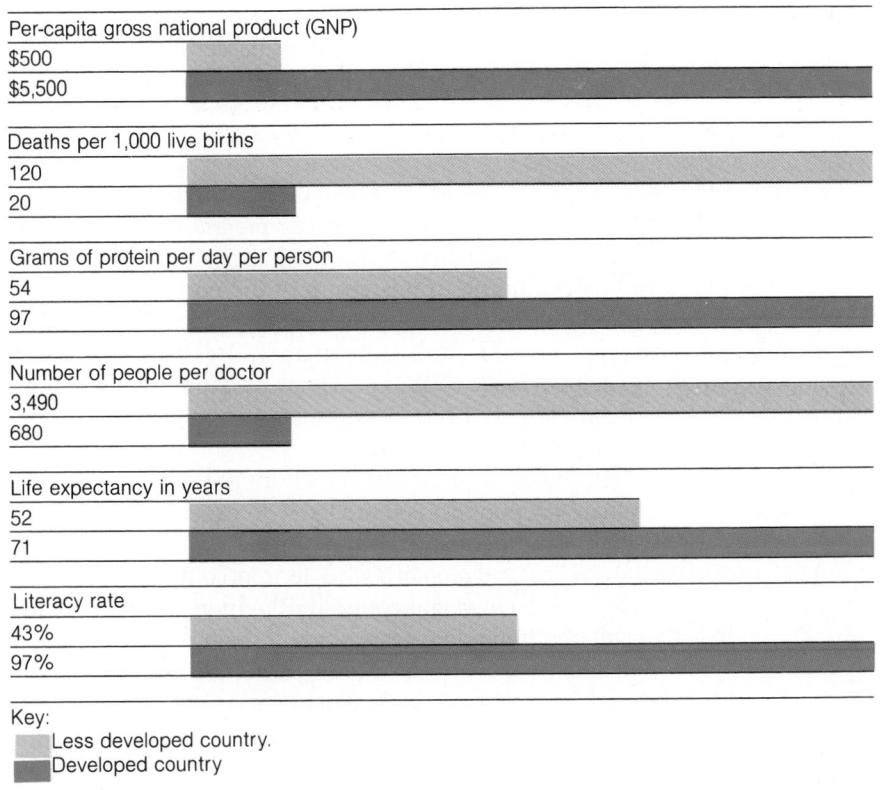

Per-capita gross national product (GNP)
$500
$5,500

Deaths per 1,000 live births
120
20

Grams of protein per day per person
54
97

Number of people per doctor
3,490
680

Life expectancy in years
52
71

Literacy rate
43%
97%

Key:
Less developed country.
Developed country

■ **FIGURE 17–1**

The Gap between Developed and Less Developed Countries

Notice that the poorer nations have higher infant mortality rates, lower daily protein intakes, fewer doctors available, shorter life expectancies, and lower literacy rates than richer nations. In short, the quality of life suffers from poverty.

Source: U.S. Presidential Commission on World Hunger, *Overcoming World Hunger: The Challenge Ahead*, abridged ed. (Washington, D.C.: Government Printing Office, June 1980), p. 4.

tion; the greed of others; unemployment; the lack of productive resources such as land, tools, and credit; and numerous other factors. If it is at all possible to provide adequate nutrition for all the earth's hungry people, it can only be achieved when the economic, political, and social structures that create a gap between rich and poor, and thereby limit food production, distribution, and consumption, become the targets of change.

Worldwide, about 40,000 to 50,000 people die each day as a result of undernutrition. Millions of children die each year from the diseases of poverty: parasitic and infectious diseases such as dysentery, whooping cough, measles, tuberculosis, cholera, and malaria. These diseases interact with poor nutrition to form a vicious cycle in which the outcome for many is death. It is estimated that 1 child dies of these causes every 2 seconds[3]—15 have died in the 30 seconds it took you to read this paragraph.

Hungry people receive such small quantities of food that they develop multiple nutrient deficiencies. Their undernutrition may result from a lack of food energy or it may result from a lack of both food energy and protein. Such distinctions can easily be made on paper, and the extremes are evident in individuals; but for the most part, the differences blur.

The malnutrition that comes from living with hunger is one of the major factors influencing life expectancy. According to the *1986 World Population Data Sheet*, life expectancy at birth in the United States and Canada is now about 76 years.[4] In Japan, Iceland, and Sweden, it is about 77 years. Worldwide, life expectancy averages about 62 years, but in Africa it is approximately 50, and in the small African country of Sierra Leone it is only 34.

Hunger and malnutrition can be found living with people of all ages, sexes, and nationalities. Even so, these problems hit some groups harder than others.

Children at Risk

When nutrient needs are high (as in times of rapid growth), the risk of undernutrition increases. If family food is limited, pregnant and lactating women, infants, and children are the first to show the signs of undernutrition. Effects of hunger can be devastating to this group of the population.

As Chapter 14 pointed out, to support normal fetal growth and development, women must gain weight during pregnancy. Healthy women in developed countries gain an average of about 27 pounds. Studies among poor women show a weight gain of only 11 to 15 pounds.[5] As a consequence, they give birth to babies with low birthweights.

Birthweight is a potent indicator of an infant's future health status. A low-birthweight baby (less than 5½ pounds) is more likely to experience complications during delivery than a normal baby, and has a statistically greater-than-normal chance of having physical and mental birth defects, of contracting diseases, and of dying early in life. Low birthweight contributes to more than half of the deaths, worldwide, of children under five years of age. Low-birthweight infants suffering undernutrition after their births incur even greater risks. They are more likely to get sick, to be unable to obtain nourishment by sucking, and to be unable to win their mothers' attention by energetic, vigorous cries and other healthy behavior. They can become apathetic, neglected babies, and this compounds the original malnutrition problems.

Breastfeeding permits infants in many developing countries to achieve weight and height gains equal to those of children in developed countries until about six months of age, but then the majority of these children fall behind in their growth and development because of the inadequate addition of supplementary foods to their diets. Visitors to developing countries may overlook the undernutrition of children because they do not realize that when they see children they think are three or four years old, that the children are actually eight or nine years old. Failure of children to grow is a warning of the extreme malnutrition that may soon follow.

Replacing breast milk with infant formula in environments and economic circumstances that make it impossible to feed formula safely may lead to infant undernutrition. Breast milk, the recommended food for infants, is sterile and contains antibodies that enhance an infant's resistance to disease. Formula in bottles, in the absence of sterilization and refrigeration, is an ideal breeding ground for bacteria. More than 1.2 billion people in developing countries do not have access to safe drinking water.[6] Mixing contaminated water with formula powder and feeding this to infants often cause infections leading to diarrhea, dehydration, and failure to absorb nutrients. In countries where poor sanitation is prevalent, breastfeeding should take priority over feeding formula. Failure to breastfeed an infant who lives in a house without indoor plumbing incurs twice the risk of perinatal mortality as breastfeeding an infant who lives in a house with good sanitation.[7]

Even if infants are protected by breastfeeding at first, they must be weaned. The weaning period is one of the most dangerous periods for children in

weaning period: the time during which an infant's diet is changed from breast milk to other nourishment.

developing countries, for a number of reasons. For one, newly weaned infants often receive nutrient-poor diluted cereals or starchy root crops. For another, the infants' foods are often prepared with contaminated water, making infection almost inevitable.

Mortality statistics reflect the hazards to infants and children. The infant mortality rate ranges from about 34 (Sri Lanka) to over 185 (Afghanistan) in the poorest of the developing countries, as compared with averages of 7 to 16 in the developed countries. The death rate for children from one to four years old is no more favorable; it ranges from 20 to 30 times higher in developing countries than in developed countries.[8]

infant mortality rate: the number of deaths during the first year of life per 1,000 live births.

Cultural Traditions

Women are more susceptible than men to hunger and undernutrition for a number of reasons. In addition to their increased needs during the childbearing years, many women in developing countries are responsible, even during their pregnancies, for most of the physical labor required to procure food for their families. The poor nutrition of some women results from both their families' lack of access to food and unequal distribution of the food supply within their own families. A woman will feed her husband, children, and other family members first, eating only whatever is left. Furthermore, each time she becomes pregnant, her body's nutrient reserves are drained.

Social beliefs may also limit women's food intakes. In the Indian Punjab, the director of a program aimed at relieving undernutrition in local villages found that an undernutrition rate of 10 to 15 percent persisted even after a major effort to provide supplementary foods to families. The majority of those affected were young girls, unable to demand their share and unrecognized by other family members as deserving a fair share. In other areas of India, a child may be forbidden to eat curds and fruit because they are "cold," or bananas because they "cause convulsions."[9]

Severe malnutrition occurs in African countries, Central America, South America, the Near East, and the Far East. Cases have also been reported on the Indian reservations and in other areas of the United States. First, we will look at hunger in the United States, and then we will consider hunger in the developing countries.

■ Hunger in the United States

The United States is the wealthiest nation in the world, consumes 40 percent of the world's resources, and is home to only 6 percent of the world's people. Still, it does not meet the food needs of its poor.

Since the early 1980s, numerous studies on hunger have been conducted throughout the United States.* Almost without exception, these studies find

*Groups that have conducted studies include the U.S. Conference of Mayors, the National Council of Churches, the Citizens' Commission on Hunger in New England, Bread for the World, the President's Task Force on Food Assistance, the Physician Task Force on Hunger, and the Food Research and Action Center.

hunger to be a serious and rapidly growing problem. Approximately 20 million people in the United States—12 million children and 8 million adults—are suffering from chronic hunger, with the problems getting worse in all regions of the country. America has become a soup kitchen society to an extent unmatched since the bread lines of the Great Depression. Malnutrition and other health problems associated with chronic hunger—stunted growth, failure to thrive, low-birthweight babies, infant mortality, and anemia—are either reported to be escalating for the first time in many years, or slowing in their long-term rates of improvement. In some of these conditions, the United States compares poorly with other industrialized countries (see Figure 17–2).

Who Are the Hungry in the United States?

Through the late 1960s, hunger was evident among the chronic poor: migrant workers, Native Americans, southern blacks, unemployed minorities, and some of the elderly. These groups were hungry during the 1970s as well, as were the newly unemployed blue-collar workers. Now, hunger is reaching into other segments of the population, without regard for age, marital status,

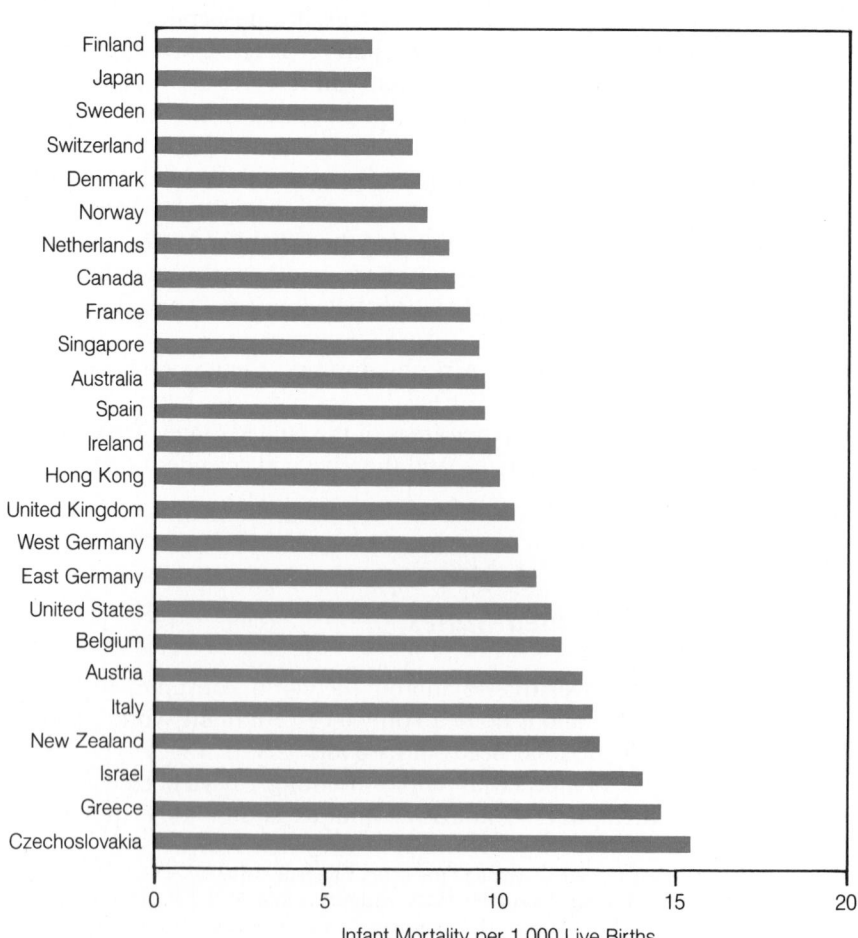

■ **FIGURE 17–2**
Infant Mortality Rate
Infant mortality rate reflects infant deaths in the first year of life per 1,000 live births and serves as an indicator of a nation's health status. Frequently, these babies weigh less than 5 lb at birth because of the mothers' poor nutrition status. The United States ranks 18th among 25 industrialized nations with a population of 2.5 million or more.

Source: Adapted with permission from ''Hunger in the U.S.,'' by J. Larry Brown. Copyright© 1987 by Scientific American, Inc. All rights reserved.

previous employment or successes, family ties, or efforts to change the situation. The U.S. farm economy has been burdened by chronic price-depressing surpluses, and available resources are failing to reach many groups. One in 12 goes hungry at least two days a month. The millions who experience hunger today in the United States include:

- *The young.* One in five U.S. children lives in poverty; an estimated 500,000 children suffer from malnutrition.[10]
- *The new poor.* Changes in the nation's economy during the 1980s have hurt millions of people who were once members of the middle class—displaced farm families and former blue-collar workers forced out of manufacturing (oil, natural gas, steel, and mining) into the service sector (maintenance and the hotel and restaurant industry). The auto industry, for example, has laid off some 40 percent of its workers since 1978. Only a third of them find jobs that pay as well as their old ones. A job that pays minimum wage does not lift a family above the federal poverty line, and many such jobs fail to provide fringe benefits to help meet rising health care costs. A minority of the poor in America are on welfare; most are working people.
- *The elderly.* Social Security benefits and other programs have pulled many older people out of poverty, but large numbers of older people who cannot work and have no savings or families to turn to are facing rising bills for housing, utilities, food, and health care. The United States is one of only two industrialized nations (the other is South Africa) that has no national health insurance program.
- *The homeless.* As many as 3.5 million people may now be living on the streets. More than half of the homeless are single mothers with children; many of the homeless are former residents of mental institutions.
- *Low-income women.* Many women live in poverty, struggling with burdens of providing child care and working for minimum wage.
- *Ethnic minorities.* While the majority of the poor in America are white, the median income of black and Hispanic families is lower than that of white families.

The most compelling single reason for this hunger is poverty.

In addition to those people who suffer from malnutrition as a result of hunger, many people are malnourished as a result of an illness or the treatment of an illness, as Chapter 18 describes.

Causes of Hunger in the United States

Poverty and hunger share an interdependent relationship. Nutrition surveys investigating people's nutritional health in the United States have demonstrated consistently that the lower a family's income, the less adequate the nutrition status. Nationally, most studies conducted since 1980 attribute the increases in hunger throughout the country to worsening economic conditions among the poor. Few low-income families obtain an adequate intake of nutrients.

Families with low food costs and low income who are receiving food stamps are as skilled as, or even more skilled than, others at food shopping. They have difficulty nourishing themselves not because they don't know how to shop, but because they are unable to buy sufficient amounts of nourishing foods. Thus it appears that income confers the ability to obtain a nutritionally adequate diet, and indeed, the numbers of households that meet or exceed the RDA rise and

■ TABLE 17–1
Nationwide Food Consumption Survey Findings

Notice that with the exception of iron, as income increases, the incidence of inadequate nutrient intakes diminishes.

	Percentage of Persons with Nutrient Intakes at or below 70% of RDA[a]			
Nutrient	Income to $6,000	Income $6,000 to $9,999	Income $10,000 to $15,999	Income $16,000 and Over
Vitamin A	36%	33%	32%	29%
Vitamin B$_6$[b]	59%	51%	49%	48%
Vitamin C	30%	29%	27%	23%
Calcium	49%	43%	39%	39%
Iron	29%	31%	33%	33%
Magnesium	48%	40%	36%	35%

[a]Data represent the percentage of persons in each income group with intakes at or below 70% of the RDA in use at the time. Example: 36% of all those surveyed whose incomes were at or below $6,000 per year had vitamin A intakes below 70% of the RDA.
[b]Vitamin B$_6$ intakes may not be as deficient as they appear. People with minimally adequate protein intakes need less than the RDA of vitamin B$_6$ to handle the amount of protein they consume.
Source: USDA Nationwide Food Consumption Survey, 1977–1978.

fall with income. Table 17–1 shows typical findings for six nutrients. People with lower incomes had lower intakes of five of them (iron intakes were low for all income levels). Many are suffering from overt malnutrition, and many more have subclinical malnutrition that is growing worse.

Repeated cuts in government aid have contributed to the poverty that causes hunger. Table 17–2 depicts increases in poverty between 1980 and 1984 among a number of population groups. Why are these increases in poverty occurring? For one thing, major reductions in federal spending for antipoverty programs have taken place throughout the 1980s. Federal expenditures for human services programs were cut by $110 billion in an attempt to reduce the national debt during the period from 1982 to 1985. Programs were eliminated, eligibility requirements were tightened, no adjustments were allowed for inflation, and budgets for the remaining programs were slashed. Some of the most severe reductions came in programs directly

■ TABLE 17–2
Increases in U.S. Poverty, 1980 to 1984

Category	National Rate of Poverty Increase
Infants and children under six years old	+63%
The "working poor"[a]	+56%
Poor married couples (two-parent families)	+47%
Young adults living independently	+13%
Single-parent families (usually headed by women)	+10%
The elderly	−3%

[a]Families who receive 75% of their income from jobs, as opposed to public assistance benefits.
Source: U.S. Bureau of the Census, *Statistical Updates* (Washington, D.C.: Government Printing Office, 1985).

affecting those deepest in poverty, including Aid to Families with Dependent Children (AFDC), food stamps, low-income housing assistance, and child nutrition. Funding for the school lunch program was cut by one-third.[11] Cuts in college financial aid effectively blocked a pathway out of poverty taken by many in the past.

While poverty is the major cause of hunger in the United States, other causes also contribute, including:

- Alcoholism and chronic substance abuse, often contributing to increased poverty and malnutrition among not only the afflicted individuals, but their families as well.
- Mental illness, loneliness, isolation, depression, and despair resulting in people's loss of concern for their own physical well-being.
- The reluctance of people, particularly of the elderly, to accept what they perceive as "welfare" or "charity."
- Delays in receiving requested food stamps and other public assistance benefits.
- An increase in the number of single mothers without the means to care for their children.
- Poor management of limited family financial resources.
- Health problems of old age, precipitating an inability to purchase and prepare food.
- Lack of nutritional adequacy and balance in the food available to hungry people through emergency feeding programs and food assistance organizations; programs take what they can get and pass it on to hungry people.
- Lack of access to assistance programs because of intimidation, ineligibility, complicated paperwork, and other reasons.
- Insufficient community food resources for the hungry.
- Insufficient community transportation systems, which are needed to deliver food to hungry people who have no transportation.[12]

Health experts saw similar situations back in the 1930s and 1960s. Let us first look at how programs were developed to handle the problems of hunger and poverty in those times, then turn to the ways those programs are working now.

Historical Background of Food Assistance Programs

During the 1930s, Congress was concerned about the plight of farmers who were losing their farms, as well as the economic depression facing U.S. families. It was then that Congress established the authority to buy and distribute excess food commodities. A few years later, Congress created the Food Stamp Program to enable low-income people to buy food. Then, in 1946, it passed the National School Lunch Act as a response to testimony from the surgeon general that "70 percent of the boys who had poor nutrition 10 to 12 years ago were rejected by the draft." Still, in the 1960s, it was evident that large numbers of people were going hungry in the United States, and that some of them suffered seriously from malnutrition as a result.

As a result of the evidence accumulated during the 1960s and 1970s showing that hunger was a problem in the United States, the problems of poverty and hunger became national priorities. Old programs were revised and new programs were developed in an attempt to prevent malnutrition in those people found to be at greatest risk. The Food Stamp Program was expanded to serve more people. School lunch and breakfast programs were enlarged to support children nutritionally while they learned. Feeding programs were started to reach senior citizens. A supplemental food and nutrition program (WIC Program) was established for pregnant and breast-feeding women, infants, and children who were of low-income and were nutritionally at risk, in order to provide food and nutrition education during the years when nutrition has the most crucial impact on growth, development, and future health.

The result of these efforts was that hunger diminished as a serious problem for this country. That the food assistance programs made a difference was documented in several studies, including comparative observations made ten years apart. In a baseline study in the late 1960s, a Field Foundation report stated:

> Wherever we went and wherever we looked we saw children in significant numbers who were hungry and sick, children for whom hunger is a daily fact of life, and sickness in many forms, an inevitability. The children we saw were . . . hungry, weak, apathetic . . . visibly and predictably losing their health, their energy, their spirits . . . suffering from hunger and disease, and . . . dying from them.

Ten years later, in 1977, a report by the same group stated:

> Our first and overwhelming impression is that there are far fewer grossly malnourished people in this country today than there were ten years ago . . . This change does not appear to be due to an overall improvement in living standards or to a decrease in joblessness in those areas . . . But in the area of food there is a difference. The Food Stamp program, school lunch and breakfast programs, and the Women-Infant-Children programs have made the difference.[13]

Now, however, hunger is on the rise due to rising poverty and cuts in government aid. Let us take a closer look at the functions of the U.S. food assistance programs in order to understand why federal budget cuts exacerbate the problem of hunger in this country.

Food Assistance Programs Today

In the absence of any national nutrition-monitoring device, we can only get a sense of the numbers of people who are too poor to feed themselves adequately by looking at the group officially counted as poor by the U.S. Census Bureau. The poverty line was developed in 1965 by taking the cost of an emergency short-term diet—called the Thrifty Food Plan—and multiplying it by 3.3 (because a 1955 survey had shown that low-income people spent about one-third of their incomes on food). This became the "poverty line" and has been adjusted every year since then, based on changes in the Consumer Price Index. Besides being out of date, the food budget used in the 1965 calculation reflects a diet that is just barely adequate—one designed for short-term use when funds are extremely low. This means that everyone whose income is below the poverty line has less money than is needed to buy even a short-term, emergency diet.

Regardless of its inadequacies, the official poverty line defines eligibility for participation in most federal assistance programs. The portion of the needy population that falls above the poverty line is automatically ineligible for programs like food stamps or free and reduced-price school meals. Given such criteria, one can conclude that the programs now in place do not reach all people in need and do not provide enough to allow those they do reach to escape poverty.

Federally subsidized nutrition programs:
- Food Stamp Program.
- School Lunch Program.
- School Breakfast Program.
- WIC Program.
- Child Care Food Program.
- Home-delivered meals.
- Congregate feeding for the elderly.

The Food Stamp Program The U.S. Department of Agriculture (USDA) issues food stamp coupons through state social services or welfare agencies to households—people who buy and prepare food together. The number of stamps a household receives varies according to the household size and income (see Figure 17–3). Recipients may use the coupons like cash to purchase food and seeds at stores authorized to accept them. They cannot buy tobacco, cleaning items, alcohol, or nonedible products with coupons.

In 1984, 46.5 million people were living at income levels at or near the poverty line. These people were all potentially eligible to receive food stamps, yet only 21 million people participated in the program. Reasons for nonparticipation include embarrassment about receiving assistance, complex rules

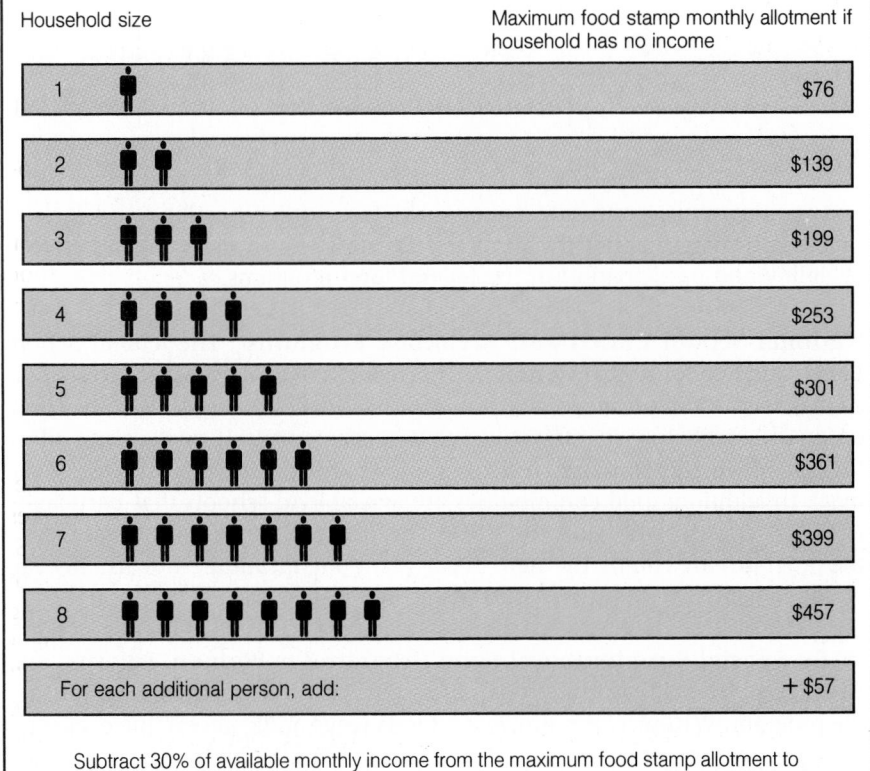

Household size	Maximum food stamp monthly allotment if household has no income
1	$76
2	$139
3	$199
4	$253
5	$301
6	$361
7	$399
8	$457
For each additional person, add:	+ $57

Subtract 30% of available monthly income from the maximum food stamp allotment to determine the coupon allotment. For example, a four-person household with $300 in available income must subtract 30% of $300, or approximately $100. Maximum monthly allotment for a family of 4 = $253 − $100 = $153 food stamp allotment.

■ **FIGURE 17–3**
Food Stamp Allotments Based on the Thrifty Food Plan (October 1983)

Source: Adapted from B. Shollenberger and B. Howell, *Underfunded and underfed: Food programs and hunger in America*, (Washington, D.C.: Bread for the World, 1984), Background paper no. 75, with permission from Bread for the World, Washington, D.C.

■ **FIGURE 17–4**
Eligibility and Participation in Federal Food Programs

Source: Adapted from B. Shollenberger and B. Howell, Underfunded and underfed: Food programs and hunger in America, (Washington, D.C.: Bread for the World, 1984), Background paper no. 75, with permission from Bread for the World, Washington, D.C.

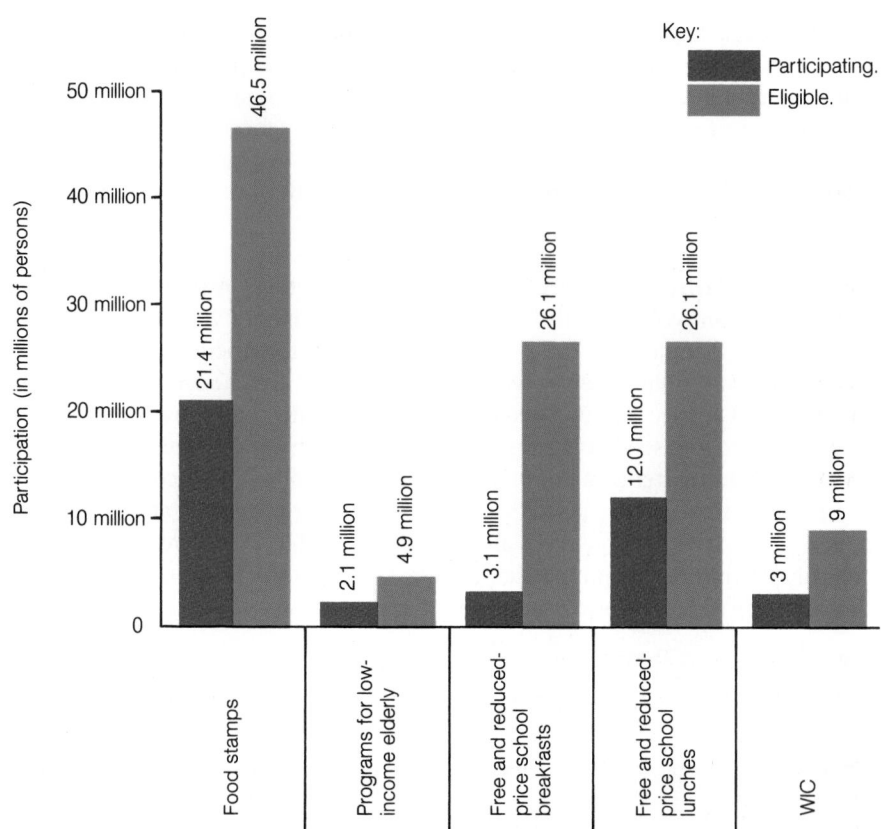

and requirements, confusing paperwork, caseworker hostility, and lack of public information about the program. Figure 17–4 shows the gap between eligibility and participation in the federal food programs.

National School Lunch and Breakfast Programs The federal School Lunch and School Breakfast programs provide financial assistance to schools so that every student can receive a nutritious lunch, breakfast, or both. These programs enable low-income students to receive meals at no cost and allow the schools to charge other students somewhat less than the full cost of the meal. In addition, food commodities are available to schools that participate in the programs. Nationally, the USDA runs the programs; on the state level, the programs are run by the state department of education. They usually can be implemented with little cost to the school district.

WIC—Special Supplemental Food Program for Women, Infants, and Children The USDA funds WIC, and state health departments administer the program. WIC provides nutritious foods (eggs, milk, cereal, juice, cheese, legumes, peanut butter, and infant formula) to infants, children up to age five, and pregnant and breastfeeding women who qualify financially and who are at nutritional risk. The WIC Program serves both a remedial and a preventive role. Services provided include:

- Food packages or vouchers for food packages to provide specific nutrients known to be lacking in the diets of the target population.
- Nutrition education.
- Health care.

The Child Care Food Program   The federal Child Care Food Program provides funds to organized child care programs. All eligible children, centers, and family day care homes have a right to participate. Meal reimbursements cover most of the meal and administration costs. Sponsors may also receive USDA commodity foods.

Nutrition for the Elderly   The federal Nutrition Program for Older Americans (Title III) is intended to improve older people's nutrition status and enable them to avoid medical problems, continue living in communities of their own choice, and stay out of institutions. Its specific goals are to provide:

- Low-cost, nutritious meals.
- Opportunities for social interaction.
- Homemaker education and shopping assistance.
- Counseling and referral to other social services.
- Transportation services.

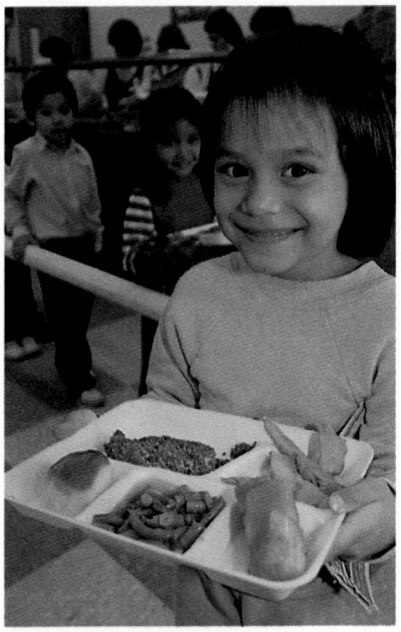

School lunches provide children with nourishment for little or no cost.

A part of Title III is the congregate meal program. Administrators try to select sites for congregate meals so as to feed as many of the eligible elderly as possible. Volunteers may also deliver meals to those who are homebound either permanently or temporarily; these efforts are known as Meals on Wheels. The home-delivery program ensures nutrition, but its recipients miss out on the social benefit of the congregate meal sites; every effort is made to persuade them to come to the shared meals, if they can.

All persons 60 years and older are eligible to receive meals from these programs, regardless of their income level. Priority is given to those who are economically and socially needy.

Despite all of these programs, since 1980, hunger and the public demand for emergency food assistance have increased in every region of the country. The need for emergency food increased by 28 percent between 1984 and 1985, and then by another 25 percent in 1986. The worsening economic conditions of the poor are attributed to the federal economic policies of the 1980s. Much of the increased public demand for food assistance is being found among the "new poor"—those who, until recently, had been employed, productive, and financially stable. Many seeking emergency food assistance are families with children. Food stamps are often no longer able to meet the food needs of the poor.

Emergency food services:
- Soup kitchens.
- Church charities.
- Surplus food giveaways.
- Food banks.
- Food pantries.

To help remedy the lack of federal solutions, concerned citizens are working through community programs and churches to provide meals to the hungry. Second Harvest, the nation's largest supplier of surplus food, distributed over 100 million pounds of goods to 80 food banks around the nation in 1985 (see Figure 17–5). However, even the dramatic increases in the number of food banks, food pantries, soup kitchens, and other emergency food assistance programs across the nation cannot keep pace with the growth in the number of hungry people seeking food assistance. Each day's worth of

■ **FIGURE 17–5**
Demand for Emergency Food Assistance

Distribution of food by the Second Harvest National Food Bank Network rose from 2.5 million pounds in 1979 to 100 million pounds in 1985, reflecting the efforts of private organizations to cope with the rise in hunger. Second Harvest services state food banks.

Source: Adapted with permission from "Hunger in the U.S.," by J. Larry Brown. Copyright© 1987 by Scientific American, Inc. All rights reserved.

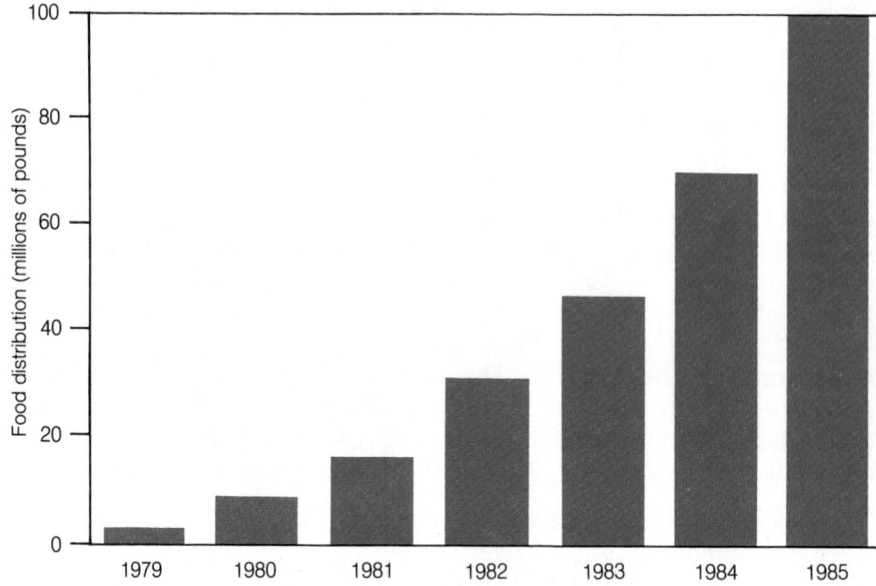

Last-resort food sources:
- Garbage scavenging and eating out of dumpsters.
- Food thefts or thefts to buy food.

meals lasts only for that day, leaving the problem of poverty unsolved, as before; moreover, one out of every five needy people is not even receiving meals. These people are left to scavenge garbage, to steal food or money to buy food, or to continue to starve.

The Plight of the Farmers

Not only on the receiving end, but also on the producing end, changes in the domestic economy are adverse. U.S. farmers today lack significant control over what products they produce, what prices they must pay for supplies, and what prices they receive in return for their commodities. Just prior to 1980, the USDA urged farmers to increase corn and soybean production for export. To do so, farmers borrowed heavily to expand their production capabilities. Since that time, the costs to farmers for seed, fertilizer, equipment, and loans have steadily risen while crop prices have declined. Today, thousands of U.S. farmers are hungry, frustrated, and at the point of desperation concerning their debt.*

The number of hungry farm families is not known, but agencies that provide aid to the rural poor say the demand for food assistance is increasing. Ironically, farm families do not generally grow fruits, vegetables, and other crops and animals to feed themselves. With modern practices aimed at efficiency, most farmers raise two or three crops—for example, feed corn, sorghum, and wheat—and buy most of the food they eat themselves from the grocery store. As a result, when crop prices drop, farmers struggle to survive under the sagging prices and realize no significant profits. Eventually, the

---

*Presently, as many as 13,000 are losing their farms each month. Select Committee on Hunger, *Farm Crisis: Growing Poverty and Hunger among America's Food Producers* (Washington, D.C.: Government Printing Office, 1987), p. 163.

farmers go out of business entirely from lack of profits, just as would happen in any other type of business in the United States.

Hunger on the domestic scene presents one picture; hunger within a developing country presents a somewhat different picture. The following section displays that scene, and the close of the chapter arrives at some conclusions about both.

◼ Hunger in Developing Countries

World hunger is more extreme than domestic hunger. In fact, most people would find it hard to imagine the severity of poverty in the developing world:

> Many hundreds of millions of people in the poorest countries are preoccupied solely with survival and elementary needs. For them, work is frequently not available, or pay is low, and conditions barely tolerable. Homes are constructed of impermanent materials and have neither piped water nor sanitation. Electricity is a luxury. Health services are thinly spread, and in rural areas only rarely within walking distance. Permanent insecurity is the condition of the poor. . . . In the wealthy countries, ordinary men and women face genuine economic problems. . . . But they rarely face anything resembling the total deprivation found in the poor countries.[14]

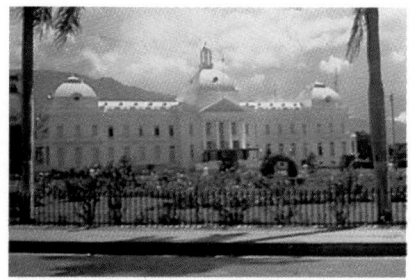

Table 17–3 reveals the human dimensions of the world hunger problem; Table 17–4 shows some of its many causes. World hunger is a problem of supply and demand, of inappropriate technology, of environmental abuse, of demographic distribution, of unequal access to resources, of extremes in dietary patterns, and of unjust economic systems. Two generalizations and an important question are suggested by these tables:

◼ The underlying causes of global hunger and poverty are complex and interrelated.

◼ Hunger is a product of poverty resulting from the ways in which governments and businesses manage national and international economies.

◼ The question that remains to be answered is, Why are people poor?

A diagram of poverty-hunger relationships is presented in Figure 17–6. Hunger and poverty, as with many current problems, have their roots in numerous human and natural factors. Some of these factors include colonialism, economic systems, corporate systems, population pressures, resource distribution, and agricultural technology.

The Role of Colonialism

The colonial era caused hunger and malnutrition for millions of people in developing countries. Much of this same activity, although no longer called colonialism, still continues today. A look at Africa might help to characterize the situation.

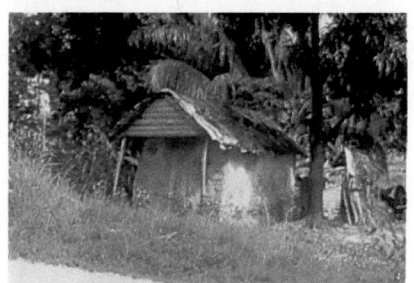

The stark contrasts between rich and poor within a single developing country are depicted here in the homes of the people. The ruler maintains a palace, while the majority of the population live in city tenements or rural huts.

■ **TABLE 17–3**
The Realities of Hunger

- The United Nations reports that there are 520 million malnourished people in the world.

- Each year, 15 to 20 million people die of hunger-related causes, including diseases brought on by lowered resistance due to malnutrition. Of every four of these, three are children.

- Over 40% of all deaths in poor countries occur among children under five years old.

- The United Nations (UNICEF) states that 17 million children died last year from preventable diseases—one every two seconds, 40,000 a day. (A vaccination immunizing one child against a major disease costs 7 cents.) At least 250,000 children are permanently blinded each year simply through lack of vitamin A.

- More than 500 million people in poor countries suffer from chronic anemia due to inadequate diet.

- Every day, the world produces 2 lb of grain for every man, woman, and child on earth. This is enough to provide everyone with 3,000 kcal/day, well above the average need of 2,300 kcal.

- A person born in the rich world will consume 30 times as much food as a person born in the poor world.

- The poor countries have nearly 75% of the world's population, but consume only about 15% of the world's available energy.

- Almost half the world's people earn less than $200 a year—many use 80 to 90% of that income to obtain food.

- Of the nearly 5 billion people on earth, more than 1 billion drink contaminated water. Water-related disease claims 25 million lives a year. Of these, 15 million are under five years of age.

- There are 800 million illiterates. In many countries, half of the population over 15 is illiterate. Two-thirds of these are women.

Source: *World Hunger: Facts*, available from Oxfam America, 115 Broadway, Boston, MA 02116; Office on Global Education, Church World Service, 2115 N. Charles St., Baltimore, MD 21218.

England, Holland, Germany, and other nations originally colonized the African continent to gain a source of raw materials for industrial use. They provided few opportunities for education, and they disrupted traditional family structures and community organization. They greatly diminished the ability of the African people to provide their own food. They created a governing infrastructure designed merely to move Africa's minerals, metals, cash crops, and wealth to Europe.

Throughout much of Africa, land that first grew forests was cleared by small landowners to grow beans, grains, or vegetables for their own use. With colonialism, fertile farmland was taken over by wealthy Africans and foreign investors. They forced the rural poor onto lands that would be suited for adequate food production only with irrigation and fertilizer, which were beyond the means of the poor. The lands were used to grow cotton, sesame, sugar, cocoa, coffee, tea, tobacco, and livestock for export. As more and more raw materials were exported, more and more food and manufactured products were needed as imports. Imported goods cost money—also beyond the reach of the poor.

■ TABLE 17–4
Causes of the World Food Problem

Worldwide Problems

1. Natural catastrophes—drought, heavy rains and flooding, and crop failures.
2. Environmental degradation—soil erosion and inadequate water resources.
3. Food supply-and-demand imbalances.
4. Inadequate food reserves.
5. Warfare and civil disturbances.
6. Migration—refugees.
7. Culturally based food prejudices.
8. Declining ecological conditions in agricultural regions.

Problems of the Developing World	Problems of the Industrialized World
1. Underdevelopment.	1. Excessive use of natural resources.
2. Excessive population growth.	2. Pollution.
3. Lack of economic incentives— farmers using inappropriate methods and laboring on land they may lose or can never hope to own.	3. Inefficient, animal-protein diets.
	4. Inadequate research in science and appropriate technology.
	5. Excessive government bureaucracy.
4. Parents lacking knowledge of basic nutrition for their children.	6. Loss of farmland to competing uses.
5. Insufficient government attention to the rural sector.	

Problems Linking Industrial and Developing Worlds

1. Unequal access to resources.
2. Inadequate transfer of research and technology.
3. Lack of development planning.
4. Insufficient food aid.
5. Excessive food aid.
6. Need for nutrition education.
7. Inappropriate technological research.
8. Inappropriate role of multinational corporations.
9. Insufficient emphasis on agricultural development for self-sufficiency.

Source: Adapted from C. G. Knight and R. P. Wilcox, *Triumph of Triage? The World Food Problem in Geographical Perspective*, resource paper no. 75–3 (Washington, D.C.: Association of American Geographers, 1976), p. 4.

The production of grains for food use has declined per capita for the last 20 years in Africa, while sugarcane production has doubled and tea production, quadrupled. The African country of Chad recently harvested a record cotton crop while in the same year experiencing an epidemic of famine. Sixty percent of national earnings for the African countries of Ghana, Sudan, Somalia, Ethiopia, Zambia, and Malawi are derived from cash crops that finance both luxury imported goods for the minority and international debts. Huge amounts of soybeans and grains are fed to livestock to produce protein foods the poor cannot afford to purchase.

International Trade and Debt

Over the years, developing countries have seen the prices of imported fuels and manufactured items rise much faster than the prices they receive for their

■ FIGURE 17–6
Behind Hunger Stands Poverty
Poverty contributes to hunger in many important ways. Oftentimes, people who are poor are powerless to change their situation because they have less access to vital resources such as education, training, food, health services, and other vehicles of change (as indicated by the arrows pointing down). On the other hand, people in power have access to numerous resources for development (as indicated by the arrows pointing up).

North-South Dialogue: the discussion of global economic change between the developed countries and the developing countries to address the economic imbalance felt by the developing world in the international trade market. (The more developed countries, with the exceptions of New Zealand and Australia, are geographically located north of the more southern, developing countries.)

New International Economic Order (NIEO): the proposals called for by the developing countries, requesting structural changes in the international economic system.

export goods on the international market. Their export commodities include items such as bananas, coffee, and various raw materials. The combination of high import costs with low export profits often pushes a developing country into accelerating international debt that sometimes leads to bankruptcy.

Debt and trade are closely related to the progress a country can make toward achieving adequate diets for its people. As import prices increase relative to export prices, more of a country's total money base moves abroad. As more and more of a country's money moves abroad, the country is forced to borrow money, usually at high interest rates, to continue functioning at home. Many of its financial resources must then go to pay the interest on the borrowed money, thus draining its economy further. Creditor nations may not demand much, or any, capital back, but they do require that interest be paid each year, and the interest can be equal to most of a country's gross national product. Large and growing debts can slow or halt a nation's attempt to deal effectively with its problems of local hunger. As more and more of its financial resources (money paid for imports and cash crops exported) are being used to pay off interest on the country's trade debts, less and less money is available to deal with hunger at home.[15] Each year, the debt crisis worsens and leads to further problems with hunger.

Currently, the developed and developing countries in the United Nations are discussing ways to lighten this burden of international debt. These discussions are known as the North-South Dialogue and represent what is referred to as a New International Economic Order (NIEO). Proposals of the NIEO include ways of rescheduling interest payments or even totally forgiving the debts of a developing country. Little consensus has been reached on the merits of these proposals. Some fear the loss of profits that the lender nations and multinational banks will sustain. Others feel that the loans were ill-advised to begin with and that the lenders have collected sufficient interest already, often many times the original value of the loans. In any case, the NIEO may have identified one of the means necessary to help solve debtor countries' hunger problems. A key step is to resolve their dilemma regarding the tremendous financial drain caused by the international debt of the developing nation. With such resolution, more of the countries' financial resources may become available for the tasks of development, particularly development that would lead to less hunger. Undoubtedly, the debate between the developing and developed world will continue. The outcome of these North-South discussions are expected to be as crucial to the future of both sides as are the discussions between the East and West regarding world peace and disarmament.

The Role of Multinational Corporations

The competition for farmland on which to grow cash crops or food crops provides a classic example of the plight of the poor. Typically, large landowners and multinational corporations hire indigenous people for below-subsistence wages to work in the fertile farmlands growing crops to be exported for profit, leaving little fertile land for the local farmers to use to grow food. The local people work hard cultivating cash crops for others, not food crops for themselves. The money they earn is not even enough to buy the products they help produce. They do not adequately share in the profits realized from the marketing of products grown with their labor. The results: imported foods—bananas, beef, cocoa, coconuts, coffee, pineapples, sugar, tea, winter tomatoes, and others—fill the grocery stores of developed countries, while the poor who labored to grow these foods have less food and fewer resources than when they farmed the land for their own use. Additional cropland is diverted for nonfood, cash crops—tobacco, rubber, cotton, and other agricultural products. These practices have also had an adverse effect on the financial status of many U.S. farmers. The foreign cash crops often undersell the same U.S.-grown produce. The U.S. farmer cannot compete against these lower-priced imported foods and may be forced out of business.

multinational corporations: international companies with direct investments and/or operative facilities in more than one country. U.S. oil and food companies are examples.

Export-oriented agriculture thus uses the labor, land, capital, and technology that is needed to help local families produce their own food. For example, the effort required to produce bananas for export could be reallocated to provide food for the local people. It has been suggested that one solution to the world food problem is not that the developed countries should *give* more food aid, but that they should *take* less food away from the poor countries.[16] The practice of raising food and cash crops for export on land from which thousands of small farmers have been displaced, vividly symbolizes the exploitation of the poor.

Countless examples can be cited to illustrate how natural resources are diverted from producing food for domestic consumption to producing luxury crops for those who can afford them. A few such examples are included in the list that follows, and Figure 17–7 provides many more.

■ **FIGURE 17–7**
The Diversion of Natural Resources
Before you finish eating breakfast this morning, you have depended on more than half the world. This is the way our universe is structured.

Source: Illustration by M. Evans and T. Peterson. Poster available from Seeds, 222 East Lake Dr., Decatur, GA, 30030. Reprinted with permission, *Seeds*.

Tungsten filament from Bolivia. A U.S. child will consume 30-50 times more goods in his/her lifetime than one born in Bolivian highlands.

Clothes from Costa Rica. Workers earn less than 40 cents an hour.

Teak furniture from Honduras. Honduras is the second poorest nation in the western hemisphere; 75 percent of Hondurans live in small, rural villages and earn an average $6 a month.

Baseball and glove from Haiti. Poorest nation in hemisphere; in a village of 6,000, average source of water is two taps. Infant mortality one-of-five.

Rubber from Thailand. Per capita, Thais make $528 a year.

Assembled in Taiwan. Workers earn less than 25 cents an hour.

Bastnaesite from Burundi. Life expectancy in Burundi is 42 years.

Electricity from coal mined in Clear Fork Valley, Ky. About half of the residents live below U.S. poverty line; two-thirds have no flush toilets.

Meat, tuna, bananas from Somalia. Somalia exported $90 million in livestock, bananas, meat, tuna and hides in 1979; the U.S. is one of its three principal trading partners. Somalia has one of the greatest per capita food shortages in the world.

Coffee from Guatemala. Two-thirds of population has annual income of $42.

Pineapples from Philippines. One-half children under four are afflicted by serious deficiency of proteins.

Cocoa and fish from Ecuador. 60 percent of children are malnourished. Sugar from Dominican Republic.

Other common items supplied by Third-World nations: tea from Bangladesh; copper wiring from Chile; aluminum from Jamaica; tin from Malaysia; dog food from fishmeal from Peru; cork (for bulletin board) from Algeria; natural gas from Mexico.

- Africa is a net *exporter* of barley, beans, peanuts, fresh vegetables, and cattle (not to mention luxury crop exports such as coffee and cocoa), yet it has a higher incidence of protein-energy malnutrition among young children than any other continent.
- Mexico now exports to the United States over half of the U.S. supply of several winter and early spring vegetables, while infant deaths associated with poor nutrition are common.
- Half of Central America's agricultural land produces food for export, while in several of its countries the poorest 50 percent of the population eat only half the protein they need. (The richest 5 percent, on the other hand, consume two to three times more than they need.)[17]

Besides diverting acreage away from the traditional staples of the local diet, some multinational corporations may also contribute to hunger as a result of their marketing techniques. Their advertisements lead many consumers with limited incomes to associate products like cola beverages, cigarettes, infant formulas, and snack foods with good health and prosperity. These promotions are tragically inappropriate for these people. A poor family's nutrition status suffers when its tight budget is pinched further by the purchase of such goods. Even worse is the case of inappropriate use of infant formula. Use of formula leads to a mother's weaning her infant. Then, when her money runs out and she cannot afford to buy more formula, her breast milk has ceased to flow, and she cannot resume breastfeeding. The result, all too often, is malnutrition, sickness, and death of the infant.

The United Nations has commissioned several studies in the hopes of establishing an international code of conduct for multinational corporations.[18] More of these powerful organizations could have an immense impact on national economies for good, rather than for ill. U.S. consumers can often influence these multinational corporations because they are shareholders in them. These corporations could increase the credit and capital available to the developing world; and these resources, if properly used, could help to eliminate hunger. The multinational corporations also possess the scientific knowledge and organizational skills needed to help develop improved food and agricultural systems. However, experience shows that sustained outside pressure may have to be applied to some of these corporations to help ensure that human needs do not become subordinate to political and financial gains.

The Role of Overpopulation

The current world population is approximately 5 billion, and for the year 2000 the projected United Nations figure is 6 billion. The earth may not be able to adequately support this many people (see Highlight 17). The world's present population is certainly of concern as is the projected increase in that population. As important as the population question is, it is only one cause of the world food problem. Poverty seems to be at the root of both problems—hunger and overpopulation.

Three major factors affect population growth: birth rates, death rates, and standards of living. Low-income countries have high birth rates, high death rates, and low standards of living.

■ TABLE 17–5
Effect of Hunger on Population Growth Rate

	Hungry Countries	Nonhungry Countries
Average infant mortality rate	113 per 1,000	35 per 1,000
Total infant deaths per year	10.6 million	1.4 million
Size of population	2.3 billion	2.3 billion
Average rate of population increase	2.4% per year	1.0% per year
Total births per year	86.4 million	38.6 million

Source: Adapted from *The Ending Hunger Briefing Workbook*, 1982, p. 26, 30, available from The Hunger Project, 2015 Steiner St., San Francisco, CA 94115.

The transition of population growth rates from a slow-growth stage (high birth rates and high death rates), through a rapid-growth stage (high birth rates and low death rates), to a low-growth stage (low birth rates and low death rates) is known as the **demographic transition**.

Fernando is a child of 5 in Bolivia. His father, a hard-working copper miner, and his mother care for him and his six brothers and sisters. Fernando has rickets, is anemic, is small in stature and weak in body. Because of the lack of clean water in his village, he and other members of his family suffer from continual diarrhea. If Fernando is lucky enough to become an adult, he will remain small in stature and weak in body. If Fernando dies soon, his parents will feel impelled to bring another child into the world in the hope that a new child will live to adulthood and be able to care for the parents in old age.

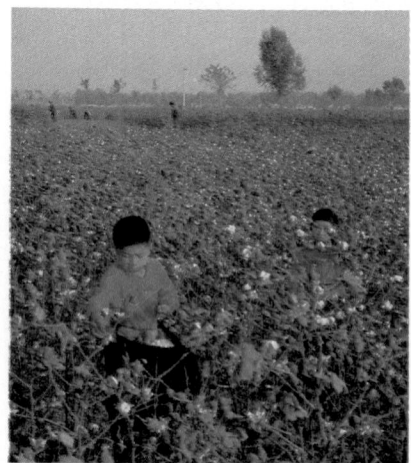

Families in developing countries depend on their children to help provide for daily needs.

When a people's standard of living rises, giving them better access to health care, family planning, and education, the death rate falls. In time, the birth rate also falls. As the standard of living continues to improve, the family earns sufficient income to risk having smaller numbers of children. A family depends on its children to cultivate the land, to secure food and water, and to make the adults secure in their old age.[19] If a family is confronted with ongoing poverty, parents will choose to have many children to ensure that some will survive to adulthood. Children represent the "social security" of the poor. Improvements in economic status help relieve the need for this "insurance," and so help reduce the birth rate. Table 17–5 shows the relationships between infant mortality rate and population growth rate, and it reveals that hunger and poverty in a nation reflect both the level of national development and the people's sense of security.[20]

In many countries where economic growth has occurred and all groups share resources relatively equally, the rates of population growth have decreased. Examples include parts of the Central American country of Costa Rica, India's island neighbor Sri Lanka, the island of Taiwan, and the Asian peninsula-country of Malaysia. In countries where economic growth has occurred but the resources are unevenly distributed, population growth has remained high. Examples are Brazil, Mexico, the Philippines, and Thailand, where a large family continues to be a major economic asset for the poor.[21]

As the world's population continues to grow, it threatens the world's capacity to produce adequate food in the future. As the highlight that follows this chapter describes, the activity of billions of human beings on the earth's limited surface is seriously and adversely affecting out planet: wiping out many of the varieties of plant life, heating up our climate, using up our freshwater supplies, and destroying the protective ozone layer that shields life from the sun's damaging rays—in short, overstraining the earth's ability to support life. Population control is one of the most pressing needs of this time in history. Until the nations of the world resolve the population problem, they must all deal with its subsequent problems and make efforts to support the life of the populations that presently exist.

Distribution of Resources

Land reform—giving people a meaningful opportunity to produce food for local consumption for example—can combine with population control to increase everyone's assets. Some background information is important to understand this relationship:

- Much of the world's agriculture is primitive. More than 50 percent of all food consumed in the world is still produced by hand.
- In many countries, up to 90 percent of the population live on rural land.
- Most governments dictate the day-to-day lives of their people, and their policies need not be equitable.
- Securing enough food on a day-to-day basis is a problem for as many as a billion human beings.
- Even the best land in many parts of the world does not support the growing of food, even by the wealthy.[22]

The problem of unequal distribution of resources exists not only between the rich and the poor within nations, but also between rich and poor nations. For wealthy nations to simply give to the poor nations would be to weaken the poor nations further. Instead, wealthy nations must foster self-reliance in poor nations. This move toward self-reliance will initially require some economic sacrifices on the part of wealthy nations, but will ultimately benefit large numbers of hungry people.

Poor nations must be allowed to increase their agricultural productivity. Much is involved, but to put it simply, poor nations must gain greater access to five things simultaneously: land, capital, water, technology, and knowledge.[23] Equally important, each nation must adopt the political priority of improving the conditions of all its people. International food aid may be required temporarily during the development period, but eventually this aid will be less and less necessary.

If you give a man a fish, he will eat for a day. If you teach him to fish, he will eat for a lifetime.

Agricultural Technology

Governments can learn from recent history the importance of developing local agricultural technology. A major effort made in the 1960s—the green revolution—demonstrated the potential for increased grain production in Asia. It was an effort to bring the agricultural technology of the industrial world to the developing countries; but the high-yielding strains of wheat and rice that were selected required irrigation, chemical fertilizers, and pesticides—all costly and beyond the economic means of too many of the farmers in the developing world.

There is much to be gained from continued work in the area of crop improvement. Instead of transplanting industrial technology into the developing countries, small, efficient farms and local structures for marketing, credit, transportation, food storage, and agricultural education should be developed. International research centers need to examine the conditions of tropical countries and orient their research toward appropriate technology—labor-intensive rather than energy-intensive agricultural methods.

For example, labor-intensive technology, such as the use of manual grinders for grains, is appropriate in some places because it makes the best use of human, financial, and natural resources. A manual grinder can process 20 pounds of grain per hour, replacing the mortar and pestle, which in the same time can pound a maximum of only 3 pounds.[24] The specific technology that is appropriate for use varies from situation to situation.

green revolution: the development and widespread adoption of high-yielding strains of wheat and rice in developing countries. The popular term *green revolution* is also used to describe almost any package of modern agricultural technology delivered to developing countries.

appropriate technology: a technology that utilizes locally abundant resources in preference to locally scarce resources. Developing countries usually have a large labor force and little capital; the appropriate technology would therefore be labor intensive.

Labor-intensive technology is most often the appropriate technology in developing countries.

Environmental concerns must be taken more seriously as well. As important as the amount of land available for crop production is the condition of the soil and the availability of water. Soil erosion is now accelerating on every continent at a rate that threatens the world's ability to continue feeding itself. Erosion of soil has always occurred; it is a natural process. But in the past, it has been compensated for by processes that build the soil up—such as the growth of trees.

Where forest has already been converted to farmland and there are no trees, farmers should alternate soil-devouring crops with soil-building crops, a practice known as crop rotation. An acre of soil planted one year in corn, the next in wheat, and the next in clover loses 2.7 tons of topsoil each year, but if it is planted only in corn three years in a row, it will lose 19.7 tons a year.[25] When farmers must choose whether to make three times as much money planting corn year after year or to rotate crops and go bankrupt, many choose the short-term profits. Ruin may not follow immediately, but it will follow.[26]

◼ *Agenda for Action*

Although the problem of world hunger may seem overwhelming, it can be broken down into many small, local problems. Significant strides can then be made toward solving them at the local level. Even if the problem of poverty itself is not immediately or fully solved, progress is possible. For example, infants and children need not be raised in middle-class homes to be protected from malnutrition. Slight modifications of the children's diets can be immensely beneficial. Encouraging examples are provided by recent experiences in Sierra Leone and Nepal.

In Sierra Leone, a food product was developed from rice, sesame (benniseed), and peanuts that were hand pounded and cooked to make a flour meal. The local children found it tasty—and whereas they had been malnourished before, they thrived when this product supplemented their diets. The village women formed a cooperative to reduce the household drudgery of preparation, and they rotated the work on a weekly or monthly basis.[27] The government also established a manufacturing plant to produce and market the mixture at subsidized prices. The success of the venture lies in the involvement of the local people in identifying the problem and devising a solution that meets the needs of the people.

A similar success story is told in Nepal. A supplementary food made from soybeans, corn, and wheat, mixed in a 2:1:1 proportion, yielded a concentrated "superflour" of high biological value suitable for infants and children. A nutrition rehabilitation center tested this superflour by giving undernourished children and their mothers two cereal-based meals a day, and giving the children three additional small meals of superflour porridge daily. Within ten days the undernourished children had gained weight, lost their edema, and recovered their appetites and social alertness. The mothers, who saw the remarkable recoveries of their children, were motivated to learn how to make the tasty supplementary food and incorporate it into their local foodstuffs and customs.

These two examples offer hope, but the real issue of poverty remains to be addressed. One-shot intervention programs—offering nutrition education,

In Nepal, the women worked together in a first step toward self-sufficiency.

food distribution, food fortification, and the like—are not enough. It is difficult to describe the misery a mother feels when she has received education about nutrition but is unable to grow or purchase the foods her family needs. She now knows *why* her child is sick and dying but is helpless in *applying* her new knowledge.

Focus on Children

There is hopeful news for children in developing countries and in neglected parts of the United States. GOBI is a plan set forth by UNICEF that can cut the number of hunger-related child deaths from 40,000 to 20,000 a day. GOBI is an acronym formed from four simple, but profoundly important, elements of UNICEF's "Child Survival" campaign: growth charts, oral rehydration therapy (ORT), breast milk, and immunization.

GOBI: an acronym formed from the elements of UNICEF's Child Survival campaign—**G**rowth charts, **O**ral rehydration therapy, **B**reast milk, and **I**mmunization.

UNICEF: the United Nations International Children's Emergency Fund.

The use of growth charts requires a worldwide education campaign. A mother can learn to weigh her child every month and chart the child's growth on a specially designed paper growth chart. She can learn to detect for herself the early stages of hidden malnutrition that can leave a child irreparably retarded in mind and body. Then at least she can know she needs to take steps to remedy the malnutrition—if she can.

The importance of oral rehydration therapy (ORT) is that most children who die of malnutrition don't starve to death—they die because their health has been compromised by dehydration from infections causing diarrhea. Until recently, there was no easy way of stopping the infection-diarrhea cycle and saving their lives. Oral rehydration therapy is the administration of a simple solution that mothers can make up themselves, using locally available ingredients, which increases a body's ability to absorb fluids 25-fold.[28] International development groups also provide mothers with packets of premeasured salt and sugar to be mixed with water in rural and urban areas. A safe and sanitary supply of drinking water is a prerequisite for the success of the ORT program. Contaminated water continues to turn the infection-diarrhea cycle.

oral rehydration therapy (ORT): the treatment of dehydration (usually due to diarrhea caused by infectious disease) with an oral solution; ORT as developed by UNICEF is intended to enable a mother to mix a simple solution for her child from substances that she has at home.

The promotion of breastfeeding among mothers in developing countries has many benefits. Breast milk is hygienic, is readily available, is nutritionally sound, and provides infants with immunologic protection specific for their environment. In the developing world, its advantages over formula feeding can mean the difference between life and death.

An important contributor to children's malnutrition in developing countries is the high bulk and low energy content of the available foods. The diet may be based on grains such as wheat, rice, millet, sorghum, and corn, as well as on starchy root crops such as the cassava, sweet potato, plantain, and banana. These may be supplemented with legumes (peas or beans), but rarely with animal proteins. Infants have small stomachs, and most cannot eat enough of these staples (grains or root crops) to meet their daily energy and protein requirements. They need to be fed more nutrient-dense foods during the weaning period. The most promising weaning foods are usually concentrated mixtures of grain and locally available pulses—that is, peas or beans—because they are both nourishing and inexpensive.[29] Mothers are advised to continue breastfeeding while they introduce weaning foods.

pulses: a term used for legumes, especially with reference to legumes that serve as staples in the diet of Third World countries.

As for immunizations (the *I* of GOBI), they could prevent most of the 5 million deaths each year from measles, diphtheria, tetanus, whooping cough, poliomyelitis, and tuberculosis. However, adequate protein nutrition is necessary in order for vaccinations to be useful so that the vaccine itself is not used by the body as a source of protein. UNICEF's goal is to immunize all of the world's children by 1990. It used to be difficult to keep vaccines stable in their long journeys from laboratory to remote villages. However, a new measles vaccine has been discovered that does not require refrigeration. The result: universal measles immunization for young children is now possible.

Focus on Women

Women make up 50 percent of the world's population. Any solution to the problems of poverty and hunger is incomplete and even hopeless if it fails to address the role of women in developing countries (see Table 17–6), for women and their children represent the majority of those living in poverty.

In many countries, over 90 percent of the population live in rural areas. The life of a woman living in rural poverty is oppressive. Women are often overworked and underfed, yet they are often expected to carry most of the

■ TABLE 17–6
Women and Development: Fiction and Fact

- *Men produce the world's food; women prepare it for the table.*
  In the Third World, where three-fourths of the world's people live, rural women account for more than half the food produced.
- *Women work to supplement the family's income.*
  Women are the sole breadwinners in one-fourth to one-third of the families in the world. The number of women-headed families is rapidly increasing.
- *When women receive the same education and training as men, they will receive equal pay.*
  So far, earning differentials persist even at equivalent levels of training. In professional fields, for example, comparisons of men's and women's salaries show a large gap between them even when samples are matched for training and experience.
- *Men are the heavy workers, and where food is short, they should have first priority.*
  As a rule, women work longer hours than men. Many carry triple work loads—in their household, labor force, and reproductive roles. Rural women often average an 18-hour day. Anemia resulting from a primary or secondary nutrient deficiency is a serious health problem for women in the Third World.
- *In modern societies, women have moved into all fields of work.*
  Relatively few women have entered occupations traditionally dominated by men. Most women remain highly segregated in low-paid jobs.
- *Women contribute a minor share of the world's economic product.*
  Women are a minority in the conventional measures of economic activity because these measures undercount women's paid labor and do not cover their unpaid labor. The value of women's work in the household alone, if given economic value, would add an estimated one-third to the world's GNP.

Source: Reproduced with permission from *Women . . . A World Survey* by R. L. Sivard. Copyright© 1985 by World Priorities, Inc., Washington, D.C.

burden of their families' survival. In many cultures, they are the last to get food, despite long hours spent each day procuring water and firewood, and pounding grains by hand (see Figure 17–8). In many countries, women in the rural areas are not only the primary food producers, but also are responsible for child care and food preparation. Often they have to work as harvesters on other people's lands as well. Husbands are frequently required to be absent from their homes—not by choice, but because they have gone to live in the cities in search of work or to find employment on distant commercial farms—growing export crops.

Development projects are often large in scale and highly technological, and they frequently overlook women's needs. Typically, only men have access to education and training programs (see Figure 17–8). Yet women play a vital role in the nutrition of their nations' people. Their nutrition during pregnancy and lactation determines the future health of their children. If women are weakened by malnutrition themselves, or ignorant about how to feed their families, the consequences ripple outward to affect many other individuals. The importance of the role women play in these countries is increasingly

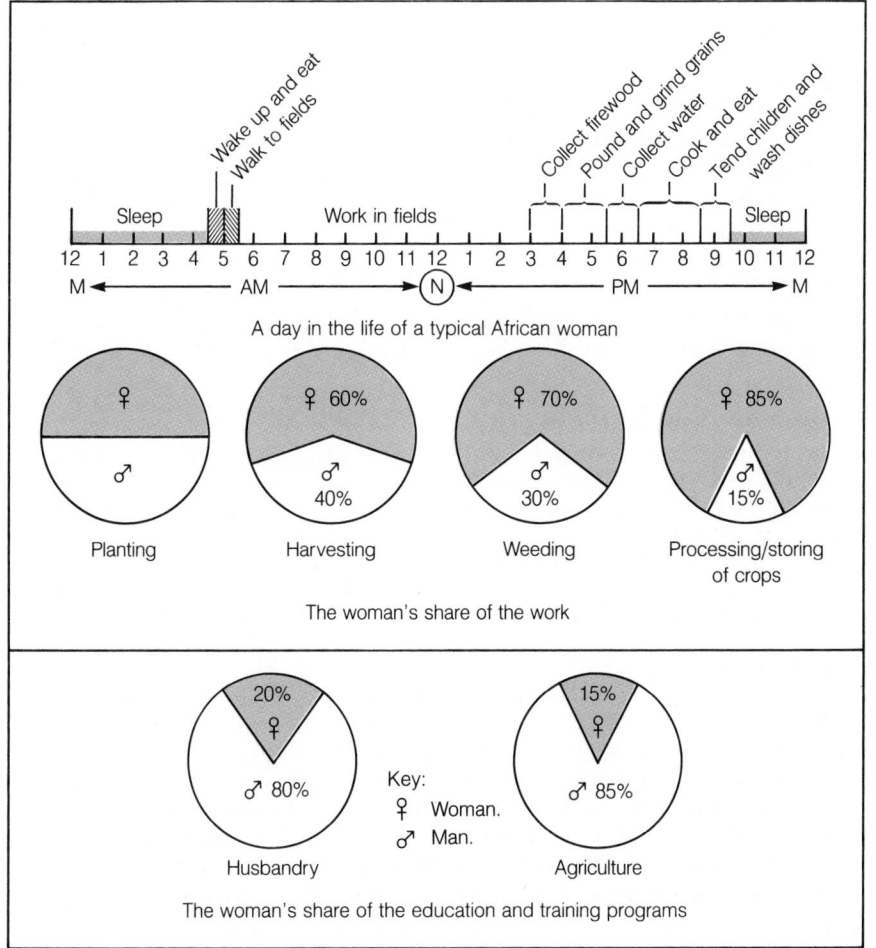

■ FIGURE 17–8
Women and Development

Source: Adapted from T. Flynn, Women in development, *Seeds* (Sprouts edition), May 1988.

appreciated, and many countries now offer development programs with women in mind.

Seven basic strategies are at the heart of women's programs:

- Removing barriers to financial credit—so that women can obtain loans for raw materials and equipment to enhance their role in food production.
- Providing access to time-saving technologies—seed grinders, for example.
- Providing appropriate training—for the purpose of self-reliance.
- Teaching management and marketing skills—to avoid exploitation.
- Making health and day-care services available—to provide a healthy environment for these women's children.
- Forming women's support groups—to foster strength by means of cooperative efforts.[30]
- Providing information and technology to promote planned pregnancies.

The recognition of women's needs by some development organizations is an encouraging trend in the efforts to contend with the world hunger crisis. Examples from Sierra Leone and El Salvador follow:[31]

Balu Kamara is a farmer in Sierra Leone in West Africa, where farming is difficult, particularly for women. There women have little money and must take out loans to buy seed rice and to pay for the use of oxen. The price of rice is so low, though, that at the end of the growing season the women do not earn enough money to repay their loans. Yet, as the economy worsens, it is up to the women to carry the burdens; it is up to the women to stretch what resources are available to feed their families regardless of hardships.

Balu is the leader of the Farm Women's Club, a basket cooperative the women formed to make and sell baskets so they could pay their debts and continue farming. Finding time to weave baskets is difficult. Yet the women and their cooperative are succeeding. On the value of the Farm Women's Club, Balu says, "We have access to credit and a cash income. We have the opportunity to learn improved methods of agriculture and marketing and to increase our belief in ourselves and ease our families through the hungry season."

A few years ago, Natividad de Mercedes became a displaced person in war-torn El Salvador. Because of fighting near the home, she, her husband, and their six children had to flee. They lost nearly everything. Now she and her family live in a one room hut in a small community for displaced families, but they hope to buy a small plot of land someday, build a home, and produce food to eat and sell.

Because Natividad's husband receives only a sporadic income, it is Natividad's job that enables her family to save money and feel hopeful about their future. She is the president of a bakery enterprise in her small El Salvadoran community. The bakery began in 1986 with assistance from OEF International, an organization that works on projects with low-income women in developing countries. Critics of the project considered "displaced women" a lost cause and felt the project would fail. They were wrong. Natividad says of the bakery's importance, "There is a big difference in my life here because now I am earning money to feed my children." The bakery also benefits the entire community by providing employment, food, and strong examples of what displaced women can do.

■ **TABLE 17–7**
Presidential Commission on World Hunger: Conclusions

- The major world hunger problem today is the prevalence of chronic undernutrition—which calls for a political, as well as a technical, solution.
- The world hunger problem is getting worse rather than better.
- A major crisis of global food supply—of even more serious dimensions than the present energy crisis—appears likely by the year 2000, unless steps are taken now to facilitate a significant increase in food production in the developing nations.
- The rising global demand for food must be met within resource limits—of land, water, energy, and agricultural inputs.
- There is no ideal food, no perfect diet, no universally acceptable agricultural system waiting to be transplanted from one geographic, climatic, or cultural setting to another. Assistance programs must focus on self-reliance and respond to the needs of each country. Needs and requirements cannot be generalized.
- In addition to action by the industrialized nations, decisive steps to build more effective national food systems must be taken by the developing countries.
- The outcome of the war on hunger, by the year 2000 and beyond, will be determined not by forces beyond human control, but by decisions and actions well within the capability of nations and people working individually and together.

Source: Adapted from Presidential Commission on World Hunger, *Overcoming World Hunger: The Challenge Ahead* (Washington, D.C.: Government Printing Office, 1980), pp. 180–185.

■ *Personal Action*

To summarize what is known about the world food situation, examine the conclusions of the Presidential Commission on World Hunger (Table 17–7). The members of the commission stressed that worldwide efforts to overcome hunger and malnutrition and to foster self-reliant development must be intensive.

The problems may appear so great that they seem approachable only by way of worldwide political decisions. But many individuals are working to improve the chances of the future well-being of the world and its people through a number of national and international organizations.*

Solutions to the hunger problem depend on people's being willing to take action and to work together. Regardless of the type and level of involvement a person chooses, each person can make a difference. The government programs regarding domestic hunger described in this chapter need people's support in a number of ways. Individual people can:

- Assist in these programs as volunteers.
- Help develop means of informing low-income people of food-related services and programs for which they are eligible.

Hunger exists not because we can't end it, but simply because we haven't.—World Runners

---

*For information, contact Bread for the World, 802 Rhode Island Ave. NE, Washington, DC 20018, or Oxfam America, 115 Broadway, Boston, MA 02116; or request a copy of *A Guide to World Hunger Organizations* from Seeds, 222 East Lake Dr., Decatur, GA 30030.

- Help increase the accessibility of existing programs and services to those who need them.
- Document the needs that exist in their own communities.
- Join with others in the community who have similar interests (support groups that speak for the poor).
- Lobby to draw political attention to the need for more job opportunities and a higher minimum wage.

Besides individual actions, any person who is concerned about the problems of poverty and undernutrition in the United States can exercise the right to affect the political process. Anyone can decide what local, state, and national governments should do to help, and communicate these ideas to elected officials for needed legislative changes. Individuals who volunteer their efforts and express their convictions to improve food assistance programs can also make a difference.

Individuals can also help change the world through the personal choices they make each day.[32] Our choices have an impact on the way the rest of the world's people live and die. As mentioned earlier, our nation, with 6 percent of the world's population, consumes about 40 percent of the world's food and energy resources. The world food problem depends partly on the demands we place on the world's finite natural resources. In a sense, therefore, we contribute to the world food problem. People in affluent nations have the freedom and means to choose their lifestyles; people in poor nations do not. We can find ways to reduce our consumption of the world's nonrenewable resources; we can use only what is absolutely required. The admonition, so familiar in childhood, to "clean your plate," as if that would alleviate the suffering of some starving stranger, could well be replaced with the mandate simply to "consume less food."

It is ironic that whereas other societies cannot secure enough clean water for people to drink, our society produces bottles of soda that contain 1 kcalorie of artificial sweetener in 12 ounces of water and that cost 800 kcalories of energy, each, to produce. Choosing a diet at the level of necessity, rather than excess, would reduce the resource demands made by our industrial agriculture. It would also produce humanitarian and economic benefits. In fact, those who study the future are convinced that the hope of the world lies in everyone's adopting a simple lifestyle. As one such person put it, "the widespread simplification of life is vital to the well-being of the entire human family."[33] Personal lifestyles do matter, for a society is nothing more than the sum of its individuals. As we go, so goes our world.

■ Study Questions

1. Describe the reasons for poverty.
2. List some reasons why women in developing countries are more susceptive than men to hunger and undernutrition.
3. What are the health problems associated with chronic hunger in the United States?
4. List factors (other than poverty) that contribute to the hunger problem in the United States.
5. Describe how economic policies of the 1980s have contributed to the U.S. hunger problem.
6. Describe how activities of colonalism in Africa have contributed to poverty and hunger.
7. Describe how overpopulation contributes to the world hunger problem.
8. Describe the UNICEF child survival campaign GOBI.

Notes

1. L. Schwartz-Nobel, *Starving in the Shadow of Plenty* (New York: Putnam, 1981), pp. 35–36.

2. K. Markandaya, *Nectar in a Sieve*, 2nd American ed. (New York: John Day, 1955), pp. 121–122.

3. D. R. Gwatkin, How many die? A set of demographic estimates of the annual number of infant and child deaths in the world, *American Journal of Public Health* 70 (1980): 1286–1289.

4. Population Reference Bureau, *1986 World Population Data Sheet* (Washington, D.C.: Population Reference Bureau, 1986).

5. M. Cameron and Y. Hofvander, *Manual on Feeding Infants and Young Children*, 2nd ed. (New York: Protein Advisory Board of the United Nations, 1976), p. 1.

6. L. Crawford, Water, l'eau, bolok, agua, maji, *Seeds*, May–June, 1989, pp. 12–15.

7. J. P. Habicht, J. DaVanzo, and W. P. Butz, Mother's milk and sewage: Their interactive effects on infant mortality, *Pediatrics* 81 (1988): 456–461.

8. World Bank, *World Development Report 1981*, (New York: Oxford University Press, 1981), Table 21.

9. Dr. Carol Dyer's findings related to social and cultural beliefs about food in India are from A. Berg, *The Nutrition Factor* (Washington, D.C.: Brookings Institute, 1973), p. 46.

10. Physician Task Force on Hunger in America, *Hunger in America: The Growing Epidemic* (Middletown, Conn.: Wesleyan University Press, 1985), p. 17.

11. Physician Task Force on Hunger in America, 1985.

12. Department of Health and Rehabilitative Services and the Florida Task Force on Hunger, *Hunger in Florida: A Report to the Legislature*, Tallahassee, Fla.: Department of Health and Rehabilitative Services, (April 1986), pp. 32–33.

13. N. Kotz, *Hunger in America: The Federal Response* (New York: Field Foundation, 1979), p. 17.

14. Independent Commission on International Issues, *North-South: A Program for Survival* (Cambridge, Mass.: MIT Press, 1980), pp. 49–50.

15. The Hunger Project, *Ending Hunger: An Idea Whose Time Has Come* (New York: Praeger, 1985), pp. 314–315.

16. G. Kent, Food trade: The poor feed the rich, *Food and Nutrition Bulletin* 4 (1982): 25–33.

17. F. M. Lappe and J. Collins, *Food First: Beyond the Myth of Scarcity* (Boston: Houghton Mifflin, 1978), p. 15.

18. Interreligious Taskforce on U.S. Food Policy, *Identifying a Food Policy Agenda for the 1980s: A Working Paper* (Washington, D.C.: Interreligious Taskforce on U.S. Food Policy, January 1980), p. 30.

19. The story of Fernando, told in the margin, is from D. Burgess, The future of hungry children abroad, *Journal of Current Social Issues*, Summer 1975, p. 36.

20. J. Kocher, Not too many but too little, in J. D. Gussow, *The Feeding Web: Issues in Nutritional Ecology* (Palo Alto, Calif.: Bull Publishing, 1978), pp. 81–83.

21. M. R. Langham, L. Polopolus, and M. L. Upchurch, *World Food Issues* (Gainesville, Fla.: University of Florida Press, 1982), pp. 18–20.

22. R. R. Spitzer, *No Need for Hunger* (Danville, Ill.: Interstate Printers and Publishers, 1981), pp. 20–23.

23. E. O'Kelly, Appropriate technology for women, *Development Forum*, June 1976, p. 2.

24. National Agricultural Lands Study, *Soil Degradation: Effects on Agricultural Productivity*, Interim Report no. 4 (Washington, D.C.: U.S. Department of Agriculture, November 1980), as cited by L. R. Brown, World population growth, soil erosion, and food security, *Science* 214 (1981): 995–1002.

25. Brown, 1981.

26. T. Peterson, Hunger and the environment, *Seeds*, October 1987, pp. 6–13.

27. *National Conference on Primary Health Care* (Kathmandu: Ministry of Health, Health Services Coordination Committee, World Health Organization, and UNICEF, 1977), pp. 9, 25, as cited by M. E. Frantz, Nutrition problems and programs in Nepal, *Hunger Notes* 2 (1980): 5–8.

28. Oral rehydration therapy, *World Health* (Geneva: World Health Organization), June 1985.

29. P. Pellet, The role of food mixtures in combating childhood malnutrition, in *Nutrition in the Community*, ed. D. McLaren (New York: Wiley, 1978), pp. 185–202.

30. Oxfam America, *Facts for Action: Women Creating a New World*, no. 3 (Boston: Oxfam America, 1986), p. 3.

31. Bread for the World, *Women in Development* (Washington, D.C.: Bread for the World, 1988).

32. The case for optimism, in E. Cornish and members and staff of the World Future Society, *The Study of the Future: An Introduction to the Art and Science of Understanding and Shaping Tomorrow's World* (Washington, D.C.: World Future Society, 1977), pp. 34–37.

33. D. Elgin, *Voluntary Simplicity: Toward a Way of Life That Is Outwardly Simple, Inwardly Rich* (New York: Morrow, 1981), p. 25.

The Environment and World Hunger

Imagine for a moment that you can stride across the globe, 100 miles at each step. Here you see a towering city of skyscrapers and cathedrals, bustling with life and human enterprise. There is a vast chain of silent, snow-covered mountains. Now you stand in a meadow blazing with brilliant flowers, humming with bees. Next, a huge valley checkered with farm fields and pastures, where rumbling tractors are harvesting fruits, vegetables, and grain. Now, a filthy city slum on a polluted river where masses of people are abjectly poor, starving, and sick. Now, an endless prairie, where countless head of cattle are grazing as far as the eye can see. Now, a forest of 100-foot-tall trees draped with vines and orchids, resounding with bird songs, frog croaks, insect clicks, and dripping rainwater. Next, a railroad crossing, where a powerful locomotive is pulling 100 boxcars filled with grain, tobacco, and toys. Now, a broad river, carrying tons of water from the mountains to the sea, alive with fish, bordered first by woodlands, then by villages, then crossed by bridges and carrying ships laden with cargo destined for a busy port at its mouth. Now, a noisy industrial complex, with factories spewing forth smoky plumes of odorous waste. Now, a sandy beach, where ocean waves surge and fall back, seabirds wheel overhead, and dolphins play offshore.

All of these scenes are parts of our world, and all affect us for well or for ill—the dolphins as well as the cathedrals, the rainforest insects as well as the slums and factories. Until recently, there has been a sort of balance among them in the sense that parts of the earth were occupied by dense urban populations with their cities and factories; parts by rural

Good planets are hard to find.

populations with their farms and ranches; and parts by untouched wilderness. Such a balance is essential, not only to the earth's well-being, but to the well-being of every human being on it. We need the agricultural areas to produce the food, and the wilderness areas to bring forth the oxygen, generate the rain, and renew the soils upon which the human food supply depends.

Areas of dense human habitation require uninhabited areas to balance them in another sense. Cities are the world's greatest generators of sewage, trash, and industrial waste, which they cannot handle themselves.[1] They deposit these materials in the land, waterways, and air around them. The larger each city, the larger the rural and wilderness areas it depends on, both to produce its food and to handle its waste. (A city resembles a fetus, in a way; it is totally dependent on the mother—earth—to nourish it. It must not grow too large, or it will overwhelm her capacity to do so.)

There is thus an optimal population size for the earth to bear—that size at which the air, water, and wilderness

can renew themselves and support human life indefinitely. This optimal population size depends, among other things, on how people behave. The more resources each person demands, the fewer people there can be. For example, if everyone on earth must own and drive a car every day, then each requires much more of the earth's support than if he or she walked or rode bicycles.

It is not possible to say exactly how many people would be ideal for our well-being. Our population size may well exceed that number by now. As this book goes to press, we number 5 billion, and each year, the number of people added to the population is greater than the number added the year before.[2] Furthermore, by the year 2000, half of all the people on earth will be living in cities. People in cities often lose their sense of connection with the earth and fail to realize how dependent they are on it. People who live in rural areas may fail to see the picture, too, and may think that to solve their hunger and poverty problems they, too, need to move into cities—or clear more land. A growing population thus spreads across the land, converting forests to pastures, pastures to parking lots, and parking lots to industrial developments. Even though each conversion may bring economic benefits, at least for a short time to some people, these conversions are now becoming intolerable for the world's people in general. The process could be viewed as beneficial to people in general only so long as *elsewhere* on earth, there was enough rural and forested land to continue replenishing the resources on which we all, ultimately, depend: air, water, and food. Now we are eating into the few remaining "elsewheres"—the rural and forested lands that are vital to sustain our lives—and so we must stop.

Many indicators are simultaneously revealing that this is so. Two major ones: first, a sudden, recent downturn in the world's food supply; second, significant changes in the world's climate. The two are related.

The world's food supply is often measured in grain output, for grain is the world's single largest crop. Between 1950 and 1984, the world's grain supply increased tremendously, encouraging world leaders to believe that continued expansion would be possible. Then in 1984, the picture suddenly changed. Grain output leveled off, and in 1987 it began to fall off sharply (see Figure H17–1). Whereas at the start of 1987, stored grain surpluses were sufficient to feed the world for 101 days, at the end of 1988, they were sufficient to feed the world for only 54 days.[3] Droughts accounted for much of the decline in reserves.

In the past, when people's grain supplies have fallen short, they have had two options, to dip into the world's stored surpluses, or to increase grain outputs. Now the stored grain surpluses are dwindling, and outputs cannot increase much more. Grain outputs have been increased in the past by farming more land, but now nearly all of the land that is suitable for farming is already under cultivation. Farming *unsuitable* land (such as the land on steep, erodible mountainsides or in rainforests) results in losses of soil and water to an extent that cannot be sustained for more than a few years. Furthermore, human habitation and industrial development are claiming the very same land, labor, and water that might be recruited for agricultural development. Thus remedies for grain shortages that have worked in the past are now failing, because they are based on the fallacy that the world's resources are infinite. The truth is that these resources are limited, and that we stand within sight of their exhaustion. Soil, water, trees,

and even usable air—all are being depleted. The world's multiplying people are demanding more resources per year than the earth can replenish.

There is a way to stop this process, and it is urgent that we all learn about it now. Since the vital resources, everywhere, are soil, water, and trees, this highlight begins by showing the roles they play in making life possible for human beings on earth. Then, since the world's population is growing, whether we want it to or not, the discussion goes on to make the distinction between two kinds of development—one that we cannot live with and the other that we can live with, at least until we get our numbers under control. The kind of development that we cannot live with is exploitative development, which uses up resources such as soil, water, and trees without restoring them. The kind of development that will tide us over is sustainable development, which involves the use of renewable resources at a pace equal to the pace of their return; it does not plunder and leave desolation behind. Let us begin at the beginning, then, with soil, water, and trees.

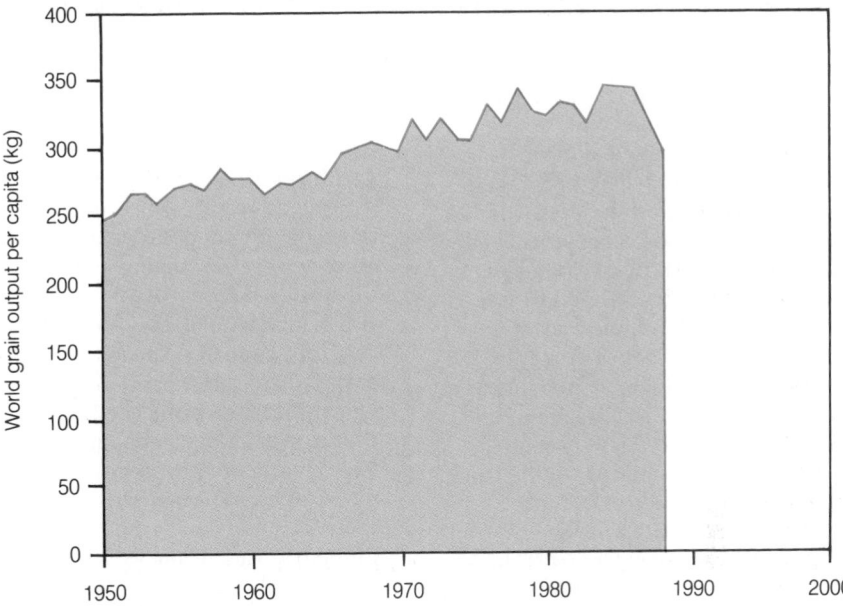

■ FIGURE H17–1
World Grain Output, 1950 to 1988
There was a steep decline in grain output after 1984. The statistics used are per capita, but total grain output also fell equally steeply.

Source: U.S. Department of Agriculture, as presented by L. R. Brown, *The Changing Food Prospect: The Nineties and Beyond*, Worldwatch paper 85 (Washington, D.C.: Worldwatch Institute, 1988), Figure 10.

The Soil

The thin cloak of soil that covers the earth provides the support in which growing plants, including food plants, need to spread their roots; it also holds the moisture from which plants draw their water. Not all plants must have soil to grow in; some trees, for example, may be able to gain a footing on bare rock or thin soil because they can sink their taproots directly into the groundwater. Grasses and agricultural crops do need soil, however, and the thicker it is, the better. Below the soil lies rock or clay in which such plants cannot grow.

Soil is both lost and created all the time. It is lost by being blown away by wind or by being washed down slopes into waterways, ultimately sinking irretrievably into the ocean. Balancing these losses, soil is created by the wind's and water's action on rocks. Soil creation is slow, and in recent times, losses have predominated. These losses are largely due to deforestation—for where trees are removed, both water and wind quickly remove soil cover, leaving bare rock or clay. Then no new vegetation can grow to shelter the land surface from further erosive rain and wind.

Soil loss worldwide is increasing every year. At present, it amounts to 25 billion tons a year, enough to fill Yankee Stadium 175,000 times.[4] Soil loss due to human misuse of the land today is taking place so fast that *a quarter of the world's farmable land is fated to become permanent wasteland.*

One way to bolster failing cropland where soil loss has occurred is to irrigate and fertilize. These measures are not sustainable, however; they are exploitative: they use up or destroy nonrenewable resources. Irrigation depletes the ground water and adds salt to the soil. Fertilizer, as usually applied, pollutes the water. In recognition of this fact, some nations are attempting to reverse the process of soil loss in the only self-sustaining way—by returning vulnerable areas to forest and grassland before it is too late. (China is now planting 4.5 million hectares—over 10 million acres—a year in reforestation projects, the world's largest such effort.)[5]* Reforestation reduces the amount of land presently being farmed, but with a difference: the plants and trees are preserved, and they help to replenish clean air and conserve water.

The Water

In addition to the soil, food-producing plants must have water to grow. Under natural circumstances, in much of the world, rainfall supplies that water, but agricultural crops often need more water, or more constantly

---

*A hectare is about 2½ acres, a metric unit used internationally to measure land areas.

Miniglossary

acid rain: rain that has picked up chemicals from the air that convert to acid when combined with water; a form of pollution.

agroforestry: agriculture within a tropical rainforest, as practiced by the indigenous people, which rotates crops beneath the forest canopy and is notable for not destroying the forest.

aquifer: a water-bearing layer of permeable rock, sand, or gravel beneath the earth's surface; the vast underground freshwater reservoir from which human populations usually draw their water.

carrying capacity: the total number of living organisms that a given environment can support without deteriorating in quality.

chlorofluorocarbons (CLOR-oh-FLOR-oh-car-bons; trade name **Freon**): chemical compounds containing chlorine, fluorine, and carbon. They are produced by industrial processes and, when released, rise into the outer atmosphere, where they react with ozone to destroy it; see *ozone layer*.

diversity: variety, the existence of differences. The term is used here in the sense of *biological* or *species* diversity, referring to the existence of many different species of plants and animals that have evolved on earth over millions of years. Once lost, these species cannot be regenerated.

evapotranspiration: the process by which plants (mainly trees) move water from below the ground into the air, renewing the clouds from which rain falls.

  evapo = evaporation
  transpire = to breathe out

exploitative development: economic development that uses up limited resources such as soil, water, and trees without replacing them. For contrast, see *sustainable development*.

fossil fuel: gas, oil, and coal, which come from the fossil remains of ancient trees and other plants.

---

available water, than rainfall can supply. Farmers then turn to irrigation—diverting rivers or pumping water up from underground. Irrigation of crops was first practiced thousands of years ago in the Middle East; now it has spread throughout the world. In 1900, 40 million hectares were irrigated; in 1950, that area had more than doubled, to 94 million; and in 1980, it had much more than doubled again, to 250 million hectares.

Irrigation sometimes solves a major water shortage problem, but in some cases the solution is only temporary or creates other serious problems. In much of the United States, water from underground that was deposited in prehistoric times (fossil water) is being used; this water will run out. Alternatively, water is taken from aquifers that are rechargeable by rains and rivers, but the water may be taken out so fast that recharging can't keep pace (overpumping), drawing down water tables. In many parts of the world, probably including yours, the land surface is sinking, even below sea level, due to the overpumping of underground water in this fashion. Along coastlines, receding underground freshwater opens the way for saltwater intrusion, ruining wells and making it impossible to grow crops.

Demands other than irrigation are

Miniglossary (continued)

fossil water: water that has been trapped below the ground since prehistoric times, and is not replenished by rainfall or river flows; not part of the cycle of rainfall and withdrawal that characterizes aquifers. Fossil water is tapped by sinking wells deep into the earth.

Freon (FREE-on): the trade name for a propellant and refrigerant (see *chlorofluorocarbons*).

greenhouse effect: the heating effect that occurs in a closed space that is warmed by sun. In a greenhouse, the glass keeps heat from escaping and facilitates plant growth. In the air surrounding the earth, accumulating gases are doing the same thing, but to excess, warming the earth to the danger point.

hectare: a metric measure of land area, equivalent to about 2½ acres.

overpumping: pumping water from below the ground more rapidly than rain and rivers can restore it, lowering the water table and ground level.

ozone: a photochemical oxidant, toxic when in direct contact with lung tissue; an air pollutant. See also *ozone layer*.

ozone layer: a layer of ozone that forms in the outer atmosphere when sunlight strikes oxygen; it protects living things on earth from harmful ultraviolet radiation from the sun.

photosynthesis: green plants' use of the sun's energy, captured by their chlorophyll, to combine carbon dioxide and water into energy-containing molecules such as sugars, starches, and fibers.

recycle: to use materials over again in the same process as before.

sustainable development: economic development that does not use up resources but recycles them, and betters people's economic well-being, not only in the short term, but also in the long term. For contrast, see *exploitative development*.

water table: the level below the ground where freshwater can be found.

---

competing for water use. Cities are growing, and they require water for domestic and industrial use. Industry uses water for transporting, dissolving, washing, rinsing, cooling, flushing away waste, and many other purposes—diverting huge quantities of water from its original, natural uses, polluting it, and returning it to pollute more water as it returns to the earth.

As mentioned, the trend earlier in this century was towards an increase in irrigated land. Now that trend has reversed. Irrigated areas have *decreased* virtually everywhere in the last ten years, as the consequence of several intensifying trends—increasing populations, overpumping, rising costs of pumping, and dwindling water supplies. For example, the United States is irrigating 7 percent less land and China, 11 percent less, than ten years ago. Further reductions in irrigation are predicted.[6] It appears that no significant expansion of irrigation will be possible henceforth; the only hope for providing water to larger land areas in the future is to reduce the wastage of the water already being used, so that it will spread further.[7]

Human overpopulation is also threatening the purity of the water supply. The more intense human activity is, the more polluted the water becomes. Among the harmful agents affecting the water supply are many contributed by agriculture (such as fertilizers and pesticides) and many contributed by industry (such as toxic and radioactive wastes and acid rain). A third contributor is human domestic throwaways and waste materials, such as garbage, plastics, and sewage. All three of these polluting influences are intensified by both the mere increase in numbers of people and by increases in their demands for consumer goods.

Trees play a major role in replenishing freshwater, just as they help replenish the soil. By preserving soil, they help the earth hold moisture; but more than that, they return vast amounts of underground water to the atmosphere by a process known as evapotranspiration. Transpired water is pure, and it forms clouds that will fall again as rain (freshwater) rather than running down rivers to join the ocean (and become unusable saltwater).

The Trees

Trees have covered much of the earth since prehistoric times. They provide a deep layer of vegetation in which many processes take place that support and renew the environment that in turn sustains the life of other plants and animals. Consider the trees in a rainforest, for example. They may be more than 100 feet tall, and measure 20 feet across at the base. They support a mass of vegetation and animal life. They create shade and hold moisture. By evapotranspiration, they create rain clouds, and these rain clouds frequently release drenching torrents. The rainforest trees generate oxygen by photosynthesis, permitting all living things in the forest to breathe. They drop tons of leaf litter, bark, branches, and animal droppings to the ground beneath them, where quantities of molds, fungi, and bacteria break down this litter as fast as it falls, keeping the system in balance. (Only an inch of soil lies below the litter, and beneath that is often impermeable clay. That is why tropical forestlands are so unsuitable for clearing and agricultural use.) The rainforest is most useful, from the point of view of basic human needs, to generate oxygen and rain.

Rainforests are important in other senses too, though. They have covered the earth for millions of years, and they hold a treasure trove of biological diversity. Millions on millions of species of animals and plants not yet known to science thrive in their honeycombs of multitudinous spaces. Within 1 acre of such forests dwell 800,000 pounds of living things.[8]

When an acre of forest is cleared—for example, to plant grass and grow beef—its soil's fertility is used up within about eight years. Unprotected by tree cover, the soil quickly washes or blows away, leaving bare clay. When a whole region's forest is gone, rain ceases to fall, and the land becomes uninhabitable—not only for cattle, but for all other life, including human beings.

Eight years of supposed value to human beings is a short time, compared with the hundreds of thousands of years it took for that rainforest system to evolve. Within that eight-year time span, the acre will produce only 50 pounds of cattle per year—400 pounds total. Of that, 200 pounds is usable meat, enough to yield 800 four-ounce hamburgers. The trade-off: 55 square feet of forest, representing half a ton of forest life, lost permanently for each hamburger.[9]

This is a prime example of exploitative development. The natural cycle of a system that could have renewed itself and brought forth agricultural products indefinitely has been brought to a halt. In its place is a system that requires massive inputs of fertilizer, pesticides, and irrigation from "elsewhere" to keep it going from one year to the next. Not only is the world running out of "elsewheres," but even with these inputs, the system soon fails, leaving wasteland behind.

The loss of rainforests worldwide in these last years of the 20th century is one of the most devastating effects of the developing world's galloping increase in population and accelerating demands for resources. Some 27 million acres (11 million hectares) of tropical forests and other woodlands are being cleared *each year*, mostly by large-scale, misguided "development" projects.[10] These projects make sense only from the point of view of a very few people who make money from them in the short term. They do not help the people they displace, for as the land's richness degenerates beyond supporting even basic food crops, the people are forced to cut deeper and deeper into the forest while continuing to live in poverty and desperation.

Cutting the forest is extremely costly biologically as well. The tropics occupy only 6 percent of the earth's surface today, yet they are home to more than 60 percent of the species diversity of this planet. That diversity reflects a vast storehouse of genetic blueprints specifying plants and animals with the potential to adapt to widely varying conditions. The diversity is a kind of bank of information that can permit different species to take over and carry on even if climatic changes or diseases render the world's currently dominant species unable to survive. It also has direct economic value for human beings; about 25 percent of the medicines now produced commercially in the United States are derived in whole or in part from tropical plants. Hundreds of lifesaving medical substances have been developed from plants found only in the world's rainforests. To lose those resources that remain before they are ever even identified and studied would be to lose forever a potentially vast storehouse of the future's scientific knowledge.[11]

Left alone, rainforests are more valuable than when "developed" for high-technology agriculture. They are valuable, however, by a measure other than dollars gained for a few years by those who invest in their destruction. The forests can, for example, support human agriculture indefinitely if handled in the age-old ways developed by the forests' original people. The natives in such an area, living on small, cleared patches beneath the undisturbed forest canopy, were able to grow 5,000 pounds of shelled corn *and* 4,000 pounds of root and vegetable crops each year on each acre for five to seven years. Then they would allow the plots to return to forest and clear others. They rotated their crops of citrus, rubber, cacao, avocado, and papaya in a system known as agroforestry, which could be continued indefinitely. If the government of the country wanted to solve its people's hunger problem, it could do no better than to encourage sustainable agricultural methods such as these. Food production systems practiced by traditional rainforest Indians are, without exception, more productive than the pasturelands that often replace them.[12] Other appropriate uses of the forests are to grow commercial, exportable crops beneath the canopy rather than cutting it down—crops such as rubber, nuts, fruits, oils, and many others.[13] For example, the rubber tappers in the Amazon River basin are conserving the rainforest while making a living growing rubber.[14] The contrast between traditional exploitative development and sustainable development is shown in Figure H17–2.

Still, the destruction of rainforests proceeds without halt. In fact, as of this writing the destruction is accelerating. In China, a forested area the size of Italy has become a desert in the last 30 years—due to firewood cutting, timbering, and clearing for agricultural use. Floods and droughts are both common, now, in this 129,000-square-mile area. In Indonesia, 600,000 hectares of closed forests are lost each year. In Southeast Asia and sub-Saharan Africa, two-thirds of the wildlife habitat has

■ **FIGURE H17–2**
Traditional Versus Sustainable Development

Sustainable development. People must support the earth if the earth is to support them.

Trees plus soil

Forever

10 years

Traditional development. People drain the earth's resources, and the earth ceases to support them.

now disappeared.[15] The loss of tropical rainforests is now bringing about the greatest destruction of life-forms that has ever occurred on earth. The shaving off of the earth's protective layer of vegetation deprives people of needed firewood, causes mud slides that bury whole villages, and worse, contributes to global environmental consequences—our atmosphere itself is deteriorating.

The Atmosphere

Human beings, and indeed all animals, require oxygen to obtain the energy they need to support their lives. While using oxygen, they exhale carbon dioxide; and they depend on green plants to consume the carbon dioxide and return oxygen to the air. People's fuel-burning processes such as cooking, heating homes, and running cars or factories do the same thing: they consume oxygen and release carbon dioxide. Green plants, too, require energy to support their lives, and they sometimes obtain it the same way as animals do—by consuming oxygen and releasing carbon dioxide (for example, during the metabolic activities that they engage in at night or underground). However, during the day, thanks to their capacity for photosynthesis, green plants can use the sun's energy directly, something that animals, of course, cannot do. Using the sun's energy, plants reverse the flow of materials: they *consume* carbon dioxide and *release* oxygen.

Green plants use the carbon dioxide they consume in two ways. One way is to store it in sugar and starch molecules (for example, in their seeds) that they can later metabolize as fuel (for example, when seeds need to grow in the dark, underground). They return all of this carbon dioxide to the atmosphere. The other way they use carbon dioxide is as the building material for their own structural elements—the fibers of roots, stems, and leaves. This carbon dioxide they keep for as long as they are alive.

It is that second way in which plants use carbon dioxide that is particularly significant in relation to trees—and especially rainforest trees—because they are so big and (in forests) so numerous. For as long as they are standing, trees are withholding a giant bank of carbon from the atmosphere. When they are felled, however, no matter whether they are burned or left to rot, they release that carbon back to the atmosphere in carbon dioxide. The destruction of rainforests actually threatens the earth's atmosphere in three ways: it adds directly to the air's carbon dioxide content, it takes away the trees that are the means for carbon dioxide removal, and it permits dedication of the land to carbon dioxide–*producing* activity such as human habitation or industry.

Now that we human beings have

become so numerous on earth, we—and especially our fuel-burning activities—are among the earth's major carbon dioxide producers. (When human beings burn fossil fuels such as gasoline and oil, they are burning plants that stored that carbon dioxide from the air of long ago.) The more of us there are, and the more intense our use of fossil fuels, the more plants (especially forests) we need to surround us and compensate for our production of carbon dioxide with their consumption of it.

The Greenhouse Effect

The amount of carbon dioxide in the atmosphere has remained about the same for hundreds of thousands of years—until this century. Carbon dioxide has been an important component of the air, necessary to life on earth as we know it. It blocks the escape of heat into the outer atmosphere, and it helps to keep the earth warm. Without it, the earth would have been 54 degrees Fahrenheit colder for all those years, and life as we know it would have been impossible. In the 30 years between 1958 and 1988, however, the concentration of carbon dioxide in the earth's air has increased by 25 percent, mostly as the result of increased burning of oil and coal. The result is that the earth appears to be warming up—the so-called greenhouse effect.[16]

The greenhouse effect is expected to increase the earth's average temperature by 3 to 8 degrees Fahrenheit in the next half-century (before 2050)—an amount that may not sound like much, but that is expected to have major effects. Many scientists believe that these effects are already occurring. Worldwide, summer heat is setting new high-temperature records. Rainfall appears to be declining across the corn and wheat belts in the United States, Europe, the Soviet Union, and the rest of Asia, resulting in more-frequent droughts than in the past, with loss of crops

and rangelands. Water tables, already falling due to the human demands for water mentioned earlier, are further depleted by global warming. Inland, rivers are shrinking, creating hardship for areas that depend on their water. Along the coastlines, saltwater is invading, depriving both vegetation and people of needed freshwater. The oceans are expanding as they warm up, and the polar ice caps are melting, so the sea level is rising. Governments are faced with the choice of seeing coastal cities and shores going underwater or building dikes and levees to hold the water back. Forests and agricultural crops, adapted for thousands of years to a certain climate, are stressed by rising temperatures and are yielding to diseases and insect pests. Whole species of animals and plants, including agricultural crops that human beings depend on, will become extinct if the earth's seasonal average temperatures change by only a few degrees.

Carbon dioxide is thought to cause about half of the heating caused by the greenhouse effect. Thinning of the ozone layer in the outer atmosphere causes a quarter of the global warming—a topic discussed in the next section.[17] Agricultural practices, including deforestation, account for much of the rest. The burning of felled rainforest trees alone accounts for up to 20 percent of greenhouse gas emissions worldwide.[18]

Ozone Depletion

Another atmospheric effect of air pollution is taking place far out, in the outer atmosphere. Where intense sunlight strikes the outer atmosphere, a layer of gas known as the ozone layer continuously forms from oxygen and breaks down again. The ozone layer has for millions of years screened out 99 percent of the ultraviolet rays of the sun, allowing just enough through to support plant growth. Life probably did not begin until after the earth's protective ozone layer was formed.

Now, air pollution from human activities all over the earth appears to be eating away at the ozone layer. At the South Pole, during each antarctic summer, when the sunlight there is intense and the air is cold and still, a hole in the layer forms. Every year it is growing larger. After each antarctic summer, the remaining ozone from the rest of the earth's atmosphere diffuses and re-covers the hole, but at the cost of thinning the ozone layer over the rest of the earth. As a result, more ultraviolet radiation is reaching the earth's surface each year. This radiation causes skin cancers in animals and people, and it damages plants and crops. As it increases, this radiation may become so intense as to induce more mutations in plants, animals, and microbes than they can repair.

Chief among the pollutants that destroy ozone are compounds known as chlorofluorocarbons (the trade name of one product made from them is *Freon*). The chlorofluorocarbons that destroy ozone are used to cool refrigerators, freezers, and air-conditioning systems; to create foams (including some Styrofoams); and to expel liquids under pressure from aerosol cans (such as deodorants). People and nations have been taking action to reduce chlorofluorocarbon output, but since it takes these molecules up to 40 years to reach the outer ozone layers, their destruction of ozone may continue long after their production has ceased. At the current rate of increase, according to several independent predictions, the ozone layer will be seriously depleted within 100 years. Skin cancer rates, already on the increase, are expected to rise proportionately—to 1 in 90 by the year 2000 and 1 in 3 by the year 2075.[19] But individual cases of cancer do not even constitute the biggest threat. Ultraviolet rays in excess of the norm disrupt the genetic material in all living tissues, damaging all future generations of forests, agricultural crops, grasslands, gardens, and animal life on land and in the seas as well.

Acid Rain

As mentioned, air pollution cannot help but affect the water and soil. One problem arising from air pollution is acid rain. Each time it rains, the air is scrubbed of its pollutants; they fall to the earth. Many of them, when combined with water, form acids, which affect living things profoundly. It doesn't matter what compound forms the acid—it can be a compound of carbon, sulfur, or nitrogen. The effects are similar, because the acid part is always the same: a tiny, charged particle of hydrogen. This chemical busybody disrupts cell membranes, distorts the proteins that do the work of living cells, and changes the characteristics of fluids so that they cannot support normal life processes.

There has always been air pollution, and there has always been acid rain. But in the last 100 years, the air's acid burden has grown greater, primarily because of increased burning of coal and petroleum. Millions of acres in many areas of the world, including U.S. mountain ranges, the Black Forest in West Germany, and many parts of China, have been deforested by acid rain. In the soil, acid particles promote the release of toxic compounds into water supplies; in the air, they damage human lungs directly.

Air pollution reduces the effectiveness of the remaining forests in their air-cleansing work of photosynthesis. In polluted air, trees, crops, and other vegetation grow slowly and are vulnerable to disease.

In summary, to grow our food we need land areas rich in fertile soil with adequate water and sun. To hold and replenish the soil and recycle the water into rain, we need forests. The forests need soil and water, too, and all need oxygen and protection by the ozone layer from the damaging rays of the sun. The earth's balance among

these elements, which has made life possible for millennia, is now threatened by three simultaneous trends:

1. The spread of industrialization.
2. The destruction of natural environments.
3. The multiplication of people.

The effects of each trend compound those of the others, because, as we emphasized, every person in an industrialized society devours the earth's resources and pollutes the environment much more heavily than a person in a primitive society. Figure H17–3 shows a simplified picture of the burdens we human beings place on the earth.

If the population growth rate remains steady, in less than 50 years, the number of people on earth will reach the maximum that the earth can support—close to 10 billion people.[20] At that level, life for most people will barely be possible, and conditions will be much worse than they are today. Already millions are starving; agricultural and grazing lands are eroding or being irreversibly paved over; soils are becoming more salty; water shortages are worsening; rainfall is diminishing in many areas; ocean pollution and overfishing are leading to smaller catches and less variety; and widespread extinctions of plants and animals are occurring.[21]

As population growth continues, development must proceed, but it must be sustainable development. If we can slow down our burning of fossil fuels and stabilize the atmosphere, we can buy ourselves time in which to develop alternative sources of energy and get our numbers under control.

Role of U.S. Consumers

The U.S. population is not growing nearly as fast as that of the rest of the world. However, that fact does not relieve U.S. citizens of responsibility in the growing worldwide crises. Take

deforestation, for example. Even though we consumers may not personally be clearing rainforest land, our demands for products are driving the process. We panel and furnish our homes and offices with teak and mahogany from giant trees harvested by Japanese and Danish companies from deep within virgin rainforest lands. We eat more than 330 million pounds of beef purchased by U.S. companies from Central American countries alone—an amount that represents 90 percent of that region's beef exports.[22] We create the demand largely through our appetite for hamburgers from innumerable fast-food restaurants. As long as consumers keep buying the teak, mahogany, and beef, the trees continue to fall.

The money to convert Central America's rainforests to grasslands comes largely from international banks, which have supplied billions of dollars to finance cattle ranching in Central and South America since 1970. The banks claim that increased beef production is bettering Central Americans' nutrition, but in reality, it is doing nothing of the kind. As beef production in Central America has increased, the people there have eaten less and less beef, for two reasons. First, foreign companies are willing to pay higher prices than the people can afford to pay. Second, the population has increased, so more people are competing for the beef that remains within the country. Even an American house cat eats more beef than the average Central American.[23]

Some argue that the conversion of rainforest to ranchland in Central America benefits economic development: it brings money in, and it encourages international trade. So it does, but it is exploitative development, and supporters fail to ask, "Bring in money to whom?" Within the country, the money is going to wealthy speculators, not to the people who live or work on the land. Speculators prefer to finance the

The Earth *before* Human Impact

THE AIR

Animals and people take up oxygen (○) and release carbon dioxide (●).

The sun's rays, passing through clear air, provide energy for plants and algae to free oxygen (○) from carbon dioxide (●).

Green plants on land and algae in the ocean take up carbon dioxide (●) and return oxygen (○) to the atmosphere.

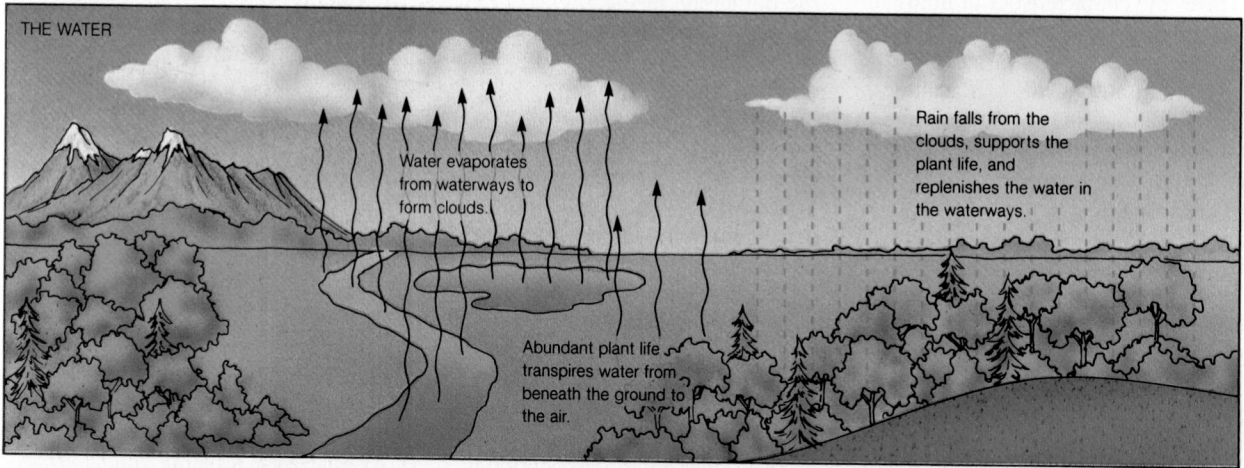

THE WATER

Water evaporates from waterways to form clouds.

Rain falls from the clouds, supports the plant life, and replenishes the water in the waterways.

Abundant plant life transpires water from beneath the ground to the air.

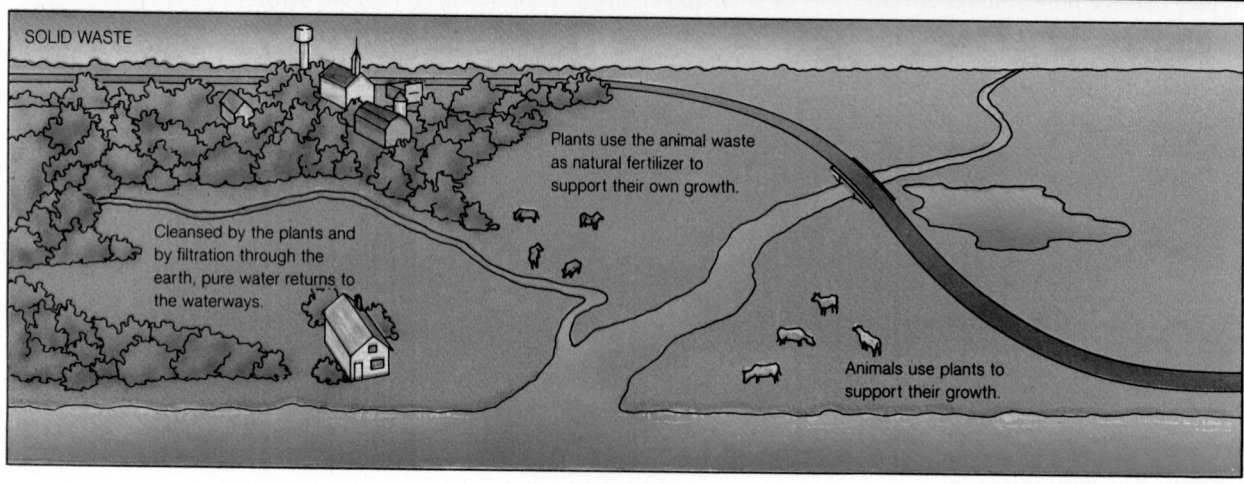

SOLID WASTE

Plants use the animal waste as natural fertilizer to support their own growth.

Cleansed by the plants and by filtration through the earth, pure water returns to the waterways.

Animals use plants to support their growth.

The Earth *with* Human Impact

Carbon dioxide (◎) and acid pollutants (●) begin to accumulate in the atmosphere.

The sun's rays deliver less energy for plants and algae to free oxygen.

Large populations take up oxygen (○) and release carbon dioxide (◎) and air pollution (●).

Green plants and algae, deprived of sunlight, diminish in quantity, capture less carbon dioxide (◎), and return less oxygen (○) to the air.

There is less water in the waterways to evaporate.

Acid rain kills plant life. This means there are fewer plants to transpire water from beneath the ground to the air. This, too, diminishes rainfall.

Air pollution causes acid rain to fall.

Dense human populations occupy land areas, and not only add waste, but also reduce the land area available to filter the waste from the water.

Human domestic and industrial activity adds plastics and toxins to the land and water.

Intensive farming contaminates soil and water with animal waste, fertilizer, and pesticides.

Contamination of the water leads to death of lakes, contaminates the world's oceans, and threatens the food supply.

production of beef that will be paid for by the U.S. market than to finance improved nutrition for the native people with no sure return in sight.

People in this country who are concerned with the destruction of tropical rainforests to raise beef ask, "Why can't we produce our own beef?" or "Why can't we import beef from elsewhere?" In fact, we do both. Only 2 percent of the beef we consume, or about 2 pounds per person (220 square feet of rainforest per person per year), comes from rainforest land, but this beef is not labeled as such. We cannot avoid using it, except by forgoing beef altogether. Even the fast-food establishments that buy beef cannot tell (without investigating) which packages are from the rainforest, because by the time they see them, they are all labeled "domestic." The problem is solvable, even simple. It requires labeling beef as to origin, but as of this writing, labeling bills have yet to be enacted into law.*

For another example of U.S. citizens' responsibility for the environmental problems of today, consider air pollution. Natural processes such as forest fires, volcanoes, and the natural rotting of organic matter have always released temporary bursts of contamination into the air, but people-generated pollution is continuous, concentrated, and in many cases growing more intense from year to year. People-generated pollutants come from four main sources: fuel burned to run cars and other forms of transportation, fuel burned to heat and cool homes and run their appliances, wastes from industrial activity, and materials being burned for disposal. These add large amounts of pollutants to the air—among them, compounds that reduce its clarity (hampering photosynthesis) and compounds such as acids that render it toxic to plants (directly damaging

them or making them vulnerable to disease).

The first two pollution sources just mentioned were fuel burned to run cars and other forms of transportation and fuel burned to heat and cool homes and run home appliances. These reflect personal, individual choices—our own lifestyle choices. The days when we could blame major industrial polluters for most of our problems are over—they still do their share, but *small consumers are now the major contributors to the pollution of our environment*. When asked at a major conference on the rainforest what we as individuals could do to help reverse the growing deforestation tragedy, several world experts said, "Convince U.S. consumers to change their own lifestyles."[24] Many avenues are open to us. We can demand that our cars be designed to get 200 miles to the gallon—already a feasible possibility. We can learn to conserve energy in many ways, without even sacrificing our luxuries; West Germany uses only half the energy per person that we use while maintaining a standard of living similar to ours.[25] We can also eat lower on the food chain—more plant foods, less beef.

Such choices will require, though, that citizens learn to live more simply (not less richly) than in the past. To do so will help considerably to reduce the burden we human beings place on the earth's carrying capacity. It can also bring each of us great personal satisfaction. Valuable suggestions for ways to accomplish this in each person's own life are offered by many inspired and creative groups of thinkers.*

As we learn to change our lifestyles, we can also encourage our political leaders to work with the leaders of other nations to take global action to conserve the environment and relieve world hunger—two efforts that must go hand in hand. This is now possible, and possible in ways it has never been before, because the world's nations are able to act as a unit, and to act quickly, for the first time in history. What makes it possible is two current trends: the explosion of scientific knowledge about environmental problems and the world's increasing use of fast communications to make that knowledge available to all governments simultaneously. Knowledge and awareness shared among people and governments can bring about rapid decision making and action.

Some of the best minds of today's world are bringing their powers to bear on the problems described here. For example, much powerful, positive thinking is coming from the Worldwatch Institute—an independent, nonprofit research institution created to analyze and focus attention on global problems.[26] Worldwatch is funded by private foundations and by the United Nations, and its papers are written for a worldwide audience of decision makers, scholars, and students. Its *State of the World* report, which comes out annually, not only keeps track of trends in all areas such as deforestation and fuel use, but also goes beyond the mere presentation of facts on environmental emergencies to analyze and compare possible solutions. *State of the World* is used as a text in more and more college courses, and is helping to make tomorrow's leaders aware of the areas on which they need to focus their attention.

An ingenious suggestion appears in *State of the World 1987*. Nations that have the greatest power to affect each problem should focus on that problem. For example, of the 83 million people added to the world's population the year before, China and India accounted for a third of the total. Those two countries should

_____

*One way to help is to join, and work with, the Rainforest Action Network, 300 Broadway #28, San Francisco, CA 94133.

_____

*One book of excellent suggestions for meeting personal responsibilities to the world is produced under the auspices of the American Friends Service Committee: J. Bodner, ed., *Taking Charge of Our Lives: Living Responsibly in a Troubled World* (San Francisco: Harper & Row, 1984). Another is produced by the Center for Science in the Public Interest, Simple Lifestyle Team, *99 Ways to a Simple Lifestyle* (Garden City, N.Y.: Anchor Books, 1977).

therefore emphasize population control the most heavily, and be supported in doing so by the others. Similarly, of all the world's increases in carbon dioxide and global warming, caused by the burning of fossil fuels, half appears to be caused by only three nations—the United States, the Soviet Union, and China. Their major efforts should be aimed at that problem. Similarly, three nations contain more than half of the remaining tropical rainforests—Brazil, Indonesia, and Zaire—so efforts at conservation should focus on them. Substantial changes can be brought about if the right efforts are made by the right groups.[27]

Finally, we need to renew our own earth consciousness and instill it in our children. After all, we do not inherit the land, we only borrow it from our children. Besides, care of the earth and its living things matters for its own sake, as well as for people's sake. The earth is truly our mother; its preservation and that of other species is a moral and ethical responsibility that concerns us in a deep, spiritual way.[28] Our native American predecessors, the Indians, have always known:

This we know. The Earth does not belong to man; man belongs to the Earth. This we know. All things are connected like the blood which unites one family. All things are connected. Whatever befalls the Earth befalls the sons of the Earth. Man did not weave the web of life, he is merely a strand in it. Whatever he does to the web, he does to himself.—Chief Seattle, 1854

Even if we worship in towering cathedrals deep within mighty cities, we must remain aware of, and responsible to, the trees, the flowers, the bees, and the dolphins, for they are as much a part of the web as we are.

NOTES

1. T. Wicker, We have battered, abused planet, *Tallahassee Democrat,* 29 November 1988.
2. National Academy of Sciences, *Resources and Man* (1969 report), as cited by L. J. Gordon, Popullution: The 1981 APHA presidential address, *American Journal of Public Health* 72 (1982): 341–346.
3. L. R. Brown, *The Changing World Food Prospect: The Nineties and Beyond,* Worldwatch paper 85, October 1988, available from the Worldwatch Institute, 1776 Massachusetts Ave. NW, Washington, DC 20036.
4. T. Peterson, Hunger and the environment, *Seeds,* October 1987, pp. 6–13.
5. Wicker, 1988.
6. The Chinese irrigated area fell from 45 million hectares in 1977 to 40 million hectares in 1985, according to data in Crook, *Agricultural Statistics;* Li Rongxia, Irrigation system in central Shaanxi, *Beijing Review,* 14–20 December 1987; Nie Lisheng, State organizes farmers to work on irrigation, *China Daily,* 16 January 1988, all as cited by Brown, 1988, p. 25.
7. Brown, 1988, p. 29.
8. C. Uhl and G. Parker, Viewpoint: Our steak in the jungle, *BioScience* 36 (1986): 642.
9. Uhl and Parker, 1986.
10. Letter (December 1988) from Conservation International, 1015 18th St. NW, Suite 1000, Washington, DC 20036.
11. Letter from Conservation International, 1988.
12. J. D. Nations and D. I. Komer, Rainforests and the hamburger society, *Environment,* April 1983, pp. 12–20.
13. First "extractive reserve" is to be created in Brazilian rainforest, *EDF Letter,* 19, no. 3 (1988): 3.
14. B. M. Rich, Development alternatives for third world conservation, *EDF Letter,* (1988): 4.
15. Wicker, 1988.
16. S. Begley, M. Miller, and M. Hager, The endless summer? *Newsweek,* 11 July 1988, pp. 18–20.
17. M. Oppenheimer, Letter to members, December 1988, Environmental Defense Fund, 257 Park Ave. South, New York, NY 10010.
18. Oppenheimer, 1988.
19. D. Rigel, research physician from New York University Medical Center, reporting to an Energy and Commerce subcommittee hearing, March 1987, as cited in Action needed to save ozone, *Tallahassee Democrat,* 10 March 1987.
20. B. Bull, Voodoo demography: What population problem? *Amicus Journal,* Fall 1984, pp. 36–40.
21. Gordon, 1982.
22. Nations and Komer, 1983.
23. Nations and Komer, 1983.
24. Tropical rainforests: Strategies for wise management, a conference, 27–31 January 1988, Florida International University, Miami, Fla.
25. Wicker, 1988.
26. Worldwatch Institute, 1776 Massachusetts Ave. NW, Washington, DC 20036.
27. *State of the World 1987: A Worldwatch Institute Report on Progress toward a Sustainable Society* (New York: Norton, 1987).
28. E. O. Wilson, *Biophilia: The Human Bond with Other Species* (Cambridge, Mass.: Harvard University Press, 1984), pp. 119–140.

Nutrition and Illness

Medicines act, as do the body's own regulatory hormones and enzymes, by altering physiological processes. These are crystals of aspirin, photographed through an electron microscope.

The earlier chapters of this book provided you with an understanding of normal nutrition—nutrition as it applies to most healthy people. Those chapters introduced the nutrients, explained how the body handles them, and described some of the many ways that nutrition influences people's lives. The knowledge and skills you gained apply to all people in general, but in health care professions, you need additional nutrition information to serve your clients well. The focus of the remaining chapters therefore shifts to providing you with an understanding of clinical nutrition—nutrition as it applies to people with illnesses.

This chapter and the next four chapters provide general nutrition information for client care, regardless of your clients' specific medical conditions. Whatever the illness, all of your clients will require nutrition care. This chapter shows the relationships between an illness and a person's nutrition status. The next two chapters explain the methods used to assess nutrition status and to provide nutrition care, and the following two chapters describe how to feed clients who require special nutrition support. These general nutrition guidelines for working with clients will prepare you for the remaining eight chapters, which examine the specific dietary care required for clients with particular medical conditions—conditions that involve trauma, upper and lower GI tract disfunction, liver disease, diabetes, heart and blood vessel abnormalities, lung disorders, kidney disease, and the wasting disorders cancer and AIDS. In addition to the nutrition regimens used to treat these disorders, you will find nutrition recommendations for preventing their development wherever appropriate. Clearly, the best treatment is prevention.

This chapter explains how illnesses in general can impair people's nutrition status and how sound nutrition can support recovery. It first reviews the stress response—for all illnesses impose stress on the body. Then it explores the relationships between nutrition and two types of defenses against illnesses—the immune system and drug therapy. It concludes by summarizing the relationships between nutrition and illness, including a look at the role of nutrition in preventing disease.

The word **illness** as used in this book refers to any medical condition that alters nutrition status. Not all such conditions are diseases. For example, major surgery can have a significant impact on nutrition status, although it is not a disease.

The Stress Response

Highlight 1 first introduced stress and defined it as any threat—physical or psychological—to a person's well-being. Surely, illnesses threaten a person's well-being, but even a healthy person visiting a physician for a regular checkup may feel anxious, triggering a mild stress response. It's all a matter of degree.

Under normal circumstances, the body efficiently maintains an internal balance, much like a finely tuned machine. Even small changes in the internal environment, such as the influx of nutrients entering the body following a meal, set in motion a series of metabolic events to restore homeostasis—that is, to bring the body back to a state of equilibrium. Occasionally, though, the body is confronted with a more severe change in the internal environment, such as a broken bone, an infection, or a burn. Because these conditions place greater stress on the body than normal, the body must employ more complicated mechanisms to reestablish balance.

Some stress is part of the body's normal and healthy functioning; this type of stress is **physiological stress.** Additional stress imposed by disease or an abnormal bodily insult such as surgery, burns, fever, or infection can overwhelm the body; such stress is **pathological stress.** One type of pathological stress is **trauma**—physical injury to the body, such as a broken bone, a gunshot wound, or surgery.

Chapter 23 describes the nutrition care of clients with severe stresses such as infection, surgery, and burns.

The concept of homeostasis was first introduced in Highlight 1, which described the body's response to stress. Stress triggers chains of coordinated events involving the entire body—from the pupils of your eyes to the blood vessels in your toes—that help the body to regain its equilibrium.

The body's response to stress depends on the intensity and duration of the insult. Taking a final exam, for example, is a fairly minor stress when compared with the stress of an illness such as cancer. Prolonged fasting (or starvation) presents a greater stress to the body than taking an exam, of course, but still, by comparison, it is relatively mild and readily resolved. In contrast, major surgery (such as open-heart surgery) represents a severe stress that requires many metabolic changes to regain equilibrium. Understanding the initial metabolic changes that occur during a relatively uncomplicated stress such as starvation lays the foundation for understanding the complex changes brought about by severe stresses. The metabolic changes are similar in all stresses, but their rates and intensities differ.

The Stress of Starvation

Chapter 7 introduced the body's metabolic response to the stress of fasting. After a short period of fasting (or other stress), the body draws on its stored carbohydrate, fat, and protein to meet its energy needs. Liver glycogen (the available stored form of carbohydrate) breaks down to maintain blood glucose concentrations to fuel the body's cells. However, glycogen stores are limited, and this source of glucose is depleted fairly soon after fasting begins.

Meanwhile, the body mobilizes its fatty acids to provide fuel. In contrast to the glycogen stores, fatty acid stores are plentiful. However, some of the body's cells (such as the brain cells) depend on glucose for fuel, and the body cannot convert fatty acids into glucose. The glycerol portion of a triglyceride can be used to make glucose, but this process retrieves as glucose only about 5 percent of a typical triglyceride's kcalories, leaving the triglyceride's fatty acids to be converted to ketones or otherwise metabolized (see pp. 175–176). Consequently, the body must find another source of glucose. That source is amino acids, which the body supplies by breaking down its protein tissue. Amino acids provide most of the glucose needed to mount a stress response.

Unlike glucose and fat, protein is not stored by the body. The body uses its proteins as parts of cell membranes and other organelles, as enzymes, as hormones, as immune system factors, and as other blood proteins and body components. Thus, the loss of too much protein from body tissues compromises the function of vital organ systems including the heart, lungs, and GI tract and can interfere with the immune response and normal metabolic processes.

To help meet its need to conserve and maintain vital proteins, the body gradually adapts to another energy source as starvation continues. Fat continues to break down, and as it does, the liver begins to synthesize ketones (see pp. 182–183). The brain and other tissues begin to use the ketones as an energy source, reducing the body's need for glucose. (The brain still needs some glucose, though.) At the same time, the body reduces its total energy needs by slowing its metabolic rate. As the metabolic rate falls, the body temperature also falls, and the person feels fatigued. All of these changes reduce energy needs. The net effect: the body conserves all of its fuel sources and minimizes its use of glucose.

In **fasting,** a person voluntarily stops eating food, whereas in **starvation,** not eating is involuntary. The body, however, makes no distinction between the two—metabolically, fasting and starvation have the same consequences.

Not all amino acids can be used to make glucose. The most important amino acids in glucose production are alanine and glutamine; they are synthesized in the body from the branched-chain amino acids.

■ **FIGURE 18–1**
Metabolic Response to Starvation

During this whole process, other nutrients play significant roles as well. Vitamins and minerals serve as cofactors in the metabolic reactions that are occurring. Depletion of these nutrients can interfere with the ability of vital organs to operate under the stress of starvation. Figure 18–1 summarizes the body's responses just described.

Severe Stress

Severe stresses such as infection and traumas such as surgery or fractures generate a chain of metabolic events similar to those that occur in starvation, with some important differences. Unlike the reduction in the metabolic rate that occurs during uncomplicated starvation, the metabolic rate rises markedly (hypermetabolism) during severe stress. An accelerated breakdown of body energy reserves (catabolism) also occurs. These metabolic responses are mediated by hormonal changes, many of which are listed in Table 18–1. Common hallmarks of the stress response during the period following injury include elevated blood glucose levels (hyperglycemia), negative nitrogen balance, increased retention of fluid and sodium, and increased excretion of potassium (see Figure 18–2 on p. 578).

While the general metabolic responses to all kinds of stress are similar, the body also responds uniquely to each type of stress. Consider that to mend a broken bone requires a different response than to heal a wound or to fight an infection. The body's response also depends on the severity of stress. For example, the response would be less dramatic for a well-nourished person

hypermetabolism: accelerated metabolic activity.

catabolism: metabolic breakdown of body energy reserves (see p. 171).

■ **TABLE 18–1**
Hormonal Changes That Occur During Severe Stress

Hormone	Alteration	Metabolic Effect
Catecholamines	Increase	Glucagon release increases. Insulin-to-glucagon ratio decreases.[a] Glycogen breakdown increases. Glucose production from amino acids increases. Mobilization of free fatty acids increases.
Cortisol	Increases	Mobilization of free fatty acids increases. Glucose production from amino acids increases. Utilization of glucose by many cells except brain decreases.
Glucagon	Increases	Glucose production from amino acids increases. Glycogen breakdown increases.
Insulin	Decreases	Storage of glucose, amino acids, and fatty acids decreases.
Antidiuretic hormone	Increases	Retention of water increases.
Aldosterone	Increases	Retention of sodium increases.

Note: These changes are part of the immediate stress response. As adaptation occurs and recovery is in progress, hormone levels gradually return to normal.

[a]Whenever the ratio of insulin to glucagon decreases, the net effect is that catabolism predominates. In the immediate stress response, hormones affect the muscle cells making them unable to use blood glucose even during hyperglycemia. Skeletal muscle breaks down to supply glucose.

undergoing minor elective surgery (a moderate stress) than it would be for a malnourished person with extensive burns (a severe stress). A severely malnourished person does not have the nutrient reserves necessary to continue meeting the increased metabolic demands of a severe injury. The result is exhaustion, which may in turn result in complications such as infection or organ failure. This further compromises the person's physical state and makes recovery more difficult.

When several stresses occur at the same time, body tissues break down to a greater degree, amplifying the loss of vital protein. Multiple stresses can occur easily in one person—for example, a person may undergo surgery, receive no food following surgery, and then develop an infection with a fever.

As draining as the stress response might sound, medical researchers believe that the initial metabolic changes provide a positive service. These changes help to prevent injury, repair damaged tissues, and maintain vital organ function. They facilitate the body's mobilization of its resources so it can regain homeostasis.

Such metabolic changes constitute an adaptation that is sustained for as long as necessary or until exhaustion leads to death. Gradually, the rate of catabolism returns to normal, blood glucose levels fall, and nitrogen balance is slowly restored. The amount of time it takes for the body to return to normal depends on the degree of stress and the individual's state of health, including nutritional health. Figure 18–3 on p. 579 illustrates the phases of the stress response. Clearly, the better nourished people are at the onset of a period of stress, the better they will be able to carry the metabolic burdens stress imposes.

The **acute,** or **flow, phase** of the stress response is the catabolic period immediately following the onset of stress. During the **adaptive phase,** the body adjusts to the stress to minimize losses. If adaptation succeeds, **recovery** follows. If adaptation fails, **exhaustion** follows.

■ **FIGURE 18–2**
Metabolic Response to Severe Stress

Severe stress

Rapid depletion of liver glycogen and mobilization of fatty acids for energy.

Early depletion of liver glycogen stores.

Metabolic rate rises markedly.

Body protein tissues break down rapidly.

Recovery   Exhaustion

Eventually, stress resolves, and the metabolic rate returns to normal or shifts to that seen in starvation.

If stress does not resolve before energy stores are severely compromised, death follows.

Catabolism
Flow / Acute phase
difference between Severe Stress & starvation

★ difference between Severe stress & STARVATION

Protein-Energy Malnutrition (PEM) and the Stress Response

Chapter 6 provided a description of protein-energy malnutrition (PEM), and Chapter 17 discussed malnutrition as a consequence of hunger in the United States and around the world. This section takes another perspective, exploring malnutrition's relationships with illness. Such malnutrition knows no geographical, financial, age, or gender boundaries. It can strike a wealthy person in a hospital in an industrialized nation just as it can hit a poor person without access to any health care in a Third World country; it affects children and adults, men and women alike.

In fact, PEM in U.S. hospitals is a serious problem. One study of hospitalized people found that 55 percent were likely to be malnourished.[1] Furthermore, only 1 in 20 of these people received nutrition therapy either prior to developing complications or early in hospitalization. You may well wonder how hospitals that can provide the latest in medical technology could neglect basic nutrition care. All health care professionals should learn to recognize the signs of PEM and the ways it interferes with a person's recovery. (Chapter 19 describes the nutrition-assessment procedures used to detect PEM.)

While strong nutritional health supports a person in withstanding the stress of illness, poor nutritional health constitutes a stress that doubles the person's burden. Consider how the body must work to counteract the compound stresses of PEM and a serious illness. Because requirements for protein and energy rise remarkably during stress, the body's ability to respond depends, to a large extent, on available energy reserves and protein status. If the person is

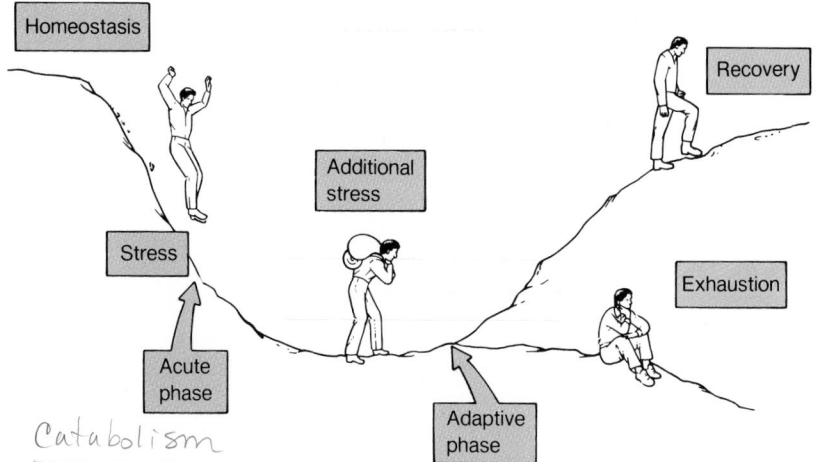

Homeostasis

Stress

Acute
phase

Catabolism

Additional
stress

Adaptive
phase

Recovery

Exhaustion

■ **FIGURE 18–3**
Phases of a Stress Response
During the initial stress response, hypermetabolism sends nutrient reserves on a downhill course. As adaptation occurs, nutrient balances are gradually restored. If depleted of nutrients, the person will be unable to make the uphill trip and may not recover (exhaustion). A person who is carrying a heavier load (additional stress) will plunge downhill faster and have a more difficult climb.

malnourished and hasn't received adequate protein or energy for a while, the body uses its protein tissues to meet its energy needs. As a result, the body loses functional protein from skeletal muscles, from organs, and from circulating pools of protein (such as albumin and immune factors).

For the well-nourished person, *some* loss of protein is acceptable, since sufficient protein will remain to support vital functions. However, for the person experiencing prolonged stress or malnutrition, the protein loss can be critical. Think about the consequences of protein loss on an accident victim who sustains multiple fractures and burns. What if the protein losses reflected breakdown of lung cells and immune factors? The loss of a critical number of functioning lung cells combined with a reduced synthesis of immune factors can lead to deterioration of lung function and depression of the immune system. The result: pneumonia—on top of multiple fractures and burns. You can see how easily stresses can multiply if they are allowed to go unchecked.

Organs that undergo rapid cell replacement—such as the GI tract—are among the first to suffer the consequences of PEM. The intestinal microvilli gradually shrink and become nonfunctional; up to 90 percent of them can be lost. Then, even with adequate nourishment, the GI tract will have serious difficulty absorbing nutrients. Consequently, PEM worsens.

Within the cells, PEM hinders the synthesis of enzymes and other protein molecules that the body needs for proper metabolism and maintenance of the cells' structures. The rapid synthesis and degradation of these protein molecules helps the body to adapt promptly to changes in the environment. Losing this ability to adapt leaves the body vulnerable and defenseless. PEM thus interferes with the body's ability to heal wounds, mount an immune response, and maintain the function of vital organs and skeletal muscles.

Nutrition is only one of many factors that influence a person's ability to respond to illness, but it is an important one. Other important factors are the severity of the stress, the number of organ systems involved, and the responses of the individual to other therapies. All of these factors working together determine whether a person will regain health. To summarize the role of nutrition described so far, adequate nutrition helps fight illness by providing the energy and nutrient reserves needed to fuel the metabolic

To understand the relationship of protein-energy malnutrition to serious illness, think of energy stores and protein status as money in the bank. Illness can be compared to a major expense that arises unexpectedly. The person who has saved enough money can pay off the expense without too much difficulty. However, if more and more expenses arise, the money may run out. The person with little or no savings is unable to pay even a small expense.

■ **TABLE 18–2**
Major Components of the Immune System

First Line of Defense

Skin.
GI tract.
Mucus.
Tears, sweat, sebaceous gland secretions.
Digestive enzymes.

Second Line of Defense

Granulocytes.
Macrophages.

Third Line of Defense

Sensitized T-lymphocytes.
Antibodies.

changes associated with stress. But adequate nutrition does more. It also supports a healthy immune system.

■ *Nutrition and Immunity*

The body's natural system of defense against invaders—the immune system—enables the body to fight off certain diseases. The immune system's response to the hormonal and metabolic changes that accompany stress, however, is to suppress its disease-fighting activity. If malnutrition accompanies stress, the immune system is forced to work without adequate nutrient support, further impairing its activity. Impaired immunity raises the risk of disease, disease impairs nutrition, and poor nutrition impairs immunity, creating a synergistic cycle that must be broken to recover from disease (Figure 18–4).

Much like a bodyguard, your immune system alertly and silently defends you against the thousands of enemy attacks mounted against you every day. Your remarkable capacity to survive an environment teeming with disease-causing organisms is a tribute to your immune system's effectiveness.

The immune system has no central organ of control, but rather depends on the interactions and secretions of various organs and white blood cells. Table 18–2 describes the major components of the immune system, and the accompanying miniglossary defines related terms.

The immune system is called into play when a foreign substance penetrates the body's first lines of defense—the skin, the GI tract, and the mucous membranes. Normally, these formidable barriers successfully prevent entry of invaders into the body. The skin is thick, coated with protective waxes, and it is constantly shedding its outermost layers while its associated glands secrete sweat and oily secretions that are toxic to some types of bacteria.

The remarkably efficient cells of the GI tract rarely allow microorganisms to pass into the body, even though over 500 species of bacteria normally reside in the intestines.[2] Some bacteria in the intestines prevent other more harmful bacteria from entering the body.

Mucous membranes coat all of the body's openings—eyes, nose, mouth, lungs, GI tract, and genitourinary tract—and secrete protective mucus. The

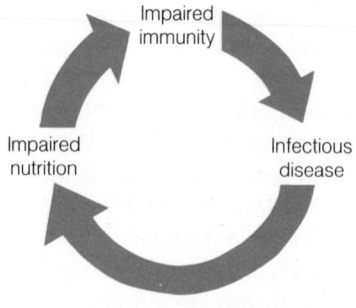

The vicious cycle of malnutrition and infection.

The ideal situation, in which nutrtion supports immunity against diseases.

■ **FIGURE 18–4**
Nutrition and Immunity

Miniglossary of Immunity Terms

acquired immunity: immunity directed at specific organisms (also called **specific immunity**). The lymphocytes mediate this type of immunity, which depends on prior exposure, recognition, and reaction to invading organisms. Two types of specific immunity are **cell-mediated immunity** and **humoral immunity.**

antibody: a protein of the type known as immunoglobulins, produced by the B-cells in response to invasion of the body by a foreign protein.

antigen: a substance that induces the formation of antibodies.

cell-mediated immunity: immunity conferred by the reaction of T-cells to an invading organism.

humoral immunity: immunity conferred by antibodies secreted by B-cells and carried to the invaded area by way of body fluids.

immune system: the body's natural defense system against foreign materials that have penetrated the skin or mucous membranes.

immunity: the body's ability to recognize and eliminate foreign materials.

immunoglobulin: a protein capable of acting as an antibody.

lymphocytes: white blood cells that participate in acquired immunity.

monokines: proteins secreted by phagocytes that activate metabolic and immune responses to infections.

nonspecific immunity: immunity directed at many kinds of organisms. Phagocytosis, the skin, and mucous membranes confer this type of immunity.

phagocytes: cells that have the ability to ingest and destroy foreign substances.

phagocytosis (FAG-oh-sigh-TOE-sis): the process by which some cells (phagocytes) engulf and destroy foreign materials.

   phagein = to eat
   kytos = cell
   osis = intensive

---

sticky mucus catches foreign materials and expels them as it flows out of the body. Moreover, it contains antimicrobial chemicals and enzymes that are lethal to invading organisms. If an invader does gain entry into the body (through a cut in the skin, for example), then the organs and cells of the immune system race into action.

Cells of the Immune System

The immune system depends primarily on the white blood cells (see Figure 18–5 on p. 582). The three types of white blood cells—the phagocytes and two types of lymphocytes—swarm over the entire body, but their primary residence is the lymph tissue. Figure 18–6 on p. 583 identifies the sites of immune system cell production. You may take comfort in knowing that of the 100 trillion cells that make up the human body, one in every hundred is a white blood cell.[3]

Phagocytes, the scavengers of the immune system, are the first to arrive at the scene if an invader gains entry. When a phagocyte spots a foreign

■ **FIGURE 18–5**
Immune System Cells, Action, and Results

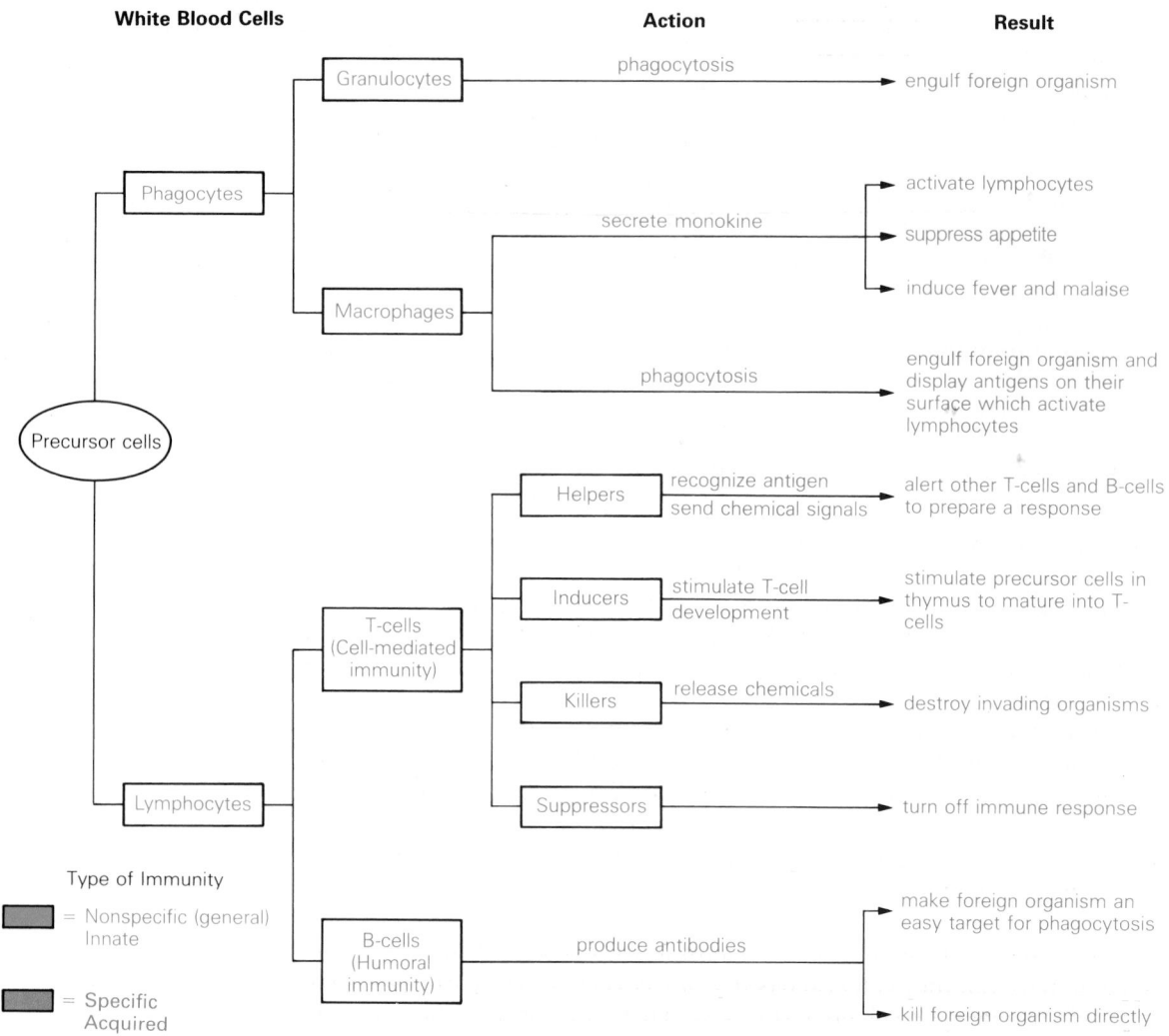

The monokine **interleukin-1** (in-ter-LOO-kin) activates lymphocytes and is also responsible for the fever-induced anorexia that commonly accompanies an infection. The monokine **cachectin** also induces anorexia. The monokine **gamma-interferon** (in-ter-FEAR-on) induces the fever and malaise that frequently occur during an infection.

substance, it engulfs (ingests) and digests that substance in a process called phagocytosis (see Figure 18–7). Phagocytes also secrete proteins called monokines, which activate the metabolic and immune responses to infection.

Among the phagocytes are some that perform the special task of facilitating recognition, the hallmark of immunity. Immunity depends on these phagocytes' being able to recognize foreign materials and destroy or otherwise neutralize them. As a phagocyte engulfs an invading organism, it detaches a portion of the invading cell (an antigen) and displays that portion on its own cell surface. The presence of the antigen on the cell's surface activates a special group of lymphocytes (described next) into action. This way, if the phagocytes cannot work fast enough to rid the body of the invader, lymphocytes will be ready to aid in the body's defense.

The lymphocytes are of two distinct types: T-cells and B-cells. (*T* stands for the thymus gland, which is where the T-cells are stored for a while; *B* stands

Nutrition and Illness **583**

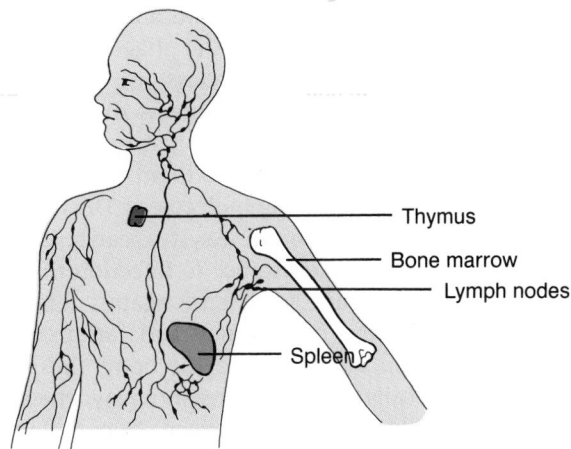

■ **FIGURE 18–6**
Sites of Immune System Cell Production
Immune system cell production takes place in the thymus, lymph nodes, spleen, bone marrow, and the areas lining the GI tract. (The patches of tissue in the GI tract are not shown.)

Thymus

Bone marrow

Lymph nodes

Spleen

for bursa, an organ in the chicken associated with the first identification of the B-cells.) The T-cells participate in cell-mediated immunity, so named because the T-cells travel directly to the invasion site and battle foreign organisms. They recognize the antigens displayed on the surfaces of their partner phagocyte cells and multiply in response. Then they release powerful chemicals to destroy all particles with this antigen on their surfaces; and as they begin to win the battle against infection, they release signals to slow down the immune response.

Unlike the phagocytes, which are capable of inactivating many different types of invaders, T-cells are highly specific. Each T-cell can attack only one type of antigen. This specificity is remarkable, for nature creates millions of antigens. After enough T-cells have been made to destroy an antigen, some lymphocytes retain the necessary information to serve as memory cells so that the immune system can produce the same type of T-cells again should the identical infection recur.

T-cells actively defend the body against fungi, viruses, parasites, and a few types of bacteria; they can also destroy cancer cells. T-cells participate in the rejection of newly transplanted tissues, which is why they must be inactivated by drugs when tissue transplantation is necessary.

The B-cells are important in a different type of immunity—humoral immunity, so named because it is the cells' secretions, not the cells themselves, that mount the defensive effort. B-cells respond to infection by rapidly dividing and then producing antibodies. Antibodies then travel to the site, where they

■ **FIGURE 18–7**
Phagocytosis
During phagocytosis, a foreign substance is engulfed by a white blood cell and eventually surrounded and digested by the cell.

stick to the surfaces of the foreign particles and kill or otherwise inactivate them, making the foreign particles easy for the phagocytes to ingest.

The antibodies are members of a class of proteins known as immunoglobulins—literally, large globular proteins that produce immunity. Antibodies react selectively to a specific foreign organism just as T-cells do, and the B-cells retain a memory of how to make them. (Figure 6–9 on p. 148 illustrates how antibodies attack invading molecules.) The next time the same foreign organism is encountered, the immune system can respond with greater speed. B-cells play a bigger role in resistance to infection than do T-cells.

In summary, the body's first line of defense against foreign materials is provided by the skin, the mucous membranes, and various body secretions. Should a microorganism gain entrance into the body, the immune system recognizes it as foreign and calls the phagocytes into play. Phagocytes produce chemicals that activate T-cells, and display antigens from the unwelcome cells on their surfaces so that the invader can be recognized and destroyed by T-cells. At the same time, the B-cells secrete specific antibodies that can directly kill invading organisms and also make them easier targets for attack by phagocytes. These changes in the immune system make it capable of responding quickly and forcefully to future exposures. Figure 18–8 summarizes the functions of the immune system cells.

The Role of Nutrition

To function at its best, the immune system must have nutrients available. For this reason, people who suffer from malnutrition develop more infections than well-nourished people. In Third World countries, infection leads to mortality and morbidity in children with PEM. In industrialized nations, malnutrition and infections present serious problems in people who have severe medical problems, undergo complicated surgeries, suffer major trauma, or have advanced cancer. Table 18–3 shows how general malnutrition affects immune system components.

Nutrient imbalances impair a variety of immune system functions and components, including the skin and exterior barriers, as well as the activities of the cells of the immune system. Table 18–4 on p. 586 shows how specific

■ **TABLE 18–3**
Effects of General Malnutrition on Immune System Components

Immune System Component	Effects of Malnutrition
Skin	Thinned, with less connective tissue.
GI tract	Likelihood of bacterial translocation compounded when intestines are injured.
Mucous membranes	Microvilli flattened; antibody secretions reduced.
Lymph tissues	Thymus gland, lymph nodes, and spleen reduced in size; T-cell areas depleted of lymphocytes.
Phagocytosis	Kill time delayed.
Cell-mediated immunity	Circulating T-cells reduced.
Humoral immunity	Circulating immunoglobulin levels normal; antibody response may be impaired.

■ **FIGURE 18-8**
Functions of Cells of the Immune System

Phagocytes	Lymphocytes	
	T-cells (cell-mediated immunity)	B-cells (humoral immunity)
Participate in phagocytosis.	Recognize antigens.	Produce antibodies.
Activate lymphocytes.	Stimulate other cells to respond.	Kill invaders or make them easy targets for phagocytosis.
Induce fever.	Release killer chemicals.	
Display antigens.	Suppress immune response.	
Suppress appetite.		

The immune system has several lines of defense.

nutrient deficiencies affect immune system functions. Cell-mediated immunity, a function of the T-cells, appears to be markedly depressed by malnutrition. People with severe malnutrition consistently have low levels of circulating lymphocytes and reduced size of the thymus, spleen, lymph nodes, and lymph-associated areas of the intestinal tract. The areas of the lymph tissues that house the T-cells are depleted of lymphocytes. Malnutrition seems to affect T-cell function more than B-cell function.

Because malnutrition impairs T-cell function, laboratory tests can help to identify people with malnutrition. Useful in nutrition assessment are *antigen skin testing* and the *total lymphocyte count*. Chapter 19 describes these tests.

■ TABLE 18–4
Effects of Selected Nutrient Deficiencies on the Immune System

Nutrient Deficiency	Effects
Protein-energy (PEM)[a]	Suppressed T-cell function, cell-mediated immunity, and phagocyte function.
Protein[a]	Suppressed T-cell function, cell-mediated immunity, and phagocyte function.
Lipid	Suppressed T-cell and B-cell functions.
Vitamin A	Suppressed T-cell and B-cell functions and cell-mediated immunity.
Vitamin B$_6$	Suppressed T-cell and B-cell functions, cell-mediated immunity, and phagocyte function.
Folate and vitamin B$_{12}$	Suppressed T-cell function and cell-mediated immunity.
Pantothenic acid	Suppressed T-cell function and cell-mediated immunity.
Vitamin C	Suppressed cell-mediated immunity.
Vitamin E	Suppressed B-cell function and cell-mediated immunity.
Iron	Suppressed T-cell function and cell-mediated immunity.
Zinc	Suppressed T-cell function and cell-mediated immunity.

Note: This table compiles data from both animal and human studies.

[a]You will notice that PEM and protein deficiency have the same effects on the immune system. However, in PEM, the most noticeable effect is suppressed T-cell function, whereas in protein deficiency alone, the most noticeable effect is suppressed phagocyte function.

translocation: the passage of microorganisms from the interior of the intestines to the inside of the body. Translocation of bacteria can occur from direct injury to the intestines, or from indirect injuries such as reduced blood flow to the intestines, burn injuries, or certain drugs.

nucleotides: nitrogen-containing components of RNA and DNA. They can be synthesized in the body and therefore are not essential in the diets of healthy individuals. However, in severely stressed individuals, a dietary source may be helpful.

immunonutrition: nutrition support directed at maintaining or enhancing the function of the immune system.

Although malnutrition clearly diminishes immune function, it is less clear how nutrition therapy can help to restore it. When given nutrition therapy, severely stressed people show signs of weight gain and positive nitrogen balance, but benefits to the immune system are inconsistent.[4] Delivering nutrients into the GI tract appears to help the intestinal cells maintain a barrier, preventing bacteria from entering the body. Feeding the person by vein fails to confer this benefit. The translocation of bacteria into the body may trigger hypermetabolism and infection, which can ultimately lead to multiple organ failure.[5] The need for research to determine the most appropriate mixture of nutrients to restore immune function is indicated. Some preliminary studies point to arginine (a nonessential amino acid), dietary nucleotides, and omega-3 fatty acids as holding some promise in stimulating immune function.[6] Accordingly, a product containing arginine, nucleotides, and a balance of lipids, in addition to the other essential nutrients, is currently being marketed for maintaining immune function in severely stressed people. Whether this immunonutrition formula will be successful, though, remains to be seen.

The body's natural defenses against insults to its internal environment are vulnerable to poor nutrition. Thus, poor nutrition impairs the individual's ability to mount both a stress response and an immune response when confronted with illness, trauma, and infection. In addition, nutrition affects the way the body responds to man-made weapons against disease, namely drugs.

Nutrition and Drug Therapy

Most people think of drugs as medicines that help them recover from illnesses, or as illegal substances that lead to addiction. Actually, both uses of the term *drug* are correct, because any substance taken into a living organism that modifies one or more of its functions is, technically, a drug. All drugs affect users physiologically, and their uses involve side effects and risks. This discussion focuses on medical drugs, both nonprescription, or over-the-counter (OTC), drugs and prescription drugs.[7] (Highlight 7 described the relationships between nutrition and the drug alcohol; Chapter 15 examined the influence of illicit drugs and tobacco on nutrition.)

When people use drugs, they set in motion a series of actions within the body—some desirable, others not. To help explain the far-reaching chemical effects of nutrient-drug interactions on body systems, this discussion will begin with a look at a class of drugs called monoamine oxidase (MAO) inhibitors.

Physicians sometimes prescribe MAO inhibitors to treat people with some forms of severe depression. MAO inhibitors block the action of the enzyme monoamine oxidase. Normally, monoamine oxidase converts tyramine, a substance found in some foods (see Table 18–5), into an inactive form. When people take MAO inhibitors, tyramine remains active and stimulates the

■ TABLE 18–5
Foods Restricted in Tyramine-Controlled Diet

Beverages	Chianti, sherry, sauterne, champagne, imported beer, nonalcoholic beer, ale.[a]
Cheeses	Aged cheeses, American, Camembert, cheddar, gouda, gruyere, mozzarella, parmesan, provolone, romano, roquefort, Stilton;[b] cheese-filled breads, crackers, and desserts.
Meats	Liver; dried, salted, smoked, or pickled fish; meat processed with tenderizers; sausage; pepperoni; dried meats; meat extracts.
Vegetables	Fava beans; Italian broad beans; sauerkraut; fermented pickles and olives.
Other	Brewer's yeast; monosodium glutamate; all aged and fermented products; caffeine and chocolate in large amounts.

Note: The tyramine contents of foods vary from product to product according to the methods used to prepare, process, and store food. The amount of tyramine a person consumes depends on the quantity of the food eaten. In some cases, as little as 1 oz of cheese can cause a severe hypertensive reaction in people taking monoamine oxidase inhibitors. The items listed in this table contain significant enough quantities of tyramine that they are not allowed. In general, the following foods contain small enough quantities of tyramine that they can be consumed in small quantities: ripe avocado, banana, yogurt, sour cream, acidophilus milk, buttermilk, raspberries, and peanuts.

[a]Most wine and domestic beer can be consumed in small quantities.
[b]Unfermented cheeses, such as ricotta, cottage cheese, and cream cheese are allowed.

Foods and beverages that may interfere with the effectiveness of nicotine gum:
- Apple juice.
- Beer.
- Coffee.
- Colas.
- Grape juice.
- Ketchup.
- Lemon-lime soda.
- Mustard.
- Orange juice.
- Pineapple juice.
- Soy sauce.
- Tomato juice.

prostaglandins: powerful, hormonelike substances; defined on p. 123.

release of norepinephrine. This action can lead to severe hypertension and headaches. If blood pressure rises high enough, it can be fatal. For this reason, people taking MAO inhibitors should restrict their intakes of foods rich in tyramine.

Nicotine gum provides another example of how specific food items alter a drug's intended action. Physicians prescribe nicotine gum to help people quit smoking cigarettes. Recently, researchers discovered that acidic foods and beverages limit the effectiveness of nicotine gum. The acidity from these foods and beverages changes the chemical balance in the mouth, thus preventing the nicotine from being absorbed through the lining of the mouth into the blood.[8] The blocking action of acidic foods may help to explain why nicotine gum is only successful in about one-fourth of the people who use it to quit smoking. For maximum effectiveness, people should refrain from ingesting foods and beverages during or immediately after chewing nicotine gum. Other side effects of this food-drug interaction—nausea and hiccups—develop when the unabsorbed nicotine arrives in the stomach. In the end, then, the combination of acidic foods and nicotine gum both interferes with the drug's effectiveness and creates uncomfortable side effects.

Nutrient interactions and risks are not unique to prescription drugs. Consider the action of a drug that is familiar to everyone: aspirin. Consumers around the world reach for 90 billion aspirin tablets a year, usually to relieve headaches, pain, and fever.[9] One action of aspirin is to retard the production of certain prostaglandins. Some prostaglandins help to produce fevers, some sensitize pain receptors, some cause contractions of the uterus, some stimulate digestive tract motility, some control nerve impulses, some regulate blood pressure, some promote blood clotting, and some cause inflammation. When aspirin interferes with these body responses, it reduces fever and inflammation, relieves pain, and opposes blood clotting, among other things.

You cannot use aspirin for one specific purpose without incurring all the other effects. A person who is prone to strokes and heart attacks might take aspirin to prevent blood clotting, but aspirin also slows blood clotting in people who take it only for pain. For them, the anticlotting effect may be dangerous, since it can cause abnormal bleeding. A single two-tablet dose doubles the bleeding time of wounds, an effect that lasts from four to seven hours. For this reason, clients must refrain from taking aspirin before surgery.

These examples illustrate that all drugs have side effects—some of which may be neutral, and some of which may be harmful. Among the side effects are the ways drugs influence the body's handling of nutrients. Using aspirin as an example again, aspirin competes with the B vitamin folate for its protein carrier, thus hindering the body's use of the vitamin. Aspirin may also cause iron-deficiency anemia by inducing bleeding in the GI tract.

Hundreds of medical drugs interact with nutrients, creating the possibility of imbalances whenever a person takes them. Drugs can profoundly affect nutrition status, and, conversely, nutrients can profoundly affect the body's responses to drugs. Drug-nutrient interactions do not always pose significant problems, however. One recent study found clinically significant drug-nutrient interactions in only 2 of 493 cases that were reviewed.[10] The researchers attributed the low incidence of interactions to the hospital's established drug-nutrient interaction policy. This policy guided health care professionals in preventing, recognizing, and treating the most common and clinically significant interactions.

Adverse drug-nutrient interactions occur more commonly if drugs are taken over long periods, if several drugs are taken simultaneously, or if poor nutrition status is present or impending. Understandably, elderly people and people with serious illnesses that raise nutrient needs are most at risk, for they are most likely to be in poor nutrition status, to suffer chronic disorders, to use many drugs, and to take them over long periods.

Nutrients and drugs may interact in many ways:

- Drugs can alter food intake, and the absorption, metabolism, and excretion of nutrients.
- Foods and nutrients can alter the absorption, metabolism, and excretion of drugs.

Table 18–6 summarizes the mechanisms by which these interactions occur and provides specific examples. The number of drug-nutrient actions that have been identified is mind-boggling, and it continues to grow. It would be difficult, if not impossible, to remember and apply all of this information in a

---

TABLE 18–6
Mechanisms and Examples of Food-Drug Interactions

Drugs Can Alter Food Intake by:

- Altering the appetite (amphetamines suppress the appetite).
- Interfering with taste or smell (methotrexate changes taste sensations).
- Inducing nausea or vomiting (digitalis does both).
- Changing the oral environment (phenobarbital causes dry mouth).
- Irritating the GI tract (cyclophosphamide induces mucosal ulcers).
- Causing sores or inflammation of the mouth (methotrexate can cause painful mouth ulcers to form).

Drugs Can Alter Nutrient Absorption by:	Foods Can Alter Drug Absorption by:
- Changing the acidity of the digestive tract (antacids can interfere with iron absorption). - Altering digestive juices (cimetidine can improve fat absorption). - Altering motility of the digestive tract (laxatives speed motility, causing the malabsorption of many nutrients). - Inactivating enzyme systems (neomycin may reduce lipase activity). - Damaging mucosal cells (chemotherapy can damage mucosal cells). - Binding to nutrients (antacids bind phosphorus).	- Changing the acidity of the digestive tract (candy can change the acidity, thus dissolving slow-acting asthma medication too quickly). - Stimulating secretion of digestive juices (griseofulvin is absorbed better when taken with foods that stimulate the release of digestive enzymes). - Altering motility of the digestive tract (aspirin is absorbed more slowly when taken with food). - Binding to drugs (tetracycline binds to calcium in dairy foods, limiting drug absorption). - Competing for absorption sites in the intestines (dietary amino acids interfere with levodopa absorption this way).

Drugs Can Alter Nutrient Metabolism by:	Foods Can Alter Drug Metabolism by:
- Acting as structural analogs (as anticoagulants and vitamin K do). - Interfering with metabolic enzyme systems (phenobarbital competes for folate coenzymes).	- Interfering with a drug's action (phenobarbital action is limited by large amounts of folate in the diet). - Contributing pharmacologically active substances (tyramine from cheese and monoamine oxidase inhibitors).

Drugs Can Alter Nutrient Excretion by:	Foods Can Alter Drug Excretion by:
- Altering reabsorption in the kidneys (some diuretics increase the excretion of sodium and potassium). - Displacing nutrients from their plasma protein carriers (aspirin displaces folate).	- Changing the acidity of the urine (vitamin C can alter urinary pH and limit the excretion of aspirin).

clinical setting. Instead, health care professionals would serve their clients well to:

- Be aware of groups of people who are at high risk for developing drug-related nutrient deficiencies.
- Keep in mind that drug-nutrient interactions can and do occur.
- Be familiar with the nutrient interactions of drugs commonly used to treat the disorders of their clients.
- Be prepared to look up the nutrition effects of drugs their clients are taking.

For example, nurses working with people who have heart disease will want to become familiar with the drug-nutrient interactions that can occur with medications used to treat heart disease. Better yet, they might keep a reference handy, such as Table E–1 in Appendix E, to check the possibility of drug-nutrient interactions. Chapters 23 through 30 list drugs commonly used to treat the specific disorders discussed in each chapter along with their possible nutrient interactions.

People may mistakenly believe that OTC drugs are harmless, but they can be dangerous if they mask serious problems by covering up the symptoms. For example, a person who repeatedly takes antacids for stomach discomfort may be ignoring the signs of an ulcer. And hidden ingredients in some OTC drugs can be undesirable—such as the significant amounts of sodium or calcium found in some antacids that aggravate certain medical conditions. The availability of OTC drugs allows people to treat themselves for minor ailments, but they should keep aware of the potential dangers and seek professional care if symptoms persist.

The Relationships between Nutrition and Illness

Figure 18–9 summarizes and illustrates some of the relationships between nutrition and illness. Nutrient deficiencies or imbalances can predispose an individual to illness or interfere with recovery from illness. A malnourished person easily falls victim to an illness, as the earlier section on PEM described.

On the other hand, an illness can lead a well-nourished person to malnutrition. The extent of damage a particular illness inflicts on nutrition status depends on the type, the severity, and the duration of the illness. Disorders that markedly raise a person's metabolic rate over long periods raise nutrient requirements and, thereby, the risk of deficiencies. A person who is unable to eat or to retain nutrients due to severe vomiting, diarrhea, or malabsorption is also at high risk. An illness can:

- Alter food intake by causing a loss of appetite or by interfering with a person's ability to chew and/or swallow food.
- Alter the body's digestion of food or absorption of nutrients.
- Alter the body's metabolism of nutrients.
- Alter the body's excretion of nutrients.

Any or all of these effects can occur during illness. In addition, secondary effects of an illness, including immobility, emotional stress, diagnostic tests, medical procedures, and drug therapy can all further impair nutrition status.

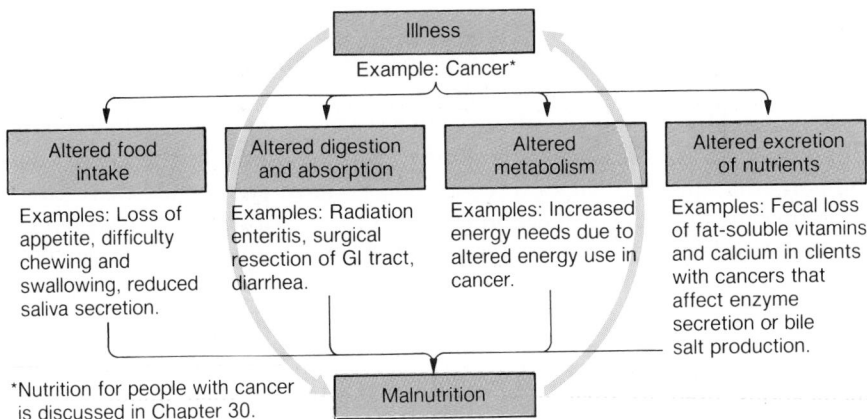

■ **FIGURE 18–9**
Interrelationships between Illness and Malnutrition
Illness, and the treatment of an illness, can contribute to malnutrition. Malnutrition can enhance the chance of becoming ill. Thus a vicious cycle is set in motion.

Oftentimes when an ill person is weak or for other reasons is confined to bed, the resultant immobilization can affect nutrition status. First, the body loses nitrogen and calcium. Bones lose calcium when the weight-bearing and muscle tension produced by normal activity do not occur. Then, in prolonged immobilization, blood and urine levels of calcium may rise, causing calcium stones to form in the bladder and kidney. Because physical activity is the best treatment, the person should be encouraged to be active as soon as possible. Moderate exercise during a hospital stay appears to maintain the function of the vital organ systems necessary to recover from illness.[11] However, it should be noted that people who are extremely ill or suffering from severe stress may be unable to tolerate exercise.

When a person remains confined to bed for a long time, bedsores may develop. Bedsores occur when the weight of the body exerts constant pressure on the skin, thus reducing blood flow to the area. Eventually, the skin breaks down and dies. The tissues and muscles under the skin, and even the bones, may also begin to break down. In addition to inadequate oxygen to the area, several nutrition risk factors have been associated with bedsores, including negative nitrogen balance, anemia, vitamin and mineral deficiencies, underweight, and overweight. Those who are severely underweight risk developing bedsores because there is too little fat to pad the area between the skin and the bone. Those who are overweight have adequate or excessive padding between the bone and the skin, but the pressure of excess weight on bony areas makes them more susceptible to bedsores.[12]

The best treatment for bedsores is to prevent their development by regularly turning and repositioning the bedridden person to alleviate pressure. In addition, special care should be taken to ensure that people with bedsores or those at risk for developing them receive diets that fully meet their nutrient needs.

In addition to the physical stresses of illness and immobilization, your clients may be responding to the psychological stresses of fear and anxiety. They may be faced with life-threatening illnesses. They may be unfamiliar with their surroundings, the people who are caring for them, and the procedures they are being asked to follow. These feelings stimulate stress hormone activity and suppress GI activity. Consequently, your clients may lose their appetites. The best nutrition care you can offer at such times is to alleviate their fears and anxieties. Of course, this may be easier said than

bedsores: the breakdown of skin and underlying tissues caused by constant pressure on and lack of oxygen to that area of the skin. Bedsores are often called **pressure sores** or **decubitus** (dee-CUE-beh-tus) **ulcers.**
de = down
cumbere = to lie

done, but friendly words of assurance and explanations of procedures go a long way. By relieving clients' emotional stresses, you can improve their nutrient intakes and hasten their physical recoveries.

Nutrition also can aid an individual in recovery from disorders that require physical or occupational therapy. Proper nutrition supplies the energy and supports the muscular strength required to perform therapeutic exercises.

Diagnostic tests and medical procedures may require that a person not eat in order to obtain accurate test results. Thus, during the very time when an individual's nutrient needs increase due to illness, food intake is restricted. Little can be done to prevent this situation, except to ensure that intake is not restricted any longer than is absolutely necessary. Providing a nutrient-rich diet when the person is eating becomes imperative. Feeding the person by vein (see Chapter 22) is an alternative in some cases.

Before leaving this chapter on nutrition and illness, it is appropriate to include a brief discussion on the role of diet in disease prevention. Prevention of diseases deserves emphasis for your clients, for yourself, and for all others interested in maintaining a healthy life. While caring for your clients, you will want to motivate them, as well as yourself, to develop habits that will postpone or deter the illnesses that have brought them in for medical care.

■ *Diet and Disease Prevention*

As an earlier section of this chapter pointed out, nutrition supports the immune system. If your immune system fails, you suddenly become vulnerable to every disease-causing agent that comes your way; infectious disease invariably follows. Several decades ago, infectious diseases such as tuberculosis, smallpox, and polio were widespread and much feared. Children's lives were often snuffed out by these diseases, and the average life expectancy was low. Today, the infectious diseases are less threatening, thanks to science's discoveries of the microbial agents that cause them and of the means to control them. Our water supply is treated to prevent the spread of infection, vaccinations protect us individually, and consequently most children live well into their later years. Only one infectious disease, acquired immune deficiency syndrome (AIDS), threatens large numbers of people, largely because it escapes the public health measures that are so effective against other infectious diseases. (Chapter 30 describes AIDS and its connections with nutrition.)

Our Nation's Health Status

Thanks to control of infectious diseases, the average life expectancy today is longer than ever before, and most of the diseases people now fear are of a different nature. Table 18−7 shows today's top ten killer diseases, as identified by the 1988 *Surgeon General's Report on Nutrition and Health*. Seven of them are the degenerative diseases of adulthood: diseases of the heart and blood vessels, cancer, diabetes, lung diseases, and liver disease. (The other three are accidents and suicide, which threaten young lives especially, and pneumonia/

■ TABLE 18–7
The Ten Leading Causes of Illness and Death, United States, 1987

Rank	Cause of Death	Number	Percentage of Total Deaths
1[a]	Heart diseases	759,400	35.7
	(Coronary heart disease)	(511,700)	(24.1)
	(Other heart disease)	(247,700)	(11.6)
2[a]	Cancers	476,700	22.4
3[a]	Strokes	148,700	7.0
4[b]	Unintentional injuries	92,500	4.4
	(Motor vehicle)	(46,500)	(2.2)
	(All others)	(45,700)	(2.2)
5	Chronic obstructive lung disease	78,000	3.7
6	Pneumonia and influenza	68,600	3.2
7[a]	Diabetes mellitus	37,800	1.8
8[b]	Suicide	29,600	1.4
9[b]	Chronic liver disease and cirrhosis	26,000	1.2
10[a]	Atherosclerosis	23,100	1.1
	Total	2,125,100	100.0

[a]Causes of death in which diet plays a part.
[b]Causes of death in which excessive alcohol consumption plays a part.

Source: National Center for Health Statistics, *Monthly Vital Statistics Report*, vol. 37, no. 1, 25 April 1988, as cited in *The Surgeon General's Report on Nutrition and Health: Summary and Recommendations*. DHHS (PHS) publication no. 88-50211 (Washington, D.C.: Government Printing Office, 1988), Table 2, p. 4.

influenza, which strikes older people whose defenses against them are impaired.) Other degenerative diseases that don't make the top ten, but that significantly impair the quality of life for millions of adults, are adult bone loss (discussed in Chapters 10 and 15), dental disease (discussed in Highlight 10), and GI disorders (discussed in Chapters 3, 4, 24, and 25).

Of the ten leading causes of illness and death, five are associated directly with nutrition and three with excessive alcohol intake, which, of course, affects nutrition adversely (see footnotes to Table 18–7). Taken together, these eight conditions account for about three-fourths of the nation's total of about 2 million deaths each year. (Adult bone loss, dental disease, and GI diseases are also nutrition related, as explained elsewhere in this book.)

Nutrition plays three roles in relation to these degenerative diseases: poor nutrition can accelerate their development, healthful nutrition can help prevent or forestall them, and nutrition therapy can ease their impact if they do occur. Poor nutrition is preventable, and the surgeon general urges that the nation's people make whatever dietary changes they can in the effort to improve their health status and outlook.

People's Choices and Their Risks of Disease

In contrast to the infectious diseases, each of which has a distinct microbial cause, such as the tuberculosis bacterium or the polio virus, the degenerative diseases of adulthood tend to have clusters of suspected causes known as risk factors. Among them are environmental, behavioral, social, and genetic factors, and combinations of these interacting with one another. In many cases one disease or condition intensifies the risk of another.

risk factors: factors known to be related to (or correlated with) a disease but not proven to be causal.

One pivotal risk factor is obesity, which aggravates the risk of almost every other disease. To follow just one possible chain of causes and effects, obesity contributes to impaired glucose tolerance and diabetes, these problems contribute to hypertension (and obesity aggravates it), and hypertension worsens the risk of stroke, especially in people with diabetes. The urgency of successful weight control pervades this text, whatever disease may be under consideration.

People's behaviors, including food behaviors, are interwoven with all of these conditions. The choice to eat high-fat foods, for example, is a choice to increase the probability of becoming obese, and thereby of contracting any of several diseases: cancer, hypertension, diabetes, atherosclerosis, diverticulosis, or others. Figure 18–10 shows the interrelationships of some of the risk factors with today's major degenerative diseases, and it highlights the food-related behaviors among them.

The exact contribution diet makes to each disease is hard to estimate. Many experts agree that diet accounts for about a third of all cases of coronary heart disease, but they argue that it may cause any amount from one-tenth to nine-tenths of all cases of cancer. Evidence is indirect and cannot be quantified, but strongly implicates an important role for diet. Moreover, diet advocates reason that because diet is largely under people's own control, if a dietary change can't hurt and might help, why not make it?

To make such choices is doubtless more important for some people than for others, since some people are genetically predisposed to certain diseases. A way to begin deciding whether the diet recommendations presented in this text are important to you is to examine your family history to see which diseases are common to your forebears. In addition, on your next physical examination, note which test results are out of line. Table 18–8 on p. 596 presents a summary of the signs to watch for in both categories.

Table 18–8 lists areas where you can make the personal investment that will bring the greatest probable rewards. Accepting that you have certain unchangeable "givens," you can look to the things that can change, and choose the most influential among them. For example, a person with diabetes and heart disease in the immediate family is urgently advised to avoid becoming obese. For another example, a person with hypertension is urged to control weight, to exercise regularly, to eat a nutritious diet, and to abstain from smoking.

The 1988 *Surgeon General's Report* makes clear the points just mentioned. Its major concern is our high intake of foods rich in fat, which often crowd more beneficial foods out of the diet—foods rich in complex carbohydrates and fiber. These recommendations for the improvement of our nutrition closely parallel those of the *NRC Recommendations* presented in Chapter 2.

As the following chapters unfold details about each of today's major diseases, watch for the reasons why each of the surgeon general's recommendations is important. Look for the diseases that respond to diet, and for ways the responses are similar. Dietary excesses increase the likelihood of all of the major diseases of today, particularly excess food energy and fat intakes. Dietary deficiencies also increase the likelihood of all of them, particularly deficiencies in fiber, vitamin, and mineral intakes.

Not all diet recommendations apply equally to all of the diseases (salt has a special relationship with hypertension, for example), but fortunately for the consumer, the dietary recommendations to help prevent these diseases do not

■ FIGURE 18–10
**Diet/Lifestyle Risk Factors and
Degenerative Diseases**

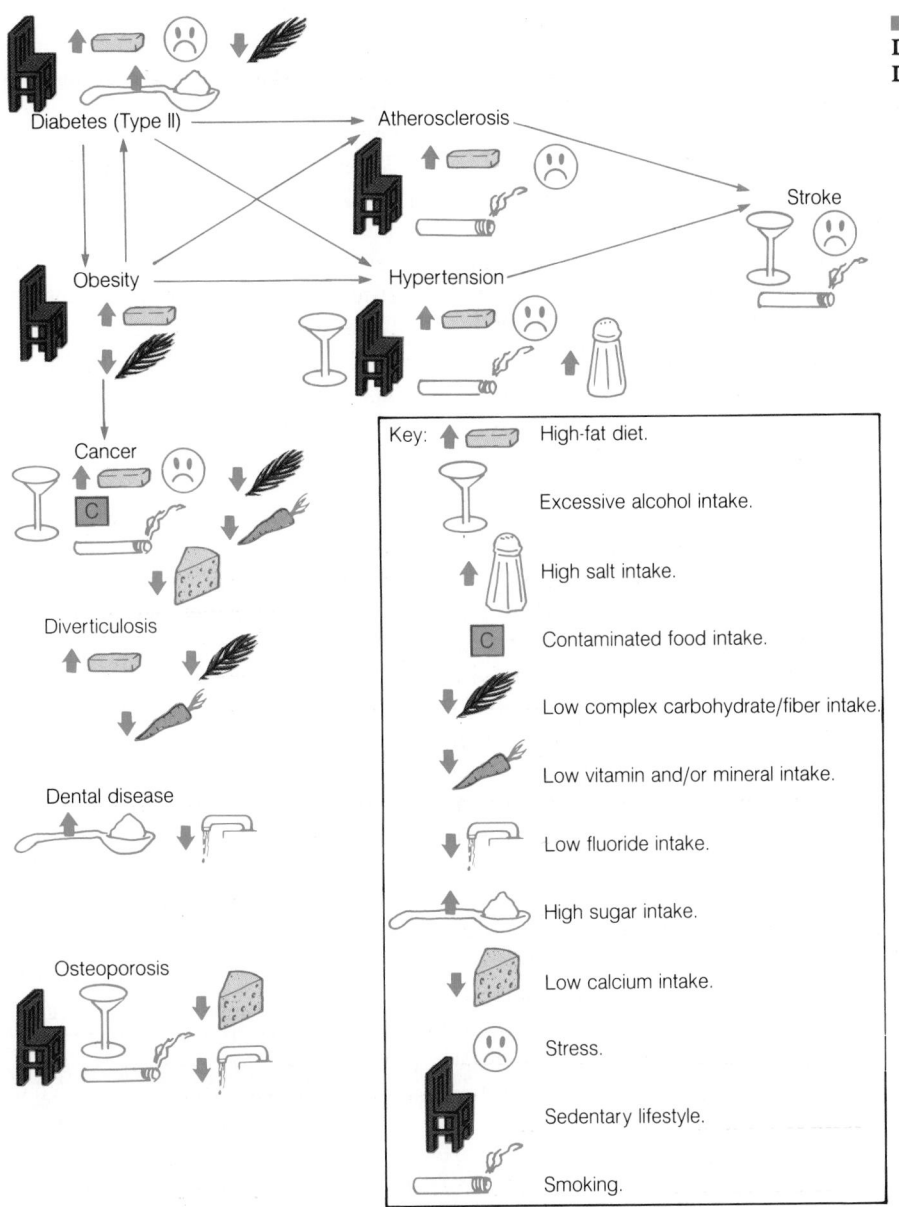

Key:

High-fat diet.

Excessive alcohol intake.

High salt intake.

Contaminated food intake.

Low complex carbohydrate/fiber intake.

Low vitamin and/or mineral intake.

Low fluoride intake.

High sugar intake.

Low calcium intake.

Stress.

Sedentary lifestyle.

Smoking.

■ **TABLE 18–8**
Priorities for People with Personal, Genetic, and Lifestyle Risk Factors

Lifestyle Changes Recommended for All People	Especially Important If Your Family History Indicates:	And/Or If Your Medical History Indicates:
Fats and cholesterol: reduce consumption of fat (especially saturated fat) and cholesterol.	Diabetes, obesity, cancer, or any form of cardiovascular disease (atherosclerosis, hypertension, heart attacks, strokes)	Glucose intolerance, high blood cholesterol or triglycerides, high blood pressure
Energy and weight control: achieve and maintain a desirable body weight.	Diabetes, obesity, cancer, or any form of cardiovascular disease (atherosclerosis, hypertension, heart attacks, strokes)	
Carbohydrate: increase consumption of complex carbohydrates and fiber.	Diabetes, obesity, cancer, or any form of cardiovascular disease (atherosclerosis, hypertension, heart attacks, strokes)	Glucose intolerance, high blood cholesterol or triglycerides, high blood pressure
Salt/sodium: reduce intake of salt/sodium.	Hypertension, diabetes, or any form of cardiovascular disease (atherosclerosis, hypertension, heart attacks, strokes)	High blood pressure
Alcohol: to reduce the risk for chronic disease, take alcohol only in moderation (no more than two drinks a day), if at all.	Liver disease (cirrhosis), cancer, any form of cardiovascular disease (atherosclerosis, hypertension, heart attacks, strokes), or osteoporosis	Glucose intolerance, high blood cholesterol or triglycerides, high blood pressure, any sign of adult bone loss

Other Issues for Some People	Especially Important If Your Family History Indicates:	Recommended Diet Especially for:
Fluoride: community water systems should contain fluoride at optimal levels for prevention of tooth decay; if such water is not available, use other appropriate sources of fluoride.	Osteoporosis or dental problems	Girls and women
Sugars: limit the consumption and frequency of use of foods high in sugars.	Susceptibility to dental caries	Children
Calcium: increase consumption of foods high in calcium, including low-fat dairy products.	Osteoporosis or cancer	Girls and women
Iron: be sure to consume good sources of iron.	Iron-deficiency anemia	Low-income families, children, teens, girls, and women

Source: *The Surgeon General's Report on Nutrition and Health: Summary and Recommendations*, DHHS (PHS) publication no. 88-50211 (Washington, D.C.: Government Printing Office, 1988), Table 1, p. 3.

contradict one another. The 1988 *Surgeon General's Report* remarked that for the two out of three Americans who do not smoke or drink excessively, "Your choice of diet can influence your long-term health prospects more than any other action you might take."[13] Indeed, healthy adults have a great opportunity to make use of the fruits of recent research on the prevention effects of a nutritious diet: the opportunity to preserve their health into their later years.

Attention to nutrition during times of wellness maintains a person's health. Attention to nutrition during times of illness, along with other medical treatments, supports a person's recovery. As you read the following chapters, keep in mind that each of your clients will be in a different state of health, with different nutrient needs and food preferences. The next chapter describes ways of assessing a person's nutrition status and using this information to determine nutrient needs.

Nutrition and Illness

One of the most interesting aspects of the study of nutrition is its application to you personally. The earlier chapters of this book included many self-study exercises in which you were invited to inspect your own diet for adequacy and energy balance; you may have performed these exercises or others (such as a computerized diet analysis) to evaluate your food habits and nutrition. This chapter now begins a series of self-studies on the subject of clinical nutrition.

Performing these exercises can benefit you in two ways. For one thing, many of the recommendations made for therapeutic diets are similar to those for preventive diets for a given condition. (The diet recommended for atherosclerosis, for example, is also considered ideal for preventing heart disease.) In these cases, learning how to design a therapeutic or preventive diet, and practicing following it for a day, which is what these exercises instruct you to do, can benefit you by influencing you to alter your own regular diet in a therapeutic or preventive direction.

For another thing, they say that "no one understands a problem like one who has been through it." Assuming this adage is at least partly true, the self-studies should help you to empathize with your clients' problems with their diets. Your practice in living with a therapeutic diet, if only for a day, may challenge you to find creative and pleasing solutions to such problems.

Begin by recording a few notes in a personal journal under the heading of "Self-Study 18." Review your own diet history or that of someone you know intimately in relation to the subject of this chapter—nutrition and illness. Answer these questions, but write freely in whatever style pleases you; this is personal, remember. Describe a time when you (or someone you know closely) were seriously ill. How did your illness affect your appetite and the way you ate? How long did this go on, and how did it affect your strength and ability to fight your way back to health? How do you suppose your nutrition status was affected during this time? Had the situation continued longer or been more stressful, what might have been the health effects? In short, relate personally to the subject of this chapter. If you are doing this exercise for class credit, ask your instructor for a page limit for this and succeeding assignments.

Study Questions

1. What is the stress response, and what is its purpose?
2. How does the stress response differ from the body's response to starvation?
3. Describe the effect of nutrition status on the body's ability to respond to stress.
4. How does the immune system defend the body against disease-causing organisms?
5. Describe the conditions that increase the risk of drug-induced nutrient deficiencies. Based on your answer, which groups of people would most likely be at risk?
6. In what ways can drugs and foods interact? Give some examples of how drugs can interfere with food intake and of how nutrients can interfere with drug action.
7. Discuss the possible dangers of OTC drugs.
8. What effects does immobilization have on nutrient balances, and how can these effects be minimized?
9. What is a bedsore? How can bedsores be prevented and treated?
10. Describe the relationships between illness and nutrition, including those relating to disease prevention.

Notes

1. Congressional Briefing on the Cost Effectiveness of Nutrition Support hosted by the American Dietetic Association, 23 January 1986. Report based on a study conducted by Arthur Anderson and Company and Ross Laboratories.
2. J. W. Alexander, Nutrition and translocation, *Journal of Parenteral and Enteral Nutrition* (supplement) 14 (1990): 170–174.
3. P. Jaret, Our immune system: The wars within, *National Geographic* 169 (1986): 702–734.
4. M. D. Lieberman and coauthors, Effects of nutrient substrates on immune function, *Nutrition* (supplement) 6 (1989): 88–91.
5. Alexander, 1990.
6. A. Barbul, Arginine and immune function, *Nutrition* (supplement) 6 (1989): 53–58; F. B. Rudolph and coauthors, Role of RNA as a dietary source of pyrimidines and purines in immune function, *Nutrition* (supplement) 6 (1989): 45–52; J. E. Kinsella and coauthors, Dietary polyunsaturated fatty acids and eicosanoids: Potential effects on the modulation of

inflammatory and immune cells: An overview, *Nutrition* 6 (1989): 24–44.

7. Parts of this discussion are adapted with permission from F. S. Sizer and E. N. Whitney, *Life Choices: Health Concepts and Strategies* (St. Paul, Minn.: West, 1988), pp. 197–225.

8. J. E. Henningfield and coauthors, Drinking coffee and carbonated beverages blocks absorption of nicotine from nicotine polacrilex gum, *Journal of the American Medical Association* 264 (1990): 1560–1564.

9. C. Dolan, What soothes aches, makes flowers last, and grows hair? *The Wall Street Journal* February 19, 1988.

10. V. L. Franse, N. Stark, and T. Powers, Drug-nutrient interactions in a Veterans Administration medical center teaching hospital, *Nutrition in Clinical Practice* 3 (1988): 145–147.

11. J. A. Windsor and G. L. Hill, Weight loss with physiologic impairment: A basic indicator of surgical risk, *Annals of Surgery* 207 (1988): 290–296; J. D. Albert and coauthors, Preservation of functional aerobic capacity with daily submaximal exercise during intravenous feeding in hospitalized normal man, *World Journal of Surgery* 12 (1988): 123–131.

12. E. D. Durr, Nutritional intervention for patients with pressure sores, *Nutritional Support Services* 6 (1986): 28–29.

13. *The Surgeon General's Report on Nutrition and Health: Summary and Recommendations*, DHHS (PHS) publication no. 88-50211 (Washington, D.C.: Government Printing Office, 1988).

Health Messages on Food Labels

Scientists and consumers alike know more about the links between diet and disease than ever in the past. With this knowledge come demands for still more information on disease prevention. Surveys show that many consumers rely on food labels to tell them about substances they want to avoid for health reasons and for information about nutrition.[1] The same surveys also show that many people find food labels confusing and misleading.

Highlight 16 described the information food labels must display, paying particular attention to the nutrition information that people can obtain from labels. Nutrition *information* does just as the term implies—informs people about the nutrients in a food. Nutrition *claims* make statements about specific nutrients (for example, "a significant source of vitamin A") or statements designed to appeal to people who want to include more of, or limit, specific nutrients in their diets. For example, a label that states "sodium-free" is making a nutrition claim.

Government regulating agencies continually require improvements in the ways labels convey nutrition information and nutrition claims. No doubt, nutrition labeling has come a long way toward providing people with information they can use to promote their health; but in some ways, it still falls short. People have to first *know* that high-fat diets may aggravate heart disease, or that high-fiber diets may help prevent cancer, in order to choose foods appropriately for a healthy diet. This is where health messages on food labels, the topic of this highlight, enter the picture.

The Food and Drug Administration (FDA) recognizes the public's right to accurate health and nutrition

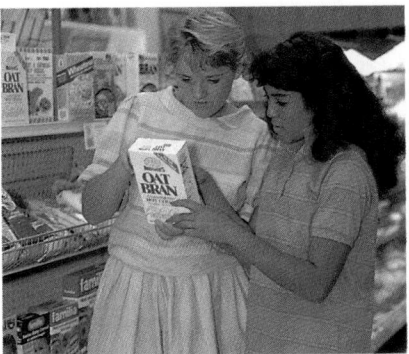

Consumers read food labels to learn more about the possible connections between diet and health.

information and the potential that food label statements have to improve people's understanding of the health benefits that result from eating a sound diet. To that end, the FDA has proposed major changes in its food label policy, the most controversial of which involves health messages on food labels.

Past and Present Perspectives

Health messages make statements on reducing the risk, or forestalling the premature onset, of certain chronic serious diseases (coronary heart disease, high blood pressure, cancer, and osteoporosis) through changes in the diet.[2] Unlike nutrition labeling (intended to make consumers aware of the nutrients in a food), which FDA has encouraged for some time, health-related messages were, until 1987, strictly prohibited. The policy forbidding health messages on labels was instated at a time when consumer fraud was widespread and relationships between diet and disease were scientifically unproven.[3] Such a policy prevented potentially harmful claims from being made, but it also forbade the providing of useful

information. As research began to substantiate relationships between diet and disease prevention, the strict policy stance became impracticable.

As of 1987, the FDA began permitting some scientifically based health statements on labels, subject to approval.[4] Currently, the FDA permits labels to emphasize the importance of the total diet without undue emphasis on the role of diet in disease prevention. The label of a high-fiber cereal may state, for example, that "a high-fiber diet may reduce your risk of some kinds of cancer." The statement is true, and it is phrased in terms of total diet, not in terms of the particular cereal in the box.

This guideline is useful but not useful enough. It fails to guide consumers adequately in making sound food choices. A cereal bearing such a statement may indeed provide abundant fiber, but it may also provide large quantities of fat, and yet this information is not required to receive equal billing on the label.

As more and more consumers seek low-kcalorie, low-fat, low-cholesterol, low-sodium, high-fiber foods, food manufacturers who strive to produce the foods that consumers will buy, are clamoring for permission to tell people *why* their products promote health. Food companies' demands for more leeway regarding health messages on food labels often conflict with FDA's and the scientific community's concerns about deceptive and misleading statements. The goal of regulations surrounding health messages is to find a common ground amongst the controversy that will best serve consumers. To that end, the FDA has proposed a formal health message policy based on three factors:[5]

- The growing amount of scientific evidence showing that people can reduce their risk of diseases such as

---

Miniglossary

nutrition information: a list of amounts of specific nutrients in a food.
nutrition claims: statements about specific nutrients, or statements that appeal to people who want to include more of, or limit, specific nutrients in their diets.
health messages: statements on reducing the risk, or forestalling the premature onset, of certain chronic serious diseases through changes in the diet.

---

cancer and coronary heart disease by eating more or less of certain foods.

- People's interest in learning more about how to improve their diets to stay healthier.
- Food industry interest in marketing and promoting products for their potential health benefits.

The FDA has two concerns pivotal to the health-message policy change for food labels. First, the FDA wants to protect people's health by preventing manufacturers from presenting health messages in such a way that some people might forgo needed medical treatment based on information they read on food labels. Second, the FDA wants to encourage the use of responsible, helpful health messages without relinquishing the power to control misleading ones.[6]

Developing Criteria

To develop criteria for health-related statements on food labels, the FDA considered these primary concerns, and the comments and suggestions from individuals, consumer groups, health and medical professional groups, and food industry representatives. The current health-message proposal cites the following specific criteria:

- The label statement must be truthful and not misleading, must not imply that the food should be used as a treatment, and must not overemphasize or distort the role of

food in promoting good health. (In determining whether food label statements mislead consumers, the proposal instructs the FDA to examine both what is said and what is left unsaid.)

- The label statement must limit its description to the value that a dietary component (or reduced consumption of the component), as part of a total dietary pattern, may have in either reducing the risk, or forestalling the premature onset, of a disease condition. Such a statement must be based on available scientific evidence from well-designed studies.
- The label statement must be consistent with generally recognized medical and nutrition principles.
- The label statement must be based on, and consistent with, the conclusions set forth in an applicable scientific summary and consumer health-message summary accepted by the FDA. (The FDA proposes to establish scientific summaries and consumer health-message summaries to ensure scientific and practical support for health messages, and to make scientific support available in comprehensive form to consumers. The health message carried on a label would be described in detail in these documents.)
- The label statement must include a reference to the appropriate consumer health-message summary. (This reference will direct interested consumers to more complete and balanced information about the food

component-disease interaction referred to on the label.)

- A health message on a food label mandates that manufacturers meet full nutrition labeling requirements.[7]

In addition, the current proposal limits health messages to six specific areas identified in *The Surgeon General's Report on Nutrition and Health: Summary and Recommendations* and the National Research Council's *Diet and Health: Implications for Reducing Chronic Disease Risk*. The six topic areas include calcium and osteoporosis; dietary fiber and cancer; lipids and cardiovascular disease; lipids and cancer; sodium and hypertension; and dietary fiber and cardiovascular disease. By initially limiting health messages to these six areas, the FDA made its goal to develop responsible health messages a manageable task.

Finally, the FDA proposes to establish a Public Health Service (PHS) Committee. This committee would develop model label statements for manufacturers to use on their products. Under the current proposal, manufacturers would not be permitted to develop their own health-related statements, but would be required to use messages developed by the PHS committee. The model statements would be based on scientific summaries and consumer health-message summaries (mentioned earlier) submitted to the FDA and the PHS Committee for review. The purpose of the proposal (to develop scientific summaries, consumer health messages, and model label statements) is to regulate the content of health messages, thereby ensuring that the health message contains appropriate information regarding diet and disease interactions.

The criteria set forth in the current proposal represent the many concerns expressed by consumer groups, health and medical professionals, and food manufacturers. Despite the extensive criteria proposed so far, some issues still remain unresolved. For example, what standards will be used to establish substantiation of a health message? Even in areas where scientific evidence supports a relationship between specific dietary components and disease conditions, questions surround the validity of data.

Another unsettled issue concerns whether the FDA should require manufacturers who promote the health benefits of their products to identify the possible health risks as well. As a case in point, must canned soup labels that state "low in fat and cholesterol" also warn of their high salt content?

Clearly, many health-message issues remain to be settled. Some experts argue that health messages on food labels may mislead consumers and may encourage manufacturers to fortify foods solely for the sake of being able to make a health claim. Most experts, however, agree that food labels undoubtedly provide an important vehicle for health information, and that this information must be well-substantiated and related to current public health problems.[8]

The final version of the FDA's health-message proposal has yet to be issued as this text goes to press. In the meantime, nutrition information and health messages on food labels continue to confuse and mislead consumers. As one senator who is pushing for Congress to pass a bill requiring nutrition labeling on all packaged foods says, "What you don't know can hurt you."[9]

Health care professionals can help people learn to decide for themselves whether a label states the "whole truth and nothing but the truth." Food labels can mislead consumers in a number of ways, for example:

- The label statement may highlight benefits without mentioning risks.
- The label statement may reach conclusions that go beyond what scientific data actually demonstrate.
- The label may suggest that the product reduces the risk of developing a disease whereas the

evidence actually reveals that the total diet is involved in producing such an effect.
- The statement may be truthful, but its emphasis, or other aspect, may cause the consumer to perceive it inaccurately.[10]

Strategies for Choosing Nutritious Foods

Regardless of how confusing labels may be, the following guidelines can help shoppers find nutritious, healthy foods:

- Choose fresh produce, especially dark green and yellow-orange fruits and vegetables like spinach, broccoli, cantaloupes, apricots, and sweet potatoes. These foods supply vitamin A and C in abundance—nutrients that correlate with a low risk of cancer. Such foods also contain valuable minerals and fiber that benefit health.
- Choose from the variety of legumes (dried beans and peas such as pinto beans, split peas, lima beans, and black beans) available in grocery stores. Legumes make an economical, low-fat, nutrient- and fiber-rich food choice.
- Choose whole-grain breads and cereals over refined, processed varieties. Whole-grain products, such as brown rice or oatmeal, provide more fiber and less salt and sugar than flavored, processed rice or sweetened cereals.
- Choose low-fat or nonfat milk and cheese.

Consumers make some of their healthiest food choices without having to read labels.

- Choose fish and poultry rather than high-fat, marbled red meats when shopping in the meat department.

In short, the foods that consumers find around the outer edge of the supermarket aisles usually offer more nutrients than the ones along the center aisles. By filling the grocery cart with produce, low-fat dairy foods, whole-grain breads, fish, and legumes, consumers will find little room left for the less nutritious, highly processed, packaged foods.

Clearly, the health-message issue goes beyond the simple alternative of whether labels should or shouldn't deliver health messages. The question now being asked is how labels can best deliver such messages. Consumers are working earnestly to promote their health. They want nutrition and health information, and they read labels for guidance in making their food selections. They deserve all the help they can get, beginning with accurate and responsible health messages on labels. Health care professionals working to enhance life's quality can do their share by assisting consumers in reading labels wisely.

NOTES

1. *A Consumer's Guide to Food Labels,* HHS publication no. (FDA)88-2083 (Rockville, Md.: Department of Health and Human Services, 1988); Food label importance, *FDA Consumer,* May 1990, p. 3.

2. Food and Drug Administration, Food labeling; health messages and label statement; reproposed rule, *Federal Register* 55 (1990): 5176–5192.

3. D. A. Kessler, The federal regulation of food labeling: Promoting food to prevent disease, *New England Journal of Medicine* 321 (1989): 717–725.

4. T. P. Labuza, A perspective on health claims on food labeling, *Cereal Foods World* 32 (1987): 256–267.

5. Selling nutrition: Should food packages carry health messages? *FDA Consumer,* November 1987, pp. 22–25.

6. Food and Drug Administration, 1990.

7. Food and Drug Administration, 1990.

8. Nutrition on food labels (ADA timely statement), *Journal of the American Dietetic Association* 89 (1989): 266–268.

9. Senator Howard Metzenbaum, Congress wants to take up the label-reading habit, *Tallahassee Democrat,* July 30, 1989.

10. Food and Drug Administration, 1990.

19

Nutrition Assessment

Contents

To the nutrition assessor, blood cholesterol concentrations are an important clue to health status. They indicate high or low heart disease risk depending on which of cholesterol's carriers predominates—low- or high-density lipoproteins. To the photographer, however, cholesterol acetate crystals are simply one of nature's creations rendered into art.

Take a moment to imagine you are in a foreign country—a country where you do not understand the language. As you walk down the street, you see signs that describe and direct. But they are meaningless to you, for you have yet to learn how to read, speak, or think in this new language. Similarly, many health care providers travel through hospitals looking at signs of malnutrition without recognizing them. They look at a person's pale complexion and lack of appetite and see only a disease; they see a person's poor posture and lethargic attitude and attribute that to old age. They have yet to learn to think "nutrition." Malnutrition is easy to miss if you are not looking for it. Caring for people requires that you at least consider the *possibility* that ill health may be due not just to a disease but perhaps to nutrient deficiencies. To overlook nutrition is to provide less than adequate care. The signs of malnutrition are there if you know where to look and how to read them.

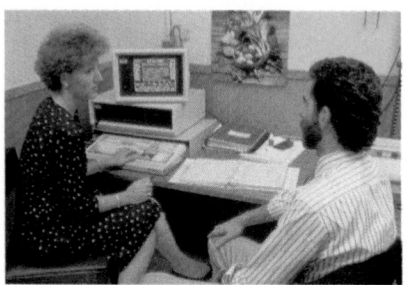

Successful nutrition intervention requires logical and systematic planning.

Appropriate nutrition assessment can detect the development of malnutrition. Health care professionals who are alert to the signs of malnutrition can then act to prevent, retard, or reverse its progress. To meet the challenge requires an organized process, and that is the topic of this chapter. An appropriately nourished individual is better equipped to fight illness and respond to therapy as quickly as possible, benefiting the individual and helping to minimize health care costs.

■ *The Nutrition Care Process*

In consideration of the unique needs of each individual, how can health care professionals effectively provide successful nutrition intervention? To do so requires a systematic and logical approach, such as the nutrition care process. To identify and solve nutrition problems, dietitians follow these five steps:

nutrition care process: an organized approach to nutrition intervention that consists of five steps (assessing, analyzing, planning, implementing, and evaluating).

- ■ Assess nutrition status.
- ■ Analyze assessment data to determine nutrient requirements.
- ■ Develop a plan of action for meeting nutrition needs, including client education.
- ■ Implement the nutrition care plan.
- ■ Evaluate the effectiveness of the nutrition care plan through ongoing assessment, and make appropriate changes.

This chapter is devoted to the first two of these steps: most of it to the assessment of nutrition status and a last short section on the estimation of nutrient needs.

While all members of the health care team share responsibility for developing and implementing nutrition care plans, the dietitian, physician, nurse, and client assume the primary roles. The dietetic technician, social worker, pharmacist, physical therapist, and occupational therapist also make valuable contributions (see Highlight 20). The greater the participation of team members, the more realistic and attainable the care plan will be. The emphasis of this chapter is on people in the hospital, but the same principles apply to people seen in outpatient clinics, community centers, nursing homes, private practice, or their own homes.

nutrition care plan: a strategy for translating nutrition assessment data into a plan for meeting the client's nutrient and nutrition education needs.

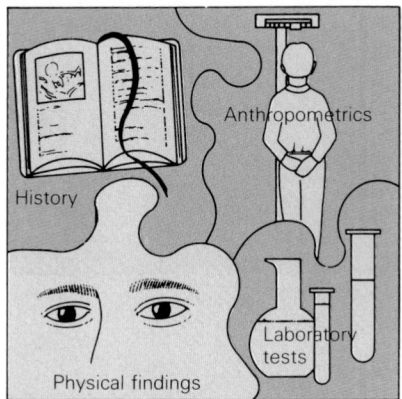

Taken as a whole, the information gathered during a nutrition assessment helps define the individual's nutrition status.

Nutrition Assessment

Nutrition assessment evaluates a person's health from a nutrition perspective. Dietitians and other health care professionals perform nutrition assessments to identify the individual's state of nutritional health. Nutrition assessment techniques apply to people who are healthy as well as to those who are ill. For the healthy person, a nutrition assessment identifies aspects of the diet that can be improved to achieve optimal health. For the ill person, a nutrition assessment alerts the health care team to nutrition factors that could hinder the response to medical treatment and recovery from illness.

Nutrition assessment evaluates many factors that influence or reflect nutrition status. The assessor (usually a skilled dietitian or other qualified health care professional) gathers information from many sources, including:

- Historical data.
- Anthropometric measurements.
- Biochemical analyses (laboratory tests).
- Physical examinations. *Appearance*

Each of these methods involves collecting data in a variety of ways, and interpreting each finding in relation to the others in order to create a total picture. The accurate gathering of this information and its careful interpretation provide the basis for a meaningful evaluation. The following sections describe each method in detail.

Historical Data

Clues about present nutrition status become evident with a review of a person's historical data (see Table 19–1). Even when data are subjective, they reveal important facts about a person. A thorough history identifies risk factors associated with poor nutrition status (see Table 19–2) and provides a sense of the whole person. Form 19–1 (on pp. 606–607) shows the kinds of questions

■ TABLE 19–1
Historical Data Used in Nutrition Assessments

Type of History	What It Identifies
Health history	Health-related factors that affect nutrition status
Socioeconomic history	Personal, financial, and environmental influences on food intake
Drug history	Medications that affect nutrition status
Diet history	Nutrient intake excesses or deficiencies
24-hour recall	
Usual intake	
Food diary	
Food frequency checklist	

■ **TABLE 19–2**
Risk Factors for Poor Nutrition Status

Health History
- Acquired immune deficiency syndrome (AIDS)
- Alcoholism
- Anorexia
- Cancer
- Chewing or swallowing difficulties (including poorly fitted dentures, dental caries, and missing teeth)
- Circulatory problems
- Constipation
- Crohn's disease
- Dementia
- Diabetes
- Diarrhea
- Diseases of the GI tract
- Drug addiction

- Fever
- Heart disease
- Hormonal imbalance
- Hyperlipidemia
- Hypertension
- Infection
- Kidney disease
- Liver disease
- Lung disease
- Mental retardation or deterioration
- Multiple pregnancies
- Nausea
- Neurologic disorders
- Overweight
- Pancreatic insufficiency

- Paralysis
- Physical disability
- Pregnancy
- Radiation therapy
- Recent major illness
- Recent major surgery
- Recent weight loss or gain
- Smoking of cigarettes
- Surgery of the GI tract
- Trauma
- Ulcerative colitis
- Ulcers
- Underweight
- Vomiting

Socioeconomic History
- Eating alone
- Inadequate food budget
- Inadequate food preparation facilities

- Inadequate food storage facilities
- Poor education

- Poor self-concept
- Transportation unavailable

Drug History
- Analgesics
- Antacids
- Antibiotics
- Anticancer agents
- Anticonvulsant agents
- Antidiarrheal agents

- Antidepressant agents
- Antihypertensive agents
- Antihyperlipemic agents
- Antiulcer agents
- Catabolic steroids
- Diuretics

- Immunosuppressants
- Laxatives
- Oral contraceptives
- Sulfonylurea agents
- Vitamin and other nutrient preparations

Diet History
- Anorexia nervosa
- Bulimia
- Excessive food intakes
- Frequently eating out

- Inadequate food intake
- Intravenous fluids (other than total parenteral nutrition) for ten or more days

- No intake for ten or more days
- Poor appetite
- Restricted or fad diets

asked to collect such information. As you can see, many aspects of a person's life influence nutrition status and provide clues to possible problems.

An adept history taker uses the interview not only to gather facts, but also to establish rapport. This section briefly reviews the major areas of nutrition concern in a person's history: health, socioeconomic, drug, and diet. Chapter 20 describes the communication skills used by an effective history taker.

Health History   *medical HX.*

The assessor can obtain health histories from records completed by the attending physician, nurse, or other health care provider. In addition, conversations with the client can uncover valuable health-related informa-

Traditionally, histories have been called *medical histories*. However, given that their contents describe a client's health status, and that current trends in the medical profession are emphasizing health promotion and disease prevention, the term *health histories* seems more appropriate.

■ **FORM 19–1**
Historical Data

Name _____   Date _____
Address _____   Date of last medical checkup _____
_____   Age _____ Sex _____
_____   Height _____ Weight _____
Phone _____   Usual weight _____
Reason for admission _____   Ideal weight _____
_____

Health History

1. Have you been told that you have (check any that apply):

   ____ Diabetes   ____ Heart disease   ____ Ulcers
   ____ GI disorders   ____ Lung disease   ____ Cancer
   ____ High blood pressure   ____ Kidney disease   ____ Other
   ____ Hardening of arteries   ____ Liver disease   _____

2. Do you have complaints about any of the following:

   ____ Lack of appetite   ____ Diarrhea   ____ Nausea
   ____ Difficulty chewing or swallowing ____ Indigestion   ____ Vomiting
   ____ Constipation   ____ Fever   ____ Other

3. For females:

   Are you pregnant? _____ How many months? _____
   How many pregnancies have you carried to term? _____
   When was your last child born? _____
   Are your menstrual periods normal? _____ If not, please explain: _____

Socioeconomic History

1. Last grade of school completed _____ Still in school? _____
2. Are you employed? _____ Occupation _____
3. Does someone else live with you? _____ Who? _____
4. Do you use tobacco in any way? _____ How much? _____
5. Where do you eat most of your meals? _____
6. Do you have a refrigerator? _____ Stove? _____
7. How often do you shop for food? _____

Drug History

1. Do you take medication, either prescribed by a doctor or over-the-counter?

Name of drug	Reason for taking	Dose	Frequency	Duration of intake
_____	_____	_____	_____	_____
_____	_____	_____	_____	_____
_____	_____	_____	_____	_____

2. Have you noticed any side effects from taking these medications? ____ If so, please explain: _____
3. Do you take vitamins or any kind of supplements? _____ Which ones? _____
   How often? _____ For what reason? _____

continued

■ FORM 19–1
Historical Data (continued)

Diet History

1. Have you recently lost or gained more than 10 lbs? _____ If yes, explain the surrounding circumstances (including associated illness, dietary changes, and time frame): _____
2. Do you eat at regular times each day? _____ How many times per day?_____
3. Do you usually eat snacks? _____ When?_____
4. What foods do you particularly like? _____ Dislike?_____
5. Are there foods you don't eat for other reasons? _____
6. Do you have difficulty eating? _____
7. How would you describe your feelings about food? _____
8. How do your eating habits change when you are emotionally upset? _____
9. Are you, or any member of your family, on a special diet? ____ If yes, who and what kind? _____
10. Do you drink alcohol? _____ How much? _____ How often?_____
11. How would you describe your exercise habits? _____ Type of exercise _____
    Intensity _____ Duration _____ Frequency _____
12. Are there any other facts about your lifestyle that you think might be related to your nutritional health?_____
    Explain _____

Note: Use the appropriate form to record food intake data (Form 19–2, 19–3, or 19–4).

tion previously overlooked because no one thought to ask or because the client was not thinking clearly when asked.

An accurate, complete health history can reveal conditions that place a client at risk for malnutrition (review Table 19–2). Diseases and their therapies can have either immediate or long-term effects on nutrition status by interfering with ingestion, digestion, absorption, metabolism, or excretion of nutrients.

Socioeconomic History

Socioeconomic factors profoundly affect nutrition status. A person's ethnic background and educational level, as well as other household members, influence food availability and food choices. An understanding of the community environment is also important in assessing nutrition status. For example, knowing the food habits of the major ethnic groups within the locale, regional food preferences, and nutrition resources and programs available in the community prepares the interviewer with an understanding of local customs and resources. Local health departments and social agencies often can provide such information.

Level of income also influences the diet. In general, the quality of the diet declines as income falls. At some point, the ability to purchase the foods required to meet nutrient needs is lost; an inadequate income puts an adequate diet out of reach. Agencies use poverty indexes to identify people at risk for poor nutrition and to qualify people for government food assistance programs.

Low income affects not only the power to purchase foods but also the ability to shop for, store, and cook them. A skilled assessor will note whether a person has transportation to a grocery store that sells a sufficient variety of low-cost foods, and whether the person has access to a refrigerator and stove.

Drug History

The many interactions of foods and drugs require that health care providers pay special attention to any client who takes drugs routinely. Hundreds of drugs interact with nutrients, making imbalances or deficiencies likely. Nausea and vomiting, common side effects of drugs, interfere with food intake. Tables in Chapters 23 through 30 and Table E-1 in Appendix E contain extensive lists of drug-nutrient interactions.

If a person is taking any drug, the assessor records the name of the drug; the dose, frequency, and duration of intake; the reason for taking the drug; and signs of any adverse effects in the nutrition care plan. Chapter 18 discusses nutrient-drug interactions in more detail.

Diet History

A diet history provides a record of a person's food intake. The accurate recording of such data requires skill. Trained dietitians often use food models or photos and measuring devices to help clients identify the types of foods and quantities consumed. The assessor also needs to know how the foods are prepared. In addition to asking about foods, assessors will ask about beverage consumption, including those beverages containing alcohol or caffeine. Food choices are an important part of the lifestyle and often represent an expression of personal philosophy. The assessor who asks nonjudgmental open-ended questions about food intake encourages trust and increases the likelihood of accurate information (see Chapter 20 for a discussion on developing communication skills).

Tools for obtaining food intake data include the 24-hour recall, the usual intake record, the food frequency checklist, and the food diary. The assessor compares food intakes with standards, usually nutrient recommendations or food guides. The question to answer is how closely the person's diet meets the recommendations. Are the types and amounts of proteins, carbohydrates, and fats (including cholesterol) appropriate? Is caffeine or alcohol consumption excessive? Are intakes of any vitamins or minerals (including sodium and iron) excessive or deficient?

Besides identifying possible nutrient imbalances, diet histories provide valuable clues about how a person will accept diet changes should they be necessary. Information about what and how a person eats provides the background for realistic and attainable nutrition goals.

24-Hour Recall The 24-hour recall provides data for one day only and is commonly used in nutrition surveys to obtain estimates of the typical food intakes of large numbers of people in given populations. The assessor asks the client to recount everything eaten or drunk in the past 24 hours or for the previous day. (Form 19–2 shows a typical 24-hour recall form.) Its usefulness is limited in that it does not provide enough accurate information to allow generalizations about an individual's usual food intake. This limitation is

■ FORM 19–2
Food Intake for a 24-Hour Recall or Usual Intake Pattern

Name and address _____ Date _____

_____

_____

Did you take a vitamin/mineral supplement? _____

If yes, what kind? _____ Dose _____

Please record the amount and type of foods and beverages consumed today. [Or:
Please record the amount and type of foods and beverages you typically consume
each day.]

Food	Amount (c, tbsp, or piece)	Description (how cooked, how served)

partially overcome when 24-hour recalls are collected on several nonconsecutive days.[1]

An advantage of the 24-hour recall is that it is easy to obtain. It is also more likely to provide accurate data, at least about the past 24 hours, than a person's estimates of average intakes over long times. However, the previous day's intake may not be typical; the person may be unable to report portion sizes accurately; and the person may even conceal or forget facts about foods eaten. As a result, sometimes the information gathered in a 24-hour recall does not truly reflect a person's usual intake.

Usual Intake To obtain data about a person's usual intake, an inquiry might begin with, "What is the first thing you usually eat or drink during the day?" Similar questions follow until a typical daily intake pattern emerges. This method is similar to the 24-hour recall and uses the same form (Form 19–2). A person's usual intake pattern can provide much useful information, especially in verifying food intake when the past 24 hours have been atypical. A person whose intake varies widely from day to day, however, may find it difficult to answer such general questions, and in such a case, the data may be useless in estimating nutrient intake.

Food Frequency Checklist Another approach is to use a food frequency checklist. The purpose of this record is to ascertain how often an individual

■ **FORM 19–3**
Food Frequency Checklist

The following information will help us to understand your regular eating habits so that we may offer you the best service possible. If you have any doubt about some items, be sure to underestimate the "goodness" of your habits rather than to overestimate.

1. How many times *per week* do you eat the following foods? Circle the appropriate number:

PER WEEK

Poultry .... 0 < 1 1 2 3 4 5 6 7 8 9 > 9___
Fish .... 0 < 1 1 2 3 4 5 6 7 8 9 > 9___
Hot dogs .... 0 < 1 1 2 3 4 5 6 7 8 9 > 9___
Bacon .... 0 < 1 1 2 3 4 5 6 7 8 9 > 9___
Lunch meat .... 0 < 1 1 2 3 4 5 6 7 8 9 > 9___
Sausage .... 0 < 1 1 2 3 4 5 6 7 8 9 > 9___
Pork or ham .... 0 < 1 1 2 3 4 5 6 7 8 9 > 9___
Salt pork .... 0 < 1 1 2 3 4 5 6 7 8 9 > 9___
Liver .... 0 < 1 1 2 3 4 5 6 7 8 9 > 9___
Beef or veal .... 0 < 1 1 2 3 4 5 6 7 8 9 > 9___
Other meats (which?) _____ .... 0 < 1 1 2 3 4 5 6 7 8 9 > 9___
Cooked dry beans or peas .... 0 < 1 1 2 3 4 5 6 7 8 9 > 9___
Eggs .... 0 < 1 1 2 3 4 5 6 7 8 9 > 9___
Fast foods .... 0 < 1 1 2 3 4 5 6 7 8 9 > 9___

2. How many times *per day* do you eat the following foods? Circle the appropriate number:

PER DAY

Bread, toast, rolls, muffins .... 0 < 1 1 2 3 4 5 6 7 8 9 > 9___
Milk (including on cereal) .... 0 < 1 1 2 3 4 5 6 7 8 9 > 9___
Yogurt or tofu .... 0 < 1 1 2 3 4 5 6 7 8 9 > 9___
Cheese or cheese dishes .... 0 < 1 1 2 3 4 5 6 7 8 9 > 9___
Sugar, jam, jelly, syrup, honey .... 0 < 1 1 2 3 4 5 6 7 8 9 > 9___
Butter or margarine .... 0 < 1 1 2 3 4 5 6 7 8 9 > 9___

3. How many times *per week* do you eat the following foods? Circle the appropriate number:

PER WEEK

Fruits or fruit juices .... 0 < 1 1 2 3 4 5 6 7 8 9 > 9___
Vegetables other than potatoes .... 0 < 1 1 2 3 4 5 6 7 8 9 > 9___
Potatoes and other starchy vegetables .... 0 < 1 1 2 3 4 5 6 7 8 9 > 9___
Salads or raw vegetables .... 0 < 1 1 2 3 4 5 6 7 8 9 > 9___
Cereal (which kind?) _____ .... 0 < 1 1 2 3 4 5 6 7 8 9 > 9___
Pancakes or waffles .... 0 < 1 1 2 3 4 5 6 7 8 9 > 9___

continued

eats a specific type of food per day, week, or month. The assessor uses a long list of foods or types of foods, asking clients to state how often they eat them. This information helps pinpoint food groups, and therefore nutrients, that may be excessive or deficient in the diet. That a person ate no vegetables yesterday may not seem particularly significant, but that the person never eats

■ FORM 19–3
Food Frequency Checklist   (continued)

PER WEEK
Rice or other cooked grains ....0 < 1 1 2 3 4 5 6 7 8 9 > 9___
Noodles (macaroni, spaghetti) ....0 < 1 1 2 3 4 5 6 7 8 9 > 9___
Crackers or pretzels ....0 < 1 1 2 3 4 5 6 7 8 9 > 9___
Sweet rolls or doughnuts ....0 < 1 1 2 3 4 5 6 7 8 9 > 9___
Peanut butter or nuts ....0 < 1 1 2 3 4 5 6 7 8 9 > 9___
Milk or milk products ....0 < 1 1 2 3 4 5 6 7 8 9 > 9___
TV dinners, pot pies, other prepared meals ....0 < 1 1 2 3 4 5 6 7 8 9 > 9___
Sweet bakery goods (cake, cookies) ....0 < 1 1 2 3 4 5 6 7 8 9 > 9___
Snack foods (potato or corn chips) ....0 < 1 1 2 3 4 5 6 7 8 9 > 9___
Candy ....0 < 1 1 2 3 4 5 6 7 8 9 > 9___
Soft drinks (which?) _____ ....0 < 1 1 2 3 4 5 6 7 8 9 > 9___
Coffee or tea ....0 < 1 1 2 3 4 5 6 7 8 9 > 9___
Frozen sweets (which?) _____ ....0 < 1 1 2 3 4 5 6 7 8 9 > 9___
Instant meals such as breakfast bars or diet meal
beverages (which?) _____ ....0 < 1 1 2 3 4 5 6 7 8 9 > 9___
Wine ....0 < 1 1 2 3 4 5 6 7 8 9 > 9___
Beer ....0 < 1 1 2 3 4 5 6 7 8 9 > 9___
Whiskey, vodka, rum, etc. ....0 < 1 1 2 3 4 5 6 7 8 9 > 9___

4. What specific kinds of the following foods do you eat most often? Include the
   name of the food; whether it is fresh, canned, or frozen; and how it is prepared.

   Fruits and fruit juices _____
   Vegetables _____
   Milk and milk products _____
   Meats and meat alternates _____
   Breads and cereals _____
   Desserts _____
   Snack foods _____

5. Please list the names of any liquid, powder, or pill forms of vitamin or mineral
   products you take, and state how often you take them. Please list also any diet
   supplement you use (such as protein milk shakes or brewer's yeast), how much
   you use, and how often you use it. _____
   _____

6. Is there anything else we should know about your food/nutrient intake? _____
   _____

vegetables should ring a bell warning of possible nutrient deficiencies. If used
with the usual intake or 24-hour recall approach, the food frequency checklist
permits double-checking the accuracy of the information obtained. Form
19–3 is a food frequency checklist.

■ FORM 19–4
Food Diary

Name				Date	
Time	Place	With Whom	Emotional State	Hungry or Not Hungry	Food Eaten (amount)

(etc.)

Food Diary Another tool for history-taking is the food diary, which includes not only food eaten, but time of day, place, others present, and mood. The assessor instructs the person keeping the diary to write down the required information immediately after eating. (Form 19–4 provides an example.) A food diary can help both the assessor and the client to determine factors associated with eating that may affect dietary balance and adequacy.

Food diaries work especially well with cooperative people but require considerable time and effort on their part. A prime advantage of the food diary is that the diary keeper assumes an active role and may for the first time become aware of personal food habits and begin to assume responsibility for them. It also provides the assessor with an accurate picture of the diary keeper's lifestyle and factors that affect food intake. For these reasons, a food diary can be particularly useful in outpatient counseling for such nutrition problems as overweight, underweight, or food allergy. The major disadvantages stem from poor compliance in recording the data and conscious or unconscious changes in eating habits that may occur while the person is keeping the diary.

After collecting food intake data, the assessor must estimate nutrient intakes, either informally or by using food composition tables. An informal estimate is possible only if the assessor has enough prior experience with formal calculations to "see" nutrient amounts in reported food intakes without calculations. Even then, such an informal analysis is best followed by a spot check for key nutrients by actual calculation.

The formal calculation can be performed either manually (by looking up each food in a table of food composition, recording its nutrients, and adding them up) or by using a computer diet analysis program. The assessor then compares the intakes with standards such as the RDA.

Used with skill, diet histories can be superbly informative about a client's nutrient intakes. The skillful assessor uses them with their limitations in mind. For example, a computer diet analysis tends to imply an accuracy greater than is possible to obtain from data as uncertain as those that provide the starting information. Nutrient contents of foods listed in tables of food composition or stored in computer databases are averages, and for some nutrients, complete data are not available. In addition, the available data on nutrient contents of foods do not reflect the amounts of nutrients a person actually absorbs. Iron is a case in point: its availability from a given meal may vary from as high as 50 percent to less than 2 percent, depending on the relative amounts of heme iron, nonheme iron, vitamin C, meat, fish, and poultry eaten at the meal and the presence of inhibitors of iron absorption such as tea, coffee, and nuts. Chapter 11 explains how to calculate iron absorption from a meal.

Furthermore, there is uncertainty about portion sizes. The person who reports eating "a serving" of greens may not distinguish between ¼ cup and 2 whole cups; only trained individuals can accurately report serving sizes. Children tend to remember the serving sizes of foods they like as being larger than serving sizes of foods they dislike.[2]

Thus there are many opportunities for error when comparing reported nutrient intakes with nutrient needs. Most history takers learn to use shortcut systems to obtain rough estimates of nutrient intakes and then use calculation methods to pinpoint suspected nutrient deficiencies or imbalances.

An estimate of nutrient intakes from a diet history, combined with other sources of information, allows the assessor to confirm or eliminate the possibility of suspected food intake problems. The assessor must constantly remember that nutrient intakes in adequate amounts do not guarantee adequate nutrient status for an individual. Likewise, insufficient intake does not always indicate deficiency, but it does alert the assessor to a possible problem. Each person digests, absorbs, metabolizes, and excretes nutrients in a unique way; individual needs vary. Intakes of nutrients identified by diet histories are only pieces of a puzzle that must be put together with other indicators of nutrition status in order to extract meaning.

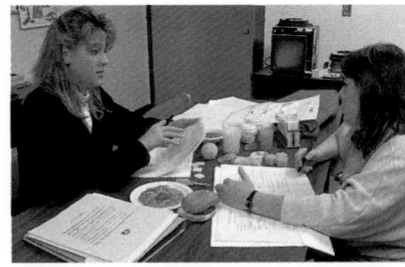

Clients complete diet histories most accurately when guided by a dietitian who is equipped with plastic models of foods to illustrate portion sizes.

Anthropometric Measurements

Anthropometrics are physical measurements that provide an indirect assessment of body composition and development (see Table 19–3 on p. 614). They primarily serve two purposes: first, to evaluate the progress of growth in pregnant women, infants, children, and adolescents; and second, to detect undernutrition and obesity in all age groups.

In using anthropometry, health care providers compare measurements taken on an individual with standards specific for gender and age or with previous measures of the individual. The standards derive from measurements taken on populations; measurements taken periodically and compared with previous measurements reveal changes in an individual's status.

anthropometric: relating to measurement of the physical characteristics of the body, such as height and weight.
anthropos = human
metric = measuring

■ TABLE 19–3
Anthropometric Measurements Used in Nutrition Assessments

Type of Measurement	What It Reflects
Abdominal girth measurement	Abdominal fluid retention
Height-weight	Overnutrition and undernutrition; growth in children
%IBW, %UBW,[a] recent weight change	Overnutrition and undernutrition
Head circumference	Brain growth and development in infants and children under two
Midarm circumference	Muscle mass and subcutaneous fat
Fatfold	Subcutaneous fat and total body fat
Midarm muscle circumference	Muscle mass (i.e., protein status)

[a]%IBW = percent ideal body weight; %UBW = percent usual body weight. These concepts are discussed in the text.

Anthropometric measurements are easy to take and require minimal equipment. However, mastering the correct techniques requires proper instruction and practice to ensure reliability.

Height and weight are well-recognized anthropometrics; other anthropometrics include fatfold measurements and various measures of lean tissue. Some measures are useful in specific situations. For example, a head circumference measurement may help to assess brain development in an infant and an abdominal girth measurement supplies information about abdominal fluid retention in individuals with liver disease.

Measures of Growth and Development

Height and weight are among the most common and useful anthropometric measurements. Length measurements for infants and children up to age three and height measurements for children over three are particularly valuable in assessing growth, and therefore nutrition status (as described in Chapters 14 and 15). For adults, height measurements alone are not critical but help to estimate desirable weight and to interpret other assessment data. Once adult height has been reached, changes in body weight provide useful information in assessing overnutrition and undernutrition.

Lying still with legs straight for a length measurement can be a trying experience.

Height For infants and children younger than three, health care professionals may use special equipment to measure length. The assessor lays the barefoot infant on a measuring board that has a fixed headboard and movable footboard attached at right angles to the surface. Often it takes two people to obtain an accurate measurement: one to hold the infant's head against the headboard and keep the legs straight, and the other to do the measuring. This method provides the most accurate measure possible, but many health care providers use a less exacting method. They may simply hold the infant straight, with its head against the headboard or other vertical support, then mark the blanket with a chalk or pen at the infant's heel, and then measure the distance from the headboard to the mark. Even more informally and less accurately, with the infant lying on a flat surface, they may extend a nonstretchable measuring tape along the side of the infant from the top of the head to the heel of the foot.

The procedure for measuring a child who can stand erect and cooperate is the same as for an adult. The best way to measure standing height is with the person's back against a flat wall alongside an affixed, nonstretchable measuring tape or stick. The person stands erect, without shoes, with heels together. The person's line of sight should be horizontal, with the heels, buttocks, shoulders, and head touching the wall. The assessor uses a block, book, or other inflexible object to ensure that the top of the head is measured at a right angle to the wall. The assessor carefully checks the height measurement and immediately records the result in either inches or centimeters. Such a practice prevents forgetting the correct measurement.

The measuring rod of a scale is an acceptable but less accurate means to measure height because of its movability. The assessor follows the same general procedure, asking the person to face away from the scale and to take extra care to stand erect.

Unfortunately, many health care providers merely ask clients how tall they are rather than measuring their height. Self-reported height is often inaccurate and should be used only as a last resort when measurement is impractical (in the case of an uncooperative client, an emergency admission, or the like).

Standing "at attention" allows for an accurate height measurement.

Weight For measuring weight, beam balance and electronic scales are most accurate. To measure infants' weights, assessors use special scales that allow infants to lie or sit. Weighing infants naked, without diapers, is standard procedure. To weigh children who can stand, health care providers use the same procedure as for an adult. To make repeated measures useful, standardized conditions are necessary. Each weighing should take place at the same time of day (preferably before breakfast), in the same amount of clothing (without shoes), after the person has voided, and on the same scale. Special scales are available for weighing people who are bedridden. Bathroom scales are inaccurate and inappropriate in a professional setting. As with all measurements, the assessor records observed weight immediately, in either pounds or kilograms.

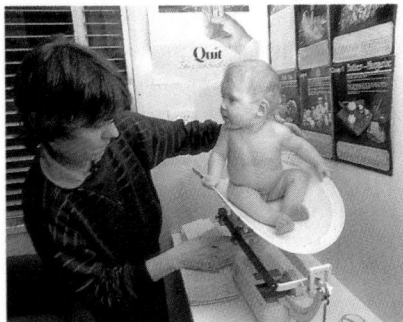

Special scales allow infants to sit and watch while they are being weighed.

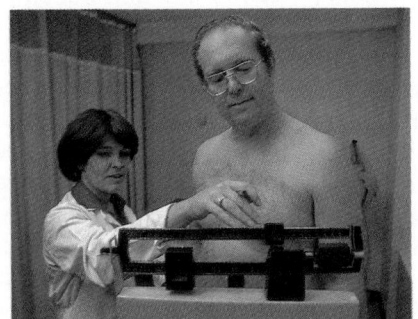

Beam balance scales provide accurate weight measurements for adults.

Head Circumference   Assessors may also measure head circumference to confirm that infant growth is proceeding normally or to help detect protein-energy malnutrition (PEM) and evaluate the extent of its impact on brain size. To measure head circumference, the assessor places a nonstretchable tape so as to encircle the largest part of the infant's or child's head: just above the eyebrow ridges, just above the point where the ears attach, and around the occipital prominence at the back of the head. For accuracy in recording, the assessor immediately notes the measure in either inches or centimeters.

Analysis of Measures   Growth retardation is an important sign of poor nutrition status. Obesity is also an important sign requiring intervention.

Health professionals generally evaluate physical development by monitoring the growth rate of a child and comparing this rate with standard charts. Standard charts compare weight to age, height to age, and weight to height; ideally, height and weight are in roughly the same percentile. Although individual growth patterns may vary, in general, a child's growth curve will stay at about the same percentile throughout childhood. In children whose growth has been retarded, nutrition rehabilitation will ideally induce height and weight to increase to higher percentiles. In overweight children, the goal is for weight to remain stable as height increases, until weight becomes appropriate for height.

To evaluate growth in infants, an assessor uses charts such as the ones shown in Figure 19–1. (All of the growth charts are located in Appendix E.) The assessor follows these steps to plot a weight measurement on a percentile graph:

- Select the appropriate chart based on age and gender. (When length is measured, use the chart for birth to 36 months; when height is measured, use the chart for 2 to 18 years.)
- Locate the child's age along the horizontal axis on the bottom or top of the chart.
- Locate the child's weight in pounds or kilograms along the vertical axis on the lower left or right side of the chart.
- Mark the chart where the age and weight lines intersect, and read off the percentile.

To assess length, height, or head circumference, the assessor follows the same procedure, using the appropriate chart. Head circumference percentile should be similar to the child's height and weight percentiles.

With height, weight, and head circumference measures plotted on growth percentile charts, a skilled clinician can begin to interpret the data. Percentile charts divide the measures of a population into 100 equal divisions. Thus half of the population falls above the 50th percentile, and half falls below. The use of percentile measures allows for comparisons among people of the same age and gender. For example, a six-month-old female infant whose weight is at the 75th percentile weighs more than 75 percent of the female infants her age.

Head circumference is generally measured in children under two years of age. Since the brain is rapidly growing before birth and during early infancy, extreme and chronic malnutrition during these times can impair brain

■ **FIGURE 19–1**
Examples of Growth Charts
These charts are representative of the growth charts provided in Appendix E. They show the two charts used for girls, ages birth to 36 months. The first one gives percentiles for length and weight for age; the other, percentiles for head circumference for age and weight for length.

development, curtailing the number of brain cells and the size of head circumference. The assessor plots head circumference measurements on a percentile growth chart; head circumference percentile should be similar to the child's weight and height percentiles. Nonnutritional factors, such as certain disorders and genetic variation, can also influence head circumference.[3]

For adults, health care providers typically compare weights with weight-for-height tables (such as Table 19–4 on p. 618), which are specific for height, gender, and frame size. To determine frame sizes, the assessor can use one of the two methods of estimating frame size shown in Appendix E. The height and weight tables suggest an appropriate weight range, rather than pinpointing one ideal weight. This is a good reminder that there is no perfect weight for anyone. A quick method of estimating ideal body weight frequently used by health care professionals is shown in Table 19–5 on p. 619.

The height-weight tables are useful for identifying both undernutrition and overnutrition. A standard derived from height and weight, which is especially useful for estimating the risk to health associated with overnutrition, is the body mass index (BMI). Appendix E presents a nomogram for determining

■ TABLE 19–4
1983 Metropolitan Height and Weight Tables

Men						Women					
Height		Frame				Height		Frame			
Feet	Inches	Small	Medium	Large		Feet	Inches	Small	Medium	Large	
5	2	128–134	131–141	138–150		4	10	102–111	109–121	118–131	
5	3	130–136	133–143	140–153		4	11	103–113	111–123	120–134	
5	4	132–138	135–145	142–156		5	0	104–115	113–126	122–137	
5	5	134–140	137–148	144–160		5	1	106–118	115–129	125–140	
5	6	136–142	139–151	146–164		5	2	108–121	118–132	128–143	
5	7	138–145	142–154	149–168		5	3	111–124	121–135	131–147	
5	8	140–148	145–157	152–172		5	4	114–127	124–138	134–151	
5	9	142–151	148–160	155–176		5	5	117–130	127–141	137–155	
5	10	144–154	151–163	158–180		5	6	120–133	130–144	140–159	
5	11	146–157	154–166	161–184		5	7	123–136	133–147	143–163	
6	0	149–160	157–170	164–188		5	8	126–139	136–150	146–167	
6	1	152–164	160–174	168–192		5	9	129–142	139–153	149–170	
6	2	155–168	164–178	172–197		5	10	132–145	142–156	152–173	
6	3	158–172	167–182	176–202		5	11	135–148	145–159	155–176	
6	4	162–176	171–187	181–207		6	0	138–151	148–162	158–179	

Note: Weights at ages 25 to 29 based on lowest mortality. Weights in pounds according to frame (in indoor clothing weighing 5 lb for men or 3 lb for women; shoes with 1-inch heels). For frame size standards, see Appendix E.

Source: Reproduced courtesy of Metropolitan Life Insurance Company. Source of basic data: Society of Actuaries and Association of Life Insurance Medical Directors of America, *1979 Build Study,* 1980.

the BMI and the inside back covers show graphs of weight ranges for various heights based on the BMI. These BMI graphs provide another quick method of estimating ideal body weight within a healthy range.

The table of average weights for height is less useful in cases where a person has weighed much more or much less than the average throughout life. To assess such a person's weight, it may be more informative to compare the present weight not with an ''ideal'' body weight, but with the person's usual body weight. The percentages of a person's actual weight compared with an ideal or usual body weight are useful indicators of malnutrition (Table 19–6).

To calculate the percent ideal body weight (%IBW), an assessor compares a person's actual weight with the ideal weight. This provides a rough estimate of the degree of overnutrition or undernutrition. A %IBW greater than 115 to 120 indicates obesity; less than 90 indicates undernutrition.

A more valuable parameter for assessing weight measurements is the percent usual body weight (%UBW), which considers what is normal for a particular individual. The client, family, friends, and older medical records can provide such information. A health care provider may inadvertently overlook malnutrition in an obese person when using %IBW rather than %UBW.

To determine any recent weight change, the assessor compares the %UBW with the time period over which a change, if any, has occurred. A 5 percent weight loss might be significant if it occurred within a month, yet might be insignificant if it occurred over five months. The box on p. 620 describes how to estimate %IBW and %UBW.

■ TABLE 19–5
Quick Estimation of Ideal Body Weight

Men:

For 5 feet, consider 106 pounds a reasonable weight.

For each inch over 5 feet, add 6 pounds.

Subtract 6 pounds for each inch under 5 feet.

Add 10 percent for a large-framed individual; subtract 10 percent for a small-framed individual.

Example: A man 5 feet 8 inches tall (medium frame) would start at 106 pounds, add 48, and arrive at a reasonable weight of 154 pounds.

Women:

For 5 feet, consider 100 pounds a reasonable weight.

For each inch over 5 feet, add 5 pounds.

Subtract 5 pounds for each inch under 5 feet.

Add 10 percent for a large-framed individual; subtract 10 percent for a small-framed individual.

Example: A woman 5 feet 6 inches tall (medium frame) would start at 100 pounds, add 30, and arrive at a reasonable weight of 130 pounds.

Weight measurements in hospitalized clients are sometimes difficult to evaluate. Diseases or therapy can cause fluid retention and mask significant weight loss. In fact, starvation itself is accompanied by an expanded extracellular fluid volume.

One of the most important anthropometric measures predictive of the birthweight of a child is the mother's amount and pattern of weight gain or loss during pregnancy. Normal weight gains related to duration of the pregnancy in weeks are shown in Figure 19–2 (on p. 621). Patterns of weight gain that deviate from these require further investigation.

Measures of growth and development are well-recognized anthropometrics. Others include measures of body fat and lean tissue.

Measures of Body Fat and Lean Tissue

Significant weight changes in both children and adults can reflect overnutrition and undernutrition with respect to energy and protein. To estimate the

■ TABLE 19–6
Weight as an Indicator of Nutrition Status

%IBW	%UBW	Nutrition Status
> 120	—	Obese
110–120	—	Overweight
80–90	85–95	Mildly undernourished
70–79	75–84	Moderately undernourished
< 70	< 75	Severely undernourished

How to Estimate %IBW and %UBW

To estimate %IBW, compare the individual's current weight with the ideal body weight from standard height-weight tables; to estimate %UBW, compare the current weight with the individual's typical weight. For example, to calculate %IBW and %UBW in a 45-year-old man of medium frame who is 5'8" tall, weighs 115 lb, and has lost 15 lbs in the last month, follow these steps:

1. $\%\text{IBW} = \dfrac{\text{Actual weight}}{\text{Ideal weight}} \times 100.$

For ideal weight, use the midpoint of the weight range. In this example, the ideal weight is 153 lb.

2. $\%\text{IBW} = \dfrac{115 \text{ lb}}{153 \text{ lb}} \times 100 = 76\%.$

The man in this example is at 76% of his ideal body weight. Look to Table 19–6 to find that 76% IBW indicates that the person is *moderately* undernourished.

3. $\%\text{UBW} = \dfrac{\text{Actual weight}}{\text{Usual weight}} \times 100.$

Calculate the usual weight (130 lb) by adding the weight loss (15 lb) to the current body weight (115 lb).

4. $\%\text{UBW} = \dfrac{115 \text{ lb}}{130 \text{ lb}} \times 100 = 89\%.$

The man is at 89% of his usual body weight. When you look to Table 19–6 you will see that 89% UBW indicates that this person is *mildly* undernourished. Based on %UBW the degree of undernourishment is less severe than implied from %IBW. In addition, the recent weight change is significant; he has lost weight at a rate of almost 4 lb per week.

degree to which various body compartments (fat stores or lean tissues) are affected by overnutrition or malnutrition, several anthropometric measurements are useful (as listed earlier in Table 19–3).

Fatfold Measures Approximately half the fat in the body is located directly beneath the skin, and its thickness reflects total body fat. In some parts of the body, this fat is loosely attached; a person can pull it up between the thumb and forefinger. These sites provide an opportunity to measure fatfold thickness. In the hands of a trained person, the fatfold test is a valuable and practical diagnostic procedure. Body fat calculations determined by fatfold measures correlate well with calculations based on other, more sophisticated methods, such as underwater weighing, obtaining a radioactive potassium count, and determining total body water. Training in the use of fatfold calipers is critical to obtaining accurate measurements, however.

Prenatal gain in weight

Immediate pregravid weight ___

Height in inches without shoes (plus one inch) ___

Standard weight ___

(Record weight *with* shoes)

■ FIGURE 19–2
Prenatal Weight Gain Grid

A major limitation of the fatfold test is that fat may be thicker under the skin in one area than in another. A pinch at the side of the waistline may not yield the same measurement as a pinch on the back of the arm. This limitation can be overcome by taking fatfold measurements at several (often three) different places on the body to obtain an accurate estimate of subcutaneous fat. However, multiple measures are not always practical in clinical settings and, most often, the triceps fatfold measurement is used because it is easily accessible. To measure fatfold, a trained technician follows a standard procedure using reliable calipers, as illustrated in Figure 19–3 (on p. 622). Triceps fatfold percentiles are given in Appendix E.

Midarm Circumferences   When taken together with the *midarm* circumference, the triceps fatfold measurement enables an assessor to calculate the derived midarm *muscle* circumference. An assessor measures midarm circumference with a nonstretchable tape around the arm midway between the

■ **FIGURE 19–3**
How to Measure the Triceps Fatfold

Clavicle

Acromial
process

Midpoint

Olecranon
process

Find the midpoint of the arm:
1. Ask the subject to bend his or her arm at the elbow and lay the hand across the stomach. (If he or she is right-handed, measure the left arm, and vice versa.)
2. Feel the shoulder to locate the acromial process. It helps to slide your fingers along the clavicle to find the acromial process. The olecranon process is the tip of the elbow.
3. Place a measuring tape from the acromial process to the tip of the elbow. Divide this measurement by 2, and mark the midpoint of the arm with a pen.

Measure the fatfold:
1. Ask the subject to let his or her arm hang loosely to the side.
2. Grasp a fold of skin and subcutaneous fat between the thumb and forefinger slightly above the midpoint mark. Gently pull the skin away from the underlying muscle. (This step takes a lot of practice. To be sure you don't have muscle as well as fat, ask the subject to contract and relax the muscle. You should be able to feel if you are pinching muscle.)
3. Place the calipers over the fatfold at the midpoint mark, and read the measurement to the nearest 1.0 mm in two to three seconds. (If using plastic calipers, align pressure lines, and read the measurement to the nearest 1.0 mm in two to three seconds.)
4. Repeat steps 2 and 3 twice more. Add the three readings, and then divide by 3 to find the average.

■ **FIGURE 19–4**
How to Measure Midarm Circumference
A nonstretchable measuring tape is placed around the arm at the midpoint.

Midarm
circumference

shoulder and the elbow (see Figure 19–4). The midarm circumference measures muscle mass and subcutaneous fat. This measurement is used to calculate the midarm muscle circumference.

The midarm muscle circumference derives from a mathematical equation; it is not directly measurable. The equation assumes the arm to be circular, subtracting the fatfold measure from the midarm circumference (see Figure 19–5). The derived midarm muscle circumference permits an estimate of muscle mass and, thus, represents protein nutrition. Appendix E includes a nomogram for determining midarm muscle circumference.

Analysis of Measures The accuracy and value of anthropometric measurements are limited by the skills of the measurer, the accuracy of the equipment used for measurement, changes in body composition related to different disorders (such as fluid retention or dehydration), and misinterpretation of measurements. Triceps fatfold and midarm muscle circumference

A. The arm is visualized as an inner circle of muscle surrounded by an outer circle of fat.
B. In reality, the arm is not circular, and there is some bone, but the simplified picture is approximately correct.
C. This measurement (the fatfold) gives you two times the thickness of the fat.
D. This measurement (the midarm circumference) gives you the measure of muscle plus fat.
E. An equation then derives the *circumference of the muscle,* an index of the body's total skeletal muscle mass. The equation is:
Midarm muscle circumference (cm) = midarm circumference (cm) − [0.314[a] × triceps fatfold (mm)].

[a]This factor converts the fatfold measurement to a circumference measurement and millimeters to centimeters.

measurements can be difficult to determine for people who are obese or for elderly individuals with loose skin hanging on the upper arm. Significant changes in measurements occur slowly in adults. When changes do occur, they represent prolonged alterations in nutrient intake. Therefore, anthropometrics cannot be used to describe small changes in body composition that occur over short periods of time.[4]

Fatfold measurements and the derived midarm muscle circumference must be interpreted with extreme caution for people with severe stress. Further research is needed to determine if internal fat stores change at the same rate as triceps fatfold or if changes in total body water markedly influence fatfold measurements during severe stress.[5] It is conceivable that fatfold measure-

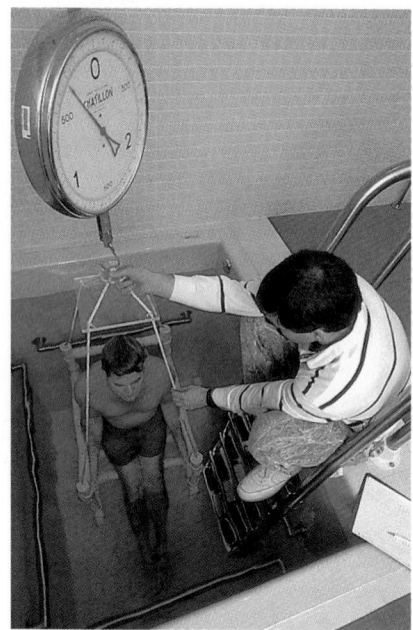

Underwater weighing is the "gold standard" for estimating percent body fat.

hydrodensitometry: measurement of body density by submerging the person underwater.

bioelectrical impedance: a method for estimating body fat using low-intensity electrical current.

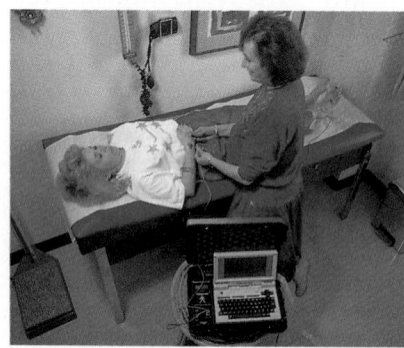

Bioelectrical impedance provides a simple and painless way to estimate body fat.

ments could remain constant in spite of internal fat stores being depleted. Any error in the fatfold measurement would affect the derived midarm muscle circumference as well. Furthermore, exercise or its lack influences muscle size independently of nutrition factors.[6]

Fatfold measurements, midarm circumference, and the derived midarm muscle circumference are reproducible measurements when standard procedures are followed. Accurately following standard procedure requires practice, however. Generally, the same person should measure the same subject routinely for best results.

Hydrodensitometry (underwater weighing) and bioelectrical impedance techniques are two additional methods for assessing total body fat. Both of these techniques are popularly used among athletes and in health clubs.

Hydrodensitometry Underwater weighing, or hydrodensitometry, measures body density. The person is weighed on a standard scale and then submerged in water. The amount of water displaced is measured. A mathematical equation using the two measurements (body weight and water displacement) allows the assessor to calculate body density and percent body fat. The assessor then uses sex-specific reference standards for men and women to evaluate the body fat measurement.

Underwater weighing generates an excellent estimate of body fat, although the technique has drawbacks. Underwater weighing requires bulky, expensive, and nonportable equipment. Furthermore, it is impractical to submerge people (especially those who are ill or fearful) underwater. Errors can result from the mathematical equation used to translate body density measurements into percent fat measurements. The standards used for comparing values to norms were developed on adults; since the young and the elderly have different body densities (for which standards are not available), assessors have difficulty interpreting data in these age groups. For all these reasons, underwater weighing is not widely used.

Bioelectrical Impedance Bioelectrical impedance techniques to determine body composition are rapidly gaining popularity. The technique is less expensive than underwater weighing, the equipment is portable, and the procedure is painless. To measure body fat using the bioelectrical impedance technique, a very low intensity electrical current is briefly sent through the body by way of electrodes placed on the wrist and ankle. Since electrolyte-containing fluids are found primarily in lean body tissues, and they readily conduct an electrical current, the leaner the person, the less resistance to the electrical current. The measurement of electrical resistance is then used in a mathematical equation to estimate the percent body fat.

In healthy adults, the bioelectrical impedance technique compares favorably with other measures of body composition.[7] However, more accurate equations need to be developed for children and adolescents, and for people who are either obese or very lean. Currently used equations may underestimate body fat in very obese people and overestimate it in those who are very lean.[8] The person's state of hydration on any given day, as well as individual differences in skin resistance, can significantly influence the technique's results.[9] In a study of people with cardiac and pulmonary disorders, body fat

■ TABLE 19–8
Routine Hospital Laboratory Tests

Test	Uses
Hematology	
Hemoglobin (Hg)	To detect anemia and determine state of hydration.
Hematocrit (Hct)	To detect anemia and determine state of hydration.
White blood cells (WBC)	To detect infection and determine total lymphocyte count.
Mean corpuscular volume (MCV)	To detect anemia and determine its causes.
Mean corpuscular hemoglobin (MCH)	To detect anemia and determine its causes.
Mean corpuscular hemoglobin concentration (MCHC)	To detect anemia and determine its causes.
Blood Chemistry	
Electrolytes	
Sodium	To check state of hydration.
Potassium	To monitor acid-base balance, renal function, and response to diuretics.
Chloride	To monitor acid-base balance and detect GI losses of chloride (from vomiting or nasogastric suctioning).
Carbon dioxide	To monitor acid-base balance.
Other	
Glucose	To detect diabetes mellitus, glucose intolerance, stress, and pancreatic tumors.
Blood urea nitrogen	To monitor renal function and determine state of hydration.
Calcium	To detect hormonal imbalances, certain malignancies, and steatorrhea (malabsorption).
Phosphorus	To detect hormonal imbalances, PEM, and cirrhosis.
Magnesium	To monitor renal function and detect PEM.
Total protein[a]	To detect PEM and various nutrient imbalances.
Albumin	To detect PEM and determine state of hydration.
Cholesterol	To assess risk of heart disease and possibility of obstructive jaundice.
Uric acid	To detect gout and determine state of hydration.
Serum creatinine	To monitor renal function and determine state of hydration.
Serum Enzymes	
Creatinine phosphokinase (CPK)	To monitor heart function.
Lactic dehydrogenase (LDH)	To monitor heart and renal function.
Alanine transaminase (ALT, formerly SGPT)	To monitor heart and liver function.
Aspartate transaminase (AST, formerly SGOT)	To monitor heart and liver function.
Alkaline phosphatase	To monitor liver function.
Serum amylase	To monitor pancreatic function.
Serum lipase	To monitor pancreatic function.

Note: This table presents a partial listing of the major uses of certain commonly performed lab tests that have implications for nutrition.
[a]More than half of the total protein is albumin.

■ TABLE 19–9
Relationship between Degree of Undernutrition and Serum Proteins

Indicator	Degree of Depletion		
	Mild	Moderate	Severe
Albumin (g/100 ml)	2.8–3.4	2.1–2.7	< 2.1
Transferrin (mg/100 ml)	150–200	100–149	< 100
Prealbumin (mg/100 ml)	10–15	5–9	< 5
Retinol-binding protein[a] (mg/100 ml)	—	—	—

Note: To convert albumin (g/100 ml) to international standard units (nmol/L), multiply by 37.06. To convert transferrin (mg/100 ml) to standard international units (g/L), multiply by 0.01.
[a]Levels of < 3 mg/100 ml suggest compromised protein status. The actual degree of depletion (mild, moderate, and severe) has not been defined.

Protein-Energy Malnutrition (PEM)

Tests available to determine protein status include serum albumin, serum transferrin, other serum proteins, and total lymphocyte count and other tests of immune function. Of these, serum albumin and total lymphocyte count are most commonly used. Physicians may also order additional tests, such as nitrogen balance studies and urinary creatinine, under special circumstances.

Serum Albumin   Albumin accounts for over 50 percent of the total serum proteins. It helps to maintain fluid and electrolyte balance and to transport many nutrients, hormones, drugs, and other compounds. Albumin synthesis depends on functioning liver cells and on an appropriate supply of amino acids. Albumin concentrations reflect the protein status of the blood and internal organs. Serum albumin concentrations tend to decline slowly, in part because albumin is plentiful in the body and it can shift from the cells to the blood when blood concentrations begin to fall. Additionally, because albumin breaks down slowly, it is slow to reflect changes in nutrition status.* Therefore, low serum albumin levels represent prolonged protein depletion. Conversely, albumin concentrations increase slowly with appropriate nutrition support, so measuring albumin as an indicator of response to nutrition therapy is of limited value.[13] Table 19–9 provides standards for determining the severity of low serum albumin concentrations.

Many other conditions besides malnutrition can depress albumin concentrations, including liver disease, advanced kidney disease (nephrotic syndrome), infection, cancer, burns, and eclampsia. Therefore, as is true for all other nutrition assessment parameters, albumin alone cannot determine protein status, but rather serves as one indicator among many.

Serum Transferrin   Transferrin is a protein that transports iron between the intestine and sites of hemoglobin synthesis and degradation. Researchers consider it a more sensitive indicator of protein malnutrition than albumin, because it responds more promptly to changes in protein intake and has a smaller body pool.**

---

*The half-life of albumin is about 20 days, an indication of a slow degradation rate.
**Transferrin has a half-life of 4 to 8 days, an indication that it is sensitive to changes in protein intake.

Most transferrin is synthesized in the liver. Transferrin levels are inversely related to iron stores: levels are high in iron deficiency and low when iron storage is excessive. Therefore, assessors may have difficulty interpreting transferrin levels when an iron deficiency is present. Liver disease, nephrotic syndrome, and burns lower the transferrin levels; pregnancy and blood loss elevate them. Standards for determining the severity of transferrin depletion are given in Table 19–9.

Other Serum Proteins   Many other serum proteins have been studied as indicators of protein status. Prealbumin and retinol-binding protein are sensitive indicators of protein status.* These proteins quickly reflect PEM and rapidly respond with appropriate refeeding. These sensitive tests are most likely to be ordered in institutions with active nutrition support programs. Other serum proteins that may be useful in nutrition assessment include serum somatomedin-C, fibronectin, fibrinogen, haptoglobin, and C-reactive protein. These indicators of protein status are less practical and more expensive to measure than albumin and transferrin and therefore are not in common use.

Skin tests provide an assessment of immune function.

Total Lymphocyte Count and Other Tests of Immune Function
Various forms of PEM and individual nutrient deficiencies depress the immune system (as Chapter 18 described). The total number of lymphocytes is reduced as protein depletion occurs, so the total lymphocyte count is one useful index in nutrition assessment. White blood cell (WBC) volume, and red and white blood cell counts are routinely measured in hospital tests, so the total lymphocyte count can be easily derived (see the box below).

Another test of immune function is antigen skin testing. Organisms (usually three or four kinds) to which most people are immune are injected just under the skin.** After 48 hours, the sites of the injections are inspected

---

How to Calculate the Total Lymphocyte Count

To calculate the total lymphocyte count, look at the laboratory report and find the complete blood count (CBC). Two figures from this report, the number of white blood cells (WBC) and the percentage of lymphocytes are used to determine the total lymphocyte count:

- Total lymphocyte count (mm^3) = WBC (mm^3) $\times$ % lymphocytes.

A person with a WBC count of 7,500 mm^3 with 15% lymphocytes would have a total lymphocyte count of:

- Total lymphocyte count (mm^3) = 7,500 mm^3 $\times$ 0.15 = 1,125 mm^3.

The standard lymphocyte count is 2,500 mm^3; values below 1,500 mm^3 are considered depleted. A lymphocyte count of 1,125 mm^3, then, suggests a moderate degree of depletion.

---

*The half-lives of prealbumin and retinol-binding protein are 2 days and 12 hours, respectively.
**Typical antigens include *Candida*, mumps, purified protein derivative (PPD), streptokinase-streptodornase (SK-SD), and *Monilla*.

induration: a raised, hardened area of skin.
durus = hard

Nitrogen balance:
    nitrogen intake = nitrogen output.
Positive nitrogen balance:
    nitrogen intake > nitrogen output.
Negative nitrogen balance:
    nitrogen intake < nitrogen output.

for raised, hardened areas (induration). In general, such areas will be apparent in the well-nourished person, but in the malnourished person, hardened areas will not appear or will be very small. However, the value of skin testing as an index of nutrition status in people who are ill has been questioned. Many factors other than nutrition can interfere with the immune response, including infections, trauma, surgery, and burns (Chapter 23); cirrhosis and hepatitis (Chapter 26); uremia (Chapter 29); and many drugs.[14]

Nitrogen Balance   Nitrogen balance studies help to estimate the degree to which protein is being depleted or repleted in the body. A simple approach to measuring nitrogen is to measure urinary urea nitrogen (UUN) in a 24-hour urine collection. During the same 24-hour period, assessors must keep an accurate record of the client's protein (nitrogen) intake to complete the balance study, as the accompanying box describes.

The kidneys must be functioning properly to obtain accurate nitrogen output measurements. In addition, abnormally high nitrogen losses (as seen in clients with severe burns) must be considered.

Nitrogen balance studies provide a prime example of the need for communication and cooperation between health care providers and departments. A nitrogen balance study is invalid if even one urine specimen is flushed or one meal's protein intake not accurately recorded. In such a case the whole procedure has to be repeated at great inconvenience to the client

---

How to Assess Nitrogen Balance

To determine nitrogen balance requires knowing the 24-hour nitrogen intake and output. To estimate nitrogen intake from dietary protein use the formula:

$$\text{Nitrogen intake} = \frac{\text{Protein intake (g)}}{6.25}.$$

Nitrogen output per day equals the measured urinary urea nitrogen (UUN) plus a factor of 4 grams to account for nitrogen lost through the lungs, hair, skin, and nails as well as nonurea nitrogen losses in the urine.

$$\text{Nitrogen output} = \text{UUN} + 4 \text{ g}.$$

Calculate nitrogen balance from the nitrogen intake and output:

$$\text{Nitrogen balance} = \text{Nitrogen intake} - \text{nitrogen output}.$$

Using the above equations, calculate nitrogen balance for a person with a protein intake of 45 g/24 hr and a UUN of 10 g/24 hr.

$$\text{Nitrogen balance} = \frac{45 \text{ g}}{6.25} - (10 \text{ g} + 4 \text{ g}).$$

$$\text{Nitrogen balance} = 7 \text{ g} - 14 \text{ g or } -7 \text{ g}.$$

The person in this example is in negative nitrogen balance; that is, nitrogen intake is inadequate to meet nitrogen needs.

and staff. Appendix E describes the proper technique for collecting a 24-hour urine specimen.

Urinary Creatinine Excretion   Creatinine is a breakdown product of the energy source phosphocreatine, or PC (described in Chapter 13). PC is present specifically in skeletal muscle. Its excretion occurs at a constant rate determined by the amount of skeletal muscle, and the amount excreted therefore reflects skeletal muscle mass. As skeletal muscle atrophies during malnutrition, creatinine excretion decreases. Creatinine excretion is also used to determine whether other urinary lab test results are appropriate to the size of the individual's skeletal muscle mass.

Creatinine is measured from a 24-hour urine collection. Generally, assessors collect three consecutive 24-hour urine specimens, average the creatinine from the three collections, and use the averaged value to calculate the creatinine-height index (see Appendix E for the creatinine-height index equation). A meat-free diet is advised for the days of the urine collection.[15] Meat contains creatinine and will raise the creatinine excretion levels.

Standards for creatinine excretion, based on sex and height, are provided in Appendix E. Assessors use these standards and the measured creatinine value to derive the creatinine-height index (see Appendix E for an example). The creatinine-height index is a percentage of the standard; generally, acceptable values are 90 to 100 percent. No standards are available for the elderly, which presents a problem since creatinine excretion declines with age. Standards for children are based on expected creatinine excretion of healthy children of normal height.

Like the nitrogen balance study, the measurement of urinary creatinine requires 24-hour urine collection, which may be difficult to obtain. The test is invalid if the client shows signs of kidney disease, since the disease might reduce the body's ability to excrete creatinine. Severe stress, fever, and infection can falsely elevate creatinine excretion. Creatinine excretion increases late in the second part of the menstrual cycle, decreasing just before and during the menstrual flow.

The biochemical tests described so far help define protein status. Biochemical tests of iron status are also in wide use because iron deficiency is the most common deficiency disease.

Iron Deficiency

Iron deficiency, the most widespread mineral deficiency, develops in stages. Chapter 11 (pp. 316–320) describes iron deficiency in detail. This section describes tests used to uncover iron deficiency as it progresses. Table 19–10 (on p. 632) shows which laboratory tests detect various stages of iron deficiency. Although other tests are more specific in detecting early deficiencies, hemoglobin and hematocrit are the commonly available tests.

Stages of iron deficiency:
 1. Iron stores diminish.
 2. Transport iron decreases.
 3. Hemoglobin production falls.

Hemoglobin   Iron forms an integral part of the hemoglobin molecule that transports oxygen to the cells. In iron deficiency, the body cannot synthesize hemoglobin. Low hemoglobin values signal depleted iron stores. Table 19–11

■ TABLE 19–10
Biochemical Tests Used to Detect Iron Deficiency

Stage	Detected By	Reflects
Stores depleted	↓ Serum ferritin	Liver and bone marrow stores
Transport iron diminished	↓ Transferrin saturation ↓ Serum iron ↑ Total iron binding capacity	Iron-binding capacity, serum iron
Hemoglobin production limited	↑ Erythrocyte protoporphyrin ↓ Hemoglobin ↓ Hematocrit ↓ Mean corpuscular volume	Detectable anemia, microcytosis

provides hemoglobin values used in nutrition assessment. Because hemoglobin concentrations drop fairly late in the development of iron deficiency, and because other nutrient deficiencies and medical conditions can also alter hemoglobin concentrations, its usefulness in evaluating iron status is limited.

Hematocrit The hematocrit is the percentage of red blood cells in the total blood volume. Hematocrit is commonly used to diagnose iron deficiency, even though it is an inconclusive measure of iron status. To measure the hematocrit, a clinician spins a volume of blood in a centrifuge to separate the red blood cells from the plasma. The packed red cell volume is the hematocrit and is expressed as a percentage of the total blood volume. Table 19–12 provides values used to assess hematocrit status. Low values indicate incomplete hemoglobin formation, which is manifested by microcytic (abnormally small-celled), hypochromic (abnormally lacking in color) red blood cells.

Low hemoglobin and hematocrit values alert the assessor to the possibility of iron deficiency. However, many nutrients and other conditions can affect hemoglobin and hematocrit. The other tests of iron status help pinpoint true iron deficiency.

■ TABLE 19–11
Standards for Hemoglobin Test Results

Age	Sex	Deficient (g/100 ml)	Acceptable (g/100 ml)
< 2 yr	(M-F)	< 9.0	10.0 or >
2–5 yr	(M-F)	< 10.0	11.0 or >
6–12 yr	(M-F)	< 10.0	11.5 or >
13–16 yr	(M)	< 12.0	13.0 or >
	(F)	< 10.0	11.5 or >
> 16 yr	(M)	< 12.0	14.0 or >
	(F)	< 10.0	12.0 or >
trimester 2		< 9.5	11.0 or >
trimester 3		< 9.0	10.5 or >

Note: To convert hemoglobin values (g/100 ml) to international standard units, multiply by 10.

■ TABLE 19–12
Standards for Hematocrit Test Results

Age	Sex	Deficient	Acceptable
< 2 yr	(M-F)	< 0.28	0.31 or >
2–5 yr	(M-F)	< 0.30	0.34 or >
6–12 yr	(M-F)	< 0.30	0.36 or >
13–16 yr	(M)	< 0.37	0.40 or >
	(F)	< 0.31	0.36 or >
> 16 yr	(M)	< 0.37	0.44 or >
	(F)	< 0.31	0.38 or >
trimester 2		< 0.30	0.35 or >
trimester 3		< 0.30	0.33 or >

Note: To convert hematocrit values (%) to international standard units, multiply by 0.01.

Serum Ferritin   In the first stage of iron deficiency, iron stores diminish. Serum ferritin measures provide a noninvasive estimate of iron stores. Such information is most valuable to iron assessment. Table E-9 in Appendix E shows serum ferritin cutoff values that indicate iron store depletion in children and adults. In infants, the reliability of serum ferritin for diagnosing iron deficiency is uncertain, since normal serum ferritin values are often present in conjunction with iron-responsive anemia.

A decrease in transport iron characterizes the second stage of iron deficiency. This is revealed by an increase in the iron-binding capacity of the protein transferrin and a decrease in serum iron. These changes are reflected by the transferrin saturation, which is calculated from the ratio of the other two values as described in the following sections.

Total Iron-Binding Capacity (TIBC)   Iron travels through the blood bound to the protein transferrin. TIBC is a measure of the total amount of iron that transferrin can carry. Lab technicians measure iron-binding capacity directly.

TIBC values greater than 400 μg/100 ml indicate iron deficiency.

Serum Iron   Lab technicians can also measure serum iron directly. Elevated values indicate iron overload; reduced values indicate iron deficiency. Table E-10 in Appendix E shows acceptable and deficient values for serum iron.

Transferrin Saturation   The percentage of transferrin that is saturated with iron is an indirect measure; the mathematical equation derives it from the serum iron and total iron-binding capacity measures, as follows:

$$\%\text{Transferrin} = \frac{\text{Serum iron} \times 100}{\text{Total iron-binding capacity}}.$$

Table E-11 in Appendix E shows deficient and acceptable transferrin saturation values for various age groups.

The third stage of iron deficiency occurs when the supply of transport iron diminishes to the point that it limits hemoglobin production. It is characterized by increases in erythrocyte protoporphyrin, a decrease in mean corpuscular volume, and decreased hemoglobin concentration and hematocrit.

Erythrocyte Protoporphyrin The iron-containing portion of the hemoglobin molecule is heme. Heme is a combination of iron and protoporphyrin. Protoporphyrin accumulates in the blood when iron supplies are inadequate for the formation of heme. Lab technicians can measure erythrocyte protoporphyrin directly in a blood sample. The cutoffs for abnormal values of erythrocyte protoporphyrin are shown in Table E-12 in Appendix E.

Mean Corpuscular Volume (MCV) A direct or calculated measure of the mean corpuscular volume (MCV) determines the average size of a red blood cell (RBC). Such a measure helps to classify the type of nutrient anemia. In iron deficiency, the red blood cells are smaller than average. The cutoffs for abnormal values of MCV that indicate iron deficiency are also shown in Table E-12 in Appendix E.

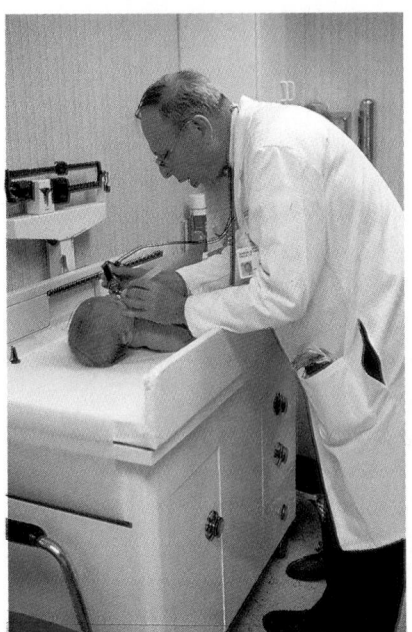

A peek inside the mouth provides clues to a person's nutrition status.

See p. 151 for definitions of PEM terms.

■ *Physical Examinations*

The assessor can also use a physical examination to search for signs of nutrient deficiency or toxicity. Like the other assessment methods, such an examination requires knowledge and skill. Many physical signs are nonspecific; they can reflect any of several nutrient deficiencies, as well as conditions not related to nutrition (see Table 19–13). For example, cracked lips may be caused by sunburn, windburn, dehydration, or any of several B vitamin deficiencies, to name just a few possible causes. For this reason, physical findings are especially unreliable, by themselves, for diagnosis of a nutrition problem. Instead, their value is in revealing possible problems for other assessment techniques to confirm, or in confirming other assessment measures.

With this limitation understood, physical symptoms can be most informative; they communicate much information about nutrition health. Many tissues and organs can reflect signs of malnutrition. Physical signs of malnutrition appear most rapidly in parts of the body where cell replacement occurs at a high rate, such as in the hair, skin, and digestive tract (including the mouth and tongue). The summary tables in Chapters 8, 9, 10, and 11 list additional physical signs of vitamin and mineral malnutrition.

■ *Classification of Protein-Energy Malnutrition*

Health care providers use these assessment methods to determine a client's nutrition status. With this information in hand, they can suggest appropriate dietary modifications to correct imbalances. One form of malnutrition that can pervade any illness is protein-energy malnutrition (PEM). Many of the upcoming chapters refer to PEM repeatedly, and so this special section focuses on its classification. Health care providers classify PEM as either kwashiorkor, marasmus, or kwashiorkor-marasmus mix.

The person with kwashiorkor has normal or above-standard anthropometric measurements with below-normal indices of blood and organ proteins. Because the individual with kwashiorkor may be obese, malnutrition may easily be overlooked. Such a case illustrates clearly why the various compo-

■ TABLE 19–13
Physical Findings Used in Nutrition Assessments

Body System	Acceptable Findings	Malnutrition Findings	What It Reflects
Hair	Shiny, firm in the scalp	Dull, brittle, dry, loose; falls out	PEM
Eyes	Bright, clear pink membranes that adjust easily to light	Pale membranes; spots; redness; adjust slowly to darkness	Vitamin A, the B vitamins, zinc, and iron status
Teeth and gums	No pain or caries, gums firm, teeth bright	Missing, discolored, decayed teeth; gums bleed easily and are swollen and spongy	Mineral and vitamin C status
Face	Clear complexion without dryness or scaliness	Off-color, scaly, flaky, cracked skin	PEM, vitamin A, and iron status
Glands	No lumps	Swollen at front of neck, cheeks	PEM and iodine status
Tongue	Red, bumpy, rough	Sore, smooth, purplish, swollen	B vitamin status
Skin	Smooth, firm, good color	Dry, rough, spotty; "sandpaper" feel or sores; lack of fat under skin	PEM, vitamin A, the B vitamins, and vitamin C status
Nails	Firm, pink	Spoon-shaped, brittle, ridged	Iron status
Internal systems	Regular heart rhythm with a heart rate between 60 and 100 and blood pressure below 140/90; no impairment of digestive function, reflexes, or psychological development	Abnormal heart rate, heart rhythm, or blood pressure; enlarged liver, spleen; abnormal digestion; burning, tingling of hands, feet; loss of balance, coordination	PEM and mineral status
Muscles and bones	Muscle tone; posture, long bone development appropriate for age	"Wasted" appearance of muscles; swollen bumps on skull or ends of bones; small bumps on ribs; bowed legs or knock-knees	PEM and vitamin D status

Note: See Table E-13 in Appendix E for a summary of symptoms of vitamin and mineral deficiencies and toxicities.

nents of nutrition assessment (historical data, anthropometric measurements, biochemical analyses, and physical examinations) cannot be used individually to define nutrition assessment.

Marasmus takes on an appearance opposite to that of kwashiorkor. The individual with marasmus has blood and organ protein levels that appear to be adequate, while skeletal muscle and subcutaneous fat are depleted.

Kwashiorkor-marasmus mix malnutrition presents signs of depleted blood, organ, and skeletal muscle proteins as well as subcutaneous fat. The individual with this type of malnutrition has virtually no energy reserves and is in grave danger, especially if confronted with severe stress.

Above-normal anthropometric measures combined with normal blood protein levels identify a person consuming energy in excess of needs. Of course, excessive energy intake risks obesity and the many chronic diseases associated with it (see Chapter 12).

In addition to uncovering PEM and energy overnutrition, nutrition assessments help pinpoint vitamin and mineral deficiencies and toxicities, poor dietary practices, possible drug-nutrient interactions, and a host of other risk factors that alert the assessor that nutrition status could easily deteriorate. Many people enter the hospital malnourished on admission; malnutrition seriously impairs recovery from illness (see Chapter 18). Other people may enter the hospital in good nutrition status only to deteriorate during the course of hospitalization. Therefore, ongoing nutrition assessment is necessary to determine if nutrition therapy is working to correct nutrient deficiencies or maintain nutrition status.

Nutrition Screening

nutrition screening: the use of preliminary nutrition assessment techniques to identify people who are malnourished or who are at risk for malnutrition.

As you can tell from the many previous pages of text, thorough nutrition assessment requires much time and money—both guarded commodities in health care today. (Highlight 30 discusses many of the issues surrounding nutrition and cost containment.) One way to help reduce the costs of nutrition assessment is to use nutrition screening techniques.

Collecting detailed information on each person entering the hospital may not be practical or even essential. A strategic compromise is to screen clients by collecting preliminary data and to observe each client for signs of problems that may change nutrition status. A basic nutrition screening includes the following:

- Reviewing the individual's diet, drug, and medical history. Does the person's history reveal risk factors for poor nutrition status (review Table 19–2)?
- Weighing each person on admission and at regular intervals during the hospital stay. Is the person's weight for height adequate, but not excessive? Has the person been losing or gaining weight? How much? How fast?
- Checking the available lab reports. Do serum albumin, total lymphocyte count, hemoglobin, and hematocrit suggest malnutrition? Are additional tests indicated?
- Looking at the person. Are there obvious signs of malnutrition (review Table 19–13)? Is the client emaciated? Obese? Extremely pale?

In addition to the above nutrition assessment procedures, take the opportunity to:

- Check the client's tray to see if food is being eaten. If the client is to receive no food or is unable to eat, how long has it been since the client has eaten? Is the client expected to be able to eat soon? Are adequate nutrients being delivered by vein? (The box in Chapter 22 shows how to calculate the nutrient content of intravenous solutions.)
- Most important, communicate any problems that you discover and follow up to make sure the problem is being handled. Always record problems in the medical record to ensure that whoever cares for a particular client will be alert to the problem. A dietitian will perform a more in-depth nutrition assessment if a problem is detected. Be persistent if you suspect that a problem is being ignored.

Nutrition screening identifies common problems that place clients at risk for malnutrition. It is especially important in health care settings where nutrition assessments are not routinely performed on each client. One study showed that nutrition screening at admission in 33 hospitals identified risk for poor nutrition status in over 50 percent of the clients for whom enough information was available to perform the screening.[16]

To know what is wrong with a person's nutrition status is not to remedy it. All the effort expended in evaluating a person's nutrition problems will be for naught if it is not used to formulate a plan of action that will correct nutrition problems. That plan will need to include an estimation of nutrient needs.

■ *Estimation of Nutrient Needs*

Nutrition assessment generates the information necessary to estimate nutrient needs (step two of the five steps outlined on the first page of this chapter). Assessors generally estimate energy and protein needs first by any of many methods. Always keep in mind that these estimates are just that—estimates. An individual's response to the nutrition program indicates the individual's needs better than estimates can.

The energy equation provided in Table 19–14 is widely used and is known as the Harris-Benedict Equation (after the researchers who developed it).

■ **TABLE 19–14**
Estimation of Energy Needs

Basal energy expenditure (BEE)[a]
  Women
    BEE = 655 + [9.6 × wt in kg[b]] + [1.7 × ht in cm[b]] − [4.7 × age in years]
  Men
    BEE = 66 + [13.7 × wt in kg] + [5 × ht in cm] − [6.8 × age in years]
Add to BEE for activity
    20% Sedentary
    35% Moderately active
    50% Active
Add to BEE for stress
    10–15% Uncomplicated elective surgery
    20–40% Complicated surgery or fractures
    50–100% Major burn
Add to BEE for fever (if present)
    13% per degree centigrade over normal body temperature (37° C).[b]
Add to BEE for growth (if necessary)
    5% Moderate weight loss
    10–15% Severe weight loss
For people with a %IBW greater than 125, adjust the weight used in the BEE equation by following this equation:[c]
    (Actual body weight − IBW) × 25%[d] + IBW = Adjusted body weight

[a]The equation used to determine basal energy expenditure (BEE) is the Harris-Benedict Equation frequently used to estimate energy needs. Basal metabolic rate (BMR, described on p. 357) and BEE express the same thing: basal energy need. The equation for BMR is traditionally used in physiology and fitness laboratories; that for BEE, in hospitals. The two equations yield slightly different results, each suitable for the purposes intended. The increments for activity used in the hospital differ from those on p. 357 for similar reasons. All are approximations; all require judgment in their application.
[b]See Appendix D for equations to convert kg, cm, and degrees centigrade.
[c]Source: J. M. Karkeck, Adjustment for obesity, *American Dietetic Association Renal Practice Group Newsletter,* Winter 1984.
[d]Approximately 25% of body fat tissue is metabolically active.

How to Estimate Energy and Protein Needs

Marjorie is a 50-year-old woman who is 5 ft 4 inches tall and weighs 118 lbs. She is a sedentary individual who currently has the flu with a 101° F temperature.

Before using the Harris-Benedict Equation for BEE, convert weight in pounds to weight in kilograms:

$$\frac{118 \text{ lb}}{2.2 \text{ lb/kg}} = 54 \text{ kg.}$$

Then convert height in inches to height in centimeters:

64 inches × 2.54 cm/inch = 163 cm.

Then place the weight, height, and age factors into the equation for women:

BEE = 655 + (9.6 × 54 kg) + (1.7 × 163 cm) − (4.7 × 50)
BEE = 655 + 518 + 277 − 235 = 1,215 kcal.

Thus, Marjorie needs 1,215 kcal to meet her basal energy needs.
Next, to account for the activity level, multiply the BEE by 20%:

1,215 kcal × .20 = 243 kcal.

Thus, Marjorie needs an additional 243 kcal to meet her sedentary activity energy needs.
Then, before accounting for the fever, convert degrees Fahrenheit to degrees centigrade:

°C = 5⁄9 (°F − 32°).
°C = 5⁄9 (101° − 32°).

Table 19–14 shows the equation for calculating the basal energy expenditure (BEE) using the Harris-Benedict Equation and how to modify the BEE to account for various levels of activity, stress, and weight gain (see the accompanying box for an example of how to use this equation).

Indirect calorimetry offers a better determination of energy needs than estimates can provide. Using a portable machine that measures oxygen consumption and carbon dioxide production, a trained clinician can determine an individual's resting energy expenditure. Indirect calorimetry can be extremely valuable in cases where there is little room for error, such as for critically ill people. Excessive energy intake overworks the heart and leads to metabolic changes that compromise an already stressed individual.[17] On the other hand, too little energy compromises the ability to recover from the stress of surgery, heal surgical wounds, and fight infection. However, indirect calorimetry has its problems. Technical difficulties can interfere with test results, limiting the usefulness of this method.[18]

Nitrogen balance studies provide a good estimate of protein needs when conducted accurately. However, because of the difficulty in conducting nitrogen balance studies, their use is limited. Medical centers that use the

°C = ⅝ (69°).
°C = 38°.

Knowing that normal body temperature is 37° C, determine how much fever she has:

38° C − 37° C = 1° C.

To determine the percentage of the BEE needed due to fever, multiply the number of fever degrees by 13%:

1° × .13 = 13%.

Then multiply the BEE by the %BEE needed for fever:

1,215 kcal × .13 = 158 kcal.

Finally, add the values for activity and fever to the BEE to determine total energy requirements:

1,215 kcal + 243 kcal + 158 kcal = 1,616 kcal.

Remember that this equation only estimates Marjorie's energy needs; her actual needs may be higher or lower. Consequently her energy intake may have to be adjusted.

Using Table 19−15 to estimate protein needs, you will find that Marjorie needs 1.5 g/protein per kg/body wt. To determine protein needs, use the weight in kg value calculated earlier:

$$54 \text{ kg} \times \frac{1.5 \text{ g}}{\text{kg}} = 81 \text{ g protein.}$$

nitrogen balance method limit their studies to people in hypermetabolic states or to those who otherwise have nitrogen requirements that are difficult to estimate. For most people, assessors estimate protein requirements using factors such as those provided in Table 19−15.

Vitamin and mineral needs are highly variable, and they are often difficult to estimate. Exact requirements vary not only from individual to individual, but needs for certain nutrients can be dramatically altered by different states

■ TABLE 19−15
Estimating Protein Needs

State of Health	Protein needs (g protein/kg body weight)
Normal, healthy	0.8−1.0
Fever, fracture, infection	1.5−2.0
Protein depleted	1.5−2.0
Extensive burns	1.5−3.0

Note: Protein needs for other disorders are given in Chapters 23 through 30.

▶▶ CLINICAL DETECTIVE WORK

Each client presents you with a unique case. Clients come in all shapes and sizes, with a variety of life experiences and medical conditions. In a sense, you are a clinical detective, searching through the facts to find clues as to how to best care for your clients. Use the "Clinical Detective Work" exercises to hone your investigative skills.

Ms. Green, a 38-year-old computer scientist, was admitted to the hospital for testing following a car accident. Her injuries included several broken bones and a collapsed left lung. Her lab report revealed a mildly depleted serum albumin and a moderately depleted total lymphocyte count. After reviewing her health record, the health care team decided that a complete nutrition assessment was necessary. The following significant information resulted.

Health History:
Increased nutrient requirements due to the injuries sustained in the car accident.

Socioeconomic History:
Lives alone; her busy schedule seldom leaves time for her to prepare meals so she often eats at fast-food restaurants.
Money for food and facilities for food preparation are adequate.

Drug History:
One standard multivitamin-mineral daily.
No other drugs.

Diet History:
Weight loss intentional.
Very low kcalorie, low-carbohydrate diet over the past six weeks.

Anthropometric Measurements:
Height: 5 ft 9 inches.
Weight: 150 lb.
Usual weight: 175 lb.
Frame size: medium.

Lab Tests

Biochemical Analyses:
Serum albumin: 3 g/100 ml (mildly depleted).
Total lymphocyte count: 1,000 mm^3 (moderately depleted).

Physical Examination:
Hair: dull, easily plucked.
Other: none noted.

Determine Ms. Green's ideal body weight, and calculate percent ideal body weight. Calculate her percent usual body weight. Consider Ms. Green's recent weight change. What is a safe rate of weight loss (see p. 000)? How does Ms. Green's weight loss compare with the safe rate? Does her recent weight change increase her risk of poor nutrition status?

What do Ms. Green's lab values indicate with respect to her protein status? Are there any other factors in Ms. Green's health, diet, socioeconomic, or drug history, or physical findings suggestive of malnutrition?

Based on Ms. Green's nutrition assessment, you determine that she is at risk for PEM. Calculate her estimated protein and energy needs. Discuss how PEM can affect Ms. Green's health status if her nutrient needs are not met. What steps can you take to ensure that Ms. Green's nutrient needs are being met?

of health. For healthy individuals, health care providers generally use RDA levels of nutrients to estimate nutrient needs. Although the RDA figures are not intended for this purpose, they are really the only available guidelines. For those who are ill, exact vitamin and mineral needs can only be estimated. More information about vitamin and mineral needs in different disorders will be discussed in Chapters 23 through 30.

Armed with the information from the assessment and with an estimate of nutrient needs, a dietitian can develop a plan of action to either maintain or improve the individual's nutrition status. Chapter 20 provides details of how nutrition assessment information is translated into a nutrition care plan.

 SELF STUDY *Nutrition Assessment*

Students use this book for a variety of purposes. Those who are studying to be nurses may never perform nutrition assessments themselves, but may be expected to understand such assessments and keep the findings in mind when working with clients. Those who are studying to be clinical dietitians may perform such assessments routinely. Therefore different personal uses of the information in this chapter may be appropriate for different students: your instructor may require you to conduct a diet interview with a partner or client; to practice some anthropometric measures under supervision; to interpret some sample physical and laboratory data; or all of these.

Study Questions

1. What are the steps in the nutrition care process that can be used to identify nutrition problems?
2. Describe the four components of nutrition assessment and what each can reveal.
3. Describe the purpose of obtaining food intake data.
4. What are the advantages and disadvantages of the 24-hour recall, usual food intake, food diary, and the food frequency checklist?
5. How do anthropometric measurements help define nutrition status? What anthropometric measurements are frequently used in nutrition assessments?
6. How do lab tests help define nutrition status? Describe the lab tests used to uncover PEM. Which tests can be used to uncover iron deficiency?
7. What is the purpose of nutrition screening? List screening techniques.
8. Describe some ways of estimating energy, protein, vitamin, and mineral needs.

Notes

1. K. J. Morgan and coauthors, Collection of food intake data: An evaluation of methods, *Journal of the American Dietetic Association* 87 (1987): 888–896.
2. J. T. Dwyer, E. A. Krall, K. A. Coleman, The problem of memory in nutritional epidemiology research, *Journal of the American Dietetic Association* 87 (1987): 1509–1512.
3. R. S. Gibson, *Principles of Nutritional Assessment* (New York: Oxford University Press, 1990), p. 172.
4. S. B. Heymsfield and K. Casper, Anthropometric assessment of the adult hospitalized patient, *Journal of Parenteral and Enteral Nutrition* (supplement) 11 (1987): 36–41.
5. J. P. Grant, Nutritional assessment in clinical practice, *Nutrition in Clinical Practice* 1 (1986): 3–11.
6. K. N. Jeejeebhoy, A. S. Detsky, and J. P. Baker, Assessment of nutrition status, *Journal of Parenteral and Enteral Nutrition* (supplement) 14 (1990): 193–196.
7. J. D. Marshall and coauthors, Comparison of convenient indicators of obesity, *American Journal of Clinical Nutrition* 51 (1990): 22–28; R. F. Kushner and coauthors, Validation of bioelectrical-impedance analysis as a measurement of change in body composition in obesity, *American Journal of Clinical Nutrition* 52 (1990): 219–223; R. N. Baumgartner, W. C. Chumlea, and A. F. Roche, Estimation of body composition from bioelectrical impedance of body segments, *American Journal of Clinical Nutrition* 50 (1989): 221–226.
8. D. S. Gray and coauthors, Effect of obesity on bioelectrical impedance, *American Journal of Clinical*

Nutrition 50 (1989): 255–260; L. Henson, Practical clinical assessment of body composition, *Nutrition and the M.D.*, August 1988, pp. 1–3.

9. A. S. Jackson and M. L. Pollack, Practical assessment of body composition, *The Physician and Sportsmedicine* May 1985, pp. 76–90.

10. F. I. Katch and coauthors, Letter to the editor: Validity of bioelectrical impedance to estimate body composition in cardiac and pulmonary patients, *American Journal of Clinical Nutrition* 43 (1986): 972–973.

11. F. Kalfarentzos and coauthors, Comparison of forearm muscle dynamometry with nutritional prognostic index, as a preoperative indicator in cancer patients, *Journal of Parenteral and Enteral Nutrition* 13 (1989): 34–36.

12. A. E. Webb and coauthors, Hand-grip dynamometry as a predictory of postoperative complications: Reappraisal using age standardized grip strengths, *Journal of Parenteral and Enteral Nutrition* 13 (1989): 30–33.

13. J. A. Tayek, Albumin synthesis and nutritional assessment, *Nutrition in Clinical Practice* 3 (1988): 219–221.

14. Jeejeebhoy, Detsky, and Baker, 1990.

15. Gibson, 1990, p. 309.

16. S. K. Kamath and coauthors, Hospital malnutrition: A 33-hospital screening study, *Journal of the American Dietetic Association* 86 (1986): 203–206.

17. F. B. Serra, How nutrition intervention changes what getting sick means, *Journal of Parental and Enteral Nutrition* (supplement) 14 (1990): 164–169.

18. S. M. Campbell and K. A. Kudsk, "High tech" metabolic measurements: Useful in daily clinical practice? *Journal of Parenteral and Enteral Nutrition* 12 (1988): 610–612.

Computers in Nutrition Care

Computers have become valuable fixtures in our lives; we use them at home and in school, for business and for pleasure. Some people have grown so accustomed to computers that they have little appreciation for the ways computers have changed our lives. If you remain unimpressed by computers, consider the words of Christopher Evans, author of *The Micro Millennium:* "If the automobile industry had developed at the same rate as computers and over the same amount of time, you would be able to buy a Rolls-Royce today for $2.75; it would get 3 million miles to the gallon and would deliver enough power to drive the *Queen Elizabeth II* oceanliner. And, if you were interested in miniaturization, you could put half a dozen of them on a pinhead."

This highlight explores some of the ways that health care professionals use computers to provide effective nutrition care. The miniglossary on the next page defines some terms related to computers.

Computer Systems

In hospitals and other health care settings, computer systems generally consist of a main computer connected with a network of terminals conveniently located at various stations throughout the facility. For example, in the hospital, each nursing station has a terminal. Other terminals are located in various departments, such as foodservice, accounts receivable, and the pharmacy. Such an arrangement allows health care providers and administrative staff to share information and communicate with one another. Some health care settings provide departments with individual computers that do not share in a network system. While such arrangements allow health care

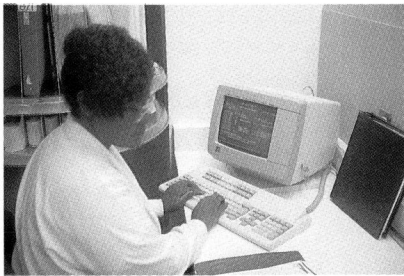

Computers assist professionals in providing effective health care.

providers to do their work, they do not provide direct communication between departments via computers.

Computer network systems can store much information and make it readily retrievable from a number of locations, dramatically saving time and reducing operating expenses. As an example, consider the computer billing system currently in use in most hospitals. Health care providers order everything for a hospital client—drugs, diet, intravenous fluids, x-rays, physical therapy treatments, and other supplies and professional services—via computer. In years past, nurses would call in various orders for each of many clients to different departments and then ensure that each client was appropriately billed for the supplies or services. You can imagine how much time this took, not only for the nurses but also for the departments receiving the orders for supplies and services.

From this example you can also see how computer systems help save time for direct client care and reduce human error. Verbal communications raise the likelihood that errors will occur. If a nurse orders an intravenous feeding by phone while worried about the client in Room 425 and the pharmacist at the other end of the line is in a noisy room, the chances of an error in communication escalate. With

printed communication (as occurs when ordered by computer), the information can be checked and verified.

Hundreds of computer software programs are available in the field of food science and human nutrition. The challenge for students, dietitians, and researchers is to determine which programs will best serve their particular needs. Publications such as *Nutrition Today, Journal of Nutrition Education,* and the *Journal of the American Dietetic Association* regularly feature articles that describe, evaluate, and recommend nutrition computer software programs. Anyone contemplating the purchase of a program would benefit from a review of the literature.

Computers in Health Care Facilities

Computers can help health care professionals with each step of the nutrition care process. Researchers have even developed a "thinking" computer program that provides a nutrition care plan based on a client's diet history, lifestyle habits, laboratory test results, and family history.[1] Given the client's medical profile, the program recommends a care plan that reflects the current knowledge of medical and dietetic experts. But although computers can perform a multitude of time-consuming tasks quickly and even make reasonable recommendations, they cannot replace health care professionals, as the following sections show.

Nutrition Assessment
Computer programs can help dietitians and other health care providers to attain a nutrition assessment in the following manner. First, a dietitian must collect the appropriate data (as described in Chapter 19). Then, the

■ ■

Miniglossary

bit: short for *binary digit;* the smallest unit of computer information.

byte: a sequence of bits.

database: the body of information stored by the computer.

diskette: a thin, flexible magnetic disk protected in a jacket and used to store or read computer information.

display screen: the televisionlike monitor, part of the terminal, that allows computer users to see what they are working on.

floppy disk: another name for a diskette.

hard copy: a printed copy of the information stored in the computer.

hardware: mechanical, magnetic, or electronic equipment used to process data. The hardware limits the type of software that can be used (see also *software*).

input: the information that is entered into the computer.

mainframe computer: a large computer capable of storing vast amounts of data. Mainframe computers can perform multiple functions very rapidly and are used by many large businesses, research centers, and universities.

microcomputer: a small computer capable of performing functions similar to mainframe computers. Microcomputers are relatively inexpensive computers frequently found in hospitals and small businesses.

output: the information that the computer prints out on paper or displays on the terminal screen.

program: the set of step-by-step instructions that tell the computer how to perform a task (see also *software*).

software: computer programs that allow the user to perform various functions. Not all software can be used with every computer; hardware and software must be compatible (see also *hardware*).

terminal: a keyboard and display screen that allow the user to access and process the information stored in a computer.

---

computer can rapidly perform the many mathematical calculations required and compare the data with the standards. Thus, in addition to storing, printing, and retrieving assessment data, computers can help with interpretation. By using computers, dietitians can efficiently identify specific nutrient needs and individuals at risk for poor nutrition status.

With the knowledge gained from an assessment, a dietitian can develop a plan of action for meeting a client's needs—both dietary and educational. Computer programs can assist here, too.

Diet Analysis

Perhaps the most commonly used of the nutrition software programs, diet analysis programs estimate the nutrients in a diet and compare intakes to dietary standards such as the RDA. To complete this task without the aid of a computer requires much time and abundant patience. With a diet analysis program, a dietitian can quickly see where a diet fails to meet recommendations. Such a program serves a dietitian both in assessment and in planning. Dietitians can design diets and compare them with the specifications of a diet order.

In the classroom, students might use

diet analysis programs to see how their diets compare to the RDA. Figure H19–1 illustrates the types of information provided by a diet analysis program.

Management

Computer programs can also assist with the management of dietary operations and resources. For example, they can help managers to determine fees for services, to distribute workloads among dietitians and staff evenly, and to monitor adherence to standards of care.[2]

Foodservice

In the foodservice department, computers can not only store recipes but they can quickly calculate the number of meals and amounts of food to prepare. They can analyze meals and products for various nutrients instantaneously, print menus, maintain a current inventory, and generate orders according to predicted needs.

Clinical Management

Computers can combine the menu files from the foodservice department with specific diet orders to generate a list of food options for each client.[3] For example, computer programs can develop diet patterns for people with diabetes or phenylketonuria and provide a list of permitted foods from which to select meals.[4]

When food is not on a client's menu, computer programs can assist dietitians in the selection of an alternative feeding program, for example, a tube-feeding formula. As you will see in Chapter 21, a dietitian must consider much information when choosing a tube-feeding formula and a method of delivery. The decisions can be overwhelming, especially when the client has several medical conditions that affect nutrient needs. Computer programs have been developed to help manage these many considerations. Similarly, computer programs help practitioners plan intravenous therapy as well. Computer

FIGURE H19–1
Sample Printout from a Diet Analysis Program

To analyze the breakfast depicted on p. 36, each item was entered into the computer using a diet analysis program. The following data show the nutrients provided by the breakfast items: the first column of numbers represents the actual quantities, whereas the second column and the graph below present each quantity as a percentage of the U.S. RDA.

```
Breakfast      (Plus % RDA for Labels - U.S. RDA)
------------------------------------------------------------------
Items analyzed:                        Code
     1 cup  Coffee-brewed              1389
     1 cup  Oatmeal cereal-prepared    1238
   .25 cup  Raisins-seedless-unpacked   330
     1 cup  Skim milk / nonfat milk      73
  1.25 cup  Strawberries-fresh          336
------------------------------------------------------------------
Weight:    941 Grams ( 33.2 oz.)      Water weight:      836 G

Calories          398     *      Vitamin B6     0.345 Mg      17%
Protein          16.9 G         37%  Vitamin B12    0.926 Mcg     15%
Carbohydrates    80.2 G    **    Folacin         59.8 Mcg     15%
Dietary Fiber    11.1 G    #     Pantothenic     1.93 Mg  *   19%
Fat-Total        3.65 G    **    Vitamin C        109 Mg      182%
Fat-Saturated   0.804 G    **    Vitamin E       0.882 Mg      9%
Fat-Mono        0.969 G    **    Calcium          369 Mg       37%
Fat-Poly         1.29 G    **    Copper          0.409 Mg  *   20%
Cholesterol      4.00 Mg   **    Iron            3.27 Mg       18%
Vit A-Carotene   9.93 RE         Magnesium        130 Mg       32%
Vit A-Preformed   149 RE         Phosphorus       498 Mg       50%
Vit A-Total       159 RE    16%  Potassium       1248 Mg  *
Thiamin-B1       0.442 Mg   29%  Selenium        30.7 Mcg
Riboflavin-B2    0.546 Mg   32%  Sodium           141 Mg  *
Niacin-B3        1.78 Mg     9%  Zinc            2.50 Mg       17%
------------------------------------------------------------------
       *  Suggested values; within recommended ranges
      ** Dietary Goals     # Fiber = 1 gram/100 kcal
```

Abbreviations: Poly/Sat = polyunsaturated to saturated fatty acid ratio; Sod/Pot = sodium to potassium ratio; Ca/Phos = calcium to phosphorus ratio; CSI = cholesterol saturated fat index (CSI = 1.01 × grams of saturated fat + 0.05 × mg of cholesterol).

```
                   Percentage of recommended amounts

              0    20    40    60    80   100   120   140
              +---+---+---+---+---+---+---+---+---+---+---+---+
Protein       ================= (37)
Vit A-Total   ======= (16)
Thiamin-B1    ============= (29)
Riboflavin-B2 ============== (32)
Niacin-B3     ===== (9)
Vitamin B6    ======= (17)
Vitamin B12   ====== (15)
Folacin       ====== (15)
Pantothenic   ======== (19)
Vitamin C     ===================================================== >>182>
Vitamin E     ===== (9)
Calcium       ================= (37)
Copper        ======== (20)
Iron          ======= (18)
Magnesium     ============== (32)
Phosphorus    ===================== (50)
Zinc          ======= (17)
```

programs can also integrate the many factors that health care providers must consider when determining whether a client is responding adequately to nutrition care, thus saving valuable time.

Clinical dietitians also use computers to compile the many reports that assist them in their daily work. For example, the computer can quickly generate lists of clients at nutrition risk (those receiving nothing by mouth, clear-liquids, full-liquids, or pureed diets for 3 or more days); those on tube-feedings; and those on special diets (such as diabetes, weight-control, protein-restricted, or modified-fat diets).

Education

Dietitians use computers to teach clients. Computer programs can inform clients of how diet influences their disease condition and of the specific foods that need to be included or excluded. For example, a program might help clients to understand the association between sodium and hypertension and how to identify the sodium content of foods. Programs are also available in the areas of weight control, diabetes, and hyperlipidemias, to name a few.

Outside the hospital, computers teach students about clinical nutrition. Clinical case studies that simulate real-life situations give students practice in dealing with clients and their special needs. The students can work at their own pace, and the instructor has a record of the students' responses. Other programs teach nutrition by giving students information and then asking them to answer questions based on the information given.

Outside the classroom, other programs educate consumers about food and nutrition in general. For example, they might provide shopping information such as how to read food labels, determine unit prices, plan meals, and reduce the amount of food wastage.

Computers as Tools

It seems that the more we use computers, the more uses we find for them. However, without a human being to interpret the information generated, computers lose their value. Our increasing dependence on computers sometimes makes it difficult to remember that computers are tools—machines programmed to perform as instructed by human beings. They possess no human qualities such as knowledge, emotions, or common sense; they cannot make judgments. If a hypertensive client who has been refusing meals and losing weight asks for a bacon, lettuce, and tomato sandwich, a dietitian might grant such a request even if the diet order specifies no bacon on a low-sodium diet. A computer could not make such a decision.

Nor can a computer see a client's reaction to dietary instructions. Computers cannot detect changes in a client's body language that might alert a professional that the client is uncomfortable with a diet plan. In short, computer programs can be a valuable tool, but they cannot replace human beings.

As much as computers save time, they also require much time. In many cases, an experienced dietitian can estimate the nutrients in a meal, within a reasonable margin of error, in less time than it takes to enter the data in a computer.

Computers are also only as error-free as the human beings who design, program, and use

them—which is to say that computers are less than perfect. Diet analysis programs illustrate the point.

A diet analysis program estimates the amounts of various nutrients in a diet and compares them to a standard such as the RDA. Accuracy depends on both the food record that is entered into the computer and the food composition values that were recorded into the database. Remember that databases are not perfect; they, too, are created by human beings. Inaccurate values in the database make the results of an analysis meaningless. Furthermore, even with complete and accurate values, the program user must interpret the results appropriately. To adequately interpret a computer diet analysis, a user must understand that nutrient values are estimates, that food composition varies, and that individual requirements for different nutrients also vary. Without such a clear understanding, individuals might have misconceptions about the data, even with the printout explanations and the accompanying computer program literature.[5]

This highlight has explored several applications of computers in nutrition care. By using computers, professionals can perform their jobs efficiently and save valuable time. No doubt computers will continue to play a significant role in the health care profession.

NOTES

1. "Smart" computers provide nutrition advice for coronary risk patients, *Journal of the American Dietetic Association* 89 (1989): 676.
2. K. M. Duffy, B. A. Fromm, and D. A. Sorensen, A computer-assisted management information system for nutrition services, *Journal of the American Dietetic Association* 89 (1989): 1296–1300.
3. M. G. Ford, The computer as an aid in clinical management, *Journal of the American Dietetic Association* 87 (1987): 497–500.
4. J. L. Balintfy and L. M. Lancaster, Computing "best fit" calorie-controlled diet patterns by microcomputer, *Journal of the American Dietetic Association* 87 (1987): 73–74; K. Anderson, B. Kennedy, and P. B. Acosta, Computer-implemented nutrition support of phenylketonuria, *Journal of the American Dietetic Association* 12 (1985): 1623–1625.
5. C. Byrd-Bredbenner and coauthors, Computer-analyzed dietary intake printouts: Guidelines for their design and student comprehension, *Journal of the American Dietetic Association* 88 (1988): 311–316.

Nutrition Care Strategies

Nutrition care attends to all nutrients equally, but for this opening photo, vitamin B$_6$ is singled out. Its feathery crystals adorned the cover of the second edition of this book.

Chapter 19 presented the first two steps in providing effective nutrition intervention. It showed how to assess a client's nutrition status and how to analyze the assessment data to determine a client's nutrient needs. This chapter begins by describing the next three steps: how to develop, implement, and evaluate nutrition care. Then, because nutrition care provides clients with both nutrients and nutrition education, the remainder of the chapter presents a general, behind-the-scenes look at the procedures and communication skills needed to feed clients and teach them about their nutrition needs.

■ Nutrition Care Plans

A dietitian uses a nutrition care plan to state what a client needs (nutritionally speaking) and how to best meet these needs. The plan clearly defines the intervention strategies necessary to meet both the client's nutrient and nutrition education needs.

Objectives of a nutrition care plan:
- To meet the client's nutrition needs.
- To educate the client.

Development of Nutrition Care Plans

The first step in developing a nutrition care plan is to study the information gleaned from analyzing the nutrition assessment data. Does the history show potential nutrition problems? Is body weight appropriate? Are lab values out of line? Are there physical signs of malnutrition? This information generates a nutrition problem list and forms the basis of the care plan. Among the problems assessors list are current and past conditions that impair nutrition status, as well as areas that may present future problems. Form 20–1 provides a sample nutrition assessment and care plan summary.

Working together, health care professionals can help each other to assess clients' situations accurately. For example, a nurse may notice that the socioeconomic history section on the assessment form says that an elderly client lives with his son's family. That statement might bring to mind the image of family members gathered around a dining table, enjoying nutritious meals and each other's company. Yet the client has mentioned to the nurse that the family is always so busy coming and going that they never eat a meal together. Sure, there's always dinner for him at 6:00 each evening, but he usually eats alone. This could explain his lack of appetite and recent weight loss. By providing the dietitian with this bit of information, the nurse adds to the dietitian's understanding of the client, and possibly enhances the nutrition care the client receives.

With a problem list in hand, a dietitian can develop a plan that specifies the objectives of the diet, the content of counseling sessions, and a tentative time frame for accomplishing each objective. If, for example, a client needs to lose weight (the objective), the dietitian might set a goal of one pound a week for three months (the time frame). That specific goal helps the dietitian to design the weight-loss program. It determines that the diet will provide 500 kcalories less than the client's energy expenditure each day; that the diet will be low in fat and high in carbohydrate; and that exercise activity should be aerobic (the areas of content).

■ FORM 20–1

Sample Nutrition Assessment and Care Plan Summary
After analyzing the assessment data as described in Chapter 19, the health care provider summarizes the findings and develops a care plan using this form.

Client: _____   Diet Order: _____

ASSESSMENT SUMMARY

Anthropometric Data: _____

_____

Biochemical Data: _____

_____

Health Data: _____

_____

Socioeconomic Data: _____

_____

Drug-Nutrient Interactions: _____

_____

Dietary Intake Data: _____

_____

Recommend Additional Screening: Yes/No _____

NUTRITION CARE PLAN SUMMARY

Problem List: 1. _____
                2. _____
                3. _____
                4. _____
                5. _____

Proposed Nutrition Care: _____

_____

Other Therapy: _____

_____

Education: _____

_____

Compliance/Understanding: _____

_____

Follow-Up: _____

_____

Date: _____   Dietitian: _____

For each nutrition problem, the dietitian specifies the strategies needed to tackle it. The strategies provide detailed plans for reaching specific goals and depend on the reason for the problem. For example, the problem of diarrhea requires an understanding of its cause before the dietitian can develop a successful strategy. If the diarrhea has developed in response to drug therapy, an appropriate strategy might be to request that the physician prescribe a different drug, or to provide the client with ample fluids and electrolytes to prevent dehydration. If the diarrhea is caused by a milk allergy, then eliminating milk and milk products from the diet is a critical problem-solving strategy.

In addition to meeting the client's nutrient needs, the nutrition care plan also provides for nutrition education. For example, the client needs instructions and suggestions for following a diet that eliminates milk and milk products.

Implementation of Nutrition Care Plans

Once care plan strategies have been developed, the next step is to implement them. This step includes providing the appropriate diet and education. Again, thanks to frequent daily contact with clients, nurses can provide clients and dietitians with information that can improve nutrition care. It is not unusual for clients to have questions after a dietary education session—quite often hours after the dietitian has left. And so, the client asks the next person to walk into the room—quite likely, the nurse. The nurse who is confident of the answers should provide them. Otherwise, the nurse should express honest uncertainty as to the answer and agree to check with the dietitian. The nurse may decide to inform the dietitian that the client needs a follow-up visit to clarify a few points.

As the care process continues, the plan may change. For example, a person admitted to the hospital for a diagnostic workup may later become a candidate for surgery. Adjustments in the care plan need to parallel the client's changing needs. Be on the alert for changes in health status so that nutrition needs will not be neglected. Suggest a new plan if the original plan falls short.

Evaluation of Nutrition Care Plans

As the planned strategies are implemented, the dietitian must begin to carefully evaluate the care plan. Are the strategies meeting the needs of the client? (If not, change strategies.) Have events occurred in the client's life that have changed nutrition status or altered nutrient needs? (If so, assess again.) Is the client able to make the suggested dietary changes? (If not, identify the obstacles and find solutions.)

The nutrition care process allows dietitians to identify nutrition needs and solve nutrition problems. But the plan is only as good as the information obtained to develop it. Nurses' and other team members' contributions can add quality information to the plan.

Part of the nutrition care plan specifies how clients will receive the nutrients they need. Most commonly, clients receive nutrients by way of meals prepared by the hospital kitchen. (Chapters 21 and 22 present alternative feeding methods.) From time to time, feeding clients in hospitals presents health care providers with unique problems. To facilitate their care of the clients, health care providers need an understanding of the general procedures underlying foodservice in health care facilities.

■ *Foodservice in Health Care Facilities*

This discussion uses the hospital as an example of a health care facility because of its familiarity to most health care providers. Other long-term care facilities such as nursing homes and mental institutions use similar foodservice systems, so the information presented applies to those settings as well. However, additional concerns arise in long-term care facilities. A person in a short-term care facility may eat poorly while hospitalized, but may make up for nutrient deficits by eating well at home. The resident in a long-term care facility continuously depends on the foodservice department to provide nutritious foods, and also to make them acceptable. It benefits no one, after all, to provide nutritious foods to a person who cannot or will not eat; the foodservice department of a long-term care facility must ensure that clients on special diets not only receive, but also eat, the appropriate foods.

The responsibility of preparing and serving food in a health care setting rests with either a chief administrative dietitian or a foodservice manager. (The accompanying miniglossary defines these and related terms.) These professionals direct all aspects of foodservice—from purchasing foods to delivering meals to clients.

The clinical dietitian works directly with clients to assess their nutrition status, to plan appropriate diets, and to provide nutrition education. In some facilities, dietetic technicians assist dietitians in both administrative and clinical responsibilities. Other dietary employees include clerks, aides, cooks, porters, and other assistants. Keep in mind that only dietitians have extensive formal training in nutrition. Other dietary employees do not have such training, and their ability to interpret diet orders or provide accurate information may be limited.

Many hospitals provide menus from which clients can select their meals. Clients who must follow a special diet receive menus that list only appropriate food selections. This system helps to ensure that clients will receive foods they enjoy and will eat. It also gives clients the feeling of having control over something in the hospital environment.

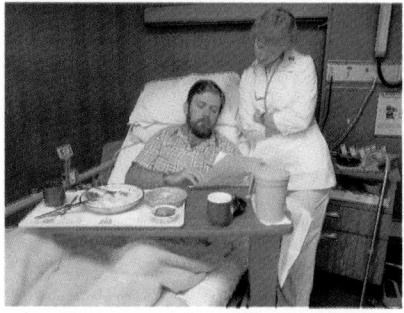

By selecting foods from a menu, clients receive meals they enjoy and gain some control over their hospital stay.

selective menu: a menu from which clients can select the foods they will receive while hospitalized.

Miniglossary of Dietitian Terms

ADA: the American Dietetic Association, the professional organization of dietitians in the United States. The Canadian equivalent is the Canadian Dietetic Association, which operates similarly.

administrative dietitian: a dietitian (see *registered dietitian,* below) who is primarily concerned with the management of a foodservice system that provides optimal nutrition and quality food. Administrative dietitians sometimes assume some clinical duties as well.

clinical dietitian: a dietitian responsible for direct client care—assessing nutrition needs, developing and implementing nutrition care plans, and evaluating and reporting the results.

dietetic technician registered (DTR): a technically skilled person with an associate's degree who meets the ADA's educational standards, and who works under the guidance of an RD (registered dietitian).

registered dietitian (RD): a trained professional with at least a bachelor's degree in nutrition and food science; a year's internship at an ADA-approved facility or the equivalent; and a passing score on the national registration exam (a four-hour qualifying exam administered over six competency areas by the ADA).

In a **centralized foodservice** system, the staff prepares and serves meals from a main kitchen. In a **decentralized foodservice** system, the staff prepares the meals in a central kitchen and then delivers them to small satellite kitchens elsewhere in the institution. These satellite kitchens then heat and distribute the meals.

Highlight 19 describes how computers assist health care providers in placing diet orders, reporting diet changes, and making special diet requests.

Some facilities do not offer selective menus; their dietary departments serve a standard house diet, adjusting the basic, balanced diet according to dietary orders as necessary. Generally, even these menus provide some flexibility, though. For example, a client can find out what foods will be served at dinner and can request simple changes, such as the substitution of one vegetable for another.

You can help your clients greatly, as well as save yourself needless aggravation and time, by learning about the foodservice system in the health care facility where you work. Some of the things you will want to know include:

- The number to call and the procedure to follow to request a physician-ordered diet, make diet changes, or report problems with a client's tray.
- The number to reach the clinical dietitian in case a client needs special nutrition advice.
- The times when the dietary department serves meals, so that you can call in any requests before these times.
- The location of the diet manual—usually available at each nursing station—and its contents.

Once you understand how the dietary department operates, you will know where to turn for help when your clients have problems with meals or nutrition.

Diet Therapy

Diet therapy strives to provide, for clients with specific diseases or disorders, the appropriate amounts of energy, protein, carbohydrate, fat, vitamins, major minerals, trace elements, and water in whatever form they can best use. For example, a person who cannot chew needs soft foods; a person whose GI tract is dysfunctional needs a formula delivered directly to the bloodstream.

Each prescribed diet has its own purpose and rationale. The purpose of weight reduction may be to improve self-image in one case, or to improve blood glucose regulation in another. The rationale of a weight-reduction diet is to provide limited food energy so that the person will use stored energy and lose body fat.

A person whose nutrition needs have been correctly identified and for whom an appropriate nutrition care plan has been designed benefits maximally from diet therapy. It is usually up to the physician and dietitian to select the diet therapy most appropriate to meet specific nutrition needs and to complement other medical therapies. As an example of how a diet must complement other therapies, a diet plan for an individual with insulin-dependent diabetes mellitus (IDDM) must coordinate meals with the times of delivery of insulin to the body.

Standard and Modified Diets

Dietitians design *regular* or *standard diets* to include all foods and provide the recommended daily allowances of all nutrients. If such diets fail to meet the specific needs of a client, modifications are made. Modifying the regular diet is much like tailoring a suit. A tailored suit is the same suit after alterations— only it fits better. So it is with the modified diet. A modified diet is a basic nutritious diet that emphasizes a variety of foods tailored to meet a particular client's needs. The tailoring may involve adjusting the consistency; adjusting the amounts of individual nutrients, energy, or fluid; altering the number of meals; or eliminating certain foods. Table 20–1 (on pp. 654–655) gives examples of modified diets used to treat diseases involving different organ systems. These diets are described further in the chapters on specific diseases, which follow.

It is helpful to think about modified diets in terms of the symptoms or conditions they relieve rather than in terms of diseases. People differ, and so do the diets they need. Two people with the same disease may need two different diets. Conversely, people in two completely different states of health may benefit from the same diet. Consider two people with cancer and a third who is pregnant. One person with cancer may be nauseated and need dietary suggestions for controlling nausea. The other person with cancer may be overweight and not experiencing nausea. The dietary suggestions you make to each cancer client will differ. However, a pregnant woman with nausea may benefit from some of the same recommendations as those for the nauseated person with cancer.

modified or therapeutic diet: a regular diet that is adjusted to meet special nutrition needs. Such diets can be adjusted in consistency, in level of energy and nutrients, in amount of fluid, in number of meals, or by the elimination of certain foods.

Diet Manuals and Diet Orders

The exact foods excluded or included on a specific modified diet differ among hospitals, generally in minor ways. These variations reflect different schools of thought regarding diet. You can familiarize yourself with a particular institution's diets by reading the diet manual.

In large hospitals, the staff of dietitians compiles a diet manual, subject to approval by the hospital administrator, several physicians, and representatives of the nursing service. A small hospital may adopt the diet manual of another hospital or an organization such as the state dietetic association. The diet manual describes the foods allowed and not allowed on each diet, the rationale and indications for use of the diets, sample menus, and information regarding the nutritional adequacy of the diets. The dietary department then uses the manual to design menus for clients.

Diets are selected for clients in several ways. Commonly, the physician prescribes the client's diet and writes the diet order in the medical record. Alternatively, the dietitian or another health care team member may suggest a diet prescription to the physician or make recommendations when changes or clarity in the diet orders appear warranted. Whenever possible, the health care team jointly recommends the most appropriate diet.

To avoid confusion, physicians order diets by the names given in the diet manual and describe exact modifications, when appropriate. For example, a physician should specify a 1,200-kcalorie weight-loss diet, rather than just a low-kcalorie diet. A "low-sodium diet" request should specify the amount of sodium; otherwise, it could be interpreted as containing any amount from 500 to 4,000 milligrams of sodium.

When a physician is not available to clarify a vague order, the dietitian may determine the exact modification and record it in the medical record. If a dietitian is not available and the dietary department receives an unclear order

diet manual: a book that describes the foods allowed and restricted on a diet, the rationale and indications for use of the diets, and sample menus.

diet order: a physician's written statement in the medical record of what diet a client should receive.

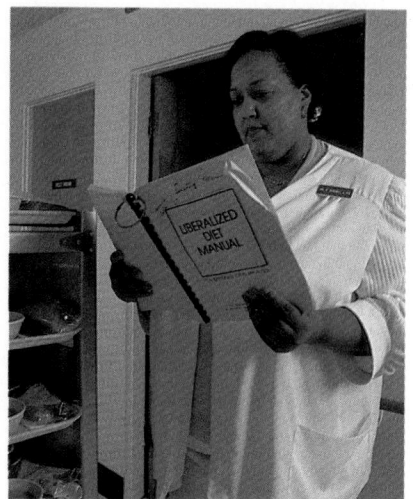
The diet manual specifies which foods to exclude or include on various modified diets.

Summary of Modified Diets by Organ System

Conditions Affecting or Involving the GI Tract, Liver, and Exocrine Pancreas[a]	Possible Diet Modifications
Broken jaw	Mechanical soft
Celiac disease	Gluten-restricted
Cirrhosis	Protein-restricted, sodium-restricted, fluid-restricted
Constipation	High-fiber, increased fluids
Cystic fibrosis	Low-fat, high-kcalorie, high-protein
Dental caries	Mechanical soft
Diarrhea	Liquid, low-fiber, regular, fluid and electrolyte replacement
Difficulty swallowing (dysphagia)	Mechanical soft, tube feeding, total parenteral nutrition (TPN)
Diverticulitis	Low-fiber
Diverticulosis	High-fiber
Dry mouth	Mechanical soft
Dumping syndrome	Carbohydrate-restricted; no concentrated sugars; small, frequent feedings; fluid and electrolyte replacement
Gallbladder disease	Low-fat, kcalorie-restricted, regular
Gastritis	Low-fiber, bland
Hepatic coma	Protein-restricted, sodium-restricted, fluid-restricted
Hepatitis	Regular, high-kcalorie, high-protein
Hiatal hernia	Small, frequent feedings; low-fat; bland; kcalorie-restricted
Ill-fitting dentures	Mechanical soft
Indigestion (dyspepsia)	Low-fiber; bland; small, frequent feedings
Inflammatory bowel disease	Low-fiber, low-fat, high-kcalorie, high-protein, fluid and electrolyte replacement, lactose-restricted, tube feeding, TPN
Lactose intolerance	Lactose-restricted
Malabsorption	Low-fat, high-kcalorie, high-protein, fluid and electrolyte replacement
Missing teeth	Mechanical soft
Nausea	Low-fiber; bland; small, frequent feedings; no liquids with meals
Oral surgery	Mechanical soft
Pancreatitis	Low-fat; regular; small, frequent feedings; tube feeding; TPN
Peptic ulcer	Bland
Periodontal disease	Mechanical soft
Plastic surgery of head or neck	Mechanical soft, tube feeding, TPN
Reflux esophagitis	Small, frequent feedings; low-fat; bland; kcalorie-restricted
Short bowel syndrome	Low-fat, high-kcalorie, high-protein, fluid and electrolyte replacement
Ulcers of mouth or gums	Mechanical soft, bland
Vomiting	Fluid and electrolyte replacement

Summary of Modified Diets by Organ System (continued)

Conditions Affecting the Endocrine Pancreas[a]	Possible Diet Modifications
Diabetes mellitus	Carbohydrate-controlled, kcalorie-restricted, fat-controlled, high-fiber
Hypoglycemia	No concentrated sweets; small, frequent feedings

Conditions Affecting the Blood Vessels, Heart and Lungs	Possible Diet Modifications
Atherosclerosis	Fat-controlled, kcalorie-restricted, sodium-restricted, high-fiber
Congestive heart failure	Sodium-restricted; kcalorie-restricted; low-fiber; bland; small, frequent feedings; fluid-restricted
Coronary heart disease	(See *Atherosclerosis* above)
Hyperlipidemias	Fat-controlled, kcalorie-restricted, carbohydrate-controlled
Hypertension	Low-sodium, kcalorie-restricted, high-potassium; fat-controlled
Myocardial infarction	Low-sodium; kcalorie-restricted; low-fiber; bland; small, frequent feedings; moderate-temperature foods; fat-controlled
Pulmonary disease	High-kcalorie, high-protein

Conditions Affecting the Kidneys	Possible Diet Modifications
Acute renal disease	Protein-restricted, high-kcalorie, fluid-controlled, sodium-controlled, potassium-controlled, fat-controlled, carbohydrate-controlled
Chronic renal disease	Protein-restricted, low-sodium, fluid-restricted, potassium-restricted, phosphorus-restricted
Kidney stones	Increased fluid intake, calcium-controlled, low-oxalate
Nephrotic syndrome	Sodium-restricted, high-kcalorie, high-protein, potassium-restricted
Urinary tract infections	Increased fluid intake, acid-ash diet

Conditions Affecting Many Organ Systems	Possible Diet Modifications
Acquired immune deficiency syndrome (AIDS)	High-kcalorie, high-protein, low-fat, low-residue, low-fiber, fluid and electrolyte replacement, lactose-resticted, mechanical soft, tube feeding, TPN
Burns	High-kcalorie, high-protein, increased fluid intake
Cancer	High-kcalorie, high-protein (see also specific related conditions: Dry mouth, Indigestion, Malabsorption, Nausea, Plastic surgery of head or neck, Ulcers of mouth or gums, Vomiting, and so on)
Food sensitivities	Elimination of offending substance
Galactosemia	Galactose-restricted
Obesity, overweight	kCalorie-restricted, high-fiber
Phenylketonuria (PKU)	Phenylalanine-restricted
Stroke	Mechanical soft, regular, tube feeding
Surgery	Regular, high-kcalorie, high-protein, increased fluids
Underweight	High-kcalorie, high-protein

[a]The pancreas produces both external (exocrine) and internal (endocrine) secretions. The external secretions (enzymes) play an important role in the digestion of food; the internal secretions (insulin and other hormones) play a primary role in the regulation of glucose metabolism.

from the nursing station, a house diet (usually specified in the diet manual) is sent.

Health care providers share responsibility for ensuring that clients receive the best possible nutrition care. The physician holds ultimate responsibility for a client's diet order, and it is easy for others to follow the order without thinking about it, but this is a mistake. Be alert to needs and prepared to communicate them so that appropriate changes will be carried out.

Similarly, the dietitian cannot always meet every client's nutrition care needs. Ideally, a dietitian visits all clients and reviews the charts of every person admitted to the hospital. But in reality, most clinical dietitians see only people on modified diets or people they have been asked to see. Some small hospitals may not even employ a full-time clinical dietitian.

In cases where many physicians, interns, and residents see clients, miscommunication regarding diet orders can easily occur. Clients may communicate their needs more clearly and more often to their nurses or other health care providers than to their physicians. Furthermore, a client's physician may not consider nutrition an important enough part of client care to warrant attention. Whatever the reason, be aware that written diet orders may be inappropriate. Examples of inappropriate diet orders include:

- The physician describes a grossly overweight individual as "well-nourished" and orders a regular diet. As a result, the dietitian does not see the client. Consequently, the client receives an inappropriate diet and no nutrition advice.
- A physician orders that a client receive no food or fluids after midnight for a lab test to be run in the morning. Due to a miscommunication, the doctor assumes that the order changes after the test, but it doesn't. The client needlessly "starves" for a day or two until someone notices the error.
- A client who routinely enjoys foods low in sugar and salt finds the foods served on the regular diet too salty. The client eats very little food and feels the hospital has totally neglected its responsibility to provide nutritious foods to its clients.

Whenever you notice inappropriate diet orders, contact the dietitian or alert the physician.

An order to give a client nothing orally (including food, beverages, and medications) reads "NPO." **NPO** stands for *nil per os*, which means "nothing by mouth." On the other hand, **PO** stands for *per os*, which means "by mouth," or "orally."

■ The Client's View of Hospital Food

What do you think of when you see or hear the words "hospital food"? What are your own experiences with hospital food, or the experiences of someone close to you? Viewing hospital food from a client's perspective will add to your understanding of nutrition care.

Most people generally look forward to eating, and in the hospital, eating may become even more enjoyable than usual, for it offers clients familiarity in an otherwise strange environment. It also provides one of the few experiences in the hospital in which clients have a choice. Consider that clients usually cannot choose when they will receive tests, how much blood they will have drawn, what nurse will care for them, or what time they will have surgery.

But for the most part, they can enjoy the opportunity to select their meals, and they can also exercise some control: they can eat them or refuse to eat them!

Of course, clients may complain about hospital food. Complaining may have little to do with the food itself, but serves instead to vent fear, frustration, anger, and physical pain. Clients need opportunities to express their feelings, and often you may find that simply listening helps to resolve some problems without the need to make any diet changes. Actual food problems need to be corrected by the dietary department, of course.

Problems with foodservice unrelated to a client's physical or mental state can interfere with appetite. For one, the hospital does not cook food the same as a client does at home—a considerable problem when the client must eat three meals a day for many days in the hospital. Unfortunately, hot meals may also be at room temperature by the time they arrive in the room. In addition, the client receives meals at specified times, regardless of hunger and often must eat alone in bed, which can be more of a chore than a pleasurable experience. Meals can also be unwelcome if they follow painful treatments. Food is so important to most people that a bad experience with it in the hospital can make them and those who work with them agitated and angry.

All this is not to say that every person in the hospital has a problem with meals. The majority of clients will eat adequate amounts of food, even if they complain about it. If their intakes decrease somewhat, the deficit will be easy to correct once they are at home eating familiar foods.

The loss of appetite can have a serious effect on the health or recovery of some people, however. These individuals lose their appetites at times when they can least afford nutrient deficits. By using the steps discussed in Chapter 19 to identify clients at risk for poor nutrition status, health care professionals can work to improve appetite and otherwise ensure that clients receive adequate nutrients.

How to Help the Client Eat

Nurses and nursing assistants most often shoulder responsibility for delivering food to the client's room. They prepare the client to eat, observe problems the client may be having with food, and communicate the client's needs to the appropriate person or department.

If a client has a poor appetite or constantly complains about the food, try to get to the root of the problem. If the client is frightened, angry, or confused, simply showing that you care may help improve the situation. Be sure the client understands how important a role nutrition plays in the recovery process. When it is permissible and possible, a friend or family member can bring favorite foods from outside the hospital if these foods will improve food intake. This may be especially useful when feeding a child.

To help improve your client's food intake, ask yourself these questions:

- Does your client understand the importance of nutrition to the recovery process?
- Does your client understand how a modified diet supports treatment?
- Does your client know which foods are allowed on the diet and which are restricted?
- Does your client understand how to mark the menu correctly?

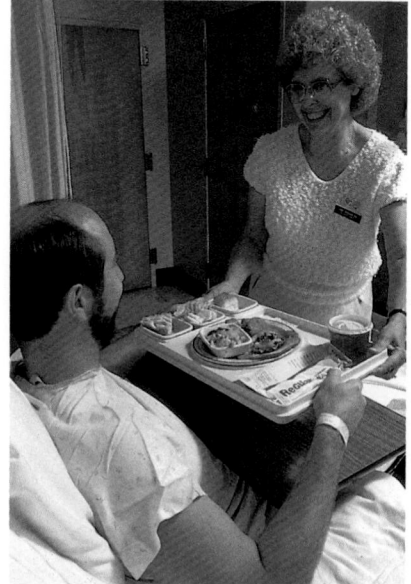

People enjoy eating when they feel comfortable and cared for.

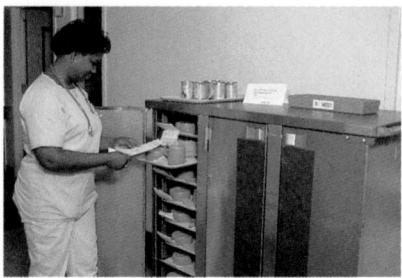

People appreciate receiving the right meal served attractively.

If clients need help in any of these areas, give the advice they need. Call a dietitian if the problem is one you cannot handle alone. The dietitian can work closely with the client to find acceptable foods.

Your own attitudes about the hospital's food can influence your client. Try to be positive; never say something like, "I couldn't eat this stuff either." Instead, say, "The dietary department really tries to make foods the way you like them. Let me call the dietitian. I'm sure we can find a solution." When a dietitian or foodservice manager is unavailable, look for the dietary department's list of alternative foods at the nursing station.

Clients can also take a few steps to make mealtimes more enjoyable for themselves. Encourage them to wash their hands and face, and to brush their teeth or rinse their mouth before eating. Help your clients get comfortable, either in bed or sitting in a chair. Adjust the extension table to a comfortable height and distance, and make sure it is clean. A clean, odor-free room also helps. Take these steps before the tray arrives so that the client can enjoy the meal at the right temperature.

When the food cart arrives on the floor, check each tray:

- Verify that the name on the tray is the client's name. A client's room number may have been incorrectly recorded, or a new client may have been admitted to a room.
- Check to see that the client receives the right diet.
- Compare the tray with the selective menu to be sure that the client has received the foods that were ordered.
- Scan the tray for overall appearance. The client will eat better if the food is served attractively. Order a new tray if foods are not appropriate.

Once you have checked the trays, serve them immediately—while warm foods are still warm and cold foods are still cold. Help clients who need assistance in opening containers such as milk cartons. Your efforts can mean a lot to clients whose illnesses, fears, and frustrations significantly interfere with the desire to eat.

How to Help the Sick Child Eat

A sick child often requires special care. Those who care for children must be sensitive to their needs and feelings. Many of the hints given in Chapter 15 for helping well children to eat are useful for working with ill children as well. Additional pointers from people experienced in working with children include:

- Notice the child's posture. Body language will tell you if a child feels fear, pain, or discomfort.
- Touch the child often and lovingly. Your touch communicates more than your words.
- As with adults, let the child choose what to eat as much as possible. Foods brought from outside the hospital can help, if permissible.
- Notice whether the child eats the food. Putting a tray of food in front of a child is not enough.
- Stay with the child during the meal, or make sure a loved person is there. The child will eat and assimilate food better if a caring person soothes away anxiety and loneliness.

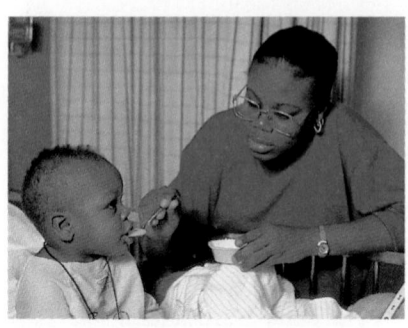

Foods taste better when you're not alone and scared.

- Encourage children to eat the most nutritious foods first before they become too full to complete the meal.
- Let children eat with other children if possible. They'll enjoy mealtimes more, accept more food, and eat for longer periods.
- Avoid painful procedures near mealtimes. The stress of pain or fear shuts down digestion and turns off interest in food.

Nutrition care contributes importantly to a child's recovery, even though its effects may not be immediately obvious.

The nutrition care plan specifies not only how to deliver nutrients but also how to deliver nutrition information. The remainder of the chapter presents ways to develop your communication skills. Much of your success in providing care depends on your ability to communicate clearly with your clients, their families, and the other professionals you work with.

Communication and Nutrition Care

Close your eyes for a moment and imagine yourself lying in a hospital bed. You are frightened and unsure of what's wrong with you or what will happen next. You have to rely on other people to do things for you. Even worse, you feel you have lost control of *yourself*. You must depend on someone else to find out what is happening inside your body and what the best treatment will be. How terrifying to be putting your health (your life) in someone else's hands (a stranger, yet)! Your body is no longer private—everyone seems to be poking, sticking, and probing it. On top of that, you hurt, and many of the examinations, tests, and procedures you must undergo also cause discomfort and embarrassment. You need time to sort through your feelings, but how can you think when every few minutes someone is coming into your room to check vital signs, draw blood, give medication, and ask endless questions that you feel you have already answered over and over?

Now open your eyes, and remember to keep them open. You now see how important communication is to your clients. Many of your clients' fears and concerns dissipate when they feel satisfied that their caretakers listen to, understand, and respond to their needs. Such actions enable your clients to retain some control over their environment, and therefore, themselves. Furthermore, if you have gained their trust and cooperation, your care will be more effective. You will be able to elicit more accurate information from clients and motivate them to follow nutrition (or other) advice.

When you speak with your clients, and when you chart information in their medical records, you communicate verbally (with words). When you touch, smile, frown, or otherwise make gestures, you communicate nonverbally. Regardless of how you communicate, to be effective, you must formulate and express your ideas clearly. Moreover, the person you are communicating with must interpret your ideas as intended. Figure 20–1 illustrates the dynamics of the communication relationship: the transfer of information from one person (sender) to another (receiver) for the purpose of eliciting a response. As you can see from the figure, the roles of sender and receiver constantly switch between the communicating parties.

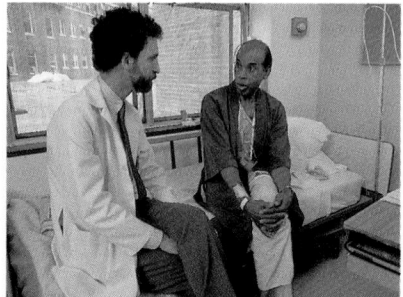

Communication makes the difference in client care.

Miscommunication can arise in many ways. Messages may not be perceived as intended if the words or actions used by a sender have a different meaning for the receiver. Values, ethnic backgrounds, and social influences affect everyone's perceptions of words and actions. For example, saying, "How do you feel today?" may seem trite to one sick person while another may think, "He really cares about me." Smiling is generally an acceptable expression of friendliness, but a smile also can be inappropriate, for example, at a time of grief.

To enhance your communication skills keep in mind the following points:

■ Establish a caring and trusting environment. Let others know that you care about them and that they can trust you.
■ Allow others to be themselves. In other words, accept and value people for who and what they are. If a listener reacts with advice, criticism, or judgment, the speaker may withhold important information, not wanting to risk belittlement.
■ Become an active listener. Let the other person do most of the talking.
■ Avoid using terminology or abbreviations that may be confusing to others. For example, a person going to surgery might be needlessly confused and frightened if told that after leaving the OR she will be taken to the RR and that she should expect to awaken with an IV and an NG tube in place. Always use common language or define terms when explaining a person's condition, diagnostic tests, or therapy.
■ Maintain eye-level contact with the other person. To do so may require that you sit down. Standing while the other person sits or lies in bed may nonverbally communicate an unfriendly and overpowering feeling.

Judgmental versus nonjudgmental responses:

Helper: Do you take any type of vitamin or mineral supplements?

Client: I take a vitamin E capsule and 2 grams of vitamin C every day.

Judgmental helper response: You know, of course, that there is no reason for taking these vitamin supplements.

Nonjudgmental helper response: For what reasons do you take these vitamin supplements?

These techniques serve you in both verbal and nonverbal communications. Nonverbal communications often "speak" as loudly as words do. To gain a person's trust and cooperation, sit at a close, yet comfortable, distance from the person and use appropriate facial expressions and gestures to clarify or emphasize important messages.

One of the most powerful nonverbal communication techniques is silence. During a pause, both parties have a chance to think about what has been said and formulate ideas. Sometimes silence indicates that a thought is complete and provides a good time to move on to another topic or to end the discussion.

The communication techniques discussed so far will serve you well whether you are communicating with clients, professors, roommates, or parents. The following sections will describe some specific ways to communicate, first with clients and then with other health care professionals.

Client Communications

Educating the client is a vital part of the care plan. Whenever possible, the client and the client's caretakers need to understand the different measures being taken. For example, prior to diagnostic tests, clients in the hospital will receive liquid diets. Explain to clients why their meal trays will contain only liquids, and caution them not to eat foods other than those they receive on the hospital tray. Such explanations help clients to feel comfortable with you and the unfamiliar procedures, thus relieving some of their anxiety.

To further help clients feel comfortable, encourage them to communicate openly and freely. Some techniques (in addition to those listed in the previous section) include:

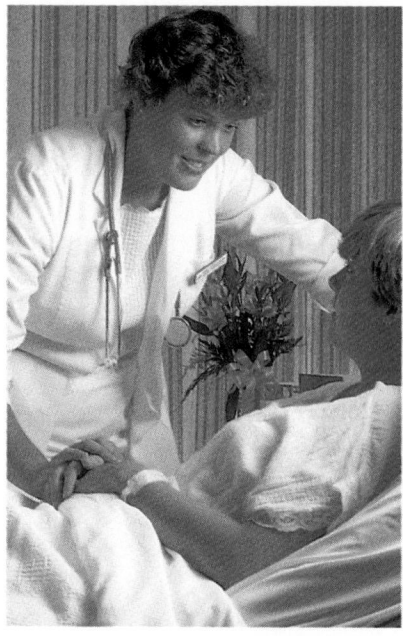

Body language speaks as loudly as words.

- *Introduction and statement of purpose.* Each time you visit a client, introduce yourself, verify the client's name, and define the purpose of your discussion. In so doing, you set the tone for the discussion and let the person know what is expected of him. At this time, it may be valuable to assure the person that all the information he gives you is confidential.
- *Appropriate use of questions.* Use open-ended questions to start a conversation. Open-ended questions ask broad questions that allow the listener a wide choice of answers. Avoid using closed-ended questions and double questions. Such questions narrowly limit a listener's responses. For example, if you ask a client if she prefers orange juice or tomato juice, you aren't giving her the chance to tell you she'd really rather have grapefruit juice or even a slice of melon.
- *Client-centered communication.* Allow the client to control the direction of the discussion. Try not to follow a set form for asking important questions; rather, use such a form as a guide, and ask questions based on what the client says.
- *Continuous feedback.* Provide the client with continuous feedback to determine whether you understand each other correctly. Table 20–2 (on p. 662) lists positive and negative feedback techniques.
- *Summary of the discussion.* Prior to ending a discussion, be sure that you both agree on what has transpired. Identify and clarify misconceptions or misunderstandings immediately. Arrange for follow-up at this time. For example, "I'll be back tomorrow," or "Let's plan to talk again next week."

Open- versus closed-ended questions:
- *Open-ended*: How do you feel about your new diet?
- *Closed-ended*: You feel fine about your new diet, don't you?

Examples of double questions:
- Do you drink orange or tomato juice with breakfast?
- Have you followed a weight-reduction or low-cholesterol diet at home?

As you practice communicating with clients, you'll develop techniques that fit your individual style. However, while learning, try all of the available techniques to discover which ones you use most comfortably and effectively.

Many of your interactions with clients will be brief and informal conversations. At times, however, it will be necessary to engage in more formal

■ TABLE 20–2
Providing Feedback

Do:	Examples:
Encourage the client to continue.	*Helper:* I see. Mm-hm. What else?
Repeat key phrases or ideas.	*Person:* I've been so distraught I've lost 10 pounds.
	Helper: You've lost 10 pounds?
Clarify what the client is saying.	*Helper:* I'm not sure I understand what you mean.
Validate the client's responses.	*Person:* I get so nervous I begin eating like a horse.
	Helper: You eat when you're nervous?
Echo the client's feelings (sometimes called reflecting).	*Person:* After 4 weeks of dieting, I just can't believe that I only lost 2 pounds.
	Helper: You feel frustrated with how slowly you lose weight.
Remain silent, when appropriate, to let the client formulate ideas.	

Don't:	Examples:
Don't talk more than listen.	
Don't interrupt the person's thoughts.	*Person:* I could stay on my diet if . . .
	Helper: If you didn't live alone.
Don't judge or moralize.	*Helper:* You have no excuse for not losing weight.
Don't use meaningless expressions.	*Helper:* I know you'll do fine.
Don't demean the person's situation or attitude.	*Helper:* You probably just don't understand how this diet works.
Don't put words into the person's mouth.	*Helper:* What did you have for breakfast today? (Assumes person eats or should eat breakfast.)
Don't give diet advice when seeking information.	*Helper:* You shouldn't eat candy on your diet. (The person may not tell you about other things he "shouldn't" be eating.)

communication. Before beginning a formal discussion with a client, be prepared. Check the chart to become familiar with the client's past and current history. Arrange for privacy, adjust the physical environment for comfort, and allow adequate time. It is difficult to discuss personal information when outsiders are present, when the room is poorly lit or stuffy-hot, or when you feel you're being rushed.

Formal communications include both soliciting and providing information. These communication methods follow specific guidelines, as the next two sections describe.

How to Solicit Information: The Interview

Almost all health professionals conduct interviews to uncover important clues that affect their clients' health. For example, a dietitian uses an interview to obtain a diet history. Interviews serve as a means of establishing a caring and trusting relationship while gathering information that will enable the health professional to deliver care effectively. The information obtained in the interview generally represents a person's lifelong habits as influenced by complex social, cultural, psychological, religious, and economic factors. No one would share this much without trusting that the interviewer truly cared and would accept the information, whatever it might be.

When preparing for an interview, review your client's records and arrange for a private, comfortable room. During the interview, follow the communication techniques described in the next section and those outlined in Table 20–3 (on the next page) for a counseling session. Before closing the interview, ask if your client has any questions and answer them, acknowledge your client's cooperation, and explain the next step for follow-up, if needed.

Chapter 19 contains forms to help dietitians conduct a diet history interview.

Tell me what kind of food you eat and I will tell you what kind of man you are. Brillat-Savarin

How to Provide Information: The Counseling Session

When the nutrition care plan involves more than a short-term dietary adjustment, the client may receive additional nutrition counseling. In outpatient clinics, nursing homes, and hospitals that do not employ a dietitian, the nurse or other health care professional may be expected to assume the full responsibility of nutrition counseling. In most hospitals, the dietitian most frequently assumes responsibility for nutrition counseling, but nurses can help to reinforce or clarify nutrition information. For example, your client might comment to you that breakfast sure is going to be different without milk in her cereal now that she's on this new low-fat diet. You can acknowledge that things will be a bit different, thus reinforcing the importance of making the necessary changes in accordance with the new low-fat diet. Then you can clarify that she need not do without all milk but that her diet can include nonfat and some low-fat milk and milk products.

Our abundant knowledge of the relationships between diet and health is purely academic until people can apply that knowledge to their lives. Nutrition counseling helps clients to benefit from the fruits of such nutrition research. Successful counselors give their clients diet and health information in a way that helps clients to integrate the needed changes into their lifestyles and provides them with the motivation needed to make these changes.

Changing behaviors is difficult, to say the least. Without commitment, it is impossible. Consider that for most of their lives, clients select foods based on taste, cost, convenience, and persuasive messages from friends and advertisements. Then one day, a nutrition counselor advises a client to make most food and beverage selections based on health. To accomplish this goal every time the choice arises—and it arises several times within each of several meals a day—requires an incredibly strong commitment.[1] Counselors may be destined to fail even before they begin if they assume that all clients are ready to make this commitment.[2] The following characteristics help counselors to identify the readiness of clients. "Ready" clients:

- Recognize the relationship between eating patterns and the risk of disease.
- Do not fear behavior change.
- Are not discouraged when discussing the need to make dietary changes.
- Are not overwhelmed by other lifestyle events.

Preparation

Successful communication begins with adequate preparation. Before beginning a counseling session, be sure to:

■ *Assess your client's needs*—nutritional, educational, and emotional. This information allows you to make the information relevant to, and appropriate for, each individual client.

■ *Assess your own knowledge* of the diet, medical condition, and treatment plans of your client. Gather the information you might need and be prepared, but don't worry that a client might ask a question or two that you can't answer.

■ *Develop objectives* for meeting your client's needs. Define specific and realistic objectives in terms of behaviors that can be observed and measured.

■ *Determine the content* of (the type and amount of information to present), as well as the methods used for, the counseling session (for example, a filmstrip, a diet booklet, food models, practice menus, or a food diary). Let the client's level of interest, motivation, and education guide you in these decisions. For example, an illiterate adult or a child might appreciate diet instructions in picture form. One person might find the in-depth details about the body's response to diet fascinating, whereas another person just wants the diet without the background.

■ *Establish a time frame* for accomplishing objectives. The time frame can be tentative and somewhat flexible to reflect the client's needs.

■ *Arrange for appropriate others* to be present at the session.

Implementation

When counseling, remember to practice the general communication skills listed in the text: establish a caring environment, allow others to be themselves, be a good listener, use familiar language and appropriate nonverbal gestures, and maintain eye contact. You will also want to use the client communications techniques already mentioned: establish identity, use open-ended questions, center the session around the client, provide positive feedback, and summarize your discussion. In addition, be sure to:

■ *Establish rapport* by spending a little time creating a trusting and caring atmosphere before beginning diet instructions.

■ *Identify and communicate the objectives* of counseling clearly. If clients know, for example, that they will be asked to explain the rationale for their diets, they may listen more closely to the explanation of the diet. Furthermore, this gives the client an opportunity to modify your expectations.

■ *Discuss the rationale for diet changes* and show your clients how nutrition supports recovery. Clients who do not understand the benefits will not be motivated to change.

■ *Answer all questions accurately,* even if it means having to explain that you will check on the information and convey it at a later time. This action clearly surpasses giving incorrect advice or ignoring a question.

■ *Stress to clients that they carry the responsibility* for their health and for making the necessary diet changes.

■ *Encourage client participation* in the counseling session. You will often hear statements such as ''You need to talk to my wife; she does the cooking.'' It does help if the family member who prepares the food participates in the counseling session and understands the diet. However, clients must accept that they—not their spouses and not the counselor—need to accept the responsibility for their diets.

■ *Be realistic* when applying principles of diet to lifestyle. Be sure that the person can actually apply the changes. The busy executive who frequently eats restaurant meals must know how to make appropriate food choices in restaurants. A person with a low income may need help with incorporating lower-cost food items into the diet, as well as tips on shopping economically. A person who follows a strictly kosher diet must know how to plan meals around the Jewish dietary laws (see Highlight 28).

■ *Make diet instructions relevant* to clients by using many examples consistent with their own eating habits. Do this by becoming familiar with diet histories, having them plan personal menus, asking them to tell you what they would select in a restaurant, or observing them make selections from the hospital cafeteria line.

■ *Encourage active participation* in the sessions and allow clients to arrive at conclusions on their own.

■ *Reinforce all positive responses* and acknowledge your client's cooperation during the session.

■ *Arrange for follow-up* if needed.

Evaluation

When a counseling session is complete, consider whether:

■ The objectives have been met.

■ The content and methods of instruction were appropriate. Ask yourself which methods worked well and which were less effective.

■ The time was adequate and whether additional counseling is needed.

■ The client's needs have changed.

■ Your counseling skills were effective. Ask yourself how you can improve your instructional techniques for future counseling sessions.

■ View diet therapy as a manageable task.

■ View diet therapy as a way to improve health.

Counselors can influence their clients' readiness by adjusting teaching styles to accommodate the individual.[3] When presenting educational material, keep in mind that the brain's capacity to process new information is limited. Present no more than three new ideas per session—generally one major concept with a couple of explanations or examples to support it. For example, you might describe the benefits of a high-fiber diet (major concept), the need to increase fiber intake gradually and with plenty of water (supporting explanations), and name several high-fiber foods (examples). Use handouts to reinforce the information presented.

Another helpful hint is to remember that learning occurs in a brain that is surrounded by emotions. Pain, anger, and resentment block messages from getting through. Under such circumstances, a counselor may fare better by rescheduling a session than forcing information on an unwilling learner. For counselors who have established caring relationships with their clients, such circumstances may be temporary and readily resolved.

Work on establishing empathy and rapport. To establish empathy, put yourself in your client's shoes: this will build the foundation for understanding between you. To establish rapport, spend a little time expressing your interest in and concern for your client. Rapport underlies trust—your trust in your client's ability to meet objectives and your client's trust in your willingness to help.

Another aid to counseling is to determine what knowledge and experience your client already possesses before actually presenting any information. This information will help you to determine what small dietary changes will make the greatest differences to your client's health. It will help you to set priorities for making changes. You can then add to the client's knowledge and experience using examples and analogies.

Finally, keep in mind that everybody learns differently. Skillful counselors learn to understand, accept, and accommodate other people's "ways of knowing." To communicate with someone like yourself is easy; to communicate with someone unlike yourself requires developing special communication skills. To improve your understanding of others' perspectives, practice listening, questioning, and establishing empathy and rapport with people you would normally not seek out as friends.

These broad concepts underlie a successful counseling session. Additional details of preparing for, implementing, and evaluating a counseling session were given in Table 20–3.

Counseling a person in the hospital requires a few special considerations. Unlike the outpatient, the hospitalized client is captive and is not necessarily discussing diet changes by choice. There is a world of difference between the hospital environment and the home environment. A person who has learned to make proper food selections from the hospital menu may feel lost about what to eat when at home. Furthermore, after the immediate danger of illness has passed, the person may soon lose the motivation to keep following a special diet. For these reasons, it is advisable to follow up once the person arrives home—through a phone call, home visit, or invited visit by the client to the counselor. If follow-up is not possible, the counselor can at least refer the client to another qualified professional.

- A little information remembered is better than a lot of information forgotten.

- Positive feelings foster learning.

- Learn what your clients know.

- Understand your client's way of understanding.

Whether nutrition counseling is effective depends on the extent to which clients change their eating habits in response to it. Clearly, nutrition counselors face a challenge: they need to use both their nutrition knowledge and their counseling skills. Counseling skills improve with practice, but even the best counselor experiences failure. In the end, clients, not counselors, must accept the responsibility for making the necessary diet changes.

From the client's point of view, communication channels with health care providers may be frustrating and confusing. A client may be attended by a primary physician, several consulting physicians, residents, interns, three shifts of nurses that change daily, student nurses, nurse's aides, dietitians, dietetic technicians, and many other health team members (laboratory technicians, physical therapists, social workers, and so on). How exasperating for an individual to communicate a need or concern to one health care provider assuming that the information will be shared, only to have to repeat the request over and over again. Whenever possible, follow through with information or items you have told the client you would deliver. Otherwise, explain why compliance with some of the requests may be difficult or impossible to handle. Jot down notes to jog your memory, if it helps. When necessary, be sure to forward requests to other departments (for example, a nurse may need to request a certain food item from the dietary department). Such actions help to close the communication gap between clients and professionals.

■ Professional Communications

Maintaining strong professional communication networks benefits both health care professionals and their clients. Conversely, miscommunication between professionals can result in inappropriate therapy and serious consequences to clients' health. Many opportunities exist for professionals to discuss clients' concerns and progress. One way professionals communicate is through the medical record.

The Medical Record and Other Records

medical record: a continuous written account of a client's health, history, diagnosis, therapy, and prognosis.

diagnosis: the disease a person has or is thought to have.
dia = through
gnosis = knowing

prognosis: the predicted course and outcome of a disease.
pro = ahead of time, before

An entry made in a POMR is generally written in the form of a **SOAP note.** SOAP stands for **S**ubjective, **O**bjective, **A**ssessment, and **P**lan.

The medical record compiles the history, the diagnosis, the therapy, and the prognosis for each client. It allows the health care team to share information with each other. Reading the medical record at regular intervals provides a continuous assessment of the client's condition and response to therapy. This information helps determine how to proceed with delivering the best possible care.

Medical records can be organized in many ways. Health care providers today commonly use the problem-oriented medical record (POMR) approach. In this approach, health care team members list each problem of the client to generate a problem list. Subsequently, each problem entered in the record addresses the actions being taken to deal with it. As new problems arise, they are added to the list.

Learn how to effectively use the record in the facility where you work. Regardless of the type of medical record approach used, be sure the client's medical record includes important nutrition-related information. Examples of important information include:

- Evaluation of the client's current diet.
- Nutrition assessment data.
- Recommended nutrition therapy.
- The client's acceptance and tolerance of the diet.
- Problems with the client's food intake.
- Documentation of diet counseling.
- Any planned follow-up or referral to another person or agency.
- The client's response to nutrition care.
- The client's response to diet counseling.

In addition to the formal medical record, various health care providers generally keep records of their own. For example, nurses keep nursing care plans, and dietitians keep nutrition care plans (as described earlier). These records contain some of the same information contained in the formal medical record. However, they also include more detailed plans and notes specifically pertinent to the individual health team member. For example, a nutrition care plan may have details regarding a client's reaction to a diet, which the dietitian will later use in preparation for diet counseling. Nursing care plans may also contain information regarding a client's nutrition needs. The direct and frequent interactions nurses have with clients generate valuable additions to the care plan.

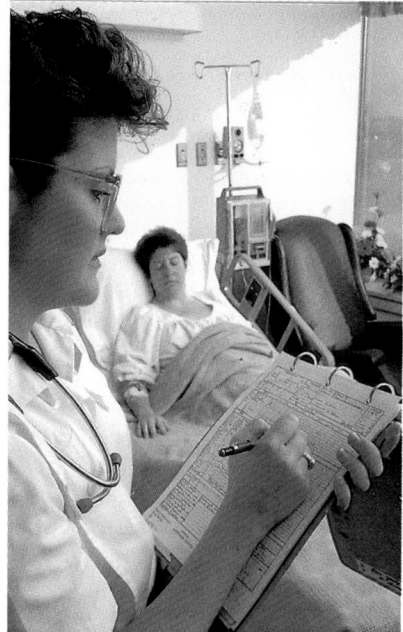

Take time to record important nutrition information in the client's medical record.

Other Communication Channels

Opportunities for verbal communication other than by way of written records also exist among health team members. Health team members in a hospital often phone or page each other when they identify problems or when questions arise. Outside the hospital, health team members may be reached in their offices or through their answering services.

Bedside rounds provide an ideal opportunity for professional communication. During rounds, teams of professionals visit and examine selected clients as a group. The health team members discuss the clients' cases either prior to or following the visits. Use these discussions to talk over nutrition problems and to exchange information about clients' concerns and attitudes.

Nurses also report to one another at the end of each shift. Use this time to pass along information regarding clients' special nutrition and diet needs and requests.

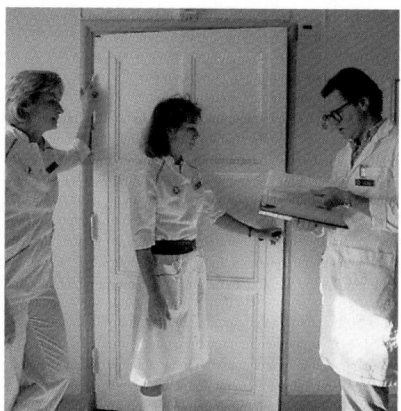

Bedside rounds provide an excellent opportunity to discuss your concerns regarding a person's nutrition status.

Nutrition care means more than providing clients with food; it also means giving them attention. This chapter has described techniques for both. The next chapter offers alternatives to feeding clients when standard oral diets cannot meet nutrient needs.

SELF STUDY *Nutrition Care*

Team up with two or three other class members and briefly (spending five minutes) review together the sections of this chapter entitled "The Client's View of Hospital Food," "Communication and Nutrition Care," and "Client Communications." Then, one of you role-play a person who is ill and having to adjust to a new diet—hospital or other—and one or more of you role-play a caretaker (nurse, dietitian, or other). (For maximum benefit from this exercise, the "ill" person may want to choose a real situation to role-play, such as that of a relative or client whose nutrition status is cause for concern.)

Let the caretaker interview the client to discover what problems are interfering with food acceptance. Discover (invent) as many problems as possible and list them in a column leaving spaces between them (see the sample form provided here). With the client's help, run through as many possible reasons for each problem as you can think of and list them in a second column. Then (again with the client's help) brainstorm solutions to each problem and list them in a third column. Performed with enthusiasm, this exercise can become a valuable memory when you are working in the clinical setting.

Problems with eating	Possible causes	Proposed solutions
Food not familiar	Client is Puerto Rican	Add permitted spice
	Food unlike wife's cooking	Request wife be allowed to bring in a meal a day
	Client drinks coffee even with dinner	Obtain decaf
	Client doesn't know how to mark menu	Educate; be present at time of menu selection if possible
Mouth is sore	From medicine—unavoidable; no change permitted	Rinse with cool water before eating
		Request soft foods
		Allow food to cool before serving

Study Questions

1. What are the steps in the nutrition care process that can be used to identify nutrition problems and take corrective measures?
2. What is the easiest way to start a conversation with a client in a health care setting? How can you facilitate communication through the use of questions? What types of questions should be used, and what type avoided? What other techniques help to maintain effective communication? How should you close a discussion with a client?
3. What is the purpose of an interview? What is the purpose of nutrition counseling? What steps can you take to make nutrition counseling more effective? Discuss each step.
4. What steps can you take before beginning a counseling session to ensure successful communication? During a counseling session, how can you encourage client participation and compliance?
5. Why is it important to evaluate a counseling session? What questions should you ask yourself about the session?
6. How can you use the medical record to communicate a client's nutrition needs to other health care professionals? What kinds of information about nutrition should you record? Where else can you find written information about a client's nutrient or nutrition-education needs?
7. Discuss some other ways that health care providers can share concerns about a client's nutrition needs.

Notes

1. S. Kayman, Applying theory from social psychology and cognitive behavioral psychology to dietary behavior change and assessment, *Journal of the American Dietetic Association* 89 (1989): 191–193.
2. A. W. Caggiula, The compliance problem: How to solve it, *Nutrition and the M.D.*, January 1990, pp. 1–3.
3. C. Achterberg, Factors that influence learner readiness, *Journal of the American Dietetic Association* 88 (1988): 1426–1428.

Team Approach to Nutrition Care

This morning's nutrition support rounds include discussions about Mrs. A, who is receiving concentrated solutions of nutrients by vein after surgery; Mr. B, who has a broken jaw and is on tube feedings; and Ms. C, who is receiving an intravenous solution. All clients in the hospital who are receiving special nutrition support require close attention. Nutrition support team members focus their efforts on client needs; they help to assure that hospital staff members use special nutrition support systems safely and appropriately. Of course, successful implementation of a nutrition care plan also requires client cooperation.

This highlight uses the nutrition support team to illustrate the workings of a health care team; the details of nutrition support are described in Chapters 21 and 22. The purpose here is to illustrate the principles of the team approach. Each health care professional on the team possesses specialized knowledge. By working as a team, the members can integrate their knowledge and provide the client with the benefits of their combined expertise. Team members also benefit—they learn how each team member contributes to the care process, and in so doing can depend on the right person to do the right job efficiently, thus saving time.

Functions of a Nutrition Support Team

The nutrition support team performs a variety of tasks. One of their tasks is to identify clients who may be at nutrition risk. Once clients at risk have been identified and special nutrition support implemented, team members monitor each client's progress. The team members maintain client records

The team approach helps to ensure safe and effective nutrition support.

and review the benefits and complications that arise from the special nutrition support measures taken. They may also serve as consultants to the hospital staff, providing nutrition information, answering questions, and solving problems as they arise.

Nutrition support team members must also keep abreast of new developments in their field. They analyze new products and review current research, which enables them to provide optimal care and to control costs.

Core members of a nutrition support team include a physician, a dietitian, a nurse, and a pharmacist. The following discussions examine some of the responsibilities of specific team members.

The Physician

Often, a physician serves as director of the nutrition support team. The responsibilities of this position include:

- Supervising the activities of other team members.
- Developing guidelines for the safe use of nutrition support.
- Monitoring the kinds and severity of complications and, when possible, correcting problems that arise.

- Conducting in-hospital educational and training programs for the professional staff.

In addition, the directing physician may serve as a consultant to other physicians, thus becoming involved with direct client management. During nutrition support rounds, the physician oversees the discussion of each client receiving special support and makes recommendations as appropriate.

The Dietitian

The dietitian is the team's nutrition expert. Generally, the dietitian assesses the client's nutrition status, either by directly measuring, recording, and evaluating nutrition parameters or by supervising others who gather the necessary data. Following an assessment, the dietitian determines a client's nutrient requirements and translates the physician's diet orders into foods or feedings.

The dietitian must have a thorough knowledge of liquid formulas in order to determine, for clients who need formulas, which products will best meet their requirements (discussed in Chapter 21). For clients requiring tube feedings, the dietitian recommends the most appropriate formula, administration schedule, and size and type of feeding tube. When clients are unable to tolerate a feeding regimen, the dietitian must be prepared to recommend alternative formulas and administration schedules. Familiarity with all enteral formulas and feeding equipment enables the dietitian to respond appropriately to questions and problems that arise.

The dietitian visits clients daily, continuously assessing nutrient intakes and nutrition status. In addition, the dietitian helps clients to understand

and cope with their unique feeding situations. The dietitian works with clients to ease the transition from parenteral nutrition or tube feeding to oral intake and assists in selecting and training clients for home parenteral and enteral nutrition support. Whenever possible, the dietitian makes home visits to all clients receiving tube feedings or special oral formulas.

The nutrition support team dietitian provides in-service training for other dietitians and nurses on such topics as nutrition assessment, the correct techniques of formula administration and care, and formula selection. And, as you might expect, the dietitian on the nutrition support team also acts as a liaison between the team and the dietary department.

The Nurse

The nurse on a nutrition support team plays a central role in client care management and client relationships. The nurse explains nutrition support techniques to clients and their families. This includes describing the need for special nutrition support, as well as explaining how to insert a catheter or feeding tube.

For clients on parenteral nutrition, the nurse ensures that hospital staff follow proper techniques of catheter care. In some hospitals, the nutrition support nurse inserts feeding tubes for clients on enteral support. In other facilities, the nutrition support team nurse supervises the staff nurses in doing so, answers their questions, and advises them on preventing complications. Like other members of the nutrition support team, the nurse assists in monitoring clients for mechanical or metabolic complications. The nurse might also administer skin tests and assess the client's reactions to them.

The team nurse also coordinates discharge from the hospital. When clients go home on special nutrition support, the nurse teaches them how to follow their feeding programs and provides them with all the supplies and equipment needed. The nurse makes arrangements for follow-up care, if necessary, and is usually available to answer the questions of clients receiving home nutrition support.

An important function of the nutrition support nurse is to act as a liaison between the team and the rest of the nursing staff. The nurse teaches the staff nurses, as a group and individually, the rationale for special nutrition support and the techniques needed to administer it. The nurse also assists in training physicians and other health care professionals.

The Pharmacist

The pharmacist on the nutrition support team ensures that intravenous fluids are prepared correctly and provides training for the hospital staff who will be handling these fluids. To best serve the client and the team, the pharmacist must be familiar with all available nutrient solutions. In addition, the pharmacist assists in writing intravenous fluid orders, formulates nutrient infusions that are not commercially available, and detects any stability problems in intravenous solutions.

The pharmacist plays a key role in anticipating and preventing possible nutrient-drug interactions and in troubleshooting when such interactions occur. This team member also shares in the responsibility of monitoring clients, helps train individuals for home parenteral nutrition, and teaches other health care professionals about nutrition support techniques.

Other Team Members

Other health care professionals can also contribute to the health care team. A physical therapist may provide an individualized exercise program to enhance a client's skeletal muscle protein synthesis or mineral uptake by bone. Such a program can help the client to gain independence by developing muscular strength. A social worker may provide practical and emotional support, particularly for people on home nutrition support programs. The social worker can also help locate funding and social services for individuals who need such assistance. Staff, IV, and infection-control nurses may also participate on the team whenever they have problems or suggestions regarding nutrition support.

How the Team Approach Works

The actual members of the nutrition support team and their duties vary considerably in different hospitals. Many times, duties overlap. For example, the dietitian and nurse may both do nutrition assessments, insert feeding tubes, or explain nutrition support techniques. As pointed out before, all team members monitor and visit clients on special nutrition support.

Research has demonstrated the benefits of the team approach to nutrition support. When hospitals use a team approach to implement and monitor appropriate nutrition support techniques, the risk of complications from these techniques decreases. Fewer complications means that everyone benefits—clients receive effective and safe nutrition support, and hospitals reduce their costs.

By using a nutrition support team, a hospital can effectively reduce the costs of specialized nutrition support.[1] Highlight 30 itemizes some of the ways the nutrition support team can contain health care costs; this highlight has already mentioned many of those ways. For example, the team identifies clients at risk; evaluates new methods of delivering nutrition support; recommends the most suitable feeding solutions and methods of feeding; purchases appropriate supplies; and monitors clients to avoid or correct metabolic and mechanical problems that can lead to costly complications. By following procedures that reduce the likelihood of complications, nutrition support teams help to limit the cost of nutrition support.[2] When compared with nutrition support initiated by an attending physician, nutrition support recommended by a nutrition support team saves on health care costs.[3]

Nutrition support rounds are just about over. The physician reports that Mrs. A will go home tomorrow. She has been gradually weaned from feeding by vein to an oral diet. Thanks to the dietitian's suggestion that Mr. B begin to "eat around the tube," he is now eating a regular diet. Ms. C's problem with an infusion pump was noted by an alert nurse, thus preventing hyperglycemia. The pharmacist provided an easy solution to the problem the team was having with fluid orders.

To appreciate the team approach, remember the old adage, "Two heads are better than one." In this case, several heads are better still. Clients benefit when they have many eyes observing for problems and many brains searching for solutions. In short, teamwork works.

NOTES

1. J. M. Mirtallo and coauthors, Cost-effective nutrition support, *Nutrition in Clinical Practice* 2 (1987): 142–151.

2. M. V. Kaminski and coauthors, Confusion of cost containment and cost effectiveness in nutritional support therapy, *Nutritional Support Services*, April 1988, pp. 27–28.

3. D. D. O'Brien and coauthors, Recommendations of nutrition support team promote cost containment, *Journal of Parenteral and Enteral Nutrition* 10 (1986): 300–302.

21

Enteral Nutrition

Contents

When delivery of adequate nutrients is
difficult, their quality becomes even
more important than usual. Egg
protein's high biological value and
ready availability make it a reasonable
choice for some enteral nutrition
formulas. Shown here is a preparation
of egg yolk protein.

As Chapter 18 describes, illness affects nutrition status and changes nutrient needs in many ways. To provide the best nutrition care for people who are ill requires that health care providers first assess and analyze nutrition needs and then translate this information into a plan of action. A part of this plan describes how to provide clients with nutrients. Most often, the nutrients can be provided by using conventional foods. In some cases, though, people cannot eat conventional foods; this chapter and the next describe how these people are fed.

■ *Supplemental Nutrition*

The majority of people in the hospital receive oral diets—either regular or modified—to provide for nutrient needs. If people cannot eat adequate amounts of ordinary foods to meet these needs, however, caretakers use other feeding strategies. These strategies include supplemental feedings, tube feedings, and intravenous nutrition. Figure 21–1 summarizes some of the factors involved in deciding the most appropriate way to feed a client.

The term **supplements** often just means *food*—snacks or drinks between meals, for example.

When a person can't eat enough food from regular meals, the first step is to supplement the diet with extra foods between meals. To encourage intake, try to give nutritious snacks that the person truly enjoys. Many clients do well with such snacks, and for people who find it easier to drink than to eat, liquid snacks are useful. Psychologically, liquids seem less filling, and they are easy for debilitated, weak, or tired people to handle.

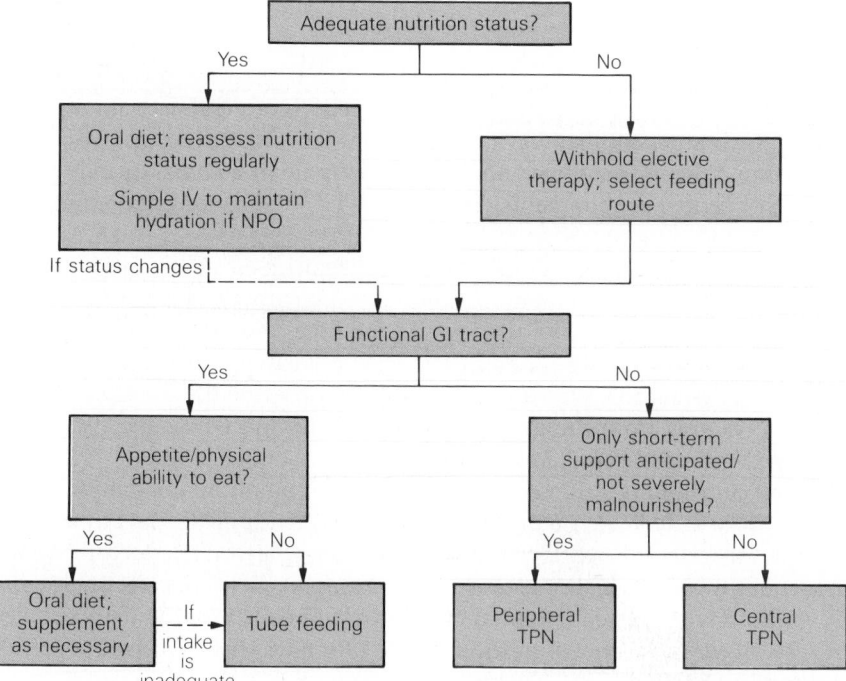

■ **FIGURE 21–1**
Selection of the Feeding Method

Both contain the same formula. Which would you rather drink?

Liquid supplements can be common drinks like milk, milkshakes, or instant breakfast drinks. Commercially prepared liquid formulas also are available (some of these formulas are listed in Appendix L). Adding powdered milk to these liquids make them high in protein, and adding a source of carbohydrate such as corn syrup or sugar can boost kcalories. Commercial products (also listed in Appendix L) can be used to raise the protein, fat, or carbohydrate content of any liquid supplement.

Even when a person enjoys a liquid supplement, palatability becomes a problem after long-term use. Help relieve boredom by using more than one type of supplemental feeding. Try adding flavorings such as chocolate, decaffeinated instant coffee, or strawberry or other fruit flavorings to the supplement. Commercially prepared flavor packets are available in a wide variety of flavors; these packets can be kept at the bedside for use as desired.

Serve liquid feedings attractively. Liquids served in a glass are far more appealing than those served from a can. Remember to serve formula cold and provide an ice bath to keep the formula cold so that it can be sipped as desired.

A liquid formula that supplies all the nutrients a client needs is called a complete formula. Such a formula should always be used when it is to be the sole source of nutrients. However, complete formulas can be (and often are) used as supplemental feedings. When used in this way, they augment the nutrient level of the diet even though they may not be given in quantities large enough to meet all nutrient needs by themselves.

complete formula: a liquid formula that supplies all the nutrients needed when given in sufficient volume.

■ Tube Feedings

An individual who has a functioning GI tract but who is unable to orally ingest enough nutrients to meet present needs is a candidate for a tube feeding. Such a person may have physical problems that make chewing and swallowing difficult, may have no appetite, may be in a coma, or may have very high nutrient requirements. Table 21–1 lists indications and contraindications for feeding people by tube.

For people who cannot eat oral diets, tube feedings are always preferred to feeding by vein, because enteral nutrition helps maintain normal gut function. When the GI tract is not used for a long time, the cellular structures of the intestine (the villi) shrink and their enzyme activity slows. In addition, enteral feedings in those who are critically ill may prevent the translocation of intestinal bacteria from the gut to the portal vein and lymphatic system, a recognized source of sepsis in individuals who are critically ill.[1]

Enteral nutrition is also associated with fewer complications than feeding by vein. It does not always require anesthetic to start; some feeding tubes can simply be inserted at bedside. Enteral nutrition is also far less costly than intravenous nutrition, an important consideration in client care (see Highlight 30). One study suggested potential cost savings of over $70,000 if 14 people who received intravenous nutrition for 280 days had received enteral nutrition instead.[2]

tube feeding: feeding a nutrient solution via a tube into the stomach or intestine.

enteral nutrition: delivering nutrients into the GI tract. Oral diets and tube feedings are types of enteral nutrition. However, the term *enteral nutrition* is frequently used interchangeably with *tube feeding.*

    enteron = intestine

■ TABLE 21–1
Indications and Contraindications for the Use of Tube Feedings

Situations in Which Tube Feedings Should Be Recommended

Protein-energy malnutrition with inadequate oral nutrient intake for 5 or more days
Less than 50% of required nutrient intake orally for 7–10 days
Severe dysphagia (difficulty swallowing)
Major burns
Major bowel resections (see Chapter 25) when used along with TPN
Low output enterocutaneous fistulas (abnormal openings between an internal organ and the skin)

Situations in Which Tube Feedings May Be Useful

Major trauma
Radiation therapy
Mild chemotherapy
Liver failure
Kidney dysfunction

Situations in Which Tube Feedings Are of Limited or Undetermined Value

Intensive chemotherapy
Immediate postoperative or poststress period if adequate oral intake is anticipated in 5–7 days
Enteritis (inflammation of the intestine due to radiation therapy, infection, or inflammatory bowel disease)
Major small bowel resections without the use of TPN

Situations in Which Tube Feedings Are Generally Not Recommended

Intestinal obstruction
Ileus (paralysis of the intestine)
Hypomotility of the intestine (lack of normal intestinal contractions)
Severe diarrhea
High output enterocutaneous fistulas
Severe acute pancreatitis (inflammation of the pancreas)
Shock
Client or legal guardian does not desire aggressive nutrition support
Prognosis does not warrant aggressive nutrition support

Source: Adapted from A.S.P.E.N. Board of Directors, Guidelines for the use of eternal nutrition in the adult patient, *Journal of Parenteral and Enteral Nutrition* 11 (1987): 435, 439.

Feeding Tube Placement

You may be wondering just how someone is fed by tube. If the thought of being "force-fed" seems terrible to you, you may feel better knowing that the administration of tube feedings has improved dramatically in recent years. More importantly, tube feedings have been used effectively to prevent and correct life-threatening disorders such as protein-energy malnutrition, thus improving the medical outlook for many people. This section describes the different tube feeding placement sites and the implications for each type of placement. The miniglossary on p. 676 describes various feeding tube placement sites.

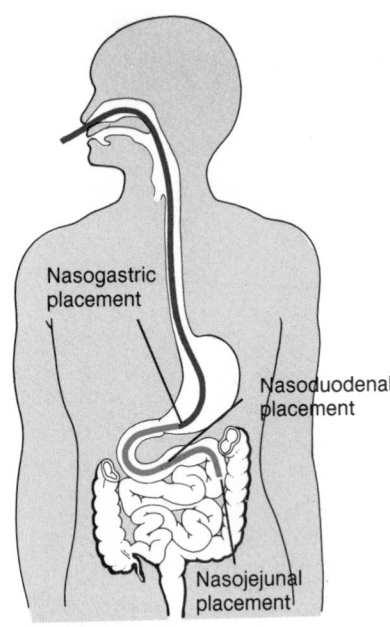

■ **FIGURE 21–2**
Transnasal Feeding Tube Placement

Nasogastric placement

Nasoduodenal placement

Nasojejunal placement

Miniglossary of Feeding Tube Placement Sites

transnasal: through the nose. A **transnasal feeding tube** is one that is passed through the nose.

naso = nose

nasogastric (NG): from the nose to the stomach.

nasoenteric: from the nose to the intestine. **Nasoenteric feedings** include both nasoduodenal and nasojejunal feedings.

nasoduodenal (ND): from the nose to the duodenum.

nasojejunal (NJ): from the nose to the jejunum.

feeding ostomy: a surgically made opening in the esophagus, stomach, or intestine through which a feeding tube is passed.

ostomy = a surgically formed opening

esophagostomy (ee-soff-uh-GOSS-toe-mee): a surgically made opening in the esophagus through which a feeding tube can be passed.

gastrostomy (gas-TROSS-toe-mee): a surgically made opening in the stomach through which a feeding tube can be passed.

jejunostomy (JEE-ju-NOSS-toe-mee): a surgically made opening in the jejunum through which a feeding tube can be passed. A **duodenostomy** (DEW-odd-eh-NOSS-toe-mee) is not used as a feeding ostomy site because the duodenum swings toward the back of the body and is not easily accessible.

■ **FIGURE 21–3**
Feeding Ostomy Sites

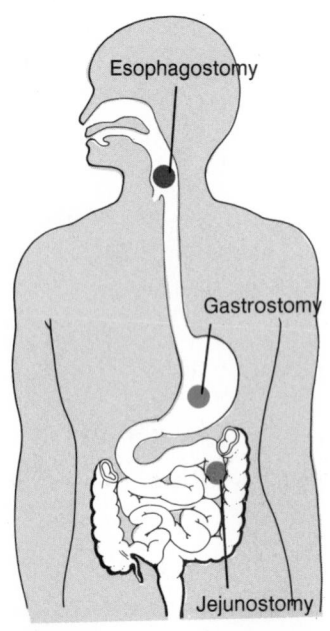

Esophagostomy

Gastrostomy

Jejunostomy

Feeding tubes are most commonly inserted through the nose and passed into the stomach or intestine. Figure 21–2 illustrates a transnasal placement. The client often remains fully alert during the procedure and helps pass the tube by swallowing. Health care professionals can insert a feeding tube transnasally with minimal discomfort to the client when the correct size and type of tube is used and the client has been emotionally prepared for the procedure. The major disadvantage of transnasal tube placement is that a client who is disoriented or uncooperative can easily pull the tube out. Furthermore, if an inappropriate tube is selected, the nasal passages and esophagus can become irritated.

When a feeding tube cannot be passed through the nose, esophagus, or stomach due to an obstruction or other medical reasons, a feeding ostomy may be created (see the miniglossary and Figure 21–3). A feeding ostomy is an opening into the esophagus, stomach, or jejunum through which a feeding tube is passed. Usually the openings are made surgically, but they can also be made at bedside with local anesthesia. Feeding ostomies are useful for clients receiving long-term tube feedings, because they are invisible under clothing and eliminate feeding tube irritation. Their disadvantages are that they involve surgery, and friction from the tube and leakage of GI secretions can cause skin irritation. Close attention to skin care is usually effective in minimizing skin irritation.

Using nasogastric, esophagostomy, or gastrostomy routes allows the digestive process to begin in the stomach. The stomach empties its contents at a controlled rate, giving the intestine time for adequate digestion and absorption. A disadvantage of these feedings, though, is that people sometimes tend to regurgitate them. If regurgitated fluids are inhaled and reach the lungs, a fatal infection (aspiration pneumonia) may develop.

■ **TABLE 21–2**
Features of Feeding Tube Sites

Site	Insertion	Potential Irritations	Risk of Regurgitation[a]	Long-term Tolerance	Chance of Removal by Uncooperative Client
Nasogastric	Nonsurgical	Nasal passages, esophagus	High	Fair[b]	Likely
Nasoduodenal	Nonsurgical	Nasal passages, esophagus	Low	Fair[b]	Likely
Nasojejunal	Nonsurgical	Nasal passages, esophagus	Low	Fair[b]	Likely
Esophagostomy	Surgery required	—	High	Good	Unlikely
Gastrostomy	Surgery required	Skin irritation	Moderate	Good	Unlikely
Jejunostomy	Surgery required	Skin irritation	Low	Good	Unlikely

[a]Relative to the other feeding sites. The absolute risk of regurgitation is small.
[b]When the appropriate type and size of tube are used.

Intestinal feedings into the duodenum or jejunum are less likely to cause regurgitation of fluids. The fluids are delivered farther down the tract, and two sphincters are working to keep them there: the pylorus and the cardiac sphincter (see pp. 46 and 47). The major disadvantage of intestinal feedings is loss of the controlled emptying action of the stomach. Formulas must be carefully selected and administered to avoid diarrhea and dehydration. Specific guidelines for selecting and administering formulas are given throughout this chapter.

Table 21–2 lists the features of the various feeding tube placement sites. As you can see, each is useful in a different set of circumstances.

Feeding Tubes

Feeding tubes in wide use today are soft, flexible, and small in diameter. They are more comfortable and safer to use than older types of feeding tubes. They remain flexible when exposed to gastric juices, whereas the older tubes would stiffen. The client on a tube feeding often becomes unaware of the tube's presence within only a few hours after its insertion.

Tubes come in lengths appropriate for placement in the stomach or intestines. Some tubes are weighted at one end, to facilitate placement and retention in the intestine, but whether the weights actually help in these respects is controversial.[3] Recent studies suggest that unweighted tubes are just as effective as weighted tubes.[4]

The inner diameter of a feeding tube is also an important consideration in choosing the appropriate tube. Generally, the smallest tube through which the feeding will flow readily is best, but it is important that the tube not be so small as to clog the tube. Unclogging a tube is difficult and attempts are frequently unsuccessful.[5] Also, insertion of a new tube can cause stress and anxiety.

Although the newer tubes greatly enhance client comfort during tube feedings, some complications are associated with their use.[6] The most common complications result from inadvertent placement of a tube in the lungs or from obstruction of the tube itself. Complications can be serious—in fact, life-threatening.

aspiration pneumonia: an infection of the lung caused by inhaling fluids regurgitated from the stomach. Aspiration pneumonia can be a fatal complication of a tube feeding.

The inner open space of a tube or hollow organ is called the **lumen.**

A typical feeding tube has an outer diameter of about 2.0 mm and an inner diameter of about 1.3 mm, as shown here.

■ *Formula Characteristics*

The number of formulas available to feed people either orally or by tube is staggering (some are listed in Appendix L). Formulas designed to meet a variety of medical and nutrition needs can be used alone or modified using other supplements to meet an even wider range of needs.

The client's specific nutrition needs, identified through a careful nutrition assessment, determine the most appropriate formula for a tube feeding. Many ways of classifying formulas have been reported, but for the purposes of this book, it is reasonable to think of two major types of formulas. Those that contain proteins, carbohydrates, and fats of higher molecular weights are called *intact formulas.* Those that contain smaller molecules of protein (including dipeptides and tripeptides), fat, and carbohydrate are called *hydrolyzed formulas.*

intact formula: a liquid diet that contains complete molecules of proteins, carbohydrates, and fats; also called **polymeric formulas.**

Intact formulas are best for people who are able to digest and absorb nutrients without difficulty; they come in the form of either protein isolate formulas or blenderized formulas. A protein isolate formula contains a purified protein. A blenderized formula can be made in a blender or purchased commercially, and usually contains pureed meat, vegetables, fruits, milk, and starches with vitamins and minerals added as necessary.

hydrolyzed formula: a liquid diet that contains broken down molecules of proteins, carbohydrates, and fats, such as amino acids or short peptide chains; also called **monomeric formulas.**

Hydrolyzed formulas are, in a sense, "predigested," and therefore only minimal further digestion is needed. People who lack digestive capabilities or who have a smaller than normal area for absorbing nutrients may benefit from these formulas.

For practical purposes, 1 ml (milliliter) is equivalent to 1 cc (cubic centimeter).

Commercially available formulas are available in ready-to-use liquid form, as a concentrate, or in powdered form. Standard formulas provide about 1 kcalorie per milliliter. Formulas containing 1.5 to 2.0 kcalories per milliliter and higher protein contents than standard formulas meet energy and protein needs in a smaller volume. Other special formulas meet the needs of people with specific diseases (such as liver, kidney, and lung diseases) who require different proportions of protein, carbohydrate, and fat.

modular formula: an incomplete liquid diet that contains specific nutrients for use as supplements.

A small number of formulas are called *modular formulas.* Some modular formulas are intact, and some are hydrolyzed. They contain different forms of individual nutrients (see Appendix L). A module can be added to another formula to alter the composition of that formula (for example, to add protein to that formula) or can be used with other modules to construct totally individualized formulas. Modular formulas can be constructed to meet specific nutrient requirements more closely than regular commercial formulas and can be less expensive in some cases.[7] However, the person formulating a modular feeding must have an in-depth nutrition knowledge to design a formula that will meet all of the individual's nutrient needs.

Osmolality

osmolality: the number of molecular and ionic particles (measured in osmoles) per kilogram of water in a solution.

Osmolality is a measurement of the concentration of molecular and ionic particles in a solution. The greater the number of particles in a solution, the greater the osmolality. The osmolality of normal blood serum is about 300 milliosmoles (mOsm) per liter. The osmolality of formulas ranges from about

250 to 800 milliosmoles. A formula that approximates the osmolality of the serum is referred to as an isotonic formula. A formula with a higher osmolality than serum is hypertonic. (The miniglossary on p. 279 defines these terms.)

A hypertonic formula can draw water into the lumen of the intestine from in and around the body cells. If the body has had time to adapt to the hypertonic solution, this process presents no problem. However, without adaptation, diarrhea, vomiting, cramps, or nausea can follow formula administration. Therefore, all else being equal, the most desirable formulas are those as near isotonic as possible.

A hydrolyzed protein formula may contain exactly the same amount of protein as an intact formula, but it contains many more particles. Hydrolyzed formulas are therefore higher in osmolality than most intact protein formulas and so are more likely to cause the GI symptoms just mentioned. They are useful, though, in cases where the gut cannot itself digest the macronutrients and has to receive them in predigested form.

↑osmolality→Hypertonic

Residue and Fiber

Dietary fiber is the portion of food that cannot be digested by enzymes in the human digestive tract. Residue is a combination of this undigested food in the colon and intestinal secretions, bacteria, and the turnover of intestinal cells. The residue content of the diet is largely responsible for fecal bulk. As you will see in later chapters, people with certain GI disorders need low residue diets. Since hydrolyzed formulas are almost completely absorbed, they leave little residue in the gut. Protein isolate formulas have a low to moderate residue content.

High-fiber diets benefit people who can tolerate them, because they help stimulate normal bowel function. People who may benefit from high-fiber tube feedings include those with diarrhea, constipation, inflammatory bowel disease, short bowel syndrome, or those who receive tube feedings for long periods of time.[8] Chapter 4 reported that certain fibers (pectins) may be digested by bacteria in the intestine to short-chain fatty acids. These fatty acids provide fuel to the lining of the intestine, enabling it to adapt more readily after large portions of the small bowel have been resected (see Chapter 25).[9] Blenderized diets are high in fiber, as are some commercially prepared formulas to which fiber has been added.

fiber: see p. 78; the portion of food that is found in the colon because people don't have the enzymes to digest it—mostly plant fibers such as cellulose, lignin, and pectin.

residue: the total amount of material in the colon; it includes dietary fiber and also undigested food, intestinal secretions, bacterial cell bodies, and shed cells from the intestinal mucosa.

Other Characteristics

Formulas can be made from many different ingredients. For example, some formulas contain lactose, while others are lactose-free. Formulas may derive their protein from a source of higher biological value (see p. 141) than other formulas. Health care providers must keep these characteristics of formulas in mind when choosing a formula for a client.

Another characteristic of formulas that varies widely is their cost. Costs vary greatly for individual products in different parts of the country and for different hospitals. However, as a general rule, hydrolyzed formulas are more costly than intact formulas, because they require more commercial modification.

Proteins → Animal Products
milk, Beef, egg, rice, corn

■ *Formula Selection*

No formula is perfect. In general, the more digestible the formula, the higher its cost and osmolality, and the lower its palatability. Because hydrolyzed formulas are more costly and more likely than other formulas to cause complications, they should be used only for people who can't digest and absorb nutrients adequately. As a rule of thumb, the formula that meets the client's nutrient needs with the least risk of complications and at the least cost is the best choice. If a formula does not meet all nutrient needs, it should be supplemented with the appropriate nutrients.

A formula given orally also needs to taste good. As a general guide, the more hydrolyzed a formula and the lower its fat content, the less tasty it will be. However, remember that people's likes and dislikes vary greatly, and what is unpalatable to one person might be perfectly acceptable to another.

Some additional factors in formula selection include:

- *The client's digestive and absorptive function.* A person who doesn't have a functioning GI tract is not a candidate for an oral or tube feeding. However, people with minimal GI function may be able to benefit from hydrolyzed formulas.
- *The placement of the feeding tube* (stomach versus intestine). Feedings delivered directly into the intestine must be easily digested, but if the GI tract is functional, they do not have to be hydrolyzed. Isotonic formulas are preferred for intestinal feedings, because the intestine is more sensitive than the stomach to hypertonic formulas.
- *Nutrient requirements.* Nutrient requirements are estimated based on careful nutrition assessment. The client's medical condition, nutrition status, and metabolic rate are all important considerations in estimating nutrient requirements.
- *Individual preferences and tolerances* (food allergies and sensitivities). Lactose-free formulas are frequently selected, because temporary and permanent lactose intolerances are common problems.

Figure 21–4 shows some of the considerations required to select the appropriate formula.

In the final analysis, the health care provider can, at best, make only an educated or informed guess about the best formula for an individual. After the selection is made, monitor each person's nutrition status and tolerance to the formula and be prepared to make or recommend a change to help ensure that individual needs are being met. As a later section in this chapter describes, the procedure for monitoring people on tube feedings includes daily weighings and weekly assessments to make sure nutrition status is satisfactory or improving.

■ *Administration of Tube Feedings*

Attention to formula preparation and administration helps ensure the successful use of tube feedings. Formulas should be prepared in a clean environment with clean equipment and by people with clean hands to reduce the risk of bacterial contamination. The person who adds new formula to the feeding bag should select only formulas made fresh within the last 24 hours; this step also reduces the risk of bacterial contamination. Unopened cans of formula are stored unrefrigerated, but once a can is opened or a powder is mixed with water, the formula must be refrigerated. Every container of formula must be labeled with the date and time of preparation, the client's name, and the client's room number. Discard unlabeled or improperly labeled containers and all opened containers of formula not used within 24 hours. Never add fresh formula to formula still in a feeding container; rinse the feeding container, the tubing attached to it, and the feeding tube itself, with water before adding fresh formula. The feeding container and all tubing except the transnasal tube should be changed every 12 to 24 hours to reduce the risk of bacterial overgrowth. Tube feedings sometimes come prepackaged in containers that can be connected directly to the feeding tube, rather than transferred to another feeding container; such systems may significantly reduce the risk of bacterial contamination.[10]

People given tube feedings often have had surgery or have not eaten for several weeks and may not be able to tolerate large volumes or highly concentrated formulas. Therefore, formulas may at first need to be diluted to one-half or one-third strength (see Figure 21–5). Initially, give the formula slowly, at about 50 milliliters per hour. If the person tolerates the formula, the rate of feeding can be increased by 25 milliliters per hour every 8 to 12 hours (see the box on p. 682). Once the final desired rate has been reached, the strength is increased. If a new rate or strength is not tolerated, back up and proceed more slowly, giving the person more time to adapt.

■ **FIGURE 21–5**
Formula Dilution

3,000 ml
Full-strength
formula

1,500 ml
Water

1,500 ml
Formula

3,000 ml
½-strength
formula

2,000 ml
Water

1,000 ml
Formula

3,000 ml
⅓-strength
formula

Formulas themselves contain considerable amounts of water. A standard formula (1.0 kcal/ml) contains about 850 ml of water per liter of formula. Higher-kcalorie formulas contain less water: formulas that contain 1.5 kcal/ml or 2.0 kcal/ml provide about 775 ml and 600 ml of water per liter of formula, respectively.

In the past, almost all people were given diluted formulas at the start of tube feedings. However, many individuals can receive undiluted formulas without problems. As a rule of thumb, people who have low serum albumin levels (less than 3.5 grams per 100 milliliters) are more likely to have problems tolerating concentrated formulas.[11]

Water is an important consideration for the individual who is fed by tube. Supplemental water is often needed to meet the client's daily fluid requirements. As a guideline, adults require from 1,500 to 2,000 milliliters (approximately 1½ to 2 quarts) of water daily. A person with a high fever may require an additional 500 to 1,500 or more milliliters. Other conditions such as excessive sweating, severe vomiting, diarrhea, blood loss, and some types of kidney disease raise water requirements. In other types of kidney, liver, and heart diseases, total water may need to be restricted.

Attention to indicators of body water balance can help determine individual water requirements. Thirst, in alert adults, is a good regulator of water needs; a person complaining of thirst generally needs water. Body weight changes can also help determine if fluid needs are being met. An unexplained body weight change of 2.2 pounds (one kilogram) can represent a fluid loss or gain of about one liter.[12] Serum electrolytes, hematocrit, and blood pressure should also be monitored regularly; high values suggest dehydration.

Water used to flush the feeding tube before and after a feeding or when the feeding apparatus is being changed not only helps prevent the feeding tube from becoming clogged but also helps keep the client hydrated. Water can also be given orally if the person can drink it.

A day's volume of a formula can be given in many ways. For example, a person can be fed four to six times daily. In such a case, the total volume of

---

An Example of Volume and Strength Progression for a Tube Feeding

Start the feeding at 50 ml/hour at half strength and then progress the feeding as follows:

- After 8 hours: 75 ml/hour at half strength.
- After 16 hours: 100 ml/hour at half strength.
- After 24 hours: 125 ml/hour at half strength.
- After 36 hours: 125 ml/hour at full strength.

A person being fed by tube. This feeding is being delivered by gravity drip.

Tube feedings can also be delivered by pump. A typical setup is shown here.

formula needed for the day is divided by 4 or 6, respectively. Feedings given intermittently allow the client greater freedom of movement between meals.

If the amount of formula necessary for each feeding is given within a few minutes, it is called a bolus feeding. Feedings given by this method may be poorly tolerated—they lead to more complaints of abdominal discomfort, nausea, fullness, and cramping. Feedings delivered intermittently (four to six times a day), but allowed to infuse over a longer period (20 to 30 minutes), are often better tolerated. This makes sense. After all, you do not gobble down a meal in just a few minutes, especially when you are not feeling well.

Feedings also can be delivered slowly, over a 16- to 24-hour period. This feeding method is called continuous drip. Continuous drip feedings can be delivered by gravity or by pumps (see Figure 21–6). Pumps (similar to those used for delivering intravenous solutions) help to control the exact rate of delivery. Continuous drip administration is useful for people who have poor tolerance to large volumes of formula. Generally, intestinal feedings (particularly jejunal feedings) are delivered by continuous drip. The box, "How to Plan a Tube Feeding Schedule" (on the next page), shows several ways to program tube feedings.

Regardless of the method used to deliver a formula, elevate the client's head to at least a 30-degree angle during the feeding and for 30 minutes following an intermittent feeding to minimize the possibility of regurgitation.

bolus feeding: delivery of a 4- to 6-hour volume of feeding solution within a few minutes.

intermittent feeding by slow drip: delivery of a 4- to 6-hour volume of feeding solution over 20 to 30 minutes.

continuous drip administration: delivery of a feeding solution continuously over a 16- to 24-hour period.

■ *Tube Feedings for Infants and Children*

Tube feedings are used to nourish children of all ages—from premature infants to adolescents. In working with such tube feedings, remember that children are not just small adults. For one thing, children are growing and their nutrient needs are changing accordingly. For another, infants' GI tracts are immature, and their intestinal motility is sluggish, even if they are healthy, so they have a limited capacity to meet nutrient needs. As with all age groups,

How to Plan a Tube Feeding Schedule

To determine a tube feeding schedule, the planner needs to know how much formula a person needs in a day to meet nutrient needs. For example, let's take a client who needs 3,000 ml of formula per day to meet his nutrient requirements. If the client is to receive the formula intermittently six times a day, then at each feeding he will need:

3,000 ml ÷ 6 feedings = 500 ml per feeding.

Alternatively, if he is to receive the same volume of formula intermittently four times a day, at each feeding he needs:

3,000 ml ÷ 4 feedings = 750 ml per feeding.

He would probably tolerate this volume of formula poorly if it were given to him within a few minutes at each feeding.

If the client is to receive the formula continuously over 24 hours, he needs 125 ml of formula each hour:

3,000 ml ÷ 24 hours = 125 ml per hour.

If the total volume of solution is to be given by continuous drip over 16 hours, he will receive 187.5 ml of formula each hour during the 16-hour administration period:

3,000 ml ÷ 16 hours = 187.5 ml per hour.

Now suppose you want to know how much water the client will receive from the formula. If the client is receiving a formula that contains 1 kcal per ml (850 ml of water per liter), you can estimate the water content as follows:

$$\frac{850 \text{ ml of water}}{1 \text{ liter of formula}} \text{ as } \frac{X \text{ ml of water}}{3 \text{ liters of formula}}.$$

X = 850 ml × 3 = 2,550 ml of water per 3 liters of formula.

Three liters of the formula provides 2,550 ml of water.

---

formula selection and choice of feeding route are determined after a thorough nutrition assessment. The accuracy of the assessment depends on the assessor's knowledge and consideration of the unique characteristics of children.

To work effectively with an infant or child, you must work effectively with the parents or guardians as well. Be sure that loved ones feel comfortable and can communicate openly with you. Encourage them to participate fully in their child's care. They may be worried about handling the child, fearing that they may cause discomfort or dislodge the feeding tube. Show parents how to handle their child, and watch them while they try your suggestions. Assure them that their support of the child makes a difference in the child's recovery, and allow them to help as much as possible.

To explain the tube insertion and feeding procedure to a young child, use dolls or stuffed toys to demonstrate. The use of very small feeding tubes minimizes feeding tube discomfort. In a baby, the use of very small diameter tubes minimizes interference with airways. In many cases, the feeding tubes are removed after each feeding. This frees the airways between feedings and reduces the risk that formula will back up into the esophagus and be aspirated into the lungs.

In infants, tubes are often inserted from the mouth to the stomach, rather than through the nose. Babies breathe through their noses, not their mouths, and insertion through the mouth therefore allows infants to breathe more easily.

Tube feedings for infants are given in very small amounts. The infant's stomach is small, and gastric emptying is slow. Aspiration pneumonia can occur readily if too much formula is in the stomach at one time. In addition, the infant can have difficulty adapting to even minor changes in a formula's composition, so the formula's concentration, infusion rate, and volume must be changed one by one, and in small increments with attentive monitoring of their effects.

Keep in mind the developmental age of each child at all times. A child being fed through a tube is missing out on the opportunity to learn feeding skills, which must be mastered at appropriate ages. Without practice, it may be difficult for a child to learn a given skill at all. In infants, the use of a pacifier during a feeding helps maintain an association of sucking and swallowing with eating and fullness. When possible, infants are given some of the tube feeding itself in a bottle or by spoon. Occupational therapists can help stimulate appropriate development in infants who are receiving long-term tube feedings.

When infusion pumps are used to administer a tube feeding to a young child, special precautions are in order. The bright lights, interesting sounds, and many controls may make the pump seem like a toy.[13] The device should be kept at a safe distance so that the child can't change the flow rate or pull the intravenous pole and infusion device over. The child could be injured, and the pump damaged.

The adolescent is more like an adult in tolerating and adapting to a tube feeding. But the teenager's psychological profile can interfere with acceptance of the tube feeding. The teenager may worry about the appearance of the tube and fear that peers will not accept her. These suggestions can help:

Parents or guardians actively involved in the care of their hospitalized child benefit their child's recovery.

- Encourage the teen to be as active as possible.
- Allow teens to dress in their own clothes, when possible. Suggest that favorite things from home be brought to their rooms (posters, stuffed toys, or bulletin boards).
- Explain the tube-feeding procedure and its importance.
- Include teens in the decision-making process whenever possible. They can help arrange their daily schedules and can help with feedings. In some cases, a teen can rinse out the feeding bag and tubing and refill the feeding bag when necessary.
- Encourage the teen to maintain contact with friends and keep up with hobbies and activities he enjoys.

Above all, be someone the teenager can trust and talk to. This advice, of course, applies to clients of all ages.

■ TABLE 21-3
Checklist for Monitoring Clients on Tube Feedings

Before starting a new or intermittent feeding:	Complete a nutrition assessment.
	Check tube placement.
	Check residual formula in stomach (if 150 ml or more, consider possible reasons for delayed gastric emptying).
Every half hour:	Check gravity drip rate, when applicable.
Every hour:	Check pump drip rate, when applicable.
Every two to four hours of continuous feeding:	Check residual.
Every four hours:	Check vital signs, including blood pressure, temperature, pulse, and respiration.
	Check glucose and acetone in urine; monitoring glucose and acetone can be discontinued after 48 hours if test results are consistently negative in a nondiabetic client.
	Refill feeding container.
Every eight hours:	Check intake and output.
	Check specific gravity of urine.
	Chart client's total intake of, acceptance of, and tolerance to, tube feeding.
Every day:	Weigh client.
	Change feeding bag and tubing.
	Check electrolytes, blood urea nitrogen, and blood glucose daily until stabilized.
Every seven to ten days:	Check all laboratory findings.
	Reassess nutrition status.
As needed:	Observe client for any undesirable responses to tube feeding; for example, nausea, vomiting, or diarrhea.
	Check tube placement (for nasogastric placement only).
	Check nitrogen balance.
	Check laboratory data.
	Clean feeding equipment.
	Chart significant details.

■ *Prevention of Tube-Feeding Complications*

People receiving the proper formula, prepared and administered correctly, seldom have problems with tube feeding. Tube feeding will probably go smoothly if a few simple measures are taken to eliminate problems. Faithful and frequent monitoring of each person is crucial to its success. Table 21-3 provides a schedule for monitoring that ensures early detection of problems.

Complications related to the formula or the way it is administered can result in GI complaints. Nausea, vomiting, diarrhea, cramps, constipation, delayed gastric emptying, and abdominal distention are among the more frequent GI complaints.[14] Metabolic complications such as dehydration, electrolyte imbalance, and elevated blood glucose levels can also occur. Table 21-4 summarizes problems associated with tube feedings, their causes, and

The term used to describe the amount of formula left in the stomach from a previous feeding is **gastric residual.** It is measured as follows: Before each feeding, any residual that may be left in the stomach is gently withdrawn through the tube using a syringe. With continuous drip administration, residual is measured every 2 to 4 hours. A volume of greater than 150 ml indicates delayed gastric emptying, and the feeding is temporarily stopped until the physician is notified.

■ **TABLE 21–4**
Causes and Prevention or Correction of Tube-Feeding Complications

Complication	Possible Causes	Preventive/Corrective Measures
Aspiration pneumonia	Regurgitation of formula, which is subsequently inhaled into lungs	Use nasoenteric, gastrostomy, or jejunostomy feedings in high-risk clients; use small-diameter transnasal tube; elevate head of bed during feeding; use continuous drip method of delivery; check gastric residual.
Clogged feeding tube	Formula too thick for tube	Select appropriate tube size; dilute formula with water; flush tubing with water before and after giving formula.
	Medications given through tube inadequately crushed or incompatible with formula	Use liquid medications whenever possible; crush tablets finely and mix with water; flush tubing with water before and after medicines are given; give medicine individually; do not mix medication with formula.
Constipation	Low-fiber formula	Provide additional fluids; use high-fiber formula; give laxatives or enemas if necessary.
	Lack of exercise	Encourage walking and other activities, if appropriate.
	Drug therapy	Change drug therapy if possible; use laxatives if indicated.
Dehydration and electrolyte imbalance[a]	Excessive diarrhea	See items under diarrhea.
	Inadequate fluid intake	Provide additional fluid.
	Carbohydrate intolerance	Use continuous drip administration of formula; monitor glucose levels in blood and urine; consider administering insulin; change amount or type of carbohydrate.
Diarrhea, cramps, distention	Excessive protein intake	Monitor blood electrolyte levels; reduce protein intake.
	Bacterial contamination	Use fresh formula every 24 hours; store opened or mixed formula in a refrigerator; rinse feeding bag and tube before adding fresh formula; change feeding bag every 24 hours; prepare formula with clean hands using clean equipment in a clean environment.
	Lactose intolerance	Use lactose-free formula in lactose-intolerant and high-risk clients.
	Hypertonic formula	Dilute formula and increase concentration gradually; use isotonic formula.
	Rapid formula administration	Use continuous drip administration of formula.
	Malnutrition/low serum albumin	Dilute formula and increase concentration gradually.
	Drug therapy	Use antidiarrheal agents; change drug therapy if possible.
	Low-fiber formula	Provide high-fiber formula.

(continued)

■ TABLE 21–4
Causes and Prevention or Correction of Tube-Feeding Complications   (continued)

Complication	Possible Causes	Preventive/Corrective Measures
Hyperglycemia	Diabetes, hypermetabolism, drug therapy	Check glucose in blood and urine; slow administration rate; provide adequate fluids; limit type or amount of carbohydrate; consider hypoglycemic drug therapy.
Nausea and vomiting	Obstruction	Discontinue tube feeding.
	Delayed gastric emptying	Check gastric residual; use continuous drip method of administration.
	Intolerance to concentration or volume of formula	Dilute formula, increasing strength gradually; use continuous drip method of administration.
	Drug therapy	Change drug therapy if possible; Use antinausea and antiemetic drugs.
	Psychological reaction to tube feeding	Address clients' concerns.
Skin irritation around feeding ostomy site	Leakage of GI secretions and friction caused by the tube	Keep site clean; inspect area for redness, tenderness, and drainage.

Note: Many of the complications presented here can be caused by the client's primary disorder rather than the tube feeding itself. In such a case, the corrective measure would include treatment of the disorder.

[a]This cluster of symptoms is sometimes called the tube feeding syndrome. Imbalances of any electrolytes are possible, and corrective measures would vary.

their prevention. A brief description of some of the more common complications follows.

Clogged Feeding Tubes

The use of small, pliable feeding tubes greatly enhances the tube-fed client's comfort. Unfortunately, though, small tubes clog more easily than large ones, especially if the formula is thick, or if formula or medication dries inside the tube. If the obstruction cannot be dislodged, the tube must be removed, and this is both inconvenient to the client and expensive.[15] To prevent clogging:

- Select the appropriate tube size.
- Always flush the tubing with water before and after administering formula. (See the upcoming section, "Drug Administration through Feeding Tubes," for more information about preventing clogging.)
- If the tube is already obstructed, try carbonated beverages, cranberry juice, pancreatic enzymes (see Chapter 24), or a meat tenderizer solution.[16]

Diarrhea

Diarrhea is the most frequently cited complication of tube feedings. Diarrhea can result from bacterial contamination of the formula, lactose intolerance, use of hypertonic formula, low serum albumin, drug therapy, or other causes.

Some people may be appalled to think that a formula could actually become contaminated in the hospital. However, contamination can and does occur. To prevent bacterial contamination:

- Use fresh formula every 24 hours.
- Store opened or mixed formula in the refrigerator.
- Rinse feeding bag and tubing before adding fresh formula.
- Change feeding bag and tubing at least every 24 hours.
- Use only formula that has been properly prepared and stored.
- Keep feeding equipment clean (see pp. 680–681).

Lactose-free formulas are available for a person who is lactose intolerant or when the possibility of lactose intolerance is high. Lactose intolerance is fairly common in any adult population; in adult blacks, Native Americans, Hispanics, Jews, and Asian populations, the incidence approaches 60 to 95 percent. Temporary lactose intolerance also can occur following surgery, radiation therapy, and chemotherapy.

For more information about lactose intolerance, see Chapters 4 and 25.

Inappropriate delivery of hypertonic solutions into the intestine also can cause diarrhea. Remember that water flows from an area of low osmolality to one of high osmolality. Thus, a concentrated solution reaching the lumen of the intestine causes water from the intestinal capillaries to move into the lumen, and diarrhea results. To prevent diarrhea:

- Dilute formulas at first, and feed slowly, especially to people with low serum albumin levels* or those who have not had any nutrients in their intestinal tract for some time.
- Increase volume and strength of the formula as indicated by the client's tolerance.
- Feed by continuous drip to allow the gut to adapt to a hypertonic formula.

A person also may develop diarrhea unrelated to the formula. Drug therapy is frequently the culprit. In this case, a careful review of the client's drug therapy is conducted, and corrective steps are taken, if possible. Oftentimes, antidiarrheal agents can be prescribed.

To correct diarrhea, **antidiarrheal agents** are given. Opiates, kaolin, and pectin are examples of antidiarrheal agents.

Dehydration and Electrolyte Imbalance

People with excessive diarrhea or those who can't handle highly concentrated formulas may become dehydrated. In most alert people, water intake is regulated by thirst. But in the unconscious or confused person, dehydration can be a dangerous problem.

One cause of diarrhea, especially for people with diabetes, may be the carbohydrate content of the tube feeding. Blood glucose may rise very high, and they begin to excrete glucose, with water, in their urine. Severe dehydration, and eventually coma, can result. To prevent such dehydration:

The rapid loss of water that is excreted with glucose in the urine is called **osmotic diuresis** (DYE-you-REE-siss). It occurs when blood glucose levels get too high.

- Monitor blood and urine glucose levels.
- Give the formula by continuous drip to prevent the delivery of large amounts of carbohydrate at any one time.
- The physician may choose to administer insulin.

*For the individual who has low serum albumin due to malnutrition or other causes, albumin may be given by vein, but this practice is controversial.

Excessive sodium in the blood is called **hypernatremia** (HIGH-per-na-TREE-me-ah). Excessive chloride in the blood is called **hyperchloremia** (HIGH-per-clo-REE-me-ah). The presence of urea and other nitrogen-containing compounds in increased amounts in the blood is called **azotemia** (AZ-oh-TEE-me-ah).

azo- = prefix indicating the presence of a nitrogen group, usually connected at either end with carbon atoms.

High-protein diets fed to people not receiving adequate fluid can result in dehydration, mental confusion, and decreasing levels of consciousness. In addition, serum sodium, chloride, and urea levels become high. To help prevent this problem:

- Monitor serum electrolytes and urea levels.

Aspiration Pneumonia

As mentioned earlier, when a formula is regurgitated and then inhaled into the lungs it can cause aspiration pneumonia, which is serious and potentially fatal. The risk of aspiration increases for people who are unconscious or comatose, severely debilitated, or restrained. To prevent aspiration:

- Use a nasoenteric placement of the feeding tube, or consider a gastrostomy or jejunostomy in people with an inadequate gag response or delayed gastric emptying.[17]
- If a transnasal tube is used, it should have a small diameter.
- Elevate the head of the bed to at least 30 degrees during feeding and for at least 30 minutes following intermittent feeding.
- Use the continuous drip method of delivery to help minimize the possibility of regurgitation.

Other GI Problems

Problems with vomiting, nausea, cramps, and distention have been mentioned earlier. To prevent these problems:

- Select the appropriate formula.
- Warm the feeding to room temperature before giving it.
- Give the formula slowly at first.
- If the person being fed by tube vomits, stop the tube feeding immediately, identify the cause, and correct the problem before restarting the feeding.

Nausea may indicate that the feeding is not moving through the intestinal tract. The presence of a large volume of formula in the stomach increases the likelihood of vomiting and aspiration. Some clients will complain of a feeling of fullness; but be sure to ask, because some people hesitate to complain. If there is a blockage, continuous feeding can lead to aspiration or a gastric rupture, another potentially lethal complication.

Unconscious, disoriented, or uncooperative clients should be given intestinal, rather than gastric, feedings. Many authorities recommend checking the gastric residual after each feeding, but others question the value of this measure.[18] It is a judgment call: check if signs indicate that blockage is a real possibility.

What to Chart

Chapter 20 emphasized the importance of the medical record as a communication tool. Document this information about tube feeding:

- Type of feeding tube.
- Tube placement.
- Client's response to tube insertion.
- Nutrients being delivered by formula.
- Administration schedule (concentration and rate).
- Method of delivery (intermittent or continuous).
- Client's tolerance to tube feeding (note any complications and any corrective actions taken).
- Client's response to tube feeding.
- Reasons (if necessary) that a tube feeding was interrupted or could not be delivered.
- Education about feeding received by client.

If a person on a tube feeding does not seem to be responding adequately, investigate to see if the tube feeding has been delivered as intended. In one study of 35 people on tube feedings, researchers found that only 16 received 100 percent of their estimated energy needs on *any* day during the period they were tube fed.[19] Intakes averaged only 61 percent of estimated energy needs. The major reasons cited for the failure to meet energy needs included inadvertent removal of the feeding tube, GI intolerances, stopping of tube feeding in order to perform medical procedures, and difficulty in positioning the tube in the appropriate feeding site (duodenum, jejunum). Furthermore, it was found that physicians typically ordered only 75 percent of clients' actual (calculated) energy needs. If these problems are prevented or corrected early, clients can benefit maximally from tube-feeding programs. Some guidelines include:

- Be alert to signs that the tube feeding is not being delivered as ordered.
- When changing the feeding bag or adding fresh formula to a bag that has been rinsed with water, check and record the amount of formula left from a previous feeding. Is the client receiving the amount of formula that has been ordered? If not, why not?
- Is the formula correctly labeled? Is it the right one?
- Has the formula been stored properly?

Be sure to correct any problems early. Appropriate charting helps all members of the health care team to maintain optimal care.

Drug Administration through Feeding Tubes

Advances in our understanding of nutrition as well as the availability of many new products to feed people by tube has resulted in a dramatic growth in the use of this feeding method. The method is especially widely used for people who are seriously ill, and of course such people are also likely to be receiving numerous medications. Often these medicines are delivered through the feeding tube, and in some cases, undesirable interactions can occur.

Crushing tablets and mixing them with water so that they will flow through the feeding tube is a common practice, but it should be avoided if possible.[20] If the particles are too large for the lumen of the feeding tube, the tube becomes clogged and may need to be reinserted at the cost of

■ **TABLE 21–5**
Selected Drugs that are Incompatible with Some Formulas

Cibalith-S syrup	Mellaril oral solution
Chlorpromazine concentrate	Mellaril concentrate
Dimetane elixir	Neo-Calglucon syrup
Dimetapp elixir	Paregoric elixir
Feosol elixir	Potassium chloride
Fleet's phosphosoda	Reglan syrup
Gevrabon liquid	Robitussin expectorant
Klorvess syrup	Sudafed syrup
Mandelamine Forte suspension	Thorazine concentrate
MCT oil	Zinc sulfate capsules

Note: These substances may be compatible with some formulas and not others.

Source: P. E. Burns, L. McCall, and R. Wirsching, Physical compatibility of enteral formulas with various common medications, *Journal of the American Dietetic Association* 88 (1988): 1094–1096; A. J. Cutie, E. Altman, and L. Lenkel, Compatibility of enteral products with commonly employed drug additives, *Journal of Parenteral and Enteral Nutrition* 7 (1983): 186–191.

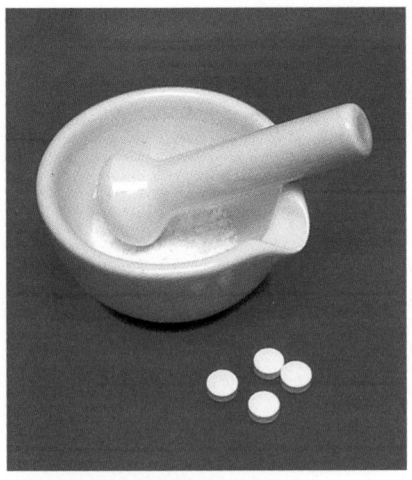

Use liquid medicines for delivery through feeding tubes whenever they are available; if not, finely crush the tablets and mix them with water.

check with Pharmacist

Drugs that may clog feeding tubes include:
- Dyazide
- Ibuprofen
- Magnesium oxide
- Metamucil
- Micro K
- Theodur Sprinkles*

considerable discomfort to the client. Also, some types of tablets and capsules are intended to release their contents slowly; they should not be crushed, or the person may be exposed to an excessive dose of the drug at one time. When administering drugs through feeding tubes, follow these guidelines:

■ Give medications orally whenever possible.
■ If a client cannot take medication by mouth, deliver a liquid form of the medication through the tube, using a syringe whenever it is available.
■ Consider giving the drug by injection or intravenously if available.
■ If tablets are the only form in which a medicine is available, crush them *finely* and mix them with water before administering them.
■ Flush the feeding tube with at least 30 milliliters of warm water or saline before and after giving any form of medicine.[21]

The location of the feeding (whether gastric or intestinal) is also of considerable importance. Some drugs are designed to dissolve in the acidic environment of the stomach. Delivered directly to the duodenum or jejunum, such drugs may not be as readily absorbed. Similarly, a drug that is absorbed optimally in the duodenum may be poorly absorbed in the jejunum. In such cases, oral, intravenous, or injectable forms of the drug should be used.

Some drugs are not compatible with feeding solutions. Common examples are highly acidic drugs; these can thicken and clump formulas, which, in turn, clog feeding tubes. Some drugs that are known to be incompatible with formulas are listed in Table 21–5. Medications should never be added directly to formulas because too little is known about the interactions of drugs with formulas. Instead, deliver medication through the tube using a syringe.

In some cases, drugs added to formulas are incompatible because the drug effects are hindered. One example is phenytoin (a drug used to control seizures). Absorption of phenytoin may be reduced by as much as 70 percent for the person who is on continuous drip tube feedings.[22] Stop tube feeding for two hours before and two hours after giving phenytoin whenever possible.

*Source: M. L. Gora, M. M. Tschampel, and J. A. Visconti, Considerations of drug therapy in patients receiving enteral nutrition, *Nutrition in Clinical Practice* 4 (1989): 105–110.

A similar interaction may occur when tetracycline is administered with tube feedings.[23] Certain electrolytes in formulas can bind tetracycline, causing it to pass unabsorbed through the intestinal tract.

An important consideration in delivering a medication through a feeding tube is the medication's osmolality. Hyperosmolar medications given too rapidly cause the same undesirable side effects as hyperosmolar formulas. If a medication is compatible with the tube-feeding formula, it can be added directly to the formula and given slowly over a longer period of time.[24] To avoid problems with hyperosmolarity:

- Mix incompatible drugs with water, and administer them slowly; rinse the feeding tube, then resume the feeding.
- Consider using injectable forms of the drugs.
- Do not mix drugs together and give them all at once; give each drug individually and flush the feeding tube with water after each one. This measure also reduces the likelihood of drug-drug interactions.

CLINICAL DETECTIVE WORK

Mrs. Innis is a 24-year-old homemaker who was involved in a car accident. She suffered from multiple fractures and some minor burns. She has been in the hospital for seven days and has no appetite. Mrs. Innis is in a hypermetabolic state, and she has lost 6 lb over the course of hospitalization. Due to the nature of her injuries, Mrs. Innis is in traction and is immobile, although the head of her bed can be elevated to 30 degrees. From the history, the dietitian determined that Mrs. Innis's nutrition status was adequate prior to hospitalization. The health care team agrees that a nasoduodenal tube feeding should be instituted before nutrition status deteriorates. The isotonic formula selected for the feeding is lactose-free, and Mrs. Innis's nutrient requirements can be met with 2,500 ml of the formula per day.

What steps can the health care team take to prepare Mrs. Innis for tube feeding? Why would nasoduodenal placement of the feeding tube be preferred to nasogastric placement for Mrs. Innis? Is the choice of formula appropriate?

The physician's orders specified that the feeding should be given intermittently six times a day. Develop a tube-feeding schedule for Mrs. Innis.

Calculate the amount of water that Mrs. Innis will receive from the tube feeding. What parameters can be monitored to ensure that Mrs. Innis is meeting fluid needs? How can the additional fluids be given?

Describe precautions that should be taken if Mrs. Innis is to receive medications through the feeding tube. After three days of feeding, Mrs. Innis develops diarrhea. Look at Table 21–5 to determine possible causes of diarrhea. Of the causes listed, which can be eliminated as possible causes of diarrhea in Mrs. Innis's case? What corrective measures can be taken to eliminate the remaining causes of diarrhea? What should be charted in the medical record about Mrs. Innis's tube-feeding program?

Drugs can trigger GI side effects similar to those associated with tube feedings. Nausea, vomiting, diarrhea, and electrolyte disturbances are a few of these possible complications. When tube feedings are being given, side effects of drugs should be considered as a possible source of problems. In some cases, a substitute drug with similar pharmaceutical action, but without the side effects, can be used to reduce GI problems.

Finally, keep in mind that tube-feeding formulas can interact with drugs in the same ways that everyday foods can (see Appendix E). Drug therapy should be carefully considered when determining nutrient requirements.

The ''Clinical Detective Work'' (on p. 693) presents a case study to help you consider the many factors involved in tube feedings. In many situations, tube feedings can provide a practical solution to feeding the person who is unable to consume adequate nutrients by mouth. However, a person without a functional GI tract cannot benefit from a tube feeding. In such a case, intravenous nutrition (the subject of the next chapter) can be a life-saving treatment option.

SELF STUDY *Enteral Nutrition*

This exercise can be conducted during fifteen minutes or more of class time or at home. Suppose that you have just been told you will have to be fed through a tube for a week or two. Record your feelings about this, and make some plans.

First, what foods will you miss most at breakfast time? At lunch? At dinner? For snacks? In what ways can you make up for these missed experiences? What requests will you make of your caretaker?

Second, what food-associated activities will you miss? Make plans to find other ways to conduct these activities. What are your plans?

Get together with one or several other class members and brainstorm for additional ideas as to how to solve these problems. Record the ideas you come up with.

Since these aspects of tube feeding are similar to those of parenteral nutrition, the next chapter has no Self-Study.

Study Questions

1. What are tube feedings? How are feeding tubes placed?
2. What are complete formulas? What are blenderized formulas? What are intact formulas? What are hydrolyzed formulas and defined formula diets?
3. What factors are considered in selecting an appropriate formula for a tube feeding? How does the digestive and absorptive function of the client narrow the formula choice? How does the feeding route influence formula selection? How do nutrient needs and individual tolerances affect the choice of formula?
4. Discuss the ways in which tube feedings can be administered to clients.
5. What special characteristics of children must be considered when an infant or child is fed by tube? Why are feeding tubes usually removed after each feeding when an infant is tube fed? How can an adolescent who is being fed by tube be helped to accept the feeding situation?
6. What are the major complications of tube feedings? What are their causes? How are they prevented or corrected?
7. Describe the problems that can occur when drugs are delivered through feeding tubes. What guidelines can be used to help prevent these problems?

Notes

1. J. W. Alexander, Nutrition and translocation, *Journal of Parenteral and Enteral Nutrition* (supplement) 14 (1990): 170–174; E. A. Deitch, J. Winterton, and M. Li, The gut as a portal of entry for bacteremia: Role of protein nutrition, *Annals of Surgery* 205 (1987): 681–884.

2. D. D. O'Brien and coauthors, Recommendations of nutrition support team promote cost containment, *Journal of Parenteral and Enteral Nutrition* 10 (1986): 300–302.

3. K. E. Fagerman and L. K. Lysen, Enteral feeding tubes: A comparison and history, *Nutritional Support Services*, September 1987, pp. 10–14.

4. D. B. Silk and coauthors, Clinical efficacy and design changes of "fine bore" nasogastric feeding tubes: A seven-year experience involving 809 intubations in 403 patients, *Journal of Parenteral and Enteral Nutrition* 11 (1987): 378–383; R. Levenson and coauthors, Do weighted nasoenteric feeding tubes facilitate duodenal intubations? *Journal of Parenteral and Enteral Nutrition* 12 (1988): 135–137.

5. L. J. Nicholson, Declogging small-bore feeding tubes, *Journal of Parenteral and Enteral Nutrition* 11 (1987): 594–597.

6. B. K. Bohnker, L. E. Artman, and W. J. Hoskin, Narrow-bore nasogastric feeding tube complications, *Nutrition in Clinical Practice* 2 (1987): 203–209.

7. S. Bell and coauthors, Modular enteral diets: Cost and nutritional value comparisons, *Journal of the American Dietetic Association* 87 (1987): 1526–1530.

8. J. C. Palacio and J. L. Rombeau, Dietary fiber: A brief review and potential application to enteral nutrition, *Nutrition in Clinical Practice* 5 (1990): 99–106; K. Shankardas and coauthors, Bowel function of long-term tube-fed patients consuming formulae with and without dietary fiber, *Journal of Parenteral and Enteral Nutrition* 14 (1990): 508–512.

9. Palacio and Rombeau, 1990.

10. L. Vaughan, M. Manore, and D. Wilson, Bacterial safety of a closed-administration system for enteral nutrition solutions, *Journal of the American Dietetic Association* 88 (1988): 35–37.

11. J. L. Rombeau, Advances in enteral feeding, an address presented at the Georgia Dietetic Association Annual Meeting, 17 July 1986.

12. C. Austin, Water: Guidelines for nutritional support, *Nutritional Support Services,* September 1986, pp. 27–29.

13. J. S. Paine, Practical aspects of nasogastric feeding in pediatric patients from a ward nursing perspective, *Nutritional Support Services,* February 1986, pp. 11–14.

14. C. L. Breach and L. G. Saldanka, Tube feeding complications, Part I: Gastrointestinal, *Nutritional Support Services,* March 1988, pp. 15–17.

15. D. W. Benson and coauthors, Clogging of feeding tubes: A randomized trial of a newly designed tube, *Nutrition in Clinical Practice* 5 (1990): 107–110.

16. S. P. Marcuard, K. L. Stegall, and S. Trogdon, Clearing obstructed feeding tubes, *Journal of Parenteral and Enteral Nutrition* 13 (1989): 81–83.

17. C. A. Monturo, Enteral access device selection, *Nutrition in Clinical Practice* 5 (1990): 207–213.

18. N. Metheny, P. Eisenberg, and M. Spies, Monitoring patients with nasally placed feeding tubes, *Heart Lung* 14 (1985): 285–286.

19. G. B. Abernathy and coauthors, Efficacy of tube feeding in supplying energy requirements of hospitalized patients, *Journal of Parenteral and Enteral Nutrition* 13 (1989): 387–391.

20. B. Wright and L. Robinson, Enteral feeding tubes as drug delivery systems, *Nutritional Support Services,* February 1986, pp. 33–37, 47.

21. M. L. Gora, M. M. Tschampel, and J. A. Visconti, Considerations of drug therapy in patients receiving enteral nutrition, *Nutrition in Clinical Practice* 4 (1989): 105–110.

22. J. Saklad, R. Graves, and W. P. Sharp, Interaction of oral phenytoin with enteral feedings, *Journal of Parenteral and Enteral Nutrition* 10 (1986): 322–323.

23. K. Fagerman, D. McGuigan, and B. Pixley, Potential interaction between enteral feeding solutions and oral tetracycline, *Nutrition and Clinical Practice* 1 (1986): 257–258.

24. P. Egging, Enteral nutrition from a pharmacist's perspective, *Nutritional Support Services,* April 1987, pp. 17–18, 34.

How People Live with Feeding Disabilities

Several years ago I had the good fortune to meet Suzanne. We needed someone to help around the office, doing such things as filing papers, typing letters, and driving to the post office, and she needed a part-time job. Suzanne was an attractive and bright student at the university, majoring in food science and nutrition. Her enthusiasm and capabilities shone through the interview and I hired her. But I had one last question to ask, Is there any task that you might not be able to do for us? You see, Suzanne had lost her left arm to cancer when she was five years old. She smiled and told me she'd always been able to figure out how to do almost anything she wanted to do—including playing first base on the city's championship softball team—with two exceptions. She couldn't clap and she couldn't climb a rope. I smiled and wondered how many people without physical or mental impairments possessed such a positive attitude and such a short list of things they could not do.

This highlight is about Suzanne and thousands of others who face obstacles in life's daily tasks—tasks as ordinary and overwhelming as eating. These obstacles can arise at any time in a person's life and from any number of conditions. An infant may be born with a physical impairment such as cleft palate, an adolescent may suffer injuries in a car accident, a middle-aged adult may lose motor control following a stroke, or an older adult may struggle with the pain of arthritis. Table H21−1 introduces some of the conditions that might lead to feeding problems.

This highlight deals primarily with the kinds of disabilities that make it difficult for people to feed themselves. Disabilities do have other nutrition-related aspects. For example, often a disability makes it difficult for a person to obtain the necessary amount of physical activity to support a healthy appetite and a sufficient nutrient intake to meet nutrient needs. As another example, a person who has lost a limb to amputation has altered energy needs. Energy needs are reduced in proportion to the weight and metabolism represented by the missing limb, but may be increased if extra effort is necessary to do ordinary things—such as walking on crutches. As another example, people with involuntary motor activity may have exceedingly high energy needs. The dietitian who calculates energy needs for people with disabilities has to take such special needs into account. The nurse and occupational therapist most often becomes involved with the nutrition of people with disabilities on the feeding end, helping people achieve as much independence in eating as possible and pointing out ways that their caretakers can help.

Ways Disabilities Can Impair Eating

When you think of the number of individual coordinated motions that are required to get food from the table to the stomach you may be amazed.

Recall what it is like for an infant to learn to feed himself. At first, the infant cannot sit upright and finds it impossible even to hold a spoon. Every single little action—from picking up the utensils, to the biting and chewing of foods, to the swallowing of them—requires coordinated actions of various body parts. Any injury or developmental disability, if it interferes with the use of these body parts, interferes with eating. The table already shown named some sixteen different conditions. For the nutrition care expert working with people who have these conditions, it is important to know which of the skills related to eating are affected. The focus is on these skills:[1]

- Ability to sit and balance oneself.
- Ability to move one's head and neck in a coordinated way.
- Movements of the jaw, lip, and tongue.
- Sucking, swallowing, chewing, and drinking actions.
- Reflexes that protect against cutting oneself, biting one's tongue, responding to noises, and all others that affect motion.
- Eye and hand movements.
- Grasping motions.

■ TABLE H21−1
Conditions Leading to Feeding Problems

The following conditions lead to feeding problems by interfering with a person's ability to suck, bite, chew, swallow, or coordinate hand-to-mouth movements.

- Amputations
- Arthritis
- Birth defects
- Cerebral palsy
- Down's syndrome
- Head injuries
- Huntington's chorea
- Hydrocephalia
- Microcephalia
- Multiple sclerosis
- Muscle weakness
- Language, visual, or hearing impairment
- Muscular dystrophy
- Neuromotor dysfunction
- Parkinson's disease
- Spinal cord injuries
- Stroke

In addition to these, a person who has problems with sight, or who cannot drive or walk or carry groceries, or who cannot plan meals and think through what to buy, also has a disability that affects eating.

As the result of any of these problems, a person with a disability has trouble maintaining adequate nutrition status.[2] As you might expect, the number-one nutrition concern for people with feeding problems is inadequate food intake, which leads to malnutrition, underweight, and, in children, poor growth.[3] In addition, many conditions that lead to feeding problems alter metabolism, and some require drug therapy, which in turn may produce additional nutrition-related problems, as Chapter 18 described.

On top of nutrition-related problems, people who have difficulty eating often encounter emotional and social problems. For example, children fail to receive the social training that mealtimes provide and older people miss the social stimulation that goes with eating in the company of others.

Independent Eating for People with Disabilities

Let us assume first that you are part of the health care team that is working with a child or adult whose disability does not necessitate constant care. This person can achieve independence in eating but needs help in arriving at that point. To evaluate and treat such a feeding problem requires the joint efforts of several health care professionals, possibly including a dietitian, a psychologist, an occupational therapist, a physical therapist, a speech pathologist, a dentist, and one or several nurses.[4] Table H21−2 (on p. 698) provides a checklist of observations health care professionals use to assess feeding problems. Because each case differs, it makes sense for everyone on the health care team to be familiar with all of these variables.

Assessing the client's nutrition status and planning a diet is the dietitian's task. The most valuable assessment tool is observation of clients during mealtimes. While observing feeding skills, the assessor can conduct a complete nutrition assessment and provide appropriate nutrition counseling.

In addition to designing a diet that will provide a balance of nutrients and the appropriate level of food energy, the dietitian needs to ensure that the diet also provides foods appropriate for the client's oral-motor capabilities. For example, people with swallowing problems prefer thickened liquids and pureed foods because these flow slowly enough to allow time to coordinate oral movements. To thicken liquids, add commercially-available thickeners or baby cereal. To puree foods easily, use a blender or a baby food grinder. If the client's abilities to eat improve, the diet can gradually progress from pureed to solid foods. The planner faces a challenge in designing a diet that coordinates the client's energy and nutrient needs, stage of development, and personal preferences.

The task of evaluating oral motor abilities and feeding skills most often falls to the occupational therapist, who can develop a care plan, educate the client, and show the caretaker, if there is one, ways to implement feeding techniques at home. As an example, it may be necessary to teach the client (or caretaker) the proper sitting position for ease of eating. The therapist may instruct the client to sit in a chair with the head and trunk in midline, the back straight and supported, the hips and knees at right angles, and the feet flat and supported on a surface. In addition to learning such behaviors, clients might benefit from the use of special feeding devices. People with disabilities can learn to use adaptive equipment to help them master self-feeding; this often improves nutrition status by making the eater independent. People who can feed themselves seem to have better appetites and eat more food than those who require assistance.[5]

Usually the occupational therapist selects the appropriate feeding devices and trains the client and caretakers in their use (see Figure H21−1 on pp. 700−701). However, everyone on the health care team should be familiar with these devices, for any of them can provide an almost magical difference in a person's ability to eat independently. Think how your own abilities were extended when you first learned to use the telephone or a computer, or to drive a car. For a person who cannot grasp an ordinary fork, a usable fork may be the key to future health.

General guidelines help therapists make selections, but each specific case presents particular needs. For example, weighted utensils can help people with tremors or spastic movements. When sporadic movements might knock dishes off the table, the therapist can recommend unbreakable dishes and suction cups, as well as aprons and bibs. Covered cups or those with slotted openings or spouts can help people gain some control when drinking beverages. Keep track of improvements in the development of utensils that help people eat. Institutions that specialize in providing equipment for people with disabilities are constantly upgrading their equipment.

Clients may need help in developing eating skills—for example, in learning to swallow. Commonly, a care plan calls for the speech therapist to step in and provide this help, for the speech therapist teaches use of the lips, tongue, and throat in speaking. The dentist may also be needed, to evaluate the client's dental health and provide instructions on oral hygiene.

Developing feeding skills requires practice. Helpers can employ strategies such as those listed in Table H21−3 (on p. 699) to help clients gain skills. For example, if a hyperreactive child is overly sensitive to oral sensations, an attendant can help by desensitizing the client gradually over time. Start by gently stroking the face with a hand,

■ **TABLE H21–2**
Feeding Evaluation

Oral ability
  Sucking
  Oral prehension
  Swallowing
  Breathing, swallowing coordinated
  Drooling
  Lips
  Tongue size, thrust, mobility
  Biting
  Munching
  Chewing
  Drinking
  Response to input

Oral structure
  Occlusion
  Teeth
  Caries
  Gingiva
  Oral hygiene
  Palate
  Pain on exam
  Hypersensitivity
  Teething stage

Body position
  General tone and movement
  Reflex activity
  Head control
  Sitting balance
  Placement of feet
  Usual feeding position

Hand use
  Palmar grasp
  Pincer grasp
  Opposition finger/thumb
  Hand-to-mouth control

Developmental feeding
  Breast _____ bottle _____ weaned _____
  Baby food _____ junior food _____ mashed table food _____ minced foods _____
  Cut table foods _____ regular table foods _____

Closes hands in on bottle
Hand to mouth/sucks on fingers
Teething biscuit/holds and brings to mouth
Finger feeds
Opposes lips to rim of cup
Attempts to grasp spoon
Grasps spoon
Dips spoon in dish
Brings spoon to mouth
Holds bottle and drinks independently
Grasps cup
Raises cup to mouth
Cup-lifting, drinking, replacing
Scoops well with spoon
Feeds independently with spoon
Straw drinking
Spears with fork
Spreads with knife

Feeding environment
  Time of feedings (note number and length of feedings)
  Atmosphere of feedings (tense, pleasant, unpleasant)
  Person responsible for feeding
  Parental and/or caretaker's attitude toward feeding
  Past successful and unsuccessful methods
  Identify positive and negative reinforcing behaviors
  Behavioral problems

Diet history, including:
  Total fluid intake
  Types of foods consumed

Medications
  Type
  Dosage
  Time given

Bowel concerns
  Regular
  Constipation
  Diarrhea

Anthropometric data
Clinical data
Laboratory findings

Source: Adapted with permission from R. B. Howard, Nutritional support of the developmentally disabled child, *Textbook of Pediatric Nutrition*, ed. R. M. Suskind (Raven Press: New York, 1981), pp. 577–582.

■ **TABLE H21–3**
Suggested Strategies for Developing Feeding Skills

Areas of Concern	Suggested Corrective Measures	
1. Inability to suck, chew, and swallow	Sucking:	Use cold substances around lips to stimulate sucking. Use a cloth soaked with water for the child to suck. Try different types of nipples. As child begins to improve in ability, change to nipple with smaller holes.
	Chewing:	Place a small amount of food between back teeth and move jaw up and down. A mirror may help demonstrate and point out various body parts. Place foods such as peanut butter on lips and encourage client to wash lips with tongue. Gradually change from pureed foods to solid foods (sprinkle crackers in soup, etc.).
	Swallowing:	Swallowing is easiest when the mouth is closed. Close jaw and lips of client together. Stroke throat upward under chin. Offer next bite of food only after child swallows. Demonstrate—let client feel *you* swallow.
2. Inability to grasp; hand-mouth coordination	To assist grasping coordination:	Allow client to finger food. Guide client in exploring mouth. Cut food into small pieces. Place your hand over client's hand and help him grasp spoon. Use adaptive equipment (plastic spoon, etc.). Make sure bowl is stabilized (suction, tape). Use plates with high straight sides, or build higher edge using aluminum foil.
	Develop activities that will help client with coordination:	Pour sand, etc. Exercise with ball. Exercise with push-pull objects. Study body parts with client, if appropriate.
	For the visually impaired:	Place meats and vegetables consistently in same areas of plate so client can find.
3. Energy imbalance: (overweight/underweight)	Obtain medical examination and assess nutrition status. Provide variety of foods.	
	For the overweight:	Cut down snacks and high-kcalorie foods. Refrain from rewarding with food. Increase exercise and leisure-time activities.
	For the underweight:	Increase number of meals per day. Include high-kcalorie foods, especially liquid supplements. Encourage proper exercise.
4. Lack of nutrition education	In working with families:	Stress the importance of proper nutrition for *all* family members. Teach proper feeding environment (good eating habits, eating positions). Provide nutrition-instruction materials.

Source: Adapted with permission from S. Calvert and F. Davies, Nutrition of children with handicapping conditions, *Dietetic Currents* 4 (1977): 13–17.

washcloth, or soft pliable toy. (This can be done playfully, making a game of it.) When the client can tolerate touch on less sensitive areas of the face such as the forehead, cheeks, and lips, then slowly and firmly rub the gums, palate, and tongue.

This discussion of ways to help clients achieve independence in feeding themselves has been brief, but the principles are clear. Accurate identification of the eating-related skills that are lacking or diminished is indispensable to deciding on a course of treatment. No matter what the disorder or condition, the skills impaired generally relate to one of the areas listed earlier. The objective is to either improve the skill or provide equipment that will help compensate for its lack. The treatment can be considered a complete success if the client becomes able to prepare, serve, and eat nutritionally adequate food daily without help.

The Roles of Helpers

The section just concluded described the best-case scenario, in which a person with a disability can learn to plan, serve, and eat meals independently. This section describes the second-best scenario, in which the person cannot operate without help, but has enough support to receive adequate nutrition. There are two parts to this. First, the same aspects of care as discussed earlier are relevant: that is, assessing needs, supplying appropriate tools, planning a proper diet, and solving all the various problems involved in delivering nutrition.

The second aspect of the care of someone with a disability relates to the caretaker, whose needs must also be met if the caretaker is to succeed in providing long-term care. Often the caretaker's needs are psychological and social, not nutritional, but they do need to be acknowledged even in a discussion primarily of nutrition.

■ **FIGURE H21–1**
Examples of Special Feeding Devices

Utensils

Rocker knife

Roller knife

A. People with only one arm or hand may have difficulty cutting foods and may appreciate using a *rocker knife* or a *roller knife.*

B. People with a limited range of motion can feed themselves better when they use *flatware with built-up handles.*

C. People with extreme muscle weakness may be able to eat with a *utensil holder.*

D. For people with tremors, spasticity, and uneven jerky movements, *weighted utensils* can aid the feeding process.

E. For people with severe limitations, *battery-powered feeding machines* require less feeding assistance from others.

Let's begin with a look at the client. Often the client who needs continuing care is one who developed the disability early or in such a way that the skills necessary for self-feeding were never achieved. For example, an infant with a central nervous dysfunction may be unable to suck

■ **FIGURE H21–1**
Examples of Special Feeding Devices (continued)
Plates

F. People who have limited dexterity and difficulty maneuvering food find *scoop dishes* or *food guards* useful.

G. People with uncontrolled or excessive movements might move dishes around while eating and may benefit from using *unbreakable dishes with suction cups*.

Cups

H. People with limited neck motion can use a *cut-out plastic cup*.

I. *Two-handed cups* enable people with moderate muscle weakness to lift a cup with two hands.

J. People with uncontrolled or excessive movements might prefer to drink liquids from a *covered cup* or glass with a *slotted opening* or *spout*.

K. A soft, flexible, long plastic straw may also ease the task of drinking.

well enough on the breast or the bottle to consume an adequate supply of nutrients to support growth. From the outset, the caretaker of such an infant must be aware of the normal infant's developmental needs and, in the case of this disabled infant, must attempt to meet those needs in as timely a manner as possible. If an infant requires a tube feeding,

caretakers should hold the infant and offer a pacifier while the feeding is going on, because the infant needs to develop a sucking reflex to whatever extent possible, and because this will associate sucking and swallowing with eating and fullness as with the normal infant. If the caretaker provides formula by tube without holding and stimulating the infant, the infant might fail to establish a loving and trusting relationship with that person, or with others, later.

The need for infants with disabilities to have their developmental needs met on schedule is so important that another example is warranted. Consider that normal infants normally develop the ability to chew and swallow during the first year of life. The timing of introduction of solid foods into a normal infant's diet depends on the infant's nutrient needs and developmental readiness. In the case of an infant with a disability, the mind may be ready but the body may not. If you withhold certain tasks from the infant until the body becomes ready, by the time you provide the opportunity to master those tasks the mind may have become closed to that mastery. Just as it is unrealistic to expect a one-year-old to ride a bicycle, so it is unrealistic to expect a developmentally disabled infant to develop a given feeding skill before the physiological capacity exists, and the timing may be delayed. And if the introduction of a variety of foods with various textures is delayed too long, the critical period when an infant's mind is especially receptive to new foods may pass, and the infant may reject new feeding techniques and foods. This can present the caretaker with a dilemma, for the alternative seems to be prolonged bottle-feeding, which can compromise nutritional and dental health. Thus, from the beginning, an infant with a developmental disability presents special problems for the caretaker. A high degree of skill and professional care is indispensable in easing these problems.

Now, consider the caretaker—for example, someone who feeds a child with cerebral palsy. In cerebral palsy, swallowing reverses so that chewed food tends to be lifted from the throat and pushed onto the rear of the tongue. If you were uninformed about this, this action might make you think the child was trying to spit out the food and you might stop feeding. The consequence might be that the child might not receive enough nutrients. (Children with cerebral palsy are highly active with involuntary motions and need more, not less, foods than other children.) To effectively feed a person who requires assistance, a caretaker needs to learn not only how to prepare and serve foods, but also what to expect at each level of development in terms of food acceptance, readiness for different textures, messiness, and self-feeding abilities.

The caretaker also needs to learn how to cope with inappropriate feeding behaviors.[6] Otherwise the emotional distress of a difficult situation can escalate during feedings and cause both the child and the caretaker to dislike mealtimes. Negative feelings during mealtimes can hinder a child's efforts to learn appropriate eating behaviors and independent selffeeding. Clearly, from this description, the obstacles imposed by developmental disabilities that affect feeding and require constant care pose a challenge both to the person with the disability and to the caretaker.

Consider the caretaker further. Children with cerebral palsy can take ten times longer to eat than other children. Some mothers have reported spending up to seven hours a day feeding these children.[7] Not only must the caretaker put in this extra time, but ideally will also make the effort to establish an emotionally pleasant atmosphere at mealtimes, reserving the task of dealing with any feelings of hostility or resentment for other times and places. Psychologists can offer counseling for caretakers; all members of the health care team need to be alert to a caretaker's emotional frustrations. In short, proper feeding of another person requires time, patience, and ingenuity from the caretaker and keen awareness, on the part of the health care team, of the caretaker's needs.

Needs similar to those of a child with cerebral palsy may arise late in life when an adult has a stroke and becomes unable to eat without help. In this case the problem is not to learn, but to relearn, the needed skills; yet many of the frustrations that the client and the caretaker experience are the same as in the case of a disabled child. As for any other disability, whether it comes on gradually or suddenly, attention to nutrition is critical and awareness of available resources and techniques is highly useful. For those who work with people with disabilities, the rewards of seeing improved independence can be gratifying.

The basic human drive to eat independently of others' assistance supports nutrition adequacy. Fortunately, some people with disabilities can obtain this independence with training. In other cases caretakers can obtain the necessary education and training to provide appropriate support. The combined approach of the health care team supports both clients and caretakers in achieving feeding independence on every level—physically, mentally, and emotionally. To whatever degree independence can be achieved, it enhances the quality of life.

NOTES

1. R. B. Howard, Nutritional support of the developmentally disabled child, *Textbook of Pediatric Nutrition*, ed. R. M. Suskind (Raven Press: New York, 1981), pp. 577–582; L. A. Wodarski, Nutrition intervention in developmental disabilities: An interdisciplinary approach, 85 (1985): 218–221; K. L. Sayler, Evaluation and management of pediatric feeding disorders, *Nutrition and the M.D.*, June 1989, pp. 1–2.

2. Position of the American Dietetic Association: Nutrition in comprehensive program planning for persons with developmental disabilities, *Journal of the American Dietetic Association* 87 (1987): 1068–1074.

3. R. K. Johnson and M. Maeda, Establishing outpatient nutrition services for children with cerebral palsy, *Journal of the American Dietetic Association* 89 (1989): 1504–1507; L. M. Thommessen and coauthors, Nutrition and growth retardation in 10 children with congenital deaf-blindness, *Journal of the American Dietetic Association* 89 (1989): 69–73; J. Krick and M. A. S. Van Duyn, The relationship between oral-motor involvement and growth: A pilot study in a pediatric population with cerebral palsy, *Journal of the American Dietetic Association* 84: (1984): 555–559.

4. L. A. Wodarski, An interdisciplinary nutrition assessment and intervention protocol for children with disabilities, *Journal of the American Dietetic Association* 90 (1990): 1563–1568.

5. S. E. Shinnar, Use of adaptive equipment in feeding the elderly, *Journal of the American Dietetic Association* 83 (1983): 321–322.

6. L. A. Wodarski, Nutrition intervention in developmental disabilities: An interdisciplinary approach, 85 (1985): 218–221.

7. R. K. Johnson and M. Maeda, Establishing outpatient nutrition services for children with cerebral palsy, *Journal of the American Dietetic Association* 89 (1989): 1504–1507.

Parenteral Nutrition

Contents

An important ingredient of parenteral nutrition formulas is salt—sodium chloride. Shown here are crystals of salt plus iodine (iodized salt). The molecules' small size and regular shape promote formation of square crystals in geometric patterns.

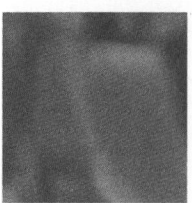

Chapter 21 described how tube feedings can nourish clients when they cannot eat conventional foods by mouth. Tube feedings are a life-saving answer as long as the client's GI tract is functional. However, without a functioning GI tract, clients must receive nutrients by an alternative, more direct route—by vein.

Intravenous Nutrition

intravenous (IV): through a vein.
Parenteral nutrition refers to the delivery of nutrients directly through a vein, bypassing the intestines.
  intra = within
  vena = vein
  para = outside
  enteron = intestine

dextrose: a form of glucose that is especially soluble in water and is therefore used in IV solutions. Dextrose contains some water, so it provides only 3.4 kcal/g, whereas glucose provides 4 kcal/g.

A variety of nutrient solutions can be administered by vein to people unable to eat or drink. These intravenous (IV), or parenteral, solutions consist of all or a combination of the essential nutrients: water, amino acids, dextrose, electrolytes (minerals), fat, vitamins, and trace elements.

In contrast to complete parenteral solutions containing all of the nutrients, simple IV solutions generally provide water, dextrose, and electrolytes. Simple IV solutions are far from complete nutritionally; instead, they help to maintain fluid and electrolyte, as well as acid-base, balances. For the well-nourished person who is expected to eat within a few days following surgery, simple IV solutions are very useful.

Generally, adults with normally functioning kidneys receive from 2½ to 3½ liters of a 5 percent dextrose solution following a major trauma or surgery. Electrolytes are replaced as needed. (The accompanying box describes how to read IV solution abbreviations.) Three liters of a 5 percent dextrose solution contribute about 150 grams glucose, or about 510 kcalories per day (see the box, "How to Calculate the Nutrient Content of IV Solutions").

People who can't eat for long periods of time, those who are malnourished, and those who have high nutrient requirements need more complete solutions than a simple IV offers. They need complete parenteral nutrition support.

How to Read IV Solution Abbreviations

Several abbreviations are used to name IV solutions, including:
  D: dextrose.
  W: water.
  NS: normal saline (0.9% sodium chloride solution).
These abbreviations are combined to specify IV solutions as follows:
  D_5W: Read as 5% dextrose in water (the subscript following the *D* tells you the percentage of dextrose in the solution).
  $D_{10}W$: Read as 10% dextrose in water.
  D_5½ normal saline: Read as 5% dextrose in a ½ normal saline solution (0.45% sodium chloride).
How would you read $D_{50}W$?

IV Fat Emulsions and Peripheral Total Parenteral Nutrition

Simple glucose solutions or those solutions containing amino acids only present a major drawback—they fall far short of meeting total nutrient needs. The problem is that the small-diameter peripheral veins become irritated and eventually collapse when highly concentrated nutrient solutions are infused. If less concentrated solutions were used, it would take 12 to 15 liters of solution a day to deliver all the needed nutrients, a volume far greater than the body can safely handle.

IV fat emulsions make it possible to deliver needed nutrients by peripheral vein for two reasons. First, they provide a concentrated source of kcalories. Ten percent fat emulsions provide 1.1 kcalories per milliliter, and 20 percent fat emulsions provide 2.0 kcalories per milliliter. Second, IV fat is isotonic to blood and does not irritate the veins as hypertonic glucose and amino acid solutions do.

IV fat is also valuable because it provides essential fatty acids, thus preventing deficiencies. IV fat can safely provide from 50 to 60 percent of the total daily energy requirement for the unstressed client.[1] Some studies suggest that in the stressed client fat may be less effective than glucose in promoting

peripheral veins: the smaller-diameter veins that bring blood to the extremities (arms and legs).

IV fat emulsions are made from egg phospholipids (see p. 112) and plant-derived oils.

How to Calculate the Nutrient Content of IV Solutions

You can have confidence in IV solutions if you know what is in them. The basic thing to remember is that the percentage of a substance in solution tells you how many grams of that substance are present in 100 milliliters. For example, in a 5 percent dextrose solution, there are 5 grams of dextrose per 100 milliliters. A 3.5 percent amino acid solution contains 3.5 grams of amino acids (protein equivalents) per 100 milliliters. A 0.9 percent normal saline solution contains 0.9 grams of sodium chloride per 100 milliliters.

A person receiving 1,500 milliliters of 50 percent dextrose and 1,500 milliliters of 7 percent amino acid solution would get, for dextrose:

$$\frac{50 \text{ g dextrose}}{100 \text{ ml}} \quad as \quad \frac{X \text{ g dextrose}}{1{,}500 \text{ ml}}$$

(50 g × 1,500 ml) ÷ 100 ml = 750 g dextrose.

And for amino acids:

$$\frac{7 \text{ g amino acids}}{100 \text{ ml}} \quad as \quad \frac{X \text{ g amino acids}}{1{,}500 \text{ ml}}$$

(7 g × 1,500 ml) ÷ 100 ml = 105 g amino acids.

To calculate the total kcalories in the mixture, simply multiply by kcalories per gram:

750 g dextrose × 3.4 kcal/g	=	2,550 kcal
105 g amino acids × 4.0 kcal/g	=	420 kcal
	Total =	2,970 kcal

peripheral total parenteral nutrition (peripheral TPN): the provision of a nutrient solution that meets nutrient needs by peripheral vein.

A typical peripheral TPN solution contains:
750 ml of 2.5% amino acid solution.
750 ml of 6.25% dextrose solution.
1,500 ml of 10% fat emulsion.

bilirubin: a pigment in the bile whose concentration in the blood may become elevated as a result of some disorders.

Hyperlipidemias and atherosclerosis are discussed in Chapter 28 and liver disease, in Chapter 26.

palpitations: rapid fluttering or throbbing of the heart.

cyanosis: a bluish or grayish color of the skin.

total parenteral nutrition (TPN): a method of meeting all nutrient needs by infusing formulas into large-diameter central veins; also called **intravenous hyperalimentation.** *Hyperalimentation* means feeding higher-than-normal amounts of nutrients either orally, enterally, or parenterally.
hyper = greater than normal
alimentation = the process of providing nutrients to the body

central veins: the large-diameter veins located close to the heart (see Figure 22–1).

IV catheter: the thin tube inserted into a vein through which nutrient solutions or medications can be given directly.

nitrogen balance.[2] Although further studies are needed to define optimal fat intake in stress, restricting fat kcalories to 30 percent of the total daily energy need is widely practiced.[3]

The use of IV fat, amino acids, and dextrose given by peripheral vein to meet all energy needs is called *peripheral total parenteral nutrition (peripheral TPN).* Vitamins, minerals, and trace elements can also be given intravenously, so that all nutrient needs can be met. Energy available from peripheral TPN solutions are not adequate for people with very high energy needs.

A typical peripheral TPN solution delivers about 2,500 kcalories per day and provides about 90 grams of amino acids. More than half of the kcalories are contributed by IV fat. People who need only short-term nutrition support (about 7 to 14 days), people with normal renal function who do not have excessive energy requirements, people in whom inserting an IV catheter into a central vein might be difficult, and people on oral or tube feedings who may need additional nutrients may benefit from peripheral TPN.

IV fat emulsions are contraindicated in some cases. Examples are newborns with markedly elevated bilirubin levels, people with some types of hyperlipidemias, people with severe liver disease, and those with severe egg allergies. Cautious use of IV fats is recommended for people with atherosclerosis, moderate liver disease, blood coagulation disorders, pancreatitis, and some types of lung problems.

Although infrequent, adverse reactions to IV fat emulsions occur in some people, particularly when IV fats are given in excessive doses or administered too rapidly. Immediate reactions may include fever, warmth, chills, backache, chest pain, allergic reactions, palpitations, rapid breathing, wheezing, cyanosis, nausea, and an unpleasant taste in the mouth. Irritation and inflammation of the vein are also possible. After long-term administration, the most commonly observed adverse effect is the deposition of a brown pigment in certain liver cells. These pigments disappear after parenteral therapy is stopped, and their effect on liver function is unknown. Other effects of long-term administration may include enlarged liver and spleen, and a decline in the number of blood platelets and white blood cells.

TPN by Central Vein

Another method used to meet all nutrient needs by vein is TPN by central vein. This may be called *central total parenteral nutrition,* but it is abbreviated simply *TPN.* In central TPN, the IV catheter is surgically placed in a large-diameter central vein (see Figure 22–1). Almost a gallon of blood rushes through one such vein, the superior vena cava, each minute. Here, highly concentrated solutions can be quickly diluted. By the time these solutions reach the peripheral veins, they are not irritating.

Enteral nutrition is always preferred to parenteral nutrition, but central TPN offers the advantage that concentrated solutions of nutrients can be delivered to people who cannot or should not be fed through the GI tract. TPN is indicated whenever long-term parenteral nutrition will be required, when nutrient requirements are high, or when people are severely malnourished. Some specific conditions that may necessitate its use are listed in Table 22–1 (on p. 708). The actual need for TPN must be determined by the individual's

■ FIGURE 22–1
The Central Veins Used for TPN
The superior vena cava is one of the largest-diameter veins and is usually used for giving TPN solutions. When it cannot be used, the internal jugular vein is the next choice, followed by the external jugular vein. Can you see why?

Labels in figure:
IV solution
External jugular vein
Subclavian vein
Catheter
Hub of catheter
Superior vena cava
Filter
IV tubing
Inferior vena cava
Internal jugular vein
External jugular vein
Internal jugular vein
Subclavian vein
Left innominate vein
Right innominate vein
Axillary vein

medical and nutrition needs. Ideally, the person should not reach a severely depleted state before TPN is initiated. It is much easier to maintain nutrition status than to try to replenish lost nutrient stores with TPN.

■ *The TPN Solution*

The actual concentrations of amino acids and dextrose that compose the final TPN solution are determined by each person's unique nutrient needs. People who are extremely malnourished or highly stressed (by burns or infection) require more energy and protein than moderately malnourished or mildly stressed individuals.

Traditionally, TPN solutions provide energy needs primarily from dextrose. IV fat is given periodically (two 500-milliliter bottles per week) to meet essential fatty acid requirements. However, the current practice is to use IV fat emulsions more frequently as an energy source. This is particularly true for people in respiratory failure, because oxidation of glucose in the body produces more carbon dioxide per kcalorie than does fat and can lead to respiratory acidosis.

Electrolytes (minerals), vitamins, and trace elements are added to the TPN solution in addition to dextrose, amino acids, and fat. Without the addition of

One liter of a typical central TPN solution contains 25% dextrose and 3.5% amino acids. Often, 3 liters of the solution are given daily and provide 3,000 kcal and 105 g protein.

respiratory acidosis: a condition of too much acid in the blood caused by failure of the lungs to ventilate properly. Excess acids are normally released from the lungs during exhalation; diseased lungs, however, are unable to perform this function adequately.

■ **TABLE 22–1**
Possible Indications for TPN by Central Vein

Major small bowel resections.

Radiation enteritis (inflammation of intestine caused by radiation).

Severe diarrhea.

Intractable vomiting.

Intensive chemotherapy.

Bone marrow transplants.

Inflammatory bowel disease (see Chapter 25).

Moderate to severe acute pancreatitis.

Severe malnutrition when GI tract is nonfunctional.

Hypermetabolic disorders, or major surgery, when it is anticipated that the GI tract will be unusable for 5–7 days.

Moderate stress if adequate nutrient intake cannot be achieved for over 7–10 days.

Enterocutaneous fistulas.

Severe nausea and vomiting associated with pregnancy (hyperemesis gravidarum) when it lasts for over 5–7 days.

Moderate malnutrition if surgical or intensive medical intervention is necessary.

When adequate enteral nutrition cannot be established within 7–10 days of hospitalization.

Source: Adapted from A.S.P.E.N. Board of Directors, Guidelines for the use of total parenteral nutrition in the hospitalized adult patient, *Journal by Parenteral and Enteral Nutrition* 10 (1986): 441–445.

these nutrients, deficiencies can arise. Essential fatty acid requirements are met by giving IV fat. Other possible additions to the TPN solution include:

■ Albumin, to raise serum albumin concentration.
■ Heparin, to prevent clots from forming on the IV catheter that might obstruct the flow of the TPN solution.
■ Insulin, to help regulate serum glucose levels.

Adding albumin, heparin, or insulin directly to the TPN solution is a controversial practice. Not all institutions consider these substances TPN additives. Where they are used, only those additives needed by each individual are given.

Insertion and Care of the TPN Catheter

The insertion of an IV catheter for TPN requires a surgical procedure. However, a qualified physician may insert the catheter at bedside rather than in an operating room; the client generally is awake but is given a local anesthetic. Unnecessary apprehension can be avoided by explaining the procedure to the client.

Because of the proximity of the catheter insertion site to the heart, the risk of introducing disease-causing microorganisms into the bloodstream and heart is great. The dressing around the catheter site must be changed frequently to keep the site clean.

The presence of disease-causing bacteria in the blood is called **sepsis**. Sepsis is a major complication of TPN.

Administration of the TPN Solution

Like a tube feeding, a TPN feeding is started slowly to give the person time to adapt to the high glucose concentration and osmolality of the TPN solution. During the first 24 hours, 1 or 2 liters of TPN solution are infused by continuous drip. An infusion pump is used to ensure a slow rate of delivery. Electrolytes and blood and urine glucose are monitored periodically. If tests indicate an unacceptably high blood glucose level or urine glucose level, the cause is investigated and treated. After the first 24 hours, the infusion rate is increased by 1 liter a day until the desired volume of solution is given within 24 hours. Table 22–2 lists the many types of complications associated with TPN, and Table 22–3 (on p. 710) summarizes how to monitor clients on TPN.

Changes in the infusion rate can cause significant hypoglycemia or hyperglycemia, which can lead to coma, convulsions, and even death, so all changes should be made gradually and with caution. When the administration of solution gets behind or ahead of schedule, the drip rate should be

[handwritten note: ↑ blood sugar? may need to give insulin]

TABLE 22–2
Complications Associated with TPN

Catheter- or Care-Related Complications

Fluid in the chest (hydrothorax).
Air or gas in the chest (pneumothroax).
Blood in the chest (hemothorax).
Catheter tip broken off, obstructing blood flow (catheter embolism).
Air leaking into catheter, obstructing blood flow (air embolism).
Hole or tear made in heart by catheter tip (myocardial perforation).
Catheter inadvertently placed in subclavian artery (arterial puncture).
Improperly positioned catheter tip.
Sepsis.
Blood clot (thrombosis).

Metabolic Complications

Elevated blood glucose (hyperglycemia).
Low blood glucose (hypoglycemia).
Dehydration.
Coma from excessive glucose load (hyperosmolar, hyperglycemic, or nonketotic coma).
Low blood magnesium (hypomagnesemia).
Low blood calcium (hypocalcemia).
High blood phosphorus (hyperphosphatemia).
Low blood phosphorus (hypophosphatemia).
Low blood potassium (hypokalemia).
Essential fatty acid deficiency.
Trace element deficiencies.
High blood ammonia levels (hyperammonemia).
Acid-base imbalances.
Elevated liver enzymes.

■ TABLE 22–3
Checklist for Monitoring Clients on TPN

Every four to six hours:	Check urinary glucose.
	Monitor vital signs (respiration, pulse, temperature).
Daily:	Monitor weight changes.
	Record intake and output carefully.
	Check urine specific gravity.
Daily until stable, and then two or three times weekly:	Monitor serum glucose.
	Monitor serum electrolytes.
	Monitor blood urea nitrogen.
Weekly:	Conduct a nutrition assessment.
	Monitor serum protein.
	Monitor serum calcium.
	Monitor serum phosphorus.
	Monitor serum ammonia.
	Monitor complete blood count.

cyclic parenteral nutrition: the periodic administration of standard TPN solutions.

adjusted to the correct hourly infusion rate, but no attempt should be made to meet the originally ordered volume. When a person is being taken off TPN, the infusion rate of the solution must be gradually tapered off; otherwise, hypoglycemia might occur.

Another way of administering TPN is called cyclic parenteral nutrition. This method of periodic administration of standard TPN solutions may help prevent a problem that has been observed when TPN is given continuously: when a person receives a TPN solution by continuous drip, insulin levels stay high. As a result, the person cannot mobilize fat stores for energy, and eventually fat may be deposited in the liver. Studies are currently being conducted to determine if cyclic infusion of TPN might correct this problem.

A person on cyclic parenteral nutrition receives a TPN solution consisting of dextrose, amino acids, and fat for 12 to 16 hours a day.[4] The infusion can be given during the night to allow the individual freedom for normal daytime activities. Cyclic administration more closely approximates a normal diet, since during sleep there usually is no nutrient intake. Liver function returns to normal when this pattern of TPN delivery is used. Additionally, it seems that fewer kcalories are necessary for maintaining nitrogen balance, probably because the person uses body fat for energy.

■ *Parenteral Nutrition in Infants and Children*

Chapter 21 addressed the special concerns that arise when infants and children are fed by tube. Many of these same concerns arise when infants and children are fed intravenously. For example, you must work with the child's parents or guardians and actively involve them in the child's care. Again, the loss of opportunities for developing feeding skills appropriate for age are a concern. Also, the infusion pump used to deliver an IV solution must be kept at a safe distance from the child, who might try to play with it as a toy. And the suggestions given in the previous chapter for helping the teenager adapt to a tube feeding apply equally to the teenager fed intravenously.

The infant fed intravenously poses additional problems. The exact nutrient needs of each infant, especially of premature infants, are difficult to determine. To formulate a synthetic mixture that will adequately promote growth without overloading an immature system is a challenge. Such mixtures might lack substances that naturally occur in foods that are needed by infants but have not yet been identified.

The renal system of an infant is immature, and it cannot adjust to changes in the blood as rapidly as an adult's renal system. Furthermore, an infant's body has a much larger percentage of fluid than an adult's, so changes in the fluid compartment of the infant's body can cause major problems. It is easy to see that when a feeding is delivered directly into a vein of an infant, too much or too little of any solution constituent can cause a problem. Too much fluid can quickly stress the infant's immature renal system; too little fluid can quickly cause dehydration. Too much glucose can rapidly lead to hyperglycemia, with severe consequences. And if the feeding is discontinued rapidly or if the tube becomes dislodged, hypoglycemia can be quickly precipitated. The list of such possible complications includes virtually every substance found in the IV solution. All members of the health care team share responsibility for identifying possible sources of all complications.

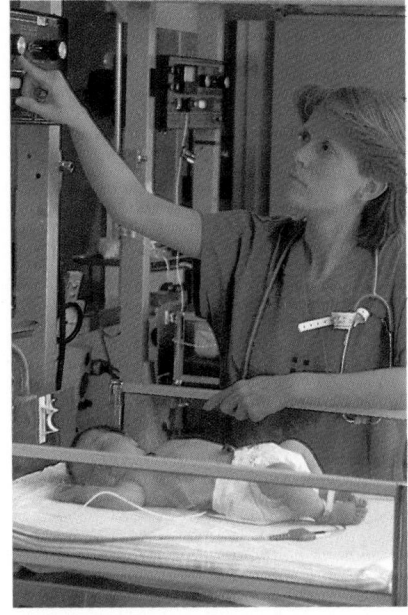

To feed an infant by IV is a challenge.

▪ *Transitional/Combination Feedings*

Once the problem causing the need for tube feedings or IV nutrition has resolved, the client can gradually shift onto an oral diet while the volume of the special feeding is tapered. Dietitians work with the health care team to ensure that the client's nutrient needs continue to be met. For example, a person on a tube feeding should be eating adequate amounts of food by mouth before the tube feeding is discontinued. The person can eat "around the tube" as the volume of the tube feeding is gradually tapered off. In many cases, the person can drink the same formula that was earlier given by tube.

The transition from IV feeding to an oral diet can be accomplished in different ways. One way is to start by placing the client on a tube feeding. Then reduce the volume of the IV nutrition solution while offering an increased volume of tube feeding, as tolerated. The person who cannot tolerate the tube feeding can still rely on TPN to meet nutrient needs. A person can also be weaned from a TPN solution while increasing oral intake, bypassing the use of the tube. Parenteral nutrition can be discontinued when 60 percent of estimated energy needs are being met by oral intake, tube feeding, or a combination of the two.[5]

The transition to enteral nutrition after a person has been on intravenous feedings for a long time is especially important. Following long periods of disuse, the intestinal villi shrink and lose some of their function. The return to enteral nutrition must be gradual to avoid problems of malabsorption and other GI discomforts. The appropriate introduction of nutrients to the GI tract stimulates the progressive return of the villi to normal structure and function.

The return to oral intake for the person who has been fed either intravenously or by tube can have a variety of psychological effects. Some people may be extremely eager to eat again, and food can be an important morale booster. Others may be apprehensive about eating, particularly if they had extensive GI problems. Appetite may be slow to return for some. In such circumstances, all members of the health care team can play important roles in the successful reintroduction of food. Recognize the person's concerns and reassure the person that you will be there to help, throughout the process.

The many decisions surrounding the provision of TPN requires careful consideration. The accompanying "Clinical Detective Work" presents a case study for your review.

 CLINICAL DETECTIVE WORK

Mr. Small has been admitted to the hospital for a diagnostic workup. He has been steadily losing weight. He appears emaciated, and states that he can't swallow and has lost his appetite. He was afraid to come to the hospital and has waited a long time before checking in. After a thorough examination, Mr. Small has been found to have an obstruction in his esophagus. The nutrition assessment reveals severe protein-energy malnutrition. Surgery will be required as soon as possible.

Mr. Small is placed on central TPN prior to surgery. He progresses well, gains weight, and undergoes surgery about two weeks after admission. During surgery, a feeding jejunostomy is made.

What factors in Mr. Small's history indicate the need for central TPN? How would you explain the need for TPN to Mr. Small?

Describe the components of a typical TPN solution. Calculate the energy and protein that would be supplied by one liter of the solution you described.

Is the placement of a feeding jejunostomy during surgery a good idea? Why or why not?

About five days after surgery, Mr. Small begins to receive feedings through the jejunostomy. His digestive and absorptive capacity are intact. When should Mr. Small be taken off central TPN? How should this be accomplished?

After several weeks, Mr. Small is ready to take some foods by mouth. How does this affect his tube feeding?

◼ *Specialized Nutrition Support at Home*

Occasionally a client must continue to receive specialized nutrition support (tube feedings or parenteral nutrition) after the primary medical condition has stabilized. In such a case, continued hospitalization is necessary primarily to receive specialized nutrition support rather than intensive medical care. An option in such a case is continuance of nutrition support at home.

The main objective of home parenteral and enteral nutrition, as with TPN and tube feedings in the hospital, is to maintain or achieve adequate nutrition status. However, nutrition support at home has an added dimension: It permits a person to get the needed nutrition care in familiar surroundings. If you have ever been in the hospital yourself, or taken a long trip, for that matter, you probably remember what comfort and relaxation you experience when you return to your own bed, know where things are, and can get things when you need them. In some cases, people who require nutrition support at home can resume many activities, such as going to work, driving, and playing sports. In general, home parenteral and enteral nutrition allows people the opportunity to lead more normal lives. Highlight 22 describes how people live with home parenteral and enteral nutrition.

An additional benefit of nutrition support at home is cost savings. It is less expensive to maintain a person on parenteral or tube feedings when that person or the family assumes responsibilities formerly performed by hospital staff. On the average, home TPN costs about half what the care would cost in the hospital, whereas for home enteral nutrition, costs are reduced by 75 percent.[6]

Since the first report of a person sent home successfully on TPN in 1969,[7] the use of nutrition support at home has expanded rapidly. The number of people benefiting from home programs continues to grow, and health care professionals who work with these programs are gaining valuable experience to improve the quality of specialized nutrition support at home. Although the exact number of people on home nutrition support programs is unknown, a 1986 survey estimates about 14,300 people are on home TPN and as many as 52,000 people are on tube feedings.[8] Many medical supply companies provide the equipment, formulations, and service necessary to support home nutrition care.

While one person may require home nutrition support for a relatively short time (for example, a few months), another may need it permanently. In addition to medical considerations, the candidate for home nutrition support and those who care for that person must have rational, stable personalities so that problems can be successfully handled as they arise. The person or those who care for the person must be capable of learning the techniques of nutrition support and of dealing with complications. Additionally, the person must have financial resources to support the program as well as access to the equipment, supplies, and professional support that are integral components of a successful home program. The members of the nutrition support team are usually the ones that decide if a client is a candidate for home parenteral and enteral nutrition.

■ FIGURE 22–2
Placement of a Home TPN Catheter
In this case, the catheter is tunneled under the skin before going into the subclavian vein; in other cases, the catheter may enter the subclavian directly.

Home Total Parenteral Nutrition (Home TPN)

People on home TPN most commonly have cancer, Crohn's disease, or ischemic bowel disease (death of a portion of the intestine). Different types of home TPN programs are in current use. Ideally, clients are given as much responsibility for their own care as they can handle. For example, a client who is capable of mixing the solutions and changing the catheter dressings is trained to do so. Typically, family members also learn the techniques so that they can assist in the procedures whenever necessary.

A special type of catheter often is inserted for home TPN; it enters the subclavian vein but is tunneled under the skin and eventually exits the body near the middle of the chest (see Figure 22–2). The use of this route makes it possible for the client to see the catheter site without using a mirror and to inspect it directly for changes, as well as to perform dressing changes.

Another system for infusing home TPN solutions is the subcutaneous port. Unlike a typical catheter that has an outside portion exposed, the port is totally implanted under the skin. Totally implanted devices appear to be associated with a lower infection rate, and they do not require a dressing except when the nutrient infusion is being delivered.[9] The port is cosmetically superior (an advantage for the adolescent), and it results in less restriction of activity (an advantage for young children and other active people). However, obese clients and those who are noncompliant or misuse the port may have a difficult time with this system.[10]

The most common method of nutrient administration is for the client to use an infusion pump set at a rate that delivers the total volume of solution needed for the day within 8 to 12 hours. Most people can tolerate solutions delivered this way. The total volume of solution can be placed in large-capacity IV bags so that the client can infuse the solution while sleeping or at any other convenient time. This method of delivery allows freedom of movement during much of the day.

The client starts the solution slowly to avoid hyperglycemia and tapers it off at the end of the feeding to avoid hypoglycemia. Each time the client disconnects the IV tubing, heparin is injected into the catheter to prevent clotting.

For people who cannot tolerate an 8- to 12-hour infusion rate, nutrients are infused over 24 hours. Those who are ambulatory can benefit from a lightweight carry case that holds a small pump and IV bags (see the photo in Highlight 22). This system allows the client to move around freely with little inconvenience.

Some people prepare their own TPN solutions from bottles of IV dextrose and amino acids. Others receive their bottles premixed. Premixed solutions are convenient, and may be essential if the client's (or family member's) ability to correctly mix the solution is questionable. The costs of premixed versus self-mixed solutions vary widely. In some cases self-mixed solutions are actually more expensive. A significant and shocking variability in the costs of home TPN solutions has been reported. In a survey of home care costs, 12 home care vendors were asked to provide price quotes for a given home TPN formula.[11] The price for self-mixed formulas ranged from $63,430 to $133,431 annually, varying by about $70,000! Similarly, the difference between the least expensive and most expensive vendor for premixed formulas was over $60,000 annually. Although the authors note that the services provided by the different vendors are not accounted for in this survey, it is obvious that health care team members need to look closely at the vendors in their area who provide home care services.

Home Enteral Nutrition

People on home enteral nutrition programs most commonly have cancer or swallowing disorders. Home enteral nutrition programs are similar to home TPN programs in many ways. Tube feeding is the choice of feeding method for the person who must continue special nutrition support at home. Enteral nutrition preserves normal bowel function, it is simpler to prepare and deliver, it is less expensive, and it has fewer complications than parenteral feedings.

The person on a home program either makes a tube feeding from blenderized table food or purchases a commercially prepared, premixed formula. Most clients prefer to purchase formula, and premixed formula should certainly be used whenever a person's ability to mix the formula is questionable.

Feeding ostomies often are placed for long-term tube feedings. Some people learn to use a transnasal tube, which they insert at each feeding. Others have a transnasal tube inserted as described in Chapter 21. When possible, an intermittent feeding schedule is arranged so that the person is free to move around between meals.

Generally, infusion pumps are used only if necessary, for they are expensive to purchase or rent. For clients on continuous drip feedings who must use pumps, small pumps, easily concealed in clothing, are available to allow more freedom of movement. Standard pumps are also available for home use.

Generally, a nurse visits the person on a tube feeding at home, and the person also sees a physician at regular intervals. In some programs, dietitians make home visits also. A qualified nurse, dietitian, or physician must be available to answer questions as they arise.

No doubt, enteral and parenteral nutrition provide life-saving alternatives for nourishing people in times of severe stress. The next chapter examines the relationships between nutrition and severe stress.

■ Study Questions

1. Describe the differences between routine IV solutions, peripheral TPN solutions, and central TPN solutions. When is each type used?
2. How have IV fat emulsions made it possible to meet energy requirements by peripheral vein?
3. What are the components of a typical TPN solution? What other additives may be present? How many kcalories are in one liter of a TPN solution containing 25 percent dextrose and 5 percent amino acids?
4. How are TPN catheters inserted? How is a TPN feeding initiated? Stopped? Why?
5. Describe some ways in which a person on tube feedings or parenteral nutrition can be weaned to ordinary table foods.
6. What are the advantages to home enteral and parenteral nutrition programs? Describe some features of home TPN that are unique to home programs.
7. Discuss how a home enteral nutrition program works.

Notes

1. M. Roesner and J. P. Grant, Intravenous lipid emulsions, *Nutrition in Clinical Practice* 2 (1987): 96–107.
2. H. Shizgal and R. Forse, Protein and calorie requirements with total parenteral nutrition, *Annals of Surgery* 192 (1980): 562–569; J. Long and coauthors, Effect of carbohydrate and fat intake on nitrogen excretion during total intravenous feeding, *Annals of Surgery* 185 (1987): 417–421.
3. R. H. Bower, Nutritional and metabolic support of critically ill patients, *Journal of Parenteral and Enteral Nutrition* (supplement) 14 (1990): 257–259; G. L. Blackburn, In search of the "preferred fuel," *Nutrition in Clinical Practice* 4 (1989): 3–5.
4. K. M. Bennett and G. H. Rosen, Cyclic total parenteral nutrition, *Nutrition in Clinical Practice* 5 (1990): 163–165.
5. M. F. Winkler, A. Pomp, M. D. Caldwell, and J. E. Albina, Transitional feeding: The relationship between nutritional intake and plasma protein components, *Journal of the American Dietetic Association* 89 (1989): 969–970.
6. Howard and coauthors, A review of the current national status of home parenteral and enteral nutrition from the provider and consumer perspective, *Journal of Parenteral and Enteral Nutrition* 10 (1986): 416–424.
7. M. E. Shils and coauthors, Long-term parenteral nutrition through an external arteriovenous shunt, *New England Journal of Medicine* 283 (1970): 341–344.
8. The Oley Foundation and A.S.P.E.N., OASIS Home Nutritional Support Patient Registry: Annual Report (Albany, NY: Aley Foundation for Home Parenteral and Enteral Nutrition, 1986).
9. S. L. Beck, N. R. Rose, and A. J. Zagoren, Home total parenteral nutrition utilizing implantable infusion ports, *Nutrition in Clinical Practice* 2 (1987): 26–29.
10. J. H. Bodzin, Homecare open forum, *Nutritional Support Services* 6 (1986): 23, 25.
11. R. J. Baptista and coauthors, The cost of home total parenteral nutrition, *Nutrition in Clinical Practice* 2 (1987): 14–22.

How People Live with Specialized Nutrition Support

Complex procedures, such as those necessary to deliver parenteral and enteral nutrition, require attention to technical details and conscientious monitoring. For these reasons it is easy to focus on the procedure and forget about the person who is the object of your care. This highlight serves to remind you of the many concerns of people on specialized nutrition support.

Coping with Nutrition Support in the Hospital

First, let us digress somewhat and talk, from personal experience, about the emotional aspects of working with people on tube feedings and parenteral nutrition. The first few experiences can be emotionally draining. One feels a deep empathy for the person who must have a catheter inserted into a vein under local anesthesia or a tube inserted through the nose and into the stomach or intestine while fully awake. The first few times you are involved with these procedures, your stomach may turn. You do your best to overcome these feelings by keeping in mind the physiological benefits the person will gain.

As you gain experience with the procedures, your fears and anxieties ease. Now the benefits stand so clearly implanted in your mind that your empathy for the person may fade somewhat. Now your mind is intent on delivering care that is as excellent as possible, technically. At this point, it is time to recall your earlier feelings. While for you these nutrition support procedures are now familiar and unthreatening, in all likelihood this is the first time your client is experiencing them. Especially for clients that are not in a health field, these procedures may be very frightening and the thought of this type of care very disturbing.

Furthermore, the person who needs special nutrition support is typically already very ill and has the usual concerns regarding illness. And now this happens. Clearly, in addition to providing your technical skill, you have the opportunity and obligation to offer moral support. Allay the client's fears. Explain carefully the procedure for inserting the catheter or tube. Give the person time to ask questions; take the time to answer them fully. Be sure clients and their caretakers understand the objective of nutrition support and how it will aid in recovery.

The person fed by tube or vein is denied the pleasure and comfort of eating food. People use food for many reasons other than nutrition (see pp. 6–8), and these aspects of food intake are denied the person on special nutrition support. Feeding becomes merely "nourishment" and not an expression of personal, social, or cultural identity. The person may also feel self-conscious about how tubing looks and may feel tied down by the feeding equipment. The conscientious health care provider will address these concerns, too.

Show understanding of the reasons the person misses eating "real" food. Find substitutes, where possible. If people can "eat around a tube" or have some foods by mouth in addition to TPN, let them select the foods they like, if possible. Sometimes a person can "drink" a favorite beverage or food (blenderized) through a tube. Even though one cannot taste a food given this way, one can derive psychological satisfaction from it.

As for the problem of feeling tied down, deal with this, too. If bedrest is not required, show the person how to manipulate the feeding equipment so as to get out of bed, walk about, and socialize. The person will soon realize

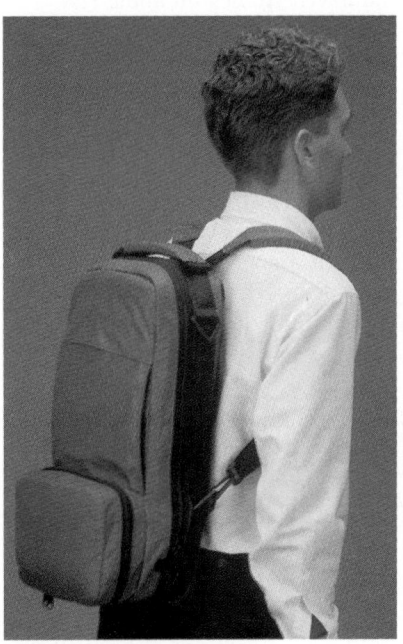

Carry cases designed to hold a battery-operated pump and a 3-liter bag of solution allow people on home TPN to lead normal lives, free from a pole-mounted apparatus.

that movement is not impossible and that exercise feels good. Opportunities for socialization gained this way can help one forget about the special feeding and lighten one's mood.

Coping with Nutrition Support at Home

The person on home parenteral or enteral nutrition, as explained in Chapter 22, has succeeded in working out a way of obtaining nutrients daily via tube feeding or through a vein. At its best, this represents a remarkably courageous adaptation to a challenging way of life. Clients can carry all their equipment and formulas in a special case so that they can move about, take care of themselves, socialize, and also sustain health at home without eating food in the usual way.

Many people in successful home programs enjoy a reasonable quality of life.[1] Home parenteral and enteral nutrition arrangements allow people to resume many activities, including employment, sexual activity, recreation, swimming, social activity, and travel. Women on home TPN successfully carry and deliver babies. Students return to college. One person on home TPN was quoted as saying, "Do I miss the taste of real food? Sure. But you get used to it. Look at the alternative. Ten years ago I would have been dead of starvation."[2]

In a 1987 survey of people on home nutrition support programs, participants were asked to rank their psychosocial concerns.[3] Depression, control, and independence were cited most frequently, followed by restricted food intake, relationship with spouse or significant others, body image, and sexual concerns. Clients also worry about the substantial costs associated with long-term nutrition support (see Chapter 22). Although techniques of home support have become safer and simpler, these changes have come at a financial cost. Financial problems can be major for the individual on expensive therapy who often cannot continue to work full time. Social workers might be able to assist clients in finding ways to handle some of these problems.

To deal with emotional problems, clients might benefit from support groups or counseling. A psychologist, Stan W. Ziegler, Ph.D., who has been on various home nutrition support programs, provides a thought-provoking and very personal testimony to the psychosocial implications of home nutrition support:

I was profoundly affected by the movie *Mask*, the story of a horribly disfigured boy who somehow fits into the world. My mask is on the inside, though, and not one that is visible to the rest of the world. If I am disfigured in some way and if some of my basic body functions are very different from that of other people, this is not something that the world looking at me knows. When the world sees me now, it sees a reasonable and healthy, if somewhat thin, looking man. The mask I wear is on my body, but more important, on the part of my mind that has been changed by all of this. If, because of my experiences, I see the world differently than most people, I have had to figure this into my perceptions of things so I do not feel too alienated. The challenge now is one of integration: to integrate my night feedings into my daily routine; to integrate my past medical experiences into my present life in a useful and growth-encouraging way; to integrate my sense of myself as a man with a serious chronic illness into my understanding of me as a whole person who doesn't live the life of a chronically ill man. Ultimately this is the challenge faced by all of your chronically ill patients on nutritional support who try to live full and useful lives.[4]

So while nutrition support provides clients with all they might need nutritionally, it also brings a few problems. Given guidance on what problems to expect and counsel on how to cope with them, however, clients can learn to accept this new way of eating as a gift of life.

NOTES

1. C. Marein and coauthors, Home parenteral nutrition, *Nutrition in Clinical Practice* 1 (1986): 179–182; J. R. Wesley, Home parenteral nutrition: Indications, principles, and cost-effectiveness, *Comprehensive Therapy* 4 (1983): 29–36; K. Ladefoged, Quality of life in patients on permanent home parenteral nutrition, *Journal of Parenteral and Enteral Nutrition* 5 (1982): 132–137.

2. D. Ingber, People who never need to eat, *Science Digest*, January 1982, pp. 34–35.

3. As cited in K. C. Hoffman, Psychosocial concerns of home nutrition therapy consumers, *Nutrition in Clinical Practice* 4 (1989): 51–56.

4. S. W. Ziegler, Living on nutrition support: One patient's perspective, *Nutrition in Clinical Practice* 4 (1989): 57–61.

Nutrition, Infection, and Trauma

This micrograph shows dozens of invasive microorganisms (oval shapes) attacking a cell (visible in the lower left-hand corner). The cells need to build up tremendous defenses against such stressful invasions, defenses that require adequate nutrition support.

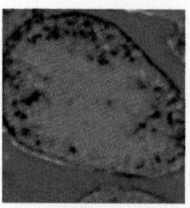

Chapter 18 described the general relationships of nutrition with stress, with the immune system, and with medications. Chapters 19 through 22 followed with general guidelines for assessing nutrition status, planning care strategies, and feeding clients. These generalities provide the basis for nutrition care. Now the chapters will begin to examine the special needs of clients with specific medical conditions. This special attention to nutrition enhances the quality of care to a level that can make a dramatic difference to recovery.

As you may recall from Chapter 18, severe stresses and traumas such as infection, surgery, and burns bring on many hormonal and metabolic changes that influence nutrient needs. In general, diets high in energy, protein, vitamins, and minerals best meet these nutrient needs. In addition, stressful conditions require close attention to fluid balance. Other types of mechanical trauma, such as bone fractures, also benefit from such a diet. As you read this chapter, notice the similarities and differences in the nutrition care of clients with various types of stresses.

Nutrition and Infection

During an **infection**, the body is invaded by a disease-causing microorganism or virus that causes illness. An infection may remain localized to one area (for example, a patch of skin) or may invade the bloodstream and, thereby, the whole body. The presence of microorganisms or their poisonous products directly in the bloodstream is known as **sepsis** or **septicemia** (sep-tee-SEE-me-ah).

Infections can develop whenever disease-causing microorganisms invade the body. They may spread throughout the body or remain localized. Infections often occur as a complication of another illness or infection. For example, the infection pneumonia may accompany measles. Infections are especially common following injuries (trauma) such as accidents, surgery, or burns.

When infectious microorganisms or their poisonous byproducts invade the bloodstream, sepsis develops. Critically ill people who develop sepsis may experience progressive failure of multiple organ systems. Such a combination frequently leads to death.

Recall from Chapter 18 that the body responds to the stress of illness with a series of metabolic changes designed to bring the body back to its normal state of equilibrium. Among the changes that occur is suppression of immune system activity. The immune system suffers even greater damage when the infection derives from the AIDS-causing virus. The AIDS virus attacks immune system cells directly, rendering them defenseless. AIDS is mentioned here to remind you that while infections can be as minor as a skin boil or food-borne illness, they can also be life-threatening. AIDS receives full attention in Chapter 30.

Infections spread easily in people already weakened by the stresses of malnutrition, surgery, or other injury. In addition, anorexia, nausea, vomiting, diarrhea, and immobilization accompany infection, placing further demands on nutrient stores. Not surprisingly, the incidence of infection is high in areas of the world where people suffer from malnutrition. Infection worsens malnutrition, and a downward spiral begins.

Nutrient Needs during Infection

Once an infection has developed, the metabolic events that follow greatly influence nutrient needs. For the most part, the body's response to infection parallels the response that occurs with other stresses: glycogen and fatty acids are mobilized for energy, the metabolic rate rises, protein tissues begin to break down, and ketones are produced as an alternative energy source. However, in infection, hypermetabolism is prolonged, body protein break down is extensive, and the body's adaptation to using ketones for energy is delayed. As a result, energy and protein losses are more severe.

The course of an infection goes something like this. Following exposure to an infective agent, a period of time (generally a few days) passes before the first symptoms of the infection appear. Shortly after this period, most infections produce a fever.

Fever may be alarming to some people, but it actually helps the body to fight harmful bacteria and viruses. Even so, fever causes discomfort and many people seek relief by using analgesic medicines such as acetylsalicylic acid (commonly known as aspirin), acetaminophen, or ibuprofen. Like other drugs, these fever-relieving medicines risk side effects and interact with foods and nutrients, as listed in Table 23–1.

After the onset of fever, the catabolic changes that characterize the stress response begin. Hyperglycemia develops. The body's losses of nitrogen (from protein catabolism) and intracellular electrolytes (potassium, magnesium, phosphorus, zinc, and sulfur) exceed intake, and negative body balances develop. If diarrhea and vomiting also occur, the body loses even more nutrients. Fever and reduced intake of food aggravates these negative balances even further. Because of associated hormonal changes, the infected individual may retain water and sodium.

The person who survives the hypermetabolic phase of an infection gradually begins to conserve nitrogen. However, this occurs after considerable weight loss and muscle wasting. Once the illness has ended, the person generally develops positive balances that restore the body to its normal composition. The time it takes for the body to reach a positive balance and the duration of the positive balance depend on prior nutrition status, the extent of nutrient deficiencies, as well as the quality and quantity of food intake.

The **incubation period** of an infection is the interval between exposure to the infection and development of related symptoms.

A **fever** is an increase of body temperature of more than 1° F above normal (98.6° F). A person who is **febrile** (FEE-brile) has a fever; **afebrile** (AY- fee-brile) means "without fever."

analgesic: a drug that relieves pain, such as aspirin, ibuprofen, or acetaminophen.
an = without
alg = pain

The **convalescent period** of an infection describes the period of recovery from illness; during convalescence the body develops positive nutrient balances.

■ TABLE 23–1
Analgesics

Drug Name	Timing with Meals	Common Side Effects That May Influence Nutrition Status
Acetaminophen	Give with food to decrease GI distress.	Side effects rarely occur.
Acetylsalicylic acid	Give with water, or with food if GI distress occurs with use.	Stomach upset, vomiting, nausea, GI bleeding, irritation of ulcers. May induce iron deficiency by causing GI bleeding. May enhance effects of anticlotting and antidiabetic medicine. Severe allergic reaction in some people.
Ibuprofen	Give on empty stomach, or with food or milk if GI distress occurs with use.	Nausea, stomach pain, heartburn, anorexia, dry mouth, diarrhea, vomiting, indigestion, constipation, abdominal cramps or pain, bloating, gas. May induce iron deficiency by causing GI bleeding.

Source: Adapted from D. E. Powers and A. O. Moore, *Food Medication Interactions*, (Phoenix, Ariz.: Food Medication Interactions, 1989).

antibiotics: drugs that kill microorganisms or interfere with their growth; also called antimicrobials.

During this time, a well-balanced diet helps to restore vital nutrient reserves and guard against the development of additional infections.

The primary task in caring for the infected person requires identification and elimination of the invading organism. Often, physicians prescribe antibiotics. Some antibiotics require specific timing with meals and may alter nutrient status (see Table 23–2). Keep your eyes open for signs of nutrient deficiencies when your clients are taking antibiotics.

Goals for Meeting Nutrient Needs

The scientific name for the centigrade temperature scale is Celsius. Conversion equations are provided on p. 3 of Appendix D.

To meet the heightened nutrient needs of infection requires a diet high in energy. Fever is a major factor in determining the energy needs of an infected person. The basal metabolic rate (BMR) increases approximately 13 percent for each degree centigrade (7 percent for each degree Fahrenheit) that the temperature rises above normal (98.6° Fahrenheit; 37° centigrade). Thus a person with 4 degrees (Fahrenheit) of fever—that is, a temperature of 102.6°—will have a BMR that is running almost a third faster than normal (4 degrees × 7 percent = 28 percent). Since the BMR requires some 1,000 to 2,000 kcalories a day (recall from Chapter 12), this person may need 300 to 600 extra kcalories a day to maintain body energy stores. In addition, the diet needs to provide extra food energy to account for activity, particularly for restless people. You might think that for an obese person the energy costs of fever and restlessness would bring about a needed loss of body fat, and indeed, fat stores can feed the body needed extra energy at such a time. However, lean tissue needs to be spared—hence even the obese person

■ **TABLE 23–2**
Antibiotics

Drug Name	Timing with Meals	Common Side Effects That May Influence Nutrition Status
Chloramphenicol	Give with water 1 hr before or 2 hr after meals.	Diarrhea, nausea, vomiting, irritation of mouth or tongue. May enhance effects of antidiabetic medicine. May raise requirements of riboflavin, vitamin B_6, and vitamin B_{12}.
Neomycin		Nausea, vomiting, diarrhea, sore mouth. Decreases absorption of fats, nitrogen, carbohydrates, folate, vitamin B_6, vitamin B_{12}, fat-soluble vitamins, calcium, and iron.
Penicillin	Give penicillin G on an empty stomach; penicillin K with or without meals.	Nausea, vomiting, diarrhea, gas, anemia, sore mouth, altered taste perceptions, anorexia.
Tetracycline	Give on an empty stomach; don't give with milk or dairy products; don't give iron-containing supplements within 3 hours of tetracycline ingestion.	Anorexia, nausea, vomiting, diarrhea, altered taste perceptions, sore mouth. Decreases absorption of fat, amino acids, calcium, iron, magnesium, and zinc. Decreases bacterial synthesis of vitamin K in intestines.

Source: Adapted from D. E. Powers and A. O. Moore, *Food Medication Interactions*, (Phoenix, Ariz.: Food Medication Interactions, 1989).

requires adequate energy from carbohydrate and fat. Chapter 19 provides an equation for estimating energy needs for obese people with fever (see p. 637).

The immune system fights infection best when supported by an optimal protein status. Generally, protein needs range from 1.5 to 2.0 grams protein per kilogram body weight per day. The accompanying box shows how to determine the energy and protein needs of a client with an infection.

Closely monitor the person with an infection to ensure that fluid intake meets fluid needs. For people with infections that are not accompanied by diarrhea, vomiting, or excessive sweating, dehydration is usually not a problem. However, in infectious diseases that do incur these fluid losses, fluid needs may be as high as 3 to 4 liters per day. On the other hand, the infected

---

How to Determine Energy and Protein Needs for an Infection

The following example illustrates how to determine the energy and protein needs of a person with an infection.

Johnny Fever is a 22-year-old male who is 5' 9'' tall, weighs 160 lb, and has a temperature of 103° F. To calculate the impact of fever on Johnny's energy needs, first determine his BMR (for males, 1 kcal/kg/hr; for females, 0.9 kcal/kg/hr).

$$1 \text{ kcal} \times \frac{160 \text{ lb}}{2.2 \text{ kg}} \times 24 \text{ hr} = 1{,}745 \text{ kcal/day}.$$

You know that BMR increases 13% per degree centigrade or 7% per degree Fahrenheit. Johnny's temperature is 4.4° F above normal, so his BMR increases by:

$$4.4° \text{ F} \times 0.07 = 31\%.$$

Therefore, his energy needs increase by:

$$1{,}745 \text{ kcal} \times 0.31 = 541 \text{ kcal}.$$

His energy needs total:

$$1{,}745 \text{ kcal} + 541 \text{ kcal} = 2{,}286 \text{ kcal}.$$

Fever has added more than 500 kcal to Johnny's daily energy needs. Energy needs may be even greater, depending on his activity level. (Alternatively, energy needs for a person with a fever can be determined based on basal energy expenditure (BEE) as described in Chapter 19 on pp. 637–639.)

Johnny's protein needs can be calculated based on the rule that he requires 1.5 to 2.0 g protein per kg body weight:

$$1.5 \text{ g} \times \frac{160 \text{ lb}}{2.2 \text{ kg}} = 110 \text{ g protein}.$$

$$2.0 \text{ g} \times \frac{160 \text{ lb}}{2.2 \text{ kg}} = 146 \text{ g protein}.$$

His protein needs range from 110 to 146 g protein daily.

person may retain water due to the hormonal changes that accompany fever. Excessive fluid in these cases can cause fluid overload.

Weigh the client daily to monitor changes in body weight. Keep in mind that the person with an infection may retain sodium and water, or conversely, may be dehydrated. Therefore, scale weight, although not useful as a reflection of tissue weight changes, is a clue to hydration status.

Little information is available regarding increased requirements for specific vitamins and minerals during infection. The need for B vitamins rises with increased intake of food energy and protein, but this greater need is usually met by the additional food intake already required to meet energy and protein needs. Physicians may prescribe multivitamin-mineral supplements throughout the course of illness to cover the possibility that vitamins may be metabolized or excreted in large amounts during hypermetabolic states.

Likewise, losses of electrolytes from infection, vomiting, or diarrhea can generally be covered through foods. Sodium may have to be restricted in people who are retaining this electrolyte.

People with infections may develop a type of anemia referred to as the anemia of infection. At the onset of an infection, the blood concentration of iron rapidly declines as iron moves into the liver for storage. This shift of iron from the blood to the liver helps fight the infection by depriving the infecting microorganisms of the body's iron, which they require to perform their metabolic functions. However, iron in storage is also unavailable to make new hemoglobin, so anemia results. This type of anemia is the body's normal response to infection and does not respond to iron, folate, or vitamin B_{12} supplements, nor to any other dietary or medical treatment. Instead, the situation corrects itself; iron returns to the blood from the liver as the infection resolves.

In general, when feeding people with infections, remember to be generous with food energy, protein, and fluids. People who experience nausea or anorexia may accept nutritionally complete liquid formulas more readily than solid foods.

anemia of infection: a condition in which iron moves from the blood to the liver to help fight infection, resulting in a decline in hemoglobin synthesis.

Nutrition and Surgery

The leading cause of death for young and middle-aged people in the United States is trauma.[1] As Chapter 18 described, trauma occurs when the body gets injured, as with a broken bone, a gunshot wound, or surgery. This section uses the trauma of surgery to describe the relationships between nutrition and trauma.

Surgery is an intentional trauma, and therefore, clients and their health care providers sometimes have enough time to prepare for it. One of the most valuable aspects of preparation is a well-designed defensive nutrition strategy, for the ability to adapt to the stress of surgery depends, in part, on a person's nutrition status. If you think about the roles nutrients play, you will see why. Consider protein: it is the material of antibodies needed to fight infection, of collagen to form scars, of all cells needed to rebuild damaged tissue, of plasma proteins that maintain fluid and electrolyte balance, of the matrix on which bones are rebuilt after fractures, and of many more crucial tissue constituents. In addition, some amino acids provide glucose when the body's glucose needs exceed its glycogen stores. Consequently, the protein-deficient person faces surgery inadequately prepared. The deficiency of any other nutrient hinders recovery in similar ways.

Of course not everyone has the privilege of planning for trauma. Some surgery must be scheduled on an emergency basis; and accidents such as car wrecks with injury happen with no advance warning whatever. Nutrition preparation for such events is not possible, except as an element of overall lifestyle. The possibility that you may have to face emergency surgery is another argument for maintaining good nutrition status at all times. Like the Boy Scouts and Girl Scouts, "Be prepared."

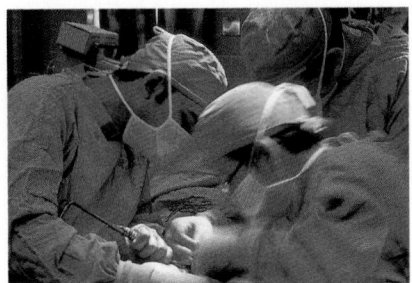

Surgery may raise nutrient needs and lower nutrient intake, digestion, and absorption.

Malnourished people undergoing surgery have a high incidence of postoperative mortality, morbidity, infections, and delayed wound healing.[2] Even a person whose nutrition status before surgery is good can become malnourished if the surgical procedure directly impairs the intake, digestion, or absorption of nutrients. Furthermore, a person who develops complications following surgery faces an even greater likelihood of becoming malnourished because of the added stress and may become especially prone to infection because stress lowers immune resistance. Studies show that preserving nutrition status improves the outcome of severe trauma.[3]

The following discussion concentrates on the nutrition needs of people undergoing surgery in general, including organ transplantation. Later chapters discuss specific nutrition needs associated with various specific surgeries wherever appropriate.

Nutrition before Surgery

Ideally, all clients enter surgery at appropriate weight, with full nutrient reserves. However, such optimal status may be difficult to achieve. The illness that necessitates the surgery, or the psychological stress associated with it, may interfere with a person's intake of food or with the body's use of nutrients. Additionally, the person may have to fast or follow a nutritionally inadequate liquid diet before undergoing diagnostic and laboratory tests, further taxing nutrition status. The health care professional who appreciates the vital roles nutrition plays in resistance and recovery will watch for signs of nutrition risk and encourage clients to eat as well as possible.

Before surgery, a well-nourished client who is expected to have an uncomplicated recovery usually receives a regular diet. A regular hospital diet provides ample food energy and protein. Given such a diet, a well-nourished person can withstand short-term starvation and some degree of protein catabolism without serious consequences.

Malnourished people require diets high in energy and high in protein prior to surgery. Such diets generally provide about 1,000 kcalories more than a person needs to maintain weight and about 1.5 grams protein per kilogram body weight daily. Most hospitals provide malnourished clients with high-kcalorie and high-protein supplements and snacks between meals; clients who understand their importance may be motivated to accept them. For people with functioning GI tracts who cannot eat enough food orally, tube feedings may be indicated; again, those who understand the need will accept them willingly. Furthermore, TPN may be initiated before surgery to boost nutrition status or to supply nutrients when use of the GI tract is contraindicated (see Chapter 22). Although it has not been proven conclusively, preoperative TPN may lower the incidence of postsurgical complications and mortality.[4] Health care providers offer a valuable service when they explain to clients the highly supportive role nutrition plays in resistance and recovery, and help them to relax, so that anxiety stress will interfere as little as possible with their bodies' digestion, absorption, and storage of nutrients prior to surgery.

Physicians may order vitamins, minerals, and trace elements according to clients' individual needs. For example, a person with iron-deficiency anemia receives iron supplementation before elective surgery, or, if surgery must be performed immediately, a blood transfusion.

Physicians generally order all foods and fluids withheld for at least eight hours before surgery. This helps to prevent regurgitation and aspiration, which can occur during anesthesia or recovery. People undergoing GI surgery receive liquids or foods low in residue for two or three days before surgery to minimize the amount of fecal material in the gut and help prevent distention after surgery. People restricted to liquid diets may receive low-residue and residue-free liquid supplements to meet their nutrient needs (described later in the chapter). These supplements can be given either orally or by tube. A person who receives these diets accepts them best if the nurse or other health care provider explains the reasons for them and serves them appropriately (see pp. 657–658).

Nutrition after Surgery

The immediate nutrition-related task for the medical team following surgery or severe accidental injury is to maintain fluid and electrolyte balance. Clients lose blood, fluid, and electrolytes and they may lose additional fluids thereafter, from fever, draining wounds, vomiting, and diarrhea. Excessive losses without replacement can lead to dehydration and shock. To replace these lost fluids and electrolytes, clients receive IV infusions after surgery or severe trauma. The intravenous, rather than the gastrointestinal, route is used because GI tract peristalsis is inactive during the immediate postoperative period; until peristalsis returns (bowel sounds can be heard), foods and fluids cannot be given orally. The physician decides how much fluid to give a client based on the person's blood pressure, pulse rate, urinary output, level of consciousness, breathing patterns, and body temperature, among other factors.

When GI tract activity resumes, the postoperative client may be ready to eat. After uncomplicated surgery, a well-nourished person who can tolerate solid foods is ready for a standard hospital diet adequate in all nutrients.

People with depleted nutrient stores and people with postsurgical complications need high-kcalorie, high-protein diets. To increase energy intake, diets include abundant fats and carbohydrates; to increase protein intake, diets include at least 1.5 grams of protein per kilogram of ideal body weight. This

Chapters 24 and 25 describe GI surgery.

shock: a sudden drop in the blood volume that disrupts the supply of oxygen to the tissues and the return of blood to the heart. Many events can lead to shock; some include major blood loss, trauma, and dehydration.

is true even for overweight people, for they, too, have high postsurgical nutrient needs and risk nutrient depletion. They may have surplus fat stores, but they may also have lost vital proteins. The period immediately following a major injury or surgery is *not* the time for a weight-reduction diet. Clients may not always feel like eating full diets after surgery, but if you know they need to, you can encourage them by explaining how the food will help them recover.

Depending on the type of surgery and the quality of the diet, supplements of some nutrients may be necessary. As mentioned, the need for many of the B vitamins increases when energy and protein intakes increase. However, diets high in food energy and protein usually contain large amounts of B vitamins as well; thus the person who consumes a variety of foods needs no supplements. Vitamin C deserves special attention; it helps form collagen, which plays an important role in wound healing. Like vitamin C, zinc also participates in wound healing. Vitamin K serves an important function after surgery in helping the blood to clot. Keep an eye open for signs of deficiencies and the possible need for supplements.

Handwritten margin note: ✱ Vit. C → forms collagen / zinc → wound healing / Vit K → Bld. clotting

Malnutrition after surgery may be further complicated by anorexia and immobilization. Imagine feeling almost too sick to move or too tired to sit up. To someone in this condition, the effort of eating even normal amounts of food three times a day seems monumental. It is even harder to eat extra foods.

Hospitals can improve clients' appetites by serving a variety of flavorful foods, at the correct temperature, in an attractive manner. You can also help clients in several ways. As with other diets, be sure clients understand the importance of eating extra food and let them know that you understand the difficulty involved. Work closely with clients to find the high-kcalorie foods they enjoy most; individualizing the diet to clients' likes will stimulate appetite. Encourage clients to select foods that require little effort to eat. For example, eating a roast beef sandwich requires less effort than cooking, cutting, and eating a steak. Drinking a high-kcalorie soup is easier than eating it with a spoon. Finally, encourage your clients to get out of bed and begin minimal exercise (such as walking) as soon as medically safe. Chapter 20 gives additional suggestions to improve clients' appetites.

People on tube feedings or TPN before surgery usually stay on special nutrition support until they are able to meet most of their nutrient needs with oral diets. People on TPN should receive nonprotein kcalories from a combination of IV fat and glucose. Glucose alone elevates blood concentrations of insulin, and high insulin levels interfere with the body's use of amino acids to make new proteins. Intravenous fat does not elevate insulin, and so facilitates recovery.

The surgeon who anticipates that a person may have difficulties in resuming oral intake may construct a feeding gastrostomy or jejunostomy during surgery. Tube feedings can then be continued until oral intake is adequate. Enteral nutrition is always preferred to parenteral nutrition (see Chapter 21).

Handwritten margin note: to stimulate action of stomach

In summary, postsurgical nutrition support aims to minimize weight loss (loss of vital body tissue) and the depletion of nutrients. Generally, the diets of people who are not receiving special nutrition support progress from clear liquids to full liquids and on to low-fiber foods and then regular foods as tolerated.

The general progression of diets after surgery from clear liquids to full liquids to low-fiber foods to regular foods is collectively called a **progressive diet**.

Liquid Diets

Liquid diets, as mentioned, are useful at the start of oral feeding after surgery. There are two classes of liquid diets: clear and full.

Clear liquid diets serve the primary function of providing fluids and electrolytes to prevent dehydration. As you might expect, they consist of foods that are relatively transparent to light, such as gelatin, tea, broth, and the like. They are liquid at body temperature, although they may be semisolid when cool (as gelatin is). The body digests and absorbs these liquids easily, and they contribute little or no residue in the GI tract. Table 23–3 lists the foods allowed on clear liquid diets and the accompanying sample menu shows an example of a day's meals.

If you take a close look at the foods allowed on a clear-liquid diet, you will see why many people find these foods unappetizing and boring. Even more disturbing, consider the nutritional quality of the diet—it is deficient in energy and most nutrients. Then consider the high energy and nutrient requirements of a stressed person. No one should stay on a standard clear-liquid diet for

■ TABLE 23–3
Foods Included on Liquid Diets

Clear-Liquid Diets	Full-Liquid Diets
Bouillon	All clear liquids
Broth, clear	Butter
Carbonated beverages	Cheese, cottage[a]
Coffee, regular and decaffeinated	Commerically prepared liquid formulas (all)
Commercially prepared clear liquid formulas	Cooked cereals, strained
Fruit drinks	Cream
Fruit ices	Custard
Fruit juices, strained	Egg, soft cooked or scrambled[a]
Gelatin	Flavorings
Hard candy	Ice cream, plain
Honey	Instant breakfast drinks
Lemonade	Margarine
Popsicles	Milk, all types
Salt	Potatoes, mashed and diluted in cream soups
Salt substitutes	Pudding
Sugar	Sherbet
Sugar substitutes	Soups, strained vegetable, meat, or cream
Tea	Sour cream
	Vegetable juices, strained
	Vegetable purees, diluted in cream soups
	Yogurt

[a]As tolerated.

Sample Clear-Liquid Diet Menu

MENU

Breakfast
Strained orange juice
Flavored gelatin
Ginger ale
Coffee or tea
Sugar

Lunch
Bouillon
Apple juice
Flavored gelatin
Coffee or tea
Sugar

Supper
Bouillon
Cranberry juice
Fruit ice
Flavored gelatin
Coffee or tea
Sugar

Between meals
Soft drinks,
gelatin, or fruit
juices as tolerated

more than a day or two, and the aware health care provider will make sure that regular food is offered as soon as possible.

A full-liquid diet includes both clear and opaque liquid foods. Table 23–3 lists the foods allowed on full-liquid diets, and the sample menu on p. 730 shows an example of a day's meals. As with clear-liquid diets it can be difficult to meet nutrient needs with a full-liquid diet.

To meet the energy and nutrient needs of people on liquid diets, health care providers use nutrition formulas. Some hospitals routinely use these formulas following surgery to prevent the severe energy and protein deficit incurred by incomplete liquid diets. The use of formulas provides other advantages. For one, formulas have a specific osmolality that reduces the likelihood of GI problems. For another, most formulas are lactose-free, which accommodates the loss of lactose tolerance often seen in GI dysfunction. For these reasons, individuals who need a liquid diet, especially if it must continue for more than a day or so, can benefit from formulas.

Often the postsurgical diet order simply says "diet as tolerated." It is up to the nurse or dietitian to keep track of the client's tolerance and readiness to advance from clear to full liquids and then to a regular diet. Sometimes the physician or other health care provider forgets to advance the diet; the alert nurse will then make the recommendation. Other times a person truly cannot tolerate foods other than clear liquids; in such cases, liquid formulas, tube feedings, or total or supplemental IV nutrition may be necessary.

If you work with people after surgery, remember to check their diets. If they must stay on liquid diets for several days, alert the dietitian or suggest to the physician that a supplemental formula be considered.

Sample Full-Liquid Diet Menu

<u>MENU</u>

Breakfast
Orange juice
Strained oatmeal
Egg, scrambled
Milk
Sugar
Margarine

Lunch
Apricot nectar
Yogurt, plain
Pudding
Milk
Coffee or tea
Sugar

Supper
Apple juice
Creamed soup
Custard
Milk
Coffee or tea
Sugar

Between meals
Milkshakes (made with plain ice cream), ice cream, eggnog, pudding, custard, or gelatin

Clients may better tolerate the shift from liquid diets to standard diets if they receive low-fiber diets during the transition. Low-fiber diets provide foods that the GI tract can easily digest and handle. (Chapter 24 describes low-fiber diets in more detail.) Standard diets provide the full spectrum of nutrients and include all foods. The accompanying "Clinical Detective Work" box provides a case study and questions to help you consider the nutrition needs of a surgical client.

Organ Transplants

Organ transplants are a special case of surgery, for when they are performed, the immune system is intentionally suppressed. Organ transplants have opened up new territory in surgical medicine, for only 50 years ago medical science knew little of the body's powerful immunological barriers or of how to circumvent the body's rejection of transplanted tissue. Much progress has been made over the years. Thanks to kidney, liver, and heart transplants, tens of thousands of people have had their lives extended.

The destruction of healthy donor cells by the recipient is called **graft-versus-host disease.**

The success or failure of an organ transplant depends on the compatibility between the transplant tissue and the recipient. Recall from Chapter 18 that the immune response begins when the body's immune system cells recognize a foreign antigen. In an organ transplant, the recipient's immune system recognizes the antigens on the transplanted tissue as foreign, thus evoking a response to attack (or reject the transplanted tissue). Medical researchers discovered that a few specific antigens evoke a greater rejection response than do others. To diminish the chances of rejection, these specific antigens from the donor and recipient are matched for compatibility. Transplants using

---

CLINICAL DETECTIVE WORK

Sally, a 20-year-old prelaw student, went to the emergency room of the university hospital complaining of nausea, fever (101° F), and severe pain in the lower right portion of her abdomen. The diagnosis was appendicitis, and Sally was taken to surgery for an appendectomy (removal of the appendix). Sally's height on admission was 5 ft 7 inches and she weighed 132 lbs. She had experienced a 5-lb weight loss in the past month, which the dietitian attributed to irregular eating habits during a heavy work schedule.

From the limited information about Sally's nutrition history presented here, what can you say about Sally's nutrition status? Does she evince any risk factors for poor nutrition status? What other data would be useful in evaluating her nutrition status?

Because Sally had emergency surgery, nothing could be done to improve her nutrition status before surgery. If surgery had been anticipated, what advice could you have given Sally about her diet? Specifically, what kind of diet would you have recommended?

Calculate her energy and protein needs and describe what kind of diet would be most appropriate for Sally after surgery. Which foods would best meet her energy, protein, vitamin, and mineral needs?

Consider Sally's nutrition-education needs. What type of nutrition advice could Sally benefit from? Who could best provide this advice?

---

well-matched organs (those with no antigen mismatches) are more successful than those using poorly matched organs (those with several antigen mismatches).[5]

In addition to antigen compatibility, drug therapy greatly improves the outcome of organ transplants.[6] Immunosuppressive drugs prevent rejection by inducing a generalized suppression of the recipient's immune response. The use of such drug therapy carries with it risks, of course. With the immune system suppressed, infections develop easily. Table 23–4 (on p. 732) provides a summary of common immunosuppressive drug side effects that may influence nutrient status.

Nutrition support during the immediate post-transplant phase involves providing the client with sufficient kcalories and protein to promote wound healing and to withstand the stress of possible rejection and infection. Long-term nutrition support focuses on the needs surrounding the specific organ that was transplanted (for example, a diet to lower triglyceride concentrations in heart transplant clients). Of course, immunosuppressive complications, such as infection, require ongoing attention and management.

People with suppressed immune systems will want to take extra precautions against food-borne illnesses. They might benefit from following food safety tips for travelers such as:

- Avoid tap water, even for teeth brushing. Avoid fruit juices and ice that may have been made from tap water.

immunosuppressants: drugs that suppress the immune response.

■ **TABLE 23–4**
Immunosuppresants

Drug Name	Timing with Meals	Common Side Effects That May Influence Nutrition Status
Azathioprine	Give with meals.	Nausea, vomiting, diarrhea, stomach pain, anorexia, sore throat, altered taste perceptions.
Cyclosporine	Give with water, juice, or milk. Give at same time each day.	Raises blood pressure. Nausea, vomiting, diarrhea, inflamed gums, anorexia. May induce anemia. May induce hyperglycemia.
Prednisone	Give with food or milk.	Fluid retention, stomach upset, peptic ulcers, blood glucose abnormalities, growth inhibition in children, decreased resistance to infection, weight gain. May decrease effects of insulin or antidiabetic medicine. May induce edema. Alters protein and carbohydrate metabolism. Decreases absorption of calcium and phosphorus.

Source: Adapted from D. E. Powers and A. O. Moore, *Food Medication Interactions*, (Phoenix, Ariz.: Food Medication Interactions, 1989).

■ Avoid dairy products that have not been pasteurized fully and refrigerated properly.
■ Avoid raw foods, including uncooked vegetables, salads, meats, fish, and shellfish.

In addition, handwashing prior to food preparation is especially important to help control the spread of infectious organisms. You may want to review Chapter 16 for other details regarding food-borne illness and its prevention.

■ *Nutrition and Burns*

A burn is sometimes called a **thermal injury**.

An extensive burn is an extreme form of trauma. Whether a burn is extensive depends on the depth of the burn as well as the amount of the body affected by the burn. Extensive burns include second- and third-degree burns covering more than 20 percent of the body surface area (BSA). Figure 23–1 shows the depth of skin affected by burns of different degrees.

The metabolic response to a burn results in major shifts in fluid and electrolyte balance, rapid tissue catabolism, and a rapid loss of body mass. The person with an extensive burn quickly uses all energy and protein reserves in the effort to survive. Moreover, most people with burns experience anorexia and depression, leading to poor food intake and further deterioration of nutrition status. Therefore, the person with extensive burns has exceptionally high nutrient needs. The burn injury itself may make eating difficult because of the associated pain or because of its physical location (for example, the hands). Immobilization and lack of exercise further intensify the catabolic decline.

Not all people with burns require aggressive nutrition support. Well-nourished people and those whose burns cover less than 20 percent BSA can do well on regular diets. People with more extensive burns or those at risk for poor nutrition status require frequent and thorough monitoring to ensure that they receive appropriate nutrition support.

Nutrient Needs during Burns

In the time immediately following a burn, dramatic changes take place in the circulatory system. Plasma proteins (mainly albumin) and electrolytes leak through the capillaries into the interstitial space and the burned area. The accumulation of fluid in the interstitial space around the burn site causes considerable edema. Plasma volume can decline to less than one-half of its normal volume in people with major burns. During this time, the primary consideration of therapy is providing enough fluid and electrolytes to maintain circulatory volume and prevent shock. Isotonic fluids are given intravenously, because the person with a severe burn generally cannot take adequate fluids by mouth. Clients receive sufficient quantities of fluid to maintain urinary output at about 50 milliliters per hour. On an average, it requires 3 to 5 liters to replace daily fluid losses; however, some clients may require over 10 liters per day. Normal bowel activity usually returns in the period following fluid replacement, eating becomes possible, and attention to adequate nutrition now takes high priority.

A person with extensive burns experiences hypermetabolism involving extreme protein catabolism and weight loss. It generally reaches a peak around the end of the first postburn week and then gradually becomes normal over the next several weeks. The duration and rate of hypermetabolism depend on the severity of the burn, reaching a maximum with a 50 percent BSA burn.

The fluid containing plasma proteins and electrolytes that leaks out through the capillaries is called the **exudate** (EX-you-date).

exsudare = to sweat out

MUST
KNOW!!

How to Determine Energy and Protein Needs for a Burn

The following examples show how to determine the energy and protein needs of people with burns.

1. Bernadette is a 39-year-old female, 5 ft 3 inches tall, who weighs 130 lb. She recently sustained a 60% BSA burn. Her *energy* needs can be estimated as follows:

$$[25 \text{ kcal} \times \frac{130 \text{ lb}}{2.2 \text{ kg}}] + [40 \text{ kcal} \times 60] = 3,877 \text{ kcal}.$$

Bernadette's energy needs are close to 3,900 kcal/day.

Alternatively, energy needs for a person with a burn can be determined based on basal energy expenditure (BEE) using the following equations.

Women: BEE = 655 + [9.6 × wt in kg] + [1.7 × ht in cm] − [4.7 × age in years]

Men: BEE = 66 + [13.7 × wt in kg] + [5 × ht in cm] − [6.8× age in years]

Add to BEE for activity:

20% sedentary
35% moderately active
50% active

Add to BEE for burn:

50 to 100% BEE

To determine Bernadette's energy needs using BEE:

$$655 + [9.6 \times \frac{130 \text{ lb}}{2.2 \text{ kg}}] + [1.7 \times 160 \text{ cm}] - [4.7 \times 39] =$$

$$655 + 567 + 272 - 183 = 1,311 \text{ kcal}.$$

Add 20% to account for sedentary activity:

$$1,311 \text{ kcal} \times 0.20 = 262 \text{ kcal}.$$

Researchers have tried to estimate the energy needs of the person with a burn. Some loss of body tissue may be inevitable, but at a minimum the person must receive at least a high enough kcaloric intake to meet all the body's needs without breaking down protein for energy. Protein is needed, instead, for the repair of burned tissue. Typically, adults will need about 4,000 kcalories and 200 grams protein per day. One common method of estimating energy needs is given here.[7]

Adults:
[25 kcal × preburn body weight (kg)] + [40 kcal × %BSA burned].

Add 100% to account for a severe burn:

1,311 kcal × 1.00 = 1,311 kcal.

Add BEE, activity, and burn values for total:

1,311 + 262 + 1,311 = 2,884 kcal.

By this method, Bernadette's energy needs are close to 2,900 kcal/day. Notice that the two methods of estimating energy result in a 1,000 kcal difference; These equations estimate that Bernadette requires between 2,900 and 3,900 kcal/day. Her actual energy needs can only be determined by monitoring her energy intake and her body's responses.

Her *protein* needs can be estimated based on the rule that she requires 1.5 to 3 g protein per kg body weight:

$$1.5 \text{ g} \times \frac{130 \text{ lb}}{2.2 \text{ kg}} = 89 \text{ g.}$$

$$3 \text{ g} \times \frac{130 \text{ lb}}{2.2 \text{ kg}} = 177 \text{ g.}$$

Bernadette's protein needs range from 89 to 177 g protein daily.

2. Bobby, an 11-month-old baby who weighs 20 lb, recently suffered a 30% BSA burn. His energy needs can be calculated as follows:

$$\left[100 \text{ kcal} \times \frac{20 \text{ lb}}{2.2 \text{ kg}}\right] + [40 \text{ kcal} \times 30] = 2,109 \text{ kcal.}$$

Bobby requires about 2,000 to 2,200 kcal/day.

To calculate his protein needs:

$$2 \times \frac{1.6 \text{ g}}{\text{kg}} \text{ (RDA for age)} \times \frac{20 \text{ lb}}{2.2 \text{ kg}} = 30 \text{ g.}$$

$$3 \times \frac{1.6 \text{ g}}{\text{kg}} \text{ (RDA for age)} \times \frac{20 \text{ lb}}{2.2 \text{ kg}} = 43 \text{ g.}$$

Bobby requires between 30 and 43 g protein daily.

Children:
[25 to 100 kcal* × preburn body weight (kg)] + [40 kcal × %BSA burned].

Always remember that these equations provide an *estimate* of requirements. While commonly used, these equations may actually overestimate energy needs for burns.[8] Alert health care professionals adjust energy intake according to the client's body weight changes or complications (such as infection).

---

*The kcalories required depend on the child's age; 100 for 1 year old, decreasing to 25 for 15 year old.

To maintain nitrogen balance, adults need to receive 1.5 to 3 grams of protein per kilogram of body weight per day.[9] The box (on pp. 734–735) provides an example of how to determine the energy and protein needs of a burn client. Children may need from two to three times the RDA for protein (as appropriate for age) per day.

Medical researchers assume that vitamin and mineral requirements increase along with energy and protein needs in people with burns, although supplemental guidelines have not been established. Even so, while physicians would prefer having specific guidelines to follow, many of them prescribe supplements to their burn clients.[10] In consideration of the high energy and protein requirements, as well as nutrients needed for tissue repair and blood and skin losses, physicians often prescribe additional B vitamins in amounts up to two times the RDA. Potentially toxic vitamins and minerals (such as fat-soluble vitamins and many trace minerals), or those that can alter normal body balances (such as calcium and phosphorus) should not exceed the RDA. Because vitamin C and zinc assist in wound healing, these nutrients may be provided in pharmacological doses.

Goals for Meeting Nutrient Needs

Traditionally, health care providers encourage clients with burns to eat as soon as the bowel becomes active. At the latest, nutrition support should begin by the fourth postburn day. However, recent animal studies suggest that enteral nutrition immediately following injury modulates the hypermetabolic response and limits weight loss.[11] Enteral nutrition helps to maintain the normal function of intestinal cells and may inhibit the translocation of bacteria across intestinal cells.[12] However, if bowel activity has not resumed by the fourth postburn day, then the client needs to receive peripheral or central parenteral nutrition support. By the seventh postburn day, energy intake should approximate energy demands.

Occasionally, people with extensive burns develop deep ulcers (usually in the duodenum) called Curling's ulcers, which can cause major bleeding. When bleeding is profuse, the person cannot be fed orally. For these individuals, TPN may be indicated.

To encourage the individual with a burn to eat, remember to offer emotional support. Understandably, food may seem unappealing to the person who faces a lengthy hospital stay, a great deal of pain, and fear of permanent disfigurement. In addition, burn therapy involves whirlpool baths and the painful cutting away of dead skin and tissue. If possible, schedule these treatments so as not to interfere with mealtimes. Give pain medications prior to meals so that mealtimes can be enjoyed.

A client may feel awkward about eating when the location of a burn interferes with self-feeding. An occupational therapist may be able to adapt feeding utensils to assist the client. Encourage the client to get up and walk around and begin physical therapy as soon as possible. This measure helps prevent further catabolism associated with injury, improves morale, and may help to stimulate the appetite.

Dead, burned skin is called **eschar** (es-CAR). As the eschar becomes loose, it is removed so that the burn wound can close as soon as possible. The removal of the eschar is called **debridement** (day-breed-MON [French] or more commonly dee-BREED-ment).
eschara = scab

Hydrotherapy, sometimes called **tanking,** is used to cleanse the burn wound and help loosen the eschar. The person is placed in a large whirlpool tub, where the wounds are gently cleansed with a special soap that helps prevent infections.

Physical therapy is important for preventing **contractures**, or loss of joint function, in people with burns. As the burn wound heals, the new skin is very tight, and it may pull the area surrounding a joint into a nonfunctional position.

[handwritten notes in margin:]
7.9 = 80 Kg.
2.2√175.
25 Cal X —Kg bdy wt
+ 40 Cal X % BSA
25 Cal X 80 =
+ 40 Cal X 40 =
106
+ 72
178 IBW

CLINICAL DETECTIVE WORK

Mr. Sampson, a 48-year-old journalist, has been admitted to the emergency room. He suffered a third-degree, 40 percent BSA burn when he was trapped in a burning building. His height on admission was 6 ft, and he weighed 175 lb. The physician ordered lab work, including serum proteins, that have not yet been reported.

Identify Mr. Sampson's immediate postinjury needs. How can these needs be met?

Do you have enough information to determine Mr. Sampson's preinjury, preburn nutrition status? If not, what information would be useful? Is information about preburn nutrition status important in this case? Why or why not?

Calculate Mr. Sampson's energy and protein needs to support burn healing. Discuss what other nutrients must be considered.

Discuss some general guidelines for providing all of Mr. Sampson's nutrient needs. What physical and emotional factors must be considered?

If Mr. Sampson cannot eat enough food to obtain adequate nutrients orally by the fourth to seventh postburn day, how should he be fed? If he developed major GI bleeding, how could he be fed? Describe the roles of physical therapy and exercise in Mr. Sampson's treatment.

The accompanying "Clinical Detective Work" presents a case study of a burn client. Use your investigative skills to answer questions about this client's nutrition needs.

Nutrition Assessment

Of course, all of the parameters of nutrition assessment discussed in Chapter 19 apply to individuals undergoing surgery or recovering from infections or burns. However, some important aspects of the assessment deserve emphasis here:

- An accurate assessment of the person's *preinjury* nutrition status will help to determine nutrient needs and complication risks.
- Careful and continuous monitoring of nutrition status will help to ensure that the diet meets nutrient needs. Remember that individuals' nutrient stores can become depleted rapidly.
- For people on oral diets, a careful history of food likes and dislikes will be invaluable in encouraging adequate oral intake.
- For people on medications, a careful evaluation of possible nutrient interactions may prevent imbalances.

- Anthropometrics must be interpreted cautiously in the period immediately following the injury. Weights may be misleading because people may be retaining or losing water. Also, the location of wounds may make anthropometric measurements impossible.
- In people with burns, expect to see low serum albumin and transferrin levels. Remember that plasma proteins leak through the capillaries to the burn wound and into the interstitial fluid. Consequently, low lab values do not serve as accurate indicators of nutrition status immediately following the burn injury.
- In all stressed individuals, serum albumin and transferrin concentrations may be low for a while. Levels that remain depressed even after nitrogen balance has been achieved, probably does not reflect nutrition status.[13]
- Results from antigen skin tests remain negative for at least 10 days following trauma.[14] Therefore, skin tests cannot be used to determine protein nutrition status during this period.

The stresses of surgery, infections, and burns place tremendous demands on the body. The body uses all that it has to fight the battle to survive and regain health. Recovery depends, in part, on the body receiving the energy and nutrients required to mount a defense, repair damaged tissues, and replenish nutrient reserves.

Study Questions

1. What factors influence nutrient needs during an infection? What nutrients are of particular concern?
2. What are some factors that can lead to poor nutrition status prior to surgery? What type of diet should be eaten in the days before and after surgery? What diet modifications are made right before and after surgery, and why?
3. Discuss the role of tube feedings and parenteral nutrition after surgery. When would these diets be indicated?
4. What is the purpose of a clear-liquid diet? What foods are allowed on this diet? Construct a sample clear-liquid diet, and consider the practical limitations of following such a diet.
5. Describe a full-liquid diet. How can liquid nutrition formulas be used to improve liquid diets?
6. What are the medical and nutrient concerns of organ transplants? How are these concerns dealt with?
7. Describe the changes in body fluids that occur immediately after a person suffers an extensive burn. What is the primary concern during this period? How are these needs met?
8. When can a person be fed by mouth after a burn? What metabolic events occur during a burn injury, and how do they affect nutrient needs?
9. Describe the energy and protein needs of an adult and a child with a burn. Calculate your own energy and protein needs based on a 50% BSA burn.
10. Discuss some major factors to keep in mind when you assess the nutrition status of a person with severe stress or trauma.

Notes

1. S. Lowry, Nutrition and trauma, *Nutrition in Clinical Practice* 3 (1988): 135–136.
2. G. P. Buzby, Perioperative nutrition support, *Journal of Parenteral and Enteral Nutrition* (supplement) 14 (1990): 197–199.
3. R. P. Bynoe, Nutrition support in trauma patients, *Nutrition in Clinical Practice* 3 (1988): 137–144.
4. F. B. Serra, How nutrition intervention changes what getting sick means, *Journal of Parenteral and Enteral Nutrition* (supplement) 14 (1990): 164–169.
5. F. H. Bach and D. H. Sachs, Current concepts: Immunology—Transplantation immunology, *New England Journal of Medicine* 317 (1987): 489–492.

SELF STUDY

Nutrition and Trauma

Suppose that you have been ill or injured in such a way as to impair your nutrition status. A member of the health care team has informed you that you will need to eat about twice as much food as you are accustomed to eating in order to replete your depleted nutrient stores or to meet the high energy needs you are currently experiencing.

Record an example of your normal food intakes for a day (use a record previously made, if it is typical). Now make a plan that doubles it: in place of 1 egg for breakfast, plan 2; in place of one bowl of cereal, plan 2; in place of 4 ounces of meat, plan 8.

How will you manage to ingest all this food, not just for one day, but day after day? Record the feelings that arise in you as you contemplate this project. Many people jest that this would be a great opportunity for anyone who habitually attempts to limit food intake: that person could finally eat to the heart's content. That might be true for a day—but for a week? A month? Try it just for a day, record your observations, and remember them when you deal with people who are presented with this challenge.

6. O. Salvathierra, Jr., Optimal use of organs for transplantation, *New England Journal of Medicine* 318 (1988): 1329–1331.

7. P. W. Curreri, Nutritional replacement modalities, *Journal of Trauma* (supplement) 19 (1979): 906–908.

8. J. P. Allard and coauthors, Validation of a new formula for calculating the energy requirements of burn patients, *Journal of Parenteral and Enteral Nutrition* 14 (1990): 115–118.

9. J. J. Cunningham, M. K. Lydon, and W. E. Russell, Calorie and protein provision for recovery from severe burns in infants and young children, *American Journal of Clinical Nutrition* 51 (1990): 553–557; S. J. Bell and J. Wyatt, Nutrition guidelines for burned patients, *Journal of the American Dietetic Association* 86 (1986): 648–653.

10. R. L. Shippee, S. W. Wilson, and N. King, Trace mineral supplementation of burn patients: A national survey, *Journal of the American Dietetic Association* 87 (1987): 300–303.

11. S. Inque and coauthors, Prevention of yeast translocation across the gut by a single enteral feeding after burn injury, *Journal of Parenteral and Enteral Nutrition* 13 (1989): 565–571; H. Saito and coauthors, The effect of route of nutrient administration on nutritional state, catabolic hormone secretion, and gut mucosal injury after burn injury, *Journal of Parenteral and Enteral Nutrition* 11 (1987): 1–7.

12. J. W. Alexander, Nutrition and translocation, *Journal of Parenteral and Enteral Nutrition* (supplement) 14 (1990): 170–174.

13. Serra, 1990.

14. Bynoe, 1988.

Ethical Issues in Nutrition Care

Chapter 23 described how infection and trauma can drastically alter nutrient needs, and how meeting these needs supports recovery in many cases. Only in recent years have we had the capability of providing nourishment to clients unable to eat by mouth. The technical advances made in the areas of enteral and parenteral nutrition have been lifesaving for many people. However, as is true with other medical technologies, the availability of special nutrition support forces health care professionals and society to face ethical issues—specifically, when is it morally and legally appropriate to discontinue use of nutrition support techniques. We must ask ourselves when such treatments are prolonging life and when they are merely delaying death.

This highlight reviews some of the ethical questions that have been raised regarding the use of nutrition support. Its intent is not to draw conclusions or to solve problems; rather, it seeks only to present the issues for your consideration.

A Look at the Problems

To put the problems into perspective, consider the circumstances under

Is it morally and legally appropriate to postpone death through high-tech methods?

> ## Miniglossary
>
> **artificial feeding:** parenteral and enteral nutrition; feeding by a route other than the normal ingestion of food.
> **comatose:** in a state of deep unconsciousness from which the person cannot be aroused.
> **competent:** having sufficient mental ability to understand a treatment, to weigh its risks and benefits, and to comprehend the consequences of refusing or accepting the treatment.
> **death:** permanent cessation of vital functions.
> **ethical:** in accordance with moral principles or professional standards.
> **legal:** established by law.
> **living will:** a document signed by a competent adult that specifically states that the person does not wish any heroic measures to be taken in the event of terminal illness or irreversible coma from which the person is not expected to recover.
> **persistent vegetative state:** exhibiting motor reflexes but without the ability to regain cognitive behavior, to communicate, or to interact purposefully with the environment.
> **terminal illness:** a progressive, irreversible disease that will lead to death in the near future.

which health care professionals generally make their decisions to feed clients. Most often, they readily provide whatever form of nutrition is necessary to support all clients who have any chance of recovering from a disease and sustaining an acceptable quality of life. Clearly, health care professionals cannot rightfully withhold nutrition support because of poor judgment or negligence. If a client were to die because nourishment was withheld, the staff and facility would be held responsible and, in all likelihood, a malpractice lawsuit would result.

The decision of whether to feed a client becomes less clear, however, when the client is not expected to recover. How aggressively do we support the person who is terminally ill or in a persistent vegetative state?

How do we respond to elderly or physically disabled clients who refuse nutrition support because they feel the quality of their lives is so poor that they do not wish to be sustained? Do we allow them such choices? Are health care professionals morally and legally obligated to comply with, or to deny, such requests? Furthermore, when clients are incompetent and unable to speak for themselves, who, if anyone, should be allowed to make such life-and-death decisions? These questions represent but a few of the unanswered concerns that have evolved along with the technology of nutrition support.

Individual Rights

The court system has ruled on several cases involving the nutrition support of both competent adults and those in a persistent vegetative state. The accompanying box presents a brief review of several landmark court decisions. In such cases, the court weighs the state's rights to preserve life, to prevent suicide, and to support the integrity of the medical profession against an individual's right to refuse medical treatments, including artificial feedings.

With respect to preserving life, the court examines the reasonable possibility that a client will return to a cognitive and discerning life, as distinguished from a biological existence. On the issue of suicide, the court considers whether refusal of treatment would allow the underlying disease to take its course; if so, eventual death is not suicide. Regarding the ethical integrity of the medical profession, the court holds that medical professionals should not be compelled to discontinue feedings against their will; if necessary, arrangements for physicians and facilities that are willing to accommodate the client's wishes must be made.

The emerging ethical, medical, and legal consensus seems to support the opinion that state interests do not outweigh those of individual rights. Individuals have a legal right to refuse medical treatment—including artificial feeding—even when medical experts consider that treatment necessary to sustain life.[1] That is, even when treatment is lifesaving and its refusal may bring an earlier death, clients' rights remain paramount.

Several court cases have argued the distinction between providing medical care and providing nourishment and hydration. They suggest that to "pull the plug" on a life-support machine is acceptable, but that to deny food and water—the basics of life—is inhumane. However, the court system has defined nutrition support as a medical procedure rather than as routine care.[2]

Many people will agree that a competent adult has the right to

Landmark Court Cases

1983–1986 Bouvia: A mentally competent 26-year-old quadriplegic woman who required assistance in eating wanted to be allowed to starve to death. Hospital officials believed that to discontinue feeding would make them party to suicide, which is illegal. A lower court rejected Bouvia's request. Two years later, her condition worsened, and she was placed on a nasogastric tube against her will. The California Second District Court of Appeals ordered removal of the tube, stating that her right to refuse treatment was absolute regardless of her motives or whether her illness was terminal.

1985–1986 Requenia: A competent 55-year-old woman refused tube feeding. The hospital objected and arranged for her transfer to another facility. When she refused to transfer, the hospital sued her to leave. The court ordered the hospital staff to honor her request to decline feeding.

1985–1986 Brophy: The wife and family of a 49-year-old man in a persistent vegetative state requested discontinuance of artificial feeding. He had made his wishes known to them prior to his illness, and it was apparent that his active life was over. When his physicians and the hospital opposed the request, the case went to probate court. The judge decided to continue feeding even though he realized that Brophy would decline artificial feeding if competent. The Massachusetts Supreme Judicial Court overruled the lower court and held that Brophy's feeding tube could be removed.

1985–1987 Jobes: The family of a 31-year-old woman in a persistent vegetative state requested discontinuance of her tube feeding. A lower court ruled that the nursing home could continue tube feeding until transfer arrangements could be made. The New Jersey Supreme Court ordered the nursing home to honor the request to discontinue feeding and to continue to provide care until her death.

1986 Corbett: The Florida Second District Court of Appeals allowed the removal of a nasogastric tube from a 75-year-old woman in a persistent vegetative state. This decision took precedence over Florida's law that specifically forbids clients to decline "provision of sustenance."

1987–1988 Gray: The family of a 49-year-old woman in a persistent vegetative state requested discontinuance of her artificial feeding. When the hospital objected, the Federal District Court of Rhode Island ordered the hospital to honor the request to discontinue feeding.

1987 Peter: The New Jersey Supreme Court found no distinction between artificial feeding and other forms of life-sustaining treatment and allowed the withdrawal of a nasogastric tube from a 65-year-old woman in a persistent vegetative state.

1988 O'Connor: The daughters of a 78-year-old woman who had multi-infarct dementia refused to allow a hospital to insert a feeding tube. They believed that their mother would not want any form of life support. The New York Court of Appeals ruled that a feeding tube must be inserted unless there was unequivocal evidence that the patient would have chosen to refuse it.

accept or refuse medical treatment. However, the controversy grows louder when the adult is comatose, incompetent, or otherwise unable to refuse or accept medical treatment—especially when the person's wishes are not known. Without knowledge of an incompetent person's wishes, the court decides in the client's "best interest."

For many families, it becomes their burden to convince the court that discontinuing feeding is in the "client's best interest." Consider the case of Nancy Cruzan, a young woman who suffered permanent and irreversible brain damage after a car crash in January 1983. Since then, she has been in a persistent vegetative state—awake but unaware. Her physicians and parents held no hope for recovery, yet given food and water, she might have lived for another 30 years. Her parents' request to discontinue tube feeding was rejected by the Missouri Supreme Court in 1987, and in 1989 the United States Supreme Court agreed to hear the case as its first "right-to-die" case. Several professional organizations— including the American Medical Association, the American Academy of Family Physicians, the American Association of Neurological Surgeons, the American College of Surgeons, the American College of Physician, and the American Society for Parenteral and Enteral Nutrition—filed briefs with the Supreme Court in support of the Cruzans.

The Missouri Supreme Court noted that Cruzan never made a definitive statement on her "right to die" wishes and decided that preserving life, no matter its quality, took precedence over all other considerations. The argument held that Cruzan's parents had no legal evidence that Cruzan would want to discontinue life-sustaining efforts; therefore they had no right to make such a request for her.

The Cruzan parents tried to convince the Supreme Court that their once independent and vivacious daughter would not want to live in a vegetative state. Their lawyer argued that Cruzan has a right to be free from medical intervention. No one questioned that Cruzan's parents knew their daughter's wishes better than anyone and had the highest and most loving motives. The question for the court to consider was: can families (or anyone) make life-and-death decisions of behalf of incompetent persons?

The Supreme Court recognized that competent adults have the right to stop life-sustaining treatments. But, in a 5-to-4 decision, the Court decided that life-sustaining treatment could not be withdrawn without "clear and convincing" evidence that the incompetent person would refuse treatment.[3] Cruzan's statements to her roommate and family regarding her desire to live or die under certain conditions were insufficient to convince the Court. In making its decision, the Supreme Court entrusted state legislatures with the task of establishing laws that address the issue of whether families (or other third parties) can authorize the withdrawal of life-sustaining treatment on behalf of incompetent persons in the absence of exacting evidence.

After another round of court battles, Cruzan's feeding tube was removed December 14, 1990. She died from dehydration two weeks later.

The financial and emotional costs involved with supporting Cruzan were phenomenal. In terms of money, health care costs to support her ran about $130,000 per year (which were paid by the state). The emotional costs are more difficult to calculate, of course. Cruzan's parents were first faced with the initial shock of their daughter's accident. Then, for several years, they held hope that with continued care their daughter would survive and regain consciousness. Then, they endured court battles over their child's fate—a fate that held grief whichever way it turned.

The Cruzan family shares this dilemma with some 10,000 other families of people who live in a persistent vegetative state. No doubt, the high court's decision has widespread implications for these people and the health professionals who care for them. In fact, this decision touches all of us, because it influences the extent to which our society views life-sustaining treatment as optional not only for our clients, but for ourselves and our families.[4] It decides how we may be allowed to die.[5]

Informed Consent

How can people protect their rights to retain or refuse treatment in the event of incompetency? How can health care professionals provide treatment in accordance with their clients' wishes? The answers rest with the attending physician, the client, and the client's family.

Physicians should encourage their competent clients to express ahead of time their preferences for medical treatments, including artificial feedings, should terminal illness or coma develop.[6] These preferences should be noted in medical records. Physicians who are unwilling to abide by these stated preferences should notify their clients immediately so that other physicians can be selected. Clients should expect that physicians and facilities will comply with their preferences, and not merely tolerate them grudgingly.[7]

In addition to informing their physicians, clients can state their preferences in legal documents known as living wills (see Form H23−1). Many states have enacted laws that authorize the use of living wills.[8]

A living will stands as a clear expression of a competent adult's wishes.[9] It may specify that no extraordinary treatments be administered in the event that the person is unable to make the necessary decisions at that time. Alternatively, a living will may declare a person's wish to have every effort made to maintain life in the event of terminal illness or irreversible loss of

To My Family, My Physician, My Lawyer And All Others Whom It May Concern

Death is as much a reality as birth, growth, and aging—it is the one certainty of life. In anticipation of decisions that may have to be made about my own dying and as an expression of my right to refuse treatment, I _____ ,

(print name)

being of sound mind, make this statement of my wishes and instructions concerning treatment.

By means of this document, which I intend to be legally binding, I direct my physician and other care providers, my family, and any surrogate designated by me or appointed by a court, to carry out my wishes. If I become unable, by reason of physical or mental incapacity, to make decisions about my medical care, let this document provide the guidance and authority needed to make any and all such decisions.

If I am permanently unconscious or there is no reasonable expectation of my recovery from a seriously incapacitating or lethal illness or condition, I do not wish to be kept alive by artificial means. I request that I be given all care necessary to keep me comfortable and free of pain, even if pain-relieving medications may hasten my death, and I direct that no life-sustaining treatment be provided except as I or my surrogate specifically authorize.

This request may appear to place a heavy responsibility upon you, but by making this decision according to my strong convictions, I intend to ease that burden. I am acting after careful consideration and with understanding of the consequences of your carrying out my wishes. *List optional specific provisions in the space below.*[a]

I sign this document knowingly, voluntarily, and after careful deliberation, this _____ day of _____ , 19 _____ .

_____
(signature)

Address _____

_____

I do hereby certify that the within document was executed and acknowledged before me by the principal this _____ day of _____ , 19 _____ .

_____
Notary Public

Witness _____
Printed Name _____
Address _____
_____
Witness _____
Printed Name _____
Address _____

Copies of this document have been given to:

_____
_____
_____
_____
_____

[a]The Living Will should clearly state your preference about life-sustaining treatment. You may wish to add specific statements that concern cardiopulmonary resuscitation, artificial or invasive measures for providing nutrition and hydration, kidney dialysis, mechanical or artificial respiration, blood transfusion, surgery (such as amputation), and antibiotics. You may also wish to indicate any preferences you have about such matters as dying at home.
Source: Reprinted by permission of Concern for Dying, 250 West 57th Street, New York, NY 10107. For a copy of "A Living Will" and other information write or call (212) 246−6962.

consciousness. Form H23−1 shows how a living will might begin and provides an address for obtaining additional information. People should make their wishes known in writing, even if their states do not have living will provisions. Each individual's preference should be known to the attending physicians and family.

Not all states authorize living wills. Even states that provide for living wills may have laws that recognize their requests only with respect to medical procedures and may specifically exclude the right to withhold or withdraw nourishment or hydration.[10] Most living wills request that no heroic measures be taken to sustain life in the event of imminent death or vegetative state, but may fail to consider whether the provision of food and water is a heroic measure. For some people, providing nourishment and hydration is ordinary care; they consider withholding or withdrawing nutrition support unjustified for any reason. For others, using artificial nutrition support to replace eating is no different than using a respirator to replace breathing—it is intrusive; they consider the refusal of nutrition support justified for people who want no heroic measures taken to sustain life. People who prefer that nourishment and hydration be discontinued need to write this specification into their living wills to ensure that their wishes be carried out.

In some states, the durable power of attorney offers clients the protection of having their wishes carried out (see Form H23−2).[11] A durable power of attorney allows a competent adult to designate another competent adult as an agent to make decisions in the event of incapacitation.

An advantage of planning ahead for future care in the case of a terminal illness or irreversible state of unconsciousness is that others are freed from the guilt and anxiety of having to make that decision. Imagine the anxiety a family member goes through in directing the health care team to stop nutrition support, knowing that it will hasten death. That decision would be far easier if the family member knew that was what the individual would want or, better yet, if a legal document took the decision out of the family's hands altogether.

When the person's wishes regarding life-sustaining measures are unknown, life support can be discontinued only if the burden of providing it clearly and markedly outweighs the benefits to the individual. Providers must also consider the pain caused by withdrawing the treatment in weighing the benefits versus the negative aspects of treatment.

Professional Considerations

The many ethical and legal problems that have evolved with the improved technology for delivering nutrients present tough challenges for individuals, their loved ones, the health care team, and the legal system.

Health care professionals can find themselves in awkward and difficult positions regarding aggressive nutrition support. On the one hand, they are obligated to provide optimal care; negligence could result in a malpractice suit. On the other hand, health care professionals are client advocates; they must respect the wishes of the people in their care. No easy answers to these dilemmas are available, yet decisions must be made. Each case must be carefully decided on its individual circumstances and actions taken as appropriate.

Most hospitals have established ethics committees to deal with ethical problems such as those presented here. Health care professionals should ensure that their disciplines are represented on such committees and become familiar with their profession's ethics guidelines.[12]

■ **FORM H23–2**
Durable Power of Attorney

Durable Power of Attorney for Health Care Decisions

To effect my wishes, I designate _____ , residing at _____
_____ (Phone #) _____ ,
(or if he or she shall for any reason fail to act, _____
_____ (Phone #) _____ ,
residing at _____)
as my health care surrogate—that is, my attorney-in-fact regarding any and all health care decisions to be made for me, including the decision to refuse life-sustaining treatment—if I am unable to make such decisions myself. This power shall remain effective during and not be affected by my subsequent illness, disability or incapacity. My surrogate shall have authority to interpret my Living Will, and shall make decisions about my health care as specified in my instructions or, when my wishes are not clear, as the surrogate believes to be in my best interests. I release and agree to hold harmless my health care surrogate from any and all claims whatsoever arising from decisions made in good faith in the exercise of this power.

I sign this document knowingly, voluntarily, and after careful deliberation, this _____ day of _____ , 19 _____ .

_____
(signature)

Address _____
_____

I do hereby certify that the within document was executed and acknowledged before me by the principal this _____ day of _____ , 19 _____ .

_____
Notary Public

Witness _____
Printed Name _____
Address _____
_____
Witness _____
Printed Name _____
Address _____
_____

Copies of this document have been given to:

_____
_____
_____
_____
_____

Source: Reprinted by permission of Concern for Dying, 250 West 57th Street, New York, NY 10107. For a copy of a durable power of attorney form and other information write or call (212) 246–6962.

NOTES

1. S. H. Miles, P. A. Singer, and M. Siegler, Conflicts between patients' wishes to forgo treatment and the policies of health care facilities, *New England Journal of Medicine* 321 (1989): 48–50; R. Steinbrook and B. Lo, Artificial feeding—Solid ground, not a slippery slope, *The New England Journal of Medicine* 318 (1988): 286–290.

2. R. Dresser, Discontinuing nutrition support: A review of the case law, *Journal of the American Dietetic Association* 85 (1985): 1289–1292.

3. Supreme Court of the United States Syllabus, *Cruzan, by her parents and co-guardians*, Cruzan et ux. v. Director, Missouri Department of Health, et al., No. 88–1503. Argued December 6, 1989—Decided June 25, 1990.

4. M. Angell, Prisoners of technology: The case of Nancy Cruzan, *New England Journal of Medicine*, 322 (1990): 1226–1228; B. Lo, F. Rouse, and L. Dornbrand, Family decision making on trial—Who decides for incompetent patients? *New England Journal of Medicine*, 322 (1990): 1228–1232.

5. The Court and Nancy Cruzan, Hastings Center Report, January/February 1990, pp. 38–50.

6. Steinbrook and Lo, 1988.

7. Miles, Singer, and Siegler, 1989.

8. B. Mishkin, Withholding and withdrawing nutritional support: Advance planning for hard choices, *Nutrition in Clinical Practice* 1 (1986): 50–52.

9. J. E. Ruark, T. A. Raffin, and the Stanford University Medical Center Committee on Ethics, Initiating and withdrawing life support—Principles and practice in adult medicine, *The New England Journal of Medicine* 318 (1988): 25–30.

10. B. Mishkin, Withholding and withdrawing nutritional support: Advance planning for hard choices, *Nutrition in Clinical Practice* 1 (1986): 50–52.

11. Mishkin, 1986.

12. American Dietetic Association, Position of the American Dietetic Association: Issues in feeding the terminally ill adult, *Journal of the American Dietetic Association* 87 (1987): 78–85.

24

Nutrition and Disorders of the Upper GI Tract

Contents

Difficulties Chewing and Swallowing

Disorders of the Esophagus

Disorders of the Stomach

Gastric Surgery

Nutrition Assessment

Highlight: How the Ulcer Diet Won the Right to Taste Good

This picture, taken through a light microscope, shows a single villus of the small intestine in which several hundred cells are visible. Each cell's location can be deduced from the presence of a blue-stained nucleus. When magnified even more, these cells turn out to be bristling with surface projections of their own, the microvilli. The opening art of the next chapter provides a close-up look at a few cells with their microvilli. Figure 3–8 on page 54 illustrates these surface features of the small intestine wall.

The remarkable GI tract serves as a conduit from the external world to the internal body environment. It wisely distinguishes nutrients from substances for which the body has no use. Indeed, a healthy GI tract allows us to ingest, digest, and absorb nutrients—functions essential to life. Conversely, a diseased GI tract can interfere with one or all of these functions, seriously impairing health. This chapter describes how some upper GI tract disorders affect food intake and how diet can ease recovery. The next chapter presents disorders of the lower GI tract and their effects on food intake and nutrition status.

Difficulties Chewing and Swallowing

The upper GI tract begins with the mouth. In the mouth, the teeth and jaw muscles work together, breaking down food to a size that can be easily swallowed and digested. A variety of dental, medical, and surgical conditions can temporarily or permanently interfere with chewing or swallowing (see Table 24−1). Without the appropriate adjustments in diet, people with these conditions might eat too little, lose too much weight, and suffer the consequences of a deteriorating nutrition status.

The process of chewing is sometimes called **mastication.**

To minimize the discomfort of chewing and swallowing, a regular diet is modified to a mechanical soft diet. Such a diet is highly individualized, yet simple. It eliminates the foods the person cannot easily chew or swallow. A person with a newly broken jaw may only be able to consume liquids; a person without teeth, however, may be able to eat pieces of baked chicken or fish, ground beef, casseroles, canned fruits, and soft cooked vegetables. The foods allowed on a mechanical soft diet may be liquid, chopped, blenderized, or regular foods with a soft consistency. Usually, the client receives all foods pureed until a dietitian or nurse determines which foods the client can tolerate in more solid forms.

mechanical soft diet: a diet that excludes all foods that are difficult to chew or swallow; also called a **dental soft diet.**

Blenderized foods are also known as **pureed** (pyoo-RAYED) foods.

Take a moment to think about a pureed diet. A typical dinner of baked chicken, boiled potatoes, and green beans might become white mush, more white mush, and a green blob. However, creative and caring people in the kitchen can make a difference. By arranging and shaping foods attractively on a plate, and adding garnishes for color, they can enhance the eye-appeal of a meal.

In many hospitals, baby foods routinely replace pureed foods. While baby foods offer nutrients, they often taste bland since manufacturers prepare them

■ TABLE 24−1
Conditions That May Interfere with Chewing or Swallowing

Achalasia	No teeth
Acquired immune deficiency syndrome (AIDS)	Oral surgery
	Periodontal disease
Broken jaw	Radiation therapy of the head and neck
Cancer or chemotherapy	
Dental caries	Sensitivity to hot or cold
Dryness of the mouth	Strokes (sometimes)
Dysphagia	Surgery of the head and neck
Ill-fitting dentures	Ulceration of mouth or gums
Missing teeth	

without salt or spices. Regardless of whether the client receives pureed foods or baby foods, the consistency creates a psychological block to eating, and malnutrition can follow.

To improve the situation, first determine whether your client truly needs pureed rather than chopped or soft foods. Second, help your client select well-balanced colorful meals. For example, substitute mashed sweet potatoes for white potatoes. Such a change adds appetizing color to the meal. Remember to serve foods attractively and at the right temperature.

Unless the physician has ordered otherwise, suggest spices that will liven the flavor of foods. Many people think that because they must follow a special diet, the foods must taste bland. Not so. A mechanical soft diet can include all seasonings and types of foods. However, people with mouth ulcers may find highly seasoned or acidic foods (such as citrus fruits and tomatoes) painful. In addition, foods that contain nuts or seeds can easily become trapped in mouth ulcers and cause discomfort.

If pureed diets consistently present a problem for a client, talk to the administrative dietitian or foodservice manager. Pureed foods should be smooth and thick—not watery or thin. Whenever possible, regular foods that have been pureed should be served instead of baby food. The use of blenders, food processors, and grinders simplifies the process of making pureed foods.

Many people who have difficulties swallowing can drink thickened liquids better than clear liquids. The slow flow allows time to coordinate movements in the mouth. Clients can use commercial products or baby cereal to thicken liquids to the appropriate consistency (see Highlight 21).

People's tolerances to food consistencies vary greatly. Talk to clients about which foods they find difficult to chew or swallow. Try to provide clients on the mechanical soft diet with foods similar to those of a regular diet. These foods will offer the most variety, improve clients' acceptance of them, and reduce the likelihood of nutrient deficiencies.

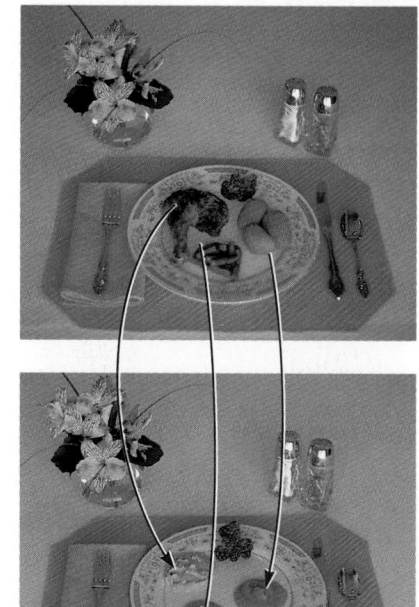

Serve colorful pureed meals at the appropriate temperature, seasoned to taste.

Disorders of the Esophagus

The upper esophagus assists in the swallowing process and transports food from the mouth to the stomach. Disorders of the esophagus can therefore impair the ability to swallow, causing dysphagia.

Dysphagia

Dysphagia can result from either psychological or physiological problems. This section discusses only those causes of dysphagia that can be helped by diet. One such cause of dysphagia is achalasia. In achalasia, nerves that control esophageal movement fail to function properly; the muscles of the esophagus cannot propel the food bolus downward toward the stomach. Additionally, the cardiac sphincter remains closed, thus preventing food from passing out of the esophagus into the stomach. Foods and fluids accumulate in the esophagus, which explains the sensation of food sticking in the throat. Eventually, either the pressure of the food causes the cardiac sphincter to open or the person regurgitates the food.

dysphagia (dis-FAY-gee-ah): difficulty in swallowing.
dys = bad
phagein = to eat

achalasia (ack-ah-LAY-zee-ah): dysfunction of the esophagus; sometimes called **esophageal dyssynergia** (ee-SOF-ah-GEE-al dis-sin-ER-gee-ah) or **cardiospasm.**
a = not
chalasis = relaxation
synergia = cooperation

■ **FIGURE 24–1**

Achalasia

In achalasia, the muscles of the esophagus do not relax enough to allow food to pass through to the stomach. The esophagus gradually enlarges.

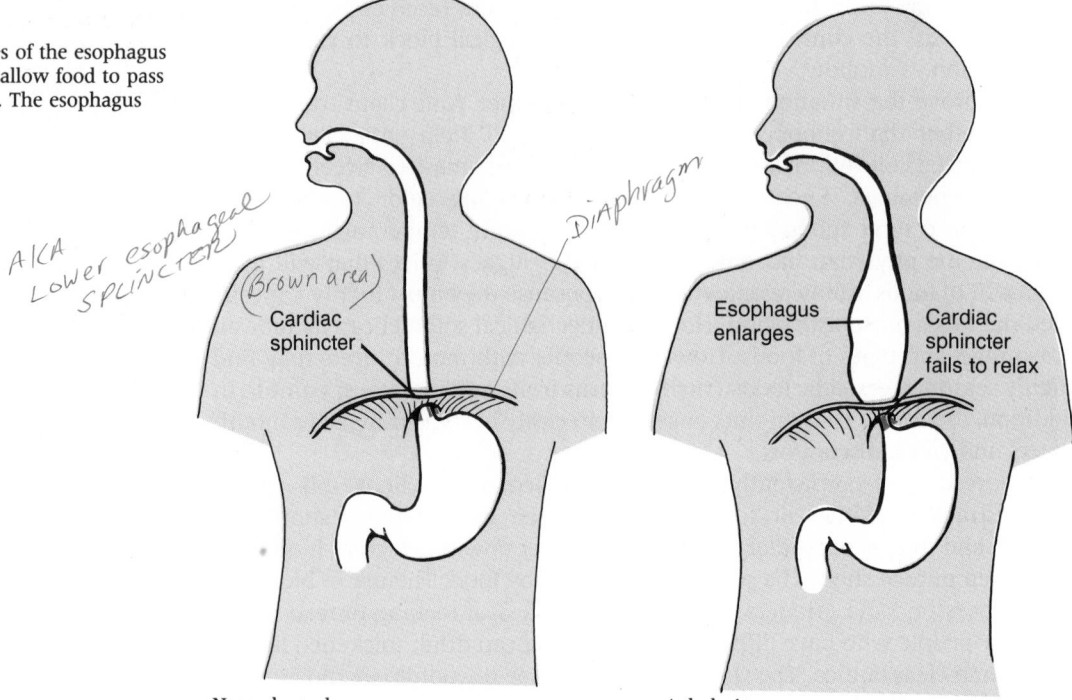

AKA Lower esophageal SPHINCTER

Diaphragm

(Brown area)

Normal esophagus   Achalasia

The **cardiac sphincter** is often called the **lower esophageal sphincter (LES)** or the **gastroesophageal sphincter.** (The passage of food through the GI tract is illustrated on p. 46.)

The fear of eating is called **sitophobia** (SIGH-toe-FOE-bee-ah).
sitos = food
phobos = fear

When an organ, such as the esophagus, becomes enlarged beyond normal dimensions, it is said to be **dilated.** The procedure of making an organ or vessel larger is called **dilation** or **dilatation.**

At first, the person with achalasia may experience only temporary and mild dysphagia. As achalasia progresses, the esophagus widens (see Figure 24–1), and the symptoms become more painful.

The person with achalasia becomes fearful of eating and begins to eat less food. By the time the person seeks medical attention, weight loss and signs of nutrient deficiencies are frequently evident. A further danger exists—the person may aspirate food stagnating in the esophagus into the lung, which could lead to a serious lung infection.

The person with achalasia may be able to tolerate liquid or semiliquid foods in small servings. Suggest liquid supplements to help meet nutrient needs. Tube feedings and parenteral nutrition may be beneficial, particularly if the person is severely malnourished or unable to consume adequate nutrients orally. However, nasogastric or gastrostomy feedings may be contraindicated; a high risk of complications, particularly aspiration pneumonia, is associated with their use in clients with achalasia.[1]

The treatment for achalasia involves either stretching or partially slitting the cardiac sphincter, making it nonfunctional. This procedure makes the person more comfortable, but it does not restore motility to the esophageal muscles. Because the cardiac sphincter remains open, reflux esophagitis is a common complication.

Reflux Esophagitis

In reflux esophagitis, the cardiac sphincter fails to close tightly. Consequently, the highly acidic gastric contents splash backward into the esophagus and irritate the esophageal mucosa.

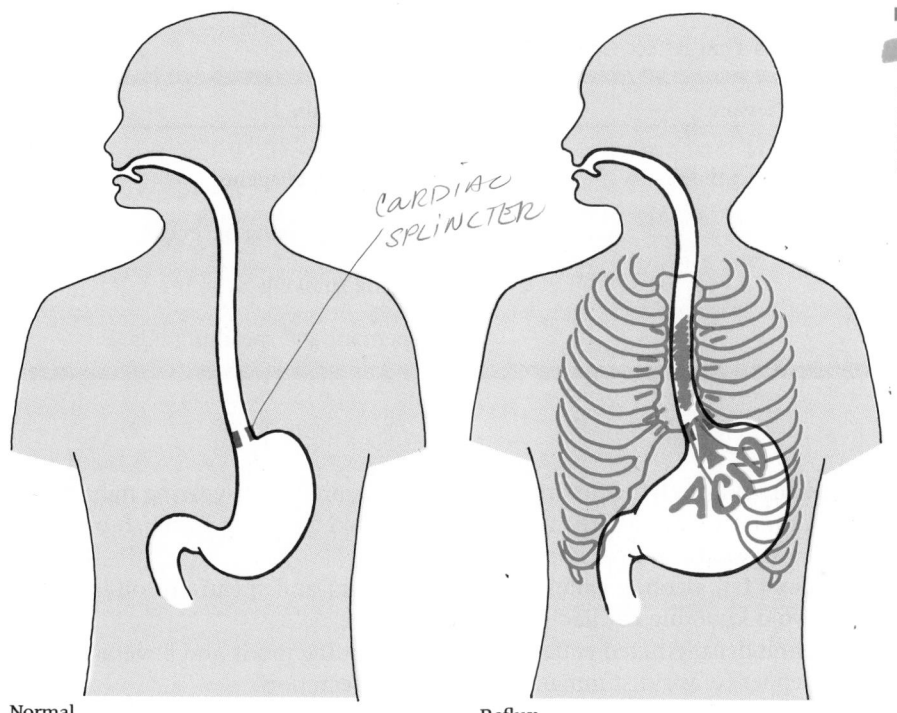

Normal

Reflux

Effect of Gastric Pressure on Reflux
Overeating and overdrinking can increase the pressure in the stomach. Whenever the pressure in the stomach exceeds the pressure in the esophagus, the chance of reflux increases.

Reflux esophagitis can occur any time cardiac sphincter pressure is not great enough to keep it closed. You can see why people treated for achalasia often develop esophagitis—their cardiac sphincters can no longer close tightly. The most common cause of reflux esophagitis is hiatal hernia (discussed in the next section).

When esophagitis becomes chronic, the inner diameter of the esophagus may become narrowed by inflammation and scarring. Dysphagia, as well as the same problems that are seen in achalasia, can result. Chronic esophagitis also can lead to the development of ulcers in the esophagus.

A burning pain called heartburn occurs when gastric juices reflux into the esophagus. At times, the pain may be so severe as to awaken a sleeping person. Heartburn usually hurts behind the sternum (see Figure 24–2), often spreading into the neck and back of the throat in waves. Because heartburn occurs when pressure in the stomach exceeds pressure in the esophagus, it more frequently flares up when a person lies down or bends over.

The best treatment of reflux esophagitis is prevention. First, encourage clients to relax and to try to enjoy their meals. Then, instruct them to avoid substances and activities that lower cardiac sphincter pressure or raise pressure in the stomach. Table 24–2 lists some foods and substances that affect cardiac sphincter pressure. Treatment for active reflux esophagitis aims at reducing gastric acidity and irritation of an already inflamed esophagus.

Diet plays an important role in the prevention and treatment of reflux esophagitis and its associated discomfort. Instruct clients to:

■ Eat small, frequent meals and drink liquids one hour before or after meals to avoid distending the stomach.

reflux esophagitis (ee-sof-ah-JIE-tis): the backflow or regurgitation of gastric contents from the stomach into the esophagus, causing inflammation of the esophagus.
re = back
fluxus = flow

A disease or condition that develops slowly, shows little change, and lasts a long time is said to be **chronic.** The term **acute** describes diseases or conditions that develop rapidly, have severe symptoms, and are of short duration.
chronos = time
acutus = sharp

heartburn: a burning sensation felt behind the sternum caused by stomach acid splashing back up into the esophagus.

The continuous reflux of gastric juices may cause scarring of the esophageal mucosa. As scar tissue forms, the diameter of the esophagus narrows, a condition referred to as an **esophageal stricture.**

■ **TABLE 24–2**
Substances That Affect Cardiac Sphincter Pressure

Elevates Pressure	Lowers Pressure
Bethanechol	Alcohol
Metoclopropamide	Anticholinergic agents
Protein	Atropine
	Caffeine-containing beverages
	Chocolate
	Cigarette smoking
	Fat
	Peppermint and spearmint oils

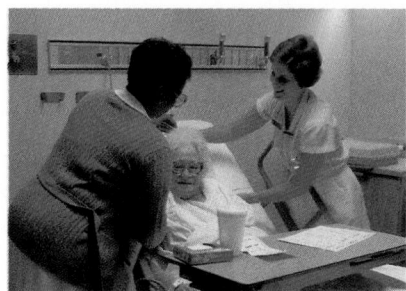

Elevate the head of the bed to minimize the likelihood of reflux from the stomach to the esophagus.

■ Refrain from lying down or bending over, and from wearing tight-fitting garments, particularly after eating, to avoid elevating stomach pressure.
■ Lose weight, if necessary.
■ Limit fat, alcohol, caffeine, and peppermint and spearmint oil intake to avoid lowering cardiac sphincter pressure.
■ Limit decaffeinated coffee, caffeine-containing foods and beverages, and pepper to avoid stimulating gastric acid secretion.
■ Avoid acidic juices such as orange, grapefruit, and tomato juice when experiencing the symptoms of reflux esophagitis to minimize esophageal irritation.

Other measures also help. Advise clients not to smoke cigarettes; cigarette smoking can reduce cardiac sphincter pressure. In addition, physicians may prescribe antacids or other drugs to neutralize gastric acidity. Advise clients to sleep with the head of the bed elevated; keeping the chest higher than the stomach helps to prevent reflux. Generally, these measures can control esophagitis. However, in some cases, surgery may be indicated if medical management fails.

Hiatal Hernia

diaphragm (DYE-ah-fram): a muscular wall separating the abdomen from the thoracic cavity.

esophageal hiatus (high-AY-tus): the opening in the diaphragm through which the esophagus passes.

hiatal hernia: a protrusion of a portion of the stomach through the esophageal hiatus of the diaphragm. There are several types of hiatal hernias, but the *sliding hiatal hernia* is the most common (see Figure 24–3).
  hiatus = to yawn

Normally, the stomach lies completely below the diaphragm. The esophagus passes through the diaphragm by way of an opening known as the esophageal hiatus. When this opening in the diaphragm weakens and allows a portion of the stomach to protrude above the diaphragm, a hiatal hernia forms. Figure 24–3 (on p. 754) shows the relationship of the upper GI tract to the diaphragm and the changes that occur in the presence of a hernia.

The symptoms of hiatal hernia result from the esophagitis that develops when acidic gastric juices reflux into the esophagus. The goals of nutrition care for hiatal hernia parallel those given earlier for esophagitis: that is, to prevent reflux, to neutralize gastric acidity, and to eliminate foods that irritate the esophagus. The accompanying "Clinical Detective Work" box provides a case study and questions to help you review the nutrition needs of a client with a hiatal hernia.

CLINICAL DETECTIVE WORK

Mrs. James, a 49-year-old accountant, recently underwent a complete physical examination. She told her physician that she had been feeling fairly well, except for heartburn, which had been occurring with increasing frequency. The attacks usually occurred after she had eaten a large meal, particularly if she lay down after eating. She told the doctor that her life was pretty hectic these days, this being the middle of the tax season.

Her past medical history shows no signs of significant health problems. The physician did advise her to stop smoking cigarettes and to lose 20 lb during her last physical, which she has yet to do. A diet history taken by the nurse shows that Mrs. James usually skips breakfast, eats lunch hurriedly while she continues to work, and eats a large dinner at about 8:00 P.M. She generally enjoys one or two alcoholic beverages in the evening before going to sleep. She drinks 6 to 8 cups of coffee during the day. Her current height and weight are 5 ft 6 inches and 155 lb. The physician diagnosed a sliding hiatal hernia after using a long tube equipped with a special optical device called a gastroscope to inspect the interior of the esophagus, stomach, and duodenum.

Can you explain to Mrs. James what a sliding hiatal hernia is and how it leads to heartburn? Describe the care plan you would develop for Mrs. James. What suggestions can you give her to help relieve the symptoms associated with the hernia? What other therapy might her physician prescribe?

Disorders of the Stomach

Turn on the television set and quite likely you will see several advertisements touting cures for indigestion, heartburn, and gas. These common GI discomforts are not diseases, but symptoms that occur for many reasons.

Indigestion, or dyspepsia, is a vague term used to describe any discomfort in the GI tract. Although it refers most often to the stomach, it can be a symptom of many disorders involving either the GI tract or other organs. Oftentimes, emotional tension triggers indigestion. You may hear a person comment that "I have a nervous stomach," or "I'm so mad my stomach feels as if it is tied in a knot." In addition to emotional factors, indigestion can be caused by underlying medical conditions, eating too much, eating too rapidly, or chewing too briefly.

Generally, a temporary bout of indigestion does not require diet modifications. When indigestion occurs frequently, however, the cause (whether

dyspepsia: vague abdominal discomfort; dyspepsia is a symptom, not a disease.
  dys = bad
  peptein = to digest

**■ FIGURE 24–3
Hiatal Hernia**

Esophagus

Esophageal hiatus *(opening in Diaphragm)*

Diaphragm

Stomach

Normally the stomach lies below the diaphragm, and the esophagus passes through the esophageal hiatus (opening in the diaphragm).

A *sliding hiatal hernia* results when part of the stomach slips through the diaphragm. This type of hiatal hernia is the most common.

physical, emotional, or dietary) needs to be identified and the following dietary advice implemented:

■ Eat slowly, at regular times, in a relaxed atmosphere, and chew food thoroughly.
■ Follow a low-fiber or soft diet (temporarily).
■ Avoid excessive amounts of fats, alcohol, and caffeine-containing foods and beverages.
■ Avoid any food known to cause indigestion.

In addition, antacids may provide relief but they must be used with caution. They can mask symptoms such as signs of an ulcer or create nutrient imbalances if used repeatedly for long periods. Antacids also contain significant amounts of sodium (those containing sodium bicarbonate) or calcium (those containing calcium bicarbonate). Although these ingredients may not be a problem for healthy individuals, they can aggravate some medical conditions. For example, sodium-containing antacids can aggravate hypertension; calcium-containing antacids can precipitate some types of kidney stones; and aluminum-containing antacids can lead to phosphorus depletion and bone disease. Like all other drugs—prescription and nonprescription alike—antacids should be taken with caution. (Antacids are also used in the treatment of ulcers and more information about their nutrient interactions is provided in a later section.)

A low-fiber diet that eliminates gas-forming foods may benefit a person with indigestion. Such a diet is frequently recommended after surgery as a person progresses from a liquid diet to a regular diet. Table 24–3 lists foods included in, and eliminated from, a low-fiber diet.

The person with persistent indigestion may habitually eat too little and become malnourished. Chronic indigestion may be a symptom of two disorders discussed later in this chapter: gastritis and peptic ulcers. Indigestion sometimes leads to nausea.

Nausea is another vague term used to describe the uncomfortable sensation that a person feels prior to vomiting. Nausea can be a symptom of many

Low-fiber diet and **soft diet** both describe the same diet. A low-residue diet is similar with the exception that it also restricts milk intake.

nausea (NAW-see-ah): inclination to vomit.

■ TABLE 24–3
Low-Fiber Diet

Foods Allowed	Foods Avoided
Meat and meat alternates Baked, broiled, or roasted beef, fish, lamb, liver, poultry, veal, crisp bacon; hard- or soft-cooked eggs	Fried poultry or meats, cold cuts, sardines, fried eggs, peanut butter
Milk and milk products Whole, nonfat, or low-fat milk; yogurt; mild cheeses	Milk drinks or yogurt containing whole fruits or berries, seeds, or skins; strongly flavored cheeses
Fruits and vegetables Cooked or canned fruits without seeds and skins; ripe bananas, orange sections, grapefruit sections; all fruit juices; cooked asparagus tips, beets, broccoli, carrots, green beans, tomato juice, wax beans, winter squash; strained peas, spinach, summer squash, or potatoes	Berries; avocado; prune juice; raw fruits except those listed; legumes, raw vegetables, and all other vegetables except those listed
Grains Refined, enriched white bread; plain muffins or rolls; white flour crackers (saltines, melba toast, zwieback); refined, ready-to-eat, or cooked cereals; noodles; macaroni; spaghetti; strained oatmeal	Whole-grain breads and cereals or those containing nuts, bran, or seeds; fried breads such as doughnuts
Miscellaneous Tea, coffee, fruit drinks, carbonated beverages, butter, cream, margarine, mayonnaise	Any dishes made with foods to be avoided; coconut

conditions from pregnancy to cancer. Certain odors, sights, or motions can trigger nausea. Generally, a nauseated person prefers not to eat. This is fine if the nausea is temporary. With persistent nausea, however (as in cancer or early pregnancy), the individual must eat or malnutrition will follow.

Dietary treatment for nausea may vary slightly depending on the cause. In general, clients with nausea should follow a low-fiber or soft diet, eat small meals, and avoid foods with odors that cause nausea. They should save liquids for between meals, slowly sip clear liquids, or suck popsicles or ice cubes made from a favorite beverage. They might prefer dry, carbohydrate-rich foods, such as toast or cereal without milk, in the morning. Loosening the clothes and getting fresh air can also help relieve nausea.

The rationale for recommending a low-fiber or soft diet to treat nausea and indigestion is weak, but it may benefit a person who believes it will help. (Recall the placebo effect described in Highlight 8.) The client may think that low-fiber foods are easier to digest, although this may not necessarily be true. Although high-fiber foods are more likely to cause gas and possible discomfort, certain low-fiber foods such as milk can also produce gas in some people.

People can experience nausea without vomiting. If nausea does lead to vomiting, other concerns arise. Highlight 3 discussed vomiting and the serious consequences of dehydration. The dangers of prolonged vomiting and dehydration warrant a review of what happens when the GI tract loses large quantities of fluid. The interstitial spaces contribute fluid to replace that lost from the GI tract. Then the capillaries of the circulatory system donate fluid to replace the lost interstitial fluid. Then the cells give fluid to resupply the circulatory system. Eventually, every cell of the body loses water and with it, electrolytes—particularly sodium, potassium, chloride, and bicarbonate. It is absolutely essential to the life of the cells that these fluids be replaced. If possible, replace fluids orally with beverages such as soft drinks, fruit "ades," or other clear liquids. Otherwise, IV feedings of saline and glucose with added electrolytes may become necessary. When vomiting continues for long periods of time, peripheral or central TPN may be indicated.

Gastritis

gastritis: inflammation of the stomach.

epigastric: the region of the body just over the stomach.
epi = above
gastric = stomach

Gastritis is a common disorder characterized by inflammation of the mucosal lining of the stomach. The person with gastritis may complain of anorexia, nausea, vomiting, belching, a feeling of fullness, and epigastric pain.

Acute gastritis most often follows ingestion of aspirin or other drugs that irritate the gastric mucosa. Alcohol abuse, food irritants, food allergies, food poisoning, radiation, stress, and infections can also cause gastritis. The dietary management of acute gastritis rests on two principles:

- Eliminate irritating foods. *BLAND DIET*
- Reduce gastric acidity.

For the person with gastritis who cannot eat because of nausea or vomiting, food may be withheld for a day or two. Then, the diet progresses from liquids to a liberal bland diet as tolerated. A bland diet is a highly individualized diet that eliminates foods that irritate the gastric mucosa, such as those named in Table 24–4. Antacids may also be given.

■ **TABLE 24–4**
Liberal Bland Diet

A liberal bland diet provides three meals a day and includes all foods except those that irritate the gastric mucosa. Substances generally contraindicated on a liberal bland diet include:

- Any foods an individual identifies as irritating to the GI tract.
- Alcohol.
- Caffeine and caffeine-containing beverages (including cola beverages, cocoa, coffee, and tea).
- Decaffeinated coffee.
- Pepper and spicy foods as tolerated.

Note: Read Highlight 24 for a more complete discussion of the liberal bland diets and its development over the years.

Chronic gastritis has the same symptoms as acute gastritis, but persists for a longer time. As gastritis progresses, the gastric cells atrophy, and gastric secretions decline. Unlike acute gastritis, chronic gastritis has no known cause. Overeating; eating too rapidly; eating when emotionally upset; eating certain foods; using alcohol, tobacco, and coffee; and having infections and nutrient deficiencies all have been implicated as possible causes, but conclusive evidence is lacking. Because so little is known about chronic gastritis, finding the appropriate diet is a matter of trial and error. A bland diet seems to relieve GI symptoms in some cases.

Peptic Ulcers

Ulcers can develop both inside and outside the body, but the term *ulcer* used alone generally refers to a *peptic ulcer*. Highlight 3 described the peptic ulcer as an erosion of the top layer of cells from the mucosa of the stomach or duodenum (occasionally they may also develop in the esophagus). This erosion leaves the underlying layers of cells exposed to gastric juices, particularly hydrochloric acid and pepsin. The erosion may proceed until the gastric juices reach the capillaries that feed the area, leading to bleeding, and the nerves, causing pain. If the erosion penetrates all the way through the mucosal lining, a major infection known as peritonitis can rapidly develop; peritonitis can be fatal.

Peptic ulcers arise from two conditions: excessive gastric secretions and a weakened mucosal defense.[2] Factors believed to influence these conditions include smoking, poor nutrition, lack of rest, drug ingestion (aspirin or glucocorticoids, for example), stress (both physiological and psychological), and genetic factors (see Figure 24–4). The "Clinical Detective Work" box on p. 758 gives the observations of two physicians and describes how their investigation uncovered the connections between stress and ulcers.

A person with an ulcer may experience a gnawing, burning pain that lasts up to several weeks. Although symptoms generally disappear for periods of time, they usually recur. People with gastric ulcers almost always have chronic gastritis.

Duodenal ulcers occur more commonly than gastric ulcers. In general, people with duodenal ulcers secrete above-normal levels of acid in their gastric juices. The sensitive duodenum becomes damaged when it receives the high-acid chyme.

Ulcers that develop following a severe physiologic stress (surgery, burns, shock, or infection) are called **stress ulcers.** Generally, once they have healed, they do not recur.

peritonitis: infection of the lining of the abdominal cavity.

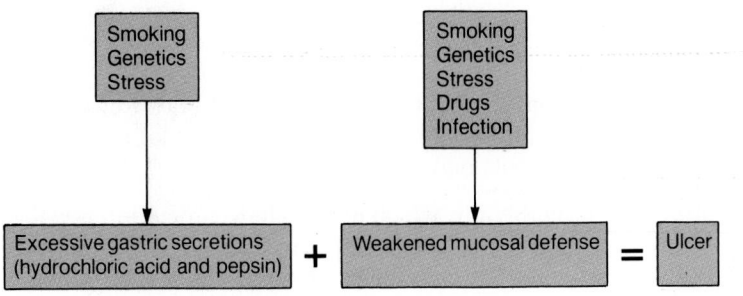

■ **FIGURE 24–4**
Ulcer Development
Ulcer formation depends on excessive gastric secretions and a weakened mucosal defense.

> ≫ **CLINICAL DETECTIVE WORK**
>
> Some interesting observations by two doctors, named Wolf and Wolff, set in motion the line of inquiry that was to culminate in today's agreement that stress is the primary factor that aggravates an ulcer. Wolf and Wolff were doctors at a hospital that admitted a most unusual client one day in 1939. This person, remembered in scientific circles only as "Tom," had had since childhood an opening from the outside of his body through the abdominal wall into his stomach. Through this fistula he had learned to feed himself, and, keeping his condition secret, he had grown to manhood and had lived a near-normal life.
>
> At the age of 53, while performing hard manual labor, he tore the edge of the opening of the fistula and was taken to the hospital where Wolf and Wolff were on the staff. The two doctors managed to gain Tom's confidence. He cooperated by allowing them to make observations of his stomach lining through the fistula. As a result, they learned that emotions called forth unique responses from the stomach. Aggressive emotions, such as anger and hostility, made the capillaries in the stomach lining flush with blood and caused the gastric juices to pour forth as if food had been introduced. However, when Tom was sad and depressed, there was no secretion of gastric juices, and the capillaries were pale pink. These emotional states and the stomach's responses to them were entirely independent of Tom's feelings of hunger.
>
> The discovery was duly reported in scientific journals. Probably the most important result of these observations was that they stimulated other doctors to experiment with their clients who had fistulas. Thus researchers began to learn exactly which foods were irritating to the lining of the stomach and which foods neutralized the acidity, instead of relying on tradition and logical thinking for this knowledge. For instance, they found that the majority of the foods that had been classified as irritating to the stomach actually were more irritating to the skin of the arm. This story should remind you to apply caution when making decisions on the basis of logic rather than evidence.

■ **FIGURE 24–5**
The Action of Cimetidine
Nerve impulses stimulate special receptor sites of cells located near the parietal cells of the gastric glands to secrete histamine. The presence of histamine at the receptor sites triggers the production of hydrochloric acid. The drug *cimetidine* blocks the receptor sites so that hydrochloric acid production diminishes.

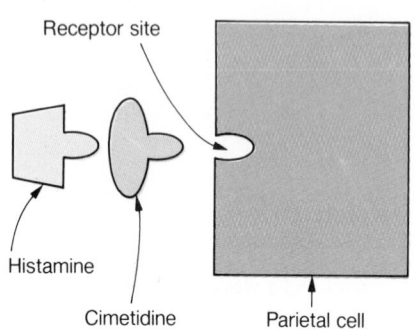

Treatment for ulcers aims at relieving pain, healing the ulcer, and minimizing the likelihood of recurrence. Both gastric and duodenal ulcers share the same treatment regimen.

Peptic ulcer therapy attempts to neutralize gastric acidity and reduce gastric acid secretion. Drug therapy has become the primary therapy for ulcers, with diet playing a minor role. Clients may be instructed to:

■ Follow prescribed drug therapy, which may include cimetidine (see Figure 24–5), or any of the other drugs listed in Table 24–5.
■ Use antacids, taken one hour after meals when gastric acid secretion is high.

■ TABLE 24–5
Antacids and Other Antiulcer Medications

Drug Name	Timing with Meals	Common Side Effects That May Influence Nutrition Status
Aluminum hydroxide	Give 1 to 3 hr after meals.	Constipation, cramps, bloating, nausea, vomiting, anorexia, chalky taste. Inactives thiamin; decreases absorption of vitamin A, phosphorous, and calcium.
Calcium carbonate	Give 1 to 3 hr after meals. Give iron supplements 1 to 2 hr before or after use. Do not take with large amounts of dairy products.	Belching, nausea, constipation, steatorrhea, chalky taste. May decrease iron absorption.
Cimetidine	Give with meals; caffeine and alcohol reduce effectiveness.	Diarrhea. Reduced gastric secretion. May induce hyperglycemia.
Dihydroxyaluminum sodium carbonate	Give 1 to 3 hr after meals.	Constipation, diarrhea, anorexia, weight loss.
Magnesium hydroxide	Give 1 hr after meals.	Constipation. May decrease absorption of vitamin A, phosphorus, and calcium; inactivates thiamin.
Magaldrate	Give on empty stomach.	Chalky taste. May decrease absorption of fat-soluble vitamins, especially vitamin A.
Ranitidine		Constipation, nausea, abdominal discomfort. (Fewer reported side effects and interactions than with cimetidine.)
Sodium bicarbonate	Give 1 to 3 hr after meals.	Belching, gas, bloating, weight gain. Decreases iron absorption.
Sucralfate	Give on empty stomach 1 hr before meals and at bedtime.	Constipation, diarrhea, nausea, cramps, dry mouth. Interferes with absorption of fat-soluable vitamins.

Source: Adapted from D. E. Powers and A. O. Moore, *Food Medication Interactions*, (Phoenix, Ariz.: Food Medication Interactions, 1989).

■ Eliminate any food that routinely causes indigestion or pain. Avoid caffeine- and alcohol-containing beverages.

■ Reduce stress, which stimulates gastric acid secretion. Learn how to handle stress without overreacting or becoming upset; learn how to relax, to get enough sleep, and to enjoy life. Regular exercise effectively reduces stress.

■ Eliminate drugs that irritate the stomach (such as aspirin and alcohol).

■ Reduce or eliminate cigarette smoking, which stimulates gastric acid secretion.

The bland diet used to treat ulcers has changed dramatically over the years, as Highlight 24 describes. People who have trouble identifying foods that cause discomfort can follow a liberal bland diet until specific food intolerances can be discerned. (Table 24–4 on p. 756 describes a liberal bland diet.)

Ulcers are painful, but the pain is intermittent. The person with an ulcer who is bothered by particular foods has one great advantage over the person with a "silent" disease or one that causes chronic pain. For this person, the pain of an ulcer is prompt to follow upon the commission of a dietary

➤➤ **CLINICAL DETECTIVE WORK**

Meet Mr. Kelly, a busy executive living a high-stress life. He entertains many business clients, so he eats most of his meals in restaurants and drinks alcoholic beverages regularly. He smokes cigarettes and gets little sleep. Mr. Kelly visited his physician after he began experiencing severe, gnawing stomach pain; the physician diagnosed a peptic ulcer.

Having assessed Mr. Kelly's medical situation, you are ready to counsel him. What changes in lifestyle would you suggest to help Mr. Kelly treat his ulcer? What diet do you recommend he follow? From the limited information you have about his eating habits, what practical suggestions can you offer Mr. Kelly? What questions could you ask Mr. Kelly to help him design an acceptable diet? How could you help him identify foods that irritate his ulcer?

indiscretion, so the client who knows this can quickly learn which foods and beverages hurt and which do not. Use this information to help clients tailor their dietary routines to their own tolerances.

The treatment of ulcers has improved so dramatically in recent years that medical management is almost always effective. Rarely, surgery may be necessary for clients who do not respond to medical treatment or for those who develop complications such as bleeding, perforation, or obstruction. The accompanying "Clinical Detective Work" box presents a case study on peptic ulcers.

■ *Gastric Surgery*

The management of gastric cancer and damage following trauma (gunshot wound or auto accident) may include gastric surgery. Figure 24–6 illustrates several types of commonly used procedures. Of course, the general nutrition care for surgical clients described in Chapter 23 applies to those undergoing gastric surgery although additional nutrition concerns arise.

After gastric surgery, people may lose a significant amount of weight as the result of limited food intake, malabsorption, increased metabolic requirements, or any combination of these. Some people have trouble regaining their preoperative weight; some people develop specific nutrient deficiencies.

One problem that may occur when a significant portion of the stomach has been removed is dumping syndrome. A typical scenario goes something like this: Mrs. Clark had a fairly extensive gastric resection about a week ago and has just begun to eat solid foods. She swallows the food, and about 15 minutes later begins to feel weak and dizzy. She looks pale, her heart beats rapidly, and she breaks out in a sweat. Shortly thereafter, she develops diarrhea. What causes this sequence of events?

Mrs. Clark has lost an important function of her stomach: its control of the rate at which food empties into the intestine. Now, food gets "dumped" rapidly

dumping syndrome: the symptoms that result from the rapid emptying of undigested food into the jejunum: sweating, weakness, and diarrhea shortly after eating and hypoglycemia later.

■ **FIGURE 24-6**

Typical Gastric Surgery Resections
(A resection is the partial removal of a structure.)

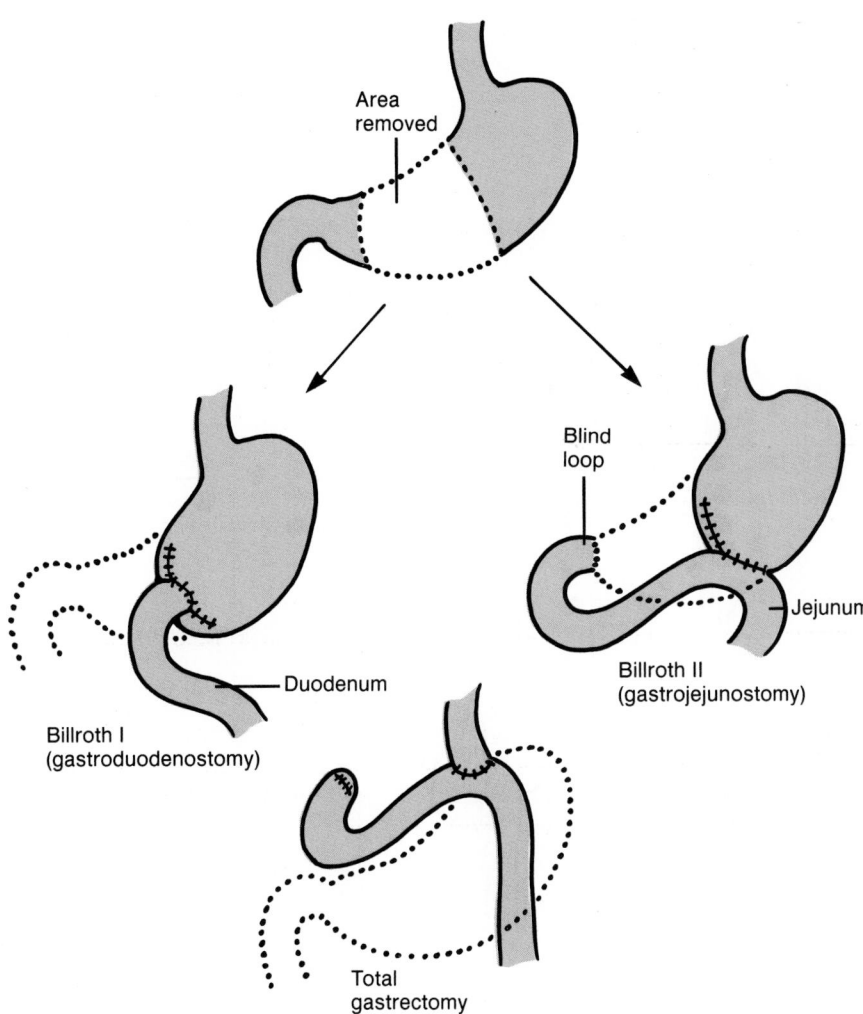

Area removed

Billroth I
(gastroduodenostomy)

Duodenum

Blind loop

Jejunum

Billroth II
(gastrojejunostomy)

Total gastrectomy

into the jejunum. (Even if the duodenum had not been bypassed during surgery, its short length would have allowed food to pass too quickly into the jejunum.) As the GI tract digests the large food particles into small nutrient units, the number of particles in the intestinal contents increases and, so, the intestinal contents become hypertonic. Water from the intestinal capillaries then moves into the lumen of the jejunum to equalize the osmolar load. Consequently, the jejunum becomes stretched, causing pain, and the volume of circulating blood diminishes rapidly, causing blood pressure to fall. Intestinal pain, weakness, dizziness, and a rapid heartbeat result. The large fluid load in the jejunum causes hyperperistalsis, resulting in diarrhea. Figure 24-7 (on p. 762) outlines the sequence of events that occurs in dumping syndrome.

Two to three hours later Mrs. Clark experiences many of the same symptoms again: dizziness, fainting, nausea, and sweating. This time the cause is different. Carbohydrates from the meal were rapidly digested and absorbed, raising blood glucose levels quickly. The pancreas responded by

Hyperglycemia

■ **FIGURE 24–7**
Dumping Syndrome
When partially digested food rapidly enters the jejunum, it creates a hyperosmolar load. Fluid from the intestinal capillaries enters the jejunum, diminishing blood volume and stimulating peristalsis. The result: low blood pressure and diarrhea.

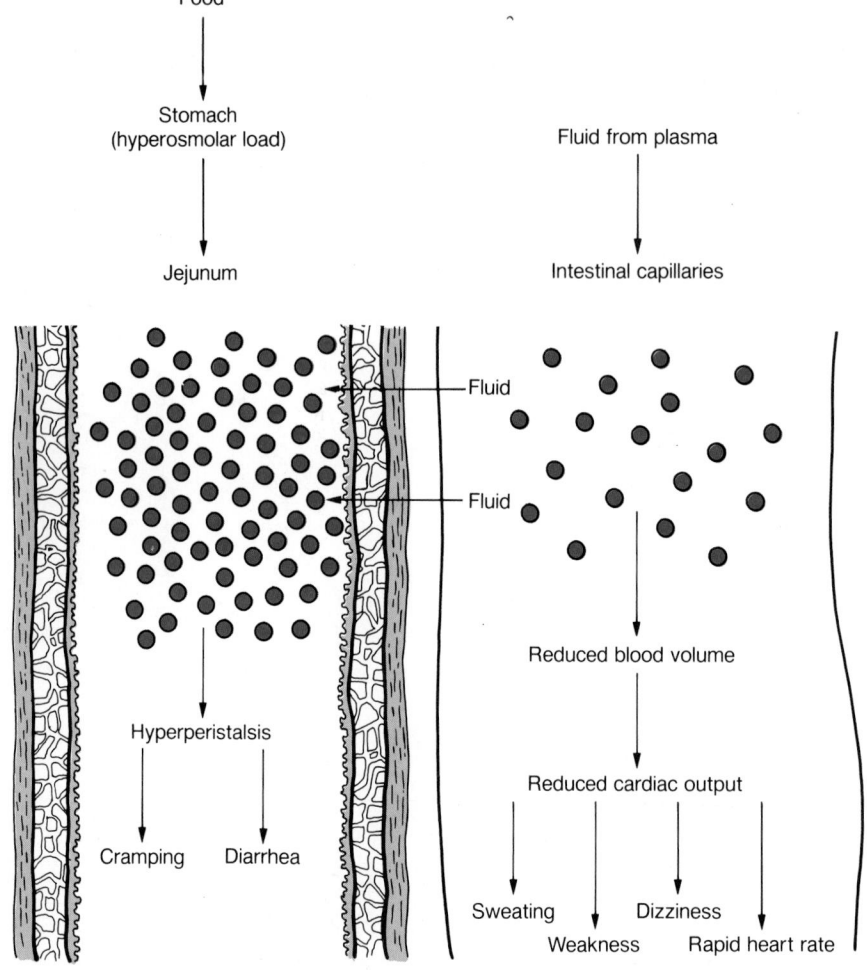

postgastrectomy diet: a diet given to prevent the symptoms of dumping syndrome and hypoglycemia that sometimes follow gastric surgery.

The type of hypoglycemia that occurs following gastric surgery is called **alimentary** (AL-ee-MEN-tah-ree) or **postgastrectomy hypoglycemia.**

overproducing insulin, making blood glucose levels fall sharply. The symptoms Mrs. Clark experiences hours after the meal are those of hypoglycemia.

Not all clients who have had gastrectomies experience the diarrhea of dumping syndrome; even fewer experience the associated hypoglycemia. Many clients who initially experience dumping syndrome gradually adapt to a fairly normal diet. However, a special diet benefits clients during the immediate postsurgical period and in prolonged or severe cases.

The postgastrectomy diet is a carbohydrate-controlled diet designed to alleviate the symptoms of dumping syndrome. Health care professionals monitor fluid and electrolyte balances carefully, correcting any imbalances that occur. The diet emphasizes foods containing protein and fat. Because proteins and fats are digested more slowly than carbohydrates, they do not attract fluid as rapidly as carbohydrates do.

Advise clients not to eat concentrated sweets (sugar, cookies, cakes, pies, or soft drinks), because the body digests these carbohydrates most rapidly. Recommend small, frequent meals to fit the reduced storage capacity of the stomach. Suggest that clients wait about 45 minutes after each meal before drinking liquids. This precaution helps slow the rate of food's passage from the stomach to the intestine. Suggest that clients lie down immediately after

Sample Postgastrectomy Diet Menu

MENU

Breakfast
1 fried egg
1 slice toast
1 tsp butter
½ c milk (take 30-60 min after meal)

Midmorning Snack
¼ c cottage cheese
1 graham cracker

Lunch
2 oz hamburger patty
¼ c mashed potatoes
1 tsp margarine
¼ small cantaloupe
½ c milk (take 30-60 min after meal)

Midafternoon Snack
2 tbsp peanut butter
3 saltine crackers

Supper
2 oz boiled ham
¼ c rice
½ c carrots
2 tsp butter
¼ c unsweetened peach slices
½ c milk (take 30-60 min after eating)

Evening Snack
¼ c tuna
1 tsp mayonnaise
1 slice bread

eating to help slow the transit of food to the intestine. Pectin, a type of dietary fiber, can be added to the diet to help prevent dumping syndrome. Table 24–6 (on p. 764) lists foods included on, and excluded from, the postgastrectomy diet. A sample postgastrectomy diet menu is provided above.

Dietitians carefully tailor the diet to meet each client's needs. Initially, visits to the client after each meal uncover food intolerances. For example, some people may be unable to tolerate any milk at all because they have developed lactose intolerance.

Gradually, many people will be able to tolerate small amounts of concentrated sweets, larger quantities of food, and some liquids with meals. Unfortunately, diet does not successfully correct the symptoms of dumping syndrome for everyone. When all dietary measures fail, additional surgery may be necessary to resolve the problem.

Other nutrition concerns arise in people with gastrectomies. For example, clients may develop iron-deficiency anemia. Blood loss from surgery, accompanied by inadequate nutrition and poor iron absorption, contributes to the problem. In addition, consider that 50 percent of iron absorption normally takes place in the duodenum. Following gastric surgery, the transit time through the duodenum may be rapid, or the duodenum may be bypassed altogether. An iron supplement helps to correct the deficiency.

Anemia also can be caused by a deficiency of vitamin B_{12} or folate. Recall from Chapter 8 that vitamin B_{12} cannot be absorbed without an intrinsic factor, which is synthesized in the stomach. Depending on the location and extent of the gastric resection, intrinsic factor production may be minimal or absent, and vitamin B_{12} absorption correspondingly impaired. To correct the deficiency, clients receive vitamin B_{12} by injection (to bypass the need for absorption) and supplemental folate orally.

■ **TABLE 24–6**
Postgastrectomy Diet

Food Item	Allowed	Excluded	Comments
Meats/meat alternates	X		Any type
Grains/starchy vegetables			
Plain breads, crackers, rolls, unsweetened cereal, rice, pasta, corn, lima beans, parsnips, peas, white potatoes, sweet potatoes, pumpkin, yams, winter squash	X		Limit to 5 servings daily
Sweetened cereal; cereal containing dates, raisins, or brown sugar		X	
Nonstarchy vegetables			
Chicory, Chinese cabbage, endive, escarole, lettuce, parsley, radishes, watercress	X		As desired
Asparagus, bean sprouts, beets, broccoli, Brussels sprouts, cabbage, carrots, cauliflower, celery, cucumbers, eggplant, green pepper, greens, mushrooms, okra, onions, rhubarb, sauerkraut, string beans, summer squash, tomatoes, turnips, zucchini	X		Limit to two ½-c servings daily; individual tolerances will vary
Vegetables prepared with sugar		X	
Fruits			
Unsweetened fruits and fruit juices	X		Limit to 3 servings daily
Sweetened fruits and fruit juices		X	
Fats	X		Any type
Beverages			
Milk (whole milk, nonfat milk, or buttermilk)	X		If tolerated
Coffee, tea, dietetic carbonated beverages	X		
Alcohol, carbonated beverages, sweetened milk, cocoa, fruit drinks		X	
Desserts			
Cakes, cookies, ice cream, sherbet		X	
Other			
Honey, jam, jelly, syrup, sugar		X	

■ FIGURE 24–8
Steatorrhea

Bile has an affinity for fats and water, so it can bring them together.

The enzymes now have access to the emulsified fat.

In blind loop syndrome, bacteria damage the bile, so that it is ineffective in fat digestion and absorption. The result is fat malabsorption and steatorrhea.

In some types of gastric resections, a portion of the small intestine is bypassed, making that portion nonfunctional. The bypassed portion is called a blind loop. Figure 24–6 (on p. 761) illustrates such a gastric resection.

Stasis occurs in the blind loop, and bacteria normally not present in that part of the intestine may begin to flourish. The bacteria compete with the body for vitamin B_{12} and folate, limiting the available supply. The bacteria also partly dismantle bile salts, making them ineffective in fat digestion and absorption. Figure 24–8 takes another look at the figure from Chapter 5 (p. 116) that shows how bile prepares fat for digestion, this time illustrating how bacteria interfere with that process. The bacterial overgrowth that occurs in a blind loop leads to fat malabsorption and steatorrhea, and to vitamin B_{12} and folate deficiencies. To correct these problems, clients receive a low-fat diet, parenteral vitamin B_{12}, and oral folate supplements. Physicians also prescribe antibiotics to inhibit bacterial growth. Sometimes the blind loop must be removed surgically.

Be aware that general malabsorption is a common problem for any client who has had a total gastrectomy or who has had the stomach surgically connected directly to the jejunum. Normally, food entering the duodenum triggers the release of the hormones secretin and cholecystokinin. These hormones, in turn, mediate the secretion of digestive enzymes and bile into the duodenum. When the duodenum is bypassed, these processes are bypassed and cannot aid digestion and absorption as usual. Malabsorption results whenever food passes rapidly through the GI tract.

Another type of gastric surgery sometimes used in the treatment of morbid obesity is gastric partitioning, or gastric stapling. During the procedure, a row of surgical staples is placed in the stomach, effectively reducing its size and making it difficult for the individual to eat large amounts of food (see Figure 24–9 on p. 766). A small opening allows food to pass slowly into the lower portion of the stomach and into the intestine for digestion and absorption.

The long-term safety and effectiveness of gastric partitioning depends, in large part, on compliance with dietary instructions. Poor dietary habits may prevent weight loss, rupture staples, or obstruct the small passage into the lower stomach. Common postsurgical complications include nausea, vomiting, dehydration, and esophageal reflux.

stasis (STAY-sis): standing still. Normal actions of the intestines keep a steady stream of secretions flowing through them. Stasis in a blind loop allows bacteria to flourish.

steatorrhea (stee-ah-toe-REE-ah): The fatty diarrhea characteristic of fat malabsorption; stools are foamy, greasy, and malodorous.
 steatos = fat
 rhea = flow

The problems of fat malabsorption and vitamin B_{12} and folate deficiencies that result from the overgrowth of bacteria in a bypassed segment of the intestine are called **blind loop syndrome.**

morbid obesity: twice or more the average desirable weight given in life insurance tables or 100 lb more than desirable weight.

gastric partitioning: surgery in which a line of surgical staples is placed in such a way as to make the upper portion of the stomach smaller; used to treat morbid obesity. Also called **gastric stapling, gastric plication,** or **gastroplasty.**

30-60 cc stomach capacity

FIGURE 24–9
Gastric Partitioning

Clients follow a liquid diet for about eight weeks after surgery.[3] Liquids reduce the risk of disrupting the line of surgical staples and flow easily through the opening to the lower stomach. Clients can tolerate only small amounts of liquids at one time because of the reduced size of the stomach; overeating or overdrinking can cause vomiting.

After about two months, the person can gradually begin to eat soft or pureed foods, and then regular foods as tolerated. Again, only small amounts of food can be eaten at one time. Clients must understand that their selection of foods and beverages influences the extent of their weight loss. If they drink high-kcalorie liquids or eat high-kcalorie foods all the time, even if only in small quantities, they will not lose weight. Their selections also affect the nutritional quality of the diet. To ensure the adequacy of an energy-restricted diet that demands small intakes requires careful planning, diligent compliance with the prescribed diet, and supplements.[4] Use the case study in the "Clinical Detective Work" box to review the needs of a client following gastric surgery.

Nutrition Assessment

As you have seen in this chapter, disorders of the upper GI tract can limit food intake and impair nutrition status. When you assess the nutrition status of people who have these disorders, keep these special points in mind:

- Obtain a thorough diet history. People who have difficulties chewing or swallowing may have poor intakes of one or several nutrients. Other disorders such as nausea, indigestion, gastritis, or peptic ulcers some-

CLINICAL DETECTIVE WORK

Mrs. Grayson was admitted to the emergency room in serious condition after suffering severe abdominal injuries in a car accident. After her initial examination, a surgeon was consulted, and Mrs. Grayson was taken to surgery immediately. A gastrojejunostomy (see Figure 24–6) was performed. Mrs. Grayson was sent to the intensive care unit following surgery and is recovering as expected. The health care team anticipates nutrition-related problems, and they are taking measures to prevent them.

Review Figure 24–6 to understand the procedure that Mrs. Grayson underwent. Consider the possibility that she might develop dumping syndrome, blind loop syndrome, and general malabsorption. Describe how these conditions might occur.

What diet will the physician prescribe for Mrs. Grayson after she begins eating orally? Describe the diet and how it progresses. What advice can you give Mrs. Grayson to prevent dumping syndrome?

Discuss the nutrition-related concerns associated with blind loop syndrome. How can these concerns be handled?

---

times indicate intolerances to certain foods. A good diet history can help to pinpoint offending foods so that they might be avoided. For the person who has undergone gastric partitioning, use diet histories to assess energy intake and eating habits.

■ Monitor body weight regularly. Disorders of the upper GI tract often lead to weight loss due to either poor food intake or to malabsorption of nutrients. Conversely, excessive eating and weight gain can interfere with efforts to control the symptoms of reflux esophagitis and with the security of gastric staples.

■ Assess biochemical parameters with caution. People with severe vomiting or those with dumping syndrome may be dehydrated, making lab values appear deceptively elevated.

This chapter has described how problems of the upper GI tract can affect dietary intake and how dietary intake, in turn, can affect these problems. The next chapter examines problems of the lower GI tract.

SELF STUDY *Diet for Upper GI Problems*

Today you cannot chew, and you are allowed no caffeine and no smoking materials. Plan a day's meals that will meet your nutritional needs and, as far as possible, also please your palate. Record the plan.

Then eat as you have planned. How did you enjoy your meals? What did you miss? How could you compensate for this lack another time? Were there any surprises in your reactions to this day's meals? How would you feel about continuing such a diet for a week or two? List all the ways in which you would attempt to help clients adjust to diets of this kind.

■ Study Questions

1. Describe some conditions of the mouth that can affect food intake. What diet would you advise in these cases? How should the diet be planned?
2. What is achalasia, and how is it managed?
3. What is a hiatal hernia? What causes the symptoms associated with a hiatal hernia? What advice can you give the person with a hiatal hernia to prevent and treat these symptoms?
4. Under what circumstances can indigestion, nausea, and vomiting be a risk to nutrition status?
5. Discuss the therapy for peptic ulcers.
6. Describe the events associated with dumping syndrome. What diet might help to prevent these symptoms? Discuss the advice you could give a person with dumping syndrome.
7. What is blind loop syndrome? What are the nutrition consequences? How are these problems avoided or corrected?
8. Discuss the dietary recommendations, and the rationale behind them, for a person who undergoes gastric partitioning.

■ Notes

1. J. V. Sitzmann, Nutritional support of the dysphagic patient: Methods, risks, and complications of therapy, *Journal of Parenteral and Enteral Nutrition* 14 (1990): 60–63.
2. A. H. Soll, Pathogenesis of peptic ulcer and implications for therapy, *New England Journal of Medicine* 322 (1990): 909–916.
3. A. S. Graney, L. B. Smith, and K. A. Hammer, Gastric partitioning for morbid obesity: Postoperative weight loss, technical complications, and protein status, *Journal of the American Dietetic Association* 86 (1986): 630–635.
4. T. Andersen and U. Larsen, Dietary outcome in obese patients treated with gastroplasty program, *American Journal of Clinical Nutrition* 50 (1989): 1328–1340.

How the Ulcer Diet Won the Right to Taste Good

At its best, diet therapy applies valid findings from nutrition science so that they benefit clients. In other words, diet therapy puts the truth to work to help people. However, gaps exist in the knowledge gained from nutrition science and in the knowledge of how to apply it. Sometimes diet modifications are based on logic rather than fact, and do not actually help clients. As researchers narrow the gaps in knowledge, it becomes necessary to alter diets accordingly. This highlight provides a dramatic example of such a dietary evolution as it presents a historical look at the changes in ulcer treatment over the years.

The Traditional Bland Diet

At the time the traditional bland diet was developed, few drugs were available to alter gastric acid secretion. Diet was therefore the cornerstone of therapy. The rationale for the bland diet, as it was originally designed, was to provide foods that did not irritate the gastric mucosa. The theory was that certain foods could neutralize or reduce gastric acid secretion, and thus help relieve the pain and damage of ulcers.

The traditional bland diet consisted of a series of diets that progressed through stages. The first stage generally provided only milk and cream, given frequently throughout the day, to coat the stomach and intestine and to buffer stomach acids. The diet then gradually progressed to include a larger quantity and variety of foods. However, even the last stage was quite restrictive, including only foods mild in flavor and low in fiber to exclude the possibility of irritating the stomach and intestinal lining. Small meals were provided several times a day, for that way, the stomach would never be empty and exposed to undiluted acid. Caffeine and alcohol were excluded, to avoid stimulating acid secretion. Table H24–1 shows a typical traditional bland diet.

If you look closely at the traditional bland diet, you will notice that some of its recommendations oppose dietary recommendations for a healthy diet. Milk and cream—mainstays of the traditional bland diet—are high in saturated fats and cholesterol, which we now know increase the risk of cardiovascular disease (see Chapter 28). In addition, some research has even shown that milk may actually impair recovery from ulcers. In one study of people with ulcers who were taking the drug cimetidine (see p. 758), the ulcers healed in 78 percent of the people who ate a normal diet but in only 53 percent of those whose main food was milk.[1]

Similarly, eliminating high-fiber foods may cause more harm than good. Health care professionals recommend high-fiber foods to maintain optimal function of the GI tract, for weight control, for blood glucose regulation, and for blood lipid control (see pp. 88–90). Unless fiber restrictions provide a greater advantage to the person with ulcers than the risks they pose, they are unwarranted and possibly harmful. Scientific facts thus seem to contradict the rationale for the traditional bland diet, which was based on theory without much research.

■ **TABLE H24–1**
Traditional Bland Diet

Stage I

3 to 4 oz milk and cream (half-and-half) every 1 to 2 hours.

Stage II

Add to the Stage I diet small feedings of low-fiber foods at frequent and regular intervals throughout the waking hours (7 to 8 feedings per 24 hours).

Foods allowed include milk; white bread; soft-cooked or poached eggs; cream of wheat; farina; boiled rice; oatmeal; strained creamed soup; white crackers; butter; margarine; small servings of tender boiled, broiled, baked, roasted, creamed, or stewed beef, chicken, fish, lamb, liver, pork, sweetbreads, turkey, or veal; plain cake, cookies, ice cream; bread, cornstarch, rice, or tapioca pudding.

Foods not allowed include all others.

Stage III

Add to the Stage II diet small feedings given six times a day as well as decaffeinated coffee.

Foods allowed include all foods except those listed below.

Foods not allowed include fried foods; most raw fruits and vegetables; dried peas and beans; broccoli, Brussels sprouts, cabbage, onions, cauliflower, cucumber, green pepper, rutabagas, turnips, sauerkraut, berries, figs; highly seasoned or cured meats, poultry, or fish; salad dressings; caffeine; alcohol; high-fiber breads and cereals; highly seasoned foods; ketchup; pepper; barbecue sauce; chili pepper; horseradish; garlic; mustard; vinegar; olives; pickles; popcorn; nuts; coconut.

■ **TABLE H24–2**
Traditional and Liberal Bland Diets Compared

Diet Modification	Traditional Bland	Liberal Bland
Frequency of feedings	Six small feedings	Three feedings
Milk	Use liberally	Use in moderation
Alcohol	Restricted	Restricted
Caffeine and caffeine-containing beverages	Restricted	Restricted
Decaffeinated coffee	Not restricted	Restricted
Pepper and spicy foods	Restricted	As tolerated
High-fiber foods	Restricted	Not restricted

A Look at the Facts

To determine what is truly best for clients with ulcers, the questions to answer are: What foods do, in reality, speed the healing of ulcers or prevent their recurrence? Do milk and low-fiber foods help? Few health care practitioners have agreed as to which foods irritated the GI tract. In the 1970s, the discrepancies prompted the American Dietetic Association (ADA) to review the literature and issue a position paper on bland diets.[2] The ADA concluded that the traditional bland diet was mostly supported by tradition and folklore, and not by scientific research. Well-controlled research studies failed to demonstrate that a bland diet benefited the healing of ulcers.

The ADA found that few of the substances commonly eliminated from traditional bland diets actually were irritating to the gastric mucosa. True irritants were a small group: black pepper, chili powder, caffeine, coffee, tea, cocoa, alcohol, and a few drugs—most notably, aspirin. The ADA also questioned the recommendation to include milk frequently and found no support for eliminating high-fiber foods. The ADA did conclude, though, that small, frequent meals were beneficial (but wait; that item changed later). Finally, the ADA recommended individualizing the diet based on specific food intolerances.

The Liberal Bland Diet

Since the publication of the ADA position paper, additional information has come to light, and further changes in the diet have been made. For one thing, *decaffeinated* coffee was found to stimulate gastric acid secretion to the same degree as caffeinated coffee; therefore, all coffee should be restricted. For another, advice to eat small, frequent meals has changed. Since food stimulates gastric acid secretion, frequent eating is contraindicated; instead, three regular meals a day are preferred.

Finally, with respect to spices, individuals who do not regularly eat spicy foods may have discomfort when they do eat such foods. However, contrary to popular belief, spicy foods do not damage the GI lining.[3] Individuals who regularly eat spicy foods are probably not at a higher risk of developing ulcers or of having ulcers recur.[4] These findings became the basis of the liberal bland diet described in Chapter 24 (see Table 24–4).

Where does that leave treatment of ulcers? Basically, the cornerstone of ulcer treatment has shifted from diet to drugs that reduce gastric acid secretion. Generally, alcohol and coffee (both with caffeine and decaffeinated) must be restricted or used judiciously. As far as foods are concerned, people with ulcers are encouraged to eat any foods they can tolerate. Also, as mentioned in Chapter 24, people can easily learn, from their own reactions, which foods cause pain—and those are, of course, the foods that cause acid secretion and further destruction of tissue. Table H24–2 illustrates the differences between the traditional bland diet and the liberal bland diet currently in use.

The vast majority of physicians and dietitians today recommend the liberal bland diet for ulcers. However, some 20 years after the basic tenets of the traditional bland diet have been disproven, some practitioners continue to prescribe restrictive diets, especially when ulcers are active.

The evolution of the bland diet provides a classic example of how new research may warrant changes in diets. Other dietary recommendations have changed over the years as well, namely for cystic fibrosis (see Chapter 25), gallbladder diseases (see Chapter 25), gout and kidney stones (see Highlight 29). In the future, the diet for people with insulin-dependent diabetes (see Chapter 27) could drastically change if a system for continuously providing insulin as needed becomes available.

To stay knowledgeable about diet therapies that really work, keep up with the research. Learning about what's new in the field of diet therapy will enhance your client care.

NOTES

1. N. Kumar and coauthors, Effect of milk on patients with duodenal ulcers, *British Medical Journal* 293 (1986): 666.
2. American Dietetic Association, Position paper on bland diet in the treatment of chronic duodenal ulcer disease, *Journal of the American Dietetic Association* 59 (1971): 244–245.
3. D. Y. Graham, J. L. Smith, and A. R. Opekun, Spicy food and the stomach, *Journal of the American Medical Association* 260 (1988): 3473–3475.
4. K. Holt and D. Hollander, Gastric mucosal injury, *Annual Review of Medicine* 37 (1986): 107.

Nutrition and Disorders of the Lower GI Tract

Contents

Gastrointestinal disorders, because they impair digestion and absorption, interfere with the nutrient supply to all other body systems. These delicate microvilli, on the surfaces of intestinal cells, are easily disrupted by digestive disorders.

As stated in Chapter 3, the intestine is "the" organ of digestion. Any disorder of the intestine, particularly if it results in malabsorption, can seriously affect nutrition status. This chapter describes disorders of the lower GI tract that influence nutrition status or are affected by diet. It begins with motility disorders, then takes up disorders of the pancreas and intestine that cause malabsorption, then those of the gallbladder, and then the colon. (Some common digestive problems, such as gas, short bouts of diarrhea, and constipation, that do not seriously impact nutrition status were already discussed in Highlight 3.)

◼ *Severe Diarrhea and Irritable Bowel Syndrome*

Two motility disorders of the GI tract are diarrhea and irritable bowel syndrome. Their causes may not always be known, but nutrition support measures may help alleviate their symptoms while a conclusive diagnosis is being made.

Diarrhea

Diarrhea that results from an accelerated movement of fluids and electrolytes from the intestinal capillaries into the lumen of the intestine is called **secretory diarrhea.** Diarrhea that results from unabsorbed water and electrolytes, increasing the osmolarity of the intestinal contents is called **osmotic diarrhea.** Fat that is not absorbed but is excreted in the stools causes **steatorrhea,** as previously mentioned. Severe, chronic diarrhea is often called **intractable diarrhea.**

Diarrhea occurs either when fluids are not absorbed as the intestinal contents move quickly through the GI tract or when water is drawn from cells lining the intestinal tract and added to the food residue. The result is frequent, watery bowel movements. A person with severe diarrhea may rapidly develop dehydration, weight loss, and multiple nutrient deficiencies. It is urgently important to prevent or correct these problems by starting nutrition support before severe depletion occurs.

Diarrhea can have many causes. Emotional and physiological stress, nervous tension, food allergies, some disorders of the GI tract, and overeating can trigger diarrhea, as can some drugs that irritate the GI tract. Spoiled food and bacterial overgrowth in the gut can also bring on diarrhea. Malnutrition can cause diarrhea. Many people on tube feedings develop diarrhea (as you may recall from Chapter 21). Infants and children frequently develop diarrhea when they are ill or given formulas that their immature GI tracts cannot tolerate.

A variety of foods and spices can cause diarrhea in different individuals and at different times. Food sensitivities, such as lactose intolerance, are a frequent cause. As Highlight 4 mentioned, aspartame and sorbitol used in large doses have been known to cause diarrhea in some people. Generally, adults who have food sensitivities that result in diarrhea are aware of the offending foods. Keeping a food diary and a record of bowel movements can help pinpoint offending foods.

Mild diarrhea that remits in 24 to 48 hours is seldom a cause for concern and does not require medical treatment unless it is very severe or the individual is already dehydrated. Eliminating food irritants and drinking clear liquids may help to alleviate mild diarrhea.

Severe diarrhea, on the other hand, can quickly lead to serious dehydration. An average-sized adult producing a large volume of watery stools can lose more than one liter of fluid and electrolytes per hour—a fluid loss that can be fatal in six hours or less.[1] The assessment section later in this chapter provides a table listing physical and laboratory findings associated with dehydration.

Chronic diarrhea is also a cause for concern. Chronic diarrhea can result from other disorders such as malabsorption or protein-energy malnutrition (PEM) or from medical treatments such as radiation therapy or drugs. The person with chronic diarrhea can become dehydrated when large amounts of water and electrolytes are lost over a long period of time.

Oral rehydration formulas may successfully prevent dehydration in some cases of severe diarrhea. Oftentimes, however, especially in seriously ill individuals, it becomes necessary to stop placing demands on the GI tract and let it rest while investigating the cause of the diarrhea. The diagnostician may order all foods and beverages withheld for 24 to 48 hours, during which time treatment primarily focuses on maintaining fluid and electrolyte balance intravenously. After a day or so of intravenous fluids, the person tries a clear liquid diet, and then progresses to a full liquid diet, a low-fiber diet, and finally a regular diet as tolerated. Once a person receives an oral diet, applesauce or scraped raw apples may be given every two to four hours. These foods contain pectin, a carbohydrate that attracts water and improves the consistency of the stools. Of course, if a food is known to have irritated the intestine, it is eliminated. The exact treatment plan depends on the cause of the diarrhea.

If the diarrhea worsens as the diet progresses, then alternate feeding programs are appropriate. Enteral nutrition is always preferred to parenteral, so a first choice is to try hydrolyzed formulas, either orally or by tube. However, some people with chronic diarrhea are unable to tolerate any type of enteral feeding. For these people, parenteral nutrition is indicated, and nothing is given by mouth (NPO).

Drug therapy also plays an important role in the treatment of diarrhea. Table 25–1 lists antidiarrheal agents and their nutrition consequences.

oral rehydration therapy formulas: formulas containing glucose and a combination of sodium and potassium salts used to prevent or treat dehydration associated with diarrhea.

i.e. Sports drinks GATORADE

■ **TABLE 25–1**
Antidiarrheal Agents

Drug Name	Timing with Meals	Common Side Effects That May Influence Nutrition Status
Diphenoxylate	May give with food.	Nausea, vomiting, bloating, anorexia, dry mouth, sore or swollen gums.
Kaolin, pectin	Mix at room temperature with milk or juice.	Constipation, dry mouth, altered taste perception.
Loperamide		Abdominal pain, constipation, bloating, dry mouth, vomiting, nausea.
Opium, belladonna, and paregoric	May give with food.	Nausea, vomiting, constipation. Sedation.

Source: Adapted from D. E. Powers and A. O. Moore, *Food Medication Interactions*, (Phoenix, Ariz.: Food Medication Interactions, 1989).

■ **TABLE 25–2**
Foods That May Produce Gas

Apples	Honey
Artichokes, Chinese	Kohlrabi
Barley	Melons
Beans	Milk
Bran	Molasses
Broccoli	Mulberries
Brussels sprouts	Nuts
Cabbage	Onions
Celery	Radishes
Cherries	Rye seeds
Coconut	Soybeans
Eggplant	Wheat
Figs	Yeast

People troubled by gas need to refrain from overindulging in foods such as beans, broccoli, cabbage, and onions.

hydrophillic colloid: a type of laxative that attracts water in the intestine to form a bulky stool, which then stimulates peristalsis. (Metamucil and Fiberall are examples of hydrophillic colloids.)

Irritable Bowel Syndrome

Irritable bowel syndrome is another common disorder characterized by a disturbance in the motility of the GI tract. The person with irritable bowel syndrome may experience a variety of symptoms including indigestion, nausea, abdominal pain, flatulence, diarrhea, constipation, or alternating diarrhea and constipation. The dietary treatment of the disorder depends on the person's symptoms.

When the primary symptom of the disorder is alternating diarrhea and constipation, adding fruits and vegetables to the diet may help.[2] People with irritable bowel syndrome who complain of gas and abdominal pain might benefit from avoiding foods that contain raffinose and stacchyose, complex carbohydrates that the body cannot digest or absorb. (Instead, bacteria in the colon metabolize these complex carbohydrates and produce gas in the process.) Table 25–2 lists some foods containing these complex carbohydrates. Excessive gas production often subsides if the person avoids gas-producing foods for about 4 to 6 weeks. Many people with irritable bowel syndrome find that adding bran or hydrophillic colloids to their meals will return their bowel function to normal. If they also have gas, though, they should use the colloids only; they should avoid the foods listed in Table 25–2 and use no bran, because bran can also produce gas.

Diarrhea's and irritable bowel syndrome's effects on nutrition status result largely from the malabsorption that they cause. Akin to these are many other states in which malabsorption occurs—the so-called malabsorption syndromes.

■ Malabsorption Syndromes

Of greatest nutrition concern are those lower GI disorders that cause malabsorption. As you know, malabsorption can seriously impair a person's nutrition status. To prevent severe malnutrition requires careful attention to diet.

■ TABLE 25–3
Risk Factors for Poor Nutrition Status in Malabsorption Syndromes

Reduced Intake	Excessive Nutrient Losses	Raised Nutrient Needs
Abdominal pain	Blind loop syndrome	Drug therapy
Anorexia	Diarrhea	Surgery
Bowel rest	General malabsorption	
Emotional stress	Short bowel syndrome	
Food intolerance	Steatorrhea *(fat malabsorption)*	
Indigestion	*fatty diarrhea*	
Nausea		

Malabsorption can occur when food is improperly digested, when the surface area of the bowel is reduced, or when normal mechanisms for absorbing nutrients are impaired. Many disorders can lead to malabsorption; several are discussed throughout the remainder of this chapter. Table 25–3 highlights the reasons why malnutrition is especially likely in malabsorption syndromes. As you can see, they contribute to poor nutrition status by reducing nutrient intakes, accelerating nutrient losses, or raising nutrient needs.

Malabsorption of fat, carbohydrate, protein, vitamins, and minerals, or any combination of these nutrients is possible. Most commonly, it is fat that is malabsorbed, because fat is digested and absorbed in a different, more involved way than either carbohydrate or protein (see Chapter 5). Unabsorbed fat is excreted from the body in the stools (steatorrhea).

The effects of fat malabsorption can be quite severe (see Figure 25–1 on p. 776). The loss of fat in the stools means the loss of valuable food energy and fat-soluble vitamins. Calcium and magnesium form soaps with unabsorbed fatty acids, so they too are lost in the stools. Vitamin D loss further adds to calcium depletion.

The loss of calcium with fatty acids can cause another problem, enteric hyperoxaluria. Oxalate, present in some foods, normally binds with calcium in the gut, and the body excretes both of them together. But when calcium binds instead to fatty acids, the oxalate remains unbound and available for absorption. Because the body does not metabolize oxalate, this increased absorption leads to increased excretion of oxalate in the urine. High urinary oxalate favors the formation of kidney stones. (Highlight 29 discusses kidney stones and presents a list of foods high in oxalate.)

The primary treatment of steatorrhea is to treat the underlying disorder. Along with this treatment, the diet restricts fat. In addition, clients receive supplements of fat-soluble vitamins in a water-miscible form that facilitates absorption. Often, the person with malabsorption receives a diet containing about 50 grams of fat per day, initially. Gradually, the amount of fat may increase if extra energy is needed and the client's tolerance allows. Table 25–4 (on p. 777) provides instructions for a fat-restricted diet, and a sample fat-restricted diet menu is shown on p. 778.

A fat-restricted diet can be difficult to follow. Fats give flavors to foods—flavors that some people may miss. Low-fat foods can also be hard to buy. Tips to lower

Fat malabsorption results in:
- Loss of food energy.
- Loss of fat-soluble vitamins.
- Loss of calcium and magnesium.

enteric hyperoxaluria (en-TER-ick HIGH-per-ok-sa-LOO-ree-ah): a condition of excess oxalate absorption that comes about because calcium is unable to bind oxalate in the gut; leads to kidney stone formation.
enteric = intestinal

water-miscible (MISS-i-bul) **vitamins**: fat-soluble vitamins that readily mix with water and can be absorbed without fat.

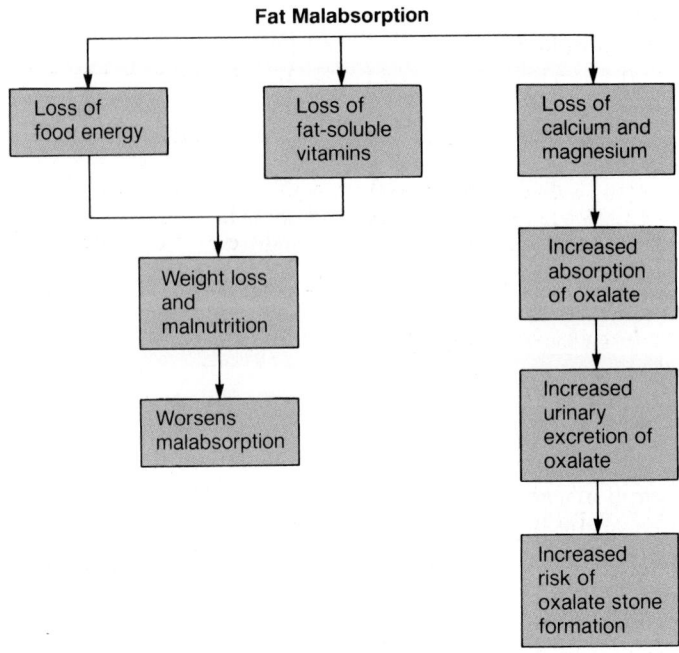

fat intake have been offered throughout the book. Suggestions include:

- Read labels and purchase low-fat foods. Nutrition labels state the fat contents of a product in grams per serving.
- Purchase low-fat meats. Fish, poultry, and veal generally contain less fat than red meats. For ground meat without too much fat, buy a lean piece of beef or pork and have the butcher grind it for you. Ground turkey can be an excellent substitute for ground beef or ground pork.
- Tempt the taste buds by cooking meats in mixtures of vegetables like tomatoes, green peppers, carrots, mushrooms, and onions.
- Remember to use herbs and spices. Unless otherwise indicated, salt is not limited on a fat-restricted diet.
- Make gravy from bouillon or broth seasoned with wine and herbs and thickened with cornstarch or flour.
- Blenderize low-fat cottage cheese or yogurt made from nonfat milk with herbs for a zesty salad dressing.
- Substitute reduced-kcalorie margarine for regular margarine, because it has half the fat. Reduced kcalorie mayonnaise and salad dressing also contain less fat.
- Use butter-salt or imitation butter flavoring to season food.
- Broil, bake, or steam foods instead of deep-fat frying whenever possible. If you panfry foods, use vegetable cooking sprays and no-stick pans instead of fat.
- Make homemade stews and soups, and refrigerate them overnight. Skim off the excess fat that forms on top before using them the next day.

Many cookbooks feature recipes low in fat.

■ TABLE 25–4
Fat-Restricted Diet (50 g)

Use
1. Nonfat milk, nonfat-milk cheeses, yogurt made from nonfat milk, sherbet, and fruit ices.
2. Low-fat egg substitutes and up to three regular eggs per week.
3. Up to 6 oz of lean meats and poultry without skin daily.
4. Up to 6 servings of fat daily. One serving is any one of the following:

 1 tsp butter, margarine, shortening, oil, or mayonnaise.
 1 strip crisp bacon.
 1 tbsp heavy cream or Italian or French dressing.
 ⅛ avocado.
 2 tbsp light cream.
 6 small nuts.
 5 small olives.

 If fat is used to cook or season food, it must be taken from this allowance.
5. All vegetables prepared without fat.
6. All fruits prepared without fat.
7. Plain white or whole-grain bread; nonfat cereals, pasta, rice, noodles, and macaroni.
8. Clear soups and cream soups made with nonfat milk.
9. Angel food cake and fruit whips made with gelatin, sugar, and egg-white meringues.
10. Jelly, jam, honey, gumdrops, jelly beans, and marshmallows.

Do not use
1. Whole milk, chocolate milk, whole milk cheeses, and ice cream.
2. Pastries, cakes, pies, sweet rolls, or breads made with fat.
3. More than one egg a day, fried or fatty meats (sausage, luncheon meats, spareribs, frankfurters), duck, goose, or tuna packed in oil (unless well drained).
4. More than 6 servings of fat.
5. Desserts, candy, or anything made with chocolate or nuts.
6. Creamed soups made with whole milk.

Suggestions
1. To make the diet still lower in fat, reduce the fat and meat (and egg) servings.
2. To raise the fat content, give additional fat or meat servings.
3. To improve acceptance of the diet, check the fat content of a well-liked food and allow that food if posible. Use the exchange system fat list for alternate suggestions for fat servings.

People with malabsorption often have difficulty getting enough food energy from a fat-restricted diet to cover their losses. It helps to use products made from medium-chain triglycerides (MCT) to supplement the diet. MCT provides as many kcalories as regular fats, but the body digests and absorbs them differently from long-chain triglycerides (see Chapter 5 and the box on the next page, "How the Body Digests and Absorbs Medium-Chain Triglycerides"). MCT can replace oil in salad dressings and in beverages, desserts, and other dishes. However, MCT does not provide essential fatty acids, so the diet must include a source of long-chain fats. Clients can obtain MCT through the dietary department of a hospital or a pharmacy; they are expensive, but their delivery of needed energy may make them worth the price.

How the Body Digests and Absorbs Medium-Chain Triglycerides

You may recall from Chapter 5 that triglycerides contain a molecule of glycerol with three fatty acids attached. Most naturally occurring triglycerides have fatty acids that contain at least 14 carbon atoms. But some fats (such as coconut oil) contain fatty acids with only 6 to 12 carbon atoms. This type of triglyceride is called a medium-chain triglyceride (MCT). Unlike long-chain triglycerides (LCT), MCT do not require pancreatic lipase or bile for digestion and absorption. MCT do not form micelles and are absorbed directly into the portal vein (like amino acids and monosaccharides) rather than into the lymphatic system (like other lipids). Thus, people who can't digest and absorb LCT can digest and absorb MCT easily. MCT can serve as a source of extra food energy but not as a source of essential fatty acids.

Pancreatitis

Pancreatic secretions contain many enzymes necessary for the digestion of protein, fat, and carbohydrate. Bicarbonate-rich juices from the pancreas provide the optimal pH necessary to activate these enzymes. Consequently, pancreatic disorders can significantly reduce the digestion and absorption of nutrients and impair nutrition status.

Sample Fat-Restricted Diet Menu

MENU

Breakfast
1 soft-cooked egg
½ c dry cereal
1 slice whole-wheat toast
1 tsp margarine
4 oz orange juice
Coffee, 1 tbsp light
    cream and sugar
Nonfat milk

Lunch
3 oz broiled chicken
½ c rice
½ c green beans
Tossed salad
1 tbsp French dressing
Fresh apple
Iced tea, sugar
2 tsp margarine

Supper
3 oz lean roast beef
½ c mashed potatoes
½ c peas
1 slice bread
1½ tsp margarine
Peaches
Nonfat milk

Snack
Fruit ice

One such disorder is pancreatitis. Biliary tract disease, surgery (often of the stomach or biliary tract), and alcoholism most often precipitate pancreatitis. Blood vessels supplying the pancreas become abnormally permeable and allow fluid and plasma proteins to leak into the spaces between the pancreatic cells. This causes localized edema and damages the pancreas. The damaged pancreas retains pancreatic secretions, including digestive enzymes, and these juices begin to digest the pancreas itself, causing severe pain. The blood picks up some of these enzymes, raising serum amylase and serum lipase levels. These elevated levels serve as indicators of pancreatitis. Typical symptoms of pancreatitis, besides severe abdominal pain, include nausea and vomiting.

pancreatitis: inflammation of the pancreas.

The goal of therapy is to reduce pancreatic secretions. Food is withheld, since food stimulates bicarbonate and enzyme secretions from the pancreas. A nasogastric tube is inserted, not for feeding, but rather to serve as a straw to suction out the stomach's secretions, so as to further reduce stimulation of the pancreas.

Clients receive intravenous fluids to maintain fluid and electrolyte balance. Edema, losses through nasogastric suction, and lack of oral intake can disrupt this balance. If pancreatitis is severe, or if the person is malnourished, TPN may be indicated. Some studies suggest that TPN does not stimulate pancreatic secretions to the degree an enteral diet would, but results of experiments in this area are unclear. Some people with pancreatitis may benefit from tube feedings of hydrolyzed formulas delivered into the jejunum.[3]

When abdominal pain subsides, active bowel sounds resume, and serum amylase levels return to normal or near-normal, a client can begin an oral diet. The diet progresses from a clear liquid diet to a low-fat diet, and, finally, to a regular diet as tolerated. At the first sign of pain, or if serum amylase levels rise, food is withheld; when these signs and symptoms subside, food can again be reintroduced. Clients may tolerate six small meals better than large, less frequent, meals.

If an acute episode of pancreatitis doesn't subside or if episodes recur at frequent intervals, the pancreatic cells can be permanently destroyed, leading to chronic pancreatitis. Chronic alcohol abuse is the most frequent cause of chronic pancreatitis.

The pancreas normally excretes enzymes far in excess of needs, so even after considerable damage has occurred, digestion may proceed normally. However, with extensive degeneration of the pancreas and chronic pancreatitis, digestion, especially of fat, becomes permanently impaired. The goals of diet therapy in chronic pancreatitis are to:

- Maintain optimal nutrition status.
- Reduce steatorrhea, if present.
- Minimize pain.
- Avoid subsequent attacks of active pancreatitis.

Health care professionals recommended a fat-restricted, bland diet for chronic pancreatitis. Small meals may be easiest to digest. The person with chronic pancreatitis usually tolerates about 50 to 70 grams of fat per day; restricting fat to less than this amount is unnecessary. Enzyme replacements taken with meals aid in the digestion and absorption of protein and fat. Absolutely no alcohol is permitted.

A bland diet eliminates foods that stimulate gastric acid secretion, which in turn stimulates the secretions of the pancreas.

Enzyme replacements are extracts of pork or beef pancreatic enzymes that help with digestion.

If steatorrhea persists, physicians prescribe fat-soluble vitamins in an easily absorbed form. Vitamin B_{12} absorption may be reduced, so injections of

> ⟩⟩ **CLINICAL DETECTIVE WORK**
>
> Mrs. Corey is a 52-year-old homemaker admitted to the hospital with severe abdominal pain, nausea, and vomiting. Laboratory tests reveal a very high serum amylase level, a low serum albumin level, and red blood cell indexes consistent with folate deficiency anemia. Mrs. Corey is diagnosed as having pancreatitis. She is 5 ft 3 inches and weighs 100 lb. Mrs. Corey's family has expressed concerns to the physician that Mrs. Corey may have a problem with alcohol abuse. The health care team is concerned not only with the diagnosis of pancreatitis, but also with Mrs. Corey's nutrition status and possible alcohol abuse.
>
> How would you describe pancreatitis to Mrs. Corey? Why are her serum amylase levels elevated? How can pancreatitis lead to poor nutrition status? Discuss factors in Mrs. Corey's medical history that put her at risk for poor nutrition status (assume alcohol abuse for the purposes of this question and review Highlight 7's description of how alcohol impairs nutrition status).
>
> If Mrs. Corey develops chronic pancreatitis, how should her diet be modified? What other measures should be taken to ensure adequate digestion and absorption?

vitamin B_{12} may be necessary. The person who needs extra food energy may benefit from products containing MCT. During active attacks of pancreatitis, diet therapy reverts to that described earlier for acute pancreatitis. The accompanying ''Clinical Detective Work'' box presents a case study for your review of pancreatitis.

Sometimes pancreatitis damages the cells that produce insulin. In these cases, clients become glucose intolerant, as in diabetes (see Chapter 27) and must follow a diabetic diet in addition to the restrictions already mentioned.

Cystic Fibrosis

cystic fibrosis: a hereditary disorder characterized by the production of thick mucus that affects many organs, including the pancreas, lungs, liver, heart, gallbladder, and small intestine.

Cystic fibrosis is the most common cause of pancreatic insufficiency in children and young adults. It is a hereditary disease that may affect many organs, including the pancreas, lungs, liver, heart, gallbladder, and small intestine. Cystic fibrosis affects 20,000 to 30,000 people in the United States alone.

Cystic fibrosis is characterized by the production of very thick mucus by glands throughout the body. Two major problems result: chronic lung disease and pancreatic insufficiency (malabsorption). The airways of the lungs become plugged with mucus, making it difficult for the person to breathe. The thick mucus tends to stagnate in the bronchial tubes, and bacteria multiply in it, making lung infections likely. Most people with cystic fibrosis die of lung infections.

Cystic fibrosis affects the pancreas in 80 to 85 percent of the cases. The thick mucus obstructs the small pancreatic ducts and interferes with the secretion of digestive enzymes and pancreatic juices. Eventually, the enzyme-

and bicarbonate-secreting cells are surrounded by mucus and are gradually replaced by fibrous tissues. Malabsorption of many nutrients, including fat, protein, vitamins, and minerals, results, often leading to malnutrition. Most children and young adults with cystic fibrosis are short and thin for their ages.

Energy needs in people with cystic fibrosis reach 150 percent of the RDA for sex and age; protein needs may be greater than twice the RDA. Energy and nutrient needs are high due to loss of nutrients through malabsorption, frequent infections, higher than normal turnover of protein and essential fatty acids, and higher than normal protein catabolism and energy expenditure.[4] Extra energy is needed simply to breathe. The combination of these factors make it nearly impossible for the individual to take in enough food energy to meet needs, thus explaining why growth failure is so common.

For the infant with cystic fibrosis, breastfeeding is recommended, as it is for any infant. The fat in breast milk is more readily and more completely absorbed by the infant than is the fat in regular infant formulas. The enhanced absorption of breast milk lipids is partially due to the presence of lipases in the breast milk that are resistant to acid and therefore can work in the infant's stomach. Another advantage is that the unique configuration of the triglycerides allows hydrolysis by the lipases. Infants who cannot be breastfed can usually tolerate regular infant formulas taken with enzyme replacements. Energy can be added to infant formulas by using carbohydrate and fat supplements, including MCT oil (see Appendix L). Infants intolerant to regular formulas receive low-fat formulas.

A child with cystic fibrosis is weaned from breast milk or infant formula to a high-kcalorie, high-protein, nutritionally balanced diet carefully tailored to the child's tolerances. In the past, diets for people with cystic fibrosis severely restricted fat. However, growth failure and essential fatty acid deficiencies commonly occur in children with cystic fibrosis. Since fat provides an important energy source and essential fatty acids, current diet recommendations do not restrict fat. Instead, clients use enzyme replacements to control steatorrhea.

Enzyme replacements lessen malabsorption but do not fully correct it. Often people with cystic fibrosis who experience persistent steatorrhea, gas, and abdominal distention can find relief from these symptoms by taking higher dosages of enzyme replacements rather than by reducing their intakes of fat. However, for those who can tolerate only small amounts of fat, or for those who need to supplement their energy intakes, products containing MCT oil can provide extra kcalories.

Abnormally high levels of electrolytes (sodium and chloride) in sweat is characteristic of cystic fibrosis. Fever, high environmental temperature, or diarrhea can rapidly precipitate electrolye depletion in people with cystic fibrosis. When these conditions exist, provide extra salt.

Vitamin supplements are prescribed; fat-soluble vitamins are given in a water-miscible form. Zinc supplements may also be prescribed. People with cystic fibrosis need regular nutrition assessments to ensure that their diet meets their nutrient needs. Height and weight measurements are particularly relevant. Despite the widespread use of unrestricted-fat diets, fat intakes in those with cystic fibrosis are often too low to meet their high needs.[5]

For the person with cystic fibrosis, maintaining adequate nutrition status is extremely important; nutrition status and the severity of pulmonary disease

fibrous: composed of fibers. The development of excess fibrous tissue is **fibrosis**.

Zinc helps ↑ appetite

Recall that water-miscible fat-soluble vitamins readily mix with water and can be absorbed without fat.

CLINICAL DETECTIVE WORK

Ryan is a 7-year-old boy diagnosed with cystic fibrosis. Symptoms of steatorrhea and failure to gain weight during infancy prompted tests that led to the diagnosis. Ryan is currently in the hospital to treat a respiratory infection. He has a temperature of 102° F. He is 43½ inches tall and weighs 38 lb.

Explain cystic fibrosis to Ryan's parents. Why are growth failure and repeated respiratory infections hallmarks of the disorder? Look at the growth chart appropriate for Ryan's age and sex in Appendix E. Plot Ryan's height and weight. What does the growth chart tell you about Ryan's growth?

What type of diet should Ryan follow? How can enzyme replacements be used effectively? What important measure should be taken to ensure that Ryan's diet is adequate?

appear to be related.[6] Home parenteral and enteral nutrition programs may help clients meet the high nutrient needs imposed by cystic fibrosis. Children might benefit from regular diets during waking hours and tube feedings or parenteral nutrition at night. In one study, researchers reported weight gains in seven of eight malnourished children with cystic fibrosis given supplemental tube feedings at night.[7] The children's lung function failed to improve, but the incidence of pneumonia declined, and the children reported feelings of improved well-being.

Such programs offer promise, but people with cystic fibrosis and their caretakers must deal with practical difficulties and emotional demands. The person with cystic fibrosis faces repeated hospitalizations and oftentimes an early death. The child's guardians must deal with many aspects of care important to the child's survival, of which nutrition is only one. Caretakers must ensure that their children receive daily respiratory therapy treatments, enzyme replacements, and often, antibiotics, to say nothing of helping them adjust to their disease, maintain some social life, and keep up with schoolwork. The accompanying "Clinical Detective Work" provides a case study of a client with cystic fibrosis.

Inflammatory Bowel Diseases

Crohn's disease: inflammation and ulceration along the length of the GI tract, often with granulomas; also called **regional ileitis** (ILL-ee-EYE-tis).

granuloma (gran-you-LOH-mah): a granular tumor or growth.
  granulum = little grain
  oma = tumor

ulcerative colitis (ko-LYE-tis): inflammation and ulceration of the colon.

Several conditions inflame the bowel and cause malabsorption. Two such disorders, Crohn's disease and ulcerative colitis, frequently lead to malnutrition.

Crohn's disease and ulcerative colitis are two distinct disorders that show similar clinical, pathologic, and biologic features. Their cause or causes remain unknown.

Crohn's Disease In Crohn's disease, cracklike ulcers and many granulomas accompany inflammation of the bowel. Symptoms most often occur in the ileum and colon, but can arise anywhere in the GI tract. The person with Crohn's disease often experiences anorexia, weight loss, fever, diarrhea, and cramping abdominal pain. The disease may be self-limited and eventually cured, but it often recurs. Inflammation and scarring may narrow the intestinal lumen, sometimes causing obstruction. The intestine may rupture and cause a severe, and sometimes fatal, infection (peritonitis). Bleeding from the ulcers can lead to anemia.

The person with Crohn's disease risks developing many nutrient deficiencies for several reasons. For one, malabsorption limits the availability of nutrients. Diarrhea can upset fluid and electrolyte balances. The person usually loses weight, and during periods when the disease is active, abdominal pain and emotional stress may diminish food intake considerably. In addition, the person with Crohn's disease may need to stop eating so that the bowel can rest, particularly when an obstruction or fistula has developed. Furthermore, the drug therapy used to treat the disease can also impair nutrition status (see Table 25–5). If the client requires surgery, nutrient needs become even greater. Because surgery removes a portion of the bowel, the procedure itself can contribute to malabsorption (see the next section of this chapter, "Malabsorption Caused by Intestinal Surgery").

fistula (FIS-too-lah): an abnormal opening between two organs or from an organ to the skin.
fistula = pipe

To restore and maintain nutrition status for the person with Crohn's disease presents many difficulties. Multiple nutrient deficiencies can develop and may reduce the effectiveness of drug therapy and threaten immune function. PEM and deficiencies of calcium, magnesium, zinc, iron, vitamin B_{12}, folate, vitamin C, and fat-soluble vitamins are commonly reported. Low serum albumin due to malnutrition and GI losses is common.

Physicians commonly prescribe antibacterial drugs (most commonly sulfasalazine) and corticosteroids to treat Crohn's disease. However, defined formula diets (given by tube) have successfully resolved active Crohn's disease without the need for TPN or steroids.[8] The upper small intestine easily absorbs defined formula diets, allowing the bowel to rest. Studies suggest that long-term use of steroids in clients with Crohn's disease may not always be necessary.

Encourage clients to accept a hydrolyzed formula orally by experimenting with different flavors and serving the formula appropriately (see Chapter 21, p. 674). If clients refuse hydrolyzed formulas orally, they can receive formulas by tube. Although hydrolyzed formulas are hypertonic and may contribute to diarrhea in some people, many people with Crohn's disease can tolerate hydrolyzed formulas administered at full strength.[9] By starting the formula at full strength, caretakers can immediately deliver all needed nutrients.

■ TABLE 25–5
Drugs Used in the Treatment of Crohn's Disease

Drug Name	Timing with Meals	Common Side Effects That May Influence Nutrition Status
Prednisone	Give with food.	(See Table 23–4, p. 732)
Sulfasalazine	Give with food or milk.	May cause anorexia, nausea, GI distress.

Source: Adapted from D. E. Powers and A. O. Moore, *Food Medication Interactions*, (Phoenix, Ariz.: Food Medication Interactions, 1989).

During the acute stages of Crohn's disease, the bowel may need complete rest. In some cases, complete bowel rest may eliminate the need for surgery.[10] When enteral nutrition significantly aggravates diarrhea, when the bowel is obstructed, or when complete bowel rest might help a fistula to close, TPN can successfully deliver needed nutrients (see Chapter 22).

If diet or drugs cannot control Crohn's disease, the diseased portion of the bowel must be removed surgically. Even after surgery, the disease may flare up in other areas of the bowel, making additional surgery necessary.

Once an acute attack of Crohn's disease subsides, the diet gradually progresses to an oral diet as tolerated. A high-kcalorie, high-protein, low-fat, low-fiber diet is often recommended. Lactose intolerance frequently develops, and the person must then eliminate milk and milk products. Supplemental vitamin-mineral preparations are frequently prescribed. Encourage clients to eat a nutrient-rich, well-balanced diet, and reassess nutrition status frequently to ensure that nutrient needs are being met. A Crohn's disease case study is presented in the accompanying "Clinical Detective Work."

Ulcerative Colitis Unlike Crohn's disease, which can occur anywhere along the GI tract, ulcerative colitis develops only in the large intestine. Ulcerative colitis is characterized by severe diarrhea, rectal bleeding, cramping, abdominal pain, anorexia, and weight loss. Diarrhea can be almost continuous, resulting in poor absorption of nutrients higher in the GI tract and great losses of fluids and electrolytes. Anemia may develop because of blood loss from rectal bleeding. Many of the dietary principles outlined for Crohn's disease apply to ulcerative colitis. A primary concern is to ensure adequate intake of fluids and electrolytes. Clients need to avoid high-fiber foods because these foods can irritate the colon. The diet includes high-kcalorie, high-protein foods and restricts fat if the client has symptoms of fat

---

≫ CLINICAL DETECTIVE WORK

Sara was first diagnosed with Crohn's disease when she was 18 years old. At that time, she weighed 120 lb and was 5 ft 7 inches tall. Her normal weight was 130 lb until she began having the symptoms of Crohn's disease. Since that time, she has been hospitalized several times for recurrent attacks of Crohn's disease. As anticipated from her weight-loss history, Sara's nutrition assessment shows that she is suffering from severe PEM. In talking with Sara, you discover that she is very particular about the foods she eats and often simply does not eat. Sara's physician has ordered a defined formula diet for Sara to be fed through a nasogastric tube.

Review Sara's weight history. What is her ideal body weight? What measures could have been taken to avoid weight loss?

What possible benefits might a defined formula diet offer Sara? Give two reasons why the physician might prefer nasogastric rather than oral feedings for Sara.

Consider Sara's long-term dietary management. What type of diet should she eventually follow? What goals for weight gain should be established?

malabsorption. Milk and milk products may need to be eliminated if lactose intolerance is present. Supplemental vitamins and minerals may be necessary.

Malabsorption Caused by Intestinal Surgery

Surgery of the intestine may be necessary for people with inflammatory bowel diseases, cancer of the intestine, obstruction, diverticulitis, or impaired blood supply to the intestine. Generally, up to 50 percent of the small intestine can be resected without serious consequences. The actual absorption of nutrients after a small bowel resection depends on three factors:

- The extent and location of the resection.
- The presence or absence of the ileocecal valve (illustrated and defined on pp. 46–47).
- The adaptive ability of the remaining bowel.

Resection of a large segment of the small intestine reduces the absorptive surface considerably. Diarrhea, weight loss, muscle wasting, protein and fat malabsorption, hypocalcemia, hypomagnesemia, and anemia often result. When several of these conditions occur at the same time, they are collectively called the *short-bowel* or *short-gut syndrome*.

People with short-bowel syndrome generally absorb carbohydrates and most water-soluble vitamins without difficulty. When more than 8 feet of the proximal jejunum have been resected, however, the absorption of fat, protein, fat-soluble vitamins, calcium, and magnesium can be impaired. When the ileum has been resected, vitamin B_{12} must be supplemented parenterally, since the ileum is the site of vitamin B_{12} absorption. Also, the reabsorption of bile salts normally occurs in the ileum. Without their reabsorption, a smaller body pool of bile salts will be available for recycling, intensifying fat malabsorption (see Figure 25–2).

short-bowel or **short-gut syndrome**: a complex of symptoms that may include diarrhea, weight loss, malabsorption, hypocalcemia, hypomagnesemia, and anemia; it can occur whenever the absorptive surface of the small bowel is reduced.

proximal: the first part or the part that is closest to the point of attachment.

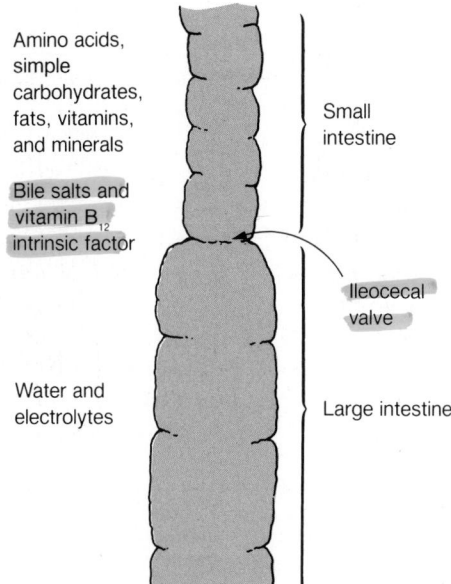

Amino acids, simple carbohydrates, fats, vitamins, and minerals

Bile salts and vitamin B_{12} intrinsic factor

Small intestine

Ileocecal valve

Water and electrolytes

Large intestine

■ FIGURE 25–2
Nutrient Absorption in the GI Tract
Absorption of 90 to 95% of nutrients takes place in the first half of the small intestine. After a resection, nutrient absorption is reduced.

The ileocecal valve controls the rate at which the intestinal contents move from the small to the large bowel. Without the valve, transit time through the small intestine is rapid, and the time available for nutrient absorption limited.

After a small bowel resection, a remarkable adaptive response occurs in the portion of the intestine that remains intact. The remaining bowel gets longer, thicker, and wider, enhancing the ability of the remaining bowel to absorb nutrients. The presence of nutrients in the remaining gut appears to stimulate this adaptation. However, when too much bowel has been resected, even adaptation will fail to compensate for the reduced surface area. People who become malnourished despite all efforts of prevention may require permanent parenteral nutrition support.

Immediately after surgery, the primary nutrition concern is to replace fluids and electrolytes. Parenteral feedings are given immediately after surgery. To ensure that energy and protein needs are met, clients receive oral feeding, tube feeding, or TPN as soon as possible. The diet gradually progresses to a high-protein, low-fat, oral diet. Fat restriction reduces steatorrhea and thus helps minimize the loss of fat, fat-soluble vitamins, calcium, and magnesium. MCT can be used to provide some of the missing food energy but some regular dietary fat is also needed to provide essential fatty acids. Research in animals suggests that adding pectin to the diet can significantly improve adaptation of the bowel following a resection, but further studies are necessary to determine whether this occurs in human beings.[11]

Resections of the large intestine are less likely to create nutrient deficiencies, because absorption of most nutrients occurs before the intestinal contents reach the colon. However, losses of fluids and electrolytes can be a problem, since they are normally reabsorbed in the colon.

An ileostomy involves the removal of the entire colon and rectum; a stoma, or opening, is made from the ileum and brought out through the abdomen to allow for defecation (see Figure 25-3). In a colostomy, only the rectum and anus are removed, and the stoma is formed from the remaining

stoma (STOH-ma): a surgically formed opening; after an ileostomy or colostomy, a stoma is formed from the cut-off end of the intestine through the abdominal wall, through which excretion of wastes occurs.

stoma = window

■ **FIGURE 25–3**
Colostomy and Ileostomy

A. Colostomy. The rectum and anus are removed, and the stoma is formed from the remaining colon.

B. Ileostomy. The entire colon and rectum are removed, and the stoma is formed from the ileum.

part of the colon. A watery stool will result from an ileostomy, whereas a more formed stool results from a colostomy.

After oral intake is initiated following surgery, people who have undergone ileostomies or colostomies generally receive bland, low-fiber diets to help promote healing of the stoma and to prevent irritation. However, encourage clients to resume normal diets as soon as possible. Add foods individually and in small amounts so that their effects can be assessed. If a new food causes problems, encourage clients to try it again a few months later.

Ostomates are often concerned about gas, odor, and loose and watery stools. Each person individually must identify the foods that cause excessively watery stools. Certain raw fruits and vegetables and highly spiced foods cause problems for some ileostomates. For example, beer and other alcoholic beverages may cause diarrhea and gas. Gas and odors can also arise from such foods as beans, onions, green peppers, cabbage, turnips, and beets.

Ostomates may restrict their fluid intake for fear of aggravating diarrhea. Explain to them the importance of drinking plenty of fluids and reassure them that excess fluid taken above and beyond the amount lost through the ostomy will be absorbed and excreted by the kidneys and will not aggravate diarrhea.

New ostomates have many adjustments to make after surgery. They may feel they have lost control over a basic and private function. The retraining required to care for the ostomy and maintain bowel function may be difficult. Ostomates may also be worried that loved ones, particularly spouses, may find them unattractive. The health care team must work closely with each person and that person's family to help everyone make the necessary adjustments and resume normal activities (see the "Clinical Detective Work" box for a case study exercise on intestinal surgery).

ostomate (OSS-toe-mate): a person who has a surgically formed opening from the bowel to the outside of the body, bypassing the anus. An **ileostomate** (ILL-ee-OSS-toe-mate) has an **ileostomy;** a **colostomate** (ko-LOSS-toe-mate) has a **colostomy.**

A health care professional specially trained to assist ostomates in learning the proper methods of caring for ostomy sites is the **enterostomal** (en-ter-oh-STOME-al) **therapist (E.T.).**

Celiac Disease

Celiac disease provides an example of how changes in intestinal mucosal cells can cause malabsorption. Celiac disease is a hereditary disorder with an incidence of about 1 in every 2,000 to 3,000 births. It is characterized by

celiac (SEE-lee-ack) **disease:** a sensitivity to gliadin that causes flattening of the intestinal villi and generalized malabsorption; also called **gluten-sensitive enteropathy** (EN-ter-OP-ah-thee) or **celiac sprue.**

CLINICAL DETECTIVE WORK

Tim is a 24-year-old accountant who recently developed a severe small bowel obstruction secondary to recurrent bouts of Crohn's disease. Medical and dietary management failed, and Tim underwent a small bowel resection of the ileum (in which the ileocecal valve remains intact). Tim was malnourished on admission, and he began TPN in the immediate postoperative period. After several days, he was placed on a nasogastric feeding.

Describe the alterations in nutrient absorption that will be affected by Tim's surgery. How can TPN help? Why is enteral nutrition important after a small bowel resection? What type of diet will be appropriate for Tim once he is on an oral diet?

gluten (GLUE-ten): a vegetable protein found in barley, rye, oats, and wheat.

gliadin (GLIGH-ah-din): a fraction of the gluten protein.

malabsorption resulting from a sensitivity to gluten, a protein found in barley, rye, oats, and wheat. A fraction of the gluten protein, gliadin, acts as a toxic substance, causing atrophy of the intestinal villi, and seriously reducing the absorptive surface of the intestinal tract. The disaccharidases (including lactase) and carrier molecules normally found on the villi disappear, and malabsorption of many nutrients, including fat, protein, carbohydrate, fat-soluble vitamins, iron, calcium, magnesium, zinc, and some water-soluble vitamins, results.

The person with celiac disease often experiences steatorrhea, diarrhea, weight loss, and malnutrition. Anemia may occur as a result of iron, folate, or vitamin B_{12} deficiency. Because protein is malabsorbed, serum protein levels can fall dramatically, inducing edema. The person may bleed easily because of clotting abnormalities precipitated by a vitamin K deficiency. Furthermore, calcium deficiency can cause tetany and bone pain.

Fortunately, when gluten is removed from the diet, the intestinal changes reverse almost completely. Generally, improvement occurs within a few weeks of strict adherence to the diet. However, lactase deficiency and lactose intolerance may be permanent. If the person fails to follow the diet, the symptoms will return.

The grains that must be restricted in celiac disease:
Barley
Rye
Oats
Wheat

The treatment for celiac disease sounds deceptively simple: eliminate gluten. Such a diet prescription is easier described than followed, since barley, rye, oats, and wheat are common in many foods, as you can see from Table 25–6. Processed foods often use wheat flour as an extender (ice cream, salad dressings, and canned foods).

■ **TABLE 25–6**
Gluten-Restricted Diet

Meat and meat alternates
Any allowed except those that are breaded, prepared with bread crumbs, or creamed.

Milk and milk products
Any allowed except milk mixed with Ovaitine, commercial chocolate milk with a cereal additive, pudding thickened with wheat flour, ice cream or sherbet containing gluten stabilizers.

Fruits and vegetables
Any allowed except those that are breaded, prepared with bread crumbs, or creamed.

Grains
Allowed: Bread, cereal, or dessert products made from arrowroot, cornmeal, soybean flour, rice flour, potato flour or gluten-free starch; gluten-free macaroni or porridge; tapioca; cornmeal, cornflakes, popcorn, hominy; rice, cream of rice, puffed rice, rice flakes; potato chips.
Not allowed: Bread, cereal, or dessert products made from wheat, rye, oats, or barley; commerically prepared mixes for biscuits, cornbread, muffins, pancakes, buckwheat pancakes, cakes, cookies, and waffles; bran; pasta, macaroni, and noodles; malt; pretzels; wheat germ; doughnuts; ice cream cones; matzoh.

Other
Not allowed: Beer; ale; certain whiskeys (Canadian rye); cereal beverages (Postum); root beer; commercial salad dressings that contain gluten stabilizers; soups containing any ingredient not allowed (such as barley or noodles).

Help people with celiac disease and those who care for them to understand what foods to avoid. Be sure they understand how to read food labels. Suggest the use of arrowroot, corn, potato, rice, and soybean flours as substitutes for wheat flour in recipes. A low-gluten wheat starch flour is also available. Families with a member who has celiac disease need a lot of support from the health care team. Books, recipes, and addresses of sources for special food products are available; share them with the family.

Disaccharidase Deficiencies

Recall from Chapter 4 how the disaccharidase enzymes split disaccharides (lactose, sucrose, and maltose) into monosaccharides (glucose, galactose, and fructose) for absorption. The disaccharidases normally reside along the intestinal villi. A deficiency of any disaccharidase results in carbohydrate malabsorption. The unhydrolyzed disaccharide remains unabsorbed in the intestine, causing the intestinal contents to become hyperosmolar. Large volumes of water are drawn into the gut to equalize the osmolarity, causing cramps, distention, and diarrhea. Bacteria in the intestine metabolize the undigested sugars to irritating acids, further contributing to cramping and diarrhea.

Lactase deficiency is the most common disaccharidase deficiency, and causes the well-known condition of lactose intolerance (discussed on p. 83). Because the intestinal cells that produce lactase are located on the delicate fringe of microvilli that form the brush border of the intestinal villi (see p. 54), any condition that damages the brush border can lead to lactose intolerance. Among disorders and conditions that lead to either temporary or permanent lactose intolerance are inflammatory bowel diseases, celiac disease, PEM, GI tract surgery, and radiation therapy.

Because people vary widely in the amount of lactose they can tolerate, a lactose-restricted diet must be individualized. People sensitive to the smallest amounts of lactose must follow a lactose-free diet as shown in Table 25–7 (on p. 790). A sample menu is also illustrated (on p. 791). As you can see, hidden lactose makes this diet difficult to follow. People on a lactose-free diet must read labels and avoid foods that include milk, milk solids, lactose, whey, and casein. They also need to check all drugs with the pharmacist because some drugs contain lactose as fillers.

Often, people with lactose intolerance can consume some lactose; the amount depends on individual tolerances. Many times people need to eliminate only milk, milk beverages, creamed foods, and ice cream from their diets. Often people with mild lactose intolerance can eat cheeses, particularly aged cheeses, and drink buttermilk, because these items contain less lactose. They generally tolerate yogurt well, some brands better than others.[12] If a client cannot use one brand of yogurt, suggest trying a different brand.

Many people can use commercially prepared products containing lactose without difficulty. Some may even be able to use milk or ice cream in limited quantities. Others add an enzyme preparation (Lact-Aid) to milk before they drink it or take enzyme tablets whenever they drink milk. The enzyme splits much of the lactose in milk to glucose and galactose. Alternatively, commercially prepared milk products that have been enzyme treated are also available.

A person born with little or no lactase activity has **primary lactose intolerance.** Lactase deficiency caused by another disease is **secondary lactose intolerance.** A lactase deficiency that develops as a person grows older is **developmental lactase intolerance.**

Be alert to the presence of lactose in a food whenever the label's ingredient list includes:
- Milk.
- Milk solids.
- Lactose.
- Whey.
- Casein.

■ TABLE 25–7
Foods to Avoid on a Lactose-Free Diet

Meat and meat alternates
Breaded or creamed meats, fish, or poultry, sausage or cold cuts containing nonfat-milk solids; omelets or soufflés made with milk; some peanut butter.

Milk and milk products
Whole, nonfat, evaporated, condensed, or dried milk; yogurt; cheese; ice cream; sherbet; whey and casein milk treated with lactobacillus/acidophilus culture; custard; pudding.

Fruits and vegetables
Any canned or frozen fruit or vegetable processed with lactose; creamed, breaded, or buttered vegetables.

Grains
Breads and rolls made with milk; prepared muffin, biscuit, waffle, pancake, cake, or cookie mixes; some dry cereals; French toast; pie crusts made with butter or margarine.

Other
Some cocoas, instant coffees, margarines, and dressings; butter; cream; creamed soups; chewing gum; chocolate; toffee; peppermint; butterscotch; caramels; some drugs and vitamin-mineral supplements; monosodium glutamate; sugar substitutes containing lactose.

Lactose-restricted diets may be deficient in calcium. Review p. 297 for nonmilk sources of calcium.

Keep in mind that people who consume little or no milk often have calcium-deficient diets. Encourage the use of milk and milk products whenever people can tolerate them; in some cases, a calcium supplement may be indicated.

These conditions, caused by abnormalities in the pancreas and intestines, are a few of the more common ones that lead to malabsorption. Clearly, all of them threaten nutrition status and require aggressive nutrition intervention to support recovery. As mentioned earlier, any other condition that leads to malabsorption requires the same attention, for the body cannot thrive, much less recover from illness, without a constant influx of nutrients and energy.

■ *Gallbladder Disorders*

While malfunction of the intestines and pancreas cause malabsorption disorders, malfunction of the gallbladder causes a different problem—stone formation. The gallbladder stores and concentrates bile produced in the liver. Sometimes the gallbladder becomes inflamed (cholecystitis), or filled with stones (cholelilithias), or a stone obstructs the outlet of the gallbladder (choledocholithiasis). Severe pain in the area of the gallbladder associated with nausea, vomiting, and flatulence are typical symptoms.

Factors implicated in gallstone formation include heredity, gender (being female), certain drugs, long-term TPN, diabetes, ileal disease or resection, and obesity. A high-fiber diet might help prevent gallstone formation, but more research is needed to confirm this possibility.

cholecystitis (KO-lee-sis-TIE-tis): inflammation of the gallbladder.
   chole = bile

cholelithiasis (KO-lee-le-THIGH-ah-sis): stones in the gallbladder. When the stones obstruct the common bile duct leading to the intestine, the condition is called **choledocholithiasis** (ko-LED-oh-ko-lee-THIGH-ah-sis).
   litho = stone

MENU

Breakfast
½ c grapefruit juice
1 soft-cooked egg
2 slices toasted Italian
bread
Milk-free margarine
Jelly
Coffee or tea

Lunch
3 oz roasted chicken
1 baked potato
Spinach salad with
homemade vinegar/oil
dressing
Milk-free roll
Milk-free margarine
Calcium-fortified soy milk
Coffee or tea

Supper
4 oz roast beef
½ c rice
½ c cooked broccoli
Milk-free bread or roll
Fresh fruit
Calcium-fortified soy milk
Coffee or tea

Low-fat diets have traditionally been prescribed for people with gallbladder diseases. The rationale was that fat in the intestine causes the gallbladder to contract, which causes pain. However, researchers have shown that the gallbladder contracts and ejects bile at the same rate after either a high- or low-fat meal.

The best advice for clients with gallbladder ailments seems not to avoid fat, necessarily, but to consume a well-balanced diet and avoid foods, or amounts of foods, that cause pain. People who cannot tolerate fat or any particular foods should adjust their diets accordingly. Obese people need to lose weight, especially if surgery is being considered.[13]

Oftentimes, people with gallstones must have their gallbladders removed (cholecystectomy). Following surgery, clients require the same care as outlined in Chapter 23 for other people after surgery.

cholecystectomy (KO-lee-sis-TEK-toe-me): surgical removal of the gallbladder.
cyst = bladder
ectomy = removal

◼ Diverticular Disease of the Colon

Diverticulosis was mentioned in Highlight 3's discussion of GI problems and Chapter 4's discussion of dietary fiber lack. In diverticulosis, pouches (called diverticula) form along the large intestine, often at points where blood vessels enter the muscle (see Figure H3–3 on p. 67 and the miniglossary on p. 68). Evidence suggests that the pouches result from high pressure in the intestinal lumen combined with weakness of the supporting muscles in the intestinal wall. Strong intestinal contractions pinch off segments of the intestine; pressure then builds in these segments and forces parts of the membrane of the intestine through the weakened intestinal muscle layer (see Figure 25–4).

■ **FIGURE 25-4**
Intestinal Pressure
A. Pressure inside the intestine normally dissipates along the length of the bowel.
B. When contractions are overly strong, segments of bowel may become pinched off. Pressure in a segment then builds because it cannot escape normally, and pouches form.

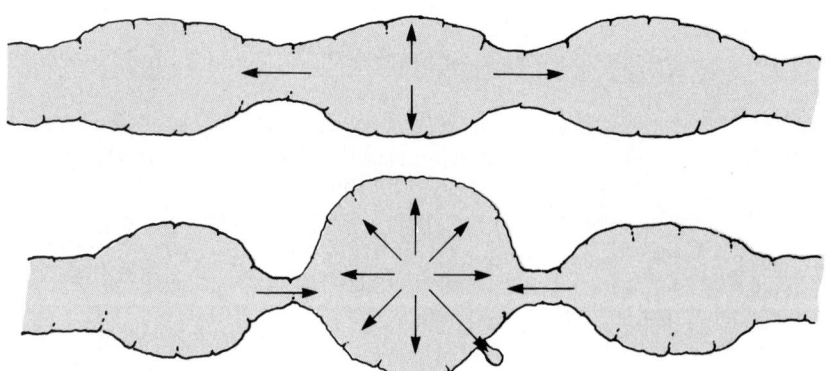

The person with diverticulosis is symptom-free and may be unaware the disorder exists. But in some people, fecal material gets trapped in the diverticula, causing inflammation and infection, a condition called diverticulitis. People with diverticulitis may complain of cramps, alternating periods of diarrhea and constipation, dyspepsia, flatus, and abdominal distention. Occasionally, a diverticulum ruptures, creating a life-threatening situation. If the diverticula become inflamed repeatedly, the intestinal wall can thicken, narrowing the intestinal lumen and creating an obstruction. An inflamed bowel segment can also stick to other pelvic organs, forming a fistula and obstructing the intestine—serious medical problems that can be fatal.

For many years, health care professionals advised people with diverticulosis to adopt low-fiber diets, believing that fiber would become trapped in the diverticula and cause irritation. However, this advice has changed dramatically. Now, health care professionals believe a high-fiber diet may actually reduce the incidence of diverticulosis. Furthermore, many people with established diverticular disease remain symptom-free while following a high-fiber diet.

Help clients adjust to a high-fiber diet by recommending that they increase their dietary fiber intake gradually and maintain an adequate fluid intake. Explain that if they increase their intake of high-fiber foods too quickly, they may experience uncomfortable symptoms such as a bloatedness, gas, and heartburn. With some warning about these symptoms, clients will be prepared to avoid them.

People with diverticulosis who have been following low-fiber diets for many years may be skeptical about switching to high-fiber foods. For this reason, always explain the rationale for including high-fiber foods. Stress the positive aspect of the change: foods once restricted can now be included. High-fiber foods have many other beneficial effects on health (see pp. 88–90). Table 4–6 on p. 97 provides a list of high-fiber foods and Appendix H lists the fiber contents of many foods. To review your knowledge of diverticular disease, read the accompanying "Clinical Detective Work" box. It presents a case study and questions to help sharpen you clinical skills.

CLINICAL DETECTIVE WORK   «

Mr. Ellis is a 69-year-old retired schoolteacher. He recently visited his doctor when he began experiencing severe cramps. He also described a change in bowel function: he is frequently constipated, although he occasionally experiences diarrhea. He further complained of indigestion and a bloated feeling. Mr. Ellis was admitted to the hospital. After an examination that included x-rays of the intestine, the physician made a diagnosis of diverticulitis, for which Mr. Ellis was treated. No food or drink was allowed by mouth, and a nasogastric tube was inserted to suction gastric contents. An IV was started to prevent fluid and electrolyte imbalances. Antibiotics were also given to prevent infection. After several days, nasogastric suction was discontinued, and oral intake was initiated. Once Mr. Ellis was tolerating adequate liquids orally, the IV was discontinued. He is now symptom-free and ready for discharge from the hospital.

Describe diverticular disease to Mr. Ellis. Be sure to distinguish between diverticulosis and diverticulitis. How do diverticula form, and what consequences does diverticula formation have?

Are Mr. Ellis's symptoms typical of people with diverticulitis? Do all people with diverticular disease have such symptoms?

What diet would you recommend Mr. Ellis follow to treat the diverticular disease? What advice can you give him about adjusting to such a diet?

■ *Nutrition Assessment*

This chapter has shown that diseases of the GI tract can affect nutrition status by interfering with food intake, affecting the absorption of nutrients, or raising nutrient needs. Remember to keep these points in mind when you interpret nutrition assessment data:

- Review Table 25–3's list of risk factors for poor nutrition status in malabsorption syndromes. Compare these factors with the client's history.
- Obtain a detailed history of weight fluctuations, food tolerances, and chronic drug use. Weight loss commonly occurs in GI tract disorders, and clients risk PEM. Likewise, the chronic drug use often necessary to treat GI tract disorders can contribute to malnutrition. A history of food tolerances will help to plan a diet that will cause the least discomfort. For people with malabsorption due to pancreatitis or cystic fibrosis, the diet history offers the opportunity to estimate tolerance for fat.
- Interpret anthropometric measurements cautiously. Anthropometric measurements will be affected by the state of hydration. Keep in mind that anthropometric measurements, including weight, may be deceptive

■ TABLE 25−8
Laboratory Tests Useful in Malabsorption Syndromes

Direct stool examination
  Stool checked for weight (greater than normal weight suggests malabsorption)
  and oily materials (excess fat in stool suggests steatorrhea).
Chemical analysis of fecal fat
  Normal fecal fat averages less than 6 g/day when the diet includes 100 g of
  fat/day.
Serum carotene
  Low serum levels accompany steatorrhea.
Serum calcium
  Low levels seen in calcium or vitamin D malabsorption. (Recall that steatorrhea
  can lead to calcium malabsorption.)
D-xylose test
  Test of carbohydrate absorption.
Chemical analysis of fecal nitrogen
  Normal fecal nitrogen is less than 2 g/day.
Schilling test
  Usual test for identifying vitamin B_{12} malabsorption.

in people who have edema. Remember that people with low serum
albumin levels (as occurs in malabsorption and weight loss) often have
edema.

■ Evaluate results from laboratory tests. Table 25−8 lists laboratory tests
  used to identify various types of malabsorption syndromes.

■ Consider that biochemical measurements may be falsely elevated in
  dehydration. Dehydration is a possibility in anyone who is experiencing
  severe diarrhea or vomiting (see Table 25−9).

■ TABLE 25−9
Physical and Laboratory Indices of Dehydration

Physical Signs
  Sunken eyes
  Hollow cheeks
  Stunned facial expression
  Dry mucous membranes
  Deep, gasping respirations
  Weak, rapid pulse
  Low blood pressure
  Skin that lacks elasticity when pinched (may not be a valid finding in the
  elderly)
  Weak cry (infants)
  Depression of anterior fontanel (infants)

Laboratory Findings
  Serum sodium, potassium, and chloride elevated
  Blood urea nitrogen (BUN) elevated
  Hemoglobin and hematocrit elevated

Note: Laboratory indices can vary depending on the cause of dehydration.

■ Look for signs of individual nutrient deficiencies in people with long-standing GI tract disorders. You must assess not only their intake, but also note any possible interferences with absorption, such as short-bowel syndrome.

This chapter has shown how diseases of the intestine can seriously impair nutrition status. With careful attention to diet and medical intervention, many people can recover from such diseases and regain full health.

SELF STUDY *Diet for Lower GI Problems*

Choose one of the following diets: the fat-restricted diet (Table 25–4), the gluten-restricted diet (Table 25–6), or the lactose-free diet (Table 25–7). Plan a day's meals that will meet the rules of this diet, will meet your nutritional needs, and will, as far as possible, also please your palate. Record the plan.

Then eat as you have planned. How did you enjoy your meals? What did you miss? How could you compensate for this lack another time? Were there any surprises in your reactions to this day's meals? How would you feel about continuing such a diet for a week or two? Permanently? List all the ways in which you would attempt to help clients adjust to diets of this kind.

■ Study Questions

1. Describe the dietary treatment of diarrhea. When is diarrhea a cause for alarm?
2. What is the irritable bowel syndrome, and how is diet used to control its symptoms?
3. Discuss various conditions that can lead to malabsorption. Why is fat frequently the biggest problem in people with malabsorption? What are the effects of fat malabsorption? What dietary modifications can be useful in treating fat malabsorption?
4. Recommend ways to make a low-fat diet palatable and easy to follow.
5. How can pancreatitis lead to the malabsorption of nutrients? Contrast the dietary treatment of the person with acute pancreatitis with the dietary treatment of a person with chronic pancreatitis.
6. What are the nutrition needs of the child with cystic fibrosis? How can the infant with cystic fibrosis be fed? What is the optimal diet for the child or adult with cystic fibrosis? How are enzyme replacements used in the treatment of cystic fibrosis?
7. What are inflammatory bowel diseases? Distinguish between Crohn's disease and ulcerative colitis. How can inflammatory bowel diseases lead to malabsorption?
8. Describe the diet therapy for a person with Crohn's disease. Discuss the possible advantages of TPN and hydrolyzed formulas for people with Crohn's disease.
9. What is the recommended diet for the person with ulcerative colitis? What is the primary concern in this disorder?
10. What factors affect absorption after small bowel surgery? Describe short-bowel syndrome and its effect on nutrition status.
11. Describe the adaptive process that occurs in the remaining intestine after a portion of the intestine is resected. What diet is most useful following intestinal resections?
12. What is an ileostomy? What is a colostomy? What diet, if any, can benefit the person who has undergone one of these procedures?
13. What protein and fraction of a protein are of particular concern in the person with celiac disease? What diet is useful in the treatment of celiac disease? Plan a day's menu for a person with celiac disease using Table 25–6 as a guide. Discuss the difficulties involved in following the diet.
14. Describe lactose intolerance. What types of foods are avoided on a lactose-restricted diet? Discuss the variability of lactose-restricted diets, and give suggestions for preventing calcium deficiency in people following these diets.
15. Discuss the role of nutrition in the prevention and treatment of gallbladder disorders.
16. What theory explains the development of diverticula in the intestine? What dangers are associated with diverticular disease? What diet is useful for treating diverticular disease? What precautions should the person trying a high-fiber diet for the first time take?

Notes

1. W. E. Woodward and T. E. Woodward, Management of dehydrating diarrhea, *Hospital Practice*, March 30, 1986.

2. A. D. Schwabe, Dietary management of irritable bowel syndrome, *Nutrition and the M.D.*, July 1987, pp. 1–2.

3. K. A. Kudsk and coauthors, Postoperative jejunal feedings following complicated pancreatitis, *Nutrition in Clinical Practice* 5 (1990): 14–17.

4. J. D. Lloyd-Still, A. E. Smith, and H. U. Wessel, Fat intake is low in cystic fibrosis despite unrestricted dietary practices, *Journal of Parenteral and Enteral Nutrition* 13 (1989): 296–298.

5. Lloyd-Still, Smith, and Wessel, 1989.

6. L. A. Lester and coauthors, Supplemental parenteral nutrition in cystic fibrosis, *Journal of Parenteral and Enteral Nutrition* 10 (1985): 289–295.

7. E. O'Loughlin and coauthors, Nutritional rehabilitation of malnourished patients with cystic fibrosis, *American Journal of Clinical Nutrition* 43 (1986): 732–737.

8. S. J. D. O'Keefe and coauthors, Steroids and bowel rest versus elemental diet in the treatment of patients with Crohn's disease: The effects on protein metabolism and immune function, *Journal of Parenteral and Enteral Nutrition* 13 (1989): 455–460; C. O'Morain, A. W. Segal, and A. J. Levi, Elemental diet as primary treatment of acute Crohn's disease: A controlled trial, *British Medical Journal* 288 (1984): 1859–1862.

9. R. G. Rees and coauthors, Elemental diet administered nasogastrically without starter regimens to patients with inflammatory bowel disease, *Journal of Parenteral and Enteral Nutrition* 10 (1986): 258–262.

10. E. Lerebours and coauthors, An evaluation of total parenteral nutrition in the management of steroid-dependent and steroid-resistant patients with Crohn's disease, *Journal of Parenteral and Enteral Nutrition* 10 (1986): 274–278.

11. M. J. Koruda and coauthors, The effect of a pectin-supplemented elemental diet on intestinal adaptation to massive small bowel resection, *Journal of Parenteral and Enteral Nutrition* 10 (1986): 258–262.

12. D. H. Whytock and J. A. DiPalma, All yogurts are not created equal, *American Journal of Clinical Nutrition* 47 (1988): 454–457.

13. R. S. Hurley and H. S. Mekhjian, Dietary habits of patients with cholelithiaisis: Do we need to instruct? *Journal of the American Dietetic Association* 87 (1987): 209–211.

Therapeutic Diets in Perspective

The clinical chapters of this book describe how health care providers use modified diets as a part of the treatment for a variety of disorders. You may have the impression that if a person has disorder A, then symptoms X, Y, and Z will appear. Then, when given diet Q, the person will recover beautifully. In reality, nothing could be farther from the truth. For one thing, the ways a disorder manifests itself and the ways a person responds to a specified diet differ from one person to the next. For another, diet therapy is only one part of treatment. In some cases, a prescribed diet is critical to recovery. In other situations, diet changes may be only slightly beneficial, or even contraindicated.

This highlight contains many judgments and a few facts—much like real clinical situations that call on professionals to make judgments when presented with a few facts. Its purpose is twofold: to help you see how important it is to adjust therapeutic diets to individual clients and to help you learn how to determine to what extent a diet may influence recovery.

Such a decision begins with an understanding of the relationships between a disorder and its associated diet. Consider the following questions:

- What are the proven benefits of the diet in question?
- What are the negative effects of the diet?
- What are the proven risks of *not* following the diet?

After you have reflected on these questions, consider the intangible, human factors of real-life situations. In addition to the diet-disease connections, you must consider the diet-client relationship.

With experience, you will learn how to exercise clinical judgment in deciding how important a diet is to a client's health, when a client's dietary indiscretions are real concerns that require further intervention, and when it may be best to leave well enough alone. The following three examples illustrate how to set priorities in order to make reasonable dietary judgments.

Ted

Last year, Ted, a busy executive who leads a hectic life, found out that he had a peptic ulcer. His doctor prescribed a traditional bland diet with six small meals a day, plenty of milk, and antacids between meals.

This diet plan upset Ted. You have established a rapport with him during his hospital stay and can empathize with his problems. He barely has time to eat three meals a day, let alone six. He hates milk. The only thing he likes about the diet is that he can still have his usual bedtime snack. Ted confided in you that he has no intention of following the diet. He was outraged when the nurses refused to bring him his morning coffee.

What should you say to Ted? Before saying anything, review the facts. Chapter and Highlight 24 provided a relevant fact or two on diet prescriptions for ulcers—for example, that the traditional bland diet is of little proven value and that eating frequent meals and drinking milk may actually increase gastric acid secretion. Couple these facts with your knowledge of Ted's intention to ignore the diet anyway, and you have identified several major factors weighing against Ted's proposed dietary regimen.

What about coffee? True, coffee, even decaffeinated, increases gastric acid secretion. But will Ted's stomach secrete even more acid if he gets worked up about not having coffee? You can't know the answer to this question, but you do know Ted, so you must draw a conclusion from what you know. All in all, it seems to you that the minuses outweigh the pluses for the diet proposed in this case.

You decide to discuss your concerns with the clinical dietitian. The dietitian contacts Ted's physician and suggests an alternative approach, which the doctor approves. The dietitian instructs Ted to follow a liberal bland diet with three meals a day. As for coffee, in talking to Ted, you reinforce what the dietitian told him: it's not recommended, and you explain why. But you add that if he does not experience pain when he drinks coffee, it is okay to have an occasional cup but to not drink it on an empty stomach.

The situation changes with a different diagnosis. Suppose that Ted doesn't have an ulcer, but rather a hiatal hernia. This time the doctor prescribes a liberal bland diet with five small meals and no eating before bedtime. Ted still fails to see how he can squeeze in two extra meals, and he balks at giving up his bedtime snack. However, now the ratio of benefits to disadvantages has changed: the diet is more justifiable. You decide to tell Ted why.

Small meals will help prevent stomach distention, which can aggravate the hiatal hernia. Furthermore, if Ted refuses to follow the diet, he may experience painful heartburn. Because lying down after a meal increases the risk of reflux esophagitis and heartburn, a bedtime snack is unwise. Coffee lowers the cardiac sphincter pressure, which also aggravates the problem.

For Ted, this diet means making a few changes in his lifestyle. He will have to find time in his busy schedule to feed himself an extra two meals. He will also need to learn to enjoy life without his morning cup of coffee and a bedtime snack.

In the case of a hiatal hernia, the benefits of the diet clearly outweigh the disadvantages. If Ted wishes to avoid the pain of heartburn and the possible complications of hiatal hernia, he will have to learn to make the necessary adjustments. The dietitian can counsel Ted on making behavior changes and selecting foods convenient for his new lifestyle. Nurses can reinforce the dietitian's suggestions.

Jennifer

Jennifer, a healthy young woman of 25, was born with phenylketonuria (PKU). Fortunately, it was diagnosed within three days' time, and her parents instituted the PKU diet immediately to promote Jennifer's normal development. Highlight 26 describes how difficult the diet is to follow and how, without strict adherence to the diet, a healthy baby develops mental retardation. Jennifer followed the diet through adolescence and then switched to a regular diet. She has led a fairly normal life since then. Now she wants to get pregnant, and her doctor has told her she must resume the PKU diet prior to conception and follow it through the pregnancy. She resents the necessity of following the diet's rules and buying its expensive special products. She remembers that the diet cramped her lifestyle and prevented her from participating fully in many social activities as a child.

What should you say to Jennifer? First, consult the facts. As Highlight 26 points out, when off the PKU diet as an adult, a woman's blood concentration of harmful byproducts soars. These toxic levels do not cause in adults the irreversible brain damage evident in young children, but they are detrimental to fetal development. Thus, to evade the doctor's orders in this case poses considerable risks—not to Jennifer herself, but to her unborn

infant. The PKU diet does not guarantee Jennifer's baby a normal mental and physical development, but it raises the chances significantly. Without it, severe disability is inevitable.

Present Jennifer with the facts, and make sure that she receives meticulous instructions about the intricacies of the diet. She will make her own decision, but you can't in good conscience support her in a choice not to comply with the doctor's orders. Inform the other members of the health care team about Jennifer's feelings so that all of you can work together to help her through a difficult time.

Other critically important diets include those that bring about life-sustaining changes in metabolism, such as diets for liver failure, renal failure, and diabetes. All efforts should focus on ensuring compliance with these diets.

A person's complaint that a diet is restrictive should signal you to look for options—which does not necessarily mean that it's all right not to follow the diet, but that most diets can be planned to accommodate the individual's lifestyle and preferences. Most foods can be worked into most diets on occasion with careful planning. Of course, "forbidden" foods should be used only infrequently, in limited amounts, and when planned. An occasional lapse from the diet rules will not be fatal, but the better the compliance with a metabolism-normalizing diet, the better the person's recovery and health are supported.

Martha

Martha, a sweet 70-year-old lady, has several different disorders that require various diet modifications. Such a situation occurs often, particularly among the elderly. Her case illustrates another set of considerations that enter into decision making about therapeutic diets. Martha's problems include:

- Obesity.
- Noninsulin-dependent diabetes.
- Hiatal hernia.
- Type IV hyperlipidemia.
- Chronic constipation.

For the first time, her doctor is recommending a special diet for her. Considering her multiple problems, the diet that might be appropriate for Martha is:

- Restricted in energy (low in kcalories).
- Low in total fat, saturated fat, and cholesterol.
- Low in concentrated sweets.
- Restricted in foods that stimulate gastric acid secretion.
- High in fiber.

Such a diet entails several problems, however. For one thing, it asks for quite a few changes from someone who has already established 70 years' worth of eating habits. For another, it could confuse someone who is trying to obey all those rules at once. Let's analyze the pros and cons in order to establish priorities before deciding what kind of diet would benefit Martha most.

An energy-restricted diet would help with four of Martha's five problems, bringing about weight loss, normalizing blood glucose, reducing abdominal pressure to improve her hernia, and bringing down her high lipids. Three of these four advantages would also be gained by making the diet low in concentrated sweets: weight loss, blood glucose control, and lower triglyceride levels. It would seem advisable, then, to help Martha work out a low-kcalorie, low-concentrated-sweets diet. Restricting concentrated sweets may even be enough to lower kcalorie intake to a reasonable level. This approach would be fairly simple and not too overwhelming to her.

After Martha has successfully incorporated these changes into her diet, perhaps another change could be made. To make Martha's diet high in fiber as well might help with her constipation problem, facilitate weight loss by displacing kcalorie-rich foods, and improve her blood glucose control—three of the five goals chosen for her. With help, Martha might incorporate these changes into her eating habits, especially if you gave her reason to hope that she would notice an improvement in her health.

What about the proposed changes in fat and cholesterol proposed for Martha's diet? A review of the facts on similar cases suggests that a fat-controlled diet for a woman Martha's age might not significantly reduce the risk of atherosclerosis. In this case, asking her to change menus

she has used for years might not be worth the trouble, although her low-kcalorie diet will probably lower her fat intake as well. As for eliminating irritating foods to help with the hiatal hernia, perhaps you might make Martha aware of the foods likely to irritate her hiatal hernia, then leave the use of these foods to her discretion.

Nurses and dietitians who care enough to provide the best nutrition therapy for their clients work hard to develop skill in giving diet advice. They won't simply give everyone who has the same "label" the same diet advice. Furthermore, because research in diet

therapy moves fast, health care professionals must keep their eyes and ears open for new information on the benefits and risks of alternatives in diet. Furthermore, they develop their clinical judgment, as all good judges do, by allowing each new fact and each new case to find its proper place in decision making.

As you read the chapters to come, keep in mind that with each client, you will encounter a variety of unique circumstances. You may find that this uniqueness makes your job a bit more difficult at times, but also more rewarding.

26

Nutrition and Disorders of the Liver

Urea's steady production in the body signifies that the liver is successfully doing its job of detoxifying ammonia. In contrast, high blood ammonia levels characterize liver disease. Shown here are crystals of urea, a small molecule that, like salt, makes pretty pictures under the electron microscope.

The liver plays many roles in the handling of nutrients. As soon as nutrients enter the body, the liver begins processing them: it receives nutrients and then metabolizes, packages, stores, or ships them out for the other organs' use. Before the body can digest and absorb fat, the liver must provide bile for emulsification. In addition, the liver helps maintain the body's well-being in other ways; for example, it neutralizes and detoxifies drugs and waste products for excretion. (To renew your appreciation for this remarkable organ, you might want to review Figure 3–13 on p. 60 and the summary of the liver's metabolic work on p. 172.)

With all these vital tasks to perform, there is little wonder that disorders of the liver profoundly affect both nutrition and general health status. A variety of conditions can lead to liver disease, including alcohol abuse, congenital disorders, toxins, infections, biliary tract obstructions, and heart disease. This chapter describes several types of liver disorders and their dietary management where appropriate. Dietary management depends to a large extent on the type and severity of the disorder.

Fatty Liver

Fatty liver develops when triglycerides accumulate in the liver and cause it to enlarge. It is not caused by an excessive intake of dietary fat, but occurs when the liver becomes unable to metabolize fat normally and either synthesizes too much, oxidizes too little, takes up too much from the blood, sends out too little back to the blood, or any combination of these errors.

Most commonly, fatty liver develops from the ingestion of toxic substances (such as alcohol, described in Highlight 7), from an inadequate intake of protein (as in kwashiorkor), or as the result of an infection or malignant disease. These conditions all compromise the liver's metabolic capabilities. Fatty liver can also develop as a complication of drug therapy (such as therapy with corticosteroids or tetracycline), or of obesity, TPN, or small bowel bypass surgery.

Fatty liver alone usually causes no harm. However, the liver's accumulation of fat suggests the presence of an underlying primary disorder that can progress to a more serious disease and death if left unattended.

Quite often, the appropriate therapy can reverse fatty liver. For example, fatty liver caused by malnutrition demands a diet adequate in protein, energy, and all other nutrients. Fatty liver due to alcohol abuse requires abstinence from alcohol and an adequate diet to replenish nutrient stores. When drug therapy is responsible, alternative drugs or other therapies must be considered. Otherwise, no specific treatment is recommended for fatty liver.

Fatty liver presents a few minor problems, but generally resolves with proper attention. In contrast, hepatitis imposes major problems that can lead to death if treatment fails.

fatty liver: see p. 187; also called **hepatic steatosis** (STEE-ah-TOE-sis).

Hepatitis

hepatitis: inflammation of the liver caused by a virus, alcohol, drug, or other toxin. Hepatitis can progress to cirrhosis.
hepat = liver
itis = inflammation

In hepatitis, the liver becomes inflamed. Inflammation may occur when any of several viruses attack the liver cells, or when excessive or chronic ingestion of alcohol, drugs, or toxins damage the liver cells. Table 26–1 shows how hepatitis can be transmitted and controlled.

During the early stages of hepatitis, the person may develop fatigue, joint and muscle pain, anorexia, nausea, vomiting, diarrhea or constipation, and low-grade fever. As hepatitis progresses, yellow bile pigments accumulate in the diseased liver and spill into the blood, causing the person to develop jaundice and produce a dark urine. In the latter stages of hepatitis, the liver enlarges and becomes tender. In severe cases, hepatitis can lead to liver failure and hepatic coma (described in a later section).

jaundice: see p. 263.

hepatic (he-PAT-ik): of, like, or pertaining to the liver.

The origin of hepatitis, the extent of liver damage, and the person's response to treatment all determine how seriously the disease will affect health. For example, hepatitis A can be so mild as to go unnoticed; hepatitis B can be so severe as to be fatal; and while hepatitis C generally has been considered a mild disease, its seriousness may have been underestimated.

As Highlight 7 clearly described, alcohol interferes with food intake, the GI tract's ability to absorb nutrients, and a number of the liver's metabolic tasks. Consequently, alcohol abuse commonly impairs nutrition status. Alcohol-induced hepatitis adds another stress to this already marginal situation. For

■ TABLE 26–1
Hepatitis Transmission and Control

Source	Transmission	Control
Alcohol	Not infectious.	Abstain from alcohol.
Hepatitis A virus	GI tract via contaminated water, food, or sewage; commonly occurs wherever seafood is harvested from contaminated water or sewage treatment is poor.	Monitor sewage treatment and commerical fisheries to reduce sources of infection.
Hepatitis B virus	Blood via contaminated blood transfusions, dialysis, or needles; virus lives in bodily fluids such as saliva and semen, and so can be transmitted through casual or sexual contact.	Vaccinate.
Hepatitis C virus[a]	Blood; most predominant cause of hepatitis associated with blood transfusion.	Improve blood screening methods.
Toxins	Not infectious.	Prevent contamination.

[a]Hepatitis C virus is responsible for the infection formerly referred to as non-A, non-B hepatitis.

Source: H. J. Alter and coauthors, Detection of antibody to hepatitis C virus in prospectively followed transfusion recipients with acute and chronic non-A, non-B hepatitis, *New England Journal of Medicine* 321 (1989): 1494–1500; J. H. Hoofnagle, Toward universal vaccination against hepatitis B virus, *New England Journal of Medicine* 321 (1989): 1333–1334; G. L. Davis and coauthors, Treatment of chronic hepatitis C with recombinant interferon alfa: A multicenter randomized, controlled trial, *New England Journal of Medicine* 321 (1989): 1501–1506.

the malnourished person with hepatitis, treatment requires abstinence from alcohol and replenishment of nutrient stores (generally by way of a high-energy, high-protein diet) with close attention to electrolyte balance. If unable to eat foods orally, clients receive an IV glucose solution temporarily. The person with hepatitis who is in good nutrition status receives a regular, well-balanced diet.

Liver cells need nutrients to help them recover from hepatitis. For the person with mild anorexia, suggest small, frequent meals, liquid supplements, or both. If nausea and anorexia persist, consider tube feedings. Intravenous feedings may be necessary if vomiting becomes a problem.

When fatty liver or hepatitis go unresolved, cirrhosis develops. Cirrhosis is the most serious and irreversible type of liver injury.

■ *Cirrhosis*

The most common cause of cirrhosis in the United States is chronic alcohol abuse, although not all alcohol abusers develop cirrhosis. Furthermore, not all people with cirrhosis have abused alcohol. Cirrhosis can develop from several other causes, including toxic chemicals, infections, biliary obstructions, and heart disease. In fact, any cause that leads to either fatty liver or hepatitis can progress to cirrhosis.

In cirrhosis, liver cells filled with fat or damaged by inflammation die, and scar tissue forms in their place. Unlike healthy liver tissue, which is soft and flexible, scar tissue is unyielding, a difference that has major consequences. The portal vein and the hepatic artery carry 1½ quarts of blood every minute through the miles of intermeshed capillaries within the liver. This huge volume of blood cannot pulse easily through the scarred tissue of a cirrhotic liver, so it backs up into the portal vein. Consequently, blood pressure in the portal vein rises sharply, causing portal hypertension. Figure 26–1 provides a diagram of the liver's circulatory system.

The rising pressure in the portal vein forces plasma out of the liver's blood vessels. The plasma fills the abdominal cavity, causing the belly to swell. This accumulation of fluid in the abdominal cavity is called ascites. Ascites tends to be a self-aggravating condition. Because the volume of blood in the circulatory system declines, less blood reaches the kidneys. The kidneys respond by calling for more aldosterone, the hormone that enlarges the blood volume by raising the body's sodium and water content. As a result of the body's sodium and water retention, swelling spreads to all body compartments. To make matters worse, the diseased liver cannot dispose of aldosterone as it normally does, so aldosterone levels remain high. Figure 26–2 (on p. 804) diagrams the sequence of events leading to ascites.

With normal blood flow through the liver blocked, pressure forces some of the blood to take a detour through smaller vessels around the liver and out to the rest of the body. These shunts, called collaterals, often develop in the area around the esophagus. Frequently, the raised pressure enlarges the collaterals so that they bulge into the lumen of the esophagus, much like varicose veins in the legs, creating esophageal varices. Eventually, the lining of the esophagus on top of the varices erodes. When the erosion penetrates into the

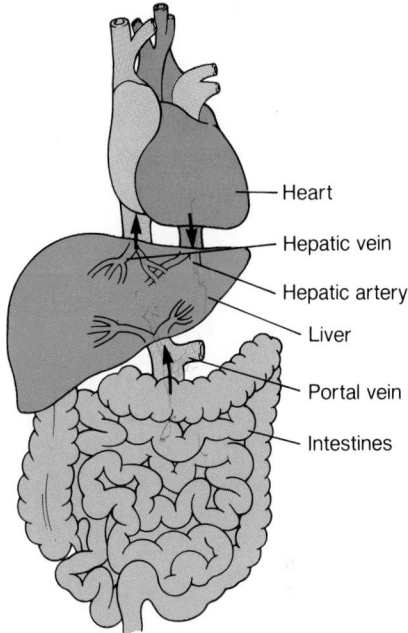

■ **FIGURE 26–1**
The Liver's Circulatory System
The **portal vein** carries nutrients from the digestive organs to the liver; the **hepatic artery** brings oxygen-rich blood from the heart to the liver; the **hepatic vein** returns blood from the liver to the heart. Note that poor circulation in the liver can raise blood pressure in the portal vein, causing portal hypertension. Veins surrounding the intestinal system, including the esophagus, can also enlarge.

Heart
Hepatic vein
Hepatic artery
Liver
Portal vein
Intestines

---

cirrhosis (seer-OH-sis): see p. 187; the type of cirrhosis associated with alcohol abuse and malnutrition is called **Laennec's** (lay-eh-NECK'S) **cirrhosis**.

portal vein: the blood vessel that carries nutrients from the GI tract to the liver.
port = entrance to an organ

hepatic artery: the blood vessel that brings oxygen-rich blood from the heart to the liver; the **hepatic vein** returns blood from the liver to the heart.

portal hypertension: elevated blood pressure in the portal vein caused by obstructed blood flow through the liver.

■ FIGURE 26–2
The Consequences of Cirrhosis

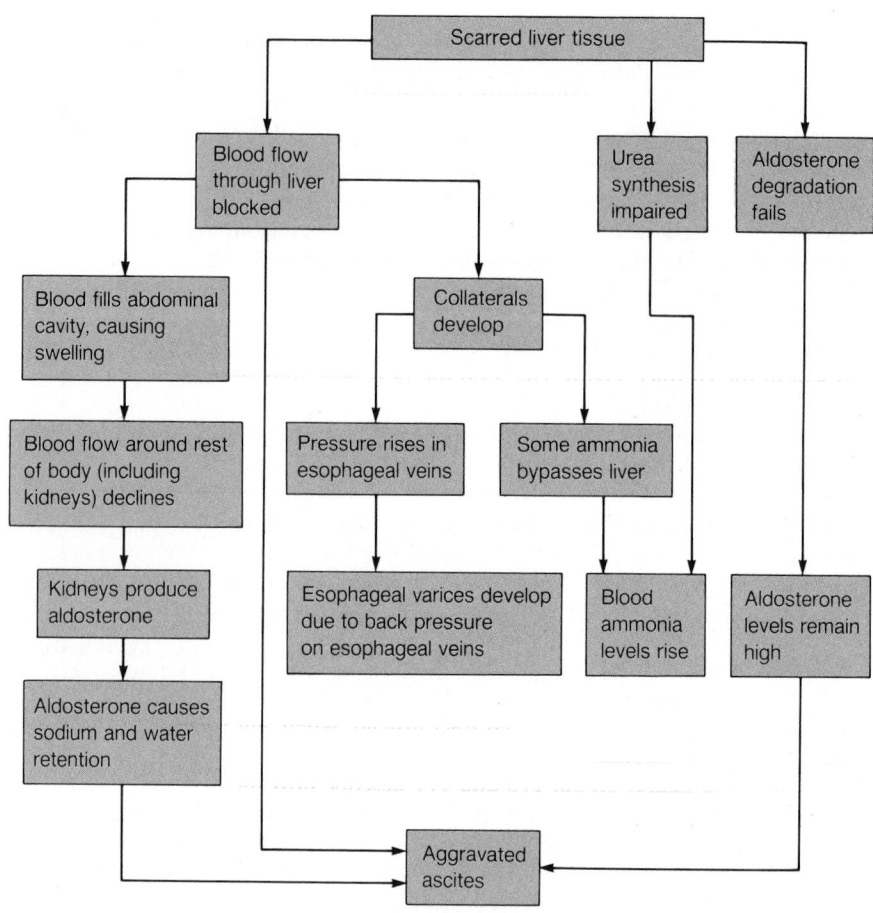

ascites (ah-SIGH-teez): a type of edema characterized by the excessive accumulation of fluid in the abdominal cavity.

collaterals: small blood vessels that develop to divert blood flow away from an obstructed organ; also called **shunts**.
   shunt = to avoid

esophageal varices (ee-SOFF-ah-GEE-al VAIR-ih-seez): tangles of distended blood vessels that protrude into the esophagus.

An elevated blood ammonia level is called **hyperammonemia**. Normal blood ammonia levels range from 80 to 100 μg/100 ml.

hepatic coma: a state of unconsciousness that results from severe liver disease; also called **hepatic encephalopathy** or **portal systemic encephalopathy**.

varices themselves, massive bleeding follows. Bleeding esophageal varices tend to recur, and such bleeding episodes can lead to death.

Normally, the healthy liver removes ammonia from circulation and converts it to urea. (For more information on this process, review p. 179, and see the accompanying discussion entitled "Ammonia Production.") A seriously diseased liver cannot synthesize urea adequately and, consequently, ammonia levels in the blood rise. Even if the liver could handle the ammonia it receives, some ammonia-laden blood bypasses the liver by way of the collaterals. Elevated blood ammonia levels insult the central nervous system, compounding the risk of hepatic coma.

Hepatic Coma

Hepatic coma is a dangerous complication of cirrhosis. Typically, the person with impending hepatic coma exhibits mental disturbances such as changes in judgment, personality, or mood. Sometimes sleep patterns change. Such a person may be unable to draw even a simple shape, such as a star. A sweet, musty, or pungent odor may develop on the breath. Flapping tremor may also

Ammonia Production

Blood ammonia comes from several sources. Recall that amino acids contain amine groups (NH_2). These amine groups generate ammonia (NH_3) during metabolic processes. These metabolic processes produce small but significant quantities of ammonia, but principally ammonia comes from the GI tract: intestinal bacteria produce ammonia, and the digestive enzymes dismantling protein generate ammonia. Therapy designed to reduce blood ammonia therefore aims at eliminating ammonia-producing bacteria and at reducing the amount of protein present in the GI tract. Figure 26–3 on the next page illustrates ammonia production in the body.

Obviously, limiting dietary protein will help to meet the goal of reducing protein in the GI tract. But even without dietary protein to digest, the enzymes in the GI tract have access to protein from the constantly shedding cells of the GI lumen. Moreover, if the person has GI bleeding from gastritis, ulcers, or esophageal varices, the blood serves as an additional source of protein. These three main protein sources in the GI tract—food, shed mucosal cells, and blood—account for about two-thirds of the ammonia that finds its way into the blood.

The GI tract also produces ammonia from urea. The kidneys filter most of the blood urea into the urine for excretion, but about 25 percent of the body's urea finds its way into the GI tract instead, where gut bacteria convert urea to ammonia.

The text and figures on pp. 178 and 179 describe how the liver and kidneys normally cooperate to remove excess nitrogen from the body. The liver performs the first step (converting ammonia to urea); the kidneys, the second (filtering urea into the urine). A diseased liver fails to do its job for two reasons—first, because, the ammonia doesn't flow into the liver as it should, and second, because the liver's dying cells can't efficiently convert the ammonia they do receive. In fact, the ammonia is directly toxic to them, as it is to all cells of the body.

You can see how this vicious cycle feeds itself: high levels of ammonia make liver function deteriorate so that less ammonia can be metabolized, and so ammonia levels continue to rise. Rising ammonia levels then make liver function deteriorate further. You can also see why blood ammonia levels rise in liver disease, whereas blood urea levels rise in kidney disease.

Many drugs used to treat liver disease work in the intestines to interrupt this vicious cycle. At the same time, a diet that supplies just enough, but not too much, protein (with its nitrogen), can help relieve the metabolic load of the liver.

---

develop in the precoma state. Just before passing into coma, the person becomes very difficult to arouse.

The exact cause of hepatic coma remains elusive, but rising blood ammonia levels play an important role. Most people in hepatic coma have elevated blood ammonia levels, although the degree of the elevation does not necessarily correlate with the severity of the coma. This poor correlation may be because *blood* ammonia levels do not reflect *brain* ammonia levels. The

flapping tremor: uncontrolled movement of the muscle group that causes the outstretched arm and hand to flap like a wing; occurs in hepatic coma and other diseases that cause encephalopathy; also called **asterixis**.

■ **FIGURE 26–3**
Ammonia Production in the Body

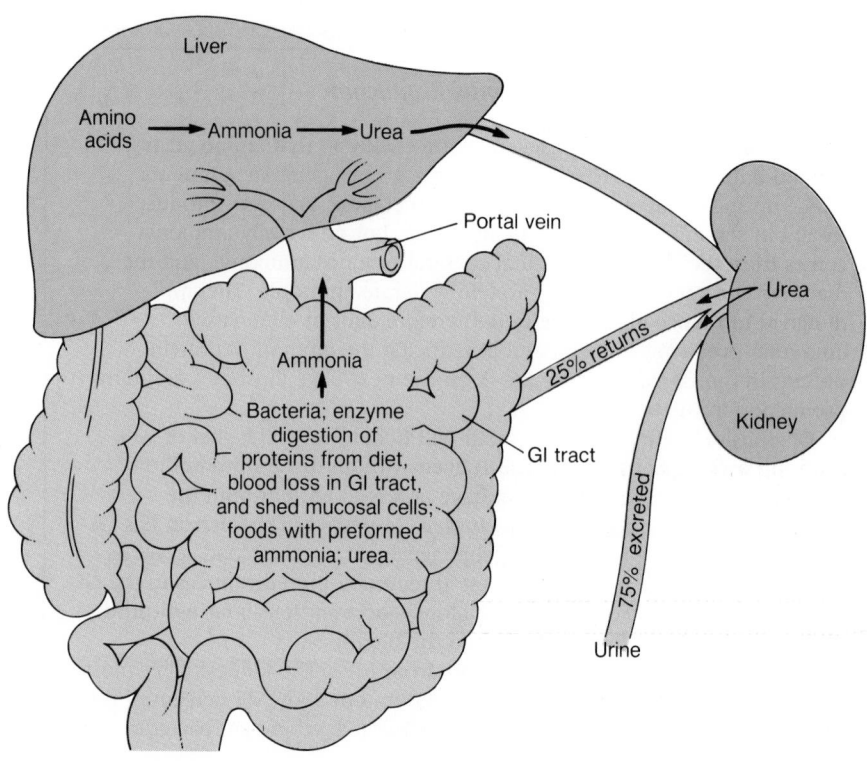

body produces greater quantities of two substances (glutamine and ketoglutarate) when brain ammonia levels are high; the degree of their elevation tends to correlate with the degree of coma. Other nitrogen-containing compounds may also be involved.

Blood amino acid patterns also change in hepatic coma. Normal catabolism of aromatic amino acids becomes impaired in liver disease. Consequently, aromatic amino acid levels rise. Elevated aromatic amino acid concentrations interfere with the formation of certain neurotransmitters (dopamine and norepinephrine) and trigger the production of false neurontransmitters; these changes may, in turn, contribute to hepatic coma.[1] Hormonal changes that accompany liver disease (specifically, elevated insulin levels) encourage the uptake of branched-chain amino acids by muscle cells. Therefore, branched-chain amino acid levels fall. Finally, altered amino acid metabolism generates high blood ammonia levels, which, as already noted, play a role in hepatic coma. Figure 26–4 provides examples of aromatic and branched-chain amino acid structures.

Diet Therapy

A diet adequate in energy and restricted in protein sets the cornerstone for cirrhosis treatment. To maintain positive nitrogen balance, clients need a diet that provides 35 to 45 kcalories per kilogram of actual body weight daily (about 2,000 to 3,000 kcalories) and just enough high-quality protein for liver cells to regenerate, but not enough to aggravate ammonia buildup.[2] The diet

■ **FIGURE 26–4**
Examples of Aromatic and Branched-chain Amino Acids

Note: Appendix C shows the structures of other aromatic and branched-chain amino acids.

Phenylalanine

Aromatic amino acids are characterized by a ring structure; tyrosine and tryptophan are other aromatic amino acids.

Valine

Branched-chain amino acids are characterized by a branched structure; other branched-chain amino acids are leucine and isoleucine.

should provide 1.0 to 1.5 grams protein per kilogram body weight.[3] The accompanying box provides dietary guidelines for liver disease.

A person with signs of impending coma requires additional dietary modifications. Protein intake must be restricted to 40 to 60 grams of high-quality protein per day. Special enteral and parenteral formulas low in aromatic amino acids and high in branched-chain amino acids can be used to provide additional protein to meet needs.* Clients also receive drugs to rid the body of excess ammonia. If coma ensues, both dietary protein and special formulas must be restricted.[4] As the client's neurological status improves, protein can be gradually increased.

Clients may better tolerate vegetable protein than meat protein, perhaps because vegetable protein contains fewer amino acids that readily form ammonia. Vegetable and dairy proteins also have fewer aromatic amino acids than do meats. In addition, diets high in plant foods contain more fiber, which

*The enteral formulas Hepatic-Aid II and Travasorb-Hepatic can be given orally or by tube; parental solutions are also available. These formulas are low in aromatic amino acids and high in branched-chain amino acids.

Dietary Guidelines for Liver Disease

In treating liver disease, health care professionals must pay attention to clients' intakes of energy, protein, and in some cases, sodium and fluid. In general, the diet should provide:

- *Energy:* 35 to 45 kcal/kg actual body weight.
- *Protein in cirrhosis:* 1.0 to 1.5 g protein/kg body weight.
- *Protein in impending coma:* 40 to 60 g/day from foods; additional protein can be supplied from special formulas.
- *Protein in severe hepatic coma:* 20 to 40 g/day at first, if tolerated, then gradually increase protein intake as condition improves.
- *Sodium and fluids:* restrict sodium to 1,000 to 2,000 mg/day and fluids to 1,500 to 2,000 ml/day if ascites has developed, then increase intake as liver function improves.

prevents constipation, thereby reducing the time available for the production and absorption of ammonia in the gut. Such diets reduce both urea nitrogen production and urinary nitrogen excretion.[5]

Because fat helps make foods more appetizing and delivers energy efficiently, fat serves an important role in the diet of a person with cirrhosis. Fat needs to be restricted only if the cirrhotic person develops steatorrhea, a clear sign of fat malabsorption. Even then, the body can usually handle MCT fat (see Chapter 25).

To protect the liver from further injury, clients with cirrhosis must completely abstain from alcohol use. A cirrhotic liver exposed to the continued onslaught of alcohol cannot manufacture the lipoproteins needed to rid itself of accumulated lipids. But without alcohol, and with enough protein as new raw material, the cirrhotic liver seems to manage well enough.

The liver's central role in the metabolism and storage of vitamins and minerals combined with coexisting conditions (such as malabsorption, alcoholism, and malnutrition), explain why vitamin and mineral deficiencies commonly occur in people with liver disorders. Virtually all people with advanced liver disease require supplementation of some vitamins, minerals, and trace elements. Physicians determine which micronutrients to supplement by monitoring serum levels and by checking for clinical signs of deficiencies.

Often, clients receive supplements of water-soluble vitamins in large amounts (up to five times the RDA). Recall from Chapter 8 how the B vitamins serve as coenzymes for the liver's many metabolic reactions and repair work. Deficiencies of folate, thiamin, and vitamin B_{12} occur most frequently.

Fat-soluble vitamins may be malabsorbed when steatorrhea develops. The body's use of vitamin A may be impaired when the diseased liver fails to synthesize adequate amounts of retinol binding protein—the protein that carries vitamin A through the blood to the tissues that need it. Vitamin D nutrition status may suffer when the diseased liver fails to activate vitamin D for the body's use. Because liver disease can prolong the time it takes for the blood to clot, clients may need vitamin D supplements.

The diuretics used to correct fluid and electrolyte imbalances associated with liver disease may lead to deficiencies of the minerals potassium, magnesium, and zinc. The GI bleeding that occurs with liver disease can lead to iron deficiencies. Calcium deficiencies can also develop as a consequence of steatorrhea, low albumin levels (albumin, manufactured in the liver, carries calcium in the blood), and impaired vitamin D metabolism.

People with ascites need to restrict their intake of fluids and sodium. The level of restriction varies with the severity of the ascites. Sodium amounts may range from 1,000 to 2,000 milligrams a day; fluids, from 1,500 to 2,000 milliliters a day. To assess changes in fluid balance, weigh the person *daily*. Rapid weight gain indicates fluid retention; sudden weight loss, in contrast, indicates successful fluid excretion. Table 26–2 shows diet patterns for various levels of sodium restriction. The menu on p. 810 provides sample protein- and sodium-restricted meals.

Dietitians face a challenge in providing a diet low in sodium that provides adequate protein and also stimulates the appetite. Many high-protein foods (for example, eggs, meat, and milk) also contain significant amounts of

The time it takes for blood to clot is called the **prothrombin time.** Both vitamin K deficiency and liver disease can prolong prothrombin time.

Foods Allowed	Number of Servings Allowed on Various Levels of Sodium Restriction			
	1,000 mg	2,000 mg	Serving Size	Sodium per Serving (mg)
Nonfat, whole, and evaporated milk	2	2	8 oz	120
Low-sodium milk	Not restricted	Not restricted	8 oz	7
Meat, fish, poultry, and unsalted cheese	4	6	1 oz	25
Egg	1	1	1	60
Bread and allowed ready-to-eat cereal	2	5	1 slice or ¾ oz	200
Low-sodium bread, cereal, and cereal products	7	4 or more	Varies	5
Fresh, frozen, or canned without salt; asparagus, bean sprouts, broccoli, Brussels sprouts, cabbage, cauliflower, cucumbers, eggplant, endive, escarole, green pepper, collard and turnip greens, lettuce, mushrooms, okra, onions, radishes, rhubarb, rutabaga, string beans, summer squash, tomatoes, watercress, zucchini, and low-sodium tomato and vegetable juices	2	Not restricted	½ c	9
Fresh, frozen, or canned without salt: corn, lima beans, parsnips, peas, potatoes, pumpkin, sweet potatoes, winter squash, and yams	1	Not restricted	½ c	5
Canned vegetables and vegetables frozen with salt	0	1	½ c	200
Salted butter and margarine	2	6	1 tsp	50
Regular mayonnaise	2	6	1½ tsp	50

Foods Not Allowed

In general, the foods listed below cannot be used unless they have been calculated into the diet; however, allowances can be made, particularly when the higher levels of sodium are allowed. For example, if a person on a 2 g sodium diet does not drink milk, you can allow 240 mg of sodium from any other food source (see Appendix H for the sodium content of foods). With this in mind, avoid the following foods:

1. Salt used in cooking or at the table.
2. Highly salted snacks, such as potato chips, corn chips, tortilla chips, salted popcorn, and pretzels.
3. Barbeque sauce; bouillon cubes (except low sodium); catsup; celery salt, seeds, or leaves; chili sauce; garlic salt; horseradish made with salt; meat extracts, sauces and tenderizers; monosodium glutamate; prepared mustard; olives; onion salt; pickles; relishes; saccharin; soy sauce; and Worcestershire sauce.
4. Commercial foods made with milk: ice cream, sherbet, malted milk, milk mixes, and milk shakes.
5. Artichokes, beets, carrots, Chinese or red cabbage, greens (except those listed with vegetables in table above), sauerkraut, and spinach.
6. Maraschino cherries, crystallized or glazed fruits, and dried fruit with sodium sulfite added.
7. Brains; kidneys; canned, salted, or smoked meats; bacon; luncheon meats; chopped or corned beef; kosher meats; shellfish; regular cheeses; egg substitutes; and regular peanut butter.
8. Salted butter or margarine, salt pork, commercial salad dressing (except low sodium), and salted nuts.
9. Leavening agents, such as baking powder and baking soda; rennet tablets; pudding mixes; and molasses.
10. Fountain beverages; instant cocoa mixes; prepared beverage mixes (including fruit-flavored powders); and commercial candy, cakes, cookies, sweetened gelatin mixes, pastries, puddings, cakes, and biscuit mixes.
11. Most commercial dry cereals or instant hot cereals. Puffed wheat, puffed rice, and shredded wheat are allowed.

Sample Protein-Restricted (60g), Sodium-Restricted (1,000 mg) Diet Menu
Foods on this low-sodium menu are cooked without salt. To raise sodium intake, add salt to foods. To reduce sodium, use unsalted butter and milk. The kcalories provided by this menu depend on how much fat is used in cooking. To raise energy intake, if needed, encourage the liberal use of fats and sugars from foods that do not contain protein (for example, butter and table sugar).

MENU

Breakfast
½ c oatmeal
½ c milk
1 egg
Butter
Coffee
Cream
Orange juice

Lunch
Sandwich with
2 oz roast beef,
2 slices bread, lettuce,
mayonnaise
Cole slaw
Cinnamon applesauce
½ c milk

Supper
2 oz baked chicken
½ c mashed potatoes
Broccoli
1 dinner roll
Butter
Fruit
½ c milk

sodium. To circumvent this problem, they sometimes use special low-sodium supplements and milk products.

The person who has bleeding esophageal varices will be unable to consume food by mouth and is often given a simple IV solution to maintain fluid and electrolyte balance. Peripheral or central TPN should be considered if the person is malnourished or unable to resume oral intake for an extended period of time.

Take a minute to try to picture the diet of a client with liver disease. Consider, for example, the foods available to a person on a 40-gram protein diet. On such a diet, the total protein allowance could be spent on just one breakfast of scrambled eggs, a couple of ounces of meat, a cup of milk, and two slices of bread.

No doubt, you can already see some problems: the amounts of food from the milk (and milk products) and meat (and meat alternates) food groups are restricted and the energy intake may be low. You can also see why fat is not restricted unless necessary: adding fat wherever possible helps to boost energy intake and satiety. Other foods that do not contain protein, such as some types of candy, jelly, and sugar, can also help, but these items obviously lack nutrients.

Imposing sodium or fluid restrictions, especially if they are strict, on a protein-restricted diet is like adding insult to injury. A person offered such a diet may give up eating altogether. You will need to offer much encouragement and advice on making foods tasty.

Diet provides critical support in the recovery from cirrhosis. Therefore, every effort must be made to ensure its acceptance. Work closely with clients and their families to individualize the diet, and serve foods attractively. Try the tactics suggested in Chapter 20 to encourage clients to eat.

The person with anorexia may accept food more willingly in small, frequent meals than in fewer large ones. If the person with cirrhosis cannot eat enough food by mouth, health care professionals should promptly begin a tube feeding or parenteral nutrition. Both types of special nutrition support have been used successfully in people with cirrhosis. In fact, as mentioned earlier, special TPN and enteral nutrition formulas are available for the person with liver disease. These formulas contain low levels of aromatic amino acids and amino acids that tend to form ammonia easily; they are enriched with branched-chain amino acids. Although these formulas theoretically should benefit the person with liver disease, their value has not been conclusively verified in clinical tests.

Physicians also use drugs such as neomycin and lactulose to lower blood ammonia levels. Neomycin kills ammonia-producing bacteria in the intestine. The action of lactulose is unknown, but perhaps it works by causing diarrhea (thus disposing of ammonia) and by converting ammonia to a form that can't be reabsorbed into the body. (Review Table 23–2 on p. 722 for nutrient interactions with neomycin.) Physicians may also prescribe diuretics (to mobilize fluids) and cholestyramine (to reduce bile acid levels). See Table 28–6 and Table 28–8 in Chapter 28 for nutrient interactions with these drugs.

The "Clinical Detective Work" on the next page presents a case study on cirrhosis. Use your clinical knowledge and judgment in answering the questions presented.

◼ *Liver Transplantation*

When the progression of liver disease reaches an irreversible stage, liver transplantation may become an option. In the United States, approximately 1,600 people receive a liver transplant each year.[6] As is true of most transplant procedures, controversy surrounds the selection of candidates for transplantation and potential donors, especially as concerns transplanting a liver lobe from a living donor.[7]

Transplantation is generally a last resort, and the decision to replace a liver requires critical judgment in timing. Delaying the decision until life-support measures are required is unacceptable, whereas making the decision while the chances for reversing the disease still exist may unnecessarily use a donor and add complications.

When surgeons remove a diseased liver and replace it with a donor liver, they must reconnect not only blood vessels but the biliary tract as well. Bile duct obstruction occurs in 10 to 15 percent of such cases. After transplantation, the donated liver adjusts its size (shrinking or growing) to accommodate the recipient's body.

In 10 to 20 percent of liver transplant cases, the graft fails to function and retransplantation is required; otherwise, death will follow. This failure is not always due to immunological rejection. In fact, the liver seems less susceptible to rejection than other organs, such as the kidneys.

CLINICAL DETECTIVE WORK

Mr. Sloan, a 48-year-old carpenter, has been in the hospital many times. He recognizes his problem with alcohol abuse, and has entered alcohol rehabilitation programs several times over the past several years. However, as of this time, he is continuing to abuse alcohol. Mr. Sloan was recently admitted to the hospital, and a diagnosis of alcoholic cirrhosis has been confirmed. At 5 ft 7 inches tall, Mr. Sloan, who once weighed 150 lb, now weighs 120 lb. He looks thin, although his abdomen is distended with ascites, and his skin is yellow. His liver disease is advanced, and he is showing signs of impending hepatic coma. Laboratory findings include:

- SGOT, 295 U/ml.
- Alkaline phosphatase, 13 Bodansky units.
- BUN, 8 mg/100 ml.
- Blood ammonia, 125 μg/100 ml.

Compare these findings with Table 26−3 to determine if they are consistent with liver disease.

Can you describe to Mr. Sloan what cirrhosis is and what its consequences are? From the limited information available, what can you determine about Mr. Sloan's nutrition status? Calculate his %IBW and %UBW (see p. 620 in Chapter 19).

What dietary changes do clients with cirrhosis generally receive? How will Mr. Sloan's diet be altered, now that he is in a precoma state?

Why is Mr. Sloan's abdomen distended? Explain the development of ascites in liver disease and how diet is adjusted.

Would you expect Mr. Sloan's blood ammonia levels to be high? Why or why not?

Describe portal hypertension, jaundice, and esophageal varices. How would Mr. Sloan's diet be changed if he were found to have esophageal varices?

■ **TABLE 26−3**
Standards for Tests Commonly Used to Diagnose Liver Disease

Test	Normal values	Values in Liver Disease
Albumin	4−6 g/100 ml	decreased
Alkaline phosphatase	2.0−4.5 Bodansky units	elevated
Ammonia	10−80 μg/100 ml	elevated
AST (formerly SGOT)[a]	0−35 U/ml	elevated
Bilirubin	0.1−1.0 mg/100 ml	elevated
BUN[a]	8−18 mg/100 ml	normal
Prothrombin time		slow

Note: To convert albumin (g/100 ml) to standard international units (g/L), multiply by 10; to convert ammonia (μg/100 ml) to standard international units, multiply by 0.5872; to convert bilirubin (mg/100 ml) to standard international units (μmol/L, multiply by 17.10; to convert BUN (mg/100 ml) to standard international units (mmol/L urea), multiply by 0.3570; to convert AST (U/ml) to standard international units (μkat), multiply by 0.01667.

[a]AST = aspartate transaminase; SGOT = serum glutamic oxalacetic transaminase; BUN = blood urea nitrogen.

As Chapter 23 mentioned, transplant recipients commonly receive the immunosuppressive drug cyclosporine. The balance between immunosuppressive drug therapy and infectious diseases is more precarious in liver transplants than in other transplants because of the liver's direct exposure to microorganisms from the GI tract.[8]

Nutrition status prior to any surgery, especially transplantation, influences recovery. Therefore, health care providers conduct a nutrition assessment prior to surgery in order to correct deficiencies before surgery and to establish the most appropriate postsurgery nutrition care plan. Because liver disease and its associated drug therapy alter many metabolic functions, assessment parameters must be interpreted with caution.

Nutrition Assessment

When you assess the nutrition status of people with disorders of the liver, keep several points in mind:

- People with diseases of the liver (especially those who abuse alcohol) are often malnourished. Obtain an accurate diet history to calculate nutrient requirements and to pinpoint inadequate nutrient intake.
- Careful diet histories can help pinpoint protein tolerance for people with advance liver disease.
- People who abuse alcohol normally derive much of their daily energy intake from alcohol. Without that energy source, as occurs during hospitalization, special care must be taken to ensure that an adequate diet meets energy needs. Routinely reassess nutrition status to ensure that dietary intake meets energy needs.
- The person with cirrhosis may retain considerable amounts of fluids. This fluid retention will affect weight measurements and, if generalized edema is present, also arm anthropometrics and laboratory results. Under these circumstances, weight measures become meaningless as an indicator of body tissue gains and losses, but can show if the person is mobilizing fluids. Weight loss, then, is a good sign that some liver function is returning.
- Another strategy useful in treating people with ascites is to measure abdominal girth. Place a tape measure around the back and over the person's abdomen directly over the umbilicus. Repeat the measurement periodically. A decreasing abdominal girth indicates fluid mobilization. In contrast, an increasing girth signals that the ascites is becoming worse.
- In people with extensive liver disease, serum albumin levels will be low. Supplying extra amino acids will not help if the liver doesn't function well enough to synthesize albumin.

The recovery of people with disorders of the liver depends in large part on attention to nutrition and nutrition assessment parameters.

No doubt, liver disorders wreak havoc on the body's metabolic work. Equally disturbing to the body's homeostasis are disorders that alter blood glucose concentrations, the topic of the next chapter.

◼ Study Questions

1. What is fatty liver, and what causes it? What diet modifications, if any, are useful for the treatment of fatty liver?
2. What is hepatitis, and what nutrition concerns arise in the person suffering from hepatitis?
3. Discuss cirrhosis, and describe how cirrhosis leads to portal hypertension, ascites, formation of collaterals, esophageal varices, and elevated blood ammonia levels.
4. Describe the dietary treatment of the person with cirrhosis and hepatic coma. Consider special dietary concerns of the person with ascites and esophageal varices.

◼ Notes

1. The false neurotransmitters produced when aromatic amino acid levels rise include tyramine, phenylethylamine, octopamine, and phenylethanolamine. J. E. Fischer, Branched-chain-enriched amino acid solutions in patients with liver failure: An early example of nutritional pharmacology, *Journal of Parenteral and Enteral Nutrition* (supplement) 14 (1990): 249–256; D. T. Hiyama and J. E.

Fischer, Nutritional support in hepatic failure: Current thought in practice, *Nutrition in Clinical Practice* 3 (1988): 96–105.
2. E. P. Shronts, Nutritional assessment of adults with end-stage hepatic failure, *Nutrition in Clinical Practice* 3 (1988): 113–119.
3. Fischer, 1990; Shronts, 1988; N. H. Mexhitis, Nutritional management in liver disease, *Nutrition in Clinical Practice* 3 (1988): 108–112.
4. E. P. Shronts and coauthors, Nutrition support of the adult liver transplant candidate, *Journal of the American Dietetic Association* 87 (1987): 441–451.
5. F. L. Weber and coauthors, Effects of vegetable diets on nitrogen metabolism in cirrhotic subjects, *Gastroenterology* 89 (1985): 538–544.
6. T. E. Starzl, A. J. Demetris, and D. V. Thiel, Liver transplantation, *New England Journal of Medicine* 321 (1989): 1014–1022.
7. P. A. Singer and coauthors, Ethics of liver transplantation with living donors, *New England Journal of Medicine* 321 (1989): 620–621.
8. Starzl, Demetris, and Thiel, 1989.

Inborn Errors of Metabolism

The discussion in Chapter 26 on the metabolic consequences of liver disorders sets the stage for a closer look at the ramifications of a genetic error in protein synthesis. Body functions, such as metabolic reactions and transports, that depend on proteins cannot proceed when proteins are made in an insufficient quantity or when they have an abnormal structure. If an enzyme is missing or malfunctioning in the metabolic pathway that converts compound A to compound B, then compound A accumulates and compound B becomes deficient. Both the excess of compound A and the lack of compound B can lead to a variety of problems and, in many cases, death. Furthermore, high concentrations of compound A become available and low concentrations of compound B make it less available for use in other metabolic pathways. These consequences, in turn, create excesses and deficiencies of other metabolites that present another array of problems. The diseases that result from these "inherited biochemical blocks in normal metabolic pathways" are known as "inborn errors" of metabolism.[1] The accompanying miniglossary defines related terms.

In some instances, the accumulated compound is not toxic and the deficient compound is not essential, and so individuals experience no problem. In all likelihood, they will never know about the error. However, in other cases, inborn errors have severe consequences, many of them causing mental retardation. Without proper diagnosis and treatment, they can be lethal. As is true of most medical disorders, the earlier the diagnosis and treatment, the better the prognosis is.

One goal of medical research is to detect genetic defects before they

---

Miniglossary

carrier: an individual who possesses one dominant and one recessive gene for a recessive trait, such as an inborn error of metabolism. Such a person may show no signs of the trait but can pass it on.

dominant: a gene that has an observable effect on an organism even when it is paired with a normal gene; see also *recessive*.

galactosemia: an inborn error of metabolism in which galactose cannot be metabolized normally to compounds the body can handle; an alternative metabolite accumulates in the tissues, causing damage.

genes: the basic units of hereditary information, made of DNA, that are passed from parent to offspring in the chromosomes. Each gene codes for a protein.

inborn error of metabolism: an inherited flaw evident as a disorder or disease present from birth.

mutation: an alteration in a gene such that an altered protein is produced.
  muta = change

phenylketonuria (PKU): an inborn error of metabolism in which phenylalanine, an essential amino acid, cannot be converted to tyrosine. Alternative metabolites of phenylalanine (phenylketones) accumulate in the tissues, causing damage, and overflow into the urine.

recessive: a gene that has no observable effect on an organism as long as it is paired with a normal gene that can produce a normal product. In this case, the normal gene is said to be *dominant*.

---

cause harm. Recent advances in medical technology allow clinicians to study the developing fetus and identify abnormal conditions during gestation. One technique, amniocentesis, analyzes amniotic fluid that has been removed by a needle or syringe puncturing the amniotic sac. This technique has proven most valuable in the identification of more than 70 different inborn errors of metabolism.[2] Analysis of the amniotic fluid and cells identifies specific enzymes and measures their concentrations, revealing abnormalities. A genetic technique called restriction enzyme analysis allows scientists to locate specific genes. Such a technique holds

promise of actually correcting a genetic defect in the future. For now, prenatal diagnosis of genetic diseases allows nutritional intervention during gestation.[3]

The primary treatment for most inborn errors of metabolism is nutrition. With an understanding of the biochemical pathway involved, a clinician can manipulate the diet to correct for excesses and inadequacies. Dietary management of genetic diseases restricts dietary precursors that occur prior to the error in the metabolic pathway, administers pharmacological doses of vitamins, or replaces needed products. The goal of therapy is to:

- Prevent the toxic accumulation of metabolites.
- Replace essential nutrients that are deficient as a result of the defective metabolic pathway.
- Provide a diet that supports growth and development.

To meet these three requirements is a major challenge that was unattainable until earlier this century. Increased knowledge about the body's many biochemical pathways, coupled with current technology to synthesize formulas of specific nutrient compositions, has greatly enhanced the treatment of inborn errors.

This discussion focuses primarily on the most common inborn error of metabolism—phenylketonuria (PKU)—which affects approximately 1 out of every 10,000 to 25,000 newborns in the United States each year.[4] The ability to detect and treat PKU has significantly improved the lives of many people and provides an example that offers hope to those suffering from other inborn errors.

PKU is only one of several inborn errors that affect amino acid metabolism. Other disorders affect not only amino acid metabolism but also carbohydrate, lipid, and vitamin metabolism. The number of possible inborn errors is limited only by the number of possible gene mutations, for genes carry the codes to make the enzymes in the body.

■ FIGURE H26–1
The Biochemical Pathway in PKU

Normally, the amino acid phenylalanine follows two pathways, one in the liver, the other in the kidney. In the liver, the enzyme phenylalanine hydroxylase adds a hydroxyl group (OH) to produce the amino acid tyrosine. Tyrosine, in turn, produces melanin, the pigmented compound found in skin and brain cells; the neurotransmitters epinephrine and norepinephrine; and the hormone thyroxin. In the kidney, enzymes convert phenylalanine to byproducts that are excreted.

In the liver:

In the kidney:

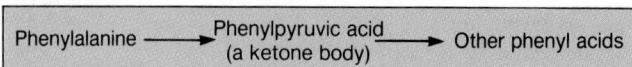

Individuals with PKU lack the liver enzyme phenylalanine hydroxylase, impairing conversion of phenylalanine to tyrosine. Phenylalanine accumulates in the liver and blood, reaching the kidney in abnormally high concentrations. In the kidney, an aminotransferase enzyme converts phenylalanine to the ketone body phenylpyruvic acid, which spills into the urine—thus the name phenylketonuria.

In the liver:

In the kidney:

Classic Phenylketonuria

Classic phenylketonuria (PKU) results from a deficiency of the enzyme phenylalanine hydroxylase. This enzyme converts the essential amino acid phenylalanine to tyrosine (see Figure H26-1). Without the enzyme, abnormally high concentrations of phenylalanine and other related compounds accumulate and damage the developing nervous system. Simultaneously, the body cannot make tyrosine or other compounds (such as the hormone epinephrine) that

normally derive from tyrosine. Under these conditions, tyrosine becomes an essential amino acid; that is, the body cannot make it, and therefore the diet must supply it. To ensure that blood tyrosine concentrations remain adequate, children with PKU receive blood tests periodically. When tyrosine levels drop, tyrosine supplements (solutions or powder added to PKU formula) are given.

PKU is a hidden disease that cannot be seen at birth, yet diagnosis and treatment beginning in the first few days of life can prevent its devastating

effects. For these reasons, all newborns in the United States receive a metabolic test to screen for PKU. Tests must be conducted after infants have consumed several meals containing protein (usually after 24 hours and before seven days). Before the 1960s, when screening became routine, infants with PKU would suffer the consequences of elevated phenylalanine concentrations. At first, the only signs are a skin rash and light skin pigmentation. Between three and six months, signs of developmental delay begin to appear. The infant

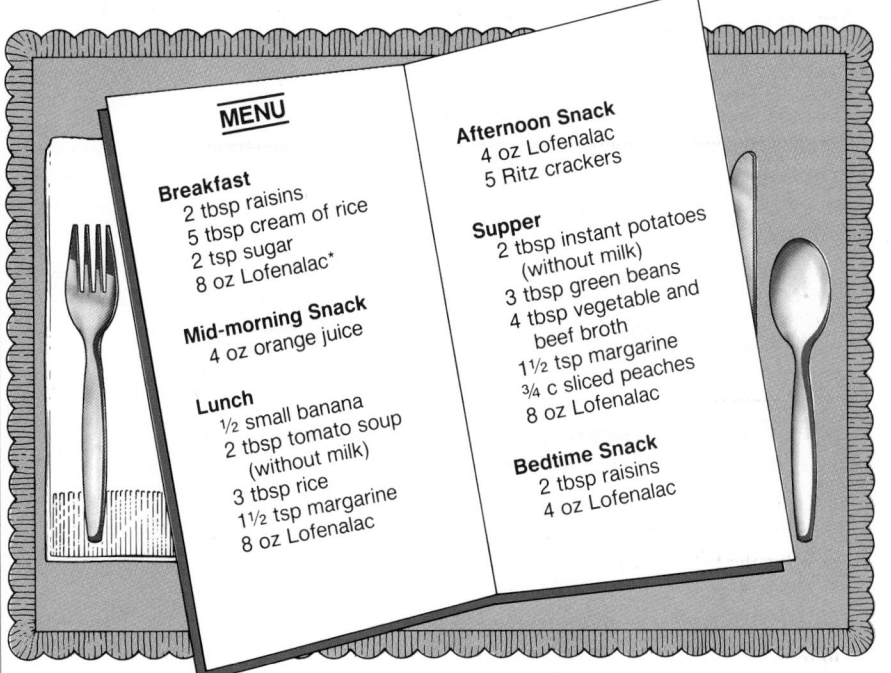

Sample Phenylalanine-Restricted Menu for a Child with PKU

MENU

Breakfast
2 tbsp raisins
5 tbsp cream of rice
2 tsp sugar
8 oz Lofenalac*

Mid-morning Snack
4 oz orange juice

Lunch
½ small banana
2 tbsp tomato soup
(without milk)
3 tbsp rice
1½ tsp margarine
8 oz Lofenalac

Afternoon Snack
4 oz Lofenalac
5 Ritz crackers

Supper
2 tbsp instant potatoes
(without milk)
3 tbsp green beans
4 tbsp vegetable and
beef broth
1½ tsp margarine
¾ c sliced peaches
8 oz Lofenalac

Bedtime Snack
2 tbsp raisins
4 oz Lofenalac

*Lofenalac is a special PKU formula that is low in phenylalanine.

becomes irritable, unable to sleep restfully, and frantic. By one year, irreversible brain damage is clearly evident, and the child has already lost 40 to 50 IQ points.[5]

Nutritional Therapy
The effect of nutrition intervention in PKU is remarkable. In almost every case, dietary management can prevent the devastating array of symptoms described. Essentially, the diet restricts phenylalanine intake to a point that maintains blood phenylalanine concentrations within a safe range. As most dietitians can attest, this is more easily said than done.

Because phenylalanine is an essential amino acid, the diet cannot exclude it completely. If phenylalanine intake is too low, children suffer bone, skin, and blood disorders; growth and mental retardation; and death.[6] Therefore, the diet must strike a balance between providing enough phenylalanine to support normal growth and health and not enough to

cause harm. It is not that children with PKU require less phenylalanine than other children, but that they cannot handle excesses without detrimental effects. To ensure that blood phenylalanine concentrations remain within a safe range, children with PKU receive blood tests periodically and alterations in their diets when necessary. With a controlled phenylalanine intake, children with PKU can lead normal, happy lives.

To control phenylalanine intake requires strict dietary management that was impossible prior to 1958, when a special low-phenylalanine formula became commercially available.[7] This type of formula is now the primary source of energy and protein for children with PKU. Their diet excludes high-protein foods such as meat, fish, poultry, cheese, eggs, milk, nuts, dried beans, or peas. Also excluded are commercial breads and pastries made from regular flour, which has a high phenylalanine

content. Basically, the diet allows foods that contain some phenylalanine, such as fruits, vegetables, and cereals, and those that contain none, such as sugar, jellies, and some candies. Clearly, it is impossible to create such a diet using only whole, natural foods, and children who depend primarily on a formula for their nourishment risk multiple trace-mineral deficiencies.[8] The accompanying menu provides a sample phenylalanine-restricted diet for a child with PKU.

Infants receive a special casein hydrolysate formula with a low phenylalanine content. It does not contain all the phenylalanine an infant requires, and so parents supplement it with measured quantities of milk, rice cereal, and baby foods as the infant develops. Other formulas and products are available that provide a synthetic mixture of amino acids without phenylalanine. This allows older children to receive their entire phenylalanine quota from foods.[9]

People with PKU must also be aware of the phenylalanine content in products containing the sweetener aspartame. Aspartame is a combination of the two amino acids aspartic acid and phenylalanine, and therefore contributes phenylalanine to the diet. Sold under the trade name NutraSweet, aspartame is an ingredient in many foods and beverages such as powdered drink mixes, instant puddings, gelatin desserts, breakfast cereals, chewing gums, and the sweetener Equal. Products sweetened with aspartame bear a warning label for people with PKU. People with PKU need to consult with their physicians or dietitians before including aspartame in their diets.

Perhaps one of the hardest parts of this diet is in the children's sense of social isolation. From birth, children with PKU are on a "special diet" and cannot eat the foods that other children are eating. Some commercially available low-protein products, such as cookies, contain very little, if any, phenylalanine and allow children to share treats with others. Teachers, friends, and family members must understand that they cannot offer food to children with PKU before receiving permission from the children's parents. Until the children are old enough to know their dietary restrictions, parents must teach them to ask before eating any food. Most parents tell their children that they will become sick if they eat the wrong foods. The threat of possible brain damage and routine blood tests motivates children and their parents to adhere to the diet.[10]

No doubt, prompt nutrition intervention during the early years of central nervous system development is critical to preventing irreversible mental retardation in the young PKU child. Of less certainty is for how long the nervous system is vulnerable to the PKU defect. In the past, researchers assumed that the child with PKU could abandon the special diet after the first few years of life, once the central nervous system had completed its development. They realized that with a regular diet, phenylalanine and associated metabolite concentrations would rise, but thought perhaps these high levels would not be damaging. While the damages are less severe than at an earlier age, elevated phenylalanine concentrations in the older child do cause problems such as short attention span, poor short-term memory, and poor eye-to-hand coordination.[11] In general, children with PKU who have discontinued their controlled diet experience problems in their school performances, mood, and behavior.[12] One study reports that IQ scores of children with PKU progressively increase the longer the diets are controlled.[13] For these reasons, clinicians now encourage children to continue the low-phenylalanine diet at least through adolescence. One approach allows children over the age of ten to have one day every month or two to eat any foods they want without having to drink the special formula.[14] To reinstitute the phenylalanine-restricted diet in adolescents after several years of unrestricted diets requires intense education and reinforcement, and even then is quite often unsuccessful.[15] Reports indicate that the reinstitution of a controlled diet does improve the person's blood phenylalanine concentrations, behavior, and IQ scores.[16]

Therapy for inborn errors goes beyond nutrition, requiring psychological counseling for the people who are affected and their families. A genetic disorder is a lifelong problem that affects the entire family. All family members are at high risk for being carriers, and they inevitably become involved in the care and management of the person with the inborn error. Therefore, families must learn how to handle the impact such a diagnosis has on the structure, development, and interactional processes of their family life.[17]

Maternal PKU
Before the development of routine metabolic screenings, special formulas, and restricted diets, children with PKU died young. Now that people with PKU are living longer and reaching reproductive age, researchers face a new set of PKU problems.

PKU, like all inborn errors, is a recessive disorder; that is, it appears only when a person inherits two defective genes—one from each parent. This can occur when both parents have PKU, when one has PKU and the other is a carrier, or when both are carriers (see Figure H26–2). Carriers are people who inherit one defective gene and one normal gene. They may be unaware that they carry a defective gene, for their symptoms are usually mild or absent. The statistical chances of two people with PKU meeting and conceiving a child would be small except for their increased contacts with each other through PKU clinics and support groups.

The risks for a PKU mother go beyond genetics. When off the diet as an adult, a woman's blood phenylalanine concentrations are high. As mentioned earlier, this causes some behavioral problems but does not cause the irreversible brain damage evident in young children. When she becomes pregnant, the fetal blood concentrations rise even higher than the mother's, and this is detrimental to fetal development.[18] A PKU mother with high phenylalanine blood concentrations is likely to give birth to an infant with mental retardation, microcephaly, congenital heart disease, and low birthweight.[19] These women frequently experience spontaneous abortions as well. These reasons, coupled with the high genetic risks of people with PKU, prompt counselors to recommend alternatives other than

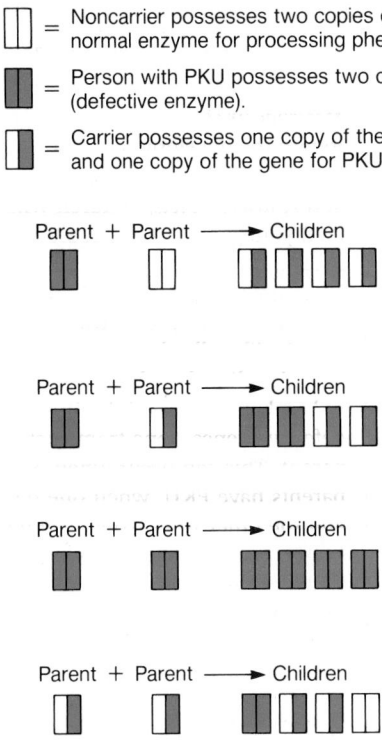

□ = Noncarrier possesses two copies of the gene producing the normal enzyme for processing phenylalanine.

■ = Person with PKU possesses two copies of the gene for PKU (defective enzyme).

▨ = Carrier possesses one copy of the gene for the normal enzyme and one copy of the gene for PKU.

Parent + Parent ⟶ Children

When a person with PKU mates with a noncarrier, all of their children will be carriers.

When a person with PKU mates with a carrier, their children will have a 50% chance of either having PKU or being a carrier.

When two people with PKU mate, all of their children will have PKU.

When two carriers mate, they can pass on either the gene for the normal enzyme or the gene for PKU. For each birth, there is one chance in four that the child will have PKU, two chances that the child will be a carrier, and one chance that the child will be PKU-free.

■ **FIGURE H26–2**
The Inheritance of PKU

pregnancy, such as sterilization, therapeutic abortion, and adoption.[20]

Dietary control of maternal PKU may protect the fetus, if implemented early enough. Women who become pregnant without planning for their pregnancies expose their fetuses to high phenylalanine concentrations during a critical time of early development. A PKU woman who departed from her restricted diet as a child must resume the low-phenylalanine diet at least one to two months prior to conception and throughout her pregnancy.[21] In fact, many physicians recommend adherence to a restricted diet throughout life. To resume a low-phenylalanine diet is not easy; the

special formulas are costly, inconvenient, and unpalatable to an adult who has been eating foods freely. Many women have forgotten that they were ever on a special diet as a child or may never have understood why. For these reasons, many PKU clinics recommend that females continue using the formula into adulthood. The low-phenylalanine diet for maternal PKU must also meet the energy, protein, vitamin, and mineral needs of pregnancy. Special PKU formulas for the pregnant PKU woman are now available.

A woman with PKU benefits from genetic and medical counseling. She must consider the possible consequences of pregnancy and the

options of contraception to prevent pregnancy and adoption if she wants children. Dietary control does not ensure a successful outcome of pregnancy, although a low-phenylalanine diet used from before conception throughout pregnancy seems promising for women with PKU.[22]

Before closing this discussion, it is appropriate to briefly describe another inborn error of metabolism to illustrate the similarities and differences between these types of disorders. To this point, the discussion has focused on PKU, an example of a defect in amino acid metabolism. The following paragraphs describe a defect in carbohydrate metabolism— galactosemia.

Galactosemia

Galactosemia is an inborn error of carbohydrate metabolism in which the body cannot use the monosaccharide galactose. Three enzymes are required for the conversion of galactose to glucose; in galactosemia, at least one of those enzymes is missing or defective. When infants with galactosemia are given milk (which contains a galactose unit in each molecule of lactose), they vomit and have diarrhea. The unmetabolized product accumulates and follows an alternative pathway to form an abnormal product that causes growth failure, liver enlargement, and other neurological abnormalities that lead to coma and death.[23] Early introduction of a galactose-restricted diet prevents or minimizes most of these symptoms. However, it may not prevent ovarian damage, some visual and speech problems, or other neurological abnormalities.

Dietary adjustment in galactosemia is simpler than in PKU for a couple of reasons. First, galactose is not an essential nutrient, as is phenylalanine. The PKU diet is a balancing act of providing just enough phenylalanine for normal growth and development, without too much left over to be toxic; the galactosemia diet needs only to exclude lactose and galactose. Second, since galactose occurs primarily in lactose (the sugar in milk), treatment depends chiefly on the careful restriction of milk and all milk products.

As scientific understanding of human genetics and biochemistry increases, more and more inborn errors are being recognized. Understanding protein structure and function makes it possible to compensate for these defects of metabolism that otherwise would destroy the quality of life. Diet cannot always be tailored to prevent the defects of inborn errors, but in many such diseases diet can make a dramatic difference in people's lives.

NOTES

1. A. E. Garrod, Inborn errors of metabolism (Croonian lectures), *Lancet* 2 (1908), as cited by M. A. Wallen and S. Packman, Nutrition and inborn errors of metabolism, in *Nutrition Update*, vol. 2, eds. J. Weininger and G. M. Briggs (New York: Wiley, 1985), pp. 71–89.

2. G. H. Lowrey, The placenta and fetal development, in *Growth and Development of Children*, 8th ed. (Chicago: Year Book Medical Publishers, 1986), pp. 53–75.

3. Wallen and Packman, 1985.

4. Committee on Genetics, Newborn screening fact sheets, *Pediatrics* 83 (1989): 449–464.

5. Wallen and Packman, 1985.

6. P. B. Acosta and coauthors, Phenylalanine intakes of 1- to 6-year old children with phenylketonuria undergoing therapy, *American Journal of Clinical Nutrition* 38 (1983): 694–700.

7. M. M. Hunt, H. K. Berry, and P. P. White, Phenylketonuria, adolescence, and diet, *Journal of the American Dietetic Association* 85 (1985): 1328–1334.

8. S. Stepnick-Gropper and coauthors, Trace element status of PKU children ingesting an elemental diet (abstract), *American Journal of Clinical Nutrition* 43 (1983): 678.

9. N. Reyzer, Diagnosis: PKU, *American Journal of Nursing* 78 (1978): 1895–1898.

10. S. Schild, Psychological issues in genetic counseling of phenylketonuria, in *Genetic Counseling, Psychological Dimensions*, ed. S. Kessler (New York: Academic Press, 1979), pp. 138–147.

11. Hunt, Berry, and White, 1985.

12. V. E. Schuett, E. S. Brown, and K. Michals, Reinstitution of diet therapy in PKU patients from twenty-two U.S. clinics, *American Journal of Public Health* 75 (1985): 39–42.

13. N. A. Holtzman and coauthors, Effect of age at loss of dietary control on intellectual performance and behavior of children with phenylketonuria, *New England Journal of Medicine* 314 (1986): 593–598.

14. R. Koch and E. Wenz, Phenylketonuria in *Annual Review of Nutrition*, eds. R. E. Olson, E. Beutler, and H. P. Broquist (Palo Alto, Calif.: Annual Reviews), pp. 117–135.

15. S. E. Hogan, G. W. MacDonald, and J. T. R. Clarke, Experience with adolescents with phenylketonuria returned to phenylalanine-restricted diets, *Journal of the American Dietetic Association* 86 (1986): 1203–1207; Schuett, Brown, and Michals, 1985.

16. Schuett, Brown, and Michals, 1985.

17. Schild, 1979.

18. P. B. Acosta, Maternal PKU. Address presented at the conference Nutrition for Pregnancy, Lactation, and Infancy, Gainesville, Fla., February 13, 1987.

19. R. R. Lenke and H. L Levy, Maternal phenylketonuria—Results of dietary therapy, *American Journal of Obstetrics and Gynecology* 5 (1982): 548–553; H. L. Levy and S. E. Waisbren, Effects of untreated maternal phenylketonuria and hyperphenylketonuria on the fetus, *New England Journal of Medicine* 309 (1983): 1269-1274.

20. Schild, 1979.

21. Lenke and Levy, 1982; Acosta, 1987.

22. E. Drogari and coauthors, Timing of strict diet in relation to fetal damage in maternal phenylketonuria, *Lancet* 2 (1987): 927–930.

23. M. A. Wallen and S. Packman, Nutrition and inborn errors of metabolism, *Nutrition Update*, vol. 2, eds. J. Weininger and G. M. Briggs (New York: Wiley, 1985).

27

Nutrition, Diabetes, and Hypoglycemia

The assessor most often "sees" glucose as printed readouts of machine-determined lab values. The microscopist, however, sees glucose as beautiful crystals like these.

Chapter 4 emphasized the importance of blood glucose in providing fuel for the brain and other tissues, and described how the body regulates blood glucose levels (pp. 90–93). Knowing this, you can understand how disorders that disturb blood glucose homeostasis can have a wide range of effects. Two metabolic disorders—diabetes mellitus and hypoglycemia—reflect two extremes of imbalance: diabetes is characterized by high blood glucose concentrations and hypoglycemia by low concentrations.

Diabetes ranks among the ten leading causes of death in the United States.[1] It is a major cause of blindness, kidney failure, leg amputations, and birth defects.[2] In addition, diabetes underlies, or contributes to, a variety of other disorders, such as atherosclerosis and hypertension. In fact, people with diabetes are twice as likely to develop these cardiovascular problems as those without diabetes.

Approximately 7 percent of the people in the United States have diabetes.[3] The most disturbing aspect of this statistic is that only about half of them have been diagnosed. Also, many other people have glucose abnormalities that put them at risk for developing the complications of diabetes. In general, the prevalence of diabetes is much higher in older age groups than in younger ones.

Like diabetes, hypoglycemia is an imbalance in glucose homeostasis. Hypoglycemia can arise in any healthy person (for example, after going without food for a longer time than usual) or it can be a symptom of a number of medical disorders. Hypoglycemia is widely misdiagnosed and people often diagnose themselves as hypoglycemic, attributing many ill effects to low blood glucose levels. A later section of this chapter sorts through the "hypoglycemias."

■ *Diabetes Mellitus*

Several disorders have been called diabetes, but by far the most common ones, and the only ones most people hear of, are the two forms of *diabetes mellitus* described here. Together, they account for 97 percent of the cases of diabetes. (The other form, diabetes insipidus, is not treated with nutrition therapy and so is not described here. It is treated with medication.)

Table 27–1 summarizes the distinguishing features of the two main forms of diabetes. In the first, less common type known as Type I, the pancreas becomes unable to synthesize the hormone insulin, so after each meal the blood glucose rises and remains elevated even though the body's cells are simultaneously starved for glucose. The person must inject insulin at intervals to assist the cells in taking up the needed glucose; therefore, Type I diabetes is called insulin-dependent diabetes mellitus (IDDM). (Insulin, being a protein, must be injected, for if it were taken orally, the GI system would digest it as it does other proteins.)

Why the pancreas fails to produce insulin in IDDM is the subject of much research. For the most part, researchers have long held genetics—specifically, immunogenetics—responsible. Perhaps immune cells mistakenly attack and destroy insulin-producing pancreatic cells.[4] More recently, researchers have

---

diabetes (DYE-uh-BEET-eez) **mellitus** (MELL-ih-tus or mell-EYE-tus): a disorder of blood glucose regulation usually caused by insufficiency or relative ineffectiveness of insulin.
mellitus = honey-sweet (sugar in the urine)

Another type of diabetes caused by inadequate secretion of antidiuretic hormone is **diabetes insipidus** (in-SIP-ih-dus).
insipid = without taste (no sugar in the urine)

insulin-dependent diabetes mellitus (IDDM) or **Type I diabetes:** the less common type of diabetes, also known as **juvenile-onset diabetes** (because it frequently develops in childhood), although some cases arise in adulthood. IDDM accounts for about 5 to 10 percent of all cases.

■ TABLE 27–1
Features of IDDM and NIDDM

	IDDM	NIDDM
Other names	Type I diabetes Juvenile-onset diabetes Ketosis-prone diabetes Brittle diabetes	Type II diabetes Adult-onset diabetes Ketosis-resistant diabetes Lipoplethoric diabetes Stable diabetes
Age of onset	< 40 (mean age, 12)	> 40
Associated conditions	Viral infection	Obesity
Insulin required?	Yes	Sometimes
Insulin receptors	Normal	Low or normal
Symptoms	Relatively severe	Relatively moderate
Prevalence in diabetic population	5 to 10%	85 to 90%

considered that environmental factors may also influence the development of diabetes.

Evidence supporting the role of environmental factors in the development of IDDM includes:[5]

■ IDDM develops after exposure to certain viruses or chemicals (in animals).
■ IDDM shows a geographical variability even greater than that seen in cardiovascular disease or cancer.
■ IDDM incidence shows extraordinary increases in a short time (less than a generation, which could not result from genetic change).
■ IDDM "low risk" populations who live in "high risk" areas begin to exhibit the risk levels of the new area.*
■ IDDM has developed from exposure to certain infections or chemicals (in human beings).

Couple this evidence with the finding that most of the people who are genetically susceptible to this form of diabetes do not develop it, and the environmental argument gains strength. Most importantly, if environmental factors do precipitate IDDM, strategies could be implemented to prevent its development.

In the second, more predominant type of diabetes mellitus known as Type II, the person's cells become resistant to insulin. The pancreas does produce insulin, but the cells respond to it less sensitively. Blood glucose first rises too high, as in IDDM, but some insulin is also available, so finally glucose moves slowly into the cells. This type of diabetes is therefore called non-insulin-dependent diabetes mellitus (NIDDM). (People with NIDDM may be given insulin or insulin-inducing agents to supplement their own supply of insulin, but this is often a temporary measure to control hyperglycemia; they do not absolutely require insulin, as do people with IDDM.)

non-insulin-dependent diabetes mellitus (NIDDM) or **Type II diabetes:** the more common type of diabetes, also called **adult-onset diabetes.** NIDDM is usually milder than IDDM, and it progresses more slowly. A type of NIDDM that develops during the teen years has been termed **maturity-onset diabetes in the young (MODY).** NIDDM accounts for about 85 to 90 percent of all cases.

---

*For example, IDDM occurs more frequently in Japanese children who live in Hawaii than in those living in Japan, and more frequently in French children living in Canada than in those living in France.

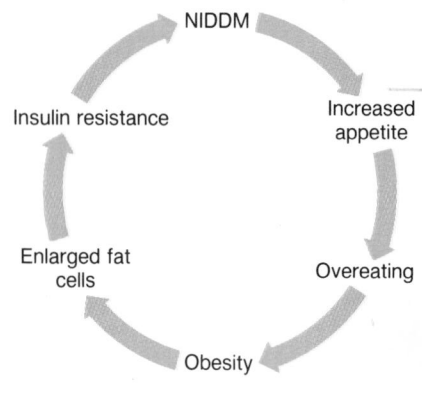

glucose tolerance: the ability of the body to respond to dietary carbohydrate by regulating its blood glucose concentration promptly to a normal level.

Glucosuria generally occurs when blood glucose levels exceed 180 mg/100 ml.

NIDDM tends to develop later in life than IDDM, and has a strong familial component. People with the disorder often become quite obese. Obesity can also precipitate diabetes, and in most people with NIDDM, precedes it.[6] The incidence of diabetes also rises with increasing age, for in all people, pancreatic cells progressively lose their function with time.[7] In some people, this age-related decline in cell function is more rapid or more severe than in others, and these are the ones who need to beware especially of weight gain.

Some borderline conditions related to diabetes mellitus exist. Health care providers keep track of those conditions by name, because they indicate a need for monitoring and preventive efforts. Some people who have mild hyperglycemia without any symptoms of diabetes are said to have *impaired glucose tolerance*. Another classification, *gestational diabetes mellitus*, occurs in some women who develop hyperglycemia while pregnant but revert to normal glucose homeostasis after childbirth. Some people develop diabetes only during times of stress (for example, after surgery or infection); they are classified as having a *previous abnormality of glucose tolerance* and need to be monitored closely to prevent full development of diabetes later in life. Another classification of diabetes that requires close monitoring, *potential abnormality of glucose tolerance*, includes people who have a higher-than-average chance of developing diabetes. These people have close relatives with diabetes, or have given birth to babies weighing over nine pounds. Finally, diabetes can develop secondary to other disorders, such as pancreatitis and cystic fibrosis (discussed in Chapter 25) or through exposure to some drugs or other chemicals.

What Happens in Diabetes

When glucose fails to gain entry into the cells, it builds up in the blood, resulting in hyperglycemia. Normally, the kidneys retain glucose rather than excrete it. But when blood glucose levels get too high, the excess "spills" into the urine (glucosuria). The box on pp. 826–827 describes how measures of glucose in the blood and urine are used to diagnose diabetes and monitor its control. Figure 27–1 provides an overview of the changes that occur in diabetes, and the accompanying miniglossary defines terms describing diabetes symptoms.

People with uncontrolled diabetes can become severely dehydrated. The rising blood glucose concentrations create an osmotic effect. Water moves from the cells into the blood. (Remember that when a solute cannot cross a cell membrane, then water crosses the membrane to the side where the solute is more concentrated.) Furthermore, as glucose spills from the blood into the urine, water leaves with it (also an osmotic effect). Thus both the intracellular fluid and the extracellular fluid become depleted. The person with diabetes produces excessive urine (polyuria) and, being dehydrated, also may experience excessive thirst (polydipsia). Polyuria and polydipsia often signal the beginning of diabetes.

In diabetes, whether insulin production is insufficient or the cells' response to insulin is ineffective, the cells are deprived of the fuels they need for energy. Recall what insulin normally does in cells. Normally, after a meal, insulin directs cellular activities that favor the storage of protein, carbohydrate, and

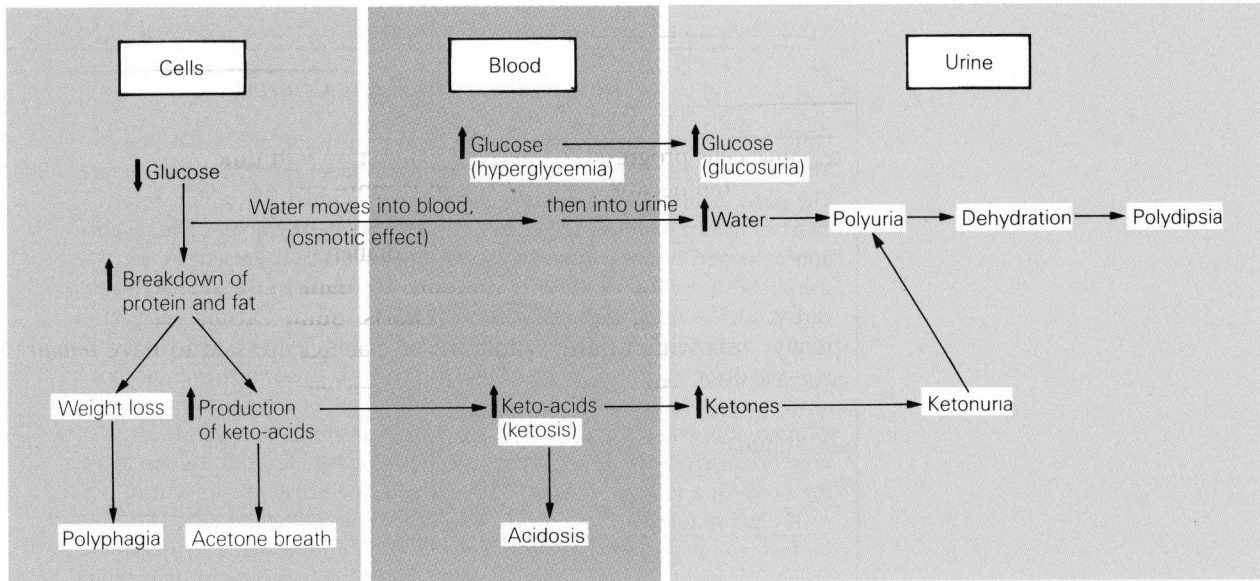

fat: insulin enhances the uptake of amino acids, glucose, and fatty acids into cells. It stimulates protein synthesis, glycogen synthesis in the liver and muscle, and fat synthesis. The net effect is a reduction in blood glucose levels. During a fast, the continued presence of some insulin prevents energy stores from being excessively mobilized.

■ FIGURE 27–1
Overview of Diabetes
As you can see, when glucose cannot enter the cells, a cascade of changes follows. The symptoms of diabetes are highlighted in white.

Miniglossary of Diabetes Symptoms

acetone breath: a distinctive, fruity odor that can be detected on the breath of a person who is experiencing ketosis (acetone is a simple ketone).

dehydration: loss of too much fluid from the body.

diabetic coma: a complication of uncontrolled diabetes precipitated by ketosis.

glucosuria (GLUE-cose-YOU-ree-ah): abnormal amount of glucose in the urine; also known as **glycosuria** (GLY-ko-SUE-ree-ah).

hyperglycemia: an abnormally high blood glucose concentration, often a symptom of both types of diabetes.

hypoglycemia: an abnormally low blood glucose concentration, a symptom that may indicate any of several diseases, including impending diabetes (NIDDM).

ketosis: the accumulation in the body of ketone bodies (ketone bodies are defined on p. 182).

ketonuria: ketones in the urine.

polydipsia (POLL-ee-DIP-see-ah): excessive thirst.

polyphagia (POLL-ee-FAY-gee-ah): excessive eating.

polyuria (POLL-ee-YOU-ree-ah): excessive urine production.

How to Measure Glucose Control

Urine tests often provide the first clue that a person may have diabetes. The person performing the test dips indicator paper into the urine sample. The paper changes color and the person then compares it with a color chart to determine the approximate concentration of glucose. The results appear as percentages, indicating how much glucose is present in the urine, thus providing an indirect measure of glucose in the blood. Health care providers often perform urine tests for glucose and ketones as part of routine examinations. High concentrations of both ketones and glucose indicate diabetes. Positive test results for ketones alone, however, do not always mean diabetes (for example, ketones may be present in people who are following low-carbohydrate diets or fasting). Nor does the presence of glucose alone clinch a diagnosis of diabetes, but it does suggest the need for a follow-up blood test—usually, a glucose tolerance test.

A glucose tolerance test works like this. First, the health care professional performing the test draws blood from the client (who has fasted overnight) to obtain the fasting glucose level. The client then drinks a measured amount of glucose in the form of a flavored beverage. Blood is drawn again at regular intervals of 30 to 60 minutes (different clinics use different intervals). Table 27–2 lists the upper limits considered normal and the values suggestive of diabetes for each time interval. At least two of the glucose levels should exceed the latter values for diabetes to be diagnosed. A person whose glucose levels fall between the upper limits of normal and the values suggestive of diabetes is diagnosed as having impaired glucose tolerance.

Once diabetes has been diagnosed, part of the treatment regimen includes monitoring glucose concentrations at regular intervals. Clients can check their urine or blood at home using the methods taught by professionals at the hospital or clinic. This enables them to be sure their insulin and diet are appropriate. Health care members will want to review records of test results at medical appointments.

■ **TABLE 27–2**
Interpretation of Glucose Tolerance Test Results

Time (minutes)	Upper Limits of Normal (mg/100 ml)	Values Suggestive of Diabetes (mg/100 ml)
0	115	140
60	200	> 200
120	140	200

Note: This is one of many variations of the glucose tolerance test.

Without these regulatory effects of insulin, amino acids and glucose may abound in the cells' fluid environment, but the cells have limited access to them and therefore must mobilize their own protein and fat supplies for energy. The liver responds to the large amounts of fatty acids being broken

In one home method of urine testing, the client drops a tablet into the urine sample and then compares the color that develops with a color chart. In another method, the client dips a piece of indicator paper briefly into the urine sample and compares the color of the paper with a color chart. Clients are instructed to check their urine at least twice a day, generally before meals and at bedtime.

Direct monitoring of blood glucose at home is more sensitive and more accurate than urine testing and is preferable to urine testing because it helps individuals maintain control of their own glucose levels. More and more people with diabetes are using these systems. Blood glucose levels must exceed 180 mg/100 ml before glucose spills into the urine. When used properly, home monitoring of blood glucose can help maintain blood glucose levels between 60 and 140 mg/100 ml.

To perform a home test of blood glucose, the client pricks a finger to get a blood sample (the same method used to determine hematocrit) and touches the blood to a paper strip. As with urine samples, the color indicates the blood glucose concentration. Meters that provide a more accurate readout of the actual glucose concentration are also available, although they are more expensive as well.

Ideally, until good blood glucose control has been established, the client performs blood tests seven times during the day: before each meal, two hours after each meal, and at bedtime. However, realizing the strain this may place on a client, many practitioners instead recommend four tests daily. The person can test at any of the seven times listed above; the times of the tests should vary daily. Once the client has established blood glucose control, one or two tests a day are sufficient for further monitoring.

Physicians will want to see clients at regular intervals to determine whether they are controlling their blood glucose adequately. One test they use to monitor control of blood glucose levels is the measurement of *glycosylated hemoglobin* (or hemoglobin A_{1c}). As blood glucose levels rise, small glucose molecules spontaneously attach to an amino acid on each hemoglobin. The altered hemoglobin remains in circulation for the life of the red blood cell (approximately 120 days), but no longer releases oxygen properly. Normally, only 4 to 8 percent of a person's hemoglobin is glycosylated, but in diabetes, because blood glucose levels remain high for periods of time, the percentage goes up to 16 percent.

Measurement of glycosylated hemoglobin allows the physician to determine how successful diabetes control has been over the past two to four months. The test has another advantage. Urine and blood glucose tests are a reflection of diabetes control only just prior to the test. A person who has been in poor control can have a normal urine and blood test just by starving or using extra insulin the day before going to the doctor. But glycosylated hemoglobin reflects control over several months, so the client can't easily outfox the test.

Diabetes care includes regular monitoring of glucose in the blood and urine.

down by making ketone bodies, which accumulate in the blood. The losses of glucose and ketone bodies (both energy sources) in the urine and the breakdown of protein lead to weight loss. This explains why the person with IDDM is likely to be thin, and may eat excessively (polyphagia). (As mentioned earlier, people with NIDDM tend to be obese rather than thin. The insulin they do have slowly takes effect, and the excess energy they have consumed is stored as fat.)

If IDDM goes uncontrolled, excessive levels of ketones persist in the blood (ketonemia). The presence of one type of ketone (acetone) is evident from a fruity odor on the breath. The ketones contain an acid group in their structure; when they build up in the blood, they lower the pH of the blood. Ketones begin to appear in the urine (ketonuria). In addition, sodium and potassium become depleted because the kidneys excrete them along with the ketones. The loss of sodium and potassium, both base formers, worsens the acidosis. When acidosis becomes severe enough, a coma may follow that is potentially fatal.

People with NIDDM diabetes generally do not develop ketosis and acidosis, since they produce enough insulin to prevent the excessive buildup of ketones. However, they are in danger of slipping into another kind of coma, hyperosmolar hyperglycemic nonketotic coma. As the name implies, this type of coma occurs when blood glucose concentrations become excessive, resulting in osmotic diuresis and dehydration.

Further Complications of Diabetes

Complications frequently arise in people with diabetes. Infections tend to develop, especially in the urinary tract, because bacteria thrive on glucose-rich blood and urine. For this reason, people with diabetes must pay special attention to hygiene.

Diabetes also affects the structures of the blood vessels and nerves, leading to impaired circulation, impaired vision, and loss of sensation in the limbs. Blood vessel disorders involve both the large blood vessels and the smaller vessels. Atherosclerosis in the large blood vessels tends to develop early in people with diabetes and is the major cause of death in NIDDM. As Chapter 28 describes, in atherosclerosis, the arteries become blocked, impairing blood flow. When the limbs (often the legs) do not receive enough blood, the cells die, and oftentimes the limbs must be amputated. People with diabetes have a 15 times higher risk of amputation due to gangrene than the nondiabetic population.[8]

Disorders of the small blood vessels (capillaries), called microangiopathies, may also develop, affecting the eyes, kidneys, or nervous system. About 85 percent of people with diabetes have retinopathy, nephropathy, or both; as mentioned in the introduction, diabetes is a leading cause of both blindness and kidney disease.

Nerve tissues also may deteriorate, causing neuropathy. In neuropathy, the individual loses sensation in the hands and feet. Consequently, injuries to these areas may go unnoticed and infections can progress rapidly. The combination of undetected injury and infection can lead to the amputation of a limb; people with neuropathy are warned to take conscientious care of their feet.

The goals of therapy for diabetes are to:

- Maintain blood glucose levels in an acceptable range.
- Prevent or delay the onset or progression of associated complications.

---

hyperosmolar hyperglycemic nonketotic coma: a complication of uncontrolled NIDDM precipitated by the presence of hypertonic blood and dehydration.

gangrene (GANG-green): death of tissue, usually due to deficient blood supply.

microangiopathies (MY-crow-ANN-gee-OP-ah-thees): disorders of the capillaries, often seen in diabetes. **Retinopathy** (RET-in-OP-ah-thee) is a type of microangiopathy affecting the capillaries of the eye; **nephropathy** (nee-FROP-ah-thee) affects the capillaries of the kidney.
  micro = tiny
  angio = blood vessel
  pathy = disease
  retino = of the retina
  nephro = of the kidney

neuropathy (new-ROP-ah-thee): any disease of the nerves.

- Encourage people to resume normal activities.
- Help people to achieve and maintain optimal body weight and nutrition status.

The person with diabetes has the same nutrient requirements as any other person of the same age, stature, and activity level. But in addition to meeting those nutrient requirements, food must help minimize fluctuations in blood glucose levels. Whether the maintenance of blood glucose within a fairly normal range can prevent the complications of diabetes remains uncertain. However, evidence seems to indicate that control of blood glucose does incur this benefit; it surely does no harm.

■ Treatment of Insulin-Dependent Diabetes Mellitus (IDDM)

A diagnosis of IDDM can be devastating to anyone. The parents of a young child with IDDM may feel overwhelmed, angry, anxious, and even guilty. To an adolescent, it may seem like the end of the world. In fact, to a person of any age, the prospect of daily insulin injections and possible complications may bring fear. In addition to insulin therapy, the person must carefully follow a new diet. Finally, to successfully control blood glucose requires the person to master the impressive task of coordinating diet, insulin, and exercise. Overwhelming as these assignments may seem at first, a person can manage them and lead an active and full life.

As mentioned, the treatment of IDDM involves coordinating three basic components: insulin, diet, and exercise. The next sections provide details.

Insulin

Because people with IDDM can't make insulin, they must receive insulin from another source.* The purification of insulin from animal sources has been life-saving, but even so, insulin therapy cannot achieve the same degree of blood glucose control as a normal-functioning body.

Commercial insulin is commonly extracted from the pancreas of cattle. Insulins made from porcine pancreatic extracts and, more recently, human insulins, are also available.** The many types of insulin are described as fast acting, intermediate acting, or long acting, depending on how quickly they begin to work and how long they remain active. Table 27–3 (on p. 830) lists examples of the various types of insulin and their actions.

The delivery of insulin mimics as closely as possible the body's normal release of insulin. Normally, the body secretes a constant, baseline amount of insulin at all times. After a meal, insulin secretion surges to help store energy

Some people develop an allergy to a particular type of insulin or an additive in the insulin called an **insulin allergy.** The person experiencing such a reaction must switch to a different type of insulin.

---

*Insulin was first used successfully in diabetic dogs by F. G. Banting and C. H. Best in 1922. Shortly after its discovery, insulin became available to thousands of persons with diabetes.
**The first dose of human insulin was given to a person in the United Kingdom in 1980. Since then, an estimated 200,000 people in the world have received human insulin. Additional research and refinement of human insulins will generate wider use of these products.

■ TABLE 27–3
Actions of Some Types of Insulin

Type	Duration of Activity	Peak of Action
Rapid acting		
Regular crystalline	5 to 7 hours	2 to 4 hours
Semilente	12 to 16 hours	2 to 8 hours
Intermediate acting		
Globin	12 to 18 hours	6 to 8 hours
NPH/lente	18 to 24 hours	8 to 14 hours
Long acting		
Protamine zinc	24 to 30 hours	16 to 24 hours
Ultralente	30 to 36 hours	18 to 29 hours

When the pancreas fails to produce insulin, people with IDDM turn to commercially available injections for the life-saving hormone.

Hyperglycemia can also result from excessive secretion of insulin antagonists (glucagon, epinephrine and glucocorticoids) in response to excessive administration of insulin. This is called **rebound hyperglycemia** or the **Somogyi** (so-MOHG-yee) **effect.**

nutrients as they flow in. The person with IDDM needs insulin both to meet baseline needs and to process energy nutrients.

To meet these insulin needs, the person with IDDM takes insulin and meals at times selected to ensure that insulin is available when nutrients from food are present and vice versa—that nutrients from food are available when the insulin is present. The physician prescribes the exact type, dosage, and administration schedule of insulin based on the individual's stage of growth, activity patterns, eating habits, and individual responses. (The accompanying box provides an example of one way insulin might be administered.) Generally, individuals receive a mixture of two or more types of insulin several times a day to approximate the normal presence of insulin in the bloodstream.

Some clients experience a temporary remission of diabetes after their initial treatment with insulin—a time referred to as the "honeymoon period." Remission may last from a few weeks to several months. Why this honeymoon occurs remains a bit of a mystery. Some researchers speculate that the constant hyperglycemia of diabetes exhausts the insulin-producing cells of the pancreas, thus impairing their function—a concept referred to as glucose toxicity.[9] With insulin treatment and relief from the glucose burden, the cells begin to function normally again—at least, temporarily. Tight control of glucose—whether by diet, insulin, or hypoglycemic agents—improves insulin secretion and sensitivity.

Insulin needs rise as body weight increases. As a rule of thumb, about 0.5 to 1.0 unit of insulin is given per kilogram of body weight per day. (Children with diabetes and their parents should be advised that higher insulin doses do not necessarily indicate a worsening of the condition.)

Activity reduces insulin needs, for exercise itself acts like insulin in lowering blood glucose levels. In contrast, insulin needs increase during stress, such as pregnancy, surgery, and infection or other illnesses. (You may recall that hyperglycemia results from the catabolic stress response, so it makes sense that insulin needs would be higher.)

The person who receives too little insulin or doesn't receive insulin when glucose from foods is available risks hyperglycemia and diabetic ketoacidosis (as described earlier). The person who receives too much insulin or has too little glucose available when insulin is high risks severe hypoglycemia.

An Example of Insulin Administration

- 30 to 45 minutes before breakfast—an injection of a mixture of rapid-acting and long-acting insulin.
- 30 minutes before lunch—an injection of rapid-acting insulin.
- 30 minutes before supper—an injection of a mixture of rapid-acting and long-acting insulin.

This hypoglycemic response is called an insulin reaction or insulin shock. An insulin reaction can result from an overdose of insulin, excessive physical activity, skipping meals, or eating too little food. People with IDDM and people who spend time with them need to learn to recognize the symptoms of hypoglycemia. As soon as someone recognizes the symptoms, the person needs to receive some form of readily absorbed glucose (½ cup of orange juice, for example). In severe cases, the person may need to receive glucose intravenously, the hormone glucagon, or both, to counteract the insulin reaction. Without treatment, the person may lapse into shock and die. (Because people lose consciousness at both extremes of glucose level, both have been called *coma,* but it is important to distinguish between coma and shock because they demand opposite treatments. The symptoms of both are listed in the margin.)

Recognizing the symptoms of insulin shock may require some training, for a person suffering from insulin shock may appear intoxicated. If the true problem goes unrecognized, the person may die. To prevent such a mistake, advise persons with IDDM to wear identification in the form of a bracelet or necklace. A card in the wallet may be inadequate, since it might go unnoticed until too late. In addition, advise individuals with IDDM to carry sugar cubes or hard candy with them, so that they can act immediately when hypoglycemic symptoms occur.

People with diabetes and those who care for them must also learn to distinguish between the symptoms of hypoglycemia and hyperglycemia. The causes and treatments for these extremes differ significantly. Hyperglycemia can result from stress (infection), too little insulin, too much food, or large amounts of concentrated sweets. The treatment involves carefully administering rapid-acting insulin (too much insulin can result in severe hypoglycemia), and correcting fluid and electrolyte imbalance by IV fluids.

Researchers continue to improve the methods of delivering insulin, trying to more closely mimic the body's normal secretion schedule and quantities. One promising method is continuous subcutaneous insulin infusion (CSII), which is available in two versions. One, referred to as the closed-loop system, involves three major components: a sensor that detects the amount of glucose in the blood, a minicomputer that calculates how much insulin (or sometimes glucose) the person needs, and a pump that delivers the insulin (or glucose). The closed-loop system responds immediately to changes in blood glucose concentration. Such a system is large, and requires that blood be continuously withdrawn. Therefore, its use is limited to a few days at a time for people who

insulin reaction: hypoglycemia that results from an overdose of insulin, strenuous physical activity, skipped meals, or inadequate intake of food; also called **insulin shock.**

Symptoms of hypoglycemia:
- Dizziness.
- Double vision.
- Nervousness.
- Shallow breathing.
- Sweating.
- Weakness.

Symptoms of hyperglycemia:
- Acetone breath.
- Confusion.
- Glucosuria.
- Intense thirst.
- Labored breathing.
- Nausea.
- Vomiting.

continuous subcutaneous insulin infusion (CSII): a system for delivering insulin that eliminates the need for insulin injections.

closed-loop CSII system: a method for delivering insulin that consists of a glucose-sensing device, a minicomputer, and a pump.

are not fully ambulatory. It may also be useful for emergency situations or when a person with diabetes undergoes surgery.

The other CSII method is the open-loop system. The open-loop system consists of a small preprogrammed pump designed to deliver anticipated insulin needs. The pump delivers insulin at a basal flow rate between meals and at a higher rate for mealtimes.

If and when researchers design a system that perfectly mimics the physiologic action of insulin, diabetes therapy will change drastically. Diet, long the cornerstone of therapy, will become a far simpler matter to the person with IDDM when insulin becomes as physiologically accessible as it is to the normally functioning body.

Diet in IDDM

To control IDDM requires a lifelong commitment to a carefully orchestrated diet, exercise, and insulin program. Therefore the plan must consider the person's lifestyle habits and food preferences. Most frequently, diet planners use the exchange patterns described in Chapter 2 (pp. 27–33). The foods in each of the exchange system's six groups are similar in food energy and in carbohydrate, protein, and fat per portion. (Thus "a bread exchange" is any portion of grain or starchy vegetable that contains about 80 kcalories of food energy, 15 grams of carbohydrate, 3 grams of protein, and trace amounts of fat. One slice of most breads, one small potato, or ⅓ cup of rice all fit that description and can be exchanged for each other in meal planning.) The person with diabetes learns that all of the food portions on any one list provide approximately the same number of kcalories and the same amounts of energy nutrients and so can be exchanged freely for one another, but that foods from one exchange list cannot be substituted for foods on another exchange list. Besides the starch/bread list, there is a milk list, a meat list, a fruit list, a vegetable list, and a fat list. Chapter 2 and Appendix G provide additional details of the exchange lists.

The diet for IDDM first focuses on providing adequate food energy to achieve or maintain a healthy body weight, and to support growth in children. To determine whether energy intake is appropriate, use the energy RDA as a guide, and take height and weight measures periodically. Then adjust the diet as necessary. (See the box on pp. 834–837, "How to Plan a Diabetic Diet Using Exchange Lists.")

In IDDM, consistency in the timing and composition of meals and snacks from day to day improves glucose control. In general, small meals with snacks between meals maintain blood glucose control best. For example, the distribution of food might provide for three meals, and a snack midmorning, midafternoon, and at bedtime, depending on the individual's blood glucose levels and insulin schedule. The individual can monitor his or her own blood glucose using commercial devices (see the box presented earlier, "How to Measure Glucose Control").

Of the total kcalories, carbohydrate should contribute 55 to 60 percent, fat should provide 25 to 30 percent, and protein intake should fall between 12 and 20 percent.[10] The diet planner divides these energy nutrients into meals that, in turn, coordinate with the insulin schedule.

Notice that the diet for IDDM does not restrict carbohydrate intake. In fact, the carbohydrate content of the diet is fairly high, and carbohydrates need to be eaten at every meal and snack to keep an even flow of glucose coming.

Encourage clients to select complex carbohydrates from whole-grain breads and cereals, dried beans and peas, fruits, and vegetables. These foods provide fiber, and evidence suggests that diets high in fiber improve blood glucose control.[11] As Chapter 4 explained, water-soluble fibers (found in legumes, oats, barley, and some fruits) slow the rate of glucose absorption from the GI tract into the blood.

Other studies show that carbohydrates from different foods raise blood glucose levels to different extents (the glycemic effect of foods). Chapter 4 described the glycemic effect and the factors that influence it (p. 93). People with diabetes might benefit from avoiding foods that raise and lower blood glucose concentrations dramatically, but, for now, research on the glycemic effect of foods provides little practical information for meal planning. Researchers need to understand how combinations of foods eaten at the same time influence blood glucose before dietitians make major revisions of the diabetic diet.

In most cases, the diabetic diet excludes concentrated sweets (except to reverse hypoglycemia). However, because the "absolutely no sugar" rule would be difficult to follow, many health care professionals allow clients (particularly children) to consume modest amounts of concentrated sweets with meals (not to exceed 5 percent of the total kcalories). Additionally, people with IDDM may need concentrated sweets before vigorous exercise or during illness (as a later section describes).

Because people with diabetes have a high risk of developing cardiovascular disease and hypertension, their diet plan should follow dietary guidelines to help protect against those conditions. Encourage the use of low-fat and nonfat milk, lean meats, and polyunsaturated fats to lower saturated fat intake and restrict sodium intake to less than 3,000 milligrams per day.[12] Chapter 28 provides more details on nutrition and disorders of the heart and blood vessels.

Exercise

In addition to insulin therapy and diet, the management of diabetes requires attention to exercise, partly because, as mentioned, exercise produces an insulinlike effect and so can improve diabetes control. Exercise programs can also help significantly to strengthen the heart, control blood pressure, and provide many other benefits to the cardiovascular system that people with diabetes especially need (see Chapter 13 for more on the benefits of exercise). For the person with IDDM, regular exercise may lower insulin requirements. For those with NIDDM, exercise can improve glucose tolerance.[13]

For nondiabetic people, blood glucose levels generally vary little during exercise. In contrast, blood glucose levels can vary markedly when people with IDDM exercise. Those with mild hyperglycemia may experience a fall in blood glucose levels during exercise, whereas those with marked hyperglycemia may experience a still greater rise in blood glucose levels. For this reason, physicians generally advise people with IDDM to refrain from

How to Plan a Diabetic Diet Using Exchange Lists

Most often, the dietitian assumes the responsibility of planning the diabetic diet. A careful look at the individual's diet history helps to plan a diet that will meet both the person's needs and the needs imposed by the disease.

At first, using exchange lists to plan diets may take hours. However, with practice, dietitians learn to prepare complete diet plans in a matter of minutes by using a few shortcuts. This diet plan follows the shortcut steps. (Chapter 12 and its "Self Study" provide a more detailed method for determining ideal body weight, energy needs, grams of energy nutrients, and meal plans.)

1. *Estimate desirable body weight.*

Males: Allow 106 lb for the first 5 ft, then add 6 lb for each inch over 5 ft.

Females: Allow 100 lb for the first 5 ft, then add 5 lb for each inch over 5 ft.

Adjustment: Add 10% for large-framed individuals; subtract 10% for small-framed individuals.

Children: Refer to growth charts in Appendix E.

This example uses a large-framed man, 5 ft 10 in tall:

106 lb + (6 lb × 10 inches) = 166 lb.
166 lb × 10% = 16.6 lb.
166 lb + 16.6 lb = 183 lb (rounded off).

2. *Calculate energy needs in kcalories.*

Multiply desirable body weight by 15 for men and active women; by 13 for most women, sedentary men, and adults over age 55; and by 10 for sedentary women, obese people, and sedentary adults over age 55.[14]

Children require about 1,000 kcal for the first year of life plus 100 kcal per year up to 2,000 kcal at age 11. From age 12 to 15, add 100 kcal per year for girls and 200 kcal per year for boys. Remember, this is an estimate, and children's needs depend more on size than on age.

In this example, the man needs the following number of kcalories to maintain a weight of 183 lb:

183 lb × 15 kcal/lb = 2,745 kcal.

3. *Determine the grams of carbohydrate, fat, and protein.*

- 55 to 60% of the kcalories from carbohydrate.
- 25 to 30% of the kcalories from fat.
- 12 to 20% of the kcalories from protein.

exercising until blood glucose falls below 300 milligrams per 100 milliliters. When blood glucose stabilizes, the physician will prescribe the type, intensity, duration, and frequency of exercise.

The person with IDDM may need to eat before, during, and after

For 2,750 kcalories, this division of nutrients translates as follows:
Carbohydrate:

55% × 2,750 kcal = 1,513 kcal.   1,513 kcal ÷ 4 kcal/g = 378 g.
60% × 2,750 kcal = 1,650 kcal.   1,650 kcal ÷ 4 kcal/g = 413 g.

(So the man needs about 380 to 415 g carbohydrate.)

Fat:

25% × 2,750 kcal = 688 kcal.   688 kcal ÷ 9 kcal/g = 76 g.
30% × 2,750 kcal = 825 kcal.   825 kcal ÷ 9 kcal/g = 92 g.
(So the man needs about 75 to 95 g fat.)

Protein:

12% × 2,750 kcal = 330 kcal.   330 kcal ÷ 4 kcal/g = 83 g.
20% × 2,750 kcal = 550 kcal.   550 kcal ÷ 4 kcal/g = 138 g.
(So the man needs about 85 to 140 g protein.)

4. *Translate the diet prescription into a meal plan.*

Table 2−5 on p. 33 provides examples of diet patterns for different energy intakes. Using that table as a guide, a dietitian might select the pattern of exchanges shown in Table 27−4, columns 1 and 2. The dietitian could then calculate the grams of energy nutrients by referring to Table 2−2 on p. 28 and come up with the next three columns in Table 27−4. Total kcalories and percentages of kcalories

■ TABLE 27−4
A Day's Exchanges for a Sample 2,750-kCalorie Diabetic Diet

Exchange Group	Number of Exchanges	Carbohydrate (g)	Protein (g)	Fat (g)
Starch/bread	14	210	42	Trace
Meat	8	—	56	24
Vegetable	5	25	10	—
Fruit	7	105	—	—
Milk	4	48	32	Trace
Fat	9	—	—	45
Total grams		388	140	69
Total kcalories		1,552	560	621
% kcalories		57%	20%	23%

Note: To translate exchanges into foods, use Figure 2−6 on pp. 30−31 or Appendix G.

(continued on the next page)

exercising. Especially important is carbohydrate, which should come from fruits, fruit juices, yogurt, crackers, and other starches.[15] As a general guideline, the exerciser should take about 10 to 15 grams of additional carbohydrate before moderate activity, or about 20 to 30 grams of carbohy-

How to Plan a Diabetic Diet Using Exchange Lists (continued)

contributed by each nutrient are shown at the bottom of the table. As you can see, the diet delivers 57 percent of its energy from carbohydrate, 20 percent from protein, and 23 percent from fat, a balance that meets recommended standards.

5. *Distribute foods into meals, being careful to distribute carbohydrates in about the same proportion to food energy in every meal.*

   To ease calculations and the distribution of food into several meals, diet planners often divide the kcalories into twice as many groups as assigned feedings. For example, let's say our client needs five feedings (three meals and two snacks). Divide the kcalories and carbohydrates into tenths before determining their distribution into meals:

   2,750 kcal ÷ 10 = 275 kcal.

   and

   378 g carbohydrate ÷ 10 = 38 g carbohydrate.

   Then distribute the exchanges into meals that will deliver smoothly graded amounts of energy and carbohydrate throughout the day. Table 27−5 gives an example in which breakfast delivers 2/10 of the energy and carbohydrate; a midmorning snack delivers another 1/10 of each; lunch delivers 3/10; supper, 3/10; and an evening snack the last 1/10.

■ TABLE 27−5
Distribution of Energy and Carbohydrate in a Sample Diabetic Diet

	Breakfast (2/10)	Midmorning Snack (1/10)	Lunch (3/10)	Supper (3/10)	Bedtime Snack (1/10)	Total
Energy (kcal)	550	275	825	825	275	2,750
Carbohydrate (g)	76	38	114	114	38	380

Note: These figures are approximations. Chances are that you will not be able to divide meals so that the kcalories and carbohydrate are distributed exactly as you would wish. (See the sample 2,750 kcal diabetic diet menu on p. 838.)

drate before vigorous activity. People with IDDM must coordinate the dose and timing of insulin injections with exercise. Vigorous exercise and warm temperatures increase blood flow, thus increasing the rate of insulin absorption and setting the stage for a hypoglycemic reaction. Reducing the insulin dosage can help to prevent this sequence of events. The best way to determine the appropriate course of action is to monitor blood glucose levels 30 minutes before and 1 hour after exercise. Table 27−7 (on p. 838) provides some general guidelines.

With this information in hand, the dietitian and client can begin to fill in the plan with real foods to create a menu (see Figure 2–6 on pp. 30–31 and Appendix G). Developing menus takes time and patience; it is a matter of trial and error until the actual plan comes "close enough" to the goals.

Exchange lists ease the task of tailoring a diet to an individual's preferences. For example, the planner can substitute one bread exchange (80 kcalories, 15 grams of carbohydrate) for 1½ fruit exchanges (90 kcalories, 15 grams of carbohydrate). If the client doesn't drink milk (90 kcalories, 12 grams of carbohydrate), the planner can substitute a half serving of bread and 1 ounce of lean meat (95 kcalories, 8 grams of carbohydrate). Adjusting the diet to the client's preferences helps to ensure diet compliance.

Table 27–6 and the sample menu (on the next page) show one possible way to approximate the goals of a 2,750 kcalorie diabetic diet. You might see ways to improve it, or you might want to try planning another day's meals to see how close you get to distributing energy and carbohydrate as recommended.

■ TABLE 27–6
Sample Worksheet for Distributing 2,750 kCalorie Diabetic Diet into Meals

Exchange List	Breakfast	Midmorning Snack	Lunch	Supper	Bedtime Snack	Total
Starch/bread	4	2	4	3	1	14
Meat	1	1	2	4		8
Vegetable			2	3		5
Fruit	1	1	2	2	1	7
Milk			1	1½	1½	4
Fat	2½		3	3		8½
Meal plan:						
kcalories	545	275	825	925	275	2,845
g carbohydrate	75	45	112	108	48	388
Meal goals:						
kcalories	550	275	825	825	275	2,750
g carbohydrate	76	38	114	114	38	380

As you can see, the meal approximates the goals, but does not meet them perfectly.

Delayed Meals and Illness

Like most people, people with IDDM occasionally miss a meal. When this happens, they need to eat some carbohydrate to protect against hypoglycemia. Usually 15 to 30 grams of complex carbohydrate will forestall hypoglycemia for one to two hours on such occasions.

In the hospital, the person with IDDM may miss a meal in preparation for diagnostic tests, following surgery, or if GI problems prevent food intake.

Sample 2,750 kCalorie Diabetic Diet Menu

MENU

Breakfast

1 soft cooked egg
2 slices whole-wheat toast
2 tsp margarine
½ banana

Midmorning Snack

1 peach
¼ c cottage cheese
1 English muffin

Lunch

Ham sandwich with 2 oz ham
  and 2 tsp mayonnaise
½ c baked beans
Broccoli/tomato salad with
  2 tbsp salad dressing
1 large pear
1 c nonfat milk

Supper

4 oz chicken
⅓ c rice
½ c cooked carrots
1 artichoke
3 tsp margarine
2 whole-wheat rolls
⅔ cantaloupe
1½ c nonfat milk

Bedtime Snack

½ c apple juice
3 c popcorn
1½ c nonfat plain yogurt

Procedures for dealing with this problem vary with each hospital. One procedure replaces at least half the prescribed carbohydrate and kcalories within three hours of the missed meal. If this cannot be done, the physician may decide to take some other measure, such as changing the insulin schedule or giving IV dextrose. Sometimes the physician will change the diet prescription to include more simple carbohydrates.

■ TABLE 27–7
Guidelines for Providing Additional Carbohydrate for Activity in IDDM

Exercise Intensity	Blood Glucose Level (mg/ml)	Additional Carbohydrate to Provide (g)
Low intensity	< 100	10–15
	> 100	None
Moderate intensity	< 100	15–20
	100–180	10–15
	180–300	None
Strenuous	< 100	35–40
	100–180	25–50
	180–300	10–15

Note: These values are estimates only. The individual should monitor blood glucose levels to more accurately determine specific needs.

Source: Adapted from M. J. Franz, Exercise and the management of diabetes mellitus, *Journal of the American Dietetic Association* 87 (1987): 872–880.

During an illness or other stress, blood glucose levels may rise, thus raising insulin requirements. This precarious time requires clients with diabetes to follow insulin and dietary instructions especially carefully. Physicians may advise clients to reduce total energy and carbohydrate intakes somewhat to limit the need for extra insulin. If appetite is poor, people with diabetes can use juice, flavored gelatin, soft drinks, or frozen fruit juice bars to meet their needs for energy and carbohydrates. The prevention of starvation, dehydration, and vomiting become main concerns.

Sugar is sometimes found in certain drugs. People with diabetes need to be aware that some liquid and chewable OTC and prescription drugs may contain sugar. Members of the health care team, too, must be alert to this possibility and take appropriate measures.

People with diabetes may require central TPN or commercial tube feedings that contain considerable amounts of simple sugars. Health care professionals must take extra care in monitoring these people and adjust insulin dosages to meet the higher carbohydrate load. Even with additional insulin, some people may be unable to tolerate the higher levels of carbohydrate in TPN. For these people, the concentration of glucose may have to be reduced and some of its energy delivered by IV fat emulsions instead (see Chapter 22). People who cannot tolerate any simple carbohydrates from tube feedings may require specially designed blenderized feedings or commercial formulas that do not contain simple sugars.

Alcohol and Dietetic Foods

The person with diabetes might ask, "Can I have alcohol?" For the person with well-controlled blood glucose, the answer is a qualified yes—on occasion (not more than once or twice a week) and in moderate amounts (less than 6 percent of the total kcalories), with the consent of the physician. Recommend that the person use alcohol only in small quantities and with, or shortly before or after, meals. Alcohol can cause hypoglycemia in any person; therefore, the person with diabetes, who is susceptible to hypoglycemia anyway, must be especially careful. Remember that the person with hypoglycemia may appear to be intoxicated anyway, thus the consumption of alcohol adds confusion to a potentially dangerous situation.

Furthermore, because alcohol delivers kcalories empty of nutrients, everyone should consume it on a limited basis, if at all. The diet planner must calculate kcalories from alcohol into the daily allowance. Most often, diet planners make room for alcohol kcalories by trading two fat exchanges for each drink of alcoholic beverage. Drinks that contain carbohydrate (drinks made with mixers, sweet wines, and liqueurs) are best avoided. If they are used, the planner must also count their carbohydrate content. Whiskey, gin, vodka, and rum do not contain carbohydrate.

1 drink = 2 fat exchanges. One drink is defined as 1½ oz liquor or 4 oz wine or 12 oz beer.

The combination of alcohol and oral hypoglycemic agents may cause flushing of the skin and a rapid heartbeat. Forewarn clients of this possible reaction.

People with diabetes often wonder about replacing sweet foods in the diet. In general, they do not need special dietetic foods. People often misinterpret *dietetic* to mean *no kcalories*, but this is not the case. Some dietetic foods may

Sweeteners that are used to take the place of sugar (sucrose) are called **alternative sweeteners.** Among them are two classes. One is the **nonnutritive sweeteners,** or **artificial sweeteners** (aspartame and saccharin), which do not contain appreciable kcalories. The other class of alternative sweeteners is the **nutritive sweeteners** (fructose, sorbitol, and xylitol) which contain the same number of kcalories as an equivalent amount of sugar (see Highlight 4).

be low in sodium instead of sugar, or they may provide reduced, but still significant, numbers of kcalories.

Some dietetic foods may be helpful, however. They include artificially sweetened soft drinks, artificial sweeteners, and water-packed canned fruits. People with diabetes may enjoy kcalorie-free soft drinks and beverages, such as artificially sweetened tea. Artificial sweeteners that do not provide significant kcalories can help make the diabetic diet acceptable.

■ *Children with Diabetes*

The overall approach to diabetes remains the same throughout life, but special problems may become apparent at different stages. Consider some of the problems of children with diabetes. Like those of all children, the energy and nutrient needs of children with diabetes keep changing throughout the growing years. Children's appetites and activities vary widely from day to day. One day a child may eat like a horse and on the next like a mouse. Children may run and play after school on a sunny day, but sit quietly in front of the television on a rainy day. Their growth and activity influence their needs for food and insulin.

To support growth and development, provide balanced meals that offer a wide variety of foods from the six exchange lists. Calculate energy needs based on age, gender, activity level, and growth status, and adjust them as necessary. Allow concentrated sweets only at times of vigorous physical activity or to treat hypoglycemia. Do not force children to finish meals, but encourage them not to skip meals either, since hypoglycemia can result. Plan meals for approximately the same times each day, and serve children the same foods as the rest of the family. Successful diet management incorporates prescribed meals into existing family lifestyles and eating patterns. Depending on insulin administration and personal preferences, children generally receive three meals with two to three snacks a day.[16] Vary snacks to prevent boredom and provide extra snacks to share with friends to prevent feelings of being different. Avoid identifying foods as "good" or "bad." Such connotations create unrealistic expectations or fears, and invite the development of manipulative eating behaviors. (The accompanying "Clinical Detective Work" presents a case study of a child with IDDM.)

Hypoglycemia that develops during the night is called **nocturnal hypoglycemia.** It is particularly dangerous, because it can go unrecognized in the sleeping person, who may go into insulin shock. Adults as well as children can develop nocturnal hypoglycemia, but children are especially susceptible.

Parents of a child with diabetes may fear that their child will develop hypoglycemia during the night, when the symptoms will go unrecognized. Snacks before bedtime may be helpful in preventing this, especially if the child engages in strenuous activity late in the day. Additionally, parents can monitor glucose levels before bedtime (especially in the newly diagnosed child) to help protect against hypoglycemia during the night.

All children develop infections of the GI and respiratory tract on occasion, and the child with diabetes may do so even more frequently. Anorexia, vomiting, or both often accompany these infections. Because hypoglycemia can easily develop under these conditions, extra care must be taken. The principles described earlier for illness apply here; hospitalization may be required if glucose levels become unmanageable.

CLINICAL DETECTIVE WORK

Kathy, a 12-year-old girl, and her parents became worried when she began losing weight, urinating excessively, and always complaining of thirst. She was diagnosed with IDDM diabetes about a year ago. Explain the metabolic events that led to the development of these diabetic symptoms.

Recently Kathy was admitted to the emergency room, complaining of nausea, vomiting, and intense thirst. The physician noted that Kathy was confused and breathing hard, and could smell acetone on her breath. Urine tests were positive for glycosuria and ketonuria, and her blood glucose level was 400 mg/100 ml. The diagnosis was diabetic ketoacidosis.

Describe how diabetes leads to ketoacidosis. Were Kathy's physical symptoms and laboratory tests consistent with this diagnosis? How would you expect the physician to manage the ketoacidosis? How can you distinguish between diabetic ketoacidosis and insulin shock?

When Kathy recovers, what advice can you offer her in order to prevent future incidents of ketoacidosis? Assume that Kathy has never been instructed on a diabetic diet. What dietary modifications would you advise her to follow?

Think about and discuss the influence of Kathy's age on her outlook and ability to cope with diabetes. What problems does her age pose? Consider some ways you might help her deal with these problems. Regarding her future, describe to her the possible role of diet in preventing the vascular complications of diabetes.

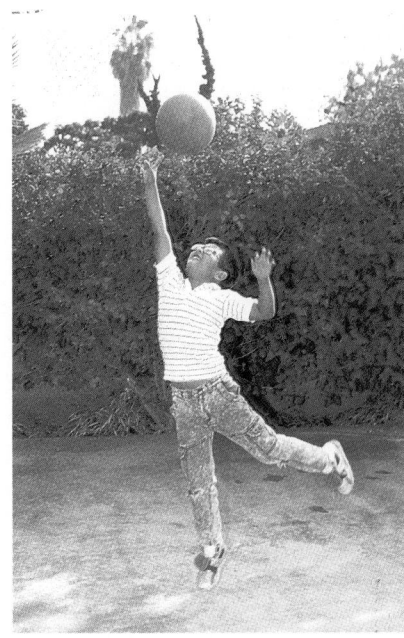

Because a child's activities vary from day to day, food and insulin needs may also change.

Treatment of Non-Insulin-Dependent Diabetes Mellitus (NIDDM)

In some ways, the treatment of NIDDM parallels that of IDDM. They share the primary goal of therapy: to maintain glucose homeostasis. However, because NIDDM develops from a resistance to insulin rather than from lack of insulin, they differ in their approach to attaining this goal. People with NIDDM can frequently control their blood glucose levels by diet alone. In other cases, drugs, in addition to diet, can maintain acceptable blood glucose levels, and exercise is important chiefly to help with weight control.

Diet in NIDDM

Diet therapy in NIDDM focuses on weight control. The majority of people with NIDDM are obese, and obesity aggravates insulin resistance.[17] Weight loss in these people can bring blood glucose levels into the normal range, ameliorate hypertension, and lower blood lipid levels.

In some centers, obese people with diabetes or severe hyperglycemia may follow a medically supervised fast temporarily or diets very low in kcalories (600 kcalories per day) until their blood glucose levels are under control. Although such programs can be successful, they can also be detrimental, either by failing to maintain weight losses or by contributing to health problems (see pp. 373–375). Weight reduction diets that provide at least 10 kcalories per pound of body weight allow a safe and gradual loss of weight. Such diets permit clients to eat enough food to obtain the nutrients they need, if they make the proper selections, and thus can be followed until the desired weight is reached.

To lose weight and control glucose levels, obese people with NIDDM need to avoid concentrated sweets and limit their energy intakes. While the timing and distribution of meals is not critical, they should limit themselves to only three meals a day, for this helps prevent excessive snacking and possible weight gain. Table 27–8 compares the key components of diet therapy in IDDM and NIDDM.

Like IDDM, the exchange list system provides the basis for the diet in NIDDM. The person at ideal weight may not need to limit energy intake but still needs to exclude concentrated sweets. Table 27–9 lists the foods to avoid on such a diet.

A program of moderate exercise offers many benefits. Exercise helps improve blood glucose control, glucose tolerance, and insulin action in NIDDM.[18] Many clinicians believe that 80 to 90 percent of all people with NIDDM who are overweight can achieve metabolic control if they follow a low-kcalorie diet combined with an exercise program of moderate intensity.[19]

■ **TABLE 27–8**
Comparisons of IDDM and NIDDM Diet Therapies

Diet Approach	IDDM	NIDDM
Reduce food energy intake	Usually not necessary	Almost invariably necessary
Keep ratio of carbohydrate, protein, and fat consistent for each feeding	Yes	No
Eat meals at regular times	Yes	Not necessary
Eat more frequent meals	Yes	No
Use food to treat or prevent hypoglycemia	Yes	No[a]
Replace carbohydrate when appetite is poor or meals are missed	Yes	No
Eat extra food for intense exercise	Yes	No
Restrict sodium to 3,000 mg/day	Yes	Yes
Follow dietary pattern of 30% kcal fat, 55% kcal carbohydrate, and 15% kcal protein	Yes	Yes
Use exchange system	Yes	Yes

Note: Philosophies vary. Not every diet therapist would follow these guidelines in every case.

[a]Food may be needed to treat or prevent hypoglycemia when oral hypoglycemic agents are given.

■ TABLE 27–9
Foods Avoided on Diets That Exclude Concentrated Sweets

Cakes	Fruit juices, sweetened	Pies
Candy	Gelatin, sweetened	Popsicles
Cereals, sweetened	Granola	Puddings
Cookies	Honey	Sherbet
Cranberry sauce	Ice cream	Soft drinks
Doughnuts	Jam	Sweet rolls
Frappés	Jelly	Sugar
Frosting	Marmalade	Syrup
Fruits, canned, glazed, frozen or cooked with sugar	Milk, chocolate or condensed	Vegetables, glazed
	Milkshakes	Yogurt, fruit flavored (if sweetened with sugar)
Fruit drinks	Molasses	
Fruit ices	Pastries	

While exercise helps to lower blood glucose and improve insulin resistance in NIDDM, its greatest value is in contributing to weight loss.[20]

In some people with NIDDM, diet alone fails to adequately control hyperglycemia. These people may need to take insulin or drugs. Remind clients that such actions do not replace their diet; advise them to continue their diets as instructed.

Oral Hypoglycemic Agents

Physicians sometimes prescribe oral hypoglycemic agents when glucose levels remain out of control. Oral hypoglycemic agents appear to stimulate the release of insulin from the pancreas. Table 27–10 (on p. 844) provides a summary of nutrition-related information about oral hypoglycemic agents.

The use of oral hypoglycemic agents is a matter for some difference of opinion. Questions arose first from a study, conducted by competent professionals over an eight-year period, that found that clients treated with diet and tolbutamide (one type of oral hypoglycemic agent) had a significant increase in deaths from heart attacks (2½ times that of clients treated by diet alone). Many physicians consider oral hypoglycemics a last option; if their clients cannot control blood glucose levels by diet alone, these physicians would consider insulin therapy before trying oral hypoglycemics. Other physicians might prescribe oral hypoglycemics when diet therapy alone first failed. In either case, they all agree that oral hypoglycemic agents do not replace diet therapy, but serve as an adjunct to diet. (For a case study of NIDDM, see the "Clinical Detective Work" box on p. 845.)

oral hypoglycemic agents: drugs that can be taken by mouth to lower blood glucose levels in NIDDM; these drugs are ineffective in IDDM.

■ Treatment of Diabetes during Pregnancy

Women with diabetes who are contemplating pregnancy should know that untreated women with diabetes have a high infertility rate. Women who do

■ TABLE 27–10
Oral Hypoglycemic Agents

Drug Name	Timing with Meals	Common Side Effects That May Influence Nutrition Status
Chlorpropamide	Give with breakfast. Avoid alcohol.	Dyspepsia, nausea, vomiting, metallic taste, anorexia. Water intoxication, edema.
Acetohexamide	Give with meals. Avoid alcohol.	Diarrhea, nausea, vomiting, heartburn, metallic taste. May induce anemia.
Glipizide	Give 30 min before breakfast. Limit alcohol.	GI distress, nausea, diarrhea, constipation, heartburn, altered taste perceptions.
Glyburide	Give before breakfast. Limit alcohol.	GI distress, nausea, diarrhea, constipation, heartburn.
Tolazamide	Give in morning or divided during day with meals. Avoid alcohol.	Diarrhea, GI distress, nausea, vomiting, dyspepsia, heartburn, altered taste perceptions, anorexia.
Tolbutamide	(same as above)	(same as above)

Source: Adapted from D. E. Powers and A. O. Moore, *Food Medication Interactions*, 6th ed. (Phoenix Ariz.: Food Medication Interactions, 1989).

respiratory distress: a disorder of the lung membranes that results in delayed onset of respiration at birth and difficulty in breathing after birth.

perinatal (PERR-ee-NAY-tal): concerning the time before, during, or shortly after birth.

peri = around
natal = birth

The hormones that antagonize the action of insulin during late pregnancy are placental lactogen, cortisol, prolactin, and progesterone.

conceive should realize that diabetes poses special concerns for both the mother and infant. Without management of maternal diabetes, women may experience episodes of severe hypoglycemia or hyperglycemia, spontaneous abortion, and pregnancy-induced hypertension; infants may suffer increased mortality and morbidity, congenital abnormalities, and other complications. These complications include developing severe hypoglycemia or respiratory distress, both of which can be fatal. Perinatal mortality in infants born of women with diabetes exceeds 200 deaths per 1,000 births.[21]

Pregnancy in all women alters insulin resistance and elevates blood insulin levels. Insulin levels begin to rise soon after conception, and the cells respond by storing energy nutrients to provide for the developing fetus. Later in pregnancy, insulin levels continue to remain high, but the tissues become insulin resistant. Hormones that act antagonistically to insulin reach higher levels. This shift signals the body to stop storing energy fuels and to begin allowing the fetus to extract energy nutrients rapidly during the mother's fasting times.

You can see why these changes can have serious metabolic consequences for the pregnant woman with diabetes. The woman with IDDM must monitor blood glucose levels and adjust insulin dosages accordingly. Hypoglycemia may occur early in pregnancy because of the transfer of glucose to the fetus, vomiting, or reduced food intake resulting from nausea. Often, however, pregnant women with IDDM must increase their insulin dosages. If hypoglycemia occurs, they may reduce insulin dosages temporarily.

In the last half of pregnancy, insulin requirements increase. The nutrient needs of the pregnant woman with diabetes follow those of other pregnant women, and the diet plan uses the exchange lists. However, the diet should

---

CLINICAL DETECTIVE WORK

Mr. Evans was 52 years old when he was first diagnosed with NIDDM. He visited his physician after experiencing symptoms of excessive thirst, excessive urination, and excessive appetite. Mr. Evans, who stands 5 ft 11 inches tall, currently weighs 200 lb., experienced a 30-lb weight gain over the past two years. His fasting blood glucose is 235 mg/100 ml.

The health care team has evaluated Mr. Evans's case, and has decided that the first goal is to bring his blood glucose levels under control. Mr. Evans will begin a one-week fast to bring his blood glucose levels down rapidly. The dietitian has provided instructions and tips to help Mr. Evans stay on the fast. The physician and nurse have also reinforced the concepts of the fast with him.

Mr. Evans is now ready to begin eating again. He is concerned about his health, worried that he may need insulin injections, and overwhelmed with all the information he has been given over the past few weeks.

Can you explain to Mr. Evans how NIDDM differs from IDDM? Describe what factors in Mr. Evans's history might have predisposed him to NIDDM. What will be the primary objective of the diet therapy for Mr. Evans? Determine Mr. Evans's ideal body weight, and plan a diet for him. (Use the information in the box on pp. 834–837 entitled, "How to Plan a Diabetic Diet Using Exchange Lists.") What was the rationale for using a fast initially? What other measure might help Mr. Evans bring his blood glucose under control? Can NIDDM usually be controlled by diet alone? What alternative treatments might his physician consider if diet alone fails? Consider Mr. Evans' emotional state of health. How can the health care team help Mr. Evans during this difficult period?

---

always provide a bedtime snack, for two reasons. For one, a bedtime snack helps to prevent episodes of hypoglycemia that may occur in the early morning. For another, it provides a source of fuel for the developing fetus and prevents the buildup of ketones.

For the pregnant woman with NIDDM, diet is central to therapy. Physicians may prescribe oral hypoglycemic agents occasionally or insulin in some cases. Oral hypoglycemic agents must be discontinued late in pregnancy and be replaced with insulin if needed; hypoglycemic agents promote hypoglycemia in the newborn infant.

The risk of developing NIDDM or glucose intolerance increases with each pregnancy.[22] This association may not appear until many years after childbearing and cannot be explained fully by age, obesity, or family history.

Gestational diabetes (as mentioned earlier) develops during pregnancy, with subsequent return to normal glucose tolerance after childbirth. It usually appears in the later part of gestation when the tissues become insulin-resistant. Health care providers evaluate a woman's potential for gestational diabetes by checking the following risk factors associated with the condition during the first prenatal examination:

■ Previous gestational diabetes.
■ History of large infants (9 pounds or more).
■ Family history of diabetes.
■ Symptoms of diabetes and glucosuria.
■ Obesity or excessive weight gain.
■ Recurrent urinary tract infections.
■ History of spontaneous abortions.
■ Previous unexplained stillbirth.

If the history has indicated a risk, the health care provider conducts glucose tolerance tests as necessary to evaluate the risk.

As added insurance against problems with diabetes, all pregnant women have glucose tolerance tests at 24 to 28 weeks' gestation. Thereafter, at every checkup, the urine is tested for ketones. Ketonuria in conjunction with elevated blood glucose levels may point to diabetes.

Gestational diabetes requires dietary management just as NIDDM does. An important aspect of nutrition management is prevention of excessive weight gain, but weight reduction diets are not normally recommended during pregnancy. Women with gestational diabetes should not reduce their carbohydrate intakes but should choose foods rich in complex carbohydrates, such as vegetables and whole-grain breads, and limit their intakes of concentrated sweets. Optimal protein intakes are also important. Dietary recommendations encourage three meals a day plus two snacks, each containing protein, carbohydrate, and moderate fat.

Almost one-third of the women who have gestational diabetes develop NIDDM within five years. Research indicates that the incidence of NIDDM in women with previous gestational diabetes is twice as high in those who are 20 percent or more overweight, compared with those who are not overweight.

Obstetricians recommend blood glucose monitoring for all pregnant women with any type of diabetes. Establishing blood glucose control is important to the health of both mother and infant. In addition to monitoring their blood glucose, pregnant women may also monitor their urine for ketones. Ketosis in early pregnancy can lead to congenital malformations, central nervous system disorders, and a low IQ in infants.

■ Diabetes Prevention

Advise the person at risk for developing diabetes to avoid unwanted weight gain and also to exercise regularly, for exercise helps insulin move glucose into cells and forestalls the onset of diabetes. In addition, advise such a client to control all possible risk factors that might contribute to heart and blood vessel disease (atherosclerosis and hypertension, discussed in Chapter 28).

While the exchange system was originally developed for people with diabetes, it serves people in perfect health equally well. A diet constructed primarily of a balanced selection of foods from the exchange lists has all the characteristics most important in diabetes prevention. It is adequate in vitamins and minerals. Deficiencies in trace minerals, especially chromium, may hasten diabetes onset. It provides ample fiber and complex carbohydrates and is low in concentrated sugar, which helps to regulate blood glucose concentrations. And it is low in fat, helping to protect against cardiovascular disease.

A person threatened with diabetes can do no better than to adopt such a diet long before any symptoms appear. A healthy diet, combined with regular exercise and abstinence from negative practices such as alcohol abuse, may forestall the onset of diabetes.

■ Nutrition Assessment

Keep these points in mind when assessing nutrition status for clients with diabetes:

■ The most valuable nutrition assessment parameter of the person with diabetes is body weight. Obtain an accurate assessment of both current and appropriate weight. Treatment of IDDM requires providing doses of insulin according to a person's body weight and treatment of NIDDM depends primarily on weight loss. Body weight establishes the basis for calculating the total kcalories in the diet. On reassessment, kcalories may need to be adjusted frequently, particularly in the growing child.

■ Obtain an accurate diet history from the person with diabetes. This step is instrumental in planning an acceptable diet, as well as noting possible nutrient deficiencies. During reassessment, use the diet history to monitor compliance with the treatment plan. In the person with IDDM, the history will help to assess the individual's knowledge of how to adjust the diet for unusually strenuous exercise, missed meals, or illness, as well as how to prevent or treat hypoglycemia.

■ Arm anthropometrics may be difficult to obtain and interpret in some people with IDDM, especially when the midarm area has hypertrophied from repeated insulin injections. Fat measurements can be taken using other areas of the body in these cases.

■ Monitor blood glucose and lipid concentrations regularly. Also, tests for renal function should be conducted periodically.

■ Hypoglycemia

Strictly speaking, the term *hypoglycemia* simply means "low blood glucose." It may or may not be accompanied by other symptoms, some of which may be uncomfortable. The symptoms most people associate with hypoglycemia are similar to those of an anxiety attack: weakness, rapid heartbeat, sweating, anxiety, hunger, and trembling. These symptoms are not surprising, since they are caused by the "emergency hormone," epinephrine, and they do not arise in most people, most of the time. Most people, after eating, experience a rise in their blood glucose level, followed by a gradual decline, during which time the cells begin to store fuels—the physiological condition characteristic of the "fed state." When glucose stops entering the body from the small intestine, metabolism shifts gently into the reverse condition—the "fasting state," in which, rather than storing glucose, the liver starts to release it from stored glycogen for the body's use. Throughout, blood glucose remains in the normal range, and the transition occurs without notice.

In some people, however, the transition from the fed to the fasting state causes stress because of the associated effects of epinephrine. The condition in which hypoglycemia with the symptoms of anxiety arises several hours after a meal and causes distress has been named reactive hypoglycemia. This type of hypoglycemia has attracted a lot of attention, is often misdiagnosed, and has been the subject of much misguided advice. To establish a valid diagnosis requires physicians' taking blood glucose measurements during the symptomatic episodes.[23]

A different kind of hypoglycemia exists in a person who has symptoms while well advanced into the fasting state (for example, overnight). The symptoms of fasting hypoglycemia differ from those of reactive hypoglycemia: headache, mental dullness, fatigue, confusion, amnesia, and even seizures and unconsciousness. These symptoms arise from medically diverse cases that interfere with normal blood glucose regulation, such as tumors of the pancreas or liver. Table 27–11 lists the major distinguishing characteristics of fasting and reactive hypoglycemia.

Because hypoglycemia can have a multitude of causes, no one treatment is appropriate for everyone. Still, many dishonest or ill-informed practitioners "diagnose" hypoglycemia on the basis of their clients' verbal reports alone, and prescribe all sorts of "remedies" for it with transparently thin rationale. People also "diagnose" themselves so commonly that physicians have identified a special category for their condition: *non*hypoglycemia.

True hypoglycemia can be identified by directly testing the blood glucose concentration. Because blood glucose homeostasis is dynamic, several measures taken at different times of day over an extended period provide the most useful picture. Otherwise, a measurement simply reflects the status of blood glucose at that point in time, missing the variations.

The finding that a person has reactive hypoglycemia requires three simultaneous observations: (1) low blood glucose concentration and (2) the

reactive hypoglycemia: hypoglycemia experienced simultaneously with epinephrine-release symptoms two to five hours after a meal; also called **postprandial hypoglycemia.**

fasting hypoglycemia: hypoglycemia that occurs after 8 to 14 hours of fasting.

nonhypoglycemia: a term used when people think they have hypoglycemia but don't.

■ TABLE 27–11
Characteristics of Fasting and Reactive Hypoglycemia

	Fasting Type	Reactive Type
Onset of symptoms	Gradual; occurs after fasting	Sudden; occurs 2 to 5 hours after meals
Type of symptoms	Headache, mental dullness, fatigue, confusion, amnesia, seizures, unconsciousness	Anxiety, weakness, sweating, rapid heartbeat, hunger, trembling
Duration of symptoms	Persistent	Transient
Possible causes	Hormonal imbalance, drugs, tumors	Early NIDDM, gastric surgery, TPN
Clinical course	Can be serious; treat underlying problems	Less serious; treat with diet
Other names	—	Alimentary, postprandial, idiopathic, functional

simultaneous presence of symptoms (3) four to six hours after a meal or after a dose of glucose. For persons who experience reactive hypoglycemia, a judicious adjustment of the meal pattern may bring needed relief. Two findings about hypoglycemia are relevant:

- People with *normal* glucose regulation can develop the symptoms of reactive hypoglycemia if they take a large dose of simple sugar after three days of following a low-carbohydrate diet.
- Some people who appear to have reactive hypoglycemia by traditional testing, properly performed, do not have it after mixed meals—only after a simple-sugar load.

People prone to reactive hypoglycemia can generally avoid it by eating normal mixed meals rather than sugar snacks. Even people *not* prone to reactive hypoglycemia can wreak havoc with glucose regulation by depriving the body of carbohydrate and then dumping in a large dose all at once. (This book has said more against low-carbohydrate diets elsewhere; this will suffice for hypoglycemia.) The remedy, then, requires people to eat regularly, and to eat balanced meals.

Hypoglycemia may also develop as a complication of another medical problem—for example, in the person who has dumping syndrome after gastric surgery or when central TPN solutions are discontinued too quickly. Hypoglycemia also occurs in some inborn metabolic disorders and sometimes in early NIDDM.

In true hypoglycemia, diet is a key part of therapy. The diet planner develops a diet similar to the diabetic diet, which is appropriate to achieve or maintain a healthy body weight, and often uses the exchange lists for instruction. To prevent episodes of hypoglycemia, the person avoids concentrated sweets and eats four to six small meals a day. A recent survey of teaching hospitals found that 83 percent of the respondents use either a low-carbohydrate or a moderately restricted carbohydrate diet for people with hypoglycemia, even though the value of this restriction remains unproven.[24] In addition, the person limits the use of alcohol.

This chapter has described the major areas of treatment for people with glucose imbalances. Putting those treatment plans into action is often easier said than done, however. Highlight 27 tells how health care providers can help their clients live with IDDM.

■ *Study Questions*

1. Name the two major types of diabetes. Which type is more common? Describe some differences between the two types.
2. Describe the basic problem in diabetes, and tell how it leads to these symptoms: hyperglycemia, glucosuria, dehydration, polyuria, polydipsia, weight loss, polyphagia, acetone breath, ketosis, and ketonuria.
3. What is hyperosmolar hyperglycemic nonketotic coma? How is it different from the coma that can be caused by severe hyperglycemia in the person with IDDM?

4. What biochemical tests are used to diagnose diabetes? What methods can the person with diabetes use to monitor glucose levels? What is glycosylated hemoglobin, and what advantage is there in measuring it in the blood?
5. What types of complications can arise as a result of diabetes?
6. What are the goals of therapy for all people with diabetes? Describe the three components that must be coordinated for the person with IDDM?
7. What two types of insulin requirements do our bodies have, and how is commercially available insulin given to

simulate these requirements? Why is insulin not taken orally? Describe the advantage of continuous subcutaneous insulin infusion (CSII).

8. What is the recommended distribution of nutrients for the diet in the treatment of IDDM? What types of carbohydrates are recommended in the diet? What type of fat is recommended?

9. Why are the timing and composition of meals important considerations in planning a diet for a person with IDDM? How is the carbohydrate content of the diet adjusted for exercise? How is the diet adjusted if a person misses meals?

10. Describe some general guidelines for the use of alcohol in the diabetic diet. Are dietetic foods always allowed? Why or why not?

11. Consider some of the special needs of children who have diabetes. How is the diet adjusted to meet these needs? What measures can be taken to safeguard against nocturnal hypoglycemia?

12. What is the primary goal of diet therapy in the person with NIDDM? How does diet therapy for IDDM differ from NIDDM?

13. What events occur in all pregnancies that may interfere with the control of blood glucose levels in the pregnant woman with diabetes? How is the pregnant woman with IDDM managed? How is the pregnant woman with NIDDM managed?

14. What is gestational diabetes? How is it managed?

15. Describe the dietary education needs of the person with diabetes, and discuss some ways that the process can be enhanced.

16. What is hypoglycemia? What type of hypoglycemia is treated with diet? For this type of hypoglycemia, what diet is recommended?

▪ Notes

1. *The Surgeon General's Report on Nutrition and Health: Summary and Recommendations*, DHHS (PHS) publication no. 88–50211 (Washington, D.C.: Government Printing Office, 1988).

2. M. G. Kovar, M. I. Harris, and W. C. Hadden, The scope of diabetes in the United States population, *American Journal of Public Health* 77 (1987): 1549–1550.

3. Surgeon General, 1988.

4. K. A. Fackelmann, Gene test foretells Type I diabetes risk, *Science News* 135 (1989): 357.

5. R. E. LaPorte and coauthors, Preventing insulin dependent diabetes mellitus: The environmental challenge, *British Medical Journal* 295 (1987): 479–481.

6. S. Lillioja and coauthors, Impaired glucose tolerance as a disorder of insulin action, *New England Journal of Medicine* 318 (1988): 1217–1225.

7. G. F. Cahill, Beta-cell deficiency, insulin resistance, or both? *New England Journal of Medicine* 318 (1988): 1268–1270.

8. P. Sinnock and R. S. Most, Diabetes mortality and morbidity data, in *Clinical Diabetes Mellitus: A Problem Oriented Approach*, ed. J. K. Davison (New York: Thieme, 1986), pp. 620–622.

9. L. Rossetti, A. Giaccari, and R. A. DeFronzo, Glucose toxicity, *Diabetes Care* 13 (1990): 610–630; Diabetic honeymoon: Prolonged at a price? *The Lancet* June 3, 1989, pp. 1235–1236.

10. M. J. Franz, Diabetes and nutrition: State of the science and the art, *Topics in Clinical Nutrition* 3 (1988): 1–16.

11. J. W. Anderson and coauthors, Dietary fiber and diabetes: A comprehensive review and practical application, *Journal of the American Dietetic Association* 87 (1987): 1189–1197.

12. Franz, 1988.

13. M. J. Franz, Exercise and the management of diabetes mellitus, *Journal of the American Dietetic Association* 87 (1987): 28–34.

14. Franz, 1988.

15. Franz, 1987.

16. K. H. Gabbay, Treatment of diabetes mellitus, in *Pediatric Nutrition*, eds. R. J. Grand, J. L. Sutphen, and W. H. Dietz (Boston: Butterworths, 1987), pp. 539–547.

17. M. L. Wheeler, L. Delahanty, and J. Wylie-Rosett, Diet and exercise in noninsulin-dependent diabetes mellitus: Implications for dietitians from the NIH Consensus Development Conference, *Journal of the American Dietetic Association* 87 (1987): 480–485.

18. Wheeler, Delahanty, and Wylie-Rosett, 1987.

19. M. Berger, Oral agents in the treatment of diabetes mellitus, in *Clinical Diabetes Mellitus: A Problem Oriented Approach*, ed. J. K. Davison (New York: Thieme, 1986), pp. 262–273.

20. Wheeler, Delahanty, and Wylie-Rosett, 1987.

21. P. Anastasio, New concern over gestational diabetes, *Environmental Nutrition*, February 1986, pp. 1–2.

22. D. K. Silverstein, E. B. Connor, and D. L. Wingard, The effect of parity on the later development of non-insulin-dependent diabetes mellitus or impaired glucose tolerance, *New England Journal of Medicine* 321 (1989): 1214–1219.

23. J. Palardy and coauthors, Blood glucose measurements during symptomatic episodes in patients with suspected postprandial hypoglycemia, *New England Journal of Medicine* 321 (1989): 1421–1425.

24. L. Schaffer Bell, L. N. Tiglio, and M. M. Fairchild, Dietary strategies in the treatment of reactive hypoglycemia, *Journal of the American Dietetic Association* 85 (1985): 1141–1143.

HIGHLIGHT 27

How People Live with IDDM

After physicians resolve the immediate crisis and restore glucose homeostasis in newly diagnosed cases of IDDM, clients and their families must begin making adjustments to living with the disease. These adjustments require establishing new attitudes and behaviors that will provide for a healthy life. Clients with IDDM and their families have a lot to deal with, and all this new information can be overwhelming. They may find the diagnosis of diabetes and all it entails difficult to grasp and accept.

To ensure that clients receive the education and support they need to meet the many demands of diabetes care, health care professionals can provide the following:

- Instruction on insulin administration (the appropriate dose and schedule; how to draw insulin and give themselves an injection; how to rotate injection sites).
- Instruction on blood and urine testing (how to administer the tests, record and interpret results, and adjust insulin doses accordingly).
- Instruction on diet (timing of meals and which foods to include and which to exclude).
- Instruction on changes in insulin and diet to accommodate exercise or illness.
- Descriptions of the complications associated with diabetes and instructions on how to prevent or treat their development.
- Suggestions on ways to cope with fears and guilt feelings.
- Encouragement to have confidence in their own [clients'] abilities to manage the disorder.
- Individualized programs for care, education, and emotional support.

Follow-up all oral instructions with printed information clients can review at a later time.

Living with IDDM means learning to adjust meals, insulin dosages, and physical activity to maintain glucose concentrations within a normal range.

To meet all the goals of diabetes education requires support from the diabetes care team—physicians, nurses, dietitians, counselors, and physical therapists. Each member of the team covers a specific area of instruction. In addition, each one reinforces the others' instructions.

Learning about Diabetes

For best results, all newly diagnosed clients and their families should receive intensive diabetes care training and counseling, including diet instruction, before leaving the hospital.[1] Even outpatient clients with mild cases would benefit from intensive training.

Those who instruct people with diabetes need to realize that the learning process takes time. Even if clients listen attentively, one counseling session falls short of providing an adequate lesson on diabetes and its dietary management. Truly, in-depth, short-term counseling will meet with failure. Instead, plan for five to seven days of individualized sessions with clients and their families.[2] During this time, clients will learn that diabetes treatment can control the disease but cannot cure it.

The dietitian will first design an appropriate diet. When explaining the diet to the client, the dietitian will emphasize the central role diet plays in the management of diabetes. As much as possible, the dietitian will incorporate the family's typical food selections, eating habits, and lifestyles into the diet plan. Even though the diet strictly limits sweets, clients can enjoy a prudent indulgence in them to celebrate birthdays and holidays.

After an initial introduction to the world of diabetes, clients may benefit from education programs designed to expand their knowledge and promote independence.[3] Some programs encourage clients to bring friends, which makes the experience more comfortable and fun.

Children can combine education and summer vacation with camps designed especially for children with diabetes. These camps offer the chance to learn more about diabetes while ''living'' the lifestyle under supervision. Children learn to describe their meals and snacks in terms of exchange lists. They trade snack ideas, try new recipes, and get involved in preparing meals. Older children assist younger ones, and both groups benefit.

Coping with Diabetes

As one young woman with IDDM neatly put it, ''Living with diabetes isn't easy, but it isn't the end, either.''[4]

Initially, a person with IDDM might feel awkward, confused, frustrated, or freakish. Like most people, people with IDDM are unaccustomed to measuring food portions and receiving insulin injections. Even when these tasks appear to have become part of life's routine, inside, frenzied feelings may continue. Maintaining the balance between diet, insulin, and exercise demands vigilant attention.

Teenagers often have intense trouble accepting a diagnosis of diabetes at first. At a time when they are striving to develop their identity with a group, and to be as similar to their peers as possible, the intrusion of an unwelcome diagnosis may elicit denial and refusal to cooperate. Yet they must cooperate and learn to manage their food, insulin, and exercise appropriately, for their lives are at stake. The person who appreciates a teen's special views on life is best prepared to help with the adjustment. Teens especially need to know that they can manage the disease themselves—that it won't turn them back into dependent children.

Parents and other family members also face the challenge of living with diabetes. The intensity of the situation can either reinforce or disrupt family unity. Parents may resent the demands of caring for a child with a chronic illness; in addition, they may experience guilt for having those feelings. They may feel anxiety about allowing their child to follow the diabetes care regimen without their constant assistance. Especially in the case of an older child, they may press their care and control on a child who needs to develop autonomy and self-care. Parents may also become emotionally upset when they see their child feeling anxious, depressed, or withdrawn. Parents need time to explore these feelings. They might want to attend meetings for parents of children with diabetes. Such meetings offer an opportunity to share feelings, ideas, and frustrations with others in similar situations. Sometimes just knowing that you're not alone helps.

NOTES

1. K. H. Gabbay, Treatment of diabetes mellitus, in *Pediatric Nutrition,* eds. R. J. Grand, J. L. Sutphen, and W. H. Dietz (Boston: Butterworths, 1987), pp. 539–547.
2. Gabbay, 1987.
3. G. L. Grossan and M. L. Uster, Islet pilots—An educational program for children with diabetes, *Journal of the American Dietetic Association* 88 (1988): 471.
4. M. A. D'Urso, The sweet life: Firsthand report, *Health,* November 1986, p. 75.

28

Nutrition and Disorders of the Blood Vessels, Heart, and Lungs

Contents

Atherosclerosis

Hypertension

Heart Attacks

Strokes

Congestive Heart Failure

Disorders of the Lungs

Prevention of Cardiovascular and Lung Diseases

Nutrition Assessment

Highlight: Healthful Ethnic Food Choices

The fine structure of the heart muscle shows the molecular elements of which it is composed: these are bundles of heart muscle fibers cut crosswise, viewed end-on. Round openings among the fibers are blood vessels, carrying nutrients and oxygen to them and waste products away.

CVD (cardiovascular disease): a general term for all disorders of the heart and blood vessels. Atherosclerosis is the main form of CVD. When the blood supply to the heart is obstructed, **coronary artery disease (CAD)** or **coronary heart disease (CHD)** results. In **ischemic** (iss-KEE-mic) **heart disease (IHD),** the blood supply to any organ or tissue may be cut off.

With red lights flashing and siren screaming, another ambulance races toward the hospital. The victim is one of over 1 million people who will suffer from a heart attack in the United States this year.[1] For decades, our leading causes of death have been diseases of the heart and blood vessels (cardiovascular diseases, or CVD).[2] CVD accounts for more than half of the nation's adult deaths each year, mostly by way of heart attacks and strokes.[3]

Efforts to fight CVD have led to valuable discoveries and public education. We now know smoking, high blood pressure, and high blood cholesterol are the three major risk factors for CVD, and many people have changed their lifestyles accordingly. Many have quit smoking, or refused to begin. Many have been willing to change their diets, consuming less food energy, less fat, less cholesterol, less salt, and more fiber. Many are exercising more. The rate of CVD has fallen steadily since 1950 for some or all of these reasons; still, it is high.

The twin demons that lead to most CVD are atherosclerosis and hypertension. Atherosclerosis is the common form of hardening of the arteries; hypertension is high blood pressure; and each makes the other worse.

This chapter first examines the factors that lead to the development of atherosclerosis and hypertension. Then it describes the major consequences of ignoring these conditions—heart attacks and strokes. It continues with discussions on congestive heart failure and disorders of the lungs. Before closing, the chapter provides information on dietary and other lifestyle changes that can help to prevent disorders of the blood vessels, heart, and lungs, and on the assessment of clients with these disorders. The highlight that follows this chapter shows how consumers can make healthy food choices while enjoying cuisines from around the world.

atherosclerosis (ath-er-oh-scler-OH-sis): the most common form of artery disease characterized by plaques along the inner walls of the arteries. (The related term **arteriosclerosis** means *all* forms of hardening of the arteries and includes some rare diseases.)
  athero = porridge or soft
  scleros = hard
  osis = too much

plaques (PLACKS): mounds of lipid material, mixed with smooth muscle cells and calcium, which develop in the artery walls in atherosclerosis. (The same word is also used to describe an entirely different kind of accumulation of material on teeth, which promotes dental caries.)
  placken = patch

■ *Atherosclerosis*

No one is free of atherosclerosis. The question is not whether you have it, but how far advanced it is and what you can do to retard or reverse it.

How Atherosclerosis Develops

Atherosclerosis usually begins with the accumulation of soft fatty streaks along the inner walls of the arteries, especially at branch points (see Figure 28–1). These fatty deposits gradually enlarge and become hardened plaques, making the artery walls lose their elasticity and narrowing the passage through them. Most people have well-developed plaques by the time they are 30 years old.

Normally, the arteries expand with each heartbeat to accommodate the pulses of blood that flow through them. Arteries hardened and narrowed by plaques cannot expand, and so the blood pressure rises. The increased pressure puts a strain on the heart and damages the artery walls further. At damaged points, plaques are especially likely to form; thus the development of atherosclerosis is a self-accelerating process.

A. Diagrams of arteries.

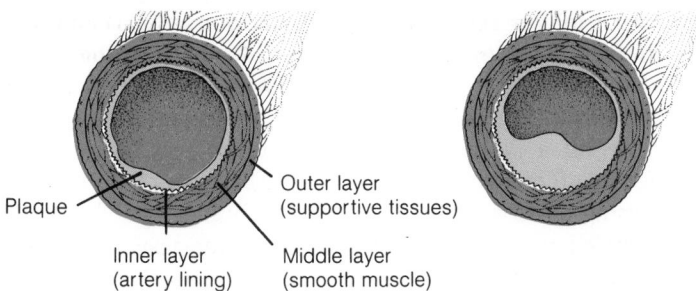

Plaque

Inner layer
(artery lining)

Outer layer
(supportive tissues)

Middle layer
(smooth muscle)

An artery (section) with plaque just
beginning to form. Plaques can
easily appear in a person as
young as 15.

The same artery, years later,
half blocked by plaque.

■ FIGURE 28–1
**The Formation of Plaques in
Atherosclerosis**
When plaques have covered 60 percent of
the coronary artery walls, the critical phase
of heart disease begins.

A healthy artery provides an open passage for the flow of blood.

Plaques along an artery narrow its diameter and obstruct blood
flow. Clots can form, aggravating the problem.

As pressure builds up in an artery, the arterial wall may weaken and
balloon out, forming an aneurysm. An aneurysm can burst, and when this
happens in a major artery such as the aorta, it leads to massive bleeding and
death.

Abnormal blood clotting also contributes to life-threatening events. Clots
form and dissolve in the blood all the time, and the balance between these
processes ensures they do no harm. That balance is disturbed in atherosclerosis. Small, cell-like bodies in the blood, known as platelets, normally cause
clots to form whenever they encounter injuries in blood vessels, but in
atherosclerosis they respond in the same way to plaques and form clots when
none are needed. Eicosanoids made from omega-6 and omega-3 fatty acids
influence the action of the platelets, and an imbalance among these com-

aneurysm (AN-you-rism): the ballooning
out of an artery wall at a point where it
has been weakened by deterioration.

aorta (ay-OR-tah): the large, primary
artery that conducts blood from the heart
to the body's smaller arteries.

platelets: tiny, disk-shaped bodies in the
blood, important in blood clot formation.
  platelet = little plate

Eicosanoids are described and defined on
p. 123.

thrombus: a stationary clot. When it has grown enough to close off a blood vessel, it is a **thrombosis.** A **coronary thrombosis** is the closing off of a vessel that feeds the heart muscle. A **cerebral thrombosis** is the closing off of a vessel that feeds the brain.

coronary = crowning (the heart)
thrombo = clot
cerebrum is part of the brain

embolus (EM-boh-luss): a thrombus that breaks loose. When it causes sudden closure of a blood vessel, it is an **embolism.**

embol = to insert

heart attack: the event in which an embolus lodges in vessels that feed the heart muscle, causing sudden tissue death. Also called **myocardial infarction.**

myo = muscle
cardial = of the heart
infarct = tissue death

stroke: the sudden shutting off of the blood flow to the brain by a thrombus or embolism.

pounds may contribute to the formation of clots. Substances released by platelets also may aggravate the growth of plaques.

A clot, once formed, may remain attached to a plaque in an artery and gradually enlarge until it shuts off the blood supply to that portion of the tissue supplied by the artery. That tissue may die slowly and be replaced by scar tissue. The stationary clot is called a thrombus, and when it has grown large enough to close off a blood vessel, it is a thrombosis. A coronary thrombosis is the closing off of a vessel that feeds the heart muscle. A cerebral thrombosis is the closing off of a vessel that feeds the brain.

A clot can also break loose, becoming an embolus, and travel along the system until it reaches an artery too small to allow its passage; there it gets caught. Then the tissues fed by this artery will be robbed of oxygen and nutrients and will die suddenly (embolism). Such a clot can lodge in an artery of the heart, causing sudden death of part of the heart muscle; we say the person has had a heart attack. When the clot lodges in an artery of the brain, killing a portion of brain tissue, we call the event a stroke.

On many occasions, it is unclear exactly what has caused a heart attack or stroke. An artery appears to go into spasms, and the blood supply to a portion of the heart muscle or brain is cut off, but examination reveals no visible cause. Much research today is devoted to asking what causes plaques to form, what causes arteries to go into spasms, what governs the activities of platelets and the synthesis of eicosanoids, and why the body allows clots to form unopposed by clot-dissolving cleanup activity.

Hypertension makes atherosclerosis worse. A stiffened artery, already strained by each pulse of blood surging through it, is more greatly stressed if the internal pressure is high. Lesions (injured places) develop more frequently, and plaques grow faster.

Atherosclerosis also makes hypertension worse. By hardening the arteries, it makes them unable to expand with each beat of the heart, so the pressure rises instead. This increased pressure leads to further hardening of the arteries, as already explained. Hardened arteries also fail to let blood flow freely through the body's blood pressure-sensing organs, the kidneys; the kidneys respond as if the blood pressure were too low—and raise it further. (Hypertension receives more attention in a later section of this chapter.)

■ TABLE 28–1
Risk Factors for Atherosclerosis

- Gender (being male)
- Glucose intolerance (diabetes)
- Heredity (history of CVD prior to age 55 in family members)
- High blood cholesterol, high LDL, and/or low HDL
- Hypertension
- Lack of exercise
- Obesity (30% or more overweight)
- Smoking
- Stress

Risk Factors for Atherosclerosis

Table 28–1 lists the risk factors for atherosclerosis. It befits a nutrition book to focus on dietary strategies to reduce these risk factors. It should be noted, though, that diet is not the only, and perhaps not even the most important, factor in the development of atherosclerosis. In fact, among the many controversies over diet and nutrition in recent years, one of the noisiest ones has been over the questions of how important diet is in heart disease; whether changes in diet can reduce the risk; and if so, whether such changes should be advocated for everyone or just for selected high-risk individuals. Form 28–1 on pp. 858–859 shows one way of calculating your risk score.

The big *diet-related* risk factors for atherosclerosis are obesity (see Chapter 12), glucose intolerance (explained in Chapter 27), hypertension (the subject of a later section in this chapter), and high blood cholesterol (discussed here). Table 28–2 provides the standards by which each of these risk factors for

■ TABLE 28–2
Standards for Atherosclerosis Risk Factors

Cholesterol[a]

Below 200 mg/dL (5.17 mmol/L) = desirable.[b]
200 to 239 mg/dL (5.17 to 6.18 mmol/L) = borderline high.[c]
240 mg/dL or higher (6.20 mmol/L) = high.[d]

Hypertension[e]

90 to 104 mm Hg = mild.
105 to 114 mm Hg = moderate.
115 mm Hg or higher = severe.

LDL[f]

Below 130 mg/dL (3.36 mmol/L) = desirable.
130 to 159 mg/dL (3.36 to 4.11 mmol/L) = borderline high.
160 mg/dL or higher (4.14 mmol/L) = high.

Obesity

BMI greater than 27.8 for men[g]
BMI greater than 27.3 for women[g]

Triglycerides

250 mg/dL or higher (2.82 mmol/L) = risk.[h]

[a]Based on the average of two cholesterol measurements that have been made within a 7- to 8-week time frame, and provided that the range between the two tests does not exceed 30 mg/dL (0.77 mmol/L). To convert cholesterol (mg/dL) to standard international units (mmol/L), multiply by 0.02586.
[b]Health care professionals recommend a follow-up checkup within 5 years.
[c]For people *without* definite cardiovascular disease (CVD) or two other CVD risk factors (one of which can be male gender), health care professionals recommend dietary changes and a follow-up checkup annually. For people *with* definite CVD or two other CVD risk factors (one of which can be male gender), health care professionals perform a lipoprotein analysis and take further action based on results.
[d]Health care professionals perform a lipoprotein analysis and take further action based on results.
[e]The diastolic pressure is the lower of the two numbers in the blood pressure reading—for example, the 70 in 105/70 mm Hg. The silver column that rises on a blood pressure instrument is a column of mercury (Hg); the height to which it is pushed is measured in millimeters (mm).
[f]To convert LDL (mg/dL) to standard international units (mmol/L), multiply by 0.02586.
[g]BMI (body mass index) is discussed on p. 362; see also Appendix E and the inside back cover.
[h]High triglycerides are not normally indicative of direct risk, but may reflect carbohydrate sensitivity, impaired glucose tolerance, or diabetes, and these conditions are risk factors for CVD. To convert triglycerides (mg/dL) to standard international units (mmol/L), multiply by 0.01129.

Source: The 1988 Report of the Joint National Committee on Detection, Evaluation, and Treatment of High Blood Pressure and the Report of the Expert Panel on the Detection, Evaluation, and Treatment of High Blood Cholesterol in Adults.

atherosclerosis is labeled "high." Additionally, the distribution of body fat shows an association with CVD independently of obesity alone. People with abdominal fat (apple shaped) have a greater risk for atherosclerosis than do people with hip and thigh fat (pear shaped).

Controversy surrounds the question of how cholesterol is linked to CVD. No one disputes that high *blood* cholesterol, particularly high LDL, predicts CVD, but researchers do dispute the hypothesis that links *diet* to CVD. The hypothesis has two parts: (1) that high blood cholesterol (LDL) is at least partly caused by a diet high in saturated fat and cholesterol; and (2) that reducing the amounts of saturated fat and cholesterol in the diet will lower blood cholesterol, thus reducing the rate of CVD.

Both parts of this hypothesis have some strong support, but pieces are missing. With respect to the first part (whether a high-fat diet elevates blood

■ FORM 28–1
Heart Disease Risk Scorecard

What is your heart disease risk score? Some of the following risk factors are powerful predictors of heart disease. Respond to each of the statements below and give yourself a score in each of the twelve categories listed. Then total your points to determine your degree of risk.

Age	If you are:		
	56 or over	1	_____
	55 or under	0	_____
Sex	If you are:		
	Male	1	_____
	Female	0	_____
Family history	If you have blood relatives who have had a:		
	Heart attack or stroke before age 60	12	_____
	History of heart disease at or before age 60	10	_____
	Heart attack or stroke after age 60	6	_____
	No history of heart disease	0	_____
Personal history	If you are:		
	50 or under and have had a heart attack, stroke, or cardiovascular surgery	20	_____
	51 or over and have had any of the above	10	_____
	None of the above	0	_____
Diabetes	If onset of diabetes appeared:		
	Before age 40 and you take insulin	10	_____
	At or after 40 and you take insulin or pills	5	_____
	After age 55 and you control it with diet	3	_____
	No diabetes	0	_____
Smoking	If you smoke:		
	2 packs/day	10	_____
	1 to 2 packs/day or quit within past year	6	_____
	6 or more cigars/day or use a pipe regularly	6	_____
	Less than 1 pack/day or quit over a year ago	3	_____
	Never smoked	0	_____
Cholesterol	If your cholesterol level is:		
	240 or higher	10	_____
	200 to 239	5	_____
	199 or lower	0	_____

cholesterol), blood cholesterol can be raised in both animals and people by raising the amounts of saturated fat and cholesterol in their diets—but whether the high blood cholesterol we see among so many people in the real world is *caused* by that aspect of their diets has been impossible to demonstrate. With respect to the second part (reducing fat and cholesterol intakes will reduce the risk of CVD), it is possible to lower blood cholesterol somewhat in both animals and people by reducing the amounts of saturated fat and cholesterol in their diets—but whether this reduces their risks of heart disease has been impossible to demonstrate.

Most investigators and organizations, including the American Heart Association, however, see links between our high-fat, high-cholesterol diet and heart disease, and they hold out the hope that continued research will

■ FORM 28–1
Heart Disease Risk Scorecard   (continued)

If you do not know your cholesterol level, answer the diet question. If you answered the cholesterol question, skip the diet question.

Diet	If you normally eat:		
	Red meat daily; more than 7 eggs weekly; and butter, whole milk, and cheese daily ..	8	_____
	Red meat 4 to 6 times weekly; margarine, low-fat dairy products, and some cheese ..	4	_____
	Poultry, fish, little or no red meat; 3 or fewer eggs weekly; some margarine, nonfat milk and milk products	0	_____
Blood pressure	If either number is:		
	160 over 100 or higher	10	_____
	140 over 90 but less than 160 over 100	5	_____
	If both numbers are less than 140 over 90	0	_____
Weight	Using the formula, 110 lb + 6 lb per inch over 5 feet for men, or 100 lb + 5 lb per inch over 5 feet for women, if you are:		
	25 lb overweight	4	_____
	10 to 24 lb overweight	2	_____
	Less than 10 lb overweight	0	_____
Exercise	If you engage in aerobic exercise more than 20 minutes:		
	Less than once a week	4	_____
	1 to 2 times a week	2	_____
	3 or more times a week	0	_____
Stress	When waiting, if you are:		
	Frustrated and easily angered	4	_____
	Impatient and occasionally moody	2	_____
	Comfortable and easygoing	0	_____
	TOTAL POINTS		_____

If you answered the blood pressure question:

High risk	36 and above
Medium risk	19 to 35
Low risk	18 and below

If you did not answer the blood pressure question:

High risk	40 and above
Medium risk	20 to 30
Low risk	19 and below

Note: A high score does not mean you will develop heart disease. It should, however, awaken you to the potential risk. Consult your physician if you have questions about your score results.

Source: Adapted from Arizona Heart Institute, Cardiovascular Risk Factor Analysis.

confirm and clarify these relationships.* The consensus seems to be that while experimental work continues, everyone over two years of age should be screened for high blood cholesterol, and those at high risk should be treated first with diet and then, if necessary, with drugs to bring their cholesterol levels down.[4]

---

*The American Heart Association provides many pamphlets and recipe booklets to consumers without charge. For suggestions on how to make recommended dietary changes, call your local American Heart Association office or write to the national office (address in Appendix F).

Low HDL
relative to LDL.

Increased risk of
heart attack.

High HDL
relative to LDL.

Decreased risk of
heart attack.

■ **FIGURE 28–2**
HDL and LDL as Predictors of Risk

HDL = **H**ealthy.
LDL = **L**ess-healthy.

hyperlipidemia (HIGH-per-LIP-ih-DEE-me-ah): elevated blood lipids. This term is often used interchangeably with **hyperlipoproteinemia** (HIGH-per-LIP-oh-PRO-teen-EE-me-ah), or elevated blood lipoproteins.

fat-controlled diet: a diet that prescribes both the amount and type of fat allowed; in contrast, a low-fat diet restricts total fat without particular concern for the type of fat.

As mentioned, the blood cholesterol of concern in atherosclerosis risk is LDL cholesterol. In general, the more elevated the LDL cholesterol, the greater the risk of coronary heart disease. (Recall from Chapter 5 that cholesterol is carried in several lipoproteins, chief among them LDL and HDL.) The HDL also carry cholesterol, but raised HDL concentrations relative to LDL represent cholesterol on its way out of the arteries back to the liver, and thus a reduced risk of developing atherosclerosis and a reduced risk of heart attack (see Figure 28–2). Cholesterol carried in LDL correlates *directly* with heart disease, whereas HDL cholesterol correlates *inversely* with risk. Ways to raise HDL include weight reduction, exercise, and dietary changes to slow the advance of atherosclerosis.

The goal of dietary measures to slow the advance of atherosclerosis is to reduce total blood cholesterol, and particularly LDL cholesterol. The measures recommended by a review panel of experts involve a two-step plan, shown in Table 28–3. If step 1 brings high blood cholesterol down, good; if not, the therapy goes on to step 2. Step 1 involves a total fat intake of less than 30 percent of kcalories, with saturated fatty acids only one-third of that and dietary cholesterol less than 300 milligrams a day. Step 2 reduces saturated fat and cholesterol further, as shown. Experts recommend that anyone attempting to lower blood cholesterol on medical advice work closely with a registered dietitian to master the practical application of these instructions.

Hyperlipidemias

Some people may have abnormal lipid profiles (high in chylomicrons, VLDL, or LDL and low in HDL) due to such poor health habits as overeating, overconsumption of fat, or underactivity, but some may have them for genetic reasons or secondary to other diseases. Disorders of blood lipid regulation known as the hyperlipidemias can cause atherosclerosis to advance rapidly. Depending on the disorder, different lipoproteins in the blood may be altered in concentration or character, and different dietary measures may be recommended to control them. Several hyperlipidemias call for a fat-controlled diet. These dietary measures may be effective when used to treat people with high blood cholesterol due to particular hyperlipidemias, but people with high blood cholesterol due to other causes may not, of course, respond.

Table 28–4 shows one of the most widely used systems for classifying hyperlipidemias. This system identifies six basic types of hyperlipidemias:

■ TABLE 28–3
Diet to Reduce Blood Lipids

	Total Fat	Saturated Fatty Acids	Polyunsaturated Fatty Acids	Monounsaturated Fatty Acids	Complex Carbohydrates	Protein	Cholesterol
Step 1	< 30%	< 10%	up to 10%	10 to 15%	50 to 60%	10 to 20%	< 300 mg/day
Step 2	< 30%	< 7%	up to 10%	10 to 15%	50 to 60%	10 to 20%	< 200 mg/day

Note: All but cholesterol are expressed as percentages of total food energy. Total food energy intake should be such as to achieve and maintain desirable weight.

Source: Adapted from N. D. Einst and J. C. LaRosa, Recommendations for treatment of high blood cholesterol: The National Cholesterol Education Program Adult Treatment Panel, *Contemporary Nutrition* 13 (1): 1988.

■ **TABLE 28–4**
The Hyperlipidemias

Type	Lipoprotein Abnormality
I	Elevated chylomicrons, triglycerides, and cholesterol
IIa	Elevated LDL and cholesterol
IIb	Elevated LDL, VLDL, cholesterol, and triglycerides
III	Elevated VLDL, cholesterol, and triglycerides
IV	Elevated VLDL; normal or elevated cholesterol and triglycerides
V	Elevated chylomicrons, VLDL, triglycerides, and cholesterol

Types I, IIa, IIb, III, IV, and V. The table also shows which lipids and lipoproteins are elevated in each type of hyperlipidemia.

The specifics of the lipid abnormalities and diet modifications may overwhelm you if you try to memorize the details. Instead, look for an overall understanding of the concepts as summarized in Table 28–5. For example, for clients with elevated chylomicrons (as in Type I) a low-fat diet is recommended—that is, a diet that limits the total amount of fat, but not necessarily the type. This makes sense, since chylomicrons initially transport all dietary fats. Clients might benefit from the use of MCT oil because medium-chain triglycerides enter the blood directly, bypassing the need for a chylomicron carrier.

The person with Type I hyperlipidemia also needs to avoid alcohol since alcohol raises serum triglyceride levels. Furthermore, Type I hyperlipidemia often develops secondary to alcohol abuse or pancreatitis, both of which require alcohol abstention.

Types IIa and IV are by far the most common, and they are associated with an increased risk of CVD. In Type IIa, dietary treatment aims at lowering blood cholesterol primarily by restricting cholesterol and saturated fat intakes and by substituting polyunsaturated fats for saturated fats. In Type IV, the focus is on lowering blood triglycerides primarily through weight loss. The

A cluster of symptoms associated with markedly elevated levels of chylomicrons in the blood is called **chylomicronemia** (KYE-lo-MY-crow-NEE-me-ah) **syndrome.** Lipid deposits in the skin and retina, as well as acute pancreatitis, are some characteristics of this syndrome.

An excessive amount of triglycerides in the blood is called **hypertriglyceridemia.** An excessive amount of cholesterol in the blood is called **hypercholesterolemia.**

■ **TABLE 28–5**
Dietary Approaches for Lowering Blood Lipids

Elevated Lipid	Major Lipoprotein Involved	Dietary Approach
Dietary triglycerides	Chylomicrons	Total fat restriction
Triglycerides	VLDL	Weight reduction Restriction of total fat to less than 20 to 30% of total kcalories
Cholesterol	LDL	Restriction of saturated fat to 10% of fat kcalories Restriction of cholesterol to 100 to 300 mg/day

Note: In heart disease, cholesterol, triglycerides, or both tend to be elevated. Since these lipids are carried through the blood in the lipoproteins, different lipoproteins are also elevated. For example, when cholesterol levels are high, LDL are elevated; when triglycerides are high, VLDL or chylomicrons are elevated. An elevation of any lipoprotein is called *hyperlipoproteinemia.*

weight-reduction diet limits the client's total fat intake. In addition, the diet moderately restricts cholesterol, substitutes polyunsaturated fats for saturated fats, and limits concentrated sweets.

As a rule, physicians do not prescribe drugs to treat hyperlipidemias until after a three-month trial period on the recommended diet has proven unsuccessful in lowering blood lipid concentrations. Drugs lower blood lipid concentrations at different sites of action. Some work in the GI tract to form insoluble complexes with bile, thus partially removing bile from the entero-hepatic cycle (p. 121). This loss of bile leads to an increased production of bile from serum cholesterol, thus lowering serum cholesterol levels. Other drugs work in the body after lipids have been absorbed by different mechanisms. For example, some drugs increase the rate of LDL breakdown while others inhibit the synthesis of cholesterol in the liver. Some drugs mainly lower triglycerides; others more effectively lower cholesterol. All of these drugs can impair nutrition status by causing GI distress and interfering with food intake (see Table 28–6).

> Drugs that lower serum lipid levels are called **antihyperlipemic agents.**

Because factors other than diet can also raise blood lipid levels, clients must make other lifestyle changes as well. They may want to exercise to help with weight loss or to stop smoking cigarettes to improve cardiovascular health. Exercise helps lower LDL cholesterol and raise HDL cholesterol levels. If heart and artery disease has already set in, a monitored exercise program may actually help to reverse it. Exercise may stimulate development of new arteries to nourish the heart muscle, and this may be a factor in the excellent recovery seen in some heart attack victims who exercise.[5] These general guidelines for treating atherosclerosis parallel the suggestions for preventing it provided later in this chapter.

Anyone concerned with atherosclerosis, and the risk of cardiovascular disease it presents, must also be concerned about hypertension. The two, together, are a threatening combination.

■ *Hypertension*

> **hypertension:** high blood pressure.

People cannot tell if they have hypertension; it presents no obvious symptoms. But for people who do have it, it threatens to impair the quality of life and bring on a premature death.

Chronic elevated blood pressure, or hypertension, is the most prevalent form of cardiovascular disease, believed to affect some 60 million people in the United States—more than a third of the entire adult population.[6] It contributes to half a million strokes and over a million heart attacks each year.[7] The higher the blood pressure is above normal, the greater the risk of heart disease. (Low blood pressure, on the other hand, is generally a sign of long life expectancy and low heart disease risk.)

How Hypertension Develops

The blood pressure is vital to life. It pushes the blood through the major arteries into smaller arteries and finally into tiny capillaries whose thin walls

■ TABLE 28–6
Drugs Used to Lower Blood Lipids

Drug Name	Timing with Meals	Common Side Effects That May Influence Nutrition Status
Cholestyramine	Give with water or other fluids; never give dry or with carbonated beverages.	Nausea, vomiting, abdominal discomfort, gas, diarrhea, constipation, heartburn, steatorrhea, anorexia, altered taste perception. May decrease absorption of calcium, fat, vitamins A, D, K, B_{12}, folate, and glucose. Depletes iron stores.
Colestipol	(same as above)	(same as above)
Clofibrate	Give with meals.	Nausea, vomiting, abdominal discomfort, loose stools, gas, aftertaste, altered taste perception, increased appetite. May decrease absorption of glucose, iron, and vitamin B_{12}. May induce anemias.
Gemfibrozil	Give ½ hour before meals.	Nausea, vomiting, abdominal discomfort, gas, constipation. May induce anemia.
Lovastatin	Give with meals.	Diarrhea, gas, constipation, abdominal pain, heartburn, nausea, indigestion, altered taste perception.
Nicotinic acid	Give with meals.	Nausea, vomiting, abdominal discomfort, diarrhea. Flushing. Decreased glucose tolerance.
Probucol	Give with meals.	Nausea, vomiting, gas, abdominal discomfort, diarrhea, anorexia, altered taste and smell perceptions.

Source: Adapted from D. E. Powers and A. O. Moore, *Food Medication Interactions,* 6th ed. (Phoenix, Ariz.: Food Medication Interactions, 1989).

permit exchange of fluids between the blood and the tissues (see Figure 28–3 on the next page). When the pressure is right, the cells receive a constant supply of nutrients and oxygen and are relieved of their wastes.

The pressure the blood exerts on the inner walls of the arteries is the result of two forces acting together: the heart's pushing the blood into the arteries, and the smallest arteries and capillaries resisting its flow. The heart's push ensures blood circulation through the whole system; the peripheral resistance and resulting pressure ensure some of the blood's components, including nutrients, are pushed through the capillary walls to feed the tissues. One other factor contributes to blood pressure: the volume of fluid in the vascular system—and that, in turn, is affected by the number of dissolved particles it

peripheral resistance: resistance to the flow of blood caused by a reduced diameter of the vessels at the periphery of the body—the smallest arteries and capillaries.

■ FIGURE 28–3
The Blood Pressure
Two major contributors to the pressure inside an artery are the heart's pushing blood into it, and the small-diameter arteries and capillaries at its other end resisting the blood's flow (peripheral resistance). Another determining factor is the volume of fluid in the circulatory system, which depends in turn on the number of dissolved particles in that fluid.

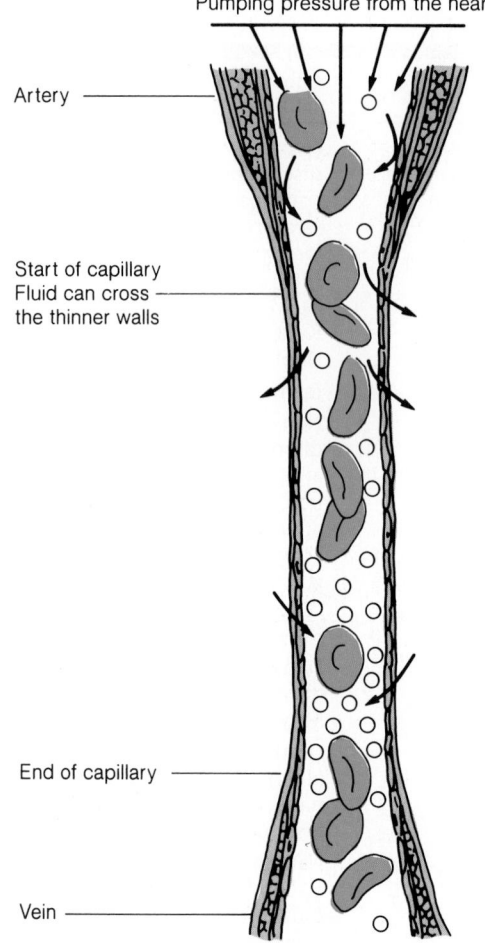

Pumping pressure from the heart

Artery

Fluid can't cross the thick wall of the artery.

Start of capillary
Fluid can cross the thinner walls

Blood pressure forces the fluid across the wall at the start of the capillary. Small molecules, oxygen, glucose, amino acids, and salts move out with the water.

Fluid is being forced out by blood pressure.

Blood proteins and cells remaining are becoming more concentrated. Blood pressure is decreasing.

Blood is now so concentrated that it attracts fluid back into the capillary.[a] Small molecules (waste products) accompany the fluid.

End of capillary

Vein

[a] The pressure that draws fluid back into the vein is osmotic pressure.

contains. By the rule of osmosis, the more dissolved particles in the blood, the more water there will be. Figures 10–3 and 10–4 on pp. 277–278 showed how the system works; Figure 28–3 shows the forces contributing to blood pressure.

The kidneys depend on the blood pressure to help them filter waste materials out of the blood into the urine (you may want to review Figure 3–12 on p. 59). The pressure has to be high enough to force the blood's fluid out of the capillaries into the kidney's filtering networks. If the blood pressure is too low, the kidneys set in motion actions to raise it, as shown in Figure 28–4. These actions constrict the peripheral blood vessels and lead to the retention of water in the body.

Dehydration sets these actions in motion, which is beneficial, because when the blood volume is low, higher blood pressure is needed to deliver substances to the tissues. By constricting the blood vessels and conserving water and sodium, the kidneys ensure normal blood pressure until the dehydrated person can drink water.

Atherosclerosis also sets this process in motion, but this is not beneficial. Atherosclerosis, by obstructing blood vessels, fools the kidneys: they react as

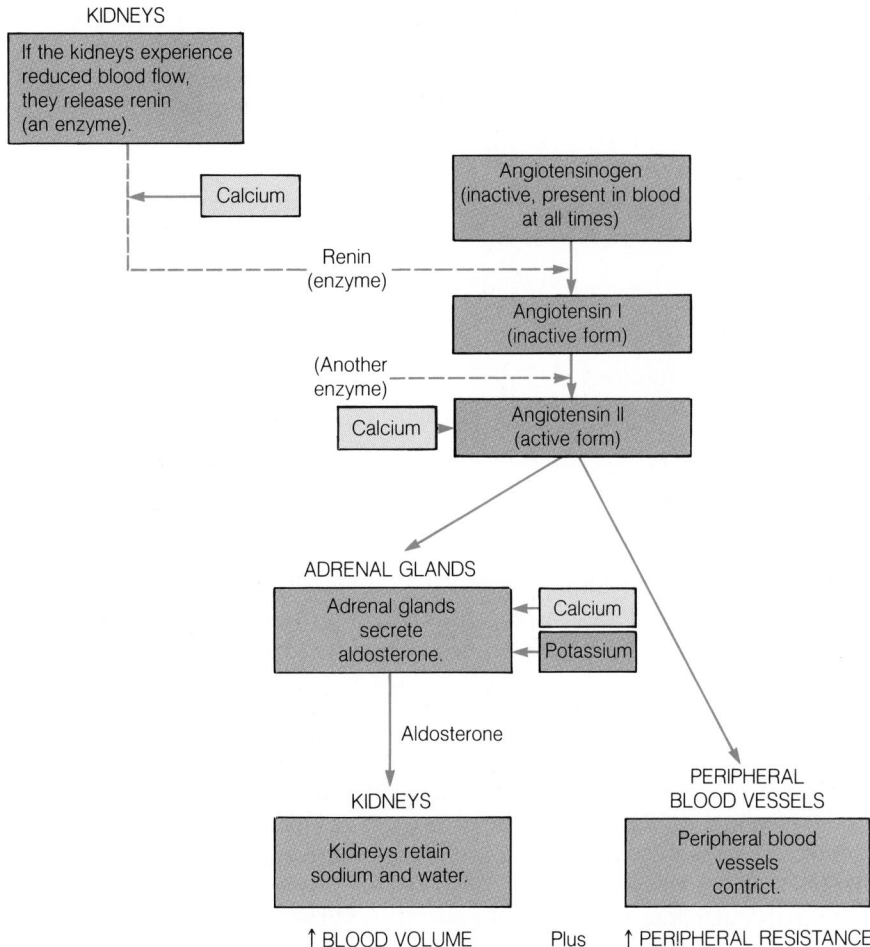

■ **FIGURE 28–4**
How the Kidneys Regulate Blood Pressure
When the kidneys experience reduced blood flow, they raise blood pressure by two means: (1) increasing blood volume and (2) increasing peripheral resistance. Calcium and potassium are two nutrients involved in this response.

if there were a water deficiency. Actually, the blood pressure may be normal initially, and the kidneys raise it too high. Such a response has harmful effects on the heart, which has to pump blood against this increased pressure. Only when the blood pressure is high, straining the heart, do the kidneys obtain enough pressure to filter the blood properly. As mentioned earlier, hypertension aggravates atherosclerosis by mechanically injuring the artery linings, making plaques likely to form; this may raise the blood pressure further, and so the problem intensifies.

Obesity makes hypertension still worse. Added adipose tissue means miles of extra capillaries through which the blood must be pumped. The combination of hypertension, atherosclerosis, and obesity puts a severe strain on the heart and arteries, leading to many forms of cardiovascular disease and death. Strain on the heart's pump, the left ventricle, can enlarge and weaken it, until finally it fails (heart failure). Pressure in the aorta may cause it to balloon out and burst (aneurysm). Pressure in the small arteries of the brain may make them burst and bleed (stroke). The kidneys can be damaged when the heart is unable to adequately pump blood through them (kidney failure).

While researchers continue looking for the cause or causes of hypertension, clearly it is urgent we do what we can to detect and treat it wherever it presents its deadly threat—or better still, prevent it. A major national effort has been made to identify and treat hypertension. Even mild hypertension can be dangerous; however, individuals who have it benefit from treatment, showing a reduced incidence of early death and illness. Sometimes diet changes alone, even without the drugs used to reduce blood pressure, can bring about these benefits without the undesirable side effects of the drugs.

Risk Factors for Hypertension

Epidemiological studies have identified several risk factors to predict the development of hypertension, including:

- *Age.* Blood pressure levels increase with age; most people who develop hypertension do so in their 50s and 60s.
- *Family background.* A family history of hypertension and heart disease raises the risk of developing hypertension two to five times.
- *Obesity.* Obese people are more likely to develop hypertension.
- *Race.* Hypertension is twice as common among blacks as among whites; it tends to develop earlier and become more severe.

Also, hypertension appears to be an insulin-resistant state. This observation holds true even in the absence of obesity and may reflect the operation of a factor common to both hypertension and diabetes. Perhaps insulin itself acts, in some way, at some times, as a causal agent of hypertension.[8] A tantalizing bit of information suggestive of the nature of this link is that insulin enhances the kidney's reabsorption of sodium.[9] Insulin also stimulates the activity of the hormones associated with the stress response, which raise blood pressure.

Of particular interest to this discussion is, What *diet-related* factors affect blood pressure? Most people might respond ''salt'' (meaning sodium), but research into sodium's role has disappointed investigators who hoped they were on the track to a single answer. Many other factors are suspect.

Weight Control   Evidence supports the positive link between obesity and hypertension already mentioned. (This is not to say that every obese person becomes hypertensive, or that all people with hypertension are overweight, but those who are obese and hypertensive should sit up and take notice.) Weight reduction in overweight people with hypertension significantly lowers blood pressure. This is so even if a person does not go all the way to achieve ideal body weight. Those who are using drugs to control their blood pressure can often reduce or discontinue use of them if they lose weight.[10] Even a 10-pound weight loss in people who have used hypertensive drugs for five years more than doubles the chance they can normalize their blood pressure without drugs.[11] Weight loss alone may be one of the most effective nondrug treatments for hypertension.[12]

Exercise, of course, is part of the energy balance equation (see Chapters 12 and 13). The more you exercise, the more energy you spend, and the less fat you accumulate (or the more you take off). But moderate exercise of the right kind also helps directly to lower the resting heart rate and blood pressure.[13]

The "right kind" of exercise is *not* the short-duration, heavy weight-lifting type. It is the aerobic, endurance type, such as walking, swimming, bicycling, or jogging. Undertaken faithfully as a daily or every-other-day routine, aerobic exercise strengthens the heart and blood vessels and permanently alters body composition in favor of lean over fat tissue. Such exercise training increases the volume of oxygen the heart can deliver to the tissues at each beat, reducing its work load. It also changes the hormonal climate in which the body does its work (it alters stress hormone secretion in such a way as to lower blood pressure). It brings about a redistribution of body water and inhibits the aggregation of platelets, thus easing blood transit through the peripheral arteries.[14] Chapter 13 gives details on this kind of exercise.

Sodium/Sodium Chloride   Salt clearly has something to do with blood pressure. In fact, for years, research on populations has seemed to indicate high sodium intakes were "the" factor responsible for people's high blood pressure; but recently that notion has been falling into disfavor. Much of the early research implicating sodium in hypertension's causation may have unwittingly uncovered the effects of sodium's silent partner, chloride, so now we talk in terms of salt.[15]

The salt concentration in the blood and other body tissues is maintained by the kidneys, the adrenal glands, the pituitary gland, and other glands. Most people can therefore safely consume more salt than they need, and rely on these control mechanisms to regulate its excretion and retention as needed. "Sodium-sensitive" individuals, however, experience high blood pressure from excesses in sodium or salt intake. People with chronic renal disease, those whose parents (one or both) have hypertension, blacks, and persons over 50 years of age are most likely to be sodium or salt sensitive.*[16]

Salt avoidance promises to help prevent hypertension in "salt-sensitive" individuals, but for others—the majority of people with hypertension—it may be an ineffective diet strategy. Salt restriction does not lower the blood pressure in half of the hypertensive people in whom it is tried.[17] It is important to look further to see what other dietary factors might be relevant.

Potassium   Some authorities believe potassium might both prevent and treat hypertension.** Even in people without high blood pressure, a high potassium intake protects against stroke and a low intake raises blood pressure.[18] So potassium in the diet seems worthy of attention. People who eat many foods high in salt often happen to be eating fewer potassium-containing foods at the same time. Table 10–4 on p. 285 showed that as the *same* food goes through several processing steps, it loses potassium and gains sodium, so its potassium-sodium ratio falls dramatically. Sodium avoidance may help in two ways, then—by reducing blood pressure in salt-sensitive individuals, and by indirectly raising potassium intakes in all individuals. A similar thing can be said of calcium, as the next paragraphs describe.

---

*Salt-sensitive individuals can be identified by measuring the renin in their blood (see Figure 28–4). Calcium and calcium channel blockers are useful in their treatment.

**People using diuretics to control hypertension should know some diuretics cause potassium excretion and can induce a deficiency. Those using these drugs must be particularly careful to include rich sources of potassium in their daily diets.

Calcium Several surveys report that people with hypertension consume less calcium than those with normal blood pressure.[19] Researchers estimate that people with the lowest calcium intakes (below 300 milligrams per day) have a two to three times greater risk of developing hypertension than people with the highest calcium intakes (1,200 milligrams per day).[20]

Calcium may be important in both prevention and treatment of hypertension. For those at risk of developing hypertension, maintaining a daily calcium intake consistent with the RDA may protect against it.[21]

For people already diagnosed with hypertension, obtaining adequate calcium in the diet may lower blood pressure. One study shows a calcium-rich diet reduced blood pressure in 44 percent of the people with hypertension studied. Even some (19 percent) of those with normal blood pressure experienced a reduction in their blood pressure.

It is recommended, therefore, that people with hypertension, or those at risk of developing it, *at least* meet the current RDA for calcium—800 milligrams a day for adults. Milk products are recommended, because they provide not only calcium, but also potassium and magnesium, which may also help keep blood pressure normal. Low-fat or nonfat milk products are the best choices, because fat contributes to hypertension, too.

Fat Fat is well known as a dietary factor contributing to atherosclerosis, but few people realize it plays an independent role in relation to blood pressure. Diets high in saturated fat are associated with hypertension. Populations consuming small quantities of animal products—vegetarians, for example—have a low incidence of hypertension (see Highlight 6 for more details).

When people restrict their total dietary fat and increase the ratio of polyunsaturated to saturated fatty acids in the diet to 1.0 or above, their blood pressure falls, regardless of whether it was their intent to make it do so.[22] This probably works at least partly by way of eicosanoids that regulate sodium excretion and peripheral blood vessel contraction and relaxation.

Alcohol Alcohol has several roles in relation to heart disease. In moderate doses, alcohol initially reduces pressure in the peripheral arteries and so reduces blood pressure, but high doses clearly raise blood pressure. In fact, of people with alcoholism, 30 to 60 percent have hypertension. Apparently, alcohol raises blood pressure directly, and presents as great a risk to cardiovascular disease as does hypertension caused by any other factor.[23] Furthermore, alcohol can induce strokes—even *without* hypertension.[24]

The surgeon general's advice on alcohol use is quite straightforward: if you drink, do so in moderation. *Moderation* means one to two drinks a day, not more.[25] The *NRC Recommendations* suggest that people do not use alcohol at all; for those who do drink, the NRC recommends limiting intake to 1 ounce pure alcohol. (For more on alcohol and nutrition, read Highlight 7.)

Other Factors Research is continuing to reveal relationships of other factors to hypertension. For example, magnesium seems to protect against it. Magnesium deficiency causes visible changes in the walls of arteries and capillaries and makes them tend to constrict, a possible mechanism for its hypertensive effect.[26] Since hypertension may also be an insulin-resistant state, it is possible that measures preventive against diabetes are also protective against hypertension.[27]

Treatment of Hypertension

The role of diet in the treatment of hypertension is fairly straightforward. The most effective dietary measure people with hypertension can take is to reduce weight if they are overweight. Because hypertensive people are at greater-than-normal risk for developing CVD, and because dietary fat and body fat contribute to hypertension, many professionals advise them to follow a fat-controlled diet. For the salt-sensitive person, it is also effective to restrict sodium, or at least salt, intake to 2 to 4 grams per day. Recommend that clients avoid foods high in salt and add no salt to foods at the table. Table 28–7 provides instructions for a no-added-salt diet.

When the body retains sodium, it excretes potassium. For this reason, people benefit from including good sources of potassium in their daily diets. When people with normal blood pressure eat foods high in sodium, ultimately their blood pressure rises—and at the same time, their potassium excretion increases. If they receive potassium simultaneously with the sodium, their blood pressure does not rise. Additionally, some diuretics used in the treatment of hypertension can lead to a potassium deficiency. Diuretics work by increasing fluid loss, thus lowering blood pressure. Table 28–8 (on pp. 870–872) includes a few of the diuretics used in the treatment of hypertension. People taking diuretics must be particularly careful to include good sources of potassium in their daily diets; their physicians may even advise them to use potassium supplements. Remind clients that whole foods of all kinds—fruits, vegetables, legumes, grains, meats, fish, and poultry—are good sources of potassium. Table 10–8 on p. 289 ranks some commonly eaten foods according to their potassium contents and Appendix H shows the potassium and sodium contents of foods. Watch for signs of hypokalemia, such as weakness (particularly of the legs), unexplained numbness or tingling sensation, cramps, irregular heartbeat, and excessive thirst and urination. Blood levels of potassium should be monitored regularly to prevent hypokalemia. A sample fat-controlled, no-added-salt, high-potassium diet menu is shown on page 873.

People may find it difficult to drastically reduce their sodium intake. Foods eaten without salt may taste unpalatable to the person who normally uses it liberally. Diet compliance is most unlikely when a person is handed an instruction sheet without additional encouragement or guidance.

In 1944, researchers found a diet consisting of rice, sugar, and fruit effective in the treatment of hypertension. Later studies revealed that the **Kempner rice diet** worked because it is very low in sodium. The diet is very restrictive, deficient in many nutrients, and no longer in use.

1 tsp of salt contains about 2 g of sodium.

hypokalemia (HIGH-po-ka-LEE-me-ah): low levels of potassium in the blood.

■ TABLE 28–7
No-Added-Salt Diet

- You may lightly salt foods during cooking, but do not add salt at the table.
- Avoid foods high in sodium, including:

  Meats—bacon; bologna; cold cuts; chipped or corned beef; frankfurters; smoked meats; sausage; salt pork or codfish; canned, salted, or smoked fish.

  Sauces, seasonings, and condiments—regular catsup; celery, garlic, and onion salt; regular chili sauce; commercial meat extracts; meat tenderizers; monosodium glutamate; olives; pickles; prepared mustard; soy and Worcestershire sauce.

  Other—regular canned or frozen soups; regular bouillon; soup mixes; pretzels, popcorn, crackers, nuts, potato chips, or other salted snack foods; sauerkraut; regular cheese; regular peanut butter.

- Low-sodium products can be substituted for regular foods.

■ TABLE 28–8
Drugs Used in the Treatment of Hypertension

Drug Name	Timing with Meals	Common Side Effects That May Influence Nutrition Status
Acebutolol	Give without regard to meals.	Constipation, gas, abdominal pain. May mask signs of hypoglycemia.
Amiloride HCl and hydrochlorothiazide	Give with food at the same time each day.	Anorexia, dry mouth, appetite changes, nausea, diarrhea, GI pain, constipation. May induce electrolyte imbalance and anemias.
Atenolol	Give without regard to meals.	Dry mouth, diarrhea, nausea. May mask signs of hypoglycemia.
Atenolol and chlorothalidone	Give on empty stomach same time each day.	Anorexia, diarrhea, nausea, vomiting, GI irritation, constipation. May induce hypokalemia, anemia.
Captopril	Give on empty stomach 1 hr before meals.	Altered taste perception, weight loss, sore mouth. May induce hypokalemia, anemias.
Chlorothiazide	Avoid natural licorice.	Nausea, vomiting, diarrhea, constipation, anorexia, dry mouth.
Chlorthalidone	Give with food 6 or more hr before bedtime. Avoid natural licorice.	Anorexia, dry mouth, GI irritation, nausea, vomiting, diarrhea, constipation.
Clonidine HCl		Dry mouth, weight gain, nausea, vomiting, constipation. May induce edema.
Deserpidine/ methyclothiazide	Give with food 6 or more hr before bedtime. Avoid natural licorice.	Dry mouth, weight gain, anorexia, nausea, vomiting, diarrhea, cramps.
Digitalis, digitoxin, digoxin	Give with water ½ hr before or 2 hr after food. Avoid natural licorice.	Nausea, vomiting. May inhibit glucose absorption.
Enalapril maleate	May give with food.	Altered taste perceptions, diarrhea, nausea, vomiting, abdominal pain.
Guanethidine sulfate	Give at same time each day. Avoid natural licorice.	Dry mouth, weight gain, diarrhea, nausea. May induce edema.
Guanfacine HCl		Constipation, nausea, vomiting, stomach cramps.
Hydralazine HCl	Give with food at the same time each day. Avoid natural licorice.	Anorexia, GI distress, constipation.

(continued)

■ TABLE 28–8
Drugs Used in the Treatment of Hypertension (continued)

Drug Name	Timing with Meals	Common Side Effects That May Influence Nutrition Status
Hydrochlorothiazide	Give with food 6 or more hr before bedtime. Avoid natural licorice.	Anorexia, dry mouth, nausea, vomiting, diarrhea, constipation. May alter insulin requirements in diabetes. May induce hypokalemia.
Indapamide	Give with food at the same time each day if GI distress.	Dry mouth, weight loss, anorexia, constipation, GI distress. May alter glucose tolerance.
Labetalol HCl	Give with food.	Altered taste perception, nausea, vomiting, indigestion. May mask signs of hypoglycemia.
Lisinopril		Diarrhea, vomiting.
Methyldopa	Avoid natural licorice.	Dry mouth, weight gain, diarrhea, nausea. May induce edema.
Metoprolol tartrate	Give with food.	Dry mouth, diarrhea, GI pain, gas, constipation, heartburn. May mask the signs of hypoglycemia.
Minoxidil	Give at same time each day.	May induce edema.
Nadolol	Give without regard to meals. Avoid natural licorice.	Dry mouth, constipation, GI distress, nausea, gas. May mask the signs of hypoglycemia.
Nifedipine	Give with food or milk.	Altered taste perception, nausea, diarrhea, constipation, cramps, gas. May induce edema.
Pindolol	Give without regard to meals.	Diarrhea, vomiting. May mask the signs of hypoglycemia. May alter glucose tolerance. May induce edema.
Prazosin HCl		Dry mouth, nausea, diarrhea, constipation, GI distress. May induce edema.

(continued)

■ TABLE 28−8
Drugs Used in the Treatment of Hypertension (continued)

Drug Name	Timing with Meals	Common Side Effects That May Influence Nutrition Status
Propranolol HCl	Give with food. Avoid natural licorice.	Dry mouth, constipation, GI distress, nausea. May mask the signs of hypoglycemia.
Rauwolfia serpentina	Give with food or milk to reduce GI irritation.	Anorexia, weight gain, dry mouth, diarrhea, nausea, vomiting, raises GI motility and gastric secretion. May lower glucose tolerance.
Spironolactone with hydrochlorothiazide	Give with food 6 or more hr before bedtime. Avoid natural licorice. Avoid salt substitutes.	Anorexia, cramps, diarrhea, nausea, vomiting. May alter serum glucose.
Terazosin HCl	Give without regard to meals at the same time each day.	Sore throat. Nausea. May induce edema.
Timolol maleate	Give with food at the same time each day.	Weight loss, nausea. May mask signs of hypoglycemia. May induce edema.
Triamterene with hydrochlorothiazide	Give with food or milk 6 or more hr before bedtime.	Dry mouth, thirst, dehydration, nausea, vomiting, diarrhea, constipation. May alter glucose levels.

Several tips can help clients adjust to a sodium-restricted diet. For one, recommend that clients reduce sodium gradually, allowing time to adjust to the flavor of unsalted foods. This suggestion implies that clients will receive regular follow-up visits, which also are important. Encourage clients to experiment with spices and herbs to add flavor to foods. Table 10−5 on p. 285 provides a list of spices and flavorings. Several cookbooks with helpful tips and low-sodium recipes are also available.

Teach clients to read labels and recognize sources of sodium (see Table 10−3 on p. 284). Local water supplies may have a high sodium content. When this water is used in food products, it may contribute significantly to sodium intake.

Medications such as antacids, antibiotics, cough medicines, laxatives, pain relievers, and sedatives may contain sodium. Some toothpastes and mouthwashes also contain large amounts of sodium; recommend that people rinse thoroughly after brushing their teeth or using a mouthwash, as well as that they avoid swallowing these compounds.

Food manufacturers have developed many low-sodium products for use with low-sodium diets. In general, clients can plan a palatable diet without

Sample Fat Controlled, No-Added-Salt, High-Potassium Diet Menu
Foods for this menu are prepared with little or no salt and a minimal amount of fat. The fats used for cooking or for flavor would be monosaturated and polyunsaturated.

using these products. Some people, however, like to use them to add variety. Clients need to be aware that many of these products are not sodium free, so the amount of sodium they do contain must be calculated into the diet. A sample fat-controlled, no-added-salt, high-potassium diet menu is shown above.

In salt substitutes, the sodium is generally replaced by potassium. Some people dislike the taste of salt substitutes but find them acceptable when used sparingly. Salt substitutes should not be used in cooking, though, because they turn bitter when heated. Often people find food more acceptable without any salt at all. The use of a potassium-containing salt substitute serves the dual purpose of increasing potassium intake while reducing sodium. Some products contain a combination of half regular table salt and half salt substitute. Although these products may be more palatable, they also can contribute a significant amount of sodium to the diet.

People with renal disease should not use potassium-containing salt substitutes.

When atherosclerosis and hypertension run their courses without treatment the consequences can be fatal. Most often, these conditions lead to heart attacks and strokes.

■ Heart Attacks

The heart receives its nutrients and oxygen not from inside its chambers, but from arteries on its surface (see Figure 28–5). As mentioned earlier, a heart attack, or myocardial infarction (MI), occurs when the supply of blood to the

---

Dietary Guidelines After an Myocardial Infarction (MI)

- Offer nothing by mouth until shock resolves; give IV fluids if necessary.
- After several hours, give a 1,000- to 1,200-kcal diet consisting of liquids or soft, bland foods of moderate temperature in small, frequent feedings.
- After 5 to 10 days, adjust the diet to meet individual needs, generally in 3 meals a day.

---

spasm: an involuntary, convulsive contraction.

rheumatic (roo-MAT-ik) **heart disease:** heart damage (often affecting the heart valves) that follows rheumatic fever (caused by a systemic bacterial infection).

■ FIGURE 28–5
The Coronary Arteries
The coronary arteries deliver nutrients and oxygen to the heart. When they become clogged, surgery may be prescribed. Coronary artery bypass surgery creates a shunt to allow blood to travel from a major artery to a coronary artery at a point beyond the obstruction.

heart muscle is cut off, causing tissue death. Most commonly, atherosclerosis contributes to heart attacks; other contributors include hypertension, abnormal blood clotting, spasms of the coronary arteries, infection of the membrane covering the heart, and rheumatic heart disease.

As an area of heart tissue dies, enzymes specific to heart cells leak out into the general circulation, much as digestive enzymes leak out of the pancreas in people with pancreatitis. Physicians use elevated concentrations of these enzymes in the blood to help diagnose heart attacks.*

The heart attack victim, like the accident victim, is in shock at first. Fluid leaves the vascular compartment and moves temporarily to the interstitial space. The person experiences this fluid shift as if it came from dehydration and complains of extreme thirst. The body does not need water during shock, however, and increasing the fluid load at such a time is unwise.

Do not offer water or food to people immediately after an MI. They commonly experience nausea at this time. If, as shock resolves, the person remains nauseated, start IV infusions to prevent dehydration.

After several hours of observation, the person can usually begin to eat (as outlined in the box above). The diet moderately restricts sodium (to about 2 grams) and food energy (to about 1,000 to 1,200 kcalories).

The diet begins with liquid or soft, bland foods that are easy to eat, given in frequent, small meals. Select foods that do not cause gas formation or abdominal distention. Abdominal distention pushes the diaphragm up toward the heart, thus adding stress on the heart muscle. Serve foods neither too hot nor too cold; temperature extremes can stimulate nerves to slow the heart rate. Many practitioners also restrict caffeine-containing beverages during the first few days after an MI, but this measure remains controversial.

After the immediate danger passes (about five to ten days), the diet changes to meet individual needs—for example, to treat hyperlipidemia, hypertension, obesity, diabetes, or the like. Oftentimes, clients need a diet to reduce weight, control fat, and moderately restrict sodium. Such a diet can be planned to provide three meals a day. People who continue to have chest pain after an MI, however, may benefit from eating small, frequent meals. Advise them to eat slowly and to avoid exercise immediately after meals.

---

*The enzymes that increase in the blood after a heart attack include serum glutamic-oxalacetic transaminase (SGOT), lactic dehydrogenase (LDH), and creatine phosphokinase (CPK).

Most of us know at least one person who seems destined for a heart attack: an overweight, hard-driving executive with hypertension who only jokes about exercising and dieting. Then one day it happens. When you visit this person in the hospital, you can hardly believe your ears.

Overnight, it seems, your friend's attitude has changed dramatically. Facing mortality, your friend places a new value on life and respects any advice the health care team offers. The time has arrived to take positive steps toward changing lifestyle habits and improving the chances for survival.

Your friend's attitude is typical of a MI victim. Like a sponge, he or she eagerly soaks up any helpful advice. You will find such clients most enjoyable to work with, for they listen carefully and try hard to follow advice.

Be sure to seize the opportunity. Offer sound and useful counsel. The person will benefit from your suggestions, and you will be rewarded by the person's interest and appreciation. Continue to offer support and encouragement as long as possible. MI clients might readily return to their old habits when their symptoms disappear if they haven't fully incorporated new healthful behaviors into their lives.

Strokes

When a stroke occurs, so that blood flow to part of the brain becomes insufficient, or when blood vessels burst and blood leaks into the brain tissue, the event is a cerebrovascular accident (CVA). Because a stroke involves the brain instead of the heart, it is a cerebrovascular, rather than a cardiovascular, disorder.

Recovery for some stroke victims is unremarkable. You may have no clue they even had a stroke. For others, recovery requires many months of rehabilitative therapy. They may suffer from temporary or permanent problems that interfere with the ability to eat or to communicate. Inability to communicate effectively makes it difficult for them to tell health care providers about foods they would like to eat or about problems they may be having with meals.

Food energy may need to be limited due to inactivity. Clients who must relearn how to walk or use other muscle groups will be better able to do so if they are not overweight. However, underweight can be a problem for physical rehabilitation also, and care should be taken to ensure the person does not become malnourished.

Many stroke victims have either temporary or permanent problems with chewing, swallowing, and the physical process of eating. Highlight 21 provides ways to overcome such problems. Tube feedings often are indicated initially until these problems are resolved. Longterm diet therapy for stroke victims depends on the underlying medical condition (such as hyperlipidemia, hypertension, atherosclerosis, or obesity).

Atherosclerosis and hypertension are not alone in limiting the flow of blood through the body; neither are heart attacks and strokes the only potentially fatal problems of the heart and blood vessels. Congestive heart failure stands out as another heart disease that threatens life.

Congestive Heart Failure

congestive heart failure (CHF): a syndrome in which the heart can no longer adequately pump blood through the circulatory system.

Many disorders—CVD, hypertension, and kidney disease—can lead to congestive heart failure (CHF). In CHF, the heart can no longer pump enough blood through the circulatory system. As a result, blood flow to the kidneys decreases. This change signals the kidneys to retain fluid. The retained fluid increases the load on the heart and further weakens it. Since the heart cannot effectively pump out blood entering the heart from the veins, peripheral, and sometimes pulmonary, edema develops. The person becomes "congested" with excess fluids. The heart enlarges and begins to beat more rapidly to try to compensate for its inability to pump. CHF threatens life, particularly when accompanied by pulmonary edema.

pulmonary edema: fluid in the lungs.

Enlargement of the heart is **cardiomegaly** (CAR-dee-oh-MEG-ah-lee). A rapid heart rate is **tachycardia** (TACK-ee-CAR-dee-ah).

  cardio = heart
  mega = large
  tachys = rapid

Heart disease that leads to protein-energy malnutrition, usually marasmus, is called **cardiac cachexia** (ka-KEKS-ee-ah). When the heart is weak, peripheral tissues fail to receive enough nutrients.

Another complication occurs because of the heart's inadequate pumping ability. The supply of nutrients and oxygen normally carried in the blood to the peripheral tissues is disrupted. Malnutrition can result, particularly as the disorder progresses. Other factors intensify the risk of malnutrition, including anorexia, altered taste sensitivity, intolerance to food odors, physical exhaustion precipitated simply by the act of eating, the diet used for treatment (some people find the diet unappealing), and the long-term use of medications that interfere with nutrition status. Undernutrition in these people often goes unnoticed, because edema masks their underweight condition. Malnutrition, in turn, can precipitate or aggravate heart failure.[28]

To provide adequate nutrients to the person with CHF is important, but to overfeed the severely malnourished person is a mistake. If refeeding occurs too rapidly, the blood volume and metabolic rate may increase to the point of overloading the already taxed heart. A gradual return to optimal intake is a wiser course.

The person with CHF may be underweight and malnourished, as just described. However, if the person is overweight, weight reduction will help to relieve stress to the heart.

People suffering from CHF can easily become exhausted when eating and may benefit from small, frequent meals and snacks. As in MI, provide small meals to reduce the abdominal distention that displaces the diaphragm toward the heart. Also, for the same reason, choose the foods least likely to form gas. Liquid formulas of high nutrient density may be useful, and if the

---

Dietary Guidelines for Congestive Heart Failure (CHF)

- Restrict sodium and fluids.
- Lose weight, if necessary.
- Eat small, frequent meals.
- Use foods least likely to cause abdominal distention.

person cannot eat enough food by mouth, tube feedings of such formulas may be necessary to prevent severe malnutrition. In some cases, TPN may be required, with particular care taken to ensure that the amount of fluid given will not overload the person.

A sodium- and fluid-restricted diet reduces the work required of the damaged heart and alleviates edema. Generally, a 2-gram-sodium diet and a fluid restriction of about 1½ to 2 liters of fluid daily can help prevent fluid overload and reduce diuretic needs. The box on the previous page outlines the dietary guidelines for CHF.

The treatment of CHF also involves the use of diuretics to promote fluid excretion and other drugs to increase the strength of heart muscle contractions (see Table 28–8). Bed rest helps to reduce the work load of the heart.

The accompanying "Clinical Detective Work" presents a CVD case study. Your careful consideration of the answers to the questions posed will help you to review the information presented to this point in the chapter.

Drugs used to increase the strength of the heart's contractions are **digitalis** (DIJ-ih-TAL-is) **glycosides.**

CLINICAL DETECTIVE WORK

Mr. Garrett, age 45, has just been diagnosed with Type IV hyperlipidemia. He is 5 ft 7 inches tall and weighs 200 lb. Mr. Garrett has a family history of CVD. His diet history shows excessive intakes of food energy, cholesterol, total fat, saturated fats, and sodium. He smokes a pack of cigarettes a day, and his lifestyle leaves him little room for exercise. Mr. Garrett also has hypertension, for which diuretics have been prescribed. He frequently forgets to take his pills, though, and his blood pressure is often quite high.

Name the risk factors for CVD in Mr. Garrett's history. Which of them can he control? Which can be helped by diet? What complications might you expect if his condition goes untreated?

What type of diet, if any, would you recommend for Mr. Garrett's type of hyperlipidemia? Explain the rationale for each diet change. How will his current diet change? What types of foods should he eat?

What type of diet, if any, would you recommend for Mr. Garrett's hypertension? What suggestions might you offer to help him make the necessary diet changes? Are these diet changes consistent with those you would recommend for Type IV hyperlipidemia? Plan a day's menu for Mr. Garrett based on the diet you would recommend for him.

What blood tests would you expect to see monitored regularly? Why?

Name at least three ways in which Mr. Garrett could benefit from losing weight. How does exercise fit into a weight loss plan?

Discuss nutrition considerations if Mr. Garrett should have a heart attack, develop congestive heart failure, or have a stroke. Describe the relationships of these disorders to hyperlipidemia and hypertension.

Disorders of the Lungs

The heart and lungs work together to ensure the delivery of oxygen to the cells of the body and to remove wastes generated by metabolic processes in these cells. Lung disorders, then, can affect nutrition status. In this section, two types of lung disorders, chronic obstructive pulmonary diseases (COPD) and respiratory failure are described, and their nutrition implications are explained.

Chronic Obstructive Pulmonary Diseases (COPD)

pulmonary (PULL-mow-na-ree): concerning or involving the lungs.

respiratory failure: failure of the lungs to perform.

chronic obstructive pulmonary diseases (COPD): disorders that cause blockage of the lungs' air passages and thus interfere with the exchange of gases between the air and the body.

emphysema (EM-fe-SEE-ma): a type of COPD in which the lungs lose their elasticity and the victim has difficulty breathing.

bronchitis (bron-KYE-tis): inflammation of the lungs' air passages.
  bronchos = wind pipe
  itis = inflammation

alveoli (al-VEE-oh-lie): air sacs in the lungs; one sac is an *alveolus.*

elastin: a flexible structural protein.

bronchioles (BRON-key-ohls): the small air passages from the trachea to the lungs.

Chronic obstructive pulmonary diseases (COPD) are conditions characterized by persistent obstruction of airflow through the lungs. The two major types of COPD are emphysema and chronic bronchitis. (Chapter 25's discussion on pancreatic disorders described cystic fibrosis, a less common form of COPD.) Like heart disease, COPD appears to be multifactorial. Smoking is the primary risk factor for COPD. Other risk factors are exposure to environmental pollution (including exposure of nonsmokers to cigarette smoke); alcohol consumption; family history of respiratory disorders; and, possibly, repeated respiratory tract infections in young children.

In emphysema, the small passages and air sacs (alveoli) within the lungs lose their elasticity. The victim can breathe air in, but has trouble exhaling it. Stale air containing an excess of carbon dioxide becomes trapped in rigid pockets in the lung, and the lung enlarges to accommodate the increased air volume. As the air pockets in the lung expand, their walls thin out; then they tend to collapse during exhalation. Emphysema is believed to be caused by the destruction of elastin, the major structural protein in healthy lungs.

The individual with chronic bronchitis suffers from a different problem. In chronic bronchitis, excessive mucus is produced and clogs the air passages (bronchioles). These passages also become inflamed, obstructing the airways further.

Regardless of the type of COPD, it gradually becomes more and more difficult for the lungs to deliver oxygen to the tissues and to remove carbon dioxide (a waste product of metabolism). No cure for COPD is available; treatment is aimed at relieving the symptoms. The prevalence of the disorder is increasing, and the search for ways to improve the length and quality of life for people with COPD continues.

At present, no known risk factors for the development of COPD are directly related to nutrition. However, malnutrition appears to play an indirect role in lung disorders. Consider that, in people who are starving, pneumonia is often the eventual cause of death. Malnutrition leads to deterioration of the lungs that interferes with their ability to exchange gases and also with their immune response. These changes significantly influence the likelihood and severity of pulmonary infections that can destroy lung tissue and lead to chronic lung disease.[29]

Regardless of whether malnutrition precedes COPD, COPD frequently results in malnutrition. Weight loss, emaciation, and infection are commonly recognized complications of COPD. People with pulmonary diseases account for many cases of malnutrition in hospitals. Nutrition status appears to correlate with the severity of pulmonary disease.

As COPD advances, the lungs lose mass and strength, and body weight decreases. Lung function is compromised, and pulmonary infections become more and more likely. Heart failure and mortality rates are higher in people with COPD who lose weight.

Some possible explanations as to why many individuals with COPD are at risk for poor nutrition status include:

- Anorexia and poor food intake.
- Increased energy expenditure associated with labored breathing.
- Steroid drug therapy that raises nutrient requirements and compromises nutrition status (see Table 23–4 in Chapter 23).
- Use of mechanical ventilators (people who require them are in a hypermetabolic state). Also, people requiring mechanical ventilation often experience weakness and discomfort which can interfere with nutrient intake.
- Repeated infections, which raise nutrient needs, and cause nutrient deficiencies. These, in turn, increase the likelihood of infection, a vicious cycle.

mechanical ventilator: a machine that "breathes" for the person who can't.

Weight loss in COPD may result from these factors, and also from an increased resting energy expenditure, which may be significantly higher in people with stable COPD who are malnourished than in people with stable COPD who are adequately nourished.[30] In one study, clients with stable COPD who weighed less than 75 percent of standard body weight reported higher energy and protein intakes than COPD clients with body weights closer to standard.[31] The authors of the study concluded that energy needs rise as the disease progresses, and that it was high needs, not poor intake, that explained weight loss in their subjects. Actually, though, both may contribute. A person with COPD may be unable to verbalize feelings of hunger and may not be able to take adequate nourishment.[32]

Repleting and maintaining nutrient stores for the person with COPD helps to maintain lung function and to prevent lung infections. However, overfeeding people with COPD can be as harmful as underfeeding them. Overfeeding produces higher carbon dioxide levels which the already stressed lungs must work hard to expel. Clients replete nutrient stores best when refed gradually. A severely depleted person may require long-term nutrition support.

Respiratory Failure

In today's intensive care units, respiratory failure is a frequent cause of illness and death. Respiratory failure can result from advanced COPD, severe stress, and many other disorders. In respiratory failure, a person's lungs are unable to exchange gases, and the person requires mechanical ventilation until able to breathe again.

Malnutrition can contribute to respiratory failure in several ways. Reduced lung muscle mass makes forceful respiratory movements impossible. Weak muscles fail to push blood along through veins and therefore experience poor circulation with consequent poor local nutrition. Poor respiration, circulation, and nutrition make pulmonary infections likely. Malnutrition manifested in low concentrations of serum proteins is reflected by a low osmotic pressure exerted by these proteins; this contributes to pulmonary edema.[33] Pulmonary edema increases the workload of the lungs. Given that the lung muscles are already weak, weaning the person from a ventilator may be increasingly difficult.

People in respiratory failure spend much energy breathing, eating, and moving in any way, especially during attempts to wean them from mechanical ventilation. High-energy, low-effort foods best support such people, and the types of energy nutrients in the foods make a difference. During metabolism, glucose generates more carbon dioxide per kcalorie delivered than does fat. Therefore, carbohydrate in excess of the body's needs taxes the lungs to rid the body of excess carbon dioxide. For this reason, authorities currently recommend that lipids supply from 50 to 60 percent of the total daily energy needs of people in respiratory failure.[34]

People in respiratory failure are often candidates for TPN. TPN solutions that contain less glucose than standard TPN solutions, and given with IV fat instead to augment energy intake, are appropriate. IV fat should be given slowly over 12 to 24 hours to permit optimal utilization.[35] Enteral formulas designed to meet the needs of people in respiratory failure have also been developed, but little information is available regarding the use of tube feedings for nutrition support of these individuals.* One study addressed this question and reported the successful use of enteral nutrition in a few people.[36]

Clearly there comes a time when lung disease has progressed too far to be reversible. As with all degenerative diseases, the best remedy is prevention. A note on prevention appears at the end of the next section.

▪ *Prevention of Cardiovascular and Lung Diseases*

For those Americans who do not smoke and do not drink excessively, the choices made about what to eat have the greatest influence on health. Each day, dietary decisions have the potential of limiting our risks for the leading causes of death—heart diseases. The following sections describe specific recommendations for the prevention of atherosclerosis, hypertension, and lung disease; notice how the sets of advice parallel and complement each other.

Prevention of Atherosclerosis

The diet to lower blood cholesterol is intended for people with high, or borderline high, cholesterol combined with other risk factors. Atherosclerotic disease is so common, however, that many experts advocate everyone's following similar advice. For those who choose to do so, pointers in the *NRC*

---

*Pulmocare (Ross Laboratories) is an enteral formula designed for use with respiratory failure.

Recommendations cited in Chapter 2 are worth emphasizing. Those relevant to atherosclerosis prevention are the first four, repeated here for reference:

- Keep total fat intake at 30 percent or less of kcalories. Keep saturated fat intake to less than 10 percent of kcalories, and the intake of cholesterol to less than 300 milligrams daily.
- Every day eat five or more half-cup servings of a combination of vegetables and fruits, especially green and yellow vegetables and citrus fruits. Also keep intake of starches and other complex carbohydrates high, by eating six or more daily servings of breads, cereals, and legumes. Carbohydrates should total more than 55 percent of kcalories.
- Maintain protein intake at moderate levels—that is, approximately the current RDA for protein, but not exceeding twice that amount, or 1.6 grams per kilogram of body weight for adults. This means limiting meat-fish-poultry intakes to about 4 to 6 ounces a day and using meat alternatives (legumes) in their place once a week or so.
- Balance food intake and physical activity to maintain appropriate body weight. An activity particularly effective in lowering LDL and raising HDL concentrations is frequent and sustained aerobic exercise; in fact, such activity may help to reverse atherosclerosis.

Saturated fats have received a lot of bad press for the role they play in raising blood cholesterol concentrations. While this is true for many saturated fats, not all saturated fats have the same effect on blood cholesterol. The saturated fats that cause cholesterol concentrations to climb include palmitic and myristic acids. Those fatty acids having no effect on cholesterol include stearic and lauric acids. The fat in milk is mostly saturated fat—and most of that is palmitic acid—so, choose nonfat and low-fat milk and milk products to reduce saturated fat intake and prevent blood cholesterol from rising. The fats in meats are mostly saturated, largely stearic acid; those in poultry and fish have a better balance between saturated and polyunsaturated fats. To keep fat intake moderate, select lean cuts of meat and poultry, trim the fat, remove the skin, and bake or broil it. In choosing dairy products look for nonfat and low-fat items and for those in which fat has been replaced by fat substitutes.

As for the other fat-contributing components of the diet, olive oil and canola oil are recommended selections among oils, for these are high in monounsaturated fatty acids—but like all fat, they should be used sparingly. Periodically, eat meals of fish, especially fatty fish, to help balance intakes of omega-6 fatty acids with the omega-3 type.

As far as cholesterol is concerned, feel free to use some eggs, but use them in moderation, unless medically advised otherwise. Eggs are an inexpensive source of high-quality protein, and while high in cholesterol, they are not as high as was once thought, and they are not high in saturated fat. Neither are shellfish as high in cholesterol as has been believed, and they do contain eicosapentanoic acid (EPA) and other omega-3 fatty acids. And eat foods high in soluble fiber—oats, oat bran, barley, and legumes—as well as fruits and vegetables, to help lower blood cholesterol.

Note that following these guidelines will do more than help ward off heart disease. Body weight has proven, in some studies, to be the most important single determinant of blood cholesterol level, but even if weight control does not reduce blood cholesterol, it will reduce blood pressure (see the next section). Exercise will also reduce blood pressure. So will eating a low-fat diet. Even if the high-fiber, high-complex-carbohydrate aspect does not reduce cholesterol, it will improve glucose tolerance (diabetes, remember from Chapter 27, is a major predictor of CVD). And even if the monounsaturated oils and the omega-3 oils from the fish do not lower blood cholesterol, they may help prevent heart disease by favoring the right eicosanoid balance so that clot formation is unlikely.

An adequate diet will protect the health of the heart muscle itself; mineral deficiencies precipitate disease of the muscle and arteries.[37] Also, plenty of whole, fresh plant foods benefit every aspect of health (not just from the heart disease angle). In addition, exercise daily. Don't smoke. Relax. Meditate or pray. Play. Happy people have lower blood cholesterol levels.

Prevention of Hypertension

The most effective single step you can take toward protecting yourself from hypertension is to find out whether you have it. At checkup time, a health care professional can give you an accurate resting blood pressure reading. (Self-test machines in drugstores and other places can mislead you by giving inaccurate readings.) If your resting blood pressure is above normal, the reading should be repeated before confirming the diagnosis of hypertension. Thereafter, it should be checked at regular intervals.

The first number in a blood pressure reading is the systolic pressure, and the second is the diastolic pressure. Resting blood pressure should probably be around 120 over 70, ideally. However, it is generally considered normal if it is less than 140 over 90. Above this level, the risks of heart attacks and strokes increase in direct proportion to increasing blood pressure, especially diastolic pressure. Return to Table 28–2 to see how to interpret your resting blood pressure.

As for dietary measures to prevent hypertension, many professionals and agencies believe enough evidence exists to warrant a recommendation to the general public to restrict salt intake moderately. They reason that, at worst, such a precaution cannot be harmful.

Probably, however, the person wishing to avoid hypertension can take many other more useful dietary measures. Start with weight control. Expend energy, so as to earn the right to eat more nutrient-dense foods—in other words, exercise. (If that benefit doesn't motivate you, then exercise to improve your circulation, reduce your weight, improve your morale, or make friends—but anyway, exercise.) Eat foods high in potassium (whole foods of all descriptions), high in calcium and magnesium (milk products and appropriate substitutes), and high in fiber (whole grains, legumes, vegetables, and fruits). The recommendations on dietary fat made earlier for atherosclerosis apply to hypertension too: limit total fat; limit saturated fat; and use monounsaturated and polyunsaturated fats, including fish oils. Vary your diet, because not all the factors affecting blood pressure have been studied yet. (Others are cadmium, selenium, lead, caffeine, and protein—some perhaps

systolic (sis-TOL-ik) **pressure:** the first figure in a blood pressure reading (the "dub" of the heartbeat), which represents the arterial pressure caused by the contraction of the left ventricle of the heart.

diastolic (dye-as-TOL-ik) **pressure:** the second figure in a blood pressure reading (the "lub" of the heartbeat), which represents the arterial pressure when the heart is between beats.

needed in greater quantities and some in less, so be moderate.)[38] Use moderation with respect to alcohol. The recommendations are similar to those made in relation to every other health goal mentioned since the start of Chapter 1.

Prevention of Lung Disease

For prevention of pulmonary disease the same common-sense guidelines apply. Don't smoke, and do obtain optimal nutrition and ample exercise. Strong, well-nourished lungs are best equipped to withstand impairment by injury and infection.

■ Nutrition Assessment

To help pinpoint areas of particular concern in the nutrition assessment of individuals with CVD or COPD, consider the following:

- For clients with CVD, pay particular attention to the total food energy intake and total fat intake if weight loss is needed. For clients with COPD, ensure an adequate energy intake to prevent weight loss.
- For clients with atherosclerosis, check the diet history for the cholesterol, saturated fat, and polyunsaturated fat content of the diet. Determine the dietary fiber intake as well.
- For clients with hypertension, in addition to energy and fat intake, examine the diet history for sodium or salt, potassium, calcium, and alcohol intake.
- Diet histories will help you determine which diet changes to recommend and how dramatic such changes might be for the individual to make. The medical history will alert you to other conditions, such as diabetes, that may alter treatment and nutrient needs.
- Generally, the only time anthropometric measurements pose a problem in people with CVD is when they have edema (such as in CHF). Weight gain, swelling in the extremities, and high blood pressure signal possible fluid retention.
- Expect abnormal lab values (for example, for albumin and transferrin) in people with either hypertension or CHF if they are retaining fluids. Monitor serum cholesterol and triglyceride levels in people with hyperlipidemia (review Table 28–2). Monitor serum potassium levels in people on diuretics.

In everyone you assess, look for factors in the history that increase the risk for CVD. Based on this information, you may be able to recommend diet and other relevant lifestyle changes before problems arise.

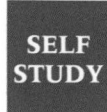

SELF STUDY *Diet to Prevent Cardiovascular Disease*

For this self-study exercise, take an optimistic, forward-looking stance. Plan a diet for a day that is truly excellent in preventive terms: low in fat, balanced in types of fat, low in cholesterol, low in salt, and rich in high-fiber and high-nutrient-density foods, including many whole foods that contain potassium, calcium, and magnesium (see the information on minerals in the earlier chapters of this book). If you are a vegetarian, include some cholesterol-lowering legumes in your main meal (tofu or other soy product, or beans). If you eat fish, plan a meal around a delicious fish dish.

Plan to make the day's meals as attractive and pleasing for yourself as you can, and eat as you have planned. Take note of your pleasures and report on them. Then keep in mind, henceforth, when advising clients, that the most healthful way to eat can also be the most enjoyable.

Study Questions

1. What is atherosclerosis? How can atherosclerosis lead to hypertension, thrombosis, heart attacks, and strokes?
2. What diet is recommended for all people to reduce the risk of heart disease? How do the recommendations change for the person with definite hyperlipidemias that involve elevated cholesterol and triglyceride levels?
3. Describe ways people can alter their diets to lower their blood cholesterol levels. Describe other measures that may be useful for lowering serum lipid levels.
4. What is hypertension? What causes hypertension?
5. Discuss the role of diet in hypertension. Describe some steps that people with hypertension can take to lower their blood pressure.
6. What is a myocardial infarction, and what events trigger an attack? Describe the diet therapy for a heart attack victim immediately after a heart attack, after several hours, and after a week. State the rationale for each diet modification you list.
7. Consider some of the ways in which a person's nutrition needs are affected by a stroke. How can nutrition affect the way a person responds to physical therapy?
8. What is congestive heart failure? Why is malnutrition common in the person with CHF?
9. Describe the diet recommended for the person with CHF. What is the rationale for each of the recommendations? Discuss some special concerns that must be considered when feeding the person with CHF by tube feeding or TPN.
10. What is COPD? Name the two major types of COPD and describe each.
11. How might nutrition play a role in the development of COPD?
12. What factors play a role in the weight loss frequently seen in people with COPD?
13. What is respiratory failure? How can malnutrition affect the course of respiratory failure?
14. Describe how the nutrient needs of the person with respiratory failure should be met.

Notes

1. *The Surgeon General's Report on Nutrition and Health: Summary and Recommendations*, DHHS (PHS) publication no. 88–50211 (Washington, D.C.: Government Printing Office, 1988).
2. *The Surgeon General's Report on Nutrition and Health: Summary and Recommendations*, 1988; Centers for Disease Control, Years of life lost from cardiovascular disease, *Journal of the American Medical Association* 256 (1986): 2794.
3. *The Surgeon General's Report on Nutrition and Health: Summary and Recommendations*, 1988; W. B. Kannel and T. J. Thom, Incidence, prevalence and mortality of cardiovascular diseases, in *The Heart*, 6th ed., ed. J. W. Hurst (New York: McGraw-Hill, 1986), pp. 557–565.
4. Lowering blood cholesterol to prevent heart disease, NIH Consensus Conference, *Journal of the American Medical Association* 253 (1985): 2080–2086; A. M. Gotto, Hypercholesterolemia: An assessment of screening and diagnostic techniques, *Modern Medicine*, April 1987, pp. 28–32.
5. K. Przyklenk and A. C. Groom, Effects of exercise frequency, intensity, and duration on revascularization in the transition zone of infarcted rat hearts, *Canadian Journal of Physiology and Pharmacology* 63 (1985): 273–278.
6. *The Surgeon General's Report on Nutrition and Health: Summary and Recommendations*, 1988.
7. Kannel and Thom, 1986.
8. E. Ferrannini and coauthors, Insulin resistance in essential hypertension, *New England Journal of Medicine* 317 (1987): 350–357; L. Landsberg, Insulin and hypertension: Lessons from obesity (editorial), *New England Journal of Medicine* 317 (1987): 378–379.
9. Ferrannini and coauthors, 1987; Landsberg, 1987.
10. M. Winston, Heart disease, in *Obesity and Weight Control*, eds. R. T. Frankle and M. Yang (Aspen: Aspen Publications, 1988), pp. 393–411.

11. H. G. Langford and coauthors, Dietary therapy slows the return of hypertension after stopping prolonged medication, *Journal of the American Medical Association* 253 (1985): 657–664.

12. S. Wassertheil and coauthors, Effective dietary intervention in hypertensives: Sodium restriction and weight reduction, *Journal of the American Dietetic Association* 85 (1985): 423–430.

13. L. G. Ekelund and coauthors, Physical fitness as a predictor of cardiovascular mortality in asymptomatic North American men, *New England Journal of Medicine* 319 (1988): 1379–1384.

14. Ekelund, 1988.

15. T. W. Kurtz, H. A. Al-Bander, and C. Morris, "Salt-sensitive" essential hypertension in men: Is the sodium ion alone important? *New England Journal of Medicine* 317 (1987): 1043–1048.

16. A. M. Altschul and J. K. Grommet, Sodium intake and sodium sensitivity, *Nutrition Reviews* 38 (1980): 393–402.

17. J. K. Huttunen and coauthors, Dietary factors and hypertension, *Acta Medica Scandinavica* (supplement) 701 (1985): 72–82.

18. G. G. Krishna, E. Miller, and S. Kapoor, Increased blood pressure during potassium depletion in normotensive men, *New England Journal of Medicine* 320 (1989): 1177–1182; L. Tobian, Potassium and hypertension, *Nutrition Reviews* 46 (1988): 273–283; F. C. Luft and M. H. Weinberger, Postassium and blood pressure regulation, *American Journal of Clinical Nutrition* 45 (1987): 1289–1294; K. T. Khaw and E. Barrett-Connor, Dietary potassium and stroke-associated mortality: A 12-year prospective population study, *New England Journal of Medicine* 316 (1987): 235–240.

19. H. Henry and coauthors, Increasing calcium intake lowers blood pressure: The literature reviewed, *Journal of the American Dietetic Association* 85 (1985): 182–185.

20. D. A. McCarron and coauthors, Blood pressure and nutrient intake in the United States, *Science* 224 (1984): 1392–1398.

21. D. A. McCarron and C. D. Morris, The calcium deficiency hypothesis of hypertension, *Annals of Internal Medicine* 107 (1987): 919–922.

22. R. Weinsier, Recent developments in the etiology and treatment of hypertension: Dietary calcium, fat, and magnesium, *American Journal of Clinical Nutrition* 42 (1985): 1331–1338.

23. A. L. Klatsky, G. D. Friedman, and M. A. Armstrong, The relationships between alcoholic beverage use and other traits to blood pressure: A new Kaiser Permanente study, *Circulation* 73 (1986): 628–636.

24. J. S. Gill and coauthors, Stroke and alcohol consumption, *New England Journal of Medicine* 315 (1986): 1041–1046.

25. A. L. Klatsky, M. A. Armstrong, and G. D. Friedman, Relationship of alcoholic beverage use to subsequent coronary artery disease hospitalization, *American Journal of Cardiology* 58 (1986): 710–714.

26. M. R. Joffres, D. M. Reed, and K. Yano, Relationship of magnesium intake and other dietary factors to blood pressure: The Honolulu heart study, *American Journal of Clinical Nutrition* 45 (1987): 469–475.

27. P. N. Hopkins and R. R. Williams, Human genetics and coronary heart disease: A public health perspective, *Annual Review of Nutrition* 9 (1989): 303–345.

28. S. M. Poindexter, W. E. Dear, and S. J. Dudrick, Nutrition in congestive heart failure, *Nutrition in Clinical Practice* 1 (1986): 83–88.

29. M. M. Rothkopf and coauthors, Nutritional support in respiratory failure, *Nutrition in Clinical Practice* 4 (1989): 166–172.

30. S. Goldstein and coauthors, Energy expenditure in patients with chronic obstructive pulmonary disease, *Chest* 91 (1987): 222–224; D. O. Wilson and coauthors, Metabolic rate and weight loss in chronic obstructive lung disease, *Journal of Parenteral and Enteral Nutrition* 14 (1990): 7–11.

31. N. L. Keim and coauthors, Dietary evaluation of outpatients with chronic obstructive pulmonary disease, *Journal of the American Dietetic Association* 86 (1986): 902–906.

32. C. N. Noller and S. Mobarhan, Enteral feeding in patients with advanced chronic obstructive pulmonary disease, *Nutritional Support Services* 6 (1986): 37–39.

33. Noller and Mobarhan, 1986.

34. Rothkopf and coauthors, 1989.

35. Rothkopf and coauthors, 1989.

36. J. N. Armstrong, Nutrition and the respiratory patient, *Nutritional Support Services* 6 (1986): 8, 10, 32.

37. Diet, metals, and hidden heart disease, *Science News*, 27 September 1986, p. 201.

38. J. Tuomilehto and coauthors, Nutrition-related determinants of blood pressure, *Preventive Medicine* 14 (1985): 413–427.

Healthful Ethnic Food Choices

Chapter 28 presented several dietary recommendations to help prevent atherosclerosis and hypertension. It even made a few suggestions as to which kinds of foods might best keep heart disease at bay: primarily, foods that are low in fat such as grain products, fruits, vegetables, lean meats, fish, poultry, and low-fat milk products. The same line of advice appears often throughout this text. But the text has stopped short of telling you exactly what foods to eat for breakfast, lunch, and dinner, Monday through Sunday. That would have been far too pushy. Such a diet plan can be designed only by you. Where to begin? Begin with the foods you enjoy eating. Then try to make improvements, little by little. This highlight inspects many of the foods people typically enjoy eating and shows how to improve menus with heart health in mind.[1]

How Foodways Arise

People eat differently, depending on many influences, including ethnic background, the local food supply, local cuisine, religious restrictions, and the other factors affecting food choices named in Chapter 1. Do some foodways support heart health better than others? This highlight presents a few of the world's many ethnic foodways to show how to successfully apply basic diet planning principles to all sorts of cuisines and foodways.

Over the years, each culture has defined which of the many plants and animals that surround it are suitable for eating. In making these decisions, the people of a culture consider these questions:

- Would eating this plant or animal injure us? If a plant or animal is found to be poisonous when eaten

Foodways and cuisines of all cultures can support heart health when dietary fat is limited.

then it is promptly deemed not edible. Even if the people only *believe* the plant or animal is harmful if eaten, it may become taboo.

- Is this plant or animal considered food for animals or for people? Most U.S. citizens generally consider insects appropriate food for anteaters or bears but not for people, while other cultures consider certain insects a delicacy. In France, corn is considered a food only for livestock, whereas in the United States, people enjoy eating corn prepared in a number of ways.
- Is this plant or animal commonly eaten by members of our culture? Some cultures may eat horsemeat, but others do not. Some people eat variety meats, such as tripe, chitterlings, or brains, but others do not.

Given these parameters within a culture's definition of foods, a person can determine whether to eat a food: if I like it, if I can afford to buy it, if it is allowed by my religion and is consistent with other values, and if it is not restricted for health reasons, this is a food I eat.[2]

So it is that plants and animals meet the criteria for foods that come to comprise a person's diet within a culture. Of course, as individual tastes

and circumstances change, people try new foods and adopt them as standard fare, thus expanding the list of foods the culture accepts.

Every country, and in fact every region of a country, has its own typical foods and ways of combining them into meals. Immigrants to North America have brought those ways with them. These foodways have evolved here into patterns called ethnic diets or cuisines. As generations have passed and people have migrated from one region of North America to another, these cuisines have melded together into combinations of the characteristics of many different diets.

Some cultures or ethnic groups have remained relatively pure, and so have their foodways. However, in the United States, many ethnic groups have mingled, so U.S. foodways reflect many subcultures. A menu in an "American-style" restaurant might list everyday foods with many different ethnic origins—spaghetti (Italian), nachos (Mexican), hot dogs with sauerkraut (German), french fried potatoes (French), peanuts (African), popcorn (Native American), and egg rolls (Chinese). These and other ethnic foods have become integral in the "American diet"; further, some ingenious cross-cultural recipes have yielded fanciful creations, such as tofu lasagne and Tex-Mex wontons.

Ethnic influences have extended the lists of foods that people accept for their own use, helping people to achieve variety in their meals. Variety helps to ensure nutrient adequacy, but only moderation will help to control energy and fat intakes—the dietary goals for heart health. How then, can people limit their fat intakes, the single most important dietary change most of us can make to improve our health, within various cuisines? Fat supports the development of more degenerative diseases than any other dietary component. It also has the greatest influence on energy intake and body fat, thus contributing more to the development of obesity than any other dietary component.[3] In short, whether a food enhances or detracts from your health often depends on the amount and kind of fat it delivers. Keep this in mind as the following sections explore the cuisines of just a few groups whose foodways have helped to shape U.S. eating habits.

Northern Europe

Immigrants from northern Europe have vastly influenced traditional American home cooking. For example, an evening meal of a hearty portion of fine roast meat, side dishes of mashed potatoes or boiled cabbage and bread, and fruit pie for dessert characterizes the cuisine of Germany, England, and Ireland. Such a meal typifies suppers across the United States as well because immigrants from those countries brought this meal plan with them to the New World. Many variations of this meal are based on the same foods prepared differently. For example, a New England dinner may include a corned (spiced and cured) cut of beef boiled together with potatoes, carrots, and cabbage.

The way people have traditionally used these foods has been to fill their plates with large portions of the meat with the vegetables on the side. Today's health advice, however, would be to load each plate with the tasty vegetables, and limit the meat to a 3-ounce portion. This way, the meal would provide plenty of carbohydrate, adequate protein, and not too much fat.

Many other familiar foodways also derive from northern Europe. The "American" breakfast of eggs with bacon and biscuits came originally from England, as did the use of tea as a beverage. We have modified the breakfast, though: the English serve baked beans with it; here, Northerners often select hash brown potatoes and Southerners often choose grits. This breakfast, like the dinner just described, allows room for improvement: today's health advice would recommend more fruit, lower-fat bread, and less fat, eggs, and meat.

Every eating style has advantages and drawbacks. The northern European style of eating provides abundant protein and ensures adequacy of all the nutrients associated with meat. However, it also delivers a lot of fat and is short on fiber and the vitamins and minerals associated with fruits and vegetables. People who adhere to foodways that resemble those of the northern

European countries can improve their nutrition by reducing meat portion sizes, by cutting down on added fats, and by choosing more whole grains, fruits, and vegetables.

The famed cuisines of France influenced the foodways of both the British Isles and Ireland, but French immigrants to the United States were relatively few in number, and most were assimilated fully into the new culture. One group, the French Arcadians from Canada who settled in southern Louisiana, preserved their French country-cooking heritage and adapted it to the local Louisiana food supply. Today their descendants, the Cajuns, have made their foodways popular with people across the nation.

A gradual blending of Arcadian and African American cultures produced the unique Cajun cuisine with both French and African influences. Many Cajun dishes use a roux made from lard, oil, or butter, flour, and salt, as a base. Cajun dishes include spicy, thick soups (gumbo, jambalaya), sausages, *Tabasco* pepper sauce, red beans and rice, dirty rice (rice made brown with chopped chicken livers and seasonings), and seafood. Many people enjoy the distinctive flavor of Cajun coffee brewed with chicory root. Especially French in nature are the puffed, sugared doughnuts known as beignets and the familiar French toast.

Some Cajun foods are perfectly suited to meeting the *NRC Recommendations* introduced in Chapter 2. Nutritionists agree with enthusiastic diners that red beans and rice is a classic dish—delicious because it is full of flavor from expert use of spice and nutritious because it is high in carbohydrate, protein, and fiber, while low in fat. Stews of seafood, tomatoes, vegetables, and rice seasoned with a little strong-flavored sausage are packed with vitamins and minerals, adequate in protein, rich in carbohydrate, while usually low in fat. To lower the fat contents of traditional dishes, roux can be prepared without

---

Miniglossary

cuisine: style of cooking or preparing food.
ethnic diets: foodways and cuisines typical of national origins, cultural heritages, or geographic locations.
foodways: the sum of the food habits, customs, beliefs, and preferences of a culture.
kosher: foods fit to eat according to Jewish dietary laws.
taboo: forbidden or banned; for food, usually a food believed to be sacred or cursed.

lard, oil, or butter by browning flour in the oven and stirring occasionally. Many Cajun foods can support efforts to meet dietary guidelines deliciously.

Southern Europe

Almost everybody enjoys one or another of the foods brought to the United States by the millions of Italian immigrants. What teenager would turn down a slice of pizza, a food native to Naples? Who wouldn't like spumone—ice cream with fruits, nuts, and flavorings?

The foods of Italy bear regional characteristics. Generally people living in the northern regions of that country consume abundant animal-derived food—meat, butter, cheese, eggs, and cream. In the southern regions, wheat pastas accompany vegetables such as artichokes, eggplants, peppers, and tomatoes; these foods are served with more beans than meat and are seasoned with olive oil, not butter. Even pasta, a favorite in both the north and south, varies by region—northern pastas are egg-based and usually ribbon shaped, while southern varieties are made without eggs and are shaped more like macaroni.

Nutritionally, Italian favorites receive high marks in balance and adequacy. Even pizza can offer something from each of the four food groups. Other Italian dishes can do equally well: eggplant parmesan served with a side dish of pasta supplies vegetables, cheese, grain, and perhaps a bit of meat in the sauce. Pastas with meaty tomato sauces and a sprinkling of cheese also meet the four food-group recommendations. However, for the sake of moderation, the eater of Italian foods must modify the recipes to reduce the fat in many original recipes. It helps especially to reduce the amounts of oil and high-fat cheeses added to the foods of southern Italian origin and to substitute low-fat ingredients for the high-fat cream and butter used in foods of the northern regions. Some Italian dishes are high in nutrient density and appealing in both taste and appearance without modifications: examples are pasta prima vera, a mixture of colorful vegetables and pasta, and minestrone, a bean and pasta soup.

West Africa

When you spread peanut butter on your bread, do you realize that you are eating an African food? Actually peanut *butter* is considered an American food, invented by George Washington Carver, an agricultural scientist. However, peanuts and peanut paste were and still are staple foods of Africa and were brought to U.S. soil by African slaves. Boiled peanuts, too, which are a southern specialty today, emerged with the origins of humankind in Africa. Similarly, okra and blackeye (cow) peas are of African origin.

Most black Americans are the descendants of ancestors who came to the United States from western Africa by force, not by choice. Although generations of blacks suffered slavery, segregation, and persecution, their unique culture strongly influenced today's general U.S. culture, especially in music, art, and foodways.

Within the possibilities allowed them, enslaved Africans held tenaciously to their familiar, ancient cuisines and adapted them to the foods they encountered in their new world. They offered their agricultural expertise to their owners, too, so that a blending of cultures took place. Slaves and owners alike ate African crops that the slaves grew on Southern agricultural plantations, often combining them with native American greens, sweet potatoes, and wild fish and game. Today's rural southern cuisine varies little between blacks and whites.

Southern cuisine offers both nutritional advantages and disadvantages. It provides ample vitamins and minerals found in green leafy vegetables, meats, and corn. Sweet potatoes are a rich source of vitamin A, naturally low in fat and high in carbohydrate. African seafood gumbo is similar to the Cajun dish already described, in being a nutritious mixture of low-fat foods. However, many foods of the rural South are perilously rich in fat and salt. Some dishes are traditionally flavored with lard or are fried in other fats. Biscuits, a favored bread, are made with almost as much shortening as flour and are often served with butter or fat-rich gravy. Preferred meals also include large servings of high-fat, high-salt meats, such as fried chicken, pork cuts or sausages, and spareribs, greatly overemphasizing protein and fat in the diet while slighting carbohydrates— whole grains, fruits, and vegetables. Vegetables may be cooked to extinction of their vitamin contents in pots swimming with salted meats such as salt pork or bacon. The trick to choosing health-promoting rural southern food is to prepare vegetables without salt and without overcooking them, to eat plenty of the beans, rice, and cornbread (go easy on the butter), and lighten up on fatty meats, biscuits, and gravies.

Mexico

Mexican restaurants typically offer beautiful plates of complex food mixtures—tortillas filled with meats and cheeses, some fried and crisp and others baked and soft, along with flavored rice and refried beans, with sour cream, guacamole (avocado sauce), and salsa (tomato sauce). These foods are of Mexican origin, but they are not the day-to-day fare of Mexican families, although they are typical of festive foods prepared for special occasions. A typical Mexican meal is simple, consisting of a stew of beans, meat, and potatoes served with tortillas or bread and tomato salsa. A Mexican breakfast might include tortillas and eggs with a beverage while lunch and supper might consist of beans and rice or a stew served with a lettuce and tomato salad or a cooked vegetable.[4]

As familiar as the hamburger place, taco stands sell fast food to millions of U.S. diners each day. If carefully chosen, these foods can make valuable contributions to the diet. Many Mexican dishes (even the fast-food type) provide beans in abundance. Beans are high in nutrient density and fiber while low in fat, although the refried variety may be cooked with lard. If you aren't careful in choosing, though, you can obtain an extraordinarily high-fat meal, such as a fried tortilla shell filled with commercial-grade, high-fat ground beef and topped with cheese and sour cream. Just as tasty, but higher in nutrient density, are soft tortillas filled with beans, lettuce, and salsa with a side order of rice.

For the special-occasion dinner described earlier, avoid adding sour cream, and skip the fried varieties of stuffed tortillas. Try instead a dish called fajita—lean meats, marinated and sizzled on a grill, wrapped in soft tortillas with chili salsa toppings. Salsa is rich in vitamins and zest but adds no fat burden to the meal. As for guacamole, even though avocados are high in fat you needn't avoid them altogether. The type of fat avocados contain is not implicated in disease causation, although they are fattening and should be limited by people who tend to gain weight.

You may be beginning to see that it is not the ethnic frame itself, but the diner's choices within the frame, that decide whether a meal will benefit the diner's health. One cuisine, though, reliably presents many interesting dishes that meet nutrient needs extraordinarily well—the Chinese cuisine.

China

Tried and true, the diet of China has supported the health of people there for thousands of years. The foodways of China reflect that economy is essential in a land crowded with more than 1,000 people per acre and where only 10 percent of the land can be used to grow food. China's population numbers well over a billion people, of whom about 75 percent are involved in agriculture. Contrast this to the United States: population density—113 per acre; land in farms—about 50 percent; population—250 million; farmers—1 to 2 percent.

There seems to be little malnutrition or obesity among Chinese people, even though they consume 20 percent more kcalories of food each day than do people in the United States. On the whole, Chinese people eating traditional foods consume three times the fiber of people eating the American way, take in about half the fat, and have blood cholesterol values about half of what they are in the United States.[5] It seems worthwhile to study the fine points of a diet so conservative of resources yet so superbly supportive of health—not to convince you to eat all Chinese meals but perhaps to encourage you to adopt some of the governing principles and to apply them to foods of all origins.

Chinese meals do not follow the separate meat-vegetable-starch pattern common in much of the United States. The vegetables and meats are cooked together. The total amount of meat (or fish or egg) in a Chinese dish is very small by Western standards; instead, there is abundant rice at almost every meal. The Chinese also usually partake of soup or tea throughout each meal. Meals center on a staple starch food (every diner has a personal rice dish) with other foods chosen according to each person's appetite (from serving dishes).

Vegetables and fruits provide tremendous variety in the Chinese diet. The nutrients in the foods are undiluted by fat and sugar. Nor do alcohol kcalories have a significant place, although the Chinese do make and drink a wine on special occasions.

The subtle flavors that make Chinese dishes appealing come largely from the fat-free seasonings and sauces used in their preparation. Among the seasonings are ginger root, almonds, scallions, sesame seed oil, rice wine, and garlic. Among the sauces are soy, hoisin, oyster, bean, and plum sauce. Most sauces add tasty flavors but no fat, unlike our gravies, butter, or sour cream. The Chinese mode of cooking in a wok employs little oil: cooks use just a tablespoon or two in an entire dish. The cholesterol content of most Chinese meals is usually minimal except for dishes such as egg foo yung and those made with lobster sauces that contain eggs. Chinese dishes do have a nutrition drawback, though: they tend to be high in sodium. Diners can enjoy a low-sodium meal if foods are prepared without salt or monosodium glutamate (MSG) and soy is used judiciously.

Cooking foods the Chinese way tends to preserve nutrients. The water in which the rice is cooked may absorb nutrients, but then it soaks back into the rice rather than being drained away, so the rice retains the nutrients. All food is cut into bite-sized pieces before cooking so that it will be easy to eat with chopsticks; cooking finely cut-up food requires only short times and so destroys few nutrients. No extra water is used, and none is thrown away, so nutrients are not lost that way either.

The Chinese diet and cooking techniques are also land-efficient, as they must be in view of the scarcity of agricultural land and fuels. Nearly all of the food energy comes from plants rather than animals. A million kcalories in wheat or rice can be produced on less than 1 acre of land; a million kcalories in beef require 17 acres. In a world in which fuel and land are becoming increasingly scarce, the Chinese way of eating offers a model to all nations.

Many other cuisines and foodways are of interest. Table H28−1 lists some of

■ TABLE H28–1
Characteristics of Selected Ethnic Diets

Group and Place of Origin	Staple Foods	Foods Excluded	Strengths and Weaknesses of the Diet
Hispanic Americans from Cuba, Haiti, Puerto Rico	Steamed white rice; many varieties of beans; wheat breads; starchy vegetables such as cassavas, yuccas, yams, breadfruit, plantains, and green bananas; green peppers; tomatoes; garlic; dried, salted fish; chicken; pork; lard; olive oil; sugar; jams and jellies; sweet pastries; sugared fruit juices; coffee	Green leafy vegetables; milk as a beverage for adults; fish other than dried and salted	Provides adequate protein, many other nutrients, and fiber; may provide too much fat, especially animal fat; may lack calcium
Hispanic Americans from Mexico, Central America	Many varieties of beans; steamed rice; corn products such as tortillas made from lime-soaked cornmeal; chili peppers; tomatoes; mangoes; prickly pear fruit; potatoes; meat and sausages; fish; poultry; eggs; milk cheeses; milk custards and bread puddings; lard; sweet chocolate and coffee drinks; cakes; cookies; pastries	Green leafy vegetables; yellow vegetables; milk as a beverage for adults	Is high in kcalories and fat, especially saturated fat, and high in sugar; most nutrients can be obtained, but with many kcalories
Black Americans from West Indies, Central or South America, and recent African immigrants	Dumplings or gruel made from millet, corn, wheat, rice, or barley; starchy roots such as cassavas, yams, plantains, and bananas; coconuts; peanuts; fresh fruits; hot peppers; tomatoes; onions; okra; palm oil; fruit wine; tea; coffee; honey; molasses	Milk and milk products (meat and fish limited use)	Is low in calcium, iron, and vitamin B_{12}; is potentially low in protein, depending on availability of foods; is low in fat and salt; is high in fiber
Southern black Americans from West Africa (many generations in United States)	Hominy grits; biscuits; cornmeal and corn bread; rice; legumes; potatoes; onions; tomatoes; hot peppers; green leafy vegetables; okra; sweet potatoes; squashes; corn; cabbage; melons; peaches; pecans; smoked pork; fresh meats and poultry; fish; thick stews; butter, shortening, and lard; sugar; bread puddings; pies and sweets	Milk and milk products; yeast breads	Provides ample nutrients of meat; provides excess protein; is high in kcalories; provides excess fat, especially saturated fat; is high in salt; is low in calcium
Chinese Americans from China (diets vary sometimes with region)	Rice and rice gruel; wheat noodles; corn; green vegetables, especially from the cabbage family; squashes; cucumbers; eggplant; leafy vegetables; various shoots, including bamboo, mung, and soy; sweet potatoes; radishes; onions; peas and pods; mushrooms; roots; many local, seasonal vegetables; pickled vegetables; sea vegetables; plums; peaches; tangerines; kumquats and other citrus fruits; litchis; longans; mangoes; papayas; pomegranates; soybean products such as tofu (soybean curd), soy sauces, bean noodles, and soy milk; tiny portions of meat, fish with bones, or poultry; seafood; soup or tea as beverage; sugar as seasoning	Milk and most milk products	Depending on availability of protein-rich foods, protein and iron may be low; is low in fat; is high in fiber and many nutrients; see text for further discussion of the Chinese diet

them, with a brief description of some foods that characterize each.

Religious Dietary Traditions

A discussion of ethnic foodways would be incomplete without mention of foodways practiced by the world's major religious groups. Religions help people to answer the questions, ''Why am I here?'' ''What purpose do I serve?'' ''What is the reason for my existence?'' To ask such universal questions seems to be essential to human mental and emotional health.[6] According to many religions, ritual and ceremony surrounding food can provide nourishment for the spirit as well as for the body. Special foodways also help give religious groups, like national groups, their distinct identity.

■ **TABLE H28–1**
Characteristics of Selected Ethnic Diets (continued)

Group and Place of Origin	Staple Foods	Foods Excluded	Strengths and Weaknesses of the Diet
Japanese Americans from Japan	Rice; vegetables; pickled vegetables; soy as miso (soup), tofu, bean paste, and soy sauce; fruits; salads; fish with bones; sugar as seasoning; sea vegetables; seafood; ginseng	Milk and milk products	Provides abundant nutrients with little fat; is high in salt
Korean Americans from South Korea	Rice; noodles; many leafy vegetables; kimchi (extremely hot pickled cabbage); sea vegetables; hot peppers; seasonal fruits; mushrooms; small fish with bones; large servings of grilled beef; chicken; fresh or dried squid, octopus, and lobster; fish with bones; mussels; eggs; lard and vegetable fat for frying; sesame oil; nuts and seeds; ginger; sugar as seasoning	Milk and milk products	Is high in fat and adequate in protein; is monotonous in winter (kimchi is served at each meal, to the exclusion of other vegetables); without the traditional small fish with bones, calcium can be lacking
Vietnamese Americans from Vietnam	Rice, rice noodles; French bread and croissants with butter; hot peppers; curries of asparagus and potatoes; salads; tropical fruits and vegetables; lemons and limes; small portions of poultry; eggs; fish pâtés; nuoc nam (a strong, fermented fish sauce); sweets, candies, sweetened drinks; coffee; tea	Milk and milk products	Can be low in iron or calcium
Native Americans (Indians)	*Southeast:* Corn; cornmeal; coontie (flour from a palmlike plant); fry breads; swamp cabbage (now illegal to harvest); pumpkins; squashes; papayas; beef, alligator, snake, wild hog, duck, fish, and shellfish. *Northeast:* blueberries; cranberries; beans; corn; pumpkins; fish; lobster; wild game; maple syrup. *Midwest:* bison; beans; corn; melons; squashes; tomatoes. *Southwest:* corn (many colors and varieties); beans; squash; pumpkins; chili peppers; melons; pinenuts; cactus. *Northwest:* salmon; caviar; other fish; otter; seal; whale; bear; elk; other game; wild fruits; acorns (and other wild nuts); wild greens.	Milk and milk products	Varies with region; may be low in calcium.

The Jewish laws set forth an extensive set of dietary rules. Orthodox Jews obey these laws worldwide: they eat only foods that are kosher. Many people, on hearing the word *kosher*, think of foods such as pickles, bagels and lox, corned beef, or matzoh crackers. However, kosher is not a cuisine but is instead a set of restrictions placed on the selection, preparation, and service of animal-derived foods. Jewish cuisines vary among Jews whose families emigrated from different countries. Jews from Eastern Europe, Germany, the Soviet Union, the Middle East, or India eat differently, but all may apply the kosher rules to their foods.[7]

The laws of kosher permit some foods and exclude others. Orthodox Jews may eat beef but not pork; fish but not shellfish; and must use special handling methods for permitted foods. Kosher rules forbid blood as food, so rules govern the methods of animal slaughter, cuts that may be eaten, and preparation rituals. To identify processed foods that have been made according to kosher laws, look for the insignia "U" or "K" on the label. This insignia means a rabbi has deemed the food kosher.

Kosher law prohibits Jews from consuming milk and meat in the same meal. This law leads some kosher cooks to replace milk with nondairy creamer in meals that include meat. Nutritionally, however, creamers do not replace milk, and they carry more saturated fat. A better choice is to use soy "milk" products formulated to resemble the nutrient and cooking qualities of milk products.

In addition to kosher laws for daily meals, holidays call for traditional feasts to use foods rich with religious symbolism. For example, a traditional Passover dinner includes a special salad of apples, nuts, cinnamon, and wine that symbolizes the mortar that Jewish slaves used to build Egyptian pyramids and palaces.

Just as with other cuisines, Jewish cuisines and kosher foods can be evaluated according to dietary standards. A Jewish meal of European cuisine might be improved by reducing the schmaltz (chicken fat) used in cooking, or by frying latke (potato pancakes) in nonstick pans, not in oil. Bagels with lox (a form of salmon) without cream cheese are an excellent breakfast choice—bagels are naturally low in fat, and lox are rich in omega-3 fatty acids. A person dining on European Jewish cuisine would do well to keep servings of meat (usually beef) to 3- to 4-ounce serving sizes, and to fill in the meal with grains such as noodle pudding (without butter), fruits, and vegetables. For Indian Kosher cuisines, emphasize grains and legumes over fats.

Occasionally someone suggests that the laws of kosher originated for reasons of health, that kosher food was "clean" and therefore kept people safe from foodborne illnesses. However, religious commitment is the sole intent of those who keep kosher; the rules of kosher offer no special benefits to health.

Food symbolism abounds in most other religions as well. Among Christians, a revered expression of faith is the sacrament of eating a bite of bread or bread wafer and taking a sip of grape juice or wine, symbolizing the last supper of Jesus Christ. During certain days of Lent, the period prior to Easter, many Christians eat only vegetarian dishes, giving up meat until Easter dinner. Eastern Orthodox Christians observe many fast days on which they consume no animal products at all. Some Christian faiths prohibit or promote certain dietary habits. The Mormon faith does not allow alcohol, coffee, or tea. Many Seventh-day Adventists consume no meat (but include eggs and milk products) and also shun alcohol, coffee, and tea. In addition, Seventh-day Adventist doctrine advises followers to avoid strong spices such as mustard or pepper and discourages between-meal snacks. Other faiths, such as Islam, Muslim, Hinduism, and Buddhism, prohibit some dietary practices while promoting others.

Whatever the cuisine, to keep total fat down, consumers have to learn to select low-fat foods. If they are to limit the percentage of kcalories from fat to 30 percent, then they need to limit foods such as cream, butter, margarine, mayonnaise, cream cheese, and the like; foods high in hidden fat, such as meat marbled with fat and whole milk; and the many others

identified in Chapter 5. Consumers can follow a low-fat, low-salt diet in any of their chosen foodways.

Dietitians know that to honor a person's cultural or religious foodways honors the person. When counseling others, be sure to learn about their foodways first. This knowledge will guide you in making suggestions that will fit into the person's life. Sometimes, respecting a person's foodways can provide nourishment of self-esteem, and that can support the changes needed to nourish the body toward health.

NOTES

1. Adapted with permission from E. M. N. Hamilton, E. N. Whitney, and F. S. Sizer, Cultural and religious cuisines: Which ethnic group has the best way to eat? in *Nutrition Concepts and Controversies* (St. Paul, MN: West, 1991).

2. Adapted from P. G. Kittler and K. Sucher, *Food and Culture in America* (New York, 1989: Van Nostrand Reinhold), p. 13.

3. S. R. Rolfes, A matter of fat, *Nutrition Clinics*, May–June 1990 (available from J. B. Lippincott, East Washington Square, Philadelphia, PA 19105).

4. S. J. Algert and T. H. Ellison, Mexican American Food practices, customs, and holidays, *Ethnic and Regional Food Practices* (series) (Chicago and Alexandria, VA: American Dietetic Association and American Diabetes Association, 1989).

5. L. Roberts, Diet and health in China, *Science* 240 (1988): 27.

6. L. S. Chapman, Developing a useful perspective on spiritual health: Love, joy, peace and fulfillment, *American Journal of Health Promotion*, Fall 1987, pp. 12–17.

7. C. Higgins and H. S. Warshaw, Jewish food practices, customs, and holidays, *Ethnic and Regional Food Practices* (series) (Chicago and Alexandria, VA: American Dietetic Association and American Diabetes Association, 1989).

Nutrition and Disorders of the Kidneys

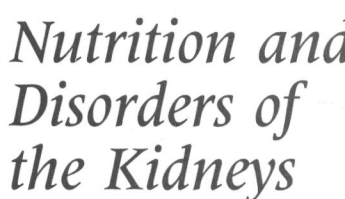

Contents

Shown here is one of the delicate structures in the kidney—a glomerulus (diagrammed in Figure 29–1 on p. 895). The coil of capillaries with blood cells within them (black) lies within the cup-shaped glomerulus (orange); surrounding kidney tissue is shown here as blue.

The kidneys certainly illustrate the old adage that good things come in small packages. Each kidney is only about the size of a fist, yet together they shoulder much of the responsibility for maintaining chemical homeostasis for the entire body. Probably the best way to appreciate the kidneys' vast importance is to learn first what they do normally, and then what happens when they fail.

What the Kidneys Do

nephron (NEF-ron): the working unit of the kidney, consisting of a glomerulus and a tubule.

glomerulus (glow-MARE-you-lus): a cup-shaped membrane enclosing a tuft of capillaries within a nephron.

tubule: a tubelike structure that surrounds the glomerulus and descends through the nephron. Pressure gradients between the glomerulus and the tubule returns needed materials to the blood and sends wastes to the bladder.

The two bean-shaped kidneys sit just above the waist on each side of the spinal column. Within the kidneys, nephrons busily work at cleansing the blood (see Figure 29–1, which redisplays a figure first shown in Chapter 3). The figure illustrates the relationships of various kidney parts and shows how the nephrons filter wastes from the blood. Each of the approximately one million nephrons (per kidney) consists of a tuft of capillaries enclosed by a cup-shaped membrane called the glomerulus, and an associated tubule. The kidneys filter out substances the body doesn't need, eliminating these waste products in the urine. Some of these substances include urea, creatinine, and uric acid. When the blood contains more water or electrolytes than it needs, these excesses are also eliminated in the urine. Other substances the body needs, such as plasma proteins and red blood cells, remain in the blood. Through this filtering process, the kidneys serve several homeostatic functions: they maintain fluid, electrolyte, and acid-base balance; and they remove metabolic waste products from the body.

Some 1,200 milliliters of blood pass through the kidneys every minute—about one-quarter of the heart's total output. Blood rushes through the glomeruli at about 650 milliliters per minute, and from this blood, some 90 to 120 milliliters of fluid filter across the glomerular membranes to enter the tubules. The fluid entering the tubules, called the filtrate, is watery looking, because it lacks red blood cells. The rate at which the nephrons form filtrate, known as the glomerular filtration rate (GFR), provides an index of kidney function.

glomerular filtration rate (GFR): the rate at which the nephrons form filtrate. Normally, GFR is between 90 and 120 ml/min.

As the filtrate travels down the tubules, its composition continually changes. In the end, substances the body needs return to the general circulation, and waste products (including excess metabolites) leave the body in the urine. Thus the kidneys help to maintain chemical homeostasis.

The work of the kidneys includes more than just waste elimination. The kidneys help regulate blood pressure by secreting the enzyme renin and by responding to the hormone aldosterone (review Figure 28–4 on p. 865). The kidneys also produce another hormone, erythropoietin, which stimulates red blood cell production. Finally, the kidneys convert vitamin D to its most active form, which supports normal calcium absorption, calcium and phosphorus metabolism, and bone maintenance. When you consider all the vital functions the kidneys perform, it is easy to see how serious the consequences must be when the kidneys fail.

The kidneys:
- Maintain fluid, electrolyte, and acid-base balance.
- Eliminate metabolic waste products.
- Help regulate blood pressure.
- Produce a hormone that stimulates red blood cell production.
- Activate vitamin D and so help regulate calcium and bone metabolim.

Blood vessel carrying blood into glomerulus

Glomerulus

Capillaries of glomerulus

Blood vessel carrying blood away from glomerulus

Tubules

Blood vessel carrying blood back to body

Blood vessel carrying blood alongside tubule

To the bladder

■ **FIGURE 29-1**

A Nephron, One of the Kidney's Many Functioning Units

Blood flows into the glomerulus, and some of its fluid is filtered into the tubules (1). As the filtrate descends through the tubules, substances the body needs are returned to the blood through the intricate network of capillaries that surround the tubules (2). The waste materials that remain pass from the tubules on to the bladder (3).

■ *Renal Failure*

Renal failure occurs when the nephrons lose function to such an extent that they cannot perform their normal homeostatic and hormonal roles. It can occur suddenly (acute renal failure) or over a period of time (chronic renal failure). Healthy kidneys may fail suddenly, due to acute insults. In some cases, the kidneys recover, and so acute renal failure is only temporary. In other cases, acute renal failure leads to more serious problems. Long-term kidney disease leads to chronic renal failure, which is generally irreversible.

Renal failure may develop from damage to the kidneys themselves, as in nephritis, renal artery obstruction, nephrotic syndrome (described in a later section), kidney stones (see Highlight 29), and renal tubular disorders. It can also result from other diseases, such as diabetic nephropathy (Chapter 27), hypertension (Chapter 28), atherosclerosis (Chapter 28), and septic shock (Chapter 23).

renal failure: failure of the nephrons to maintain normal function.

nephritis (nef-RYE-tis): inflammation of the kidney. **Pyelonephritis** (PIE-eh-low-neh-FRY-tis) is an inflammation of the kidney and bladder, and **glomerulonephritis** (glow-MARE-you-low-neh-FRY-tis) is an inflammation of the glomerular capillaries.

Impairment of renal blood flow because of renal artery damage is called **nephrosclerosis** (NEF-row-skle-ROW-sis). It can be caused by hypertension or atherosclerosis.

As nephrons fail, the composition of the blood and urine changes. Therefore, laboratory tests of these fluids provide a useful evaluation of renal function. Clearance tests measure the GFR, which declines as renal failure progresses. The body's principal nitrogen-containing metabolic waste products—blood urea nitrogen (BUN), creatinine, and uric acid—accumulate in the blood when renal function is impaired. Consequently, laboratory tests for the person with renal failure show high levels of BUN, creatinine, and uric acid.

As renal failure progresses to a severe stage, the buildup of toxic waste products in the blood (uremia) can precipitate a complex of symptoms known as the uremic syndrome. The person with uremia experiences a wide array of symptoms in virtually every body system: fatigue, weakness, diminished mental alertness, muscular twitches, muscle cramps, anorexia, nausea, vomiting, stomatitis, and an unpleasant taste in the mouth. The skin may itch uncomfortably, and in later stages, GI ulcers and bleeding commonly develop.

uremia (you-REE-me-ah): the buildup of toxic waste products in the blood, associated with renal insufficiency.

uremic syndrome: a complex of symptoms seen late in renal failure, caused by uremia.

When urea (which can be excreted through sweat) crystallizes and becomes visible on the skin, the condition is called **uremic frost.**

▪ Chronic Renal Failure

In chronic renal failure, the nephrons gradually and progressively deteriorate. In the early stages, the nephrons enlarge in an attempt to maintain normal function. The nephrons work so efficiently that the kidney can lose about 80 percent of them before experiencing seriously impaired renal function. The GFR may fall to one-tenth of the normal rate—10 to 12 milliliters per minute—before symptoms appear. This explains why renal failure is often far advanced before anyone even detects its presence.

The early stages of renal failure generally go undetected, and so clients make no dietary adjustments. However, when treatment begins, diet plays a significant role. Dietary restrictions aim at preventing hypertension, edema, congestive heart failure, and uremia. The physician prescribes the diet and regularly adjusts it based on the degree of renal insufficiency.

Eventually, as renal failure progresses and uremia threatens, the person must begin dialysis or receive a kidney transplant to survive. (See the box on pp. 898-899 entitled ''Dialysis'' and the later section, ''Kidney Transplants and Diet.'') This stage of renal disease is known as end-stage renal disease.

Renal failure alters the metabolism of nutrients and their end products significantly for many reasons. Among these reasons are:

The capacity of the kidney to function despite loss of some nephrons is referred to as **renal reserve.**

When the GFR falls below 4 to 5 ml/min, dialysis is usually initiated. Recall that normal GFR is between 90 and 120 ml/min.

Abnormal accumulation of nitrogen-containing substances in the blood is called **azotemia** (AZE-oh-TEE-me-ah). Normal BUN levels are 10 to 20 mg/dL. A BUN of 50 to 150 mg/dL indicates serious impairment of renal function. BUN may rise to as high as 150 to 250 mg/dL in end-stage renal disease.

end-stage renal disease (ESRD): the severe stage of renal disease in which diet alone is no longer effective in maintaining normal kidney functions.

- Failure to excrete toxic waste products.
- Inability of the renal tubules to reabsorb many needed nutrients.
- Reduced GI absorption of some nutrients.
- Reduced inactivation of many hormones, including insulin, parathyroid hormone, glucagon, and thyrotropin.
- Reduced synthesis of other important substances, such as erythropoietin and active vitamin D.
- Alteration of nutrient needs by other medical therapy (drugs and dialysis).

■ Limited food intake because of GI distress, depression, superimposed illnesses, and restrictive or unpalatable diets.

Because of these difficulties, the nutrition status of people with chronic renal failure is often compromised. Children with renal disease often fail to grow normally, and people of any age with renal disease may have the wasting syndrome—reduced muscle mass, depleted fat tissue, and lowered blood protein levels.

Diet in Renal Failure

Special attention to nutrient needs can help prevent wasting syndrome in renal failure. The objectives of dietary management of chronic renal failure are:

■ To achieve or maintain optimal nutrition status and nitrogen balance.
■ To prevent the buildup of toxic metabolic products, thus minimizing the risk of uremia.
■ To delay the progression of renal failure and to postpone the need for dialysis.
■ To prevent complications, such as growth failure, wasting syndrome, bone disease, hypertension, edema, and congestive heart failure.
■ To foster the client's well-being.

The actual diet is highly individualized; most often, it restricts protein and carefully controls total kcalories, sodium, potassium, phosphorus, and fluids.

As you read the following sections, notice how complex the renal diet is and how critical the control of certain nutrients. Keep in mind how restrictions placed on those nutrients affect food choices. Remember, when you communicate with a client, with a member of the client's family, or with another health care team member, you need to know *why* nutrients such as protein must be restricted so that your instructions to clients will be backed by your own knowledge and convictions. You most effectively serve clients when you truly understand the disease and the necessity of the renal diet.

Protein and Energy Providing the right amount of protein to the person in renal failure is like walking a tightrope. Too little protein, and the person develops malnutrition. Too much protein, and blood urea levels (the toxic waste product of protein metabolism) rise. Studies of adults with chronic renal failure have shown that people who eat unrestricted-protein diets experience a more rapid decline in renal function than people on diets containing from 0.55 to 0.60 grams of protein per kilogram of body weight per day.[1] Other studies have shown that diets containing from 0.4 to 0.6 grams of protein per kilogram of body weight per day can delay or halt the progression of chronic renal failure.[2] Even moderate protein restriction (1 gram per kilogram of body weight per day) has shown value in improving renal function in people with chronic renal failure.[3]

Clinicians disagree about when a low-protein diet becomes too low to maintain nutrition status. Some investigators believe that once the GFR falls below 4 to 5 milliliters per minute, dialysis needs to be initiated in order to

Dialysis

The kidneys are virtually irreplaceable. No perfect substitute for one's own kidneys has been found. However, although they fall short of the real thing, dialysis and kidney transplants can be lifesaving for the person with ESRD.

Dialysis removes excess fluids and wastes from the blood. The way dialysis works is actually simple. It works on the principles of simple diffusion and osmosis across a semipermeable membrane. A solution similar in composition to normal blood plasma, called the dialysate, is placed on one side of the semipermeable membrane; the person's blood flows by on the other side. The blood has a higher concentration of urea and electrolytes than the dialysate, so these substances diffuse from the blood into the dialysate. The dialysate also contains glucose; the higher the concentration of glucose in the dialysate, the more fluid will move from the blood into the dialysate by osmosis.

The membrane that covers the abdominal organs (the peritoneum) can serve as the semipermeable membrane, in which case the procedure is called peritoneal dialysis. In peritoneal dialysis, the dialysate is infused directly through a tube into the space within the person's abdomen that

dialysis (dye-AL-ih-sis): removal of waste from the blood using the principles of simple diffusion and osmosis through a semipermeable membrane.

Diffusion is illustrated on p. 57; osmosis, on p. 278.

peritoneal (PERR-ee-toe-NEE-al) **dialysis**: removal of waste from the blood using the peritoneum as a semipermeable membrane.

■ FIGURE 29–2
Peritoneal Dialysis
Peritoneal dialysis removes toxic wastes from the body through an exchange across the peritoneal membrane.

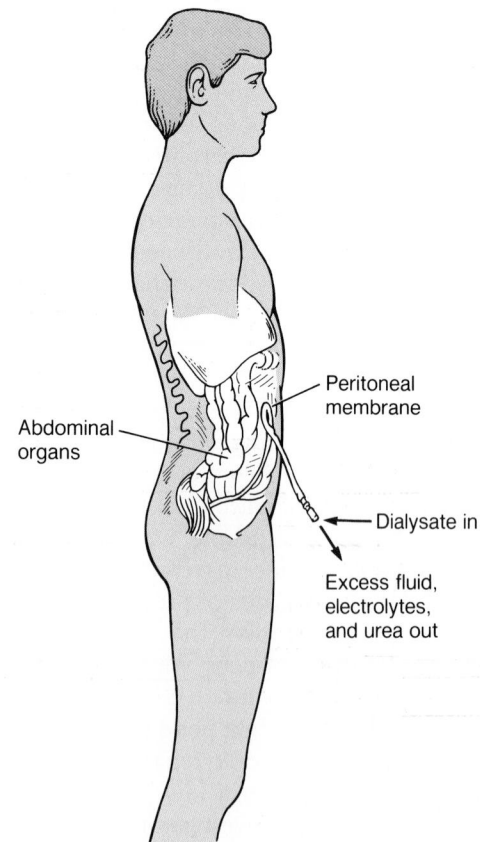

Peritoneal membrane

Abdominal organs

Dialysate in

Excess fluid, electrolytes, and urea out

surrounds the intestines (but lies outside the peritoneal membrane). The fluid is kept in the abdomen for about 30 minutes, then the fluid is drained through a tube from the abdomen by gravity (see Figure 29–2 on the previous page). The procedure is repeated with fresh aliquots of fluid. One complete exchange takes about an hour, and the total treatment takes from 24 to 72 hours.

A synthetic semipermeable membrane also can be used for dialysis. In this case, blood is conducted from the person's artery through tubing made of the semipermeable membrane, and this tubing lies in a bath of solutions that selectively remove unwanted material. After being cleansed, the blood is returned to the person's body through a vein. This procedure is called hemodialysis (see Figure 29–3). Oftentimes, the person with chronic renal failure on hemodialysis gets four- to eight-hour treatments three times a week.

Dialysis takes over two important functions of the kidney: waste removal and fluid removal. In so doing, dialysis reduces the symptoms of uremia, hypertension, and edema, as well as the risk of congestive heart failure. But the hormonal functions of the kidney are not restored. Anemia may become a problem. Hypertension may still persist, and hypotension can also be a problem if too much fluid is removed during dialysis.

hemodialysis (HE-mow-dye-AL-ih-sis): removal of wastes from the blood by passing it outside the body through tubes made of semipermeable membranes submerged in a dialysate solution.

■ FIGURE 29–3
Hemodialysis
Hemodialysis removes toxic wastes from the body by passing blood through a machine that houses semipermeable membranes that lie in a bath of dialysate.

Blood from an artery

Synthetic semipermeable membrane

Blood back to a vein

Dialysate

■ FIGURE 29–4
Keto-Acid Analogues
Urea is the waste product, normally excreted, into which many of the body's unused amino groups (NH_2) are collected:

$$O$$
$$\|$$
$$C$$
(H_2N) (NH_2) Amino groups

Urea

When you replace the amino group (NH_2) of an amino acid with a keto group ($=O$), you have made a keto-acid analogue. For example, pyruvic acid is the keto-acid analogue of the *nonessential* amino acid alanine:

Pyruvic acid
(keto-acid)

COOH
|
C=O
|
CH_3

Alanine
(amino acid)

COOH
|
HC—(NH_2)
|
CH_3

In renal failure, clients receive keto-acid analogues of *essential* amino acids in the hope that the body will replace the keto group from the analogue with an amino group from its unexcreted urea, thus making essential amino acids and reducing its blood urea burden at the same time.

provide enough dietary protein without precipitating uremia. However, others continue to prescribe diets low in protein (about 20 grams) in hopes of avoiding the need for dialysis. Virtually all of the protein in such a restrictive diet must be of high quality; thus, the diet emphasizes sources of protein with high biological value, such as eggs, milk, meat, poultry, and fish.

The rationale for a high-quality, low-protein diet is that the body can use nitrogen from excess urea in the blood, together with other metabolites (such as pyruvate), to synthesize nonessential amino acids.* In theory, by using urea in this way, the body can reduce blood urea levels while receiving an adequate protein supply at the same time. The diet aims at providing just enough essential amino acids to support normal nitrogen balance without causing BUN levels to rise. Protein adjustment depends on the kidneys' ability to excrete wastes, as measured by the GFR.

Unfortunately, the body's ability to use endogenous urea for protein synthesis is limited. Furthermore, diets so restrictive in protein are unpalatable. People have difficulty consuming adequate food energy on a very-low-protein diet, and without enough food energy, protein will be used for energy. When the body uses protein for energy, nitrogen forms additional urea, which accumulates in the blood.

Researchers expanded on the concept of using the diet to manipulate amino acid metabolism, and have developed another approach to the dietary treatment of renal failure. It involves keto-acid analogues, and Figure 29–4 illustrates the concept. Very-low-protein diets supplemented with keto-acid analogues of essential amino acids effectively maintain nitrogen balance while reducing the symptoms of uremia. One study suggests that the addition of keto-acids to a low-protein diet delays the rate of renal deterioration.[4] Another study cautions that while a low-protein diet supplemented with keto-acid analogues may slow the decline in renal function in some people, muscle mass may also be lost.[5] Additional research to define the risks and benefits of these diets continues.

Once the client begins dialysis, protein restrictions become less severe because the dialysis procedure results in protein losses. Table 29–1 summarizes nutrient needs of people with chronic renal failure and shows how these needs change for the person on dialysis.

Regardless of the protein allowance, all people with renal failure need adequate food energy to achieve or maintain ideal body weight and to prevent protein catabolism. Adults need at least 35 kcalories per kilogram of body weight per day.[6] For children, energy intake should at least meet the RDA.[7] One hundred or even more kcalories per kilogram of body weight per day is often desirable, but even 80 kcalories per kilogram of body weight per day is considered a realistic intake. Children cannot grow when energy intake falls below 40 kcalories per kilogram per day. The box on the next page shows how to determine energy and protein needs for chronic renal failure.

---

*The concept of supplying a low-protein diet high in essential amino acids to people with renal failure was first introduced by Giordano, Giovannetti, and Maggiore and is often called the G-G, or Giordano-Giovannetti, diet. See C. Giordano, Use of exogenous and endogenous urea for protein synthesis in normal and uremic subjects, *Journal of Laboratory and Clinical Medicine* 62 (1963): 231–246; S. Giovannetti and Q. Maggiore, A low-nitrogen diet with proteins of high biological value for severe chronic uraemia, *Lancet* 1 (1964): 1000–1003.

■ TABLE 29–1
Typical Nutrient Needs in Chronic Renal Failure

Nutrients	Predialysis	Hemodialysis	Peritoneal Dialysis
Energy (kcal/kg)	35–45	35–45	35–45
Protein (g/kg)	0.5–1.0	1.0–1.5	1.5–2.0
Fluid (ml)	1,000–1,500	800–1,000	800–1,000
Sodium (g)	0.5–2.0	2.0	2.0–4.0
Potassium (g)	1.5–2.5	1.5–2.5	2.0–4.0
Phosphorus (mg)	a	a	a
Supplements			
Calcium (mg)	1,200–1,600	1,000	1,200–1,600
Folate (mg)	1	1	1
Vitamin B$_6$ (mg)	5	10	10
Vitamin C (mg)	70–100	100	100
Other water-soluble vitamins	RDA	RDA	RDA
Vitamin D	As appropriate	As appropriate	As appropriate

Note: The actual amounts of these nutrients in the diet must be highly individualized based on each person's responses.
[a]The extent of phosphorus restriction depends on serum levels of phosphorus. Often, phosphate binders are used to help control these levels.

Energy from nonprotein sources becomes very important in renal failure, because renal diets provide so little protein. Most of the diet's energy should derive from complex carbohydrates; some should come from fat. No matter how the diet is designed, though, clients may have difficulty eating enough food to get energy intake high enough. To raise energy intake, clients may need to use additional fats (margarine, cream, and butter) and also concentrated sweets (hard candy and jelly).

Such dietary instructions fly in the face of most nutrition advice. Can you imagine a dietitian offering a child with renal failure a lollipop several times a day? Why would a health care professional feed a child candy? Because the child has a hard time getting enough energy to protect the protein she eats.

How to Determine Energy and Protein Needs for Chronic Renal Failure

Renee, an adult with chronic renal failure, is on peritoneal dialysis (see Table 29–1). At 155 lb, she has the following energy needs:

35 kcal/kg × 70 kg = 2,450 kcal.
45 kcal/kg × 70 kg = 3,150 kcal.

Her daily energy needs range between 2,450 and 3,150 kcal.
Renee has the following protein needs:

1.5 g/kg × 70 kg = 105 g.
2.0 g/kg × 70 kg = 140 g.

Her daily protein needs range between 105 and 140 g.

She needs energy in whatever form she will accept it. The candy contains little or no protein and few or no electrolytes to burden the kidney, but it offers sugar to help spare protein. Nothing could add more to this growing child's health or pleasure.

To provide adequate energy from nonprotein sources may sound like an easy task, but in reality it presents many challenges. While there are no simple solutions, there are reasonable compromises. Dietitians can include many of the client's favorite foods in carefully controlled amounts.

The person with renal disease frequently also has diabetes, in which case concentrated sweets should be avoided. However, small portions of foods containing sugar are often given with meals to add kcalories. Both renal disease and diabetes are associated with abnormal serum lipids and atherosclerosis (see Chapter 28); and the best treatment of lipid abnormalities in renal disease is unknown.

Fluid and Electrolytes   Renal disease causes disturbances in the sea of fluid and electrolytes that bathes the cells. Early in renal failure, the kidneys lose the ability to reabsorb sodium as normal kidneys do. Therefore, even though renal volume may be reduced somewhat, the person can maintain sodium balance on a moderate sodium intake. However, as end-stage renal disease approaches, the person excretes less urine and cannot handle normal amounts of sodium. At this point, both sodium and water must be restricted to prevent hypertension, edema, and heart failure. A typical diet will contain from 1 to 4 grams of sodium and from 500 to 3,000 milliliters of fluid daily (the equivalent of ½ to 3 quarts of liquid).

A person on dialysis who is excreting little or no urine must take extreme precautions not to exceed sodium, potassium, and fluid allowances. Fluid intake is controlled to allow a weight gain of about 2 to 2½ pounds (of fluid) between dialysis treatments. Table 29–2 lists foods considered part of the

■ TABLE 29–2
Foods and Beverages Controlled on Fluid-Restricted Diets

Beverages

Alcoholic beverages	Milk
Carbonated beverages	Tea
Coffee	Water
Juices	Any other

Foods

Frozen yogurt (melts to ½ initial volume)	Gelatin
	Popsicles
Ice cream (melts to ½ initial volume)	Sherbet (melts to ⅔ initial volume)
Ice milk (melts to ½ initial volume)	Soup

Other

Cream	Ice (melts to ⁹⁄₁₀ initial volume)
Liquid medications	

Note: All foods contain some water, but these foods are considered part of the fluid allowance on a fluid-restricted diet.

fluid allowance. Sodium becomes a special concern for the person on peritoneal dialysis, because this type of dialysis does not effectively remove sodium. Table 29–1 shows how requirements of fluid and minerals vary in renal disease.

Health care professionals determine individual needs by carefully monitoring each person's weight, blood pressure, and urine output. Body weight and blood pressure will increase if the person is retaining sodium and fluid. Urine output also provides a useful estimation of daily fluid needs. Simply add 500 milliliters for insensible water loss to the 24-hour urine output.

Potassium is another electrolyte of concern for the person with renal failure. Most people with renal failure do not have problems handling typical intakes of potassium. However, hyperkalemia can develop, and if it does, it can be fatal. Therefore, potassium is often moderately restricted to about 1½ to 3 grams per day. Table 10–8 on p. 289 lists the potassium contents of commonly eaten foods; the person with renal failure must avoid foods that are high in potassium. However, remember that individual needs vary. If the person is also on potassium-wasting diuretics, then potassium intake may need to be raised.

Phosphorus, Calcium, and Vitamin D   Normally, the body maintains a balance of phosphorus and calcium in the blood. When phosphorus rises, calcium falls, and vice versa. The parathyroid hormone (PTH) and active vitamin D play essential roles in regulating this balance, which, in turn, helps in maintaining bone structure. Bone disease frequently occurs in people with chronic renal failure, because the normal ratio of calcium to phosphorus is upset. Several factors seem to interact, leading to bone disease.

First of all, when serum phosphorus rises, the body normally excretes phosphorus in the urine. But in renal disease, the body retains phosphorus. As serum phosphorus rises, serum calcium falls. The low serum calcium concentration triggers the release of PTH, which works to raise blood calcium concentrations by promoting the renal excretion of phosphorus.

For a while, this action helps to lower serum phosphorus and to raise serum calcium, but every time the GFR falls, more PTH is needed to maintain the effectiveness of phosphorus excretion. Hyperparathyroidism develops. Finally, as the GFR continues to drop, PTH becomes ineffective in reducing the serum phosphorus concentration.

These problems are compounded by the diseased kidney's making little or no active vitamin D. Under normal conditions, active vitamin D works with PTH to help mobilize calcium from bone and increase the serum calcium concentration. With less active vitamin D available, PTH has to work harder to maintain normal serum calcium. Calcium absorption in the GI tract is also impaired, further lowering serum calcium. Besides all this, diets restricted in protein and phosphorus tend to be low in calcium as well.

The net result of this mineral imbalance is renal osteodystrophy, the defective bone development seen in renal disease. The bones become soft (demineralized) and fracture easily. Growth retardation in children is common; they need nutrition intervention before the end of puberty if they are to make up the growth deficit. The person with renal bone disease may experience bone pain related to the hyperparathyroidism. With PTH unable to reduce phosphorus levels, the phosphorus and calcium may form a salt that

Minimal urine volume is **oliguria**; no urine excretion is **anuria**.

hyperkalemia: excessive amount of potassium in the blood.

renal osteodystrophy (OS-tee-oh-DIS-tro-fee): a bone disorder resulting from calcium and phosphorus imbalances in renal disease. One type of renal osteodystrophy that leads to a softening of the bones is called **osteomalacia** (see p. 254).

A type of renal osteodystrophy that results from hyperparathyroidism and is characterized by kidney stones, decalcification and softening of bones, and, sometimes, formation of cysts and tumors is called **osteitis** (os-tee-EYE-tis) **fibrosis.**

The deposition of phosphorus and calcium salts in soft tissue is called **metastatic** (MET-ah-STAT-ik) **calcification.**

is deposited in soft tissues and blood vessels. Figure 29–5 summarizes the events leading to renal osteodystrophy.

The cycle of events leading to renal osteodystrophy is largely preventable through dietary control. To maintain serum phosphorus within the low normal range (2 to 3 milligrams per 100 milliliters), the person must avoid foods particularly high in phosphorus, such as those listed in the "not allowed" column of the renal diet table presented on pp. 908–909. The amount of phosphorus allowed depends on the degree of renal function. (Generally, a low-protein diet provides little phosphorus anyway, so this restriction is generally easy to manage.) Researchers have reported that phosphorus along with protein restriction can delay the rate of progression of advanced renal failure.[8] Often, physicians prescribe phosphate binders—aluminum-containing antacids—that work by binding phosphorus in the GI tract, thus making it unavailable for absorption.

Most people with renal disease receive calcium supplements (1,200 to 1,600 milligrams daily) to help prevent bone disease. Vitamin D (50,000 to 200,000 international units daily) may improve the absorption and utilization of calcium. If active vitamin D supplements are given, smaller doses are prescribed. The dosages must be carefully tailored to the individual to prevent hypercalcemia. (To prevent further deterioration of renal function, clients do not receive active vitamin D supplements when serum phosphorus is high.)

Other Nutrients Vitamin deficiencies frequently develop in people with renal failure. The restrictive diet is partly responsible, since diets low in potassium are also low in water-soluble vitamins. Vitamins can be lost in dialysis, and drug therapy can change nutrient needs. Uremia can affect the metabolism of nutrients. For these reasons, clients receive generous amounts of vitamin B_6 (5 milligrams), vitamin C (70 to 100 milligrams), and folate (1 milligram), along with the RDA of the remaining water-soluble vitamins. Supplementation of the fat-soluble vitamins, except for vitamin D, is usually not necessary.

People with renal failure should never take antacids, laxatives, or enemas high in magnesium; serious hypermagnesemia can result.

People with chronic renal failure frequently develop iron-deficiency anemia and need to receive iron supplements. Many factors contribute to iron deficiency in renal failure. For one thing, clients may lose blood (and iron), when it is drawn for testing. Additionally, GI bleeding is fairly common, and people on hemodialysis may lose some blood during dialysis. Finally, the intestinal absorption of iron may be impaired in people with uremia. Anemia unrelated to iron deficiency can also occur. The limited production of erythropoietin leads to reduced synthesis of red blood cells to carry oxygen. The toxins that accumulate in renal failure can shorten the life span of the existing red blood cells, thus compounding the problem.

People on dialysis may be zinc deficient. They frequently complain of anorexia and altered taste perceptions (dysgeusia), symptoms typical of zinc deficiency. Studies providing supplemental zinc to improve taste sensitivity and appetite have shown variable and inconclusive results. However, for people with uremia, oral zinc supplements may help to restore cell-mediated immunity (see Chapter 18).[9]

A deranged mental state seen in some people on dialysis and characterized by abnormal speech, muscle spasms, and convulsions—**dialysis encephalopathy**—has been associated with aluminum toxicity.

Aluminum toxicity may be a problem for people on dialysis. Contamination of the dialysate with aluminum has been linked to mental disturbances, bone fractures, and a severe anemia. Review Table 29–1 for a summary of the nutrient needs of people with renal disease.

Kidney Transplants and Diet

An alternative to dialysis in ESRD is a kidney transplant. Given a choice, many would prefer transplants; however, a suitable kidney donor can't always be found. Kidney transplants can successfully restore kidney function and normal growth. For this reason, transplants are particularly desirable in children. People who generally are not considered as candidates for kidney transplants are the elderly, people with other life-threatening conditions, or people who prefer dialysis.

Finding a suitable kidney donor is of paramount importance. Once a kidney has been transplanted, the body will treat it like any other foreign tissue and reject it unless the cells of the donor and recipient are properly matched. Without such a match, a transplant cannot take place. So many advances have been made in the area of renal transplants, particularly the availability of drugs that help guard against rejection of the new organ, that such procedures have become much safer and far more common in recent years.

After receiving the new kidney, the person must take very large doses of immunosuppressants to prevent rejection (see Table 23–4 on p. 732). Muscular weakness, GI bleeding, carbohydrate intolerance, sodium retention,

---

Dietary Guidelines for Post Kidney Transplant

- An energy intake designed to meet the client's need to gain or lose weight. (Immunosuppressants can induce weight gain.)
- A protein intake above the RDA—between 1.2 and 1.5 grams per kilogram body weight. Intakes may be adjusted downward to restore normal lab values or upward to counteract catabolic effects of immunosuppressants. (Immunosuppressants can induce protein catabolism and lead to negative nitrogen balance.)
- Restriction of sodium to 2 to 4 grams per day, about the same as for a person being prudent for the sake of heart-disease prevention. (Hypertension and edema often accompany immunosuppressant treatment.)
- A carbohydrate intake of 40 to 50 percent of energy intake with an emphasis on complex carbohydrates. (Glucose intolerance can develop in people taking immunosuppressants.)
- Adjustment of potassium intake when necessary. (Many people with renal transplants require potassium-wasting diuretics. Table 28–8 on p. 870–872 includes nutrition-related information about some diuretics.)

---

hypertension, and a characteristic puffy-faced appearance commonly accompany medical therapy. Infections and increased susceptibility to malignant tumors are also common. If the kidney is rejected or fails to function, dialysis must be reinstituted.

The person with a successful kidney transplant may have normal renal function and can enjoy a much freer choice of foods than the person on dialysis. However, the accompanying drug therapy can cause nutrition problems. Post-transplant diet modifications typically recommended are provided in the box above.[10]

People with kidney transplants may develop temporary periods of kidney rejection, or they may permanently reject their new kidneys. During these times, they must return to the prescribed diet for renal failure. Clients may find this regression difficult to accept, and need to be prepared for the possibility before it occurs. See the "Clinical Detective Work" box on the next page for a case study of a client with chronic renal failure.

Helpful Hints

No doubt you have long since arrived at the conclusion that designing renal diets is a task for a specialist. The complexities pile up, and diet planners must carefully adjust intakes of sodium, potassium, protein, kcalories, liquids, lipids, vitamins, and minerals. Then they must find food combinations that will deliver the necessary amounts of these nutrients. Not only that, these foods must be ones *the individual on the diet will accept and enjoy*. Renal dietitians face these challenges every day. Many of them use a system similar

CLINICAL DETECTIVE WORK

Mickey is a nine-year-old child who developed chronic glomerulonephritis several months after suffering from a streptococcal infection (strep throat). Mickey's renal function has declined steadily over the last three years. Mickey's mother brought him in to see his physician because the boy had been very tired, unable to eat, and complaining of stomach cramps and unpleasant taste sensations. Laboratory tests revealed the following information:

  GFR : 4 ml/min (below normal).

  BUN : 102 mg/dL (above normal).

Mickey was admitted to the hospital, and after further testing, dialysis was begun. A search for a suitable kidney donor was also begun. Mickey is 3 ft 8 inches tall and weighs 40 lb. Before coming to the hospital, Mickey was following a 30-g-protein, no-added-salt, potassium- and fluid-restricted diet. His typical energy intake is 1,100 kcal/day.

Describe chronic renal failure. Are the symptoms Mickey complained of typical of renal failure? Why did his GFR fall, and why did his BUN levels rise?

Look closely at Mickey's height and weight. How do they compare with the height and weight of a child his age without renal disease? (Use the growth charts in Appendix E.) Discuss reasons why growth may be compromised in the child with renal failure.

Think about Mickey's diet before he came into the hospital. Describe the reasons why protein, sodium, and potassium were restricted. Calculate Mickey's energy range, and compare this estimate with his actual energy intake. Consider the effect of Mickey's energy intake on his growth.

Describe ways Mickey's nutrient needs will change when he begins hemodialysis. How will his needs change if he receives a kidney transplant?

Discuss some diet strategies you can suggest to Mickey and his parents to help him comply with his diet. Consider the impact of renal disease on Mickey and his family. How can all members of the health team help support Mickey and his family during this difficult crisis?

to the exchange system to develop renal diet menus (see Table 29–3 on pp. 908-909).

With all that hard work to do, diet planners have still another task—communicating with, and especially listening to, the client. Inside that tangled web of grossly altered metabolic processes, dialysis lines, and toxic waste products is a person, often a frightened or discouraged one. One person will say he dreams of ice cream sodas, forbidden because of their high sodium content. He needs to feel understood, at least. Another says she feels guilty because her mother spends so much time preparing special foods for her. She too needs support. Another is fighting guilt and resentment because he repeatedly sneaks foods high in protein. If you have ever been "on a diet,"

■ **TABLE 29-3**
Renal Diet

Foods Allowed	Foods Avoided
Meats and Meat Alternates One serving contains 7 g protein, 30 mg sodium, 100 mg potassium, 200 mg phosphorus.	
1 medium egg; 1 oz beef, lamb, pork, veal, rabbit, venison, organ meats, chicken, turkey, duck, quail, goose, fish, or lobster; ¼ c water-packed, unsalted canned tuna or salmon; 5 small clams, oysters, scallops, or shrimp; 1 oz unprocessed cheese.	Luncheon meats, sausage, ham, frankfurters, or bacon; chipped, corned, or dried beef; salted, cured, or smoked meat or fish; sardines, caviar, or fish roe; canned or frozen dinners; processed cheeses or cheese spread.
Starch/breads One serving contains 2 g protein, 150 mg sodium, 30 mg potassium, 75 mg phosphorus.	
1 slice white, Italian, French, whole wheat, or rye bread; 1 2″ roll, muffin, biscuit, or corn muffin (made with allowed ingredients); ½ small bun, bagel, or English muffin; 2 tbsp plain flour or cornmeal; ½ c macaroni, noodles, spaghetti, or rice; 1 4″ pancake or waffle; ½ c cooked cereal; ¾ c dry cereals; 1 slice angel, pound, sponge, white, yellow, or spice cake with plain or flavored icing; 3 butter, 2 sandwich, 4 shortbread, 4 sugar, 5 lemon snap, 8 animal cracker, 3 oatmeal, or 9 vanilla wafer cookies; 2 squares graham crackers, 5 slices melba toast, 3 soda crackers, or 3 rye crisps; 1 plain, cake, or yeast doughnut; 1 sweetroll or cinnamon roll; 2″ square of coffee cake or plain danish pastry.	Pumpernickel bread; muffin, biscuit, cookie, and cake mixes; self-rising flour or cornmeal; instant or quick-cooking cereals; pretzels or salted popcorn; wheat germ, granola, or dry cereal containing nuts, coconut, dried fruit, or chocolate; boxed rice and dinner mixes such as Rice-a-Roni or Hamburger Helper.
Vegetables[a] One serving contains 2 g protein, 10 mg sodium, 200 mg potassium, 45 mg phosphorus.	
½ c asparagus, beets, broccoli, Brussels sprouts, carrots, cauliflower, celery, corn, eggplant, kale, mushrooms, mustard greens, green pepper, summer squash, English peas, rutabagas, radishes, turnips, turnip greens, mixed vegetables, bean sprouts, dialyzed[b] sweet or white potatoes; 1 c green beans, cabbage, lettuce, cucumber, onions, and okra; 1 slice tomato; ½ ear corn on the cob.	Artichokes, dried beans and peas, fresh garden peas, lima beans, sauerkraut, spinach, winter squash; V-8, tomato juice; canned tomato products; canned soup, pickles and olives; instant potatoes.
Fruits One serving contains 0.5 g protein, 2 mg sodium, 150 mg potassium, 30 mg phosphorus.	
1 medium fresh apple, apricot, pear, tangerine, plum, or nectarine; ½ c fresh cherries, pineapple, plums, or figs; 1 c fresh berries, watermelon, grapes or muscadines; ½ medium fresh grapefruit; ½ c canned or frozen applesauce, pineapple, berries, grapefruit, figs, peaches, apricots, cherries, plums, grapes, pears, fruit cocktail, and rhubarb; ½ c apple, lime, grapefruit, lemon, pineapple, grape, blackberry, and tangerine juice; ½ c apricot, peach or pear nectar; ½ c sweet cider.	Fresh peaches, rhubarb, avocado, cantalope, bananas, honeydew, oranges, muskmelon, dates, dried fruits, kumquats, loquats, mango, prunes, pomegranate, plantain, pumpkin, tangelo; orange or prune juice; coconut.
Milks and Milk Products One serving contains 4 g protein, 80 mg sodium, 165 mg potassium, 125 mg phosphorus.	
½ c whole milk, cream, half and half, vanilla ice cream, plain yogurt; ¼ c evaporated milk, cottage cheese, ricotta cheese; 1½ tbsp nonfat dry milk.	Buttermilk; low-sodium, goat, chocolate, coconut milk; instant breakfast drinks or other milk-based drink mixes; milkshakes; eggnog; puddings, ice cream containing chocolate, coconut, or nuts.
Fats One serving contains 0 g protein, 50 mg sodium, 10 mg potassium, 25 mg phosphorus.	
1 tsp regular or unsalted butter, margarine, mayonnaise, vegetable oil, cooking oil; 1 tbsp cream cheese, sour cream, or whipping cream.	Fatback, salted pork, bacon drippings; canned or packaged gravy.
Beverages[c]	
8 oz ades, carbonated beverages, instant orange-flavored drinks (such as Tang), cranberry juice cocktail, coffee, weakly brewed tea; alcohol, wine, and beer (if approved by physician).	Instant breakfast drink mixes; sports drinks; other drinks not listed in foods allowed.

■ **TABLE 29–3**
Renal Diet (continued)

Foods Allowed	Foods Avoided
Desserts and Sweets^c	
Popsicles, fruit ices, tapioca; gumdrops, jelly beans, lollipops, and hard candy; sugar, honey, jelly, marmalades, corn syrup; marshmallows.	Candy bars; cocoa; coconut; molasses; fudge; candy containing nuts or foods not allowed.
Miscellaneous^c	
Tapioca; cornstarch; frozen dessert topping; allspice, almond extract, anise, basil, bay leaves, caraway seeds, celery flakes, chives, cinnamon, cloves, cumin, curry powder, celery powder, dill, fennel, fresh garlic, garlic powder, ginger, horseradish root, lemon juice, mace, marjoram, mint, dry mustard, fresh onion, onion powder or juice, oregano, paprika, parsley, pepper, pimento, poultry seasoning, rosemary, sage, saffron, tarragon, thyme, extracts (such as vanilla or lemon); tabasco sauce; vinegar.	Regular or low-sodium baking powder or soda; celery, garlic, or onion salt; salt substitutes; monosodium glutamate (MSG); chili, meat, soy, steak, or Worcestershire sauce; meat extracts and tenderizers.

Note: The number of servings allowed from each list depends on the diet prescription. Diet planners use the renal diet lists to create a renal meal plan in the same way they use the diabetic exchange list to develop other diets (see Chapter 2).
^a Vegetables are measured the way they are eaten, either raw or cooked. They should be washed in large amounts of water and drained well. Fresh, frozen, and low-sodium and regular canned vegetables can be used; regular canned vegetables must be rinsed, drained, and parboiled for one minute.
^b Dialyzed vegetables have undergone a soaking and rinsing procedure that removes much of the sodium and potassium.
^c These foods can be used freely. They do not have to be calculated into the diet.

even though it wasn't a renal diet, you will appreciate some of the problems these people face.

The person with renal disease has to live a life that involves many frustrations. Successful treatment often hinges on compliance with diet and drug orders. All the members of the health care team need to know what is involved if they are to offer effective support.

Explain the concept of the diet several times, and evaluate the person's compliance frequently. Many people on a renal failure diet can comply with a sodium restriction by following a no-added-salt diet (see Table 26–2 on p. 809). However, caution clients to avoid low-sodium products and salt substitutes that contain potassium. Potassium can be kept in check if clients eliminate foods high in potassium (see Table 10–8 on p. 289).

Many people with renal failure experience severe thirst, making compliance with fluid restriction difficult. One method for helping people monitor their fluid intakes is to have them fill a container with water in the amount of their total fluid allowance at the start of each day. For example, they can fill a jar with 1,500 milliliters of water if this is their fluid allowance. Every time they use a liquid food or drink, have them discard an equivalent amount of water from the container. They can look at the jar to see how much fluid they have left for the day. Remind the person to save some of the fluid allowance for taking medications. Other suggestions to help control thirst include:

■ Chew gum or suck hard candy.
■ Freeze fluids so they take longer to consume.
■ Add lemon juice to water to make it more refreshing.
■ Gargle with refrigerated mouthwash.

Sample Renal Diet Menu
This diet menu provides 60 grams of protein, and controls sodium and potassium intake. To increase the kcalories in this diet, prepare food with oil or unsalted margarine (regular margarine, if allowed) and use additional sugar or syrup whenever possible. For example, canned fruit packed in heavy syrup, rather than in juice, add kcalories.

MENU

Breakfast
1 egg, fried with
    1 tbsp margarine
1 slice toast
2 tsp margarine
½ c grape juice
Coffee
Nondairy creamer
Sugar

Lunch
Sandwich with
    2 oz turkey
    2 slices bread
    1 tbsp mayonnaise
    Lettuce leaf
1 c green beans
2 tsp margarine
½ c strawberries
2 tbsp whipping cream
Sugar
½ c milk

Supper
3 oz roast beef
½ c rice
2 tsp margarine
½ c mushrooms sauteed in
    2 tsp olive oil and
    seasonings
½ c applesauce
Iced tea
2 tsp sugar

Snacks
Hard candy
Carbonated beverages

Remember the renal failure diet can be extremely restrictive, unappealing, and monotonous for clients. Try to provide exciting and appetizing changes. Special renal cookbooks can offer ideas. Incorporate favorite foods whenever possible. Encourage clients and their families to eat together and to eat the same foods whenever possible. Many times clients need to adjust only the portion sizes. Spices and seasonings such as garlic and onion powder, chili powder, curry powder, oregano, pepper, and lemon juice can add zest to many foods. The menu above provides a sample renal diet and Table 29–4 shows the diet plan used to develop the menu.

■ TABLE 29–4
Sample Renal Diet Menu Plan (60 g protein, 2 g sodium, 2 g potassium)

	Number of Servings	Protein (g)	Sodium (mg)	Potassium (mg)
Starch/breads	4	8	600	120
Meats	6	42	180	600
Vegetables	2	4	20	400
Fruits	3	1.5	6	450
Milks	1	4	80	165
Fats	16	—	800	160
Totals		59.5	1,686	1,895

Acute Renal Failure

Acute renal failure occurs suddenly as a consequence of another medical condition. The typical victim of acute renal failure is hypercatabolic and has a major illness, such as multiple trauma, severe infection, or a burn, or has suffered cardiac arrest. Suddenly the GFR drops, urine output falls, blood pressure shoots up, and toxic waste products begin to accumulate in the blood. Acidosis is common. As the body's cells break down, intracellular fluids release potassium and the kidneys fail to excrete it. Consequently, blood potassium levels rise sharply. Common clinical symptoms of acute renal failure include hiccups, anorexia, nausea, and vomiting. GI bleeding and diarrhea sometimes occur. Drowsiness, agitation, and confusion are frequently seen.

What went wrong? Many times acute renal failure develops from problems that originate outside the kidney. For example, acute renal failure can develop when blood flow to the kidney declines. This problem can occur for many reasons, including heart failure, shock, or severe blood loss after trauma (such as surgery or an accident). As less blood reaches the nephrons, the pressure gradient between the glomerulus and the tubule diminishes. As a consequence, less than normal amounts of urine are produced.

Another cause of acute renal failure that originates outside the kidney is a urinary tract obstruction. In this case, the kidney can make urine, but the urine can't exit.

Damage to the kidneys themselves can also cause acute renal failure. Infections, toxins, some drugs, and environmental pollutants can damage kidney cells.

In the early stages of acute renal failure, urine volume often diminishes markedly. Sometimes, though, too much urine is produced. Later in the course of renal failure, the kidneys cannot conserve water, and the person begins to excrete large amounts of urine and electrolytes. With recovery, kidney function gradually improves over a 3- to 12-month period.

In some cases, acute renal failure is reversible. In others, it progresses into chronic renal failure. About one-half of all people with acute renal failure die. Death from acute renal failure occurs more often in people who develop the disorder after surgery, particularly GI surgery. In these people, the mortality rate is about 80 percent.

The primary concern in acute renal failure is to treat the underlying disorder in order to prevent permanent or further damage to the kidneys. For example, if severe blood loss is the problem, a blood transfusion is given to restore blood volume. Other measures must be taken to restore fluid and electrolyte balance and minimize blood concentrations of toxic waste products. In addition to the nutrition factors mentioned in the following paragraphs, treatment may require diuretics to mobilize fluids in the oliguric phase of acute renal failure. Dialysis (either peritoneal dialysis or hemodialysis) is necessary when blood urea, creatinine, or potassium concentrations are high.

Chronic renal failure [is like] a downhill course for your patient; acute renal failure is like seeing him go over a cliff no one quite knew was there. J. L. Stark

Reduced blood flow to the kidney is a **prerenal** cause of acute renal failure.

A urinary tract obstruction is a **postrenal** cause of acute renal failure. The kidneys can make urine, but the urine cannot be excreted.

Damage to the kidney cells themselves is an **intrarenal** cause of acute renal failure.

The early phase of acute renal failure, when urine volume is reduced, is the **oliguric phase;** the phase characterized by large fluid and electrolyte losses in the urine is the **diuretic phase;** the gradual return of renal function marks the **recovery phase.**

Energy and Protein

As mentioned, the person in acute renal failure is often in a hypercatabolic state and suffering from another major illness. Add to these conditions nausea, vomiting, and confusion, and you have a person who really needs food energy but is unable to eat. It is particularly important for this person to receive enough energy to reverse the hypercatabolic state, because the breakdown of protein for energy contributes to the rising blood urea and potassium levels. The person's actual energy needs depend on the rate of catabolism; usually 35 to 50 kcalories per kilogram of body weight will meet these needs. Energy needs frequently increase to 50 to 100 percent above normal resting energy expenditure. The diet to meet these high energy needs emphasizes complex carbohydrates and some fat.

Protein needs also vary, depending on the catabolic rate. The protein requirement of people with acute renal failure is unknown. Generally, the diet restricts protein to about 30 to 40 grams per day. However, impaired wound healing, infection, muscle wasting, and negative nitrogen balance are commonly seen in these individuals; they often die. Some practitioners prefer to provide a higher protein intake, even if this might make dialysis necessary, to prevent negative nitrogen balance and its possible consequences. If dialysis is instituted, a more liberal protein intake of 70 to 85 grams may be allowed.

Fluid and Electrolytes

Clients must carefully control their total fluid intakes to avoid overhydration or dehydration. Health care professionals determine fluid requirements by carefully measuring urine output. To the volume of urine, add about 500 milliliters for water lost through the skin, lungs, and perspiration. The person who is vomiting, has diarrhea, has a high fever, or otherwise loses fluids, needs additional fluid. In the oliguric stage, the person will need small volumes of fluids. In the diuretic stage, up to 3 liters of urine may be lost daily, and large amounts of fluids will have to be provided.

Sodium may be restricted (to 500 to 1,000 milligrams) in the oliguric phase, but this may change as the person enters the diuretic phase. Likewise, potassium may be restricted (to less than 2 grams per day) in the oliguric phase but may need to be supplemented in the diuretic phase. Pay special attention to potassium in the person with acute renal failure—hyperkalemia can be life-threatening.

Drugs called exchange resins must sometimes be used to treat severe hyperkalemia. These drugs, which are placed rectally, cause sodium to be exchanged for potassium in the colon, and the potassium is then excreted in the stool. Another method that can temporarily reduce high potassium levels is to give IV dextrose and insulin. Potassium moves into the cells with glucose. However, this is only a temporary measure.

The "Clinical Detective Work" box on the next page provides a case study of a client with acute renal failure. Take a moment to review the many parameters health care providers must consider when treating such clients.

CLINICAL DETECTIVE WORK

Mrs. Calley is a 35-year-old homemaker admitted to the hospital's intensive care unit. She was first seen in the emergency room after she sustained many severe injuries in an auto accident. She had lost so much blood she almost died before reaching the hospital. In addition to her injuries, which include a fractured leg, broken ribs, a collapsed lung, and internal bleeding, she has developed acute renal failure. Mrs. Calley is 5 ft 3 inches tall and weighs 125 lb.

Mrs. Calley has a urine volume of less than 50 ml/day and has a BUN of 75 mg/dL. A test of GFR could not be performed due to the low volume of urine excreted. She is receiving blood transfusions to maintain blood volume and will undergo surgery to uncover and correct the source of the internal bleeding.

Describe the most probable reason why Mrs. Calley developed acute renal failure. What other problems can cause acute renal failure? Describe the phases of acute renal failure.

What are Mrs. Calley's dietary needs in the early phase? What waste products and electrolytes are of greatest concern? Why? What factors do you have to keep in mind in determining Mrs. Calley's energy and protein needs during her episode of acute renal failure? How will these needs change if dialysis is begun?

How will her nutrient needs change as she progresses to the second stage of acute renal failure? Contrast Mrs. Calley's current nutrient needs with the nutrient needs of a person with chronic renal failure. Describe some of the differences between the two diets.

Special Nutrition Support in Renal Failure

When clients with either acute or chronic renal failure are hypercatabolic or for other reasons are unable to eat adequately, then special nutrition support is in order. As discussed in Chapter 21, health care providers first try to supplement the diet or offer a liquid diet orally if the GI tract is functioning. Encourage clients to drink supplements between meals to increase the amount of energy received. Appendix L lists commercial formulas useful for this purpose. But remember, the person with renal failure who is restricted to a certain amount of fluid has to derive the maximum energy from a small volume: select formulas that provide more than 1 kcalorie per milliliter. Some products specially formulated for people with renal disease can be taken orally or by tube. Other formulas can be modified for renal disease. Special glucose polymer powders effectively add food energy without requiring clients to eat extra food or use their fluid allowance.[11] Remember to notice the amounts of vitamins and minerals delivered by these products; Appendix L lists the vitamin and mineral contents of some formulas.

Many people with renal failure, particularly acute renal failure, require TPN. Consequently, a growing interest in the use of TPN for people in renal failure has evolved. Mixtures of both nonessential and essential amino acids at lower concentrations than in standard TPN solutions produce favorable results. To prevent fluid overload during TPN, clinicians use 70 percent, rather than 50 percent, glucose solutions in order to deliver more kcalories in a smaller volume. Health care providers monitor and adjust electrolytes as necessary. Glucose intolerance and insulin resistance are common in both uremia and catabolic illnesses, so insulin must often be given.

◼ *Nephrotic Syndrome*

Nephrotic syndrome is not a disease, but rather a complex of symptoms caused by the loss of plasma protein into the urine. Many disorders can lead to nephrotic syndrome, including glomerulonephritis, diabetes mellitus, infections, and renal vein thrombosis.

The loss of protein in the urine is called **proteinuria** and loss of the protein albumin in the urine is called **albuminuria**.

Normally, only small plasma proteins pass through the glomerulus into the filtrate. The tubules then reabsorb these proteins and return them to the blood. But in nephrotic syndrome, the permeability of the glomerular capillaries is defective, and plasma proteins escape in the urine. Since albumin is the major plasma protein, it is also the major protein lost in the urine.

As plasma proteins are lost, blood proteins fall sharply. Together with other factors, low blood protein concentrations cause fluid to move into the interstitial space, and edema develops. As protein loss continues, lean body mass breaks down. Losses of some plasma proteins, such as immunoglobulins, render the person with nephrotic syndrome prone to infections, which can compromise nutrition status further. The loss of transferrin, the iron-carrying protein, may lead to anemia (see Figure 29–6). Serum lipids rise markedly for unknown reasons.

Note that different renal diseases require different dietary adjustments. In renal failure, dietary protein is low to moderate; in nephrotic syndrome, dietary protein is high.

Treatment of nephrotic syndrome depends largely on the underlying cause. Diet is central to preventing protein malnutrition and alleviating edema. A diet high in energy (50 to 60 kcalories per kilogram of body weight) and high in protein (about 120 grams per day) is prescribed. Sodium must be restricted because the body avidly retains sodium in nephrotic syndrome. In the early treatment, a diet low in sodium (250 milligrams) and diuretics help to mobilize the fluid that has accumulated in the interstitial space. Once edema is resolved and sodium balance achieved, the sodium restriction relaxes to about 1,500 milligrams per day—still fairly stringent. Chapters 26 and 28 provide more information on low-sodium diets. If physicians prescribe potassium-wasting diuretics, they must remember to advise clients to select foods rich in potassium.

People with nephrotic syndrome often have hyperlipidemia—most commonly, type II or V (see Chapter 28) and face the risk of atherosclerosis. Clinicians advise clients to follow the diet appropriate for the type of hyperlipidemia.

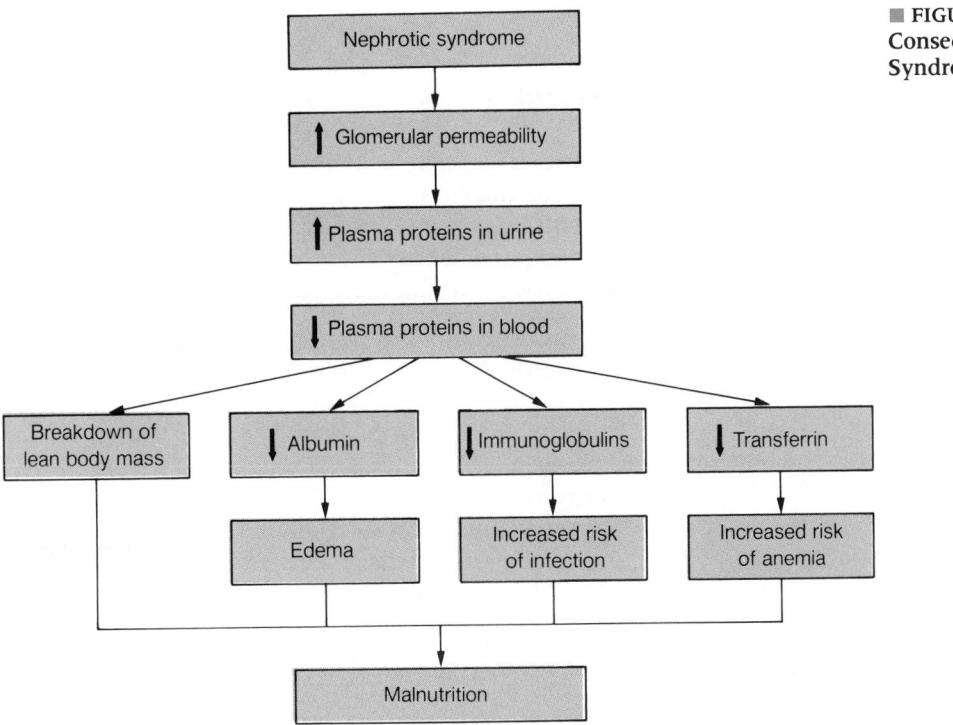

■ FIGURE 29–6
Consequences of Nephrotic Syndrome

■ *Urinary Tract Infections*

People with urinary tract infections are encouraged to eat a well-balanced diet and to drink plenty of fluids. Fluids will help prevent stagnation and the growth of bacteria. Fluids also aid in delivering antibiotics to the urinary tract, where they are needed. Many antibiotics used for urinary tract infections work better in an acid urine; therefore, people with such infections may be encouraged to use acid-producing juices and foods. However, the effects of foods on urine acidity are not clear (see Highlight 29), and drug therapy to alter urinary pH may be more effective for this purpose.

See the discussion entitled "A Note on Acid-formers and Base-formers" on p. 282.

Traditionally, people with a urinary tract infection have been advised to drink plenty of cranberry juice. This suggestion stems from the widespread belief that cranberry juice can lower urinary pH more effectively than other foods and drinks. Furthermore, cranberry juice contains a precursor of an acid that has an antibacterial action in the urine.

Unfortunately, it is impractical to use cranberry juice for these purposes. Although cranberry juice has a high acidity, it does not consistently lower urinary pH. The antibacterial potential of cranberry juice is never achieved, because the antibacterial product does not become concentrated enough in the urinary tract to be effective.

◼ *Nutrition Assessment*

The person in renal failure is at high risk for malnutrition. It therefore becomes essential that health care providers conduct nutrition assessments frequently and that problems be prevented or promptly corrected, otherwise nutrient stores will dwindle. Carefully consider:

- Diet history, to determine the usual intake of kcalories, protein, sodium, potassium, phosphorus, calcium, and vitamin D. These data will help you in adjusting the newly diagnosed person's current eating habits for better compliance in a restricted diet. For the person already following a renal diet, diet history helps to assess the person's understanding of, and compliance with, the diet.
- Anthropometric measurements, which will be significantly influenced by the state of hydration. Weight taken immediately after dialysis treatments will most accurately reflect true weight. This weight is sometimes called the "dry weight." When the person isn't on dialysis, weight may be deceptively normal or high because of water retention. Likewise, arm measurements may be affected by edema. The person with nephrotic syndrome may be dehydrated, in which case anthropometric measurements may be lower than normal.
- Weight changes and blood pressure, which are useful in assessing the state of hydration in people with renal failure. Weight gain and blood pressure elevations suggest fluid retention; weight loss and low blood pressure suggest dehydration.
- Weight and height in children, which must be routinely assessed to ensure that their diets adequately meet the needs for growth. Remember that growth failure is common in children with renal failure. Weight loss often occurs in renal failure. Wasting is common in people with nephrotic syndrome who fail to eat enough protein.
- Albumin and transferrin levels, which may be extremely low in people with nephrotic syndrome, rise when protein intake is adequate. People with renal failure also have lower transferrin levels than healthy people do; these are even lower when malnutrition accompanies renal disease.
- Serum electrolytes, BUN, and creatinine, which must be carefully monitored in renal failure.
- Serum lipids, which are frequently elevated in both chronic renal failure and nephrotic syndrome.
- Health care providers must conscientiously monitor people with chronic renal failure so that they can institute timely measures to prevent growth failure and renal osteodystrophy. Anemia also may be a problem that can be partially corrected by diet.

This chapter has devoted most of its space to the consequences of renal failure and the dietary treatments that might help to resolve them. Highlight 29 describes the development and treatment of kidney stones.

SELF STUDY *Fluid Intake Adjustments*

Restrict your fluid intake for a day to an amount less than you are comfortable with—say, 6 glasses instead of 8. Record your sensations and any measures you find useful in helping yourself live with this restriction.

On a second day, increase your fluid intake to one and a half times what you are accustomed to—say, 12 glasses instead of 8. Again, record your reactions.

This exercise should give you some insight into one of the many problems that clients with renal disease often face—living with amounts of fluid (particularly, restricted intakes) that are uncomfortable for them. By experiencing this discomfort for one or two days you can develop empathy that should stand you in good stead when offering advice and moral support to clients with renal disease.

Study Questions

1. What functions do the kidneys perform? What is the role of the kidneys in maintaining chemical homeostasis?
2. What is renal failure? Why is it often difficult to detect renal failure in the early stages? What causes renal failure?
3. What happens in the end stage of renal failure? Describe some of the symptoms associated with the buildup of toxic metabolic products in the blood.
4. When is a special diet instituted in the course of renal failure? When is dialysis or a kidney transplant considered for the person with renal failure?
5. Describe some of the reasons why the metabolism of nutrients is affected by renal failure. What are the objectives of dietary treatment of chronic renal failure?
6. Why is the protein (nitrogen) intake of the person with chronic renal failure a particular concern? Describe the use of keto-acid analogues along with a low-protein diet for the treatment of chronic renal failure.
7. What are the energy needs of adults with chronic renal failure? Of children? What are the consequences of providing too little energy in the diet of the person with chronic renal failure?
8. What fluid and electrolyte modifications are made to the diet of the person with chronic renal failure? What modifications are made concerning phosphorus, calcium, and vitamin D? Why?
9. What other vitamins and minerals need special consideration in the diet of the person with chronic renal failure? Describe why each of the nutrients you list may be a problem.
10. Discuss the nutrient needs of the person with a kidney transplant.
11. What suggestions can you give people with chronic renal failure to help them comply with their restrictive diets?
12. Describe the differences between chronic renal failure and acute renal failure. List some causes of acute renal failure.
13. What are the nutrient needs of the person in the oliguric phase of acute renal failure? How do these needs change as the person progresses to the diuretic phase?
14. Can tube feedings and TPN be used safely in the person with renal failure? What special considerations must be made when selecting an enteral or parenteral formula for the person with kidney failure?
15. What is nephrotic syndrome? What are the consequences of nephrotic syndrome? What are the protein and energy needs of the person with nephrotic syndrome? What are the fluid and electrolyte needs of these individuals?
16. What dietary advice can benefit the person with a urinary tract infection?

Notes

1. L. Oldrizzi and coauthors, Progression of renal failure in patients with renal disease of diverse etiology on protein-restricted diets, *Kidney International* 27 (1985): 553–557; A. J. Williams and coauthors, Alteration of the course of chronic renal failure by dietary protein restriction, *Proceedings of the European Dialysis and Transplant Association* 21 (1985): 604–607; S. R. Acchiardo, L. W. Moore, and S. Cockrell, Does low protein diet halt the progression of renal insufficiency? *Clinical Nephrology* 25 (1986): 289–294.
2. B. U. Ihle and coauthors, The effect of protein restriction on the progression of renal insufficiency, *New England Journal of Medicine* 321 (1989): 1773–1777; J. B. Rosman and coauthors, Early protein restriction in chronic renal failure, *Proceedings of the European Dialysis and Transplant Association* 21 (1985): 567–573; C. Giordano, Early dietary protein restriction protects the failing kidney, *Kidney International* 28 (1985): 566–570.
3. G. Zakar, Effects of dietary protein restriction on the course of early renal failure, *Proceedings of the European Dialysis and Transplant Association* 21 (1985): 600–603.

4. P. T. Frohling and coauthors, Influence of phosphate restriction, keto acids and vitamin D on the progression of chronic renal failure, *Proceedings of the European Dialysis and Transplant Association* 21 (1985): 561–566.

5. P. A. Lucas and coauthors, The risks and benefits of a low-protein-essential amino acid-keto acid diet, *Kidney International* 29 (1986): 995–1003.

6. J. D. Kopple, F. J. Monteon, and J. K. Shaib, Effect of energy intake on nitrogen metabolism in nondialyzed patients with chronic renal failure, *Kidney International* 29 (1986): 734–742.

7. F. Santos, B. I. Friedman, and J. C. Chan, Management of chronic renal failure in children, *Current Problems in Pediatrics* 16 (1986): 237–301.

8. Frohling and coauthors, 1985; D. Lumlertgul and coauthors, Phosphate depletion arrests progression of chronic renal failure independent of protein intake, *Kidney International* 29 (1986): 658–666.

9. D. Grekas and coauthors, Effect of zinc treatment on cell mediated immunity of chronic renal failure patients, *Proceedings of the European Dialysis and Transplant Association* 21 (1985): 825–829.

10. M. S. Edwards and S. Doster, Renal transplant diet recommendations of a survey of renal dietitians in the United States, *Journal of the American Dietetic Association* 90 (1990): 843–846.

11. M. A. Allman and coauthors, Energy supplementation and the nutritional status of hemodialysis patients, *American Journal of Clinical Nutrition* 51 (1990): 558–562.

Prevention and Treatments for Kidney Stones

Chapter 29 described how the kidneys work, what happens to the body when they fail, and the dietary plan for treating kidney disorders. This highlight focuses on a far more common kidney problem—kidney stones. In the United States, about one in every 10 adults (mostly men over 25 years old) suffers from kidney stones, a painful, although rarely fatal, condition. People who have experienced a kidney stone may have a recurrence, but a large percentage report only a single episode, suggesting that with proper treatment, recurrence may be preventable. This highlight reviews the role of diet in the prevention and treatment of kidney stones. The accompanying miniglossary defines related terms.

Formation of Kidney Stones

Kidney stones vary in their chemical composition. Most of them contain calcium in the form of calcium oxalate (60 percent of all stones), calcium phosphate (9 percent), or a combination of the two (11 percent). Calcium stones may form in response to a variety of underlying medical conditions. However, many calcium stones are associated with excessive urinary calcium excretion for which no underlying cause can be identified—idiopathic hypercalciuria. Quite likely, idiopathic hypercalciuria involves genetic factors that alter enzyme activity in transporting calcium across membranes.[1] Risk factors for calcium stones include low urine volume; high urine pH; excessive urinary excretion of calcium, oxalate, uric acid, or a combination; and deficiencies of substances in the urine that normally inhibit stone formation.

Less common stones are composed of uric acid, the amino acid cystine, or magnesium ammonium phosphate

---

Miniglossary

cystinuria (SIS-te-NEW-ree-ah): the presence of cystine in the urine; the symptom of an inherited metabolic disorder in which large amounts of the amino acids cystine, lysine, arginine, and ornithine are excreted in the urine. Cystinuria commonly results in kidney stone formation.

dysuria (dis-YOU-ree-ah): painful or difficult urination.

gout: a metabolic disorder that results in excess uric acid in the blood and sometimes in the urine, characterized by acute arthritis and inflammation of the joints.

hematuria (HEME-ah-TOO-ree-ah): blood in the urine.

hypercalciuria (HIGH-per-KAL-see-YOU-ree-ah): excessive urinary excretion of calcium. When the excessive urinary excretion of calcium is not related to a known underlying medical condition, it is known as **idiopathic hypercalciuria**.

hyperoxaluria (HIGH-per-OK-sa-LOO-ree-ah): excessive urinary excretion of oxalate; may occur when calcium intake is insufficient to bind oxalate in the intestine, thus allowing excessive oxalate absorption. When GI diseases cause excessive oxalate absorption and subsequent excessive oxalate excretion, it is known as **enteric hyperoxaluria**.

nidus (NIGH-dus), **nucleus**: a small bit of crystallized mineral or other substance that serves as a matrix for further crystallization.

pH: see pp. 50–51, 280–281, and Appendix B.

purine: a nitrogen-containing compound found in DNA and RNA.

renal colic: the severe pain that accompanies the movement of a kidney stone from the kidney through the ureter to the bladder.

struvite: crystals of magnesium ammonium phosphate.

supersaturation: a term that describes the concentration of a substance in a liquid at the point where it is too concentrated to stay in solution and begins to precipitate.

(known as struvite). Uric acid stones can form when the urine becomes persistently acid, contains excessive uric acid, or both. They are frequently associated with the metabolic disorder of gout. Cystine stones form when an inherited disorder of amino acid metabolism (cystinuria) causes the abnormal excretion of cystine in the urine. Sometimes called "infection stones," struvite stones form when the urinary tract becomes infected with a specific type of microorganism that hydrolyzes urea, creating an ammonia-rich alkaline urine. (You may want to review the discussion of how the body disposes of excess nitrogen on pp. 178–179.) Such infections and stones are about twice as prevalent in women as in men.

The exact mechanisms by which kidney stones form remain undefined. Why is it, for example, that all people pass crystals in the urine routinely, whereas only 10 percent develop kidney stones?[2] Practitioners widely accept three theories that help to explain how kidney stones form.

These theories form the basis for the prevention and treatment of kidney stones.

One proposed mechanism of stone formation—supersaturation—bases its explanation on the relative insolubility of stone constituents in urine. When stone constituents (such as calcium salts, uric acid, or oxalic acid) become concentrated, they form crystals that eventually precipitate and grow larger. Urine volume and pH influence the concentrations of these constituents. In general, the more concentrated a constituent in the urine, the greater the likelihood is that a stone will form.

Another mechanism holds that a small seed (sometimes called a nucleus or nidus) is responsible for the formation of some stones. Composed of a substance different from that found in the remainder of the stone, the seed develops from the crystallization of a supersaturated compound in the urine. The crystalline structure then provides a matrix upon which less-saturated minerals can attach. In some cases, calcium oxalate stones have been found to form around a uric acid seed. Treatment for this type of stone focuses on the mineral within the seed rather than on the minerals that make up most of the stone.

Finally, many practitioners believe that a deficiency of one or more naturally occurring stone inhibitors in the urine may contribute to stone formation. For example, researchers have identified a protein that inhibits the formation of kidney stones; its defective version fails to inhibit stone formation.[3] Other probable inhibitors include citrate, a type of phosphate, a type of polysaccharide, magnesium, zinc, and ribonucleic acid (RNA).[4] All of these substances have been identified as inhibitors of calcium oxalate stone formation.[5] Research has yet to provide enough knowledge about these inhibitors to influence therapy.

Diet probably does not play a role in the development of kidney stones in healthy people. In people who are

■ TABLE H29–1
Conditions Associated with Kidney Stones

Bowel diseases causing malabsorption
Cystinuria
Glucocorticoid excess
Gout
Hyperparathyroidism
Hyperthyroidism
Immobilization
Malignancies (some types)
Osteoporosis
Paget's disease
Recurrent urinary tract infections
Renal tubular acidosis
Vitamin D intoxication

susceptible to kidney stone formation, however, diet may influence the course of stone development. Studies have found differences between the diets of people with kidney stones and those without them.[6] Components generally found lacking in the diets of people with kidney stones include fiber, phytate, magnesium, phosphate, and thiamin; a nutrient found in excess is vitamin C.[7] Although the significance of these findings is unclear at this time, they appear to suggest a possible link between diet and the development of kidney stones. For people with recurrent stones, diet can effectively help to control the formation of some types of stones.

Table H29–1 summarizes some of the disorders associated with stone formation. Because so many disorders can result in stone formation, the choice of diet for the treatment and prevention of kidney stones becomes complicated. Of course, the underlying disorder and the kidney stones demand medical and dietary attention.

Treatment and Prevention of Kidney Stones

Treatment of kidney stones concentrates on the removal of existing stones, if necessary, and the prevention of recurrent stones. In some cases, kidney stones pose no problems, especially when they are

few and small. Small stones (less than 5 millimeters, or one-fifth of an inch in diameter) may not require treatment. They may pass readily through the ureters and out of the body via the urine (see Figure H29–1). Larger stones cannot exit the body as easily. When a large stone or a large broken-off piece of a stone enters a ureter, the person experiences a severe, stabbing pain, called renal colic. Typically, the pain starts suddenly in the back, just above the ribs, and follows the course of the stone down the abdomen toward the groin. When the stone reaches the bladder, the pain normally subsides. Urinary symptoms include frequent urination, urgency of urination, dysuria, and hematuria. If a stone blocks the flow of urine or causes an infection, a physician must either remove it surgically or, more commonly, use sound waves or shock waves to break the stone into pieces small enough to pass easily through the urinary tract.

Success in inhibiting stone growth or in preventing new stone formation depends, in part, on diet. Dietary regimens vary according to the type of stone, but all include one bit of advice: increase fluid intake. An increased fluid intake raises the urine

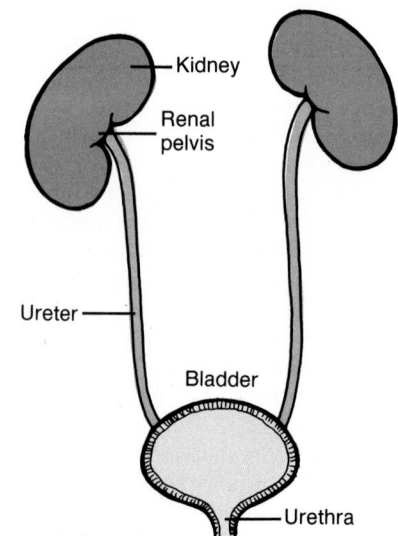

■ FIGURE H29–1
The Urinary Tract

output, thus diluting the concentration of minerals in the urine and reducing the risk of stone formation. People with kidney stones need to drink enough fluid to maintain a urine volume of at least 2 liters per day. This requires an intake of about 3 to 4 liters total, taken at regular intervals throughout the day.

For people who are susceptible to stone formation, fluid intake is particularly important during exercise. Physical exercise without fluid replacement enhances crystallization of calcium oxalate and uric acid stones.[8] Therefore, all exercisers, especially those with a history of kidney stones, need to increase fluid intake to compensate for sweat loss.

Other aspects of dietary treatment for kidney stones have been far more controversial and have changed dramatically in recent years. The remainder of this highlight discusses the role of diet in treating different types of stones. Keep in mind as you read that each of the dietary plans that follow center on fluid intake; all physicians recommend hydration to all clients who form stones.

Dietary Treatment of Calcium Stones
One of the most controversial topics in the treatment of kidney stones concerns the role of dietary calcium restriction for the person with a calcium-containing stone. On the surface, it appears reasonable that a person who is excreting large amounts of calcium in the urine should restrict dietary calcium. For years, people with calcium stones were routinely instructed to reduce their calcium intakes by eliminating milk and milk products from their diets. Such a diet may be advisable only for clients with idiopathic hypercalciuria in whom calcium absorption increases significantly when on a high-calcium diet. In this case, urinary calcium excretion rises, thus increasing the risk of calcium stone formation. For these people, then, a low-calcium diet (600 milligrams calcium per day) may be beneficial. In addition, they need to

refrain from using vitamin-mineral preparations and medicines containing calcium (such as calcium-containing antacids) or vitamin D (which enhances calcium absorption).

For clients who do not absorb calcium excessively, calcium restriction might lead to negative calcium balance and bone loss. They have high urinary calcium levels even when their dietary calcium is not high. This indicates that they are losing calcium from their bones.[9] Calcium loss from bones raises urinary calcium, thus making stone formation more, not less, likely.

Calcium restriction is also contraindicated for people who are susceptible to developing calcium oxalate stones. You may recall from Chapter 10 that calcium normally binds to oxalate in the intestinal tract.

If dietary calcium is severely limited, oxalate absorption and subsequent excretion may increase, resulting in hyperoxaluria. Hyperoxaluria increases the likelihood of calcium oxalate stone formation. Instead of restricting calcium intake, then, treatment focuses on oxalate. Of the oxalate in the urine, only a small percentage derives from the diet. Nevertheless, people with calcium oxalate stones are advised to limit their intakes of foods high in oxalate. Table H29–2 lists foods containing considerable amounts of oxalate.

Most of the oxalate in the urine comes from the body's synthesis of it. One of the oxalate synthesis pathways in the body begins with vitamin C. Consequently, megadoses of vitamin C over a prolonged time raise urinary

■ TABLE H29–2
Foods High in Oxalate

Vegetables

Baked beans canned in tomato sauce	Leeks
Beans (green, wax, or dried)	Mustard greens
Beets	Okra
Celery	Parsley
Chard, Swiss	Peppers, green
Chives	Potatoes, sweet
Collards	Rutabagas
Dandelion greens	Spinach
Eggplant	Summer squash
Escarole	Watercress
Kale	

Fruits

Blackberries	Lemon peel
Blueberries	Lime peel
Currants, red	Orange peel
Dewberries	Raspberries
Fruit cocktail	Rhubarb
Gooseberries	Strawberries
Grapes, Concord	Tangerines

Other

Chocolate	Pepper (more than 1 tsp/day)
Cocoa	Soybean crackers
Cola beverages	Soybean curd (tofu)
Draft beer	Tea
Fruit cake	Tomato soup
Grits	Vegetable soup
Peanut butter	Wheat germ

oxalate concentrations, which, in some people, can aggravate stone formation. People with hyperoxaluria must steer clear of vitamin C supplements.

While the goal of calcium stone treatment is to reduce urinary calcium excretion, diet alone rarely accomplishes this satisfactorily. Certain medications, such as thiazide diuretics, effectively reduce the excretion of calcium and oxalate, and thus the recurrence of idiopathic calcium stones. However, because thiazide diuretics can precipitate a potassium deficiency, they are generally given with a diuretic that conserves potassium.

Health care providers advise clients on thiazide diuretics to follow a moderately restricted sodium diet. A high sodium intake can offset the beneficial effects of the diuretic and can cause excessive potassium excretion.[10] Health care providers must monitor potassium levels closely, and provide potassium supplements when necessary. Sodium restriction may have another benefit: calcium excretion may be linked to sodium excretion.[11] A moderately restricted sodium diet might lower calcium in the urine, even for calcium stone formers not taking thiazide diuretics.

Other studies have shown that a diet high in animal protein may influence calcium stone development. Such diets increase the urinary excretion of calcium, oxalate, and uric acid—three risk factors for calcium stones. In addition, high animal protein diets contain large quantities of purines, which in turn raise uric acid excretion. As mentioned earlier, uric acid may form the seed for the crystallization of a calcium oxalate stone. However, researchers have yet to demonstrate that restricting dietary protein will help prevent calcium stone formation.

In summary, most people with calcium stones need not restrict their calcium intakes. On the other hand, they should not exceed 1 gram calcium per day either.[12] Some people

with calcium stones whose calcium absorption is exceptionally high might benefit from a moderately limited calcium intake (600 milligrams per day). People with calcium oxalate stones should limit their intakes of foods high in oxalate. Those on thiazide diuretics may benefit from a moderately restricted sodium intake, and possibly a potassium supplement, if potassium becomes deficient. Of course, fluid intake remains a high priority.

Dietary Treatment of Other Stones

A common practice in the treatment of kidney stones has been to design diets to alter the acidity of the urine. An acid ash diet, intended to make the urine more acid, centers on meat, cheese, eggs, whole grains, and some fruits. An alkaline ash diet, intended to reduce the acidity of the urine, emphasizes milk, vegetables, and most fruits. Diet can affect the acidity of the urine, it is true, but current methods used to calculate the effects of different foods on the acidity of the urine are inaccurate and difficult to use.[13] Until a better estimate of the effects of dietary components on urine acidity is available, drug therapy remains more reliable and more frequently used for this purpose.

Uric Acid Stones. Low-purine diets are commonly prescribed to reduce uric acid levels in the urine. A low-purine diet restricts foods that consist of large numbers of cells loaded with DNA and RNA, notably red meats, particularly organ meats, anchovies, sardines, and meat extracts. The benefits of such a diet are unproven, but it may be useful to limit excessive protein intake; health care providers advise a diet containing no more than 120 grams protein per day.[14] Drug therapy may be prescribed to inhibit uric acid production, thus reducing the uric acid levels and acidity of the urine.

Struvite Stones. No specific diet therapy is recommended for struvite "infection" stones. Effective treatment includes removal of the stones and

antibacterial drugs.

Cystine Stones. To reduce cystine in the urine, health care providers prescribe a diet restricted in the amino acid methionine, because the body makes the nonessential amino acid cystine from methionine. Drug therapy to reduce the acidity of the urine may also be beneficial.

As you can see, many connections between diet and kidney stones have been explored. Dramatic advances in the nonsurgical treatment of kidney stones have triggered a renewed interest in this area. Health care professionals will want to keep up with changes such as these so as to provide the best possible care for their clients.

NOTES

1. G. Bianchi and coauthors, Abnormal red-cell calcium pump in patients with idiopathic hypercalciuria, *New England Journal of Medicine* 319 (1988): 897–901.

2. B. Goldwasser, J. L. Weinerth, and C. C. Carson, Calcium stone disease: An overview, *Journal of Urology* 135 (1986): 1–9.

3. Mystery of kidney stone formation is solved, *Journal of the American Dietetic Association* 85 (1985): 1493.

4. S. P. Kanig and R. L. Conn, Kidney stones: Medical management and newer options for stone removal, *Postgraduate Medicine* 78, no. 6 (1985): 38–51.

5. Goldwasser, Weinerth, and Carson, 1986.

6. H. M. Griffith and coauthors, A case-controlled study of dietary intake of renal stone patients: 1. Preliminary analysis, *Urology Research* 14 (1986): 67–74.

7. H. M. Griffith and coauthors, A case-controlled study of dietary intake of renal stone patients: 2. Urine biochemistry and stone analysis, *Urology Research* 14 (1986): 75–82.

8. K. Sakhaee and coauthors, Assessment of the pathogenic role of physical exercise in renal stone formation, *Journal of Clinical Endocrinology Metabolism* 65 (1987): 974–979.

9. F. L. Coe and J. H. Parks, Recurrent renal calculi: Causes and prevention, *Hospital Practice* 21, no. 3A (1986): 49–57.

10. Coe and Parks, 1986.

11. Kanig and Conn, 1985.

12. National Institutes of Health, Prevention and treatment of kidney stones, National Institutes of Health Consensus Development Conference Statement, HHS publication no. 1988–216–941/80620 (Washington, D.C.: Government Printing Office, 1988).

13. J. Dwyer and coauthors, Acid/alkaline ash diets: Time for assessment and change, *Journal of the American Dietetic Association* 85 (1985): 841–845.

14. Goldwasser and Weinerth, and Carson, 1986.

Nutrition and Wasting Disorders: Cancer and AIDS

Cancer cells multiply within organs and spread to other organs, threatening their integrity and functions. Often, they rob the organs of needed nutrients, causing local starvation. Shown here is a cervical cancer cell.

Previous chapters have shown that malnutrition accompanies and complicates many disorders. Two of the most serious types of disorders, chronic renal disease and inflammatory bowel diseases, last for long periods of time and can eventually lead to severe protein-energy malnutrition (PEM). This chapter describes two other disorders—cancer and acquired immune deficiency syndrome (AIDS)—that often impact equally severely on nutrition status.

As different as they may appear to be at first, these two disorders, cancer and AIDS, present many similarities nutritionally. Both affect many organ systems. Both are associated with wasting, and in both, the wasting is caused not only by the diseases themselves but by their treatments as well. In both cases, malnutrition aggravates the symptoms, interferes with treatment, impairs the quality of life, and shortens life expectancy.

Cancer

cancer: a disease in which cells multiply out of control, forming masses (**tumors**) that disrupt normal functioning of one or more organs.

tumor: an unchecked new growth of tissue with no function; **benign** (bee-NINE) tumors often pose no problems; **malignant** tumors (cancers) resist treatment and are harmful. The term **neoplasm** (NEE-oh-plazm) frequently denotes a malignant tumor, or cancer. A **carcinoma** (KAR-see-NO-mah) is a cancer that affects epithelial tissue. A **sarcoma** (sar-KO-mah) is a cancer that arises from muscle, bone, or connective tissue. A **hematopoietic** (HEE-ma-toe-poy-ET-ik) **neoplasm** is a malignant tumor of the blood and immune system. A cancer that spreads from one area to another is said to **metastasize** (me-TAS-tah-size).

One out of every four people now alive will eventually contract cancer. The word *cancer* refers to any uncontrolled growth of abnormal cells. Cancer is not a single disorder; instead, there are multiple *cancers*—that is, many different kinds of tumors. They have different characteristics, occur in different locations in the body, take different courses, and require different treatments.

A growing neoplasm interferes with the normal functioning of an organ or tissue. The growth seemingly has no built-in brakes and is supported by nutrients from the diet or body reserves. The words *neoplasm, malignant tumor,* and *cancer* are often used interchangeably to describe the unchecked growth of abnormal cells.

Diet relates to cancer in several ways, and it is important to get them all in perspective. Constituents in foods may cause cancer, promote cancer, or protect against cancer. Also, for the person who has cancer, diet can make a crucial difference to recovery. Of course, nondiet factors are important in relation to cancer, too. Some cancers are programmed by genes to develop. Other, environmental factors are also involved—smoking, for example, and water and air pollution. The emphasis here is on diet, of course.

The accompanying box outlines how cancer develops. The initiating event may be either physical or chemical. The physical event may occur when radiation—either the general radiation that is always present, or medical or industrial radiation—bombards the cell and alters the genetic material. The chemical event may occur when the intrusion of a chemical—a carcinogen—into the cell alters the genetic material. In each case, the protein-making machinery of the cell changes so that the DNA produces a new, or altered, "foreign" protein—either an odd structural protein or an enzyme that produces abnormal products. The end result is that the cell is unable to halt its own multiplication; the neoplasm grows uncontrollably.

The most common cancer treatments include radiation therapy, chemotherapy, surgery, or any combination of the three, intended to annihilate all cancer cells. Through their use, cancer can sometimes be arrested, but ironically, any of these treatments can cause serious side effects that threaten health and nutrition status.

How Cancer Develops

The steps in cancer development are thought to be:

1. Exposure to a carcinogen.
2. Entry of the carcinogen into a cell.
3. Initiation, probably by the carcinogen's altering of the cellular DNA somehow.
4. Enhancement of cancer development by promoters, probably involving several more steps before the cell begins to multiply out of control; tumor formation.

Researchers think that the first three steps, which culminate with initiation, are the key ones. Consequently, many people think that they should learn to avoid eating foods that contain carcinogens. In particular, many people have learned to fear food additives. However, food additives probably have little to do with the causation of cancer. Contaminants of foods—things that get into foods by accident—may be powerful carcinogens, but the additives permitted in foods are not. Additives are not discussed in this section, but they receive attention in Chapter 16.

carcinogen (car-SIN-oh-jen): a cancer-initiating substance. A carcinogen is one kind of initiator; another is radiation.
carcin = cancer
gen = gives rise to

initiation: an event caused by radiation or chemical reaction that can give rise to cancer.

promoters: factors that favor the development of cancer once the initiating event has taken place. Other factors, **antipromoters,** oppose the development of cancer.

Radiation therapy works by disrupting the chemical bonds necessary to form DNA. For this reason, radiation most severely damages cells that are actively dividing and making new DNA, such as tumor cells. Unfortunately, though, radiation also damages all normal body cells that are dividing actively, such as the cells of the blood and the GI tract. Cancer cells divide fastest, so they are most promptly and intensely affected by radiation, but other actively dividing cells are also susceptible.

Many chemotherapeutic drugs work the same way as radiation—they destroy dividing cells by interfering with DNA or RNA synthesis. Among types of chemotherapeutic agents are antibiotics, alkaloids, alkylating agents, antimetabolites, steroids, and others. Like radiation, these drugs also affect normal cells, especially those that divide the most rapidly. The current trend in chemotherapy is to use high doses of several chemotherapeutic agents together in cycles. This method helps ensure that malignant cells will be killed. Although these treatments are often effective, they also may intensify undesirable side effects.

New treatments for cancer are on the horizon. Among the newer treatments is the bone marrow transplant, which is being used to treat leukemia, advanced breast cancers, and other blood disorders. During a bone marrow transplant, the individual with cancer receives normal bone marrow from a donor, usually a close relative. Before the bone marrow transplant is performed, the recipient is prepared for the procedure with high doses of chemotherapy and sometimes whole body radiation therapy. Although the preparatory procedure effectively kills leukemic cells as intended, it kills healthy white blood cells as well. Rendered defenseless by a lack of white blood cells, the individual becomes susceptible to infection. Many of the nutritional consequences of bone marrow transplants are those caused by chemotherapy, radiation, and infections.

radiation therapy: the use of radiation to arrest or destroy cancer cells.

chemotherapy: the use of drugs to arrest or destroy cancer cells. Drugs used for chemotherapy are called **chemotherapeutic** or **antineoplastic agents.**
chemo = chemical

bone marrow transplant: the transfer of healthy bone marrow from a donor to a recipient, used as a treatment for leukemia and other blood disorders.

leukemia (loo-KEE-me-ah): cancer of the white blood cells.

graft-versus-host disease (GVHD): destruction of healthy donor white blood cells by the recipient's immune system, which recognizes the donor cells as foreign.

A serious complication of bone marrow transplants occurs when the immune system of the recipient recognizes the marrow cells of the donor as foreign. Chapter 23 described this destruction of healthy donor cells (called graft-versus-host disease) and the immunosuppressive drugs used to help treat or prevent its occurrence (see Table 23—4 on p. 732). Antibiotics are also widely used in bone marrow recipients, to treat infections (see Table 23—2 on p. 722).

Cancer Cachexia

About two-thirds of people with cancer develop cachexia—a combination of loss of appetite with accelerated and abnormal metabolism that simultaneously reduces the supply of energy and nutrients and increases the demand for them. People with cachexia swiftly fall into a downward spiral. Their poor nutrient intakes lead to muscle wasting and general poor health, which further contribute to their inadequate intakes of nutrients. Malnutrition interferes with their quality of life, interferes with cancer therapy, and contributes to the morbidity and mortality associated with the disease process. Loss of appetite, weight loss, and depletion of lean body mass and serum proteins typify the cancer cachexia syndrome. People with cancer have the highest incidence of PEM of any group of people who are ill.

cancer cachexia (ka-KEKS-ee-ah) **syndrome:** a syndrome that frequently accompanies many types of cancer, characterized by anorexia, inadequate intake of food, malnutrition, accelerated metabolism and wasting, and general ill health.

cachectin (ka-KEK-tin) **tumor necrosis factor:** a monokine whose action leads to depletion of fat from adipose tissues and weight loss.

Cancer cachexia is a multifactorial problem. The wasting process begins early in tumor development, even before weight loss occurs.[1] Cachexia appears to be tumor-derived; that is, the tumor itself causes the changes that lead to cachexia, and removal of the tumor can reverse the cachexia.[2] Investigators continue to search for clues as to what tumor-related factors might be involved. One substance secreted during an immune response to tumors called the cachectin/tumor necrosis factor may be an important mediator of the cancer cachexia syndrome.[3] Cachectin may induce the weight loss and hyperlipidemia frequently seen in people with cancer cachexia.

Not all people with cancer develop cancer cachexia. Those with advanced cancers, particularly of the GI tract, pancreas, lung, and prostate, as well as those with some types of lymph node cancers, are more likely to suffer from this problem than those with cancer of the breast or sarcomas.

Figure 30—1 summarizes some of the known causes of the cancer cachexia syndrome and its relationship with anorexia. Anorexia is widely recognized as a major precipitating factor in cancer cachexia.

Anorexia

A person may experience anorexia and weight loss even before being diagnosed with cancer. In some cases, these complaints motivate the person to visit the doctor. (This is one reason why, in preventive medicine, an important question in the dietary interview is: Have you experienced any recent changes in appetite or body weight?) No one knows exactly what precipitates anorexia. Perhaps the tumor produces substances that cause anorexia, but evidence to date remains elusive.

A person with cancer might experience a premature feeling of fullness: "I feel hungry, but I take a few bites and I'm full." Sometimes the person feels

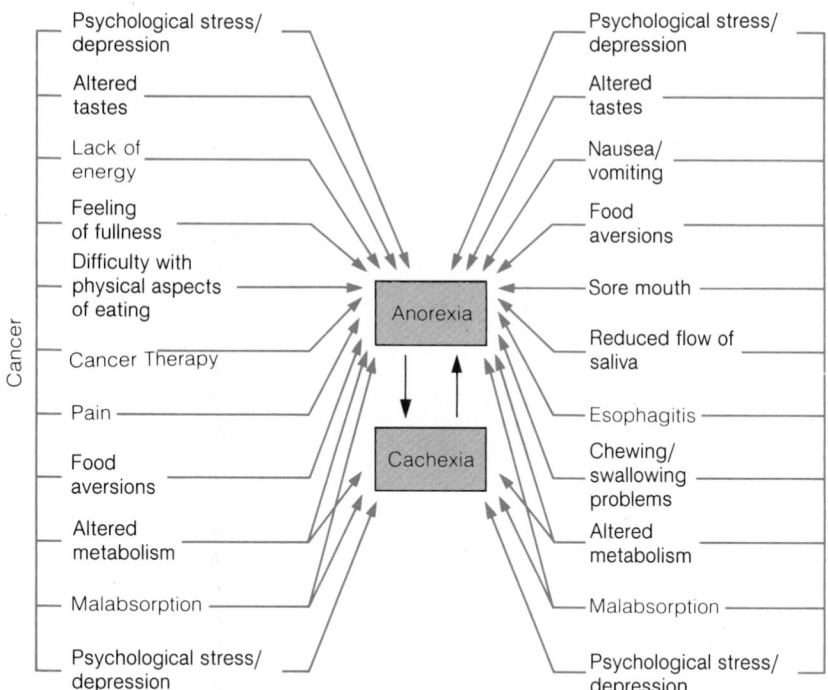

■ FIGURE 30–1

Causes of the Cancer Cachexia Syndrome

Anorexia and cachexia contribute to each other. Cancer itself and the available treatments for it make both problems worse.

full for a good reason. For example, the tumor may be pressing against the stomach or some other part of the GI tract. But for the most part, though, the reason for feeling full is unexplainable.

Some types of cancer cause anorexia when they obstruct the GI tract. For example, a tumor of the esophagus may cause a partial or complete obstruction; the person with such a tumor is unable to eat or has difficulty swallowing. A tumor obstructing the lower GI tract may cause nausea and vomiting.

People with cancer often tire easily. Consequently, they lack energy to prepare meals and eat. Many people with cancer feel the most energetic and the least full in the morning. As the day progresses, they become drained and feel full rapidly. Others may have more energy and be able to eat better later in the day.

Loss of strength is called **asthenia** (as-THEE-nee-ah).

Anorexia can be the result of pain associated with a tumor. A person in pain may have little interest in food, particularly if eating makes the pain worse.

Psychological stresses further contribute to anorexia. The very diagnosis of cancer can cause so much anxiety that eating becomes unimportant. People with terminal cancer may feel that eating simply isn't worth the effort. In addition, self-image may suffer from some of the treatments for cancer (for example, from a colostomy to treat colon cancer, hair loss that may accompany chemotherapy, or radical surgery that disfigures the body). The depression that follows interferes with food intake. As weight loss continues, depression may grow worse.

Cancer-induced causes of anorexia include:
- Early satiety.
- Fatigue.
- Pain.
- Obstructions.
- Depression.

As you can see, cancer itself is not the only factor that interferes with food intake. Therapy for cancer, whether chemotherapy, radiation therapy, surgery, or a bone marrow transplant, can also dramatically reduce food intake and contribute to wasting. The ways these treatments affect digestion, absorption,

■ TABLE 30–1
Drugs Used in the Treatment of Cancer

Drug Name	Timing with Meals	Common Side Effects That May Influence Nutrition Status
Adrenocorticosteroids	Give with food.	Increased appetite, GI upset. Glucose intolerance; negative nitrogen and calcium balance.
Asparaginase	Give parenterally.	Anorexia, nausea, vomiting. Pancreatitis, hepatitis, glucose intolerance.
Bleomycin	Give parenterally, intramuscularly, or subcutaneously.	Anorexia, nausea, vomiting, mouth ulcers, stomatitis, weight loss, altered taste perceptions.
Busulfan	Give with food.	Nausea, vomiting, diarrhea, cracking at corners of mouth, inflammation of the tongue, anemias, weight loss, dry mouth.
Carmustine	Give parenterally.	Anorexia, nausea, vomiting, esophagitis, diarrhea. Impaired liver function.
Mithramycin	Give parenterally; slow infusion reduces nausea.	Anorexia, nausea, vomiting, diarrhea, inflammation of the tongue, metallic taste.
Procarbazine	Give with food. Avoid foods containing tyramine (see Table 18–5).	Anorexia, nausea, vomiting, diarrhea, constipation, anemia, sore throat, dry mouth, difficulty swallowing.
Vinblastine	Give parenterally.	Anorexia, nausea, vomiting, diarrhea, constipation, stomatitis, sore throat, reduced bowel activity, abdominal pain, bowel inflammation.
Vincristine	Give parenterally.	Anorexia, nausea, vomiting, diarrhea, constipation, abdominal pain, mouth ulcers, anemia, thirst, weight loss, altered taste perceptions.

Source: Adapted from D. E. Powers and A. O. Moore, *Food Medication Interactions*, 6th ed. (Phoenix, Ariz.: Food Medication Interactions, 1989).

Cancer therapy can lead to anorexia by causing:
- Depression.
- Nausea.
- Vomiting.
- Altered taste perceptions.
- Mouth blindness.
- Dry mouth.
- Esophagitis.
- Stomatitis.
- Mouth ulcers.
- Food aversions.

and metabolism are described later in this chapter; consider now how they affect food intake.

People who receive radiation or chemotherapy frequently experience anorexia, nausea, vomiting, and altered taste perceptions. Chemotherapy can also inflame the lining of the mouth (stomatitis) and sometimes cause mouth ulcers, making chewing and swallowing painful. The person on chemotherapy may also experience abdominal pain or develop intestinal ulcers,

■ TABLE 30–2
Effects of Radiation and Chemotherapy on Nutrition Status

Radiation	Chemotherapy
Reduced nutrient intake	
Anorexia	Abdominal pain
Damage to teeth and bones	Anorexia
Esophagitis	Intestinal ulcers
Nausea	Nausea
Reduced salivary secretions	Taste alterations
Taste alterations	Vomiting
Thick salivary secretions	
Vomiting	
Accelerated nutrient losses	
Chronic blood loss from intestine and bladder	Diarrhea
	Malabsorption
Diarrhea	
Fistula formation	
Intestinal obstructions	
Malabsorption	
Altered metabolism	
(Secondary to malnutrition)	Fluid and electrolyte imbalance
	Hyperglycemia
	Interference with vitamins or other metabolites
	Negative nitrogen and calcium balance

which interfere with food intake. Table 30–1 (on the previous page) describes the drug-nutrient interactions of various chemotherapeutic agents.

The nutrition (and other) side effects of radiation depend on many factors, such as the type of radiation, the area of the body being irradiated, the size of the area, the dose, and the clinical and nutrition status of the person in therapy. Table 30–2 summarizes the effects of radiation and chemotherapy on nutrition status.

People receiving radiation therapy to the head and neck frequently experience altered taste perceptions and diminished taste sensitivities. As a result of this "mouth blindness," foods they once liked may taste unpleasant to them. An intolerance to meat, especially red meat, often develops. For some, food is just not sweet enough; for others, it's too sweet.

Radiation to the head and neck area also can reduce saliva production; moreover, the saliva that is available is often thick. This situation makes swallowing difficult. In addition, radiation may damage the bones of the jaws and the teeth, further interfering with the ability to chew and swallow. Radiation can also cause mouth ulcers to form, another problem that makes eating quite painful.

Radiation to the esophagus can cause esophagitis (see Chapter 24). Esophagitis often resolves when radiation therapy ends, but some people develop fibrosis or strictures, resulting in permanent swallowing problems. Fistulas can also develop, which may necessitate the use of a feeding tube or parenteral nutrition. When you consider that a person undergoing radiation therapy, particularly to the head and neck area, may suffer from several of these complications, you can see how markedly impaired nutrient intake can become.

■ TABLE 30–3
Possible Effects of Cancer Surgery on Nutrition Status

Head and neck resection
Difficulty in chewing/swallowing   Inability to chew/swallow

Esophageal resection
Reduced gastric motility   Steatorrhea (fat malabsorption)
Reduced gastric acid secretion   Fistula formation
Diarrhea   Stenosis (constriction)

Stomach resection
Dumping syndrome   Vitamin B_{12} malabsorption
Hypoglycemia   General malabsorption
Lack of gastric acid

Intestinal resection
General malabsorption   Hyperoxaluria
Steatorrhea   Fluid and electrolyte imbalance
Diarrhea   Blind loop syndrome

Pancreatic resection
General malabsorption   Diabetes mellitus

People treated with either radiation or chemotherapy may develop a strong dislike for certain foods, tastes, and odors. These aversions seem to develop for foods, tastes, or odors that are associated too closely in time with nausea. For example, if the person eats a certain food an hour before chemotherapy, and the treatment causes nausea, the person might develop an aversion to that food. This problem makes it important to maintain a food-free "window" of an hour or so before and after treatment times, if the treatments will be unpleasant.

Surgery, of course, can also cause anorexia, nausea, and vomiting; and some types of cancer surgery have additional side effects. For example, partial or total removal of the tongue, resection of the muscles of the mouth or esophagus and salivary glands, and removal of the lower jaw invariably create extensive problems with chewing and swallowing. People with these kinds of surgery may have to be maintained on tube feedings or TPN. Table 30–3 summarizes how some types of GI tract surgery for cancer can affect nutrition status.

Graft-versus-host disease also interferes with food intake by causing anorexia, nausea, vomiting, difficulty in swallowing, mouth ulcers, taste alterations, dry mouth, and esophagitis. Bone marrow transplant recipients frequently receive nourishment parenterally until their immune status improves and adequate oral intake resumes.

Many effects of cancer and cancer therapy that affect food intake are realized only when you work with a person who has a particular type of cancer. Because this is so important to understand, and to show just how varied these effects can be, we would like to share an example from a personal experience with you. Kathy was a 36-year-old, vibrant, intelligent woman who developed a malignant brain tumor that progressively affected her speech center and the right side of her body. Because this type of tumor progresses rapidly, the prognosis was poor, with an expected length of survival of six months.

As her ability to communicate declined, Kathy found it more and more difficult to express her desires and needs regarding foods she would like to eat.

Simultaneously, she became less able to prepare and physically eat foods herself because she was losing control of the right side of her body. Learning to use her left hand, particularly to handle feeding utensils, was hard for her. One solution to this problem was to serve foods she could eat with her fingers. She was an intelligent adult who did not want to be treated as a child, so the types of foods served this way had to be consistent with her need to preserve her dignity. She found breads, cheeses, fruits, and luncheon meats easy to handle, but the depression that resulted from her inability to communicate made it even more difficult for her to eat.

Another problem arose if foods were too small. Kathy lost the ability to move her tongue back and forth, and if small foods lodged in the right side of the back of her mouth, she could not feel them and could choke.

Kathy was taking a steroid medication to reduce swelling in the brain, as well as narcotics to deal with the severe headaches associated with the tumor. Both the tumor itself and the steroids caused nausea, although in Kathy's case, she ate more rather than less to alleviate the nausea. She stated that she felt much more nauseated when she had an empty stomach. The tumor and the narcotics also made Kathy sleepy, and this compounded the difficulty she had with the physical aspects of eating.

As you can see, many factors affect food intake in the person with cancer. In this case, the prognosis was poor, so the effects on long-term nutrition status were not as critical as helping Kathy preserve her feelings of self-esteem, dignity, and independence. These considerations are particularly important for the person whose disease is terminal. When time is short, you want the person to enjoy, rather than be burdened by, the routine experiences of everyday life.

Nutrient Losses

Excessive nutrient losses in the person with cancer can further impair nutrition status. As is the case with anorexia, nutrient losses can develop in response to cancer itself or the treatment for it.

Depending on the location and type of cancer, maldigestion or malabsorption of nutrients can be a problem. For example, cancer of the pancreas may cause a deficiency of pancreatic enzymes, or cancer of the liver, of bile salts. In the Zollinger-Ellison syndrome, tumors secrete the hormone gastrin which triggers the hypersecretion of gastric acid, thus inactivating digestive enzymes. Tumors of the small intestine cause malabsorption, as does a tumor that obstructs the upper small intestine, which creates a blind loop. (See Chapter 24 for a description of blind loop syndrome and how it causes malabsorption.)

Some cancers directly cause severe vomiting, diarrhea, or both, resulting in electrolyte imbalances and dehydration. For example, a tumor that obstructs the stomach or small bowel may cause vomiting.

Radiation to the small bowel often interferes with normal intestinal function, resulting in diarrhea and vomiting. Many times, intestinal function returns after radiation therapy ends, but for some people, changes may be permanent. After radiation therapy to the intestine, the structure of the intestine changes (radiation enteritis). The intestinal wall becomes thick and fibrotic, and the small intestinal arteries may become so inflamed that blood flow to some sections of the bowel is cut off. The lumen of the intestine may

Cancer-induced causes of nutrient losses include:
- Inadequate digestion.
- Malabsorption.
- Severe vomiting or diarrhea.
- Radiation enteritis.

Zollinger-Ellison syndrome: a condition caused by pancreatic tumors secreting excess gastrin, which stimulates the stomach to release great amounts of hydrochloric acid and pepsin.

radiation enteritis: changes in the structure of the small intestine caused by radiation therapy.

become narrow and obstructed, or a fistula may form. Radiation enteritis leads to malabsorption and chronic blood loss from the intestine and bladder, leading to malnutrition, as well as fluid and electrolyte imbalances.

Chemotherapy also may cause diarrhea and malabsorption because it prevents the cells of the intestine from regenerating as they normally do, thus impairing nutrient absorption. As shown in Chapters 24 and 25, surgery to the GI tract also can have many ill effects on nutrition status. (These effects were summarized in Table 30–3.)

Finally, bone marrow transplants can also lead to vomiting, diarrhea, and repeated infections, all of which incur nutrient losses. Additionally, the bone marrow recipient often develops pancreatitis, which can further impair digestion and absorption. Transplant recipients with graft-versus-host disease frequently develop intestinal lesions that resemble those seen in inflammatory bowel diseases (see Chapter 25), and these further hinder absorption. The liver may be debilitated as well, resulting in steatorrhea and a reduced production of bile salts. And on top of all this, people receiving bone marrow transplants also receive radiation or chemotherapy, with all the nutrition consequences of those treatments.

Thus, all these forms of treatment for cancer, as well as cancer itself, point in the same direction: malnutrition. In fact, death from cachexia in people with cancer is estimated at 4 to 23 percent.[4]

Metabolic Alterations

So far we have seen how a reduced intake of food and excessive losses of nutrients can contribute to cancer cachexia. If reduced availability of nutrients was the only problem in people with cancer, then weight loss would largely occur at the expense of body fat. But in cancer, muscle wasting also occurs to a great extent. This wasting is accounted for, in part, by the metabolic changes that occur in cancer.

In people with cancer, metabolic changes either raise energy needs or cause the body to use energy nutrients ineffectively. Studies suggest that some people with cancer are hypermetabolic while others are not.[5] It may be that metabolic changes vary with different types of tumors or their locations in the body. However, even in the absence of hypermetabolism, metabolic pathways are altered and nutrients are cycled in less efficient ways.

One metabolic problem is that many people with cancer are hyperglycemic, probably for two reasons. For one thing, they tend to be insulin resistant; for another, they secrete less insulin in response to glucose loads. Consequently, a diabeticlike state arises. Glucose and amino acids in the blood become less available to the cells than they normally are; this contributes to wasting. Also, hunger generally corresponds to a return of blood glucose to fasting levels, and in the person with cancer, this return may be delayed—hence the person's lack of appetite.

In normal cells, energy is derived mainly through the cycle that uses oxygen (the TCA cycle; see Chapter 7 and Appendix C) rather than through the pathway that involves no oxygen (the glycolytic pathway). The TCA cycle is the more efficient of the two and can metabolize either glucose or fat for energy. But tumor cells use the glycolytic pathway to make energy. This pathway produces less energy and relies on glucose for its source of fuel.

■ FIGURE 30–2
Two Antivitamins
Methotrexate (an antineoplastic drug) and pyrimethamine (an antimalaria drug) are structurally similar to the vitamin folate. They compete for the enzyme that normally activates folate.

As the tumor metabolizes glucose by way of glycolysis, lactic acid (lactate) is produced. Lactate then returns to the liver, where it is reconverted to glucose in an energy-requiring process. Thus the tumor places a direct demand on the body to provide energy to support its preferred metabolic pathway.

After depleting the body's glycogen stores to provide glucose, the tumor calls on muscle catabolism to begin providing amino acids to make new glucose. Additionally, tumor tissues consume nitrogen (from amino acids) at the body's expense. The muscle mass becomes progressively depleted, further contributing to negative nitrogen balance.

Changes in lipid metabolism also occur, typically hyperlipidemia and depletion of fat stores. Studies suggest that these changes may be due to a defect in the activity of lipoprotein lipase, the enzyme that helps transfer lipids from the blood to the fat cells.[6] People with cancer have an enhanced mobilization of fat stores and reduced synthesis of lipids in the fat cells. The accelerated breakdown of fat coupled with a defective clearance of lipids from the blood may work to suppress immune function.[7]

The metabolic changes associated with cancer raise energy needs. Other factors, such as emotional or physiologic stress or surgery, further raise energy needs. Also, both chemotherapy and radiation can impair the immune system and infections can easily occur, raising energy and nutrient needs still further (see Chapter 23).

Chemotherapy using vitamin antagonists (see Figure 30–2) interferes with normal metabolic pathways and creates nutrient deficiencies. This further compromises nutrition status. Anemias caused by a variety of vitamin deficiencies are frequently seen in people with cancer.

Obviously, the person with cancer risks poor nutrition status. Providing optimal nutrition care is often crucial to recovery.

■ *Nutrition Support for the Person with Cancer*

For many years, the deteriorating nutrition status that accompanies cancer was largely ignored. Many practitioners believed that emaciation and physical debilitation were an inevitable result of cancer. Others believed that if you fed the client, you also fed the tumor, so to "starve" the tumor, they would almost starve the client. Another problem was the state of the art of feeding people. The widespread use of tube feedings and TPN is a relatively recent advance.

Today, experts recognize the benefits of nutrition in cancer treatment. Attention to diet can prevent or reverse poor nutrition status. The person in good nutrition status:

- Enjoys a better quality of life. The malnourished person is less active and becomes weak, eats less, becomes weaker, and goes into a downward spiral.
- Is less susceptible to infections (see Chapter 18).
- Probably tolerates cancer therapies better (surgery, chemotherapy, and radiation therapy).

Although it makes sense to prevent PEM in the person with cancer, actual research in restoring and maintaining lean body mass has been disappointing. Despite seemingly adequate nutrition support, people with cancer cachexia often fail to replete their lean body masses. They may gain weight, but this weight often represents fat and water weight rather than lean body mass. A direct benefit of weight gain on either tumor response or survival after chemotherapy or radiation therapy cannot be proven.[8] The metabolic changes associated with cancer probably explain this finding. Research continues to seek ways to use individual nutrients and other substances to correct metabolic derangements.

As hinted at earlier, some clinicians express concern that feeding the host feeds the tumor and that a tumor might grow with nutrition support. Such an effect has not been scientifically documented in people with cancer.[9]

In weighing the value of nutrition support in cancer, it is important to remember that progressive malnutrition in people with cancer can lead to death.[10] In a study of people with head and neck cancer, adequate nutrition status was associated with a highly significant increased survival rate (almost 60 percent of adequately nourished people lived for two years), as opposed to poor nutrition status (less than 10 percent of those in poor nutrition status lived for two years).[11] In people with radiation enteritis who were unable to use their GI tracts, TPN allowed 95 percent of the people to complete the course of radiation.[12] A positive correlation between tumor response and nutrition status was identified.

In all cases, providing adequate nutrition support is essential. Whether aggressive nutrition support can actually reverse cachexia or improve response to therapy appears to depend largely on the type of cancer.

Oral Diets during Therapy

Recognizing the many obstacles affecting the appetite of the person with cancer, health care professionals are faced with an enormous challenge in

---

How to Determine Energy and Protein Needs for Cancer

Energy: Calculate the basal energy expenditure (BEE) using the Harris
          Benedict equation provided in Table 19–14 on p. 637.
          Energy needs range from 1.5 to 2.0 times the BEE.
Protein: 1.5 to 2.0 g protein per kg ideal body weight.

---

helping these individuals maintain their nutrition status. Every bit of inter-personal skill and nutrition knowledge can help, beginning with the professional's awareness of the client's predicament. Remember first of all to keep the client's feelings in mind and acknowledge them when appropriate. Point out the proven benefits of aggressive nutrition therapy in cancer treatment, and offer all the practical pointers you can to help clients help themselves. Encourage people to eat extra food between chemotherapy or radiation treatments. Minimize the likelihood of learned food aversions by suggesting that clients save favorite foods for times when they are feeling relatively good. Remind them not to eat within an hour or two before or after scheduled radiation treatments or chemotherapy. When intake from regular foods fails to meet nutrient needs, suggest liquid supplements between or with meals.

The energy and protein requirements for people with cancer are determined as shown in the box above. Table 30–4 shows diet modifications that may be necessary for different types of cancer.

■ **TABLE 30–4**
Dietary Considerations for Various Cancers

Location of Cancer	Dietary Considerations
Brain	Physical feeding disabilities (see Highlight 21); chewing and swallowing problems.
Head/neck	Chewing and swallowing problems.
Mouth/esophagus	Chewing and swallowing problems; if obstructed, tube feeding below the obstruction may be necessary.
Stomach	Nausea, vomiting; if obstructed, tube feeding below the obstruction may be necessary; if resection is performed, a postgastrectomy diet (see Chapter 24) may be needed; nutrient deficiencies due to blind loop syndrome (Chapter 24) may occur.
Intestine	If obstructed, tube feeding or TPN may be necessary; resections or inflammation may cause multiple nutrition problems (see Chapter 25); low-fat, lactose-restricted diet may be useful.
Liver	Protein-, sodium-, and fluid-restricted diet may be necessary (see Chapter 26).
Pancreas	Low-fat diet and enzyme replacements may be necessary (see Chapter 25); diabetic diet may be necessary if insulin production is affected (see Chapter 27).
Kidneys	Protein-, electrolyte-, and fluid-controlled diet may be necessary (see Chapter 29).

Note: The considerations listed here are specific to the type of cancer; they do not include the effects of treatment. Other factors described for all cancers, such as anorexia, nausea, and vomiting, are considered in addition to the interventions discussed here.

Oral food intake can be improved if the specific problems of the individual are addressed. Table 30–5 addresses these problems and offers suggestions for alleviating them.

Tube Feedings and Parenteral Nutrition

Tube feedings or TPN may be indicated (see Chapters 21 and 22) when anorexia persists, particularly during and immediately after treatment. Begin these measures before severe malnutrition sets in. As is true whenever special nutrition support is indicated, tube feedings are preferred to TPN when the GI tract is functional. People requiring head and neck resections may need long-term tube feedings and may need to continue tube feedings at home.

Animal studies suggest that defined-formula diets (formulas containing only free amino acids as a protein source) may be contraindicated when methotrexate (a chemotherapeutic drug) is administered.[13] In one study, all the animals given only free amino acids died from severe inflammation of the intestine, whereas survival improved as protein in the form of polypeptides or a regular diet was provided.[14] Further studies will need to be conducted to determine whether the results of these trials are applicable to human beings.

Although every malnourished person with cancer who cannot consume an adequate diet orally is a potential candidate for aggressive nutrition support, the answers to some important questions should be considered before tube feeding or parenteral nutrition is undertaken. What will change if the cachexia is reversed or progressive wasting is arrested? Will the person survive longer? Will quality of life improve? Will therapy be more successful? If special nutrition support can provide direct benefits, it should be undertaken. However, for the person with little hope of recovery, the yet unproven benefits of specialized nutrition support may not be worth the cost and discomfort involved. Making this decision requires good clinical judgment from the health care team as well as consideration of the client's feelings about the goals of the nutrition therapy.

Support for Recipients of Bone Marrow Transplants

The person receiving a bone marrow transplant often receives parenteral nutrition support because the GI tract is severely compromised by the preparation procedure. Appropriate nutrition benefits the healing of the GI tract and the regeneration of the immune system. As GI function returns, the person begins to receive food orally, and parenteral nutrition gradually tapers off as oral intake improves. The nutrition-related side effects of the bone marrow transplant procedure make oral intake difficult, and the individual needs encouragement from all members of the health care team.

Early oral feedings often start with lactose-free, low-residue, low-fat liquids to maximize absorption and minimize the risk of nausea, vomiting, and steatorrhea (see Appendix L). Gradually, solid foods are introduced. As individual tolerances allow, fiber and lactose can be added back to the diet. Additional fat is given if the individual does not develop steatorrhea.

Because the bone marrow recipient must take immunosuppressants following the procedure, recommendations include a high-protein, high-calcium diet. In addition, physicians often prescribe calcium and vitamin D

Suggestions for Improving Food Intake

To improve the appetite
- Explain why eating is important.
- Encourage clients to eat the most when they feel the best.
- Suggest foods that are easy to prepare and eat.
- Recommend smaller meals.
- Advise clients not to drink liquids with meals.
- Recommend the use of time-saving food preparation appliances.
- Give pain or antinausea medications when they will work best (usually before meals).
- Provide a pleasant and relaxed environment.
- Reassess clients regularly to solve feeding problems as they may arise.

To combat bitter or metallic taste perceptions
- Encourage the use of eggs, fish, poultry, and dairy products instead of meats.
- Recommend adding sauces and seasonings to meats.
- Suggest that meats be served cold or at room temperature.
- Advise clients to brush teeth or use a mouthwash before eating.

To control nausea and vomiting
- Recommend small meals.
- Advise clients to avoid spicy and high-fat foods.
- Advise clients to avoid odors that cause nausea.
- Encourage clients to save liquids for after meals. Clear liquids or Popsicles after meals help prevent dehydration.
- Suggest that clients get fresh air, loosen clothing, or lie down after meals.
- Advise clients to avoid eating their favorite foods during the times of the day when they frequently experience nausea or vomiting.
- Give antinausea drugs before mealtimes.

To alleviate problems with chewing and swallowing
- Work with clients to find the consistency of food that will be easiest to handle. Thin liquids, true solids, and sticky foods are often difficult to swallow.
- Provide fluids with meals to ease chewing and swallowing.
- Advise the client with mouth sores to try foods at cooler temperatures. They are often soothing.
- Recommend that clients experiment with tilting the head forward and backward to see if swallowing can be made easier with the head positioned differently.
- Suggest a straw for drinking.
- Advise clients with mouth ulcers to avoid foods that are spicy, acidic, or coarse or that contain seeds that can be trapped in an ulcer.
- Encourage clients who suffer from a reduced flow of saliva to rinse the mouth frequently and to avoid concentrated sweets. Artificial saliva from the pharmacy can also help. Sour candy or gum can stimulate the flow of saliva.
- Encourage good oral and dental hygiene.

To add kcalories and protein
- Add 2 tablespoons of milk powder to liquid milk, recipes, soups, puddings, and cereals.
- Add ground meats, chicken, fish, or grated cheeses to sauces, soups, casseroles, or vegetables.
- Use extra butter, margarine, or cream cheese on breads.
- Eat peanut butter on fruit, celery, or crackers.
- Use butter or margarine whenever possible (on breads, potatoes, vegetables, pasta, and rice).
- Use yogurt, sour cream, or a sour cream dip with vegetables.
- Use mayonnaise as a salad dressing and on sandwiches.
- Add whipping cream to desserts and hot chocolate, or use it to lighten coffee.
- Have snacks available at all times.
- Add nuts and dried fruits such as raisins to desserts or cereals.
- Use cream instead of milk with cereal.
- Try commercially available liquid supplements or instant breakfast mixes for meals or between-meal snacks.

supplements. Encourage individuals with persistent diarrhea to eat high-potassium foods (see Table 10–8 on p. 289). The accompanying "Clinical Detective Work" box provides a case study for cancer.

■ *Acquired Immune Deficiency Syndrome (AIDS)*

acquired immune deficiency syndrome (AIDS): an immune system disorder that leaves its victims defenseless against numerous infections. AIDS is transmitted to a person from direct contact of the person's body fluids with contaminated body fluids. It is most often transmitted through sexual intercourse, contaminated needles or blood products, or from mother to infant during pregnancy or lactation.

opportunistic infections: infections from microorganisms that normally do not cause disease in the general population but can infect people once their immune systems are compromised (as in AIDS).

human immunodeficiency virus (HIV): the virus that causes AIDS.

The devastating disorder AIDS affects young and old, rich and poor, urban and rural dwellers, men and women. An estimated fifty million people worldwide have been infected with the virus that causes AIDS and virtually all of these people will likely develop the disorder and die from it.[15] As its incidence rises sharply, prevention and treatment of AIDS becomes a critical concern of health care professionals around the world.

AIDS is an immune system disorder that renders its victims defenseless against opportunistic infections and disorders from which most people are protected. The disorder begins with infection by the human immunodeficiency virus (HIV). AIDS then progresses in stages. At first, the individual is a carrier of the virus but exhibits no symptoms. Then symptoms begin to appear. The person with AIDS frequently develops infections of the lungs, central nervous system, GI tract, and skin. Pneumonia, a special type of

■ TABLE 30–6
Causes of Malnutrition in AIDS

Anorexia
Drug therapy
Lack of energy to eat
Pain associated with eating
Fever/infection
Nausea and vomiting
Psychological factors such as fear and depression

Oral lesions
Drug therapy
Bacterial and viral infections
Kaposi's sarcoma

Nausea and vomiting
Drug therapy
Oral lesions
Inflammation of the stomach (gastritis) or esophagus (esophagitis)

Diarrhea and malabsorption
Drug therapy
Various GI infections
Low serum albumin levels and PEM

Altered metabolism
Drug therapy
Infections
Cancer

cancer (described in a later section), and severe diarrhea are common and often fatal complications.

Currently, AIDS has no cure. Treatment focuses on slowing its course and controlling its symptoms to improve the individual's comfort and quality of life. However, researchers and clinicians remain optimistic that they will be able to develop effective therapies and an AIDS vaccine. AIDS research has spurred a tremendous growth in our understanding of the immune system. This knowledge has unraveled some of the mysteries of AIDS and other immune system disorders as well.

The severe PEM and wasting associated with AIDS, much as in cancer, are multifactorial: inadequate food intake, excessive nutrient losses, hypermetabolism, and drug-nutrient interactions. The exact causes of wasting depend on the particular complications the individual develops. Repeated infections and, of course, cancer accelerate wasting dramatically. Weight loss in people with AIDS can be so severe that they require complete nursing care. Table 30–6 lists the many factors that lead to wasting in AIDS.

Anorexia

Anorexia in AIDS arises from causes similar to those in cancer. Depression over the diagnosis can destroy appetite even before symptoms of the disease appear. The individual who tests positive for AIDS must deal with the psychological impact of the diagnosis, the terminal nature of the infection,

AIDS-induced causes of anorexia include:
- Depression.
- Fever.
- Pain.
- Mouth blindness.
- Dry mouth.
- Difficulty swallowing.
- Mouth ulcers.
- Esophageal lesions and obstructions.
- Use of oxygen masks.
- Drug therapy.
- Lethargy.
- Dementia.

■ **TABLE 30–7**
Drugs Used in the Treatment of AIDS

Drug Name	Timing with Meals	Common Side Effects That May Influence Nutrition Status
Acyclovir	Give parenterally or orally with food.	Nausea, diarrhea, vomiting, anorexia.
Amphotericin B	Give parenterally.	Nausea, vomiting, fever, anemia, kidney dysfunction.
Ampicillin	Give with water 1 hr before or 2 hr after meals; do not give with fruit juice, beer, wine.	Nausea, vomiting, diarrhea, steatorrhea, anemia, inflammation of the mouth and tongue, stomatitis, altered taste perceptions, hypokalemia.
Azidothymidine (AZT)		Anorexia, nausea, vomiting, diarrhea, constipation, altered taste perceptions, mouth ulcers, edema of tongue and lips, abdominal pain, anemia.
Bleomycin	(see Table 30–1)	
Cisplatin	Give parenterally.	Anorexia, nausea, vomiting, altered taste perceptions.
Clotrimazole	Dissolve slowly in mouth and swallow saliva.	Nausea, vomiting.
Cyclophosphamide	Give during or after meals.	Anorexia, nausea, vomiting, mouth ulcers, inflammation of the colon, anemia.
Dactinomycin	Give parenterally.	Anorexia, nausea, vomiting, mouth ulcers, heartburn, anemia.
Doxorubicin	Give parenterally.	Anorexia, nausea, vomiting, diarrhea, stomach pain, sore throat, mouth ulcers, mouth blindness, esophagitis.
Erythromycin	Give on empty stomach 1 hr before or 2 hr after meals; if GI distress, give with meals, not milk, fruit juice, beer, or wine.	Nausea, vomiting, cramps, abdominal pain, diarrhea, inflammation of the mouth.
Estrogens	Give with food at same time each day.	Anorexia, nausea, vomiting, edema, weight change alters glucose tolerance.
Ethambutol hydrochloride		Anorexia, nausea, vomiting, abdominal pain.
Fluconazole	Give orally or parenterally.	Nausea, vomiting, diarrhea, intestinal inflammation.
Fluorouracil	Give parenterally. If given orally, give with water, not acidic beverages.	Anorexia, nausea, vomiting, stomatitis, diarrhea, heartburn, sore mouth, altered taste perceptions, GI bleeding, esophagitis.

thrush: a fungal infection caused by *Candida albicans;* the technical term for this infection is *Candidiasis.*

herpes virus: a virus that can lead to mouth lesions and may also affect the lower GI tract, causing diarrhea.

and the medical, personal, and financial problems that lie ahead. Understandably, food intake becomes trivial to the person overwhelmed with problems.

As the disorder progresses, fever, pain, and infections contribute to anorexia. In addition, people with AIDS often develop the common oral infection thrush. Thrush manifests itself as a thick white coating on the mouth, tongue, and sometimes the esophagus. The coating covers the taste receptors and alters taste sensations. Thrush also causes pain and reduces the flow of saliva. When the esophagus becomes infected, swallowing is extremely painful. All of these factors contribute to anorexia.

Oral infections caused by herpes virus, and common in people with AIDS, lead to painful mouth ulcers and problems with chewing and swallowing.

■ **TABLE 30–7**
Drugs Used in the Treatment of AIDS (continued)

Drug Name	Timing with Meals	Common Side Effects That May Influence Nutrition Status
Ganciclovir	Give parenterally.	Anorexia, nausea, vomiting.
Hydroxyurea	Give with food.	Anorexia, nausea, vomiting, mouth ulcers.
Isoniazid	Give 1 hr before or 2 hr after meals; may give with food to relieve GI distress.	Anorexia, nausea, vomiting, dry mouth, diarrhea, anemia, cracked lips.
Ketoconazole	Give with food to reduce nausea and vomiting.	Nausea, vomiting, abdominal pain, diarrhea, anemia. Renal and liver dysfunction.
Mercaptopurine	Give with food.	Anorexia, nausea, vomiting, stomatitis, stomach pain, diarrhea, anemia, vitamin B_6 depletion.
Methotrexate	Give on an empty stomach; give with food to reduce gastric distress. Do not give with milk.	Anorexia, nausea, vomiting, diarrhea, GI ulcers, GI inflammation, anemia, stomatitis, steatorrhea, mouth ulcers.
Metronidazole	Give with food.	Anorexia, nausea, vomiting, diarrhea, altered taste perceptions, dry mouth, constipation, stomatitis, abdominal discomfort.
Nystatin	Give orally as directed; retain drug in mouth as long as possible.	Diarrhea, nausea, and vomiting, GI pain (occasionally).
Pentamidine isethionate	Give parenterally or as an inhalant.	Nausea, vomiting, taste alterations. Kidney dysfunction, hypoglycemia or hyperglycemia, diabetes.
Pyrimethamine	Give with food.	Anorexia, nausea, vomiting, diarrhea, and anemia.
Rifampin	Give with water on empty stomach.	Anorexia, nausea, vomiting, cramps, diarrhea, altered taste perceptions, abdominal distress.
Sulfadiazine	Give with water.	Anorexia, nausea, vomiting, and diarrhea.
Trimethoprim	Give with water on empty stomach.	Nausea, vomiting, anorexia, anemia, diarrhea, stomatitis, GI distress.
Vinblastine	(see Table 30–1)	
Vincristine	(see Table 30–1)	

Source: Adapted from D. E. Powers and A. O. Moore, *Food Medication Interactions*, 6th ed. (Phoenix, Ariz.: Food Medication Interactions, 1989).

Kaposi's sarcoma, a cancer associated with AIDS, can cause lesions and obstructions in the esophagus that can further interfere with food intake.

Respiratory infections can also limit food intake in people with AIDS. The individual using an oxygen mask (which covers the nose and mouth) may have difficulty eating. Respiratory infections also cause fever and pain, which worsen anorexia.

Drugs used to treat the various complications associated with AIDS also suppress appetite and reduce food intake. As in cancer treatment, antimicrobial drugs and chemotherapy often cause anorexia, nausea, and vomiting; food aversions associated with the side effects of drug therapy can also arise. Table 30–7 describes the nutrition side effects of drugs frequently used in managing AIDS.

Kaposi's sarcoma: a type of cancer rare in the general population but common in people with AIDS.

dementia: irreversible loss of mental function.

AIDS-induced causes of nutrient losses include:
- HIV infection.
- GI tract infections.
- Cancer.
- Cancer therapy.
- Antimicrobial drugs.
- Megadoses of vitamins.
- Home remedies for AIDS.
- Low serum albumin.
- PEM.
- Reduced gastric acid secretion.
- Bacterial overgrowth.

The diarrhea and malabsorption symptoms associated with AIDS for which no known cause has been identified are called **AIDS enteropathies**.

antimicrobial agents: drugs used to kill microorganisms, including bacteria, viruses, fungi, protozoa, and parasites.

In the later stages of AIDS, lethargy and dementia become common problems that interfere with food intake. The individual may be chronically exhausted and may not care or even remember to eat.

Nutrient Losses

In addition to anorexia, the PEM associated with AIDS is accelerated by excessive nutrient losses. Diarrhea and malabsorption interfere with the absorption of nutrients. From 50 to 90 percent of people with AIDS experience chronic or recurrent diarrhea.[16] The HIV infection itself may damage the GI tract, causing malabsorption.[17] Damage to the intestinal cells also increases the risk of microbial infection.

Infections of the GI tract commonly precipitate diarrhea and malabsorption in people with AIDS. In some cases, diarrhea is unresponsive to drug therapy, and nutrient losses continue unchecked for long times. One common GI infection, cryptosporidia, is characterized by severe and prolonged diarrhea of 2 to 3 liters of stool per day. In rarer cases, up to 25 liters of stool per day may be excreted—possible only when a high fluid intake is provided to meet fluid needs.[18] Table 30–8 summarizes other infectious agents that can cause diarrhea and malabsorption in people with AIDS. Notice that some of the pathogens listed in the table come from infected foods. People with AIDS are highly susceptible to food-borne illnesses.

People with AIDS who develop cancer are at additional risk for malabsorption. Cancers of the GI tract and therapies for all cancers (as previously discussed) frequently lead to malabsorption. Other drug therapies, including antimicrobial agents, also can cause diarrhea and malabsorption (see Table 30–7). Megadoses of vitamins (especially vitamin C) and other home remedies that people with AIDS may use as self treatment have been associated with diarrhea as well.

Low serum albumin levels and PEM can further contribute to malabsorption and diarrhea in people with AIDS (see Chapter 18). Nutrient losses are also possible because people with AIDS do not secrete enough gastric acid. A high gastric pH not only limits the absorption of iron and calcium but also allows bacteria to grow in the upper GI tract, promoting infections. Bacterial

■ **TABLE 30–8**
Causes of GI Infections in AIDS

Bacterial	Protozoan
Clostridium dificile	*Cryptosporidium* species
Mycobacterium avium-intracellulare (MAI)	*Giardia lamblia*
Mycobacterium tuberculosis	*Isosporia belli*
Salmonella species	*Microsporidium* species
	Pneumocystitis carinii
Fungal	*Toxoplasma gondii*
Candida albicans	
Cryptococcus neoformans	**Viral**
	AIDS enteropathy
Parasitic	*Cytomegalovirus* (CMV) species
Nonpathogenic amoeba	Epstein-Barr
Entamoeba histolytica	Herpes simplex

overgrowth can also lead to the deconjugation of bile salts (as is seen in the blind loop syndrome) and result in fat malabsorption. Finally, although direct evidence is lacking, the effects of PEM on the immune system (see Chapter 18) added to those of HIV infection itself may hasten the course of the disease.

Metabolic Alterations

Hypermetabolism associated with infection and fever contribute to wasting in people with AIDS. The impacts of stress on metabolism are described in Chapter 18 and illustrated in Figure 18–2 on p. 578. Repeated infections significantly tax nutrition status already compromised by a reduced intake of food, diarrhea, and malabsorption. Of course, the metabolic alterations associated with cancer also apply to AIDS clients who have cancer (see pp. 932–933).

■ Nutrition Support for the Person with AIDS

Although attention to nutrition cannot change the ultimate outcome of AIDS, it is possible that good nutrition status can slow its progression and meanwhile improve the quality of life. Good nutrition status may also improve response to drug therapy. Maintaining nutrition status may make the difference between an individual's being able to stay at home or having to move to a nursing home.[19]

A positive test for HIV infection in an individual alerts the health care professional to the need for aggressive nutrition intervention. Although the person may still have no symptoms, early intervention may detect and correct subclinical deficiencies in preparation for the stresses ahead, and to establish baseline assessment parameters to assist in monitoring changes in nutrition status. Researchers suggest that weight loss, reduced percent body fat, and reduced body mass index are early signs of nutrition status deterioration in people with AIDS.[20]

For people with AIDS, as for all individuals, oral diets are appropriate as long as they are possible. Nutrient needs depend on the complications experienced in each case. The equations given in Table 19–14 on p. 637 for determining energy needs can be used for people with AIDS. Although the exact vitamin and mineral needs of people with AIDS have not been determined, at least 100 percent of the RDA for these nutrients should be provided daily. People who are unable to consume sufficient foods to comprise an adequate diet might benefit from a multivitamin-mineral supplement containing at least 100 percent of the RDA of these nutrients.[21] Many physicians prescribe a daily prenatal vitamin supplement for people with HIV infections.[22]

The same tips that help people with cancer are useful for people with AIDS. Suggestions for alleviating the problems of anorexia, altered taste sensations, nausea and vomiting, and difficulty with chewing and swallowing were described in Table 30–5. Treatment of diarrhea and malabsorption vary depending on the cause and the extent to which the intestine is affected. Appropriate drug therapy along with the provision of adequate fluids and

■ TABLE 30-9
Dietary Modifications for Managing Diarrhea and Malabsorption in HIV-Related GI Infections

Area of Intestine Affected	Diet Modifications
Total small intestine	Low fat (less than 20% of total energy), low fiber, low residue, no lactose, no caffeine; parenteral nutrition is often necessary.
Partial small intestine	Low fat (less than 20% of total energy), low residue, low lactose, no caffeine.
Large intestine	Low fat, medium-chain triglycerides (MCT), low fiber, low residue, low lactose, no caffeine.
Nonspecific involvement	Bulking agent (pectin), low lactose, fat as tolerated.

Source: Adapted from Task Force on nutrition support in AIDS, Guidelines for nutrition support in AIDS, *Nutrition* 5 (1989): 39–46.

electrolytes set the cornerstones of treatment. Salty broths and high-potassium juices can help replace fluids and electrolytes. Table 30–9 shows the dietary modifications recommended for the treatment of diarrhea and malabsorption based on the part of the intestine involved.

Susceptibility to food-borne illnesses requires that the individual with AIDS be given written and oral instructions on the safe handling of foods. Table 16–2 on pp. 498–499 describes such precautions.

Individuals unable to consume adequate oral diets to prevent nutrition complications and unintentional weight loss need aggressive nutrition support. As a guideline, aggressive nutrition support should be considered when:

■ The individual loses 5 percent of body weight within a month.
■ A weight loss of more than 10 percent has occurred over the last 6 months.[23]

As always, enteral feeding is preferred to parenteral feeding. Sometimes liquid formulas given with or between regular meals can help maintain or restore nutrition status; otherwise, tube feedings can be used. Tube feedings given at night can supplement oral diets during the day, especially for people at home. If pain or obstructions in the upper GI tract make nasogastric passage of the feeding tube difficult or painful, gastrostomy or jejunostomy feedings are indicated.

Particular care must be taken to keep tube feeding from causing diarrhea unrelated to the HIV infection. Table 21–4 on pp. 687–688 describes the causes and prevention of diarrhea associated with tube feeding. Preventing bacterial contamination of the formula is particularly important because of the susceptibility of HIV-infected individuals to GI infections.

The use of TPN in people with AIDS is controversial, especially in the final stages of the disorder. Generally, it is used only when people are expected to benefit from other therapy and need to maintain their nutrition status while undergoing that therapy. TPN may be more useful in repleting the body mass of people whose primary problems are reduced food intake or malabsorption, rather than those who have other systemic diseases.[24] People with GI tract obstructions, severe vomiting, or GI infections affecting the entire small bowel

systemic: affecting the whole body rather than one part or organ system.

CLINICAL DETECTIVE WORK

Kevin sought medical help at age 34 when he began feeling run-down and developed a painful white coating over his mouth and tongue. The presence of thrush and anemia alerted Kevin's physician to the possibility of a HIV infection. When Kevin tested positive for a HIV infection, the news was devastating both to him and to his family and friends. Fortunately, those closest to him have supported him through this difficult time, and he has a strong desire to live out his life as independently as possible. Four months after the diagnosis of HIV infection, Kevin developed a serious, continuous diarrhea that required hospitalization to classify and control. Since the diagnosis of HIV infection was made, Kevin has lost 10 lb. At 6 ft tall, he currently weighs 158 lb.

Describe how AIDS can lead to reduced food intake, nutrient losses, and hypermetabolism. From the limited information given here, what factors could have contributed to Kevin's weight loss?

Discuss nutrition strategies for dealing with thrush and diarrhea. Is Kevin's weight loss significant? What is his %IBW? What steps could be effective in preventing further weight loss?

may benefit from TPN. People with AIDS can benefit from the safe and effective use of home TPN programs.[25] The accompanying "Clinical Detective Work" box presents a case study on AIDS.

Prevention of Cancer and AIDS

Unfortunately, the prognosis for many people with some types of cancer and AIDS is bleak. While there is little hope for cure in some of these cases, there may be an opportunity for people to prevent the disease or to be in the best condition to overcome the effects of the disease.

Prevention of Cancer

We know that factors beyond our control, such as genetic predisposition, or factors within our control, such as cigarette smoking, have a strong influence on the development of cancer. We do not know to what extent diet contributes to cancer development. Some experts have estimated that diet is responsible for perhaps a third or more of all cases of cancer. But while some dietary factors may contribute to its development, others may contribute to its prevention. The following sections present the findings from research on the relationships between diet and cancer and current recommendations.

Findings on Diet and Cancer Our understanding of the relationships between diet and cancer derives from different kinds of research studies, as

NUTRITION DETECTIVE WORK

Several kinds of research have led to what we now know about diet and cancer. Studies of whole populations in different areas of the world—epidemiology—provide one source of information on diet and cancer. Another approach is to conduct case-control studies—studies of people who have cancer and of other people as closely matched to them as possible in age, occupation, and other key variables, but who do not have cancer—to see what differences in their lifestyles may account for the differing cancer incidences. Still another approach is to test possible causes of cancer on animals under controlled laboratory conditions in which all other variables can be ruled out.

The most powerful research tool, human intervention trials, are only now beginning to be employed to a limited degree in cancer research. In these trials, human subjects agree to adopt a new behavior and continue it for years, so that any effect of the behavior on cancer can be discovered. Generally, researchers have a firm suspicion from animal research that the treatment they are testing is protective, and not harmful. Currently, for example, a number of physicians have agreed to take daily supplements of the vitamin A compound carotene for many years into the future, to determine if levels greater than those in food may protect against cancer development. Each type of study has its limitations and must be interpreted with an awareness of those limitations.

described in the "Nutrition Detective Work" box above. Epidemiological studies have shown that the incidence of certain cancers varies both by geographic area and by racial group. For example, Japanese people living in Japan develop more stomach cancers and fewer colon cancers than people in the United States. However, when Japanese people come to the United States, their children develop both stomach and colon cancers at a rate like that of U.S. citizens. Japan and the United States are both industrial countries, and their environmental pollution rates are similar. However, something in the environment must account for the changed cancer pattern in immigrants, and an obvious candidate is diet.

Another finding is that vegetarians have lower mortality rates from cancer than the rest of the population, even when cancers linked to smoking and alcohol are taken out of the picture. In general, studies of populations have suggested that low cancer rates correlate with low meat and high vegetable and grain intakes. Case-control studies, in which researchers can control some of the variables, have supported the epidemiological studies, and they, too, implicate diet in cancer causation; Highlight 6 summed up the evidence.

Laboratory studies using animals confirm suspicions that fat, of all dietary components, is uniquely correlated with cancer. Fat does not initiate the cancers, however; to get the tumors started, an experimenter has to expose the animals to a known carcinogen. After that exposure, the high-fat diet makes more cancers develop and makes them develop earlier than they would with a low-fat diet. Thus fat appears to be a cancer promoter, rather than an initiator. A high-fat diet may promote cancer in any of a number of ways:

- By causing the body to secrete more of certain hormones (for example, estrogen), thus creating a climate favorable to the development of certain cancers (for example, breast cancer).
- By promoting the secretion of bile into the intestine; bile may then be converted by organisms in the colon into compounds that cause cancer.
- By being incorporated into cell membranes and changing them so that they offer less defense against cancer-causing invaders.

It may not be fat in general that has these effects, but rather certain forms of fat. The finding that linoleic acid, the polyunsaturated fatty acid of vegetable oils, is particularly implicated in cancer causation is especially important. (On the other hand, omega-3 fatty acids and monounsaturated fatty acids do not promote cancer.) The person wishing to apply this information should reduce consumption of all forms of fat. There would appear to be no harm in reducing fat intake to the point where it contributes a maximum of 30 percent of total kcalories, as recommended for cardiovascular disease prevention, and some cancer researchers suggest an even stricter limit: 20 percent of total kcalories. For the ''average American'' to accomplish this degree of fat restriction in practice means drastically reducing the amount of fat used in food preparation, and excluding many traditional foods almost entirely: butter, margarine, mayonnaise, and salad dressings. Of the fats used, olive oil and fish oils would seem to be the most desirable—as is the case for prevention of cardiovascular disease.

At the same time, it seems desirable to increase plant fiber intakes. Fiber might help protect against some cancer—for example, by promoting the excretion of bile from the body, or by speeding up the transit time of all materials through the colon so that the colon walls are not exposed for long to cancer-causing substances. That fiber does have an independent protective effect of some kind is supported by evidence from Finland. The Finns eat a high-fat diet, but unlike other such diets, theirs is high in fiber as well. Their colon cancer rate is low, suggesting that fiber has a protective effect even in the presence of a high-fat diet.

It seems apparent from all of these studies that foods contain two kinds of substances that affect people's susceptibility to cancer: promoters and antipromoters. Dietary fats act as promoters; fiber may act as an antipromoter, and indications are that many other factors in foods also act as antipromoters. If fat, a meat-rich diet, or both, are implicated in the causation of certain cancers, and if fiber, a vegetable-rich diet, or both are associated with prevention, then vegetarians should have a lower incidence of those cancers. They do, as Highlight 6 demonstrated.

A number of studies have supported special roles for plant foods in cancer resistance. One study found less frequent use of vegetables in people with colon cancer; another found, specifically, less use of cabbage, broccoli, and brussels sprouts in colon cancer victims. Stomach cancer, too, correlates with low vegetable intakes—in one study, vegetables in general; in another, fresh vegetables; in others, lettuce and other fresh greens, or vegetables containing vitamin C.

Cancers of the head and neck seem to correlate best not with diet but with the combination of alcohol and tobacco consumption. However, some dietary factors are implicated as protective, particularly fruits and raw vegetables, and specifically the fruits and vegetables that contribute carotene (the vitamin A

Cruciferous vegetables, such as cauliflower, broccoli, and Brussels sprouts, contain nutrients and nonnutrients that protect against cancer.

cruciferous vegetables: a group of vegetables named for their cross-shaped blossoms. They have been shown to protect against cancer in laboratory animals. Examples are cauliflower, cabbage, Brussels sprouts, broccoli, turnips, and rutabagas.

indoles: a family of compounds with a structure resembling that of the amino acid tryptophan, mentioned here because some of those found in cruciferous vegetables have anticancer activity.

dithiolthiones: a class of compounds important in connection with diet and cancer because some are found in plant foods and seem to exhibit anticancer activity.

protease inhibitors: compounds that inhibit the action of protein-digesting enzymes.

precursor) and the B vitamin riboflavin. Carotene and its relatives, the retinoids, are also important in preventing cancers of epithelial origin, including skin cancer.

Vitamin A regulates cellular differentiation, which goes awry in cancer. This vitamin also helps maintain the immune system. Immunity can work against cancer even after a tumor has begun to form. Lung cancer incidence can be as much as 60 to 80 percent lower in people with high vitamin A intakes than in those with low intakes. In Japan, a study of 280,000 people showed lung cancer rates to be 20 to 30 percent lower in smokers who ate yellow or green vegetables daily than in those who did not. In ex-smokers who ingested yellow or green vegetables daily, the reduction was much greater, as if the *repair* of damage done by smoking after the initiation of cancer was enhanced by something in the vegetables.

For anyone who might be tempted to think that pills containing vitamin A or carotene might provide the same benefit as green vegetables, it should be pointed out immediately that green vegetables appear to have an additional protective effect not supplied by vitamin A, vitamin C, and fiber. Among other nutrients cited as possible antipromoters are vitamin B_6, folate, pantothenic acid, vitamin B_{12}, vitamin E, iron, zinc, selenium—and more. Besides, nonnutrient substances in vegetables may also act as antipromoters, and these would not be found in vitamin pills.

Some nonnutrient compounds occur in vegetables of the cabbage family—the so-called cruciferous vegetables. These compounds, known as indoles, dithiolthiones, and other chemicals, activate enzymes that destroy carcinogens.* Another class of possible anticancer compounds occurs in beans and plant seeds. These are protease inhibitors, and they are thought to inhibit enzymes associated with the spreading of tumors.

Other vegetables and fruits contain other constituents that may activate the enzyme system that degrades carcinogens. These constituents are so widespread among plants that the single most valuable application of the information obtained to date is *not* to eat cabbages, for example, but to eat a wide variety of vegetables and fruits in generous quantities.

Recommendations for Cancer Prevention   By the early 1980s, enough evidence had accumulated to permit the making of some provisional dietary guidelines for cancer prevention. They centered on the following:

- Control total food energy intake.
- Reduce the consumption of both saturated and unsaturated fats.
- Include fruits (especially citrus fruits), vegetables (particularly carotene-rich and cruciferous vegetables), and whole-grain products in the daily diet.
- Avoid possible carcinogens by limiting consumption of foods preserved by salt curing, salt packing, or smoking.
- Minimize contamination of foods with carcinogens from any source.
- Continue to evaluate food additives for carcinogenic activity.
- Reduce the concentration of mutagens in foods when feasible.
- Consume only moderate amounts of alcohol, if any.
- Monitor drinking water with an eye out for toxic substances.

---

*The enzymes are the microsomal mixed-function oxidases, and in particular, aryl hydrocarbon hydroxylase. Among the other inducers of the mixed-function oxidase system, found in plants, are flavones, aromatic isothiocyanates, coumarin, and selenium salts.

The Committee on Diet, Nutrition, and Cancer of the National Research Council, which published these guidelines, specifically stated, however, that additives legally permitted in foods were not implicated in cancer causation.

To the recommendations made in these guidelines, we would add one other: vary your choices. Don't let your diet become monotonous. This last suggestion is based on an important concept that is specific to the prevention of cancer initiation—dilution. Whenever you switch from food to food, you are diluting whatever is in one food with what is in the others. For example, it is safe to eat *some* salt-cured or smoked meats, but don't eat them all the time. Eat many green, yellow, and orange vegetables; they are all needed in the diet for many good reasons. If you include high-fiber foods and reduce your fat intake as well, you have every reason to feel confident that you are providing your body with the best nutrition at the lowest possible risk.

Prevention of AIDS

AIDS is frightening, but it can be prevented. Its transmission requires sexual activity, blood sharing, or infection of an infant during pregnancy, birth, or breastfeeding. While diet plays no role in the transmission or prevention of AIDS, the message of prevention is important enough to warrant some mention at this time.

To fully protect yourself from contracting AIDS, abstain from IV drug use and sexual activity outside of a mutually exclusive relationship with a partner whom you *know* is not infected. Additional strategies include:

- Do not have sexual contact (including open-mouth kissing) with anyone who has symptoms of AIDS, who is a member of a high-risk group, or who has had sexual contact with a member of a high-risk group. (High-risk groups include people with AIDS-infected sex partners or multiple sex partners, IV drug users, prostitutes, and homosexuals.)
- If you do have sexual contact with any of those people mentioned above or with someone whose history is unknown to you, use a latex condom and a spermicidal agent.
- Do not share toothbrushes, razors, or other implements that could become contaminated with blood.
- Exercise caution when undergoing procedures such as acupuncture, tattooing, or ear piercing, in which needles might be contaminated.
- If you are an IV drug user, seek help for your addiction. Meanwhile, use only sterile, unused needles and dispose of them so that others will not use them. Avoid sexual contact with others.

It is urgent that every person not yet infected with AIDS adopt an aggressive, effective personal strategy to prevent it from occurring.

◼ Nutrition Assessment

Early identification of the nutrition problems of people with cancer or AIDS helps prevent severe malnutrition and may improve their responses to other therapy and enhance the quality of their lives. Some areas that deserve special consideration include the following:

- First, closely examine the diet history. Look for signs of reduced food intake, and pinpoint causes so that you can construct a viable nutrition care plan.
- Keep in mind that people with cancer and AIDS, particularly those who feel they cannot benefit from therapy, are easy targets for peddlers of nutrition "cures." They may take massive doses of vitamins and minerals or follow other home remedies that may impair nutrition status. Be sure to ask what supplements, and what amounts of them, your clients may be taking.
- Check to see what type of therapy the person has been receiving or will receive and ascertain how it may affect nutrition status. Be alert to possible drug-nutrient interactions.
- Record anthropometric measurements regularly to help determine whether energy and protein needs are being met. Monitor weight changes, noting both unintentional and significant ones. Be sure to identify problems that have led to weight loss and offer solutions whenever possible. Remember that edema may be present in certain types of cancer and can affect anthropometric measurements.
- When a client has been vomiting or has diarrhea, be alert to the possibility of dehydration. Remember that biochemical parameters in dehydrated people may falsely appear to be normal.
- Total lymphocyte counts and skin testing are not useful in assessing protein status in people with AIDS because the infection itself interferes with these immune system parameters independently of nutrition status. Similarly, these parameters are also not useful in assessing nutrition status for people undergoing bone marrow transplants or those given large doses of chemotherapy that interfere with immune function.

PEM is a frequent complication of both cancer and AIDS. Health care professionals, alert to this fact, look for signs of deteriorating nutrition status and take active steps to correct problems before they become severe.

This chapter brings to a close your introduction to normal and clinical nutrition. Congratulations! You have received an abundance of information since you first turned to page 1. The normal nutrition chapters of this text provided you with current recommendations to promote optimal health. You learned how the body transforms foods into nutrients and how those nutrients support the body's well-being. The clinical chapters of the text addressed you as a future health care professional, concerned not only with your own health, but also with the well-being of others during times of illness. They provided guidelines on diet for a variety of disorders from AIDS to ulcers. Along the way, you learned about tube feedings, pureed foods, and all kinds of modified diets.

We hope this text has served you well, and that you will remember, when selecting food for yourself or when making recommendations for others, to honor the body. It is a prized possession. Nourish it well.

Study Questions

1. What is cancer? What events are believed to lead to cancer?
2. What are some of the treatments for cancer, and how do they work?
3. What is cancer cachexia? What factors contribute to the development of cancer cachexia? Can nutrition intervention help prevent this problem?
4. Describe the anorexia that is associated with cancer. How does it differ from anorexia in other disease states? Discuss how cancer and its therapy contribute to anorexia.
5. How can cancer result in excess nutrient losses, and how do these losses contribute to the cancer cachexia syndrome?
6. What are food aversions, and how can they be dealt with?
7. Describe the metabolic changes that occur in the person with cancer, and discuss their role in the cancer cachexia syndrome.
8. What are the possible advantages of good nutrition status for the person with cancer? What methods are used to help prevent people with cancer from developing severe nutrient deficiencies?
9. In the person with cancer, what strategies can combat anorexia? Bitter or metallic taste in the mouth? Nausea and vomiting? Problems with chewing and swallowing? Mouth ulcers? Reduced flow of saliva?
10. What is AIDS? What factors contribute to the wasting associated with AIDS?
11. Describe factors that can lead to reduced food intake in people with AIDS.
12. In what ways can AIDS lead to excessive nutrient losses? How can metabolism be affected by AIDS?
13. In what ways can good nutrition status possibly alter the course of AIDS?
14. Why are people with AIDS highly susceptible to food-borne illness?

Notes

1. J. L. Peacock and coauthors, Resting energy expenditure and body cell mass alterations in sarcoma patients, *Surgical Forum* 37 (1986): 789–795.
2. K. A. Kern and J. A. Norton, Cancer cachexia, *Journal of Parenteral and Enteral Nutrition* 12 (1988): 286–298.
3. B. Beutler and A. Cerami, Cachectin: More than a tumor necrosis factor, *New England Journal of Medicine* 316 (1987): 379–385.
4. As cited in F. Bozzetti, Effects of artificial nutrition on the nutritional status of cancer patients, *Journal of Parenteral and Enteral Nutrition* 13 (1989): 406–420.
5. W. W. Souba and E. M. Copeland, Parenteral nutrition and metabolic observations in cancer, *Nutrition in Clinical Practice* 3 (1988): 183–190.
6. Kern and Norton, 1988.
7. Kern and Norton, 1988.
8. J. M. Daly and coauthors, Nutrition support in the cancer patient, *Journal of Parenteral and Enteral Nutrition* (supplement) 14 (1990): 244–248.
9. Souba and Copeland, 1988.
10. Bozzetti, 1988.
11. G. B. Brookes, Nutritional status—A prognostic indicator in head and neck cancer, *Otolaryngology Head and Neck Surgery* 93 (1985): 69–73.
12. Souba and Copeland, 1988.
13. L. P. Harvey and coauthors, Reversibility of elemental liquid diet-enhanced methotrexate toxicity by refeeding with chow, *Journal of Parenteral Nutrition* 11 (1987): 119–123.
14. O. J. McAnena and coauthors, Alteration of methotrexate toxicity in rats by manipulation of dietary components, *Gastroenterology* 92 (1987): 354–360.
15. D. P. Kotler, Protein-energy malnutrition in AIDS, *Nutrition in Clinical Practice* 5 (1990): 41–42.
16. *Nutritional Aspects of the AIDS Patient*, Department of Continuing Education in Health Sciences, UCLA Extension (Los Angeles: 1989).
17. R. Ullrich and coauthors, Small intestinal structure and function in patients infected with human immunodeficiency virus (HIV): Evidence for HIV-induced enteropathy, *Annals of Internal Medicine* 111 (1989): 15–21.
18. P. A. Cuff, Acquired immunodeficiency syndrome and malnutrition: Role of gastrointestinal pathology, *Nutrition in Clinical Practice* 5 (1990): 43–53.
19. Cuff, 1990; and Department of Continuing Education, UCLA Extension, 1989.
20. C. McCorkindale and coauthors, Nutritional status of HIV-infected patients during the early disease stages, *Journal of the American Dietetic Association* 90 (1990): 1236–1241.
21. Task Force on Nutrition Support in AIDS, Guidelines for Nutrition Support in AIDS, *Nutrition* 5 (1989): 39–46.
22. Department of Continuing Education in Health Sciences, UCLA Extension, 1989.
23. Department of Continuing Education in Health Sciences, UCLA Extension, 1989.
24. D. B. Kotler and coauthors, Effect of home total parenteral nutrition on body composition in patients with acquired immunodeficiency syndrome, *Journal of Parenteral and Enteral Nutrition* 14 (1990): 454–458.
25. T. Singer and coauthors, Risks and benefits of home parenteral nutrition in acquired immunodeficiency syndrome, *Journal of Parenteral and Enteral Nutrition* 15 (1991): 75–79.

Cost Containment and Specialized Nutrition Support

Anyone who has needed medical attention recently knows that health care costs are skyrocketing. This trend troubles everyone—health care facilities, their employees, their clients, government agencies, private insurance carriers, and taxpayers. The costs of hospitalization have risen especially fast among service industries, and this affects the delivery of nutrition care. Specialized nutrition support, being costly anyway, is being priced out of reach for many people. Once able to pay their nutrition care costs out of Medicare, people now are faced with a new system that does not always cover those costs.

Changes in How Health Care Costs Are Set

Prior to 1983, Medicare (a form of government insurance for elderly and disabled people) reimbursed hospitals for a portion of the costs incurred during an eligible client's hospital stay. Using this system, hospitals had little incentive to control costs, since they received payment for any expenses incurred. Obviously, such a system contributes to skyrocketing costs.

To help contain spiraling health care costs, the U.S. government introduced the prospective payment system to cover the medical bills of people on Medicare. Prospective payment differs significantly from the previous plan in that hospitals received a fixed payment for the care of a client with a particular diagnosis. In effect, the hospital is given a budget for each case: it receives specified amounts for delivering care for specified disorders—so much for gallbladder surgery, so much for treating a broken arm, and so on. The diagnoses that qualify for a given amount of money are grouped together; hence the term diagnosis-related group, or DRG, for

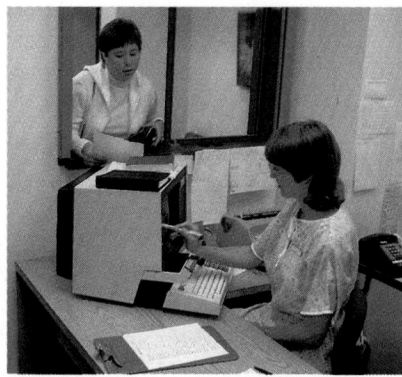

Soaring health care costs demand attention if people are to continue receiving quality care.

the categories of care funded by the system.

The DRG system motivates hospitals to cut costs, for each client's DRG determines how much money the hospital will receive when that client leaves the hospital. The payment given the hospital is independent of the actual costs the hospital incurred. If, for example, the hospital can care for a client in fewer days with fewer tests than provided for under the DRG system, the hospital makes money. If, on the other hand, a client must remain in the hospital longer or if physicians request too many tests, the hospital may lose money. The hospital can apply for exceptions to these limits. If a client must be hospitalized for much longer than normal, or incurs much higher hospital costs for a particular DRG, the hospital may receive additional support for the case. Still, in most of these cases, called outliers, the hospital's costs exceed what it receives in reimbursement; the hospital loses money. Currently, the prospective payment system affects only people on Medicare. Private insurance companies operate on a

fee-for-service basis. Clients with private insurance bolster hospital revenues when they have extended hospital stays or when they receive additional services or tests. These clients help limit the losses a hospital might incur under the DRG system, but they also contribute to rising health care costs. Additionally, private insurers are carrying a higher cost burden, which affects many consumers. For these reasons, private carriers may switch to prospective payment systems in the future if the DRG prove effective. Such a switch could severely curtail hospitals' revenues and force the elimination of some services, such as special nutrition support.

The DRG system raises other concerns among consumers and health care professionals. Isn't it possible that, in the effort to reduce hospital costs, clients will not receive full medical care? Will physicians hesitate to order tests that might be helpful to clients? Will clients be discharged from the hospital before they should be? So far, these concerns appear to be unwarranted. The Prospective Payment Assessment Commission, created by Congress to oversee the DRG system, has found no evidence of reduced quality of care created by the system.[1] Hospitals and their staffs exist to treat disease and to relieve suffering and pain. This commitment to quality care coupled with the competition among hospitals for clients, as well as the threat of malpractice suits balance the situation.

However, the verdict on the effectiveness of DRG in reducing health care costs is still out. While the rate of growth of in-hospital expenditures paid by Medicare has slowed, costs of outpatient services have risen.[2]

The Costs of Special Nutrition Support

That the DRG system sometimes fails to fully cover health care costs raises particular concerns for people who need special nutrition support. Medicare covers about a third of people on nutrition support.[3] These people are frequently critically ill and require long hospital stays.[4] One study demonstrated that people who need special nutrition support while hospitalized stayed in the hospital four times longer and needed more nursing care than individuals with similar disorders who did not need nutrition support.[5]

As Chapter 18 explained, studies suggest that appropriate nutrition support lowers mortality rates, results in fewer complications, and reduces length of hospital stays. Common sense dictates that no disease process benefits from starvation. However, the degree to which nutrition support alleviates disease is difficult to quantify. Malnourished people who need specialized nutrition support are usually quite ill. Their diseases may lead to complications or death regardless of their nutrition status. Furthermore, the severity of a given disease and the degree of malnutrition differ from case to case. Therefore, health care providers cannot prove, when one person recovers faster than another, that one factor such as nutrition was directly responsible for the difference.

Providing nutrition support, particularly total parenteral nutrition, is expensive. The average cost of parenteral nutrition runs about $365 per day.[6] Since the average person placed on parenteral nutrition needs the therapy for about 21 days, the cost of parenteral nutrition alone during an average hospitalization exceeds $7,500. The total cost of providing parenteral nutrition solutions in hospitals in 1984 was estimated at $3 billion.[7]

By comparison, enteral nutrition is a far less expensive therapy. On the average, enteral nutrition costs about $30 per day and requires about 19 days.[8] Using these figures, the average cost of enteral nutrition during a typical hospitalization runs about $570.

Studies have clearly shown that aggressive nutrition support can improve nutrition status, but few studies have documented that nutrition support speeds up recovery from disease. The effects simply have not been dramatic.[9] This does not mean that nutrition support does not help clients, but it may help in ways that are difficult to justify in terms of costs. Unfortunately, subjective improvements, like energy level and quality of life, do not come with a price tag. Although it might be cheaper to keep a person in the hospital for an extra day than to give several days of nutrition support, what price do you put on the individual's comfort and desire to go home? Nutrition support can also affect the individual's risk of becoming ill again. All of these factors are difficult to justify in a context where cost containment is a high priority.

The combination of high costs for parenteral nutrition and extended hospital stays for clients who require it puts a serious financial burden on hospitals. The Prospect Payment Assessment Committee estimated that in 1987 hospitals were reimbursed 62 cents for every dollar spent on people receiving TPN.[10] Financial pressures may force hospitals to discontinue the use of specialized nutrition support or to discourage its use.[11] Either of these measures could impair the nutrition status and support of hospital clients.

Easing the Problem

The DRG system appears here to stay—at least for now. As everyone concerned gains more experience working with the system, some practitioners remain pessimistic about its future effects on the delivery of specialized nutrition support, while others feel more optimistic. It is hoped that the government will provide additional money under the system to cover the costs of specialized nutrition support. Meanwhile, health care providers need to learn how to work within the system to justify the costs of specialized nutrition support. Research has shown that the nutrition support team can, if it tries, effectively reduce the costs of specialized nutrition support.[12]

Miniglossary

comorbidity: a condition that exists at the time a person is hospitalized that usually adds at least one extra day of hospitalization.

complication: a condition that develops during hospitalization that usually adds at least one extra day of hospitalization.

cost effective: promoting quality care at the least cost.

cost containment: measures that reduce costs.

diagnosis-related groups (DRG): classification of disorders that provides a basis for reimbursement under Medicare's prospective payment system.

Medicare: health insurance for eligible recipients that is administered from the Social Security Administration.

outliers: unusual cases in which the person develops severe complications or must be hospitalized much longer than expected for a particular DRG.

prospective payment system: a system for reimbursing medical costs for eligible recipients that is based on the person's diagnosis rather than actual costs.

Among the steps health care providers can take to keep nutrition care costs down are these:

- Identify people with malnutrition at entry into the system, so that malnutrition can be documented as a diagnosis and, in some cases, hospital reimbursement can be increased.[13]
- Recommend the most cost-efficient method of feeding (enteral versus parenteral) as well as the most suitable feeding solution.
- Evaluate and purchase nutrition support supplies that will provide the needed service at a minimum cost.
- Monitor clients who are receiving nutrition support, so as to avoid or to promptly correct metabolic, mechanical, and other problems that can lead to costly complications.
- Document the positive effects of specialized nutrition support techniques to show that costs would have been higher had nutrition support not been provided.
- Continuously evaluate new methods of delivering nutrition support that could save money.

One study compared the costs of nutrition support recommended by a nutrition support team versus those of nutrition support initiated by attending physicians.[14] In 14 cases, the team had recommended enteral nutrition but the physician initiated parenteral nutrition. Had the team's advice been followed, the potential savings to clients would have amounted to $5,000 per client or over $70,000 in all.

Teams help limit the cost of nutrition support by following procedures that reduce the likelihood of complications. One group of authors report an estimated cost savings of $400,000 a year to their hospital due to the low rate of total parenteral nutrition catheter sepsis.[15] The authors credit their nutrition support nurse with the much-lowered sepsis rate (1 percent per client catheter) compared to the rate observed in hospitals without a nutrition support nurse (33 percent per client catheter). Such documentation justifies the nurse's position and increases the probability that clients will continue to receive needed special nutrition support.

These examples illustrate how health care providers can help ensure that specialized nutrition support will continue to be safely and readily available for people who need it. Professionals must understand the problems associated with reimbursement under the DRG system and take the necessary steps to ensure that clients will receive optimal nutrition care.

NOTES

1. American Society for Parenteral and Enteral Nutrition, *PENline* (newsletter discussing the DRG system), February 1987.

2. M. Regenstein, Reimbursement for nutrition support, *Nutrition in Clinical Practice* 4 (1989): 194–202.

3. Regenstein, 1989.

4. Nutrition Services Payment Task Force, Inpatient nutrition care: Adults—enteral and parenteral nutrition, *Journal of the American Dietetic Association* (supplement) 89 (1989): 47–52.

5. T. P. Clemmer and coauthors, Impact of Medicare prospective reimbursement system on nutritional support service patients: The importance of pass throughs, *Journal of Parenteral and Enteral Nutrition* 13 (1989): 71–76.

6. Regenstein, 1989.

7. G. F. Anderson and E. P. Steinberg, Prospective payment and nutritional support: The need for reform, *Journal of Parenteral and Enteral Nutrition* 10 (1986): 3–8.

8. Regenstein, 1989.

9. J. A. Sargent, Assessing the utility and improving the effectiveness of nutritional support, *Nutrition in Clinical Practice* 1 (1986): 29–39.

10. Regenstein, 1989.

11. J. M. Mirtallo and coauthors, Cost-effective nutrition support, *Nutrition in Clinical Practice* 2 (1987): 142–151.

12. K. S. Christensen, Hospitalwide screening increases revenue under prospective payment system, *Journal of the American Dietetic Association* 86 (1986): 1234–1235.

13. D. M. Delhey, E. J. Anderson, and S. H. Laramee, Implications of malnutrition and diagnosis-related groups (DRGs), *Journal of the American Dietetic Association* 89 (1989): 1444–1451.

14. D. D. O'Brien and coauthors, Recommendations of nutrition support team promote cost containment, *Journal of Parenteral and Enteral Nutrition* 10 (1986): 300–302.

15. M. V. Kaminski and coauthors, Confusion of cost containment and cost effectiveness in nutritional support therapy, *Nutritional Support Services* 8 (April 1988): 27–28.

Appendixes

A

B

C

D

E

F

G

H

I

J

K

L

Cells, Hormones, and Nerves

This appendix is offered as an optional chapter for readers who want to enhance their understanding of the body's ways of coordinating its activities. The text presents a brief summary of the structure and function of the body's basic working unit (the cell) and of the body's two major regulatory systems (the hormonal system and the nervous system).

Contents

The Cell

The Hormones

The Nervous System

Putting It Together

cell: the basic unit of life, of which all living things are composed. Every cell is surrounded by a membrane and contains cytoplasm, within which are organelles and a nucleus; the cell nucleus contains chromosomes.

A

■ The Cell

Every body organ is made up of millions of cells and of materials produced by them. Each organ's cells are specialized to perform that organ's functions, but all cells have basic things in common (see Figure A–1). Every cell is contained within a cell membrane. Inside the membrane lies the cytoplasm, or cell "fluid," and another membrane-enclosed body, the nucleus. Inside the nucleus are the chromosomes, which contain the genetic material, DNA. The DNA encodes all the instructions for carrying out the cell's activities.

The cell membrane's functions in moving materials into and out of the cell, and some of its special proteins such as "pumps," are described in Chapter 6. Also described are specializations of the cell membrane, such as microvilli (Chapter 3), which permit cells to interact with other cells and with their environments in highly specific ways.

The role of DNA in coding for cell proteins is summarized in Chapter 6, Figure 6–7. Chapter 6 also describes the variety of proteins produced by cells and the ways they perform the body's work.

The cytoplasm contains much more than just fluid. It is a highly organized system of fibers, tubes, membranes, particles, and subcellular organelles as complex as a city. These parts intercommunicate, manufacture and exchange materials, package and prepare materials for export, and maintain and repair themselves.

Among the organelles are ribosomes, mitochondria, and lysosomes. Figure 6–7 briefly refers to the ribosomes; they assemble amino acids into proteins, following directions conveyed to them by RNA copies from the DNA in the chromosomes.

The mitochondria are made of intricately folded membranes that bear thousands of highly organized sets of enzymes on their inner and outer surfaces. Although not often referred to in this book's chapters, their presence is implied whenever the enzymes of the TCA cycle and electron transport

cell membrane: the membrane that surrounds the cell and encloses its contents; made primarily of lipid and protein.

cytoplasm (SIGH-toe-plazm): the cell contents, except for the nucleus.
cyto = cell
plasm = a form

nucleus: a major membrane-enclosed body within every cell, which contains the cell's genetic material, DNA, embedded in chromosomes.
nucleus = a kernel

chromosomes: a set of structures within the nucleus of every cell that contain the cell's genetic material, DNA, associated with other materials (primarily proteins).

organelles: subcellular structures such as ribosomes, mitochondria, and lysosomes.
organelle = little organ

ribosomes: protein-making organelles in cells; composed of RNA and protein.
ribo = containing the sugar ribose (in RNA)
some = body

■ **FIGURE A–1**
The Structure of a Typical Cell
The cell shown might be one in a gland (such as the pancreas) that produces secretory products (enzymes) for export (to the intestine). The rough endoplasmic reticulum with its ribosomes produces the enzymes; the smooth reticulum conducts them to the Golgi region; the Golgi membranes merge with the cell membrane, where the enzymes can be released into the extracellular fluid.

A

Cell membrane
Cytoplasm
Golgi apparatus
Smooth endoplasmic reticulum
Rough endoplasmic reticulum
Ribosomes
Mitochondrion
Chromosomes
Nucleus
Lysosomes

mitochondria (my-toe-KON-dree-uh); singular **mitochondrion**: the cellular organelles responsible for producing ATP aerobically; made of membranes (lipid and protein) with enzymes mounted on them.
   mitos = thread (referring to their slender shape)
   chondros = cartilage (referring to their external appearance)

lysosomes: cellular organelles; membrane-enclosed sacs of degradative enzymes.
   lysis = dissolution

rough endoplasmic reticulum (en-doh-PLAZ-mic reh-TIC-you-lum): intracellular membranes on which ribosomes are mounted, where protein synthesis takes place.
   endo = inside
   plasm = the cytoplasm

smooth endoplasmic reticulum: smooth intracellular membranes bearing no ribosomes.

Golgi (GOAL-gee) **apparatus:** a set of membranes within the cell where secretory materials are packaged for export.

chain are mentioned, for the mitochondria house all these enzymes.* Mitochondria are therefore crucial to aerobic metabolism, described in Chapter 7, and muscles conditioned to work aerobically are packed with them. Several chapter-opening photographs depict mitochondria in different kinds of cells.

The lysosomes are membranes enclosing degradative enzymes. When a cell needs to self-destruct or to digest materials in its surroundings, its lysosomes free their enzymes. Lysosomes are active when tissue repair or remodeling is taking place—for example, in cleaning up infections, healing wounds, shaping embryonic organs, and remodeling bones.

Besides these and other cellular organelles, the cell's cytoplasm contains a highly organized system of membranes, the endoplasmic reticulum. The ribosomes may either float free in the cytoplasm or may be seated on these membranes. A membranous surface dotted with ribosomes looks speckled under the microscope and is called ''rough'' endoplasmic reticulum; such a surface without ribosomes is called ''smooth.'' Some intracellular membranes are organized into tubules that collect cellular materials, merge with the cell membrane, and discharge their contents to the outside of the cell; these membrane systems are named the Golgi apparatus, for the person who first described them. The rough and smooth endoplasmic reticulua and the Golgi apparatus are continuous with one another, so secretions produced deep in the interior of the cell can be efficiently transported to the outside and released.

These and other cell structures enable cells to perform the multitudes of functions for which they are specialized. The illustrations at the start of each chapter depict further details of cell structure and function.

---

*For the reactions of glycolysis, the TCA cycle, and the electron transport chain, see Chapter 7 and Appendix C. The reactions of glycolysis take place in the cytoplasm; the end product acetyl CoA moves into the mitochondrion; and the TCA and electron transport reactions take place there. The mitochondrion then releases carbon dioxide, water, and ATP as its end products.

The actions of cells are coordinated by both hormones and nerves, as the next sections show. Among specializations of cellular organelles are receptors for hormones that deliver instructions originating elsewhere in the body. Some hormones penetrate the cell and nucleus, and attach to receptors on chromosomes, from which they activate certain genes to initiate, stop, speed up, or slow down synthesis of certain proteins as needed. Other hormones attach to receptors on the cell surface and transmit their messages from there. The hormones are described in the next section; the nerves, in the one following.

■ *The Hormones*

A hormonal system message originates in a gland and travels as a chemical compound—a hormone—in the bloodstream. The hormone flows everywhere in the body, but only its target organs respond to it, because only they possess the equipment to receive it.

The hormones, the glands they originate in, and their target organs and effects are described in this section. All the hormones you might be interested in are included, but only a few are discussed in detail. Figure A–2 identifies the glands that produce the hormones discussed in this section.

hormone: a chemical messenger. Hormones are secreted in response to altered conditions by a variety of endocrine glands in the body. Each travels to one or more specific target tissues or organs, where it elicits a specific response.

Endocrinology is the study of hormones and their effects, and the system of glands and hormones that regulates body processes is the **endocrine system.**

endocrine: with reference to a gland, one that secretes its product directly into (*endo*) the blood, like the pancreas cells that produce insulin. An **exocrine** gland secretes its product(s) out (*exo*) of the gland through a duct into a cavity; the sweat glands of the skin and the enzyme-producing glands of the pancreas are both examples. The pancreas is therefore both an endocrine and an exocrine gland.

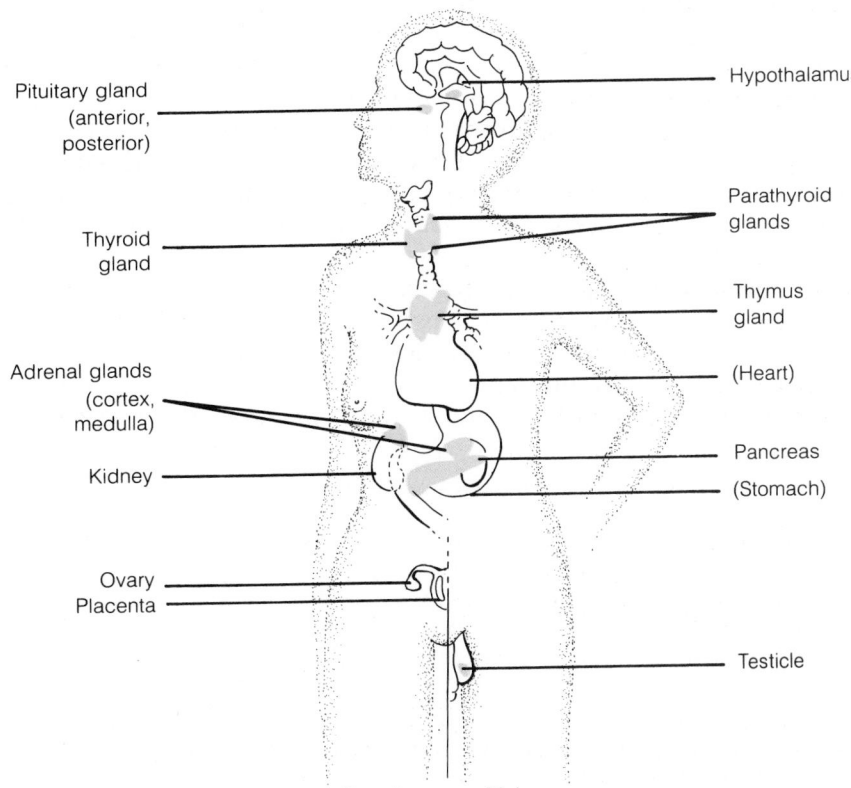

Pituitary gland (anterior, posterior)

Thyroid gland

Adrenal glands (cortex, medulla)

Kidney

Ovary
Placenta

Hypothalamus

Parathyroid glands

Thymus gland

(Heart)

Pancreas

(Stomach)

Testicle

Female   Male

■ **FIGURE A–2**
The Endocrine System

The whole picture is of a complex system in which many of the parts interact with one another. For example, several hormones are produced in the anterior pituitary gland in the brain. All of these are regulated by hormones produced in another part of the brain, the hypothalamus. Furthermore, each of the pituitary gland hormones has effects on the production of compounds elsewhere in the body. Some of these compounds are also hormones that will affect still other body parts. A hormone may travel far from its point of origin and ultimately have profound, even unexpected, effects.

Hormones of the Pituitary Gland and Hypothalamus

The anterior pituitary gland produces the hormones:

- Adrenocorticotropin (ACTH).
- Thyroid-stimulating hormone (TSH).
- Growth hormone (GH).
- Follicle-stimulating hormone (FSH).
- Luteinizing hormone (LH).
- Prolactin.
- Melanocyte-stimulating hormone (MSH).

Each of these hormones acts on one or more target organs and elicits a characteristic response. ACTH acts on the adrenal cortex, promoting the making and release of its hormones. TSH acts on the thyroid gland, promoting the making and release of thyroid hormone. GH works on all tissues, promoting growth, fat breakdown, and the formation of antibodies. FSH works on the ovaries in the female, promoting their maturation, and on the testicles in the male, promoting sperm formation. LH also acts on the ovaries, forwarding their maturation, the making of progesterone and estrogens, and ovulation; and on the testicles, promoting the making and release of androgens (male hormones). Prolactin, secreted in the female during pregnancy and after she has borne a baby, acts on the mammary glands to stimulate their growth and the making of milk. Finally, MSH acts on the pigment cells, promoting the making and dispersal of pigment.

The controls over this array of actions are sensitive and specific. Each of the seven hormones itemized above has one or more signals that turn it on and another (or others) that turn it off.

Among the controlling signals are several hormones from the hypothalamus:

- Corticotropin-releasing hormone (CRH), which promotes release of ACTH. CRH is itself turned on by stress, and turned off by ACTH when enough has been released.
- TSH-releasing hormone (TRH), which promotes release of TSH. This is turned on by large meals or low body temperature.
- GH-releasing hormone (GRH), which is turned on by insulin.
- GH-inhibiting hormone (GIH or somatostatin), which inhibits the release of GH and interferes with the release of TSH. This is turned on by hypoglycemia and/or exercise, and is rapidly destroyed by body tissues so that it does not accumulate.

The **pituitary** gland in the brain has two parts—the **anterior** (front) and the **posterior** (hind) parts.

adrenocorticotropin: so named because it stimulates (*trope*) the adrenal cortex. The adrenal gland, like the pituitary, has two parts, in this case an outer portion (*cortex*) and an inner core (*medulla*).

follicle: that part of the female reproductive system where the ovary lies and eggs are produced.

luteinizing: so called because the follicle turns orange as it matures.
  lutein = an orange pigment

prolactin: so named because it promotes (*pro*) the production of milk (*lacto*).

melanocyte (MEL-an-oh-cite): a cell containing the pigment melanin.
  cyte = cell

hypothalamus: a brain region (see Figure A–2) that is connected by a channel to the pituitary and can produce many hormones in response to signals from it or from other body conditions.
  hypo = below
  thalamus = another brain region

Hormones that are turned off by their own effects are said to be regulated by **negative feedback.** For example, when a pituitary gland hormone has caused the release of a substance from a target organ, that substance itself switches off the original hormone signal (that is, it feeds back, negatively).

somatostatin (GIH): a hormone that inhibits the release of growth hormone; the opposite of **somatotropin** (GH).
  somato = body
  stat = keep the same
  tropin = make more

■ FSH/LH–releasing hormone (FSH/LH–RH), which is turned on in the female by nerve messages or low estrogen, and in the male by low testosterone.

■ Prolactin-release-inhibiting hormone (PIH), which is turned on by high prolactin levels and off by estrogen, testosterone, and suckling (by way of nerve messages).

■ MSH-release-inhibiting hormone (MIH), which is turned on by the hormone melatonin.

Let's examine some of these controls. PIH, for example, responds to high prolactin levels (remember, prolactin promotes the making of milk). High prolactin levels will ensure that milk is made and—by calling forth PIH—will ensure that they don't get too high. But when the infant is suckling—and creating a demand for milk—then PIH is not allowed to work (suckling turns off PIH). The consequence: prolactin remains high, and milk manufacture continues. Demand from the infant thus directly adjusts the infant's supply of milk. This example shows not only how the need is met but also illustrates the cooperation between nerves and hormones that achieves this effect.

As another example, take CRH. Stress, perceived in the brain and relayed to the hypothalamus, switches on CRH. CRH, on arriving at the pituitary, switches on ACTH. Then ACTH acts on its target organ, the adrenal cortex, which responds by producing and releasing stress hormones, and the stress response is under way. Events cascading from there involve every body cell and many other hormones (see Highlight 1).

You may wonder why so many steps are required to set the stress response in motion. Having many steps makes it possible for the body to fine-tune the stress response, because control can be exerted at each step. These are just two examples of what the body can do in response to two different stimuli—producing milk in response to an infant's need, and gearing up for action in an emergency.

Two hormones produced by the posterior pituitary gland are:

■ Antidiuretic hormone (ADH), or vasopressin.
■ Oxytocin.

ADH promotes contraction of arteries and acts on the kidney to prevent water from being excreted. It is turned on whenever the blood volume is depleted, or the blood pressure is low, or the salt concentration of the blood is too high. It is turned off by correction of these deviations from normal. Oxytocin is produced in response to reduced progesterone levels, suckling, or the stretching of the cervix, and acts on two target organs. One, the uterus, contracts, thus inducing labor; the other, the mammary glands, release milk.

Hormones That Regulate Energy Metabolism

Hormones produced by a number of different glands have effects on energy metabolism:

■ Insulin, from the pancreas beta cells.
■ Glucagon, from the pancreas alpha cells.
■ Thyroxin, from the thyroid gland.

antidiuretic hormone (ADH): the hormone that prevents water loss in urine (also **vasopressin**).
  anti = against
  di = through
  ure = urine
  vaso = blood vessels
  pressin = pressure

oxytocin: the hormone of childbirth.
  oxy = quick
  tocin = childbirth

cervix: the circular muscle that guards the opening of the uterus. When a baby is about to be born, the cervix begins to stretch.
  cervic = neck

A

Norepinephrine and epinephrine were formerly called noradrenalin and adrenalin.

glucocorticoid: a hormone from the adrenal cortex affecting the body's management of glucose.
  gluco = glucose
  corticoid = from the cortex

- Norepinephrine and epinephrine, from the adrenal medulla.
- Growth hormone (GH), from the anterior pituitary (already mentioned).
- Glucocorticoids, from the adrenal cortex.

Insulin is turned on by many stimuli, including raised blood glucose, and it acts on cells to increase glucose and amino acid uptake into them and to promote the secretion of GRH. Glucagon responds to low blood glucose and acts on the liver to promote the breakdown of glycogen to glucose, the conversion of amino acids to glucose, and the release of glucose. Thyroxin responds to TSH and acts on many cells to increase their metabolic rate, growth, and heat production. The hormones norepinephrine and epinephrine respond to stimulation by sympathetic nerves and produce reactions in many cells that facilitate the body's readiness for fight or flight: increased heart activity, blood vessel constriction, breakdown of glycogen and glucose, raised blood glucose levels, and fat breakdown; they also influence the secretion of the many hormones from the hypothalamus that exert control on the body's other systems. The glucocorticoid hormones become active during times of stress and carbohydrate metabolism.

Every body part is affected by these hormones. Each different hormone has unique effects; and hormones that oppose each other can be produced in carefully regulated amounts, so each part can respond to the exact degree that is appropriate to the occasion.

Hormones That Adjust Other Body Balances

Three hormones are involved in moving calcium into and out of the body's storage deposits in the bones:

calcitonin: so called because it regulates (tones) the calcium level.

parathyroid: named for their location, the four parathyroid glands nestle in the surface layers of the two thyroid lobes in the neck.
  para = beside, next to

Vitamin D, once thought to be a nutrient, is now viewed as a hormone, because it is produced in one body organ and regulates others. For details, see Chapter 9.

erythropoietin (eh-REE-throw-POY-eh-tin): named for its red blood cell–making function.
  erythro = red (blood cell)
  poiesis = creating (like poetry)

relaxin: the hormone of late pregnancy.

- Calcitonin (CT), from the thyroid gland.
- Parathyroid hormone (PTH), from the parathyroid gland.
- Vitamin D, from the kidney.

One of calcitonin's target tissues is the bones, which respond by storing calcium from the bloodstream whenever blood calcium rises above the normal range. Calcitonin also acts on the kidney to increase excretion of both calcium and phosphorus in the urine. Parathyroid hormone responds to the opposite condition—lowered blood calcium—and acts on three targets: the bones, which release stored calcium into the blood; the kidney, which slows its excretion of calcium; and the intestine, which increases its calcium absorption. Vitamin D acts with parathyroid hormone and is essential for the absorption of calcium in the intestine.

Another hormone has effects on blood-making activity:

- Erythropoietin, from the kidney.

Erythropoietin is responsive to oxygen depletion of the blood and to anemia, and acts on the bone marrow to stimulate its making of red blood cells.

Another hormone, special for pregnancy, is:

- Relaxin, from the ovary.

This hormone is secreted in response to the raised progesterone and estrogen levels of late pregnancy, and acts on the cervix and pelvic ligaments to allow them to stretch so that they can accommodate the birth process without strain.

Other agents help regulate blood pressure:

- Renin (an enzyme), from the kidney, in cooperation with angiotensin in the blood.
- Aldosterone, a hormone from the adrenal cortex.

Renin responds to a reduced blood supply experienced by the kidney, and acts in several ways. Encountering the inactive form of angiotensin in the bloodstream, renin converts this molecule to active angiotensin I and then to the very active angiotensin II. The angiotensins constrict the blood vessels, thus raising the blood pressure. They also stimulate thirst, leading to increased water intake, another way of raising the blood pressure. The angiotensins also cause the kidneys to retain water and salt. Thus the angiotensins increase blood pressure by several means at once.

Renin and angiotensin also stimulate the adrenal cortex to secrete the hormone aldosterone. This hormone's target is also the kidney, which responds by excreting less sodium, and with it, less water. The effect is to retain more water in the bloodstream—thus, again, raising the blood pressure. (Chapters 10 and 28 provide more details.)

renin (REEN-in): an enzyme from the kidney, which works by activating angiotensin.
ren = kidney

angiotensin: a hormone involved in blood pressure regulation.
angio = blood vessels
tensin = pressure

aldosterone: a hormone from the adrenal gland, involved in blood pressure regulation.
aldo = aldehyde

A

The Gastrointestinal Hormones

Three hormones are known to be produced in the stomach and intestines in response to the presence of food or the components of food:

- Gastrin, from the stomach and duodenum.
- Cholecystokinin, from the duodenum.
- Secretin, from the duodenum.

Gastrin stimulates the stomach to make and release its acid and digestive juices and to move and churn its contents actively. Cholecystokinin signals the gallbladder and pancreas to release their contents into the intestine to aid in digestion. Secretin calls forth acid-neutralizing bicarbonate from the pancreas into the intestine, and slows the action of the stomach and its secretion of acid and digestive juices. These hormones are dealt with in more detail in Chapter 3.

testosterone: a steroid hormone from the testicles, or testes. The steroids, as explained in Chapter 5, are chemically related to, and some are derived from, the lipid cholesterol.
sterone = a steroid hormone

The Sex Hormones

The three major sex hormones are:

- Testosterone, from the testicles.
- Estrogen, from the ovary.
- Progesterone, from the ovary's corpus luteum in preparation for, and during, pregnancy.

Testosterone, in the male, in response to LH (described earlier), acts on all the tissues that are involved in male sexuality and promotes their sexual development and maintenance. Estrogens, in response to both FSH and LH,

estrogens: hormones responsible for the menstrual cycle and other female characteristics.
oestrus = the egg-making cycle
gen = gives rise to

progesterone: the hormone of gestation (pregnancy).
pro = promoting
gest = gestation (pregnancy)
sterone = a steroid hormone

A

do the same thing in the female. Progesterone, in response to raised LH and prolactin, acts on the uterus and mammary glands, stimulating them to grow and develop.

The Prostaglandins

prostaglandin: see p. 123.

The prostaglandins are a group of hormonelike substances produced by many different body organs with a multitude of diverse effects. They don't have descriptive names but are designated by letters and numbers: E_1, E_2, and so forth. One, produced in the kidney in response to angiotensin and increased epinephrine, dilates and/or constricts blood vessels, working especially on those of the kidney itself. The lung and liver rapidly inactivate this hormone so that it will not work in these organs. Another prostaglandin, produced in the neural tissue in response to certain nerve activity, alters transmission of nerve impulses. Still another, produced by many of the body's cells, alters their response to hormones. The prostaglandins are all derived from the polyunsaturated fatty acids, and account in part for the essentiality of these fatty acids in the diet.

The description of the hormones just given names the major ones and lists a function or two for each. This should suffice to provide an awareness of the enormous impact these compounds have on body processes. The other overall regulating agency is the nervous system.

■ The Nervous System

The nervous system has a central control system—a sort of computer—that can evaluate information about conditions within and outside the body, and a vast system of wiring by means of which the nervous system receives information and sends instructions. The control unit is the brain and spinal cord, called the central nervous system; and the vast complex of wiring between the center and the parts is the peripheral nervous system. The smooth functioning that results from the system's adjustments to changing conditions is homeostasis.

central nervous system: the central part of the nervous system, the brain and spinal cord.

peripheral (puh-RIFF-er-ul) **nervous system:** the peripheral (outermost) part of the nervous system, the vast complex of wiring that extends from the central nervous system to the body's outermost areas. It contains both somatic and autonomic components (defined next).

somatic (so-MAT-ick) **nervous system:** the division of the nervous system that controls the voluntary muscles, as distinguished from the autonomic nervous system, which controls involuntary functions.
soma = body

autonomic nervous system: the division of the nervous system that controls the body's automatic responses. Its two branches are the **sympathetic** branch, which helps the body respond to stressors from the outside environment, and the **parasympathetic** branch, which regulates normal body activities between stressful times.
autonomos = self-governing

The nervous system has two general functions: it controls voluntary muscles in response to sensory stimuli from them, and it controls involuntary, internal muscles and glands in response to nerve-borne and chemical signals about their status. In fact, the nervous system is best understood as two systems that use the same or similar pathways to receive and transmit their messages. The somatic nervous system controls the voluntary muscles; the autonomic nervous system controls the internal organs.

When scientists were first studying the autonomic nervous system, they noticed that when something hurt one organ of the body, some of the other organs reacted as if in sympathy with the afflicted one. They therefore named the nerve network they were studying the sympathetic nervous system. The term is still used today to refer to that branch of the autonomic nervous system that responds to pain and stress. The other branch is called the

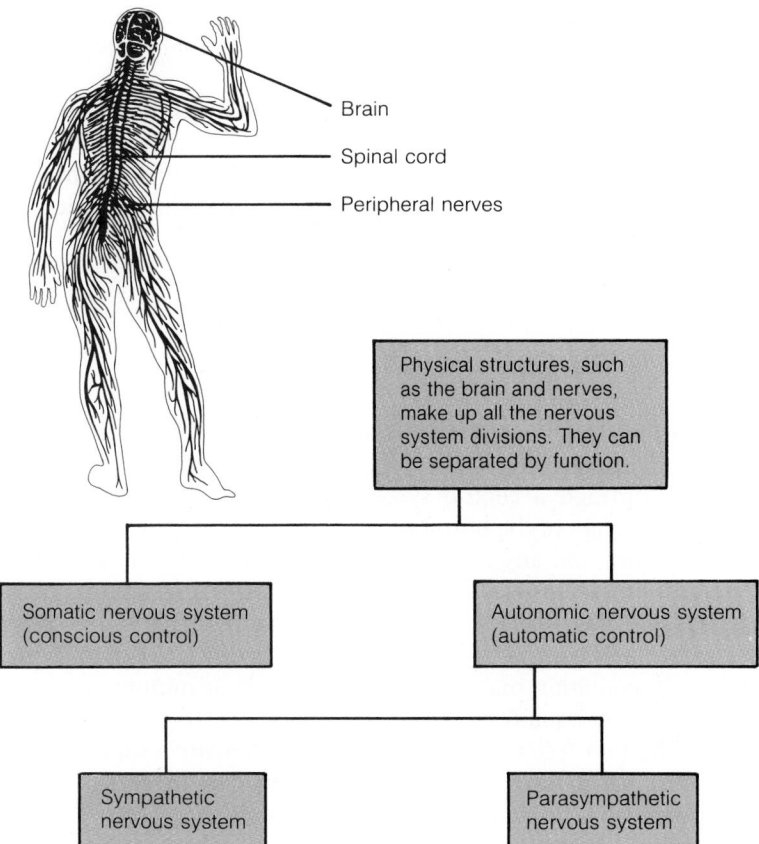

Brain

Spinal cord

Peripheral nerves

Physical structures, such
as the brain and nerves,
make up all the nervous
system divisions. They can
be separated by function.

Somatic nervous system
(conscious control)

Autonomic nervous system
(automatic control)

Sympathetic
nervous system

Parasympathetic
nervous system

A

parasympathetic nervous system. (Think of the sympathetic branch as the
responder when homeostasis needs restoring and the parasympathetic branch
as the commander of function during normal times.) Both systems transmit
their messages through the brain and spinal cord. Nerves of the two branches
travel side by side along the same pathways to transmit their messages, but
they oppose each other's actions (see Figure A–3).

An example will show how the sympathetic and parasympathetic nervous
systems work in balance to maintain homeostasis. When you go outside in
cold weather, your skin's temperature receptors send "cold" messages to the
spinal cord and brain. Your conscious mind may intervene at this point to tell
you to wrap your sweater more closely around you, but let's say you have no
sweater. Your sympathetic nervous system reacts to the external stressor, the
cold. It signals your skin-surface capillaries to shut down so your blood will
circulate deeper in your tissues, where it will conserve heat. Your sympathetic
nervous system also signals involuntary contractions of the small muscles just
under the skin surface. The product of these muscle contractions is heat, and
the visible result is goose bumps. If these measures do not raise your body
temperature enough, then the sympathetic nerves signal your large muscle
groups to shiver; the contractions of these large muscles produce still more
heat. All of this activity adds up to a set of adjustments that maintain your

homeostasis (with respect to temperature) under conditions of external extremes (cold) that would throw it off balance. The cold was a stressor; the body's response was resistance.

Now let's say you come in and sit by a fire and drink hot cocoa. You are warm, and you no longer need all that sympathetic activity. At this point, your parasympathetic nerves take over; they signal your skin-surface capillaries to dilate again, your goose bumps to subside, and your muscles to relax. Your body is back to normal. This is recovery.

■ *Putting It Together*

The hormonal and nervous systems coordinate body functions by transmitting and receiving messages. The point-to-point messages of the nervous system travel through a central switchboard (the spinal cord and brain), whereas the messages of the hormonal system are broadcast over the airways (the bloodstream), and any organ with the right receiver can pick them up. Nerve impulses travel faster than hormonal messages do—although both are remarkably swift. Whereas your brain's command to wiggle your toes reaches the toes within a fraction of a second and stops as quickly, a gland's message to alter a body condition may take several seconds or minutes to get started and may fade away equally slowly.

Together, the two systems possess every characteristic a superb communication network has to have: varied speeds of transmission, along with private communication lines or public broadcasting systems, depending on the needs of the moment. The hormonal system, together with the nervous system, integrates the whole body's functioning so that all parts act smoothly together.

Basic Chemistry Concepts

B

This appendix is intended to provide the background in basic chemistry that you need to understand the nutrition concepts presented in this book. Chemistry is the branch of natural science that is concerned with the description and classification of matter, with the changes that matter undergoes, and with the energy associated with these changes. Matter is anything that takes up space and has mass. Energy is the ability to do work.

■ Matter: The Properties of Atoms

Every substance has characteristics or properties that distinguish it from all other substances and thus give it a unique identity. These properties are both physical and chemical. The physical properties include such characteristics as color, taste, texture, and odor, as well as the temperatures at which a substance changes its state (changes from a solid to a liquid or from a liquid to a gas) and the weight of a unit volume (its density). The chemical properties of a substance have to do with how it reacts with other substances or responds to a change in its environment so that new substances with different sets of properties are produced.

A physical change is one that does not change a substance's chemical composition. For example, when ice changes to liquid water and to steam, two hydrogen atoms and one oxygen atom remain bound together in all three states. However, a chemical change does occur if an electric current is passed through water. The water disappears, and two different substances are formed: hydrogen gas, which is flammable, and oxygen gas, which supports life. Chemical changes are also referred to as chemical reactions.

Substances: Elements and Compounds

Molecules are two or more atoms of the same or different elements joined by chemical bonds. They constitute the smallest part of a substance that can exist separately without losing its physical and chemical properties. If a substance is composed of atoms that are alike, the substance is an element (for example, O_2). If a substance is composed of two or more different kinds of atoms, the substance is a compound (for example, H_2O).

Just over 100 elements are known, and these are listed in Table B–1. A familiar example is hydrogen, whose molecules are composed only of hydrogen atoms linked together in pairs (H_2). On the other hand, over a million compounds are known. An example is the sugar glucose. Each of its molecules is composed of 6 carbon, 6 oxygen, and 12 hydrogen atoms linked together in a specific arrangement (as described in Chapter 4).

The Nature of Atoms

Atoms themselves are made of smaller particles. The atomic nucleus contains protons (positively charged particles), and electrons (negatively charged particles) surround the nucleus. The number of protons ($+$) in the nucleus of an atom determines the number of electrons ($-$) around it. The positive charge on a proton is equal to the negative charge on an electron, so that the charges cancel each other out and leave the atom neutral to its surroundings.

The nucleus may also include neutrons, subatomic particles that have no charge. Protons and neutrons are of equal mass, and together they give an atom its weight. Electrons bond atoms together to make molecules, and they are involved in chemical reactions.

Each type of atom has a characteristic number of protons in its nucleus. The hydrogen atom (symbol H) is the simplest of

■ TABLE B–1
Chemical Symbols for the Elements

Number of Protons (Atomic Number)	Element	Number of Electrons in Outer Shell	Number of Protons (Atomic Number)	Element	Number of Electrons in Outer Shell
1	Hydrogen (H)	1	52	Tellurium (Te)	6
2	Helium (He)	2	53	Iodine (I)	7
3	Lithium (Li)	1	54	Xenon (Xe)	8
4	Beryllium (Be)	2	55	Cesium (Cs)	1
5	Boron (B)	3	56	Barium (Ba)	2
6	Carbon (C)	4	57	Lanthanum (La)	2
7	Nitrogen (N)	5	58	Cerium (Ce)	2
8	Oxygen (O)	6	59	Praseodymium (Pr)	2
9	Fluorine (F)	7	60	Neodymium (Nd)	2
10	Neon (Ne)	8	61	Promethium (Pm)	2
11	Sodium (Na)	1	62	Samarium (Sm)	2
12	Magnesium (Mg)	2	63	Europium (Eu)	2
13	Aluminum (Al)	3	64	Gadolinium (Gd)	2
14	Silicon (Si)	4	65	Terbium (Tb)	2
15	Phosphorus (P)	5	66	Dysprosium (Dy)	2
16	Sulfur (S)	6	67	Holmium (Ho)	2
17	Chlorine (Cl)	7	68	Erbium (Er)	2
18	Argon (Ar)	8	69	Thulium (Tm)	2
19	Potassium (K)	1	70	Ytterbium (Yb)	2
20	Calcium (Ca)	2	71	Lutetium (Lu)	2
21	Scandium (Sc)	2	72	Hafnium (Hf)	2
22	Titanium (Ti)	2	73	Tantalum (Ta)	2
23	Vanadium (V)	2	74	Tungsten (W)	2
24	Chromium (Cr)	1	75	Rhenium (Re)	2
25	Manganese (Mn)	2	76	Osmium (Os)	2
26	Iron (Fe)	2	77	Iridium (Ir)	2
27	Cobalt (Co)	2	78	Platinum (Pt)	1
28	Nickel (Ni)	2	79	Gold (Au)	1
29	Copper (Cu)	1	80	Mercury (Hg)	2
30	Zinc (Zn)	2	81	Thallium (Tl)	3
31	Gallium (Ga)	3	82	Lead (Pb)	4
32	Germanium (Ge)	4	83	Bismuth (Bi)	5
33	Arsenic (As)	5	84	Polonium (Po)	6
34	Selenium (Se)	6	85	Astatine (At)	7
35	Bromine (Br)	7	86	Radon (Rn)	8
36	Krypton (Kr)	8	87	Francium (Fr)	1
37	Rubidium (Rb)	1	88	Radium (Ra)	2
38	Strontium (Sr)	2	89	Actinium (Ac)	2
39	Yttrium (Y)	2	90	Thorium (Th)	2
40	Zirconium (Zr)	2	91	Protactinium (Pa)	2
41	Niobium (Nb)	1	92	Uranium (U)	2
42	Molybdenum (Mo)	1	93	Neptunium (Np)	2
43	Technetium (Tc)	1	94	Plutonium (Pu)	2
44	Ruthenium (Ru)	1	95	Americium (Am)	2
45	Rhodium (Rh)	1	96	Curium (Cm)	2
46	Palladium (Pd)	—	97	Berkelium (Bk)	2
47	Silver (Ag)	1	98	Californium (Cf)	2
48	Cadmium (Cd)	2	99	Einsteinium (Es)	2
49	Indium (In)	3	100	Fermium (Fm)	2
50	Tin (Sn)	4	101	Mendelevium (Md)	2
51	Antimony (Sb)	5	102	Nobelium (No)	2

B

all. It possesses a single proton, with a single electron associated with it:

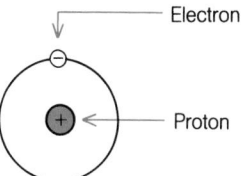

Hydrogen atom (H), atomic number 1.

Just as hydrogen always has one proton, helium always has two, lithium three, and so on. The atomic number of each type of atom is the number of protons in the nucleus of an atom, and this never changes in a chemical reaction; it gives the atom its identity. The atomic numbers for the known elements are listed in Table B–1.

All atoms except hydrogen also have neutrons in their nuclei, and these contribute to their atomic weight. The most common form of helium, for example, has two neutrons in its nucleus in addition to its two protons, for a total of four nuclear particles and an atomic weight of 4.

Besides hydrogen, the atoms most common in living things are carbon (C), nitrogen (N), and oxygen (O), whose atomic numbers are 6, 7, and 8, respectively. Their structures are more complicated than that of hydrogen. Each possesses a number of electrons equal to the number of protons in its nucleus. These electrons are found in orbits, or shells:

  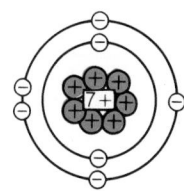

Carbon atom (C), atomic number 6.

Nitrogen atom (N), atomic number 7.

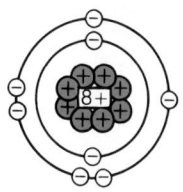

Oxygen atom (O), atomic number 8.

In these and all diagrams of atoms that follow, only the protons and electrons are shown. The neutrons, which contribute only to atomic weight, not to charge, are omitted.

The most important structural feature of an atom for determining its chemical behavior is the number of electrons in its outer shell. The first shell is full when it is occupied by two electrons; so an atom with two or more electrons has a filled first shell. When the first shell is full, the atom is in a very stable energy state, or a state of lowest energy. Electrons then begin to fill the second shell.

The second shell is completely full when it has eight electrons. A substance that has a full outer shell tends to enter into no chemical reactions. Atomic number 10, neon, is a chemically inert substance, because its outer shell is complete. Fluorine, atomic number 9, has a great tendency to draw an electron from other substances to complete its outer shell and thus is highly reactive. Carbon has a half-full outer shell, which helps explain its great versatility; it can combine with other elements in a great variety of ways to form a large number of compounds.

Atoms seek to reach a state of maximum stability or of lowest energy in the same way that a ball will roll down a hill until it reaches the lowest place. An atom achieves a state of maximum stability:

- By gaining or losing electrons to either fill or empty its outer shell.
- By sharing its electrons through bonding together with other atoms.

The number of electrons determines how the atom will chemically react with other atoms. Hence the atomic number, not the weight, is what gives an atom its chemical nature.

Chemical Bonding

Atoms often complete their outer shells by sharing electrons with other atoms. In order to complete its outer shell, a carbon atom requires four electrons. A hydrogen atom requires one.

B

Thus, when a carbon atom shares electrons with four hydrogen atoms, each completes its outer shell:

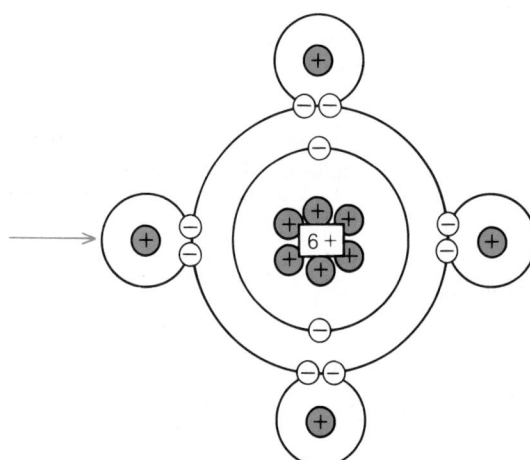

Methane molecule. The chemical formula for methane is CH_4. (Note that with the sharing of electrons, every atom has a filled outer shell.)

This electron sharing binds the atoms together and satisfies the conditions of maximum stability for the molecule. The outer shell of each atom is complete, since hydrogen effectively has the required two electrons in its first and outer shell, and carbon has eight electrons in its second and outer shell; and the molecule is electrically neutral, with a total of ten protons and ten electrons.

Bonds that involve the sharing of electrons, like the bond between carbon and hydrogen, are the most stable kind of

association that atoms can form with one another. They are sometimes called covalent bonds, and the resulting combinations of atoms are called molecules. A single pair of shared electrons forms a single bond. A simplified way to represent a single bond is with a single line. Thus the structure of methane (CH_4) could be represented like this (ignoring the inner-shell electrons, which do not participate in bonding):

$$
\begin{array}{c}
H \\
| \\
H-C-H \\
| \\
H
\end{array}
$$

Methane (CH_4).

Similarly, one nitrogen atom and three hydrogen atoms can share electrons to form one molecule of ammonia (NH_3):

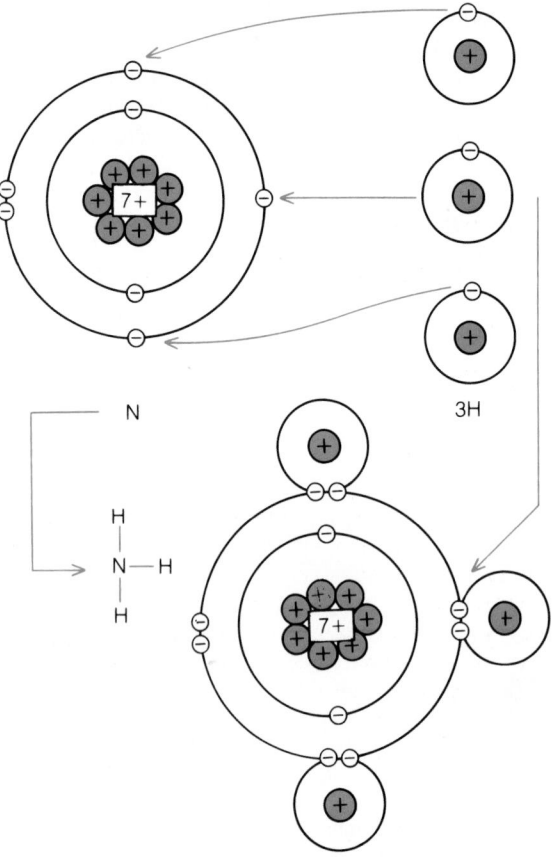

Ammonia molecule (NH_3). Count the electrons in each atom's outer shell.

One oxygen atom may be bonded to two hydrogen atoms to form one molecule of water (H_2O):

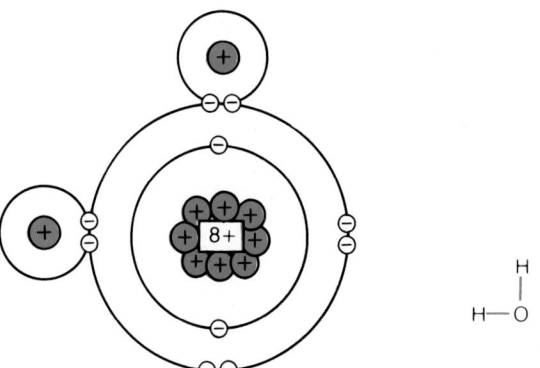

Water molecule (H_2O).

When two oxygen atoms form a molecule of oxygen, they must share two pairs of electrons. This double bond may be represented as two single lines:

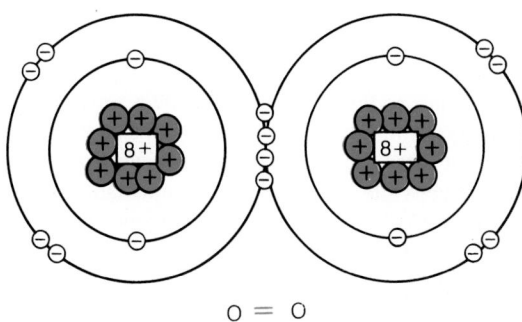

$$O = O$$

Oxygen molecule (O_2).

Small atoms form the tightest, most stable bonds. H, O, N, and C are the smallest atoms capable of forming one, two, three, and four electron-pair bonds (respectively). This fact is the basis for the simple statement in Chapter 4 that when you draw compounds containing these atoms, hydrogen must always have one, oxygen two, nitrogen three, and carbon four lines radiating to other atoms.

The stability of the associations between these small atoms and the versatility with which they can combine make them very common in living things. Interestingly, all cells, whether they come from animals, plants, or bacteria, contain the same elements in very nearly the same proportions. The atomic elements found in living things are shown in Table B–2.

■ TABLE B–2
Elemental Composition of Living Cells

Element	Chemical Symbol	Composition by Weight (%)
Oxygen	O	65
Carbon	C	18
Hydrogen	H	10
Nitrogen	N	3
Calcium	Ca	1.5
Phosphorus	P	1.0
Sulfur	S	0.25
Sodium	Na	0.15
Magnesium	Mg	0.05
Total		99.30[a]

[a]The remaining 0.70% by weight is contributed by the trace elements: copper (Cu), zinc (Zn), selenium (Se), molybdenum (Mo), fluorine (F), chlorine (Cl), iodine (I), manganese (Mn), cobalt (Co), and iron (Fe). There are also variable traces of some of the following in cells: lithium (Li), strontium (Sr), aluminum (Al), silicon (Si), lead (Pb), vanadium (V), arsenic (As), bromium (Br), and others.

■ *Formation of Ions*

An atom such as sodium (Na, atomic number 11) cannot easily fill its outer shell by sharing. Sodium possesses a filled inner shell of two electrons and a filled second shell of eight; there is only one electron in its outermost shell:

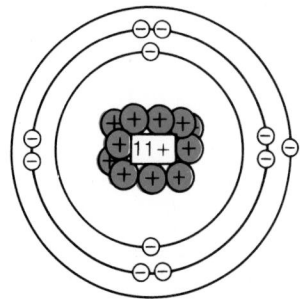

Sodium atom (Na)
11 + charges
11 − charges
————————
0 net charge
with one reactive
electron in outer shell
minus
1 electron

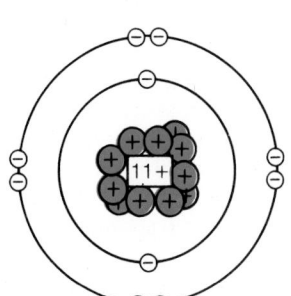

Sodium ion (Na^+)
11 + charges
10 − charges
————————
1 + net charge
and a filled
outer shell

B

If sodium loses this electron, it satisfies one condition for stability: a filled outer shell (now its second shell counts as the outer shell). However, it is not electrically neutral. It has 11 protons (positive) and only 10 electrons (negative). It therefore has a net positive charge. An atom or molecule that has lost or gained one or more electrons and so is electrically charged is called an ion.

An atom such as chlorine (Cl, atomic number 17), with seven electrons in its outermost shell, can share to fill its outer shell, or it can gain one electron to make its outer shell complete and thus give it a negative charge:

Chlorine atom (Cl)

17+ charges
17− charges
_____
0 net charges
but lacks one
electron to fill
outer shell

plus 1
electron

Chloride ion (Cl⁻)

17+ charges
18− charges
_____
1− net charge
and a filled
outer shell

A positively charged ion such as a sodium ion (Na^+) is called a cation; a negatively charged ion such as a chloride ion (Cl^-) is called an anion. Cations and anions attract one another to form salts:

Sodium chloride (Na^+Cl^-)

28+ charges
28− charges
_____
0 net charge
and filled outer shells

Na⁺

Cl⁻

With all its electrons, sodium is a shiny, highly reactive metal; chlorine is the poisonous greenish-yellow gas that was used in World War I. But after they have transferred electrons, they form the unreactive white salt familiar to you as table salt, or sodium chloride (Na^+Cl^-). The dramatic difference illustrates how profoundly the electron arrangement can influence the nature of a substance. The wide distribution of salt in nature attests to the stability of the union between the ions. Each meets the other's needs (a good marriage).

When dry, salt exists as crystals; its ions are stacked very regularly into a lattice, with positive and negative ions alternating in a sort of three-dimensional checkerboard structure. In water, however, the salt quickly dissolves, and its ions separate from one another, forming an electrolyte solution in which they move about freely. Covalently bonded molecules rarely dissociate like this in water solution. The most common exception is when they behave like acids and release H^+ ions, as discussed in the next section. Molecules and ion pairs (salts) behave very differently in many ways.

An ion can also be a group of atoms bound together in such a way that the group has a charge and enters into reactions as a single unit. Many such groups are active in the fluids of the body. The bicarbonate ion is composed of five atoms—one H, one C, and three O—and has a net charge of −1 (HCO_3^-). Another important ion of this type is a phosphate ion with one H, one P, and four O, and a net charge of −2 (HPO_4^{-2}).

Whereas many elements have only one configuration in the outer shell and thus only one way to bond with other elements, some elements have the possibility of varied configurations. Iron is such an element. Under some conditions iron loses two electrons, and under other circumstances it loses three. If iron loses two electrons, it then has a net charge of $+2$, and we call it ferrous iron (Fe^{++}). If it donates three electrons to another atom, it becomes the $+3$ ion, or ferric iron (Fe^{+++}).

Fe^{++} Fe^{+++}

Ferrous iron (Fe^{++})   Ferric iron (Fe^{+++})
(had 2 outer-shell   (had 3 outer-shell
electrons but has   electrons but has
lost them)   lost them)
26 + charges   26 + charges
24 − charges   23 − charges
———————   ———————
2 + net charge   3 + net charge

(Note: It is important to remember that a positive charge on an ion means that negative charges—electrons—have been lost and not that positive charges have been added. If you could add two protons to an iron atom, they would go to the nucleus, adding 2 to its atomic number. Then it would no longer be iron, atomic number 26, but nickel, atomic number 28—and it would gain two more electrons to balance its positive charges.)

◼ Water, Acids, and Bases

The water molecule is electrically neutral, having equal numbers of protons and electrons. However, when a hydrogen atom shares its electron with oxygen, that electron will spend most of its time nearer the large, positively charged oxygen nucleus (see Figure 10-3 on p. 277). This leaves the positive proton (nucleus of the hydrogen atom) exposed on the outer part of the water molecule. We know, too, that the two hydrogens both bond toward the same side of the oxygen. These two ideas explain the fact that water molecules are polar: they have regions of more positive and more negative charge.

Polar molecules like water are drawn to one another by the attractive forces between the positive polar areas of one and the negative poles of another. These attractive forces, sometimes known as polar bonds or hydrogen bonds, occur among many molecules and also within the different parts of single large molecules. Although very weak in comparison with covalent bonds, polar bonds may occur in such abundance that they become exceedingly important in determining the structure of such large molecules as proteins and DNA.

Water (H_2O).

Water (H_2O). The arrows on the diagram of the polar molecule show displacement of electrons toward the O nucleus; thus the negative region is near the O and the positive region, near the H.

Water molecules have a slight tendency to ionize, separating into positive (H^+) and negative (OH^-) ions. In pure water, a small but constant number of these ions is present, and the number of positive ions exactly equals the number of negative ions.

An acid is a substance that releases H^+ ions (protons) in water solution. Hydrochloric acid (HCl) is such a substance because it dissociates in water solution into H^+ and Cl^- ions. Acetic acid is also an acid, because it dissociates in water to acetate ions and free H^+:

Acetic acid dissociates into an acetate ion and a hydrogen ion.

The more H^+ ions released, the stronger the acid.

Chemists define degrees of acidity by means of the pH scale. The pH scale runs from 0 to 14. A pH of 1 is extremely acidic, 7 is neutral, and 13 is very basic. There is a tenfold difference between points on this scale. A solution with pH 3, for example, has *ten times* as many H^+ ions as a solution with pH 4. At pH 7, the concentrations of free H^+ and OH^- are exactly the same—1/10,000,000 moles per liter (10^{-7} moles per liter).* At pH 4, the concentration of free H^+ ions is 1/10,000 (10^{-4}) moles per liter. This is a higher concentration of H^+ ions, and the solution is therefore acidic.

---

*A mole is a certain number (about 6×10^{23}) of molecules. The pH of a solution is defined as the negative logarithm of the hydrogen ion concentration of the solution. Thus if the concentration is 10^{-2} (moles per liter), the pH is 2; if 10^{-8}, the pH is 8; and so on.

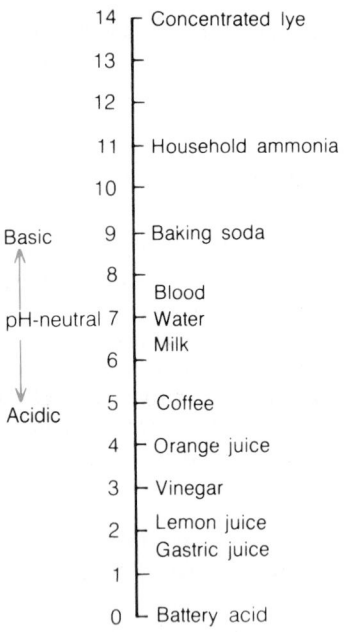

Ammonia captures a hydrogen ion from water. The two dots here represent the two electrons not shared with another atom. These are ordinarily not shown in chemical structure drawings. Compare this with the earlier diagram of an ammonia molecule.

A base is a substance that can soak up, or combine with, H^+ ions, thus reducing the acidity of a solution. The compound ammonia is such a substance. The ammonia molecule has two electrons that are not shared with any other atom; a hydrogen ion (H^+) is just a naked proton with no shell of electrons at all. Thus the proton readily combines with the ammonia molecule to form an ammonium ion and so is withdrawn from the solution as a free proton and no longer contributes to its acidity. Many compounds containing nitrogen are important bases in living systems. Acids and bases neutralize each other to produce substances that are neither acid nor base.

pH	
14	Concentrated lye
13	
12	
11	Household ammonia
10	
9	Baking soda
8	
	Blood
7	Water
	Milk
6	
5	Coffee
4	Orange juice
3	Vinegar
2	Lemon juice
	Gastric juice
1	
0	Battery acid

Basic ↑
pH-neutral 7
Acidic ↓

The pH scale.

Note: Each step is ten times as concentrated in base (¹/₁₀ as much acid, H^+) as the one below it.

Chemical Reactions

A chemical reaction, or chemical change, results in the disappearance of substances and the formation of new ones. Almost all such reactions involve a change in the bonding of atoms. Old bonds are broken, and new ones are formed. The nuclei of atoms are never involved in chemical reactions—only their outer-shell electrons take part. At the end of a reaction there is always the same number of atoms of each type as there was at the beginning. For example, two hydrogen molecules can react with one oxygen molecule to form two water molecules. In this reaction two substances (hydrogen and oxygen) disappear, and a new one (water) is formed, but at the end of the reaction there are still four H atoms and two O atoms, just as there were at the beginning. The only difference is in how they are linked.

Diagrams:

Hydrogen

Hydrogen

Oxygen

Water

Water

Hydrogen and oxygen react to form water.

Formulas: $2H_2$ + O_2 ⟶ $2H_2O$

In many instances chemical reactions involve not the relinking of molecules but the exchanging of electrons or protons among them. In such reactions the molecule that gains one or more electrons (or loses one or more hydrogen ions) is said to be reduced; the molecule that loses electrons (or gains protons) is oxidized. (A hydrogen ion is equivalent to a proton.) Oxidation and reduction take place simultaneously, because an electron or proton that is lost by one molecule is accepted by another. The addition of an atom of oxygen is also oxidation, because oxygen (with six electrons in the outer shell) accepts two electrons in becoming bonded. Oxidation, then, is loss of electrons, gain of protons, or addition of oxygen (with six electrons); reduction is the opposite—gain of electrons, loss of protons, or loss of oxygen. The addition of hydrogen atoms to oxygen to form water can thus be described as the reduction of oxygen *or* the oxidation of hydrogen.

If a reaction results in a net increase in the energy of a compound, it is called an endergonic, or "uphill," reaction (energy, *erg*, is added into, *endo*, the compound). An example is the chief result of photosynthesis, the making of sugar in a plant from carbon dioxide and water using the energy of sunlight. Conversely, the oxidation of sugar to carbon dioxide and water is an exergonic, or "downhill," reaction, because the end products have less energy than the starting products. Oftentimes, but not always, reduction reactions are endergonic, resulting in an increase in the energy of the products. Oxidation reactions often, but not always, are exergonic.

Chemical reactions tend to occur spontaneously if the end products are in a lower energy state (are more stable) than the reacting compounds were. These reactions often give off energy in the form of heat as they occur. The generation of heat by wood burning in a fireplace and the maintenance of human body warmth both depend on energy-yielding chemical reactions. These downhill reactions occur easily, although they may require some activation energy to get them started, just as a ball requires a push to get started rolling downhill.

Uphill reactions, in which the products contain more energy than the reacting compounds started with, do not occur until an energy source is provided. An example of such an energy source is the sunlight used in photosynthesis, where carbon dioxide and water (low-energy compounds) are combined to form the sugar glucose (a higher-energy compound). Another example is the use of the energy in glucose to combine two low-energy compounds in the body into the high-energy compound ATP (see Chapter 7). The energy in ATP may be used to power many other energy-requiring, uphill reactions. Clearly, any of many different molecules can be used as a temporary storage place for energy.

Neither downhill nor uphill reactions occur until something sets them off (activation) or until a path is provided for them to follow. The body uses enzymes as a means of providing paths and controlling chemical reactions (see Chapter 6). By controlling the availability and the action of its enzymes, the body can

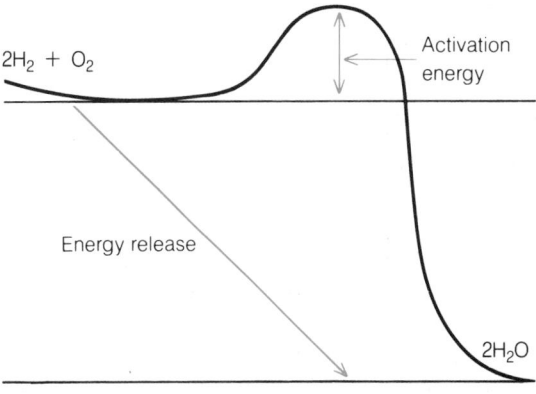

Energy Change as Reaction Occurs

$2H_2 + O_2$

Activation energy

Energy release

$2H_2O$

Start of reaction → End of reaction

Reactants → Products

$2H_2 + O_2 \rightarrow 2H_2O$

"decide" which chemical reactions to prevent and which to promote.

■ *Formation of Free Radicals*

Normally, when a chemical reaction takes place, bonds break and re-form with some redistribution of atoms and rearrangement of bonds to form new, stable compounds. Normally, bonds don't split in such a way as to leave a molecule with an odd, unpaired electron. However, weak bonds can split this way, and when they do, free radicals are formed. Free radicals are highly unstable and quickly react with other compounds, forming more free radicals in a chain reaction.

H—O—O—H   H—O• + •O—H

or   Heat or light   or

R—O—O—H   R—O• + •O—H

Hydrogen peroxide or any hydroperoxide (R is any carbon chain with appropriate numbers of H).   Free radical.

Free radicals are formed. The dots represent single electrons that are available for sharing (the atom also needs another electron to fill its outer shell).

A physical event such as the arrival of an energy-carrying particle of light or other radiation starts the process by breaking a weak bond so that free radicals are formed. A cascade may ensue in which many highly reactive radicals are generated, resulting finally in the disruption of a living structure such as a cell membrane.

$$
\text{H—O•} \quad + \quad
\begin{array}{c}
\text{H} \\
| \\
\text{H—C—H} \\
| \\
\text{H}
\end{array}
\longrightarrow \quad \text{H—O—H} \quad + \quad
\begin{array}{c}
\text{H} \\
| \\
\text{H—C•} \\
| \\
\text{H}
\end{array}
$$

	or		or
	R—H		R•
Free radical.	Compound with weak bond (perhaps an unsaturated fatty acid).	New stable compound (water or an alcohol).	Free radical.

Destruction of biological compounds by free radicals. The free radical attacks a weak bond in a biological compound, disrupting it and forming a new stable molecule and another free radical. This can attack another biological compound, and so on.

Oxidation of some compounds can be induced by air at room temperature in the presence of light. Such reactions are thought to take place through the formation of compounds called peroxides:

Peroxides:

H—O—O—H   Hydrogen peroxide.

R—O—O—H   Hydroperoxides (R is any carbon chain with appropriate numbers of H).

R—O—O—R   Peroxide.

Some peroxides readily disintegrate into free radicals, initiating chain reactions like those just described.

Free radicals are of special interest in nutrition because the antioxidant properties of vitamin E are thought to protect against the destructive effects of these free radicals (see Chapter 9). Vitamin E on the surface of the lungs reacts with (and is destroyed by) free radicals, thus preventing them from reaching underlying cells and oxidizing the lipids in their membranes.

Biochemical Structures and Pathways

C

The diagrams of nutrients presented here are meant to enhance your understanding of the most important organic molecules in the human diet. The names used are those agreed on by the American Institute of Nutrition and other scientific organizations in 1987.[1] Following the diagrams of nutrients are sections on the major metabolic pathways mentioned in Chapter 7—glycolysis, the TCA cycle, and the electron transport chain—and a description of how alcohol interferes with these pathways. Discussions of the urea cycle and the formation of ketone bodies complete the chapter.

Carbohydrates

Monosaccharides

Glucose (alpha form). The ring would be at right angles to the plane of the paper. The bonds directed upward are above the plane; those directed downward are below the plane. This molecule is considered an alpha form because the OH carbon 1 points downward.

Glucose (beta form). The OH on carbon 1 points upward.
Fructose, galactose: see Chapter 4.

Disaccharides

Maltose.

C

Lactose (alpha form).

Sucrose.

Polysaccharides

As described in Chapter 4, starch, glycogen, and cellulose are all long chains of glucose molecules covalently linked together.

Amylose

Amylopectin

Starch. Two kinds of covalent linkages occur between glucose molecules in starch, giving rise to two kinds of chains. Amylose is composed of straight chains, with carbon 1 of one glucose linked to carbon 4 of the next. Amylopectin is made up of straight chains like amylose but has occasional branches arising where the carbon 6 of a glucose is also linked to the carbon 1 of another glucose. On amylopectin, some of the H have been left off, for simplicity's sake. (See the rules for simplified chemical structures on p. 75).

Glycogen: like amylopectin but with longer chains and many more branches.

Cellulose.

Mucopolysaccharides

Repeating units of hyaluronic acid.
Such structures are typical of mucopolysaccharides.

Hyaluronic acid

Lipids

Saturated Fatty Acids Found in Natural Fats

Saturated Fatty Acid	Chemical Formula	Source
Butyric	C_3H_7COOH	Butterfat
Caproic	$C_5H_{11}COOH$	Butterfat
Caprylic	$C_7H_{15}COOH$	Coconut oil
Capric	$C_9H_{19}COOH$	Palm oil
Lauric	$C_{11}H_{23}COOH$	Coconut oil
Myristic[a]	$C_{13}H_{27}COOH$	Nutmeg oil, butterfat
Palmitic[a]	$C_{15}H_{31}COOH$	Animal and vegetable fat
Stearic[a]	$C_{17}H_{35}COOH$	Animal and vegetable fat
Arachidic	$C_{19}H_{39}COOH$	Peanut oil

[a]Most common saturated fatty acids.

Unsaturated Fatty Acids Found in Natural Fats

Unsaturated Fatty Acids and their Chemical Formulas	Number of Carbons	Number of Double Bonds	Standard Notation[a]	Omega Notation[b]	Source
Palmitoleic $C_{15}H_{29}COOH$	16	1	16:1;9	16:1ω7	Butterfat
Oleic $C_{17}H_{33}COOH$	18	1	18:1;9	18:1ω9	Olive oil
Linoleic $C_{17}H_{31}COOH$	18	2	18:2;9,12	18:2ω6	Linseed oil
Linolenic $C_{17}H_{29}COOH$	18	3	18:3;9,12,15	18:3ω3	Linseed oil
Arachidonic $C_{19}H_{31}COOH$	20	4	20:4;5,8,11,14	20:4ω6	Lecithin
Eicosapentanoic $C_{19}H_{29}COOH$	20	5	20:5;5,8,11,14,17	20:5ω3	Fish oils

Note: A fatty acid has two ends, designated the methyl (CH_3) end and the carboxyl, or acid (COOH), end.

[a]Standard chemistry notation begins counting carbons at the acid end. The notation identifies first how many carbons the fatty acid contains, followed by a colon and another number which indicates the number of double bonds, then a semicolon followed by a number or numbers which indicate the positions of the double bonds. Thus linoleic acid, an 18-carbon fatty acid with two double bonds between carbons 9 and 10 and between carbons 12 and 13 is noted 18:2;9,12.

[b]Because fatty acid chains are lengthened by adding carbons at the acid end of the chain, chemists use the omega system of notation to ease their task of identifying them. The omega system begins counting carbons at the methyl end and notes the position of the double bond nearest the methyl end. Thus linoleic acid with its first double bond at the sixth carbon from the methyl end would be noted 18:2ω6 in the omega system.

Protein: Amino Acids

The common amino acids may be classified into the seven groups listed below.* Amino acids marked with an asterisk (*) are essential, because human beings cannot synthesize them.

*A discussion of the designated abbreviations for the common amino acids presented here is found in Nomenclature policy: Abbreviated designations of amino acids, *Journal of Nutrition* 117 (1987): 15.

1. Amino acids with aliphatic side chains, which consist of hydrogen and carbon atoms (hydrocarbons).

$$H-\underset{\underset{NH_2}{|}}{\overset{\overset{H}{|}}{C}}-\overset{\overset{O}{\|}}{C}-OH \qquad \text{Glycine (Gly).}$$

$$CH_3-\underset{\underset{NH_2}{|}}{\overset{\overset{H}{|}}{C}}-\overset{\overset{O}{\|}}{C}-OH \qquad \text{Alanine (Ala).}$$

$$\begin{array}{c} CH_3 \\ \diagdown \\ CH_3 \diagup \end{array} CH-\underset{\underset{NH_2}{|}}{\overset{\overset{H}{|}}{C}}-\overset{\overset{O}{\|}}{C}-OH \qquad \text{Valine* (Val).}$$

$$\begin{array}{c} CH_3 \\ \diagdown \\ CH_3 \diagup \end{array} CH-CH_2-\underset{\underset{NH_2}{|}}{\overset{\overset{H}{|}}{C}}-\overset{\overset{O}{\|}}{C}-OH \qquad \text{Leucine* (Leu).}$$

$$\begin{array}{c} CH_3 \\ \diagdown \\ CH_2 \\ \diagup \\ CH_3 \end{array} CH-\underset{\underset{NH_2}{|}}{\overset{\overset{H}{|}}{C}}-\overset{\overset{O}{\|}}{C}-OH \qquad \text{Isoleucine* (Ile).}$$

2. Amino acids with hydroxylic (OH) side chains.

$$HO-CH_2-\underset{\underset{NH_2}{|}}{\overset{\overset{H}{|}}{C}}-\overset{\overset{O}{\|}}{C}-OH \qquad \text{Serine (Ser).}$$

$$CH_3-\underset{\underset{OH}{|}}{CH}-\underset{\underset{NH_2}{|}}{\overset{\overset{H}{|}}{C}}-\overset{\overset{O}{\|}}{C}-OH \qquad \text{Threonine* (Thr).}$$

3. Amino acids with side chains containing acidic groups or their amides, which contain the group NH_2.

$$HO-\overset{\overset{O}{\|}}{C}-CH_2-\underset{\underset{NH_2}{|}}{\overset{\overset{H}{|}}{C}}-\overset{\overset{O}{\|}}{C}-OH \qquad \text{Aspartic acid (Asp).}$$

$$HO-\overset{\overset{O}{\|}}{C}-CH_2-CH_2-\underset{\underset{NH_2}{|}}{\overset{\overset{H}{|}}{C}}-\overset{\overset{O}{\|}}{C}-OH \qquad \text{Glutamic acid (Glu).}$$

$$NH_2-\underset{\underset{O}{\|}}{C}-CH_2-\underset{\underset{NH_2}{|}}{\overset{\overset{H}{|}}{C}}-\overset{\overset{O}{\|}}{C}-OH \qquad \text{Asparagine (Asn).}$$

$$NH_2-\underset{\underset{O}{\|}}{C}-CH_2-CH_2-\underset{\underset{NH_2}{|}}{\overset{\overset{H}{|}}{C}}-\overset{\overset{O}{\|}}{C}-OH \qquad \text{Glutamine (Gln).}$$

4. Amino acids with basic side chains.

$$NH_2-CH_2-CH_2-CH_2-CH_2-\underset{\underset{NH_2}{|}}{\overset{\overset{H}{|}}{C}}-\overset{\overset{O}{\|}}{C}-OH \qquad \text{Lysine* (Lys).}$$

$$NH_2-\underset{\underset{NH}{\|}}{C}-NH-CH_2-CH_2-\underset{\underset{NH_2}{|}}{\overset{\overset{H}{|}}{C}}-\overset{\overset{O}{\|}}{C}-OH \qquad \text{Arginine (Arg).}$$

$$\begin{array}{c} H-C=C-CH_2-\underset{\underset{NH_2}{|}}{\overset{\overset{H}{|}}{C}}-\overset{\overset{O}{\|}}{C}-OH \\ \underset{N}{|} \qquad \underset{N}{|} \\ \diagdown \underset{C}{} \diagup \overset{|}{H} \\ \overset{|}{H} \end{array} \qquad \text{Histidine* (His).}$$

$$NH_2-CH_2-CH_2-CH_2-\underset{\underset{NH_2}{|}}{\overset{\overset{H}{|}}{C}}-\overset{\overset{O}{\|}}{C}-OH \qquad \text{Ornithine (Orn).}$$

5. Amino acids with aromatic side chains, which are characterized by the presence of at least one cyclical (ring) structure.

Phenylalanine* (Phe).

Tyrosine (Tyr).

Tryptophan* (Trp).

7. Imino acids.

Proline (Pro)*

---

*Proline has the same $H_2N-C-COOH$ structure as the other amino acids, but its amino group has given up a hydrogen to form a ring, as shown.

6. Amino acids with side chains containing sulfur atoms.

Cysteine (Cys).

Cystine (Cys-Cys).

Methionine* (Met).

Vitamins and Coenzymes

Vitamin A: retinol.

Vitamin A: retinal.

Vitamin A: beta-carotene.

Thiamin hydrochloride. Chloride ions (Cl⁻) are shown nearby because two of the nitrogens in this compound have donated their spare outer-shell electrons to bond with positively charged ions (see Appendix B). Thus the whole molecule is positively charged (+2) and will attract two negatively charged ions (Cl⁻) into its vicinity. When crystallized out of water solution, this complex precipitates as the salt thiamin hydrochloride. This chemical name usually appears on vitamin bottles containing thiamin.

Thiamin pyrophosphate (TPP). TPP is a coenzyme that includes the thiamin molecule as part of its structure.

Riboflavin. This molecule is a part of two coenzymes—flavin mononucleotide (FMN) and flavin adenine dinucleotide (FAD).

Flavin mononucleotide (FMN).

Flavin adenine denucleotide (FAD).

Nicotinic acid   Nicotinamide

Niacin (nicotinic acid and nicotinamide). These molecules are a part of two coenzymes—nicotinamide adenine dinucleotide (NAD^+) and nicotinamide adenine dinucleotide phosphate ($NADP^+$).

**Nicotinamide adenine dinucleotide (NAD⁺) and
nicotinamide adenine dinucleotide phosphate (NADP⁺).**
NAD has also been called coenzyme I and DPN; NADP has been
called coenzyme II and TPN. NADP has the same structure as NAD
but with a phosphate group attached at the dagger (†).

Reduced NAD⁺ (NADH). When NAD⁺ is reduced by the
addition of H⁺ and two electrons, it becomes the coenzyme NADH.
(The dots on the H entering this reaction represent electrons—see
Appendix B.)

**Vitamin B₆ (a general name for three compounds—
pyridoxine, pyridoxal, and pyridoxamine).**

Pyridoxal phosphate and pyridoxamine phosphate. These are the coenzymes necessary for transamination and other important processes.

Vitamin B$_{12}$ (cyanocobalamin). The arrows in this diagram indicate that the spare electron pairs on the nitrogens attract them to the cobalt.

Folate (folacin or folic acid). This molecule consists of a double ring combined with a single ring and at least one glutamate (a nonessential amino acid marked in a box).

Tetrahydrofolic acid, the active coenzyme form of folate. (The four hydrogens added to folate are circled. An intermediate form, dihydrofolate, has two of these hydrogens added.)

Pantothenic acid

Coenzyme A (CoA). This molecule is made up in part of pantothenic acid.

Biotin.

Vitamin C (ascorbic acid). The oxidized form of vitamin C is dehydroascorbic acid. (The dots on the H indicate that two hydrogen atoms, complete with their electrons, are lost when ascorbic acid is oxidized and gained when it is reduced again.)

Vitamin C

Dehydroascorbic acid

7-dehydrocholesterol

Ultraviolet light on the skin

Vitamin D_3

Carbon #7

+O
Liver

25-hydroxy-D_3

Carbon #25

+O
Kidney

1,25-hydroxy-D_3

Carbon #1

Active vitamin D and its precursors, beginning with 7-dehydrocholesterol. (The carbon atoms at which changes occur are numbered.)

C

Tocotrienols contain double bonds here.

Vitamin E (alpha-tocopherol). The number and position of the methyl groups (CH$_3$) bonded to the ring structure differentiate among the tocopherols.

Vitamin K, a naturally occurring compound.

Menadione, a synthetic compound that has the same activity as natural vitamin K.

Adenosine triphosphate (ATP), the energy carrier. The cleavage point marks the bond that is broken when ATP splits to become ADP + P.

Adenosine diphosphate (ADP).

Energy of falling water
dissipated without doing work.

Energy of falling water coupled
with the turning of a series of
water wheels.

Analogy for a coupled reaction. The
breakdown of glucose is coupled with the
making of ATP—or the breakdown of ATP
is coupled with the activation of glucose
(making glucose-P).

Glycolysis

Figure C–1 depicts the events of glycolysis. First, a phosphate is attached to glucose at the carbon that chemists call number 6. The product is called, logically enough, glucose-6-phosphate.

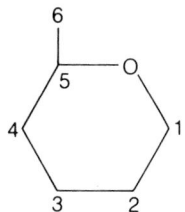

This is the way chemists number the
carbons in a glucose molecule.

In the next step, glucose-6-phosphate is rearranged by an enzyme, and a phosphate is added in another coupled reaction with ATP. (A coupled reaction is a chemical event in which an enzyme complex catalyzes two reactions simultaneously. It often involves the breakdown of one compound to two and the synthesis of another from two.)

The product this time is fructose-1,6-diphosphate. At this point the six-carbon sugar has a phosphate group on its first and sixth carbons and is ready to break apart. Two ATP molecules have been used to accomplish this.

The breakdown of glucose is coupled with
the making of ATP (simplified). Actually,
two ATP are used to prepare glucose for the
reactions, and four ATP are gained in
catabolism to two molecules of pyruvate.

(From this point to the production of pyruvate, we will use letters in place of compound names. The names are in Figure C–1, for those who wish to know them.)

C

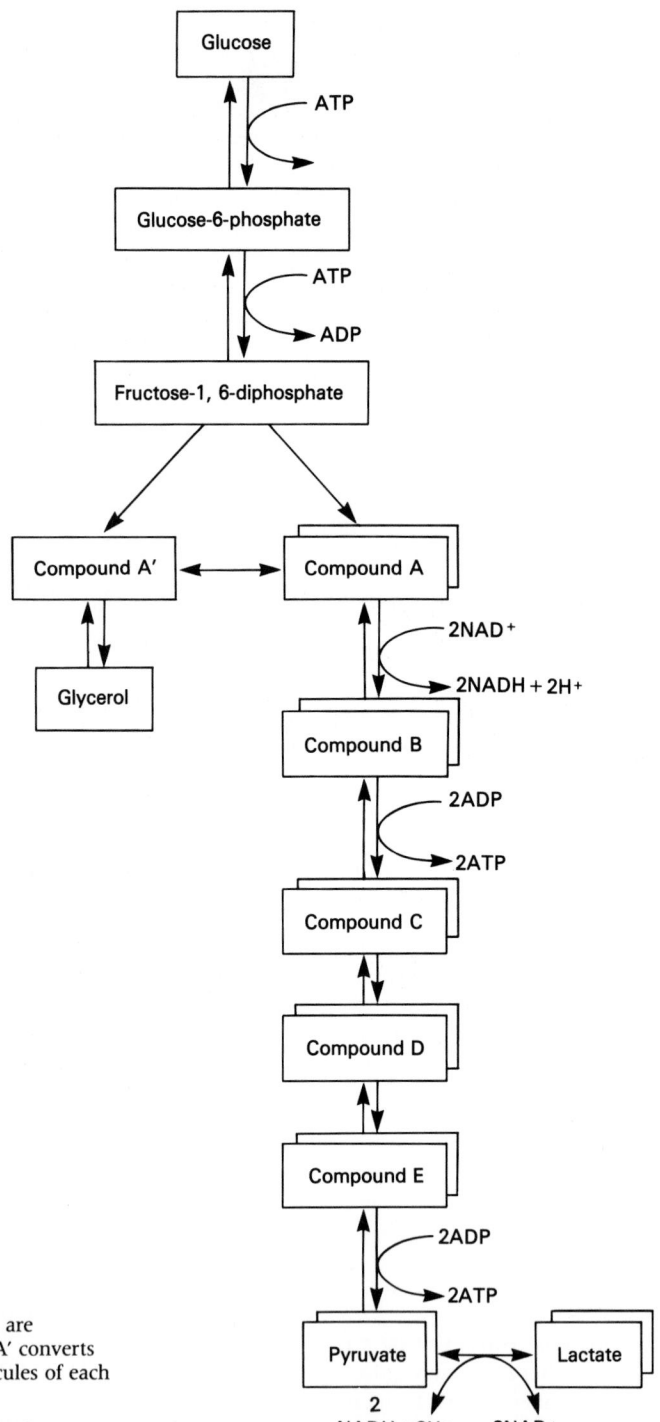

Glycolysis
Two molecules of compound A are
produced (because compound A' converts
to A), and therefore, two molecules of each
succeeding compound.

- A = glyceraldehyde-3-phosphate.
- A' = dihydroxyacetone phosphate.
- B = 1,3-diphosphoglyceric acid.
- C = 3-phosphoglyceric acid.
- D = 2-phosphoglyceric acid.
- E = phosphoenol pyruvic acid.

When fructose-1,6-diphosphate breaks in half, the two three-carbon compounds (A and A′) are not identical. Each has a phosphate group attached, but only one converts directly to pyruvate. The other compound, however, converts easily to the first. (Compound A′ is usually ignored, except for its role as the point of entry for the synthesis of glycerol; we say that two molecules of compound A are derived from one glucose molecule.)

In the step from compound A to compound B, enough energy is released to convert NAD^+ to $NADH + H^+$. Also, in the steps from B to C and from E to pyruvate, ATP is regenerated. Remember that there are effectively two molecules of compound A produced from glucose; therefore, four ATP molecules are generated from each glucose molecule. Two ATP were needed to get the sequence started, so the net gain at this point is two ATP and two molecules of $NADH + H^+$.

So far, no oxygen has been used; the process has been anaerobic. But at this point, oxygen is needed. If oxygen is not immediately available, pyruvate converts to lactic acid, to soak up the hydrogens from the $NADH + H^+$ that was generated. Lactic acid accumulates until oxygen becomes available. However, in the energy path from glucose to carbon dioxide, this side step usually is not necessary. As you will see later, each $NADH + H^+$ moves to the electron transport chain to unload its hydrogens onto oxygen. The associated energy produces two ATP, making the total yield eight ATP for the process from glucose to pyruvate.

The TCA Cycle

The tricarboxylic acid, or TCA, cycle (Figure C–2) is the name given to the set of reactions involving oxygen and leading from acetyl CoA to carbon dioxide (and water). To link glycolysis to the TCA cycle, pyruvate is converted to acetyl CoA. The TCA cycle is not restricted to the metabolism of carbohydrate. It also includes fat and protein. Any substance that can be converted to acetyl CoA directly, or indirectly through pyruvate, may enter the cycle.

The step from pyruvate to acetyl CoA is exceedingly complex. We have included only those substances that will help you understand the transfer of energy from the nutrients. When pyruvate is in the presence of oxygen, it loses a carbon in the form of carbon dioxide, and is attached to a molecule of CoA. In the process, NAD^+ picks up two hydrogens with their associated energy, becoming $NADH + H^+$.

The step from pyruvate to acetyl CoA.
(TPP is a helper compound containing the B vitamin thiamin.)

As the acetyl CoA breaks down to carbon dioxide and water, its energy is captured in ATP. Let's follow the steps by which this occurs (see Figure C–2).

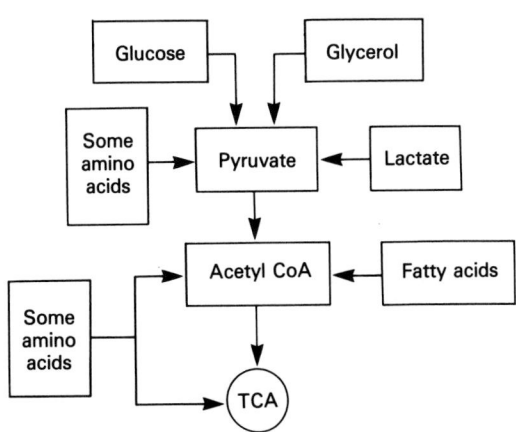

Any substance that can be converted to acetyl CoA directly, or indirectly through pyruvate, may enter the TCA cycle.

C

C

■ FIGURE C–2
The TCA Cycle

1. The two-carbon acetyl CoA combines with a four-carbon compound, oxaloacetate. The CoA comes off, and the product is a six-carbon compound, citrate.
2. The atoms of citrate are rearranged to form isocitrate.
3. Now NAD^+ reacts with isocitrate. Two H and two electrons are removed from the isocitrate. One H becomes attached to the NAD^+ with the two electrons; the other H is released as H^+. Thus NAD^+ becomes $NADH + H^+$. (Remember this $NADH + H^+$. It is carrying the H and the energy released from the last reaction. But let's follow the carbons first.) A carbon is combined with two oxygens, forming carbon dioxide (which diffuses away into the blood and is exhaled). What is left is the five-carbon compound alpha-ketoglutarate.
4. Now two compounds interact with alpha-ketoglutarate—a molecule of CoA and a molecule of NAD^+. In this complex reaction, a carbon and two oxygens are removed (forming carbon dioxide); two hydrogens are removed and go to NAD^+ (forming $NADH + H^+$); and the remaining four-carbon compound is attached to the CoA, forming succinyl CoA. (Remember this $NADH + H^+$ also. You will see later what happens to it.)
5. Now two molecules react with succinyl CoA—a molecule called GDP and one of phosphate (P). The CoA comes off, the GDP and P combine to form the high-energy compound GTP (similar to ATP), and succinate remains. (Remember this GTP.)
6. In the next reaction, two H with their energy are removed from succinate and are transferred to a molecule called FAD (an electron-hydrogen receiver like NAD^+) to form $FADH_2$. The product that remains is fumarate. (Remember this $FADH_2$.)
7. Next a molecule of water is added to fumarate, forming malate.
8. A molecule of NAD^+ reacts with the malate; two H with their associated energy are removed from the malate and form $NADH + H^+$. The product that remains is the four-carbon compound oxaloacetate. (Remember this $NADH + H^+$.)

We are back where we started. The oxaloacetate formed in this process can combine with another molecule of acetyl CoA (step 1), and the cycle can begin again. (The whole scheme is shown in Figure C–2.)

So far, what you have seen is that two carbons are brought in with acetyl CoA and that two carbons end up in carbon dioxide. But where is the energy and the ATP we promised you?

Each time a pair of hydrogen atoms is removed from one of the compounds in the cycle, it includes a pair of electrons. This chemical bond energy is thus captured into the compound to which the H become attached. A review of the eight steps of the cycle shows that energy is thus transferred into other compounds in steps 3, 4, 6, and 8. In step 5, energy is stored when GDP and P are bound together to form GTP. Thus the compounds $NADH + H^+$ (three molecules), $FADH_2$, and GTP store energy originally found in acetyl CoA. To see how this energy ends up in ATP, we must follow the electrons further. Let us take those attached to NAD^+ as an example.

The Electron Transport Chain

The six reactions described here are those of the electron transport chain. Since oxygen is required for these reactions, and ADP and P are combined to form ATP in several of them (ADP is phosphorylated), these reactions are also called oxidative phosphorylation.

An important concept to remember at this point is that an electron is not a fixed amount of energy. The electrons that bond the H to NAD^+ in NADH have a relatively large amount of energy. In the series of reactions that follow, they lose this energy in small amounts, until at the end they are attached (with H) to oxygen (O) to make water (H_2O). In some of the steps, the energy they lose is captured into ATP in coupled reactions.

1. In the first step of the electron transport chain, NADH reacts with a molecule called a flavoprotein, losing its electrons (and their H). The products are NAD^+ and reduced flavoprotein. A little energy is lost as heat in this reaction.
2. The flavoprotein passes on the electrons to a molecule called coenzyme Q. Again they lose some energy as heat, but ADP and P bond together and form ATP, storing much of the energy. This is a coupled reaction: $ADP + P \longrightarrow ATP$.
3. Coenzyme Q passes the electrons to cytochrome *b*. Again the electrons lose energy.
4. Cytochrome *b* passes the electrons to cytochrome *c* in a coupled reaction in which ATP is formed: $ADP + P \longrightarrow ATP$.
5. Cytochrome *c* passes the electrons to cytochrome *a*.
6. Cytochrome *a* passes them (with their H) to an atom of oxygen (O), forming water (H_2O). This is a coupled reaction in which ATP is formed: $ADP + P \longrightarrow ATP$.

The entire electron transport chain is diagrammed in Figure C–3. As you can see, each time NADH is oxidized (loses its electrons) by this means, the energy it loses is parceled out into three ATP molecules. When the electrons are passed on to water at the end, they are much lower in energy than they were originally. This completes the story of the electrons from NADH.

As for $FADH_2$, its electrons enter the electron transport chain at coenzyme Q. From coenzyme Q to water there are only two steps in which ATP is generated. Therefore, $FADH_2$ coming out of the TCA cycle yields just two ATP molecules.

■ **FIGURE C–3**
The Electron Transport Chain

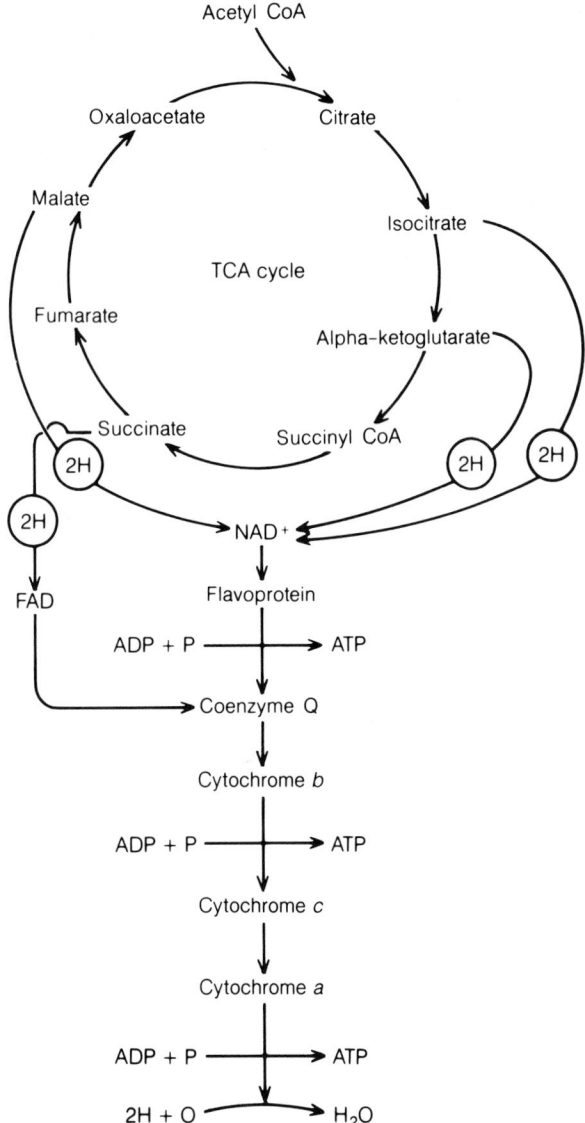

One energy-receiving compound of the TCA cycle (GTP) does not enter the electron transport chain but gives its energy directly to ADP in a simple phosphorylation reaction, yielding one ATP.

It is now possible to draw up a balance sheet of glucose metabolism (see Table C–3). Glycolysis has yielded 4 NADH + H$^+$ and 4 ATP molecules and has spent 2 ATP. The 2 acetyl CoA going through the TCA cycle have yielded 6 NADH + H$^+$, 2 FADH$_2$, and 2 GTP molecules. After the NADH + H$^+$ and FADH$_2$ have gone through the electron transport chain, there are 34 ATP. Added to these are the 4 ATP

from glycolysis and the 2 ATP from GTP, making the total 40 ATP generated from one molecule of glucose. After the expense of 2 ATP is subtracted, there is a net gain of 38 ATP.*

■ **TABLE C–3**
Balance Sheet for Glucose Metabolism

	Expenditures	Income
Glycolysis:		
1 glucose	2 ATP	4 ATP
1 fructose-1,6-diphosphate		2 NADH + H$^+$
2 pyruvate		2 NADH + H$^+$
TCA cycle:		
2 isocitrate		2 NADH + H$^+$
2 alpha-ketoglutarate		2 NADH + H$^+$
2 succinyl CoA		2 GTP
2 succinate		2 FADH$_2$
2 malate		2 NADH + H$^+$
Total ATP collected:		
From glycolysis	2 ATP	4 ATP
From 2 NADH + H$^+$		4–6 ATP[a]
From 8 NADH + H$^+$		24 ATP
From 2 GTP		2 ATP
From 2 FADH$_2$		4 ATP
Totals:	2 ATP	38–40 ATP
Balance on hand from 1 molecule of glucose:		36–38 ATP

[a]Each NADH + H$^+$ from glycolysis can yield 2 or 3 ATP. See accompanying text.

The TCA cycle and the electron transport chain are the body's major means of capturing the energy from nutrients in ATP molecules. Other means, such as anaerobic glycolysis, contribute, but the aerobic processes are the most efficient. Biologists and chemists understand much more about these processes than has been presented here.

Alcohol's Interference with Energy Metabolism

Highlight 7 provides an overview of how alcohol interferes with energy metabolism. With an understanding of the TCA cycle, a few more details may be appreciated. During alcohol metabolism, the enzyme alcohol dehydrogenase oxidizes alco-

---

*The total may sometimes be 36 or 37, rather than 38, ATP. The NADH + H$^+$ generated in the cytoplasm during glycolysis pass their electrons on to shuttle molecules, which move them into the mitochondria. One shuttle, malate, contributes its electrons to the electron transport chain before the first site of ATP synthesis, yielding 3 ATP. Another, glycerol phosphate, adds its electrons into the chain beyond that first site, yielding 2 ATP. Thus sometimes 3, and sometimes only 2, ATP result from the NADH + H$^+$ that arise from glycolysis. It depends on the cell.

hol to acetaldehyde while it simultaneously reduces a molecule of NAD$^+$ to NADH + H$^+$. The related enzyme acetaldehyde dehydrogenase reduces another NAD$^+$ to NADH + H$^+$ while it oxidizes acetaldehyde to acetyl CoA, the compound that enters the TCA cycle to generate energy. Thus whenever alcohol is being metabolized in the body, NAD$^+$ diminishes, and NADH + H$^+$ accumulates. Chemists describe the consequence by saying that the body's "redox state" is altered, because NAD$^+$ can oxidize, and NADH + H$^+$ can reduce, many other body compounds. During alcohol metabolism, NAD$^+$ becomes unavailable for the multitude of reactions for which it is required.

As the previous sections just explained, for glucose to get completely metabolized, the TCA cycle must be operating, and NAD$^+$ must be present. If these conditions are not met (and when alcohol is present, they may not be), the pathway will be blocked, and traffic will back up—or an alternate route will be taken. Think about this as you follow the pathway shown in Figure C–4.

In each step of alcohol metabolism in which NAD$^+$ is converted to NADH + H$^+$, hydrogen ions accumulate, resulting in a dangerous shift of the acid-base balance toward acid (Chapter 10 explains acid-base balance). The accumulation of NADH + H$^+$ depresses TCA cycle activity, so pyruvate and acetyl CoA build up. This condition favors the conversion of pyruvate to lactic acid, which serves as a temporary storage place for hydrogens from NADH + H$^+$. The conversion of pyruvate to lactic acid restores some NAD$^+$, but a lactic acid

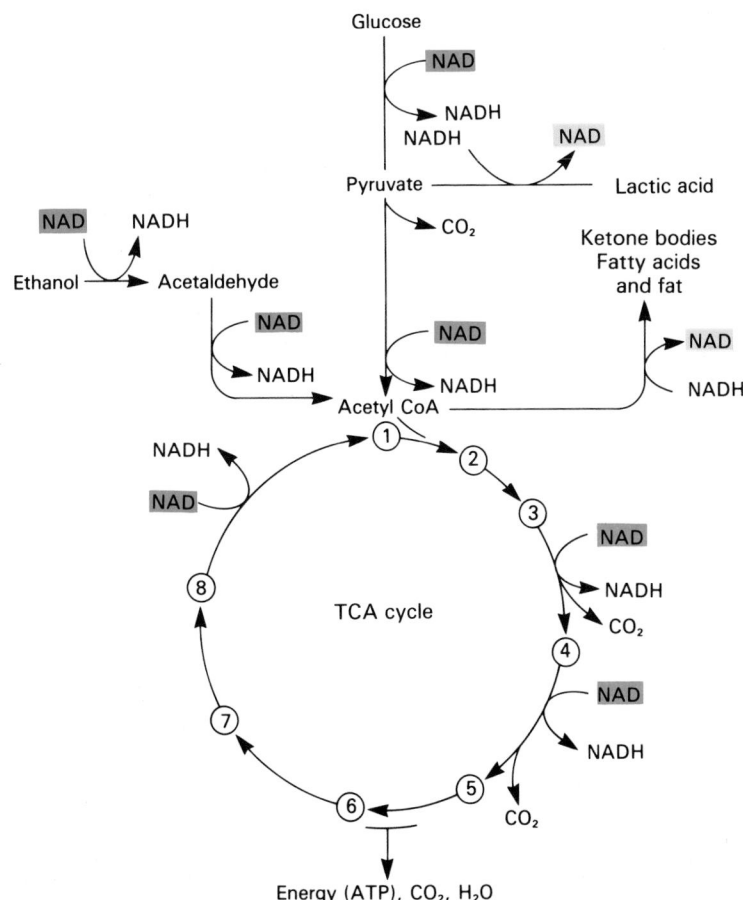

■ **FIGURE C–4**
Ethanol Enters the Metabolic Path
This is a simplified version of the glucose-to-energy pathway showing the entry of ethanol into it. The coenzyme NAD (which is the active form of the B vitamin niacin) is the only one shown here; however, many others are involved.

buildup has serious consequences of its own. It adds to the body's acid burden and interferes with the excretion of uric acid, causing goutlike symptoms. Molecules of acetyl CoA become building blocks for fatty acids or ketone bodies. The making of ketone bodies consumes acetyl CoA and generates NAD^+; but some ketone bodies are acids, so they push the acid-base balance further toward acid.

The presence of alcohol cascades through the pathways of metabolism, wreaking havoc along the way. These consequences have physical effects, which Highlight 7 describes.

The Urea Cycle

Chapter 7 sums up how waste nitrogen is eliminated from the body by stating that ammonia molecules combine with carbon

dioxide to produce urea. This is true, but it is not the whole story. Urea is produced in a multistep process within the cells of the liver.

Ammonia, freed from an amino acid or other compound during metabolism anywhere in the body, arrives at the liver by way of the bloodstream and is taken into a liver cell. There, it is first combined with carbon dioxide and a phosphate group from ATP to form carbamyl phosphate:

$$CO_2 + NH_3 \xrightarrow{\text{ATP ADP}} H_2N-C(=O)-O-P(=O)(O^-)-O^-$$

Carbon dioxide   Ammonia

Carbamyl phosphate   Phosphate group

Figure C–5 shows the cycle of four reactions that follow. In the first step, carbamyl phosphate combines with the amino

■ FIGURE C–5
The Urea Cycle

acid ornithine, losing its phosphate group. The compound formed is citrulline.

In the second step, citrulline combines with the amino acid aspartic acid, to form argininosuccinate. The reaction requires energy from ATP. (ATP has been shown, before, to lose one phosphorus atom in a phosphate group, P, becoming ADP. In this reaction, it loses two phosphorus atoms joined together, PP, and becomes adenosine monophosphate, AMP.)

In the third step, argininosuccinate is split, forming another acid, fumarate, and the amino acid arginine.

In the fourth step, arginine loses its terminal carbon with two attached amino groups and picks up an oxygen from water. The end product is urea, which the kidneys excrete in the urine. The compound that remains is ornithine, identical to the ornithine with which this series of reactions began, and ready to react with another molecule of carbamyl phosphate and turn the cycle again.

Formation of Ketone Bodies

Normally, fatty acid oxidation proceeds all the way to carbon dioxide and water. However, in ketosis (discussed in Chapter 7), an intermediate is formed from the condensation of two molecules of acetyl CoA: acetoacetyl CoA. Figure C–6 shows the formation of ketone bodies from that intermediate. In step 1, acetoacetyl CoA condenses with another acetyl CoA to form a six-carbon intermediate, beta-hydroxy-beta-methyl glutaryl CoA. In step 2, this intermediate is cleaved to acetyl CoA and acetoacetic acid. This product can be metabolized either to beta-hydroxybutyric acid (step 3a) or to acetone (3b).

The three last-named compounds are the three so-called ketone bodies of ketosis. Two are real ketones (they have a C=O group between two carbons); the other is an alcohol that has been produced during ketone formation—hence the term *ketone bodies* to describe the three of them, rather than ketones. There are many other ketones in nature; these three are the ones characteristic of ketosis in the body.

■ FIGURE C–6
Formation of Ketone Bodies

Notes

1. Nomenclature policy: Generic descriptors and trivial names for vitamins and related compounds, *Journal of Nutrition* 117 (1987): 7–14; Nomenclature policy: Abbreviated designations of amino acids in the *Journal of Nutrition* 117 (1987): 15.

Aids to Calculation

Contents

Many mathematical problems have been worked out for you as examples at appropriate places in the text. This appendix aims to help with the use of the metric system and with those problems not fully explained elsewhere.

Conversion Factors

Conversion factors are useful mathematical tools in everyday calculations, like the ones encountered in the study of nutrition. Skill in the use of conversion factors is especially desirable as the United States and Canada "go metric."

A conversion factor is a fraction in which the numerator (top) and the denominator (bottom) express the same quantity in different units. For example, 2.2 pounds (lb) and 1 kilogram (kg) are equivalent; they express the same weight. The conversion factor used to change pounds to kilograms or vice versa is:

$$\frac{2.2 \text{ lb}}{1 \text{ kg}} \text{ or } \frac{1 \text{ kg}}{2.2 \text{ lb}}.$$

Because both factors equal 1, measurements can be multiplied by the factor without changing the value of the measurement. Thus the units can be changed.

The correct factor to use in a problem is the one with the unit you are seeking in the numerator (top) of the fraction. Following are two examples of problems commonly encountered in nutrition study; they illustrate the usefulness of conversion factors.

Example 1 Convert the weight of 130 pounds to kilograms.

1. Choose the conversion factor in which the unit you are seeking is on top:

$$\frac{1 \text{ kg}}{2.2 \text{ lb}}.$$

2. Multiply 130 pounds by the factor:

$$130 \text{ lb} \times \frac{1 \text{ kg}}{2.2 \text{ lb}} = \frac{130 \text{ kg}}{2.2} = \begin{array}{l} 59 \text{ kg (rounded off to the} \\ \text{nearest whole number).} \end{array}$$

Example 2 How many grams (g) of saturated fat are contained in a 3-ounce (oz) hamburger?

1. Appendix H shows that a 4-ounce hamburger contains 7 grams of saturated fat. You are seeking grams of saturated fat; therefore, the conversion factor is:

$$\frac{7 \text{ g saturated fat}}{4 \text{ oz hamburger}}.$$

2. Multiply 3 ounces of hamburger by the conversion factor:

$$3 \text{ oz hamburger} \times \frac{7 \text{ g saturated fat}}{4 \text{ oz hamburger}} = \frac{3 \times 7}{4} = \frac{21}{4}$$

$$= 5 \text{ g saturated fat (rounded off to the nearest whole number).}$$

Percentages

A percentage is a comparison between a number of items (perhaps your intake of energy) and a standard number (perhaps the number of kcalories recommended for your age and sex—your energy RDA). The standard number is the number you divide by. The answer you get after the division must be multiplied by 100 to be stated as a percentage (*percent* means "per 100").

Example 3 What percentage of the RDA for energy is your energy intake?

1. Find your energy RDA (Appendix I). We'll use 2,100 kcalories to demonstrate.
2. Total your energy intake for a day—for example, 1,200 kcalories.
3. Divide your kcalorie intake by the RDA kcalories:

    1,200 kcal (your intake) ÷ 2,100 kcal (RDA) = 0.573.

4. Multiply your answer by 100 to state it as a percentage:

    0.573 × 100 = 57.3 = 57% (rounded off to the nearest whole number).

In some problems in nutrition, the percentage may be more than 100. For example, suppose your daily intake of vitamin A is 3,200 RE and your RDA (male) is 1,000 RE. Your intake as a percentage of the RDA is more than 100 percent (that is, you consume more than 100 percent of your vitamin A RDA). The following calculations show your vitamin A intake as a percentage of the RDA:

3,200 ÷ 1,000 = 3.2.
3.2 × 100 = 320% of RDA.

Sometimes the comparison is between a part of a whole (for example, your kcalories from protein) and the total amount (your total kcalories). In this case, the total number is the one you divide by.

Example 4 What percentages of your total kcalories for the day come from protein, fat, and carbohydrate?

1. Using Appendix H and your diet record, find the total grams of protein, fat, and carbohydrate you consumed—for example, 60 grams protein, 80 grams fat, and 285 grams carbohydrate.
2. Multiply the number of grams by the number of kcalories from 1 gram of each energy nutrient (conversion factors):

    $60 \text{ g protein} \times \dfrac{4 \text{ kcal}}{1 \text{ g protein}} = 240 \text{ kcal.}$

    $80 \text{ g fat} \times \dfrac{9 \text{ kcal}}{1 \text{ g fat}} = 720 \text{ kcal.}$

    $285 \text{ g carbohydrate} \times \dfrac{4 \text{ kcal}}{1 \text{ g carbohydrate}} = 1,140 \text{ kcal.}$

    240 + 720 + 1,140 = 2,100 kcal.
3. Find the percentage of total kcalories from each energy nutrient (see example 3):

- Protein: 240 ÷ 2,100 = 0.114 × 100 = 11.4 =11% of kcal.
- Fat: 720 ÷ 2,100 = 0.342 × 100 = 34.2 = 34% of kcal.
- Carbohydrate: 1,140 ÷ 2,100 = 0.542 × 100 = 54.2 = 54% of kcal.
- 11% + 34% +54% = 99% of kcal (total).

The percentages total 99 percent rather than 100 percent because a little was lost from each number in rounding off. This is a reasonable error.

▪ *Ratios*

A ratio is a comparison of two or three values in which one of the values is reduced to 1. A ratio compares identical units and so is expressed without units. For example, the P:S ratio is a comparison of the grams of polyunsaturated fat to the grams of saturated fat in the diet.

Example 5 Find the P:S ratio of your diet.

1. Using Appendix H and your diet record, find the grams of polyunsaturated fat and the grams of saturated fat that you consumed. Say they are 32 grams polyunsaturated fat and 25 grams saturated fat.
2. Divide the polyunsaturated fat grams by the saturated fat grams:

    Polyunsaturated fat (g) ÷ saturated fat (g).

    32 g ÷ 25 g = 1.28.
3. The P:S ratio is usually expressed as correct to one decimal place: 1.28 = 1.3.

The P:S ratio of your diet is 1.3:1 (read as "one point three to one" or simply "one point three"). A ratio greater than 1 means that the first value (in this case, grams of polyunsaturated fat) is greater than the second (saturated fat). If it were less than 1, you would know that the second value was the greater.

Research is beginning to find that diets low in saturated fats and high in monounsaturated fatty acids may protect against heart disease. Consequently, the polyunsaturated to monounsaturated to saturated (P:M:S) ratio may be more meaningful than the P:S ratio.[1]

▪ *Weights and Measures*

Length
1 inch (in) = 2.54 centimeters (cm).
1 foot (ft) = 30.48 centimeters.
1 meter (m) = 39.37 inches.

Temperature

	Celsius[a]	Fahrenheit	
Steam	100° C	212° F	Steam
Body temperature	37° C	98.6° F	Body temperature
Ice	0° C	32° F	Ice

To convert Fahrenheit temperature (t_F) to Celsius:

$$t_F = 9/5\ t_C + 32.$$

To convert Celcius temperature (t_C) to Fahrenheit:

$$t_C = 5/9\ (t_F - 32).$$

Volume

1 liter (l) = 1.06 quarts (qt) or 0.85 imperial quart.
1 liter = 1,000 milliliters (ml).
1 milliliter = 0.03 fluid ounces.
1 gallon = 3.79 liters.
1 quart = 0.95 liter or 32 fluid ounces.

---

[a]Also known as *centigrade*.

1 cup (c) = 8 fluid ounces.
1 tablespoon (tbsp) = 15 milliliters.
3 teaspoons (tsp) = 1 tablespoon.
16 tablespoons = 1 cup.
4 cups = 1 quart.

Weight

1 ounce (oz) = approximately 28 grams (g).
16 ounces = 1 pound (lb).
1 pound = 454 grams.
1 kilogram (kg) = 1,000 grams or 2.2 pounds.
1 gram = 1,000 milligrams (mg).
1 milligram = 1,000 micrograms (μg).

Notes

1. F. H. Mattson, A changing role for dietary monounsaturated fatty acids, *Journal of the American Dietetic Association* 89 (1989): 387–391.

D

Nutrition Assessment: Supplemental Information

E

Chapter 19 describes the nutrition assessment techniques health care professionals commonly use to determine clients' nutrition status. From this assessment, they identify clients' nutrition needs and develop care plans for meeting those needs. This Appendix provides additional details and alternative methods of assessing nutrition status to support a complete nutrition assessment.

▪ *Drug History: Nutrition and Drug Interactions*

Chapters 18 through 30 include a series of tables listing drugs used in the treatment of the specific diseases being discussed. Those tables provide information on how the drugs are administered with respect to timing of food intake and on common side effects that may influence nutrition status. Table E-1 (A and B) presents an expanded summary of those drug tables for your reference.

E

■ **TABLE E–1A**
Guide to Table E–1B*

Drug Name	Drug Classification in Table E–1B
Acebutolol	Antihypertensive Agents
Acetaminophen	Analgesic Agents
Acetohexamide	Antidiabetic Agents
Acetylsalicylic acid	Analgesic Agents
Acyclovir	Anti-Infective Agents
Adrenocorticosteroids	Antineoplastic Agents
Aluminum hydroxide	Antacids
Amiloride HCl	Diuretics
Amphotericin B	Anti-Infective Agents
Ampicillin	Anti-Infective Agents
Asparaginase	Antineoplastic Agents
Atenolol	Antihypertensive Agents
Azathioprine	Immunosuppressants
Azidothymidine (AZT)	Anti-Infective Agents
Belladonna	Antidiarrheal Agents
Bisacodyl	Laxatives
Bleomycin	Antineoplastic Agents
Buspirone HCl	Antianxiety Agents
Busulfan	Antineoplastic Agents
Calcium carbonate	Antacids
Captopril	Antihypertensive Agents
Carmustine	Antineoplastic Agents
Castor oil	Laxatives
Chloramphenicol	Anti-Infective Agents
Chlorothiazide	Diuretics
Chlorpromazine HCl	Antipsychotic Agents
Chlorpropamide	Antidiabetic Agents
Chlorthalidone	Diuretics
Cholestyramine	Antilipemic Agents
Cimetidine	Antiulcer Agents
Cisplatin	Antineoplastic Agents
Clofibrate	Antilipemic Agents
Clonidine HCl	Antihypertensive Agents
Clotrimazole	Anti-Infective Agents
Colchicine	Miscellaneous
Colestipol	Antilipemic Agents
Cyclophosphamide	Antineoplastic Agents
Cyclosporine	Immunosuppressants
Dactinomycin	Antineoplastic Agents
Deserpidine/methyclothiazide	Antihypertensive Agents
Dicumarol	Anticoagulants
Digitalis	Antihypertensive Agents
Digitoxin	Antihypertensive Agents
Digoxin	Antihypertensive Agents
Dihydroxyaluminum sodium carbonate	Antacids
Diphenoxylate	Antidiarrheal Agents
Doxepin HCl	Antidepressant Agents—Other
Doxorubicin	Antineoplastic Agents
Enalapril maleate	Antihypertensive Agents
Erythromycin	Anti-Infective Agents
Estrogen	Antineoplastic Agents
Ethambutol HCl	Anti-Infective Agents
Famotidine	Antiulcer Agents
Fluconazole	Anti-Infective Agents
Fluorouracil	Antineoplastic Agents

■ **TABLE E–1A**
Guide to Table E–1B*   (continued)

Drug Name	Drug Classification in Table E–1B
Ganciclovir	Anti-Infective Agents
Gemfibrozil	Antilipemic Agents
Glipizide	Antidiabetic Agents
Glyburide	Antidiabetic Agents
Guanethidine sulfate	Antihypertensive Agents
Guanfacine HCl	Antihypertensive Agents
Hydralazine HCl	Antihypertensive Agents
Hydrochlorothiazide	Diuretics
Hydroxyurea	Antineoplastic Agents
Ibuprofen	Analgesic Agents
Indapamide	Diuretics
Isocarboxide	Antidepressant Agents—MAO Inhibitors
Isoniazid (INH)	Anti-Infective Agents
Kaolin	Antidiarrheal Agents
Ketoconazole	Anti-Infective Agents
Labetalol HCl	Antihypertensive Agents
Lactulose	Laxatives
Levodopa	Miscellaneous
Lisinopril	Antihypertensive Agents
Lithium carbonate	Miscellaneous
Loperamide	Antidiarrheal Agents
Lovastatin	Antilipemic Agents
Loxapine HCl	Antipsychotic Agents
Magaldrate	Antacids
Magnesium hydroxide	Antacids
Meprobamate	Antianxiety Agents
Mercaptopurine	Antineoplastic Agents
Methotrexate	Antineoplastic Agents
Methyldopa	Antihypertensive Agents
Metoprolol tartrate	Antihypertensive Agents
Metronidazole	Anti-Infective Agents
Mineral oil	Laxatives
Minoxidil	Antihypertensive Agents
Mithramycin	Antineoplastic Agents
Nadolol	Antihypertensive Agents
Neomycin	Anti-Infective Agents
Nicotinic acid	Antilipemic Agents
Nifedipine	Antihypertensive Agents
Nystatin	Anti-Infective Agents
Opium	Antidiarrheal Agents
Oral contraceptives	Miscellaneous; see also estrogen
Paregoric	Antidiarrheal Agents
Pectin	Antidiarrheal Agents
Penicillin	Anti-Infective Agents
Pentamidine isethionate	Anti-Infective Agents
Perphenazine	Antipsychotic Agents
Phenelzine sulfate	Antidepressant Agents—MAO Inhibitors
Phenytoin	Anticonvulsants
Pindolol	Antihypertensive Agents
Prazosin HCl	Antihypertensive Agents
Prednisone	Immunosuppressants
Probucol	Antilipemic Agents
Procarbazine	Antineoplastic Agents
Propranolol HCl	Antihypertensive Agents
Pyrimethamine	Anti-Infective Agents

E

(continued)

■ TABLE E–1A
Guide to Table E–1B*   (continued)

Drug Name	Drug Classification in Table E–1B
Ranitidine	Antiulcer Agents
Rauwolfia serpentina	Antihypertensive Agents
Rifampin	Anti-Infective Agents
Sodium bicarbonate	Antacids
Spironolactone	Diuretics
Sucralfate	Antiulcer Agents
Sulfadiazine	Anti-Infective Agents
Sulfasalazine	Anti-Infective Agents
Terazosin HCl	Antihypertensive Agents
Tetracycline	Anti-Infective Agents
Thioridazine HCl	Antipsychotic Agents
Timolol maleate	Antihypertensive Agents
Tolazamide	Antidiabetic Agents
Tolbutamide	Antidiabetic Agents
Tranylcypromine sulfate	Antidepressant Agents—MAO Inhibitors
Trazodone HCl	Antidepressant Agents—Other
Triamterene	Diuretics
Trimethoprim	Anti-Infective Agents
Valproic acid	Anticonvulsants
Vinblastine	Antineoplastic Agents
Vincristine	Antineoplastic Agents
Warfarin	Anticoagulants

*This table provides an alphabetical listing of the drugs described in Table E–1B and shows where each drug can be found.
Note: The drug classifications shown here have been adapted for use in this text and are not always the formal drug classification. For example, lithium carbonate listed here as "Miscellaneous" is formally a "Miscellaneous Psychotherapeutic Agent." Also, many drugs actually have more than one classification. For example, corticosteroid hormones can be considered to be both "Immunosuppressants" and "Antineoplastic Agents." Only one classification is shown in this table for each drug.

■ TABLE E–1B
Administration and Common Nutrition-Related Side Effects of Selected Drugs

Drug Classification and Name	Administration	Common Side Effects That May Influence Nutrition Status
Analgesic Agents		
Acetaminophen	Give with food to decrease GI distress.	Side effects rarely occur.
Acetylsalicylic acid	Give with water, or with food if GI distress occurs with use.	Stomach upset, vomiting, nausea, GI bleeding, irritation of ulcers. May induce iron deficiency by causing GI bleeding. May enhance effects of anticlotting and antidiabetic medicine. Severe allergic reaction in some people.
Ibuprofen	Give on empty stomach, or with food or milk if GI distress occurs with use.	Nausea, stomach pain, heartburn, anorexia, dry mouth, diarrhea, vomiting, indigestion, constipation, abdominal cramps or pain, bloating, gas. May induce iron deficiency by causing GI bleeding.

■ TABLE E–1B
Administration and Common Nutrition-Related Side Effects of Selected Drugs (continued)

Drug Classification and Name	Administration	Common Side Effects That May Influence Nutrition Status
Antacids		
Aluminum hydroxide	Give 1 to 3 hr after meals.	Constipation, cramps, bloating, nausea, vomiting, anorexia, chalky taste. Inactivates thiamin; decreases absorption of vitamin A, phosphorous, and calcium.
Calcium carbonate	Give 1 to 3 hr after meals. Give iron supplements 1 to 2 hr before or after use. Do not take with large amounts of dairy products.	Belching, nausea, constipation, steatorrhea, chalky taste. May decrease iron absorption.
Dihydroxyaluminum sodium carbonate	Give 1 to 3 hr after meals.	Constipation, diarrhea, anorexia, weight loss.
Magaldrate	Give on empty stomach.	Chalky taste. May decrease absorption of fat-soluble vitamins, especially vitamin A.
Magnesium hydroxide	Give 1 hr after meals.	Constipation. May decrease absorption of vitamin A, phosphorus, and calcium; inactivates thiamin.
Sodium bicarbonate	Give 1 to 3 hr after meals.	Belching, gas, bloating, weight gain. Decreases iron absorption.
Antianxiety Agents		
Buspirone HCl	Give with food.	Nausea, vomiting, diarrhea, dry mouth.
Meprobamate	Give with food to decrease GI distress.	Anorexia, nausea, vomiting.
Anticoagulant Agents		
Dicumarol	Avoid excessive amounts of foods containing vitamin K (see p. 263).	Anorexia, nausea, vomiting, diarrhea, abdominal pain, mouth ulcers.
Warfarin	Avoid excessive amounts of foods containing vitamin K (see p. 263).	Nausea, vomiting, diarrhea, abdominal pain.
Anticonvulsants		
Phenytoin	Give with food to decrease GI distress. Tube feedings may reduce drug absorption and should be stopped for 2 hours before and after giving the drug, if possible.	Nausea, vomiting, swollen gums. May cause folate and vitamin B_{12} deficiencies.
Valproic acid	Give with food to decrease GI distress. Do not mix liquid form with carbonated beverages.	Anorexia, nausea, vomiting, abdominal pain.
Antidepressant Agents—MAO Inhibitors (see p. 587)		
Isocarboxide	Avoid foods containing tyramine and tryptophan. Avoid alcohol and caffeine.	Anorexia, constipation.
Phenelzine sulfate	Avoid foods containing tyramine and tryptophan. Avoid alcohol and caffeine.	Anorexia, constipation.
Tranylcypromide sulfate	Avoid foods containing tyramine and tryptophan. Avoid alcohol and caffeine.	Anorexia.
Antidepressant Agents—Other		
Doxepin HCl	Dilute oral concentrate with water, milk, or juice. Do not mix with carbonated beverages. Avoid alcohol and caffeine.	Dry mouth, constipation.
Trazodone HCl	Give with food.	Nausea, dry mouth, constipation.

(continued)

■ TABLE E–1B
Administration and Common Nutrition-Related Side Effects of Selected Drugs   (continued)

Drug Classification and Name	Administration	Common Side Effects That May Influence Nutrition Status
Antidiabetic Agents		
Acetohexamide	Give with meals. Avoid alcohol.	Diarrhea, nausea, vomiting, heartburn, metallic taste. May induce anemia.
Chlorpropamide	Give with breakfast. Avoid alcohol.	Dyspepsia, nausea, vomiting, metallic taste, anorexia. Water intoxication, edema.
Glipizide	Give 30 min before breakfast. Limit alcohol.	GI distress, nausea, diarrhea, constipation, heartburn, altered taste perceptions.
Glyburide	Give before breakfast. Limit alcohol.	GI distress, nausea, diarrhea, constipation, heartburn.
Tolazamide	Give in morning or divided during day with meals. Avoid alcohol.	Diarrhea, GI distress, nausea, vomiting, dyspepsia, heartburn, altered taste perceptions, anorexia.
Tolbutamide	(same as above)	(same as above)
Antidiarrheal Agents		
Diphenoxylate	May give with food.	Nausea, vomiting, bloating, anorexia, dry mouth, sore or swollen gums.
Kaolin, pectin	Mix at room temperature with milk or juice.	Constipation, dry mouth, altered taste perception.
Loperamide		Abdominal pain, constipation, bloating, dry mouth, vomiting, nausea.
Opium, belladonna, and paregoric	May give with food.	Nausea, vomiting, constipation. Sedation.
Antihypertensive Agents		
Acebutolol	Give without regard to meals.	Constipation, gas, abdominal pain. May mask the signs of hypoglycemia. May induce electrolyte imbalance and anemias.
Atenolol	Give without regard to meals.	Dry mouth, diarrhea, nausea. May mask signs of hypoglycemia.
Atenolol and chlorothalidone	Give on empty stomach same time each day.	Anorexia, diarrhea, nausea, vomiting, GI irritation, constipation. May induce hypokalemia, anemia.
Captopril	Give on empty stomach 1 hr before meals.	Altered taste perception, weight loss, sore mouth. May induce hypokalemia, anemias.
Clonidine HCl		Dry mouth, weight gain, nausea, vomiting, constipation. May induce edema.
Deserpidine/methyclothiazide	Give with food 6 or more hr before bedtime. Avoid natural licorice.	Dry mouth, weight gain, anorexia, nausea, vomiting, diarrhea, cramps.
Digitalis, digitoxin, digoxin	Give with water ½ hr before or 2 hr after food. Avoid natural licorice.	May inhibit glucose absorption. Nausea, vomiting.
Enalapril maleate	May give with food.	Altered taste perceptions. Diarrhea, nausea, vomiting, abdominal pain.

■ **TABLE E–1B**
Administration and Common Nutrition-Related Side Effects of Selected Drugs   (continued)

Drug Classification and Name	Administration	Common Side Effects That May Influence Nutrition Status
Antihypertensive Agents (continued)		
Guanethidine sulfate	Give at same time each day. Avoid natural licorice.	Dry mouth, weight gain, diarrhea, nausea. May induce edema.
Guanfacine HCl		Constipation, nausea, vomiting, stomach cramps.
Hydralazine HCl	Give with food at the same time each day. Avoid natural licorice.	Anorexia, GI distress, constipation.
Labetalol HCl	Give with food.	Altered taste perception, nausea, vomiting, indigestion. May mask signs of hypoglycemia.
Lisinopril		Diarrhea, vomiting.
Methyldopa	Avoid natural licorice.	Dry mouth, weight gain, diarrhea, nausea. May induce edema.
Metoprolol tartrate	Give with food.	Dry mouth, diarrhea, GI pain, gas, constipation, heartburn. May mask the signs of hypoglycemia.
Minoxidil	Give at same time each day.	May induce edema.
Nadolol	Give without regard to meals. Avoid natural licorice.	Dry mouth, constipation, GI distress, nausea, gas. May mask the signs of hypoglycemia.
Nifedipine	Give with food or milk.	Altered taste perception, nausea, diarrhea, constipation, cramps, gas. May induce edema.
Pindolol	Give without regard to meals.	Diarrhea, vomiting. May mask the signs of hypoglycemia. May alter glucose tolerance. May induce edema.
Prazosin HCl		Dry mouth, nausea, diarrhea, constipation, GI distress. May induce edema.
Propranolol HCl	Give with food. Avoid natural licorice.	Dry mouth, constipation, GI distress, nausea. May mask the signs of hypoglycemia.
Rauwolfia serpentina	Give with food or milk to reduce GI irritation.	Anorexia, weight gain, dry mouth, diarrhea, nausea, vomiting, raises GI motility and gastric secretion. May lower glucose tolerance. May alter serum glucose.
Terazosin HCl	Avoid salt substitutes. Give without regard to meals at the same time each day.	Sore throat. Nausea. May induce edema.
Timolol maleate	Give with food at the same time each day.	Weight loss, nausea. May mask signs of hypoglycemia. May induce edema.
Anti-Infective Agents		
Acyclovir	Give parenterally or orally with food.	Nausea, diarrhea, vomiting, anorexia.
Amphotericin B	Give parenterally.	Nausea, vomiting, fever, anemia, kidney dysfunction.
Ampicillin	Give with water 1 hr before or 2 hr after meals; do not give with fruit juice, beer, wine.	Nausea, vomiting, diarrhea, steatorrhea, anemia, inflammation of the mouth and tongue; stomatitis, altered taste perceptions, hypokalemia.

■ **TABLE E–1B**
Administration and Common Nutrition-Related Side Effects of Selected Drugs   (continued)

Drug Classification and Name	Administration	Common Side Effects That May Influence Nutrition Status
Anti-Infective Agents (continued)		
Azidothymidine (AZT)		Anorexia, nausea, vomiting, diarrhea, constipation, altered taste perceptions, mouth ulcers, edema of tongue and lips, abdominal pain, anemia.
Chloramphenicol	Give with water 1 hr before or 2 hr after meals.	Diarrhea, nausea, vomiting, irritation of mouth or tongue. May enhance effects of antidiabetic medicine. May raise requirements of riboflavin, vitamin B_6, and vitamin B_{12}.
Clotrimazole	Dissolve slowly in mouth and swallow saliva.	Nausea, vomiting.
Erythromycin	Give on empty stomach 1 hr before or 2 hr after meals; if GI distress, give with meals, not milk, fruit juice, beer, or wine.	Nausea, vomiting, cramps, abdominal pain, diarrhea, inflammation of the mouth.
Ethambutol HCl		Anorexia, nausea, vomiting, abdominal pain.
Fluconazole	Give orally or parenterally.	Nausea, vomiting, diarrhea, intestinal inflammation.
Ganciclovir	Give parenterally.	Anorexia, nausea, vomiting.
Isoniazid (INH)	Give 1 hr before or 2 hr after meals; may give with food to relieve GI distress.	Anorexia, nausea, vomiting, dry mouth, diarrhea, anemia, cracked lips.
Ketoconazole	Give with food to reduce nausea and vomiting.	Nausea, vomiting, abdominal pain, diarrhea, anemia. Renal and liver dysfunction.
Metronidazole	Give with food.	Anorexia, nausea, vomiting, diarrhea, altered taste perceptions, dry mouth, constipation, stomatitis, abdominal discomfort.
Neomycin		Nausea, vomiting, diarrhea, sore mouth. Decreases absorption of fats, nitrogen, carbohydrates, folate, vitamin B_6, vitamin B_{12}, fat-soluble vitamins, calcium, and iron.
Nystatin	Give orally as directed; retain drug in mouth as long as possible.	Diarrhea, nausea, and vomiting, GI pain (occasionally).
Penicillin	Give penicillin G on an empty stomach; penicillin K with or without meals.	Nausea, vomiting, diarrhea, gas, anemia, sore mouth, altered taste perceptions, anorexia.
Pentamidine isethionate	Give parenterally or as an inhalant.	Nausea, vomiting, taste alterations. Hypoglycemia or hyperglycemia, diabetes, kidney dysfunction.
Pyrimethamine	Give with food.	Anorexia, nausea, vomiting, diarrhea, and anemia.
Rifampin	Give with water on empty stomach.	Anorexia, nausea, vomiting, cramps, diarrhea, altered taste perceptions, abdominal distress.
Sulfadiazine		Anorexia, nausea, vomiting, and diarrhea.
Sulfasalazine	Give with food or milk	May cause anorexia, nausea, GI distress.

■ TABLE E–1B
Administration and Common Nutrition-Related Side Effects of Selected Drugs   (continued)

Drug Classification and Name	Administration	Common Side Effects That May Influence Nutrition Status
Anti-Infective Agents (continued)		
Tetracycline	Give on an empty stomach; don't give with milk or dairy products; don't give iron-containing supplements within 3 hours of tetracycline ingestion.	Anorexia, nausea, vomiting, diarrhea, altered taste perceptions, sore mouth. Decreases absorption of fat, amino acids, calcium, iron, magnesium, and zinc. Decreases bacterial synthesis of vitamin K in intestines.
Trimethoprim	Give with water on empty stomach.	Nausea, vomiting, anorexia, anemia, diarrhea, stomatitis, GI distress.
Antilipemic Agents		
Cholestyamine	Give with water or other fluids; never give dry or with carbonated beverages.	Nausea, vomiting, abdominal discomfort, gas, diarrhea, constipation, heartburn, steatorrhea, anorexia, altered taste perception. May decrease absorption of calcium, fat, vitamins A, D, K, B_{12}, folate, and glucose. Depletes iron stores.
Colestipol	(same as above)	(same as above)
Clofibrate	Give with meals.	Nausea, vomiting, abdominal discomfort, loose stools, gas, aftertaste, altered taste perception, increased appetite. May decrease absorption of glucose, iron, and vitamin B_{12}. May induce anemia.
Gemfibrozil	Give ½ hour before meals.	Nausea, vomiting, abdominal discomfort, gas, constipation. May induce anemia.
Lovastatin	Give with meals.	Diarrhea, gas, constipation, abdominal pain, heartburn, nausea, indigestion, altered taste perception.
Nicotinic acid	Give with meals.	Nausea, vomiting, abdominal discomfort, diarrhea. Flushing. Decreased glucose tolerance.
Probucol	Give with meals.	Nausea, vomiting, gas, abdominal discomfort, diarrhea, anorexia, altered taste and smell perceptions.
Antineoplastic Agents		
Adrenocorticosteroids	Give with food.	Increased appetite, GI upset. Glucose intolerance, negative nitrogen and calcium balance.
Asparaginase	Give parenterally.	Anorexia, nausea, vomiting. Pancreatitis, hepatitis, glucose intolerance.
Bleomycin	Give parenterally, intramuscularly, or subcutaneously.	Anorexia, nausea, vomiting, mouth ulcers, stomatitis, weight loss, altered taste perceptions.
Busulfan	Give with food.	Nausea, vomiting, diarrhea, cracking at corners of mouth, inflammation of the tongue, anemias, weight loss, dry mouth.

E

(continued)

Administration and Common Nutrition-Related Side Effects of Selected Drugs (continued)

Drug Classification and Name	Administration	Common Side Effects That May Influence Nutrition Status
Antineoplastic Agents (continued)		
Carmustine	Give parenterally.	Anorexia, nausea, vomiting, esophagitis, diarrhea. Impaired liver function.
Cisplatin	Give parenterally.	Anorexia, nausea, vomiting, altered taste perceptions.
Cyclophosphamide	Give during or after meals.	Anorexia, nausea, vomiting, mouth ulcers, inflammation of the colon, anemia.
Dactinomycin	Give parenterally.	Anorexia, nausea, vomiting, mouth ulcers, heartburn, anemia.
Doxorubicin	Give parenterally.	Anorexia, nausea, vomiting, diarrhea, stomach pain, sore throat, mouth ulcers, mouth blindness, esophagitis.
Estrogen	Give with food at same time each day.	Anorexia, nausea, vomiting, edema, weight changes. Alters glucose tolerance.
Fluorouracil	Give parenterally. If given orally, give with water, not acidic beverages.	Anorexia, nausea, vomiting, stomatitis, diarrhea, heartburn, sore mouth, altered taste perceptions, GI bleeding, esophagitis.
Hydroxyurea	Give with food.	Anorexia, nausea, vomiting, mouth ulcers.
Mercaptopurine	Give with food.	Anorexia, nausea, vomiting, stomatitis, stomach pain, diarrhea, anemia, vitamin B_6 depletion.
Methotrexate	Give on an empty stomach; give with food to reduce gastric distess. Do not give with milk.	Anorexia, nausea, vomiting, diarrhea, GI ulcers, GI inflammation, anemia, stomatitis, steatorrhea, mouth ulcers.
Mithramycin	Give parenterally; slow infusion reduces nausea.	Anorexia, nausea, vomiting, diarrhea, inflammation of the tongue, metallic taste.
Procarbazine	Give with food. Avoid foods containing tyramine (see Table 18–5).	Anorexia, nausea, vomiting, diarrhea, constipation, anemia, sore throat, dry mouth, difficulty swallowing.
Vinblastine	Give parenterally.	Anorexia, nausea, vomiting, diarrhea, constipation, stomatitis, sore throat, reduced bowel activity, abdominal pain, bowel inflammation.
Vincristine	Give parenterally.	Anorexia, nausea, vomiting, diarrhea, constipation, abdominal pain, mouth ulcers, anemia, thirst, weight loss, altered taste perceptions.
Antipsychotic Agents		
Chlorpromazine HCl	Give with food. Dilute liquid concentrate with milk, fruit juice, or semisolid foods.	Dry mouth, constipation.
Loxapine HCl	Give with food or water. Dilute liquid concentrate with orange or grapefruit juice.	Dry mouth, constipation.
Perphenazine	Give with food. Dilute liquid concentrate with milk, fruit juice, carbonated beverages, or semisolid foods; do not dilute with colas, black coffee, tea, or grape or apple juice.	Dry mouth, constipation.

E

Administration and Common Nutrition-Related Side Effects of Selected Drugs   (continued)

Drug Classification and Name	Administration	Common Side Effects That May Influence Nutrition Status
Antipsychotic Agents (continued)		
Thioridazine HCl	Give with food. Dilute liquid concentrate with fruit juice or water.	Dry mouth, constipation.
Antiulcer Agents		
Cimetidine	Give with meals; caffeine and alcohol reduce effectiveness.	Diarrhea. Reduced gastric secretion. May induce hyperglycemia.
Famotidine		Nausea, diarrhea, constipation, flatulence.
Ranitidine		Constipation, nausea, abdominal discomfort. (Fewer reported side effects and interactions than with cimetidine.)
Sucralfate	Give on empty stomach 1 hour before meals and at bedtime.	Constipation, diarrhea, nausea, cramps, dry mouth. Interferes with absorption of fat-soluble vitamins.
Diuretics		
Amiloride HCl and hydrochlorothiazide	Give with food at the same time each day.	Anorexia, dry mouth, appetite changes, nausea, diarrhea, GI pain, constipation.
Chlorothiazide	Give with food 6 or more hr before bedtime. Avoid natural licorice.	Nausea, vomiting, diarrhea, constipation, anorexia, dry mouth.
Chlorthalidone	Give with food 6 or more hr before bedtime. Avoid natural licorice.	Anorexia, dry mouth, GI irritation, nausea, vomiting, diarrhea, constipation.
Hydrochlorothiazide	Give with food 6 or more hr before bedtime. Avoid natural licorice.	Anorexia, dry mouth, nausea, vomiting, diarrhea, constipation. May alter insulin requirements in diabetes. May induce hypokalemia.
Indapamide	Give with food at the same time each day if GI distress.	Dry mouth, weight loss, anorexia, constipation, GI distress. May alter glucose tolerance.
Spironolactone with hydrochlorothiazide	Give with food 6 or more hr before bedtime. Avoid natural licorice.	Anorexia, cramps, diarrhea, nausea, vomiting.
Triamterene with hydrochlorothiazide	Give with food or milk 6 or more hr before bedtime.	Dry mouth, thirst, dehydration, nausea, vomiting, diarrhea, constipation. May alter glucose levels.
Immunosuppressants		
Azathioprine	Give with meals.	Nausea, vomiting, diarrhea, stomach pain, anorexia, sore throat, altered taste perceptions.
Cyclosporine	Give with water, juice, or milk. Give at same time each day.	Raises blood pressure. Nausea, vomiting, diarrhea, inflamed gums, anorexia. May induce anemia. May induce hyperglycemia.
Prednisone	Give with food or milk.	Fluid retention, stomach upset, peptic ulcers, blood glucose abnormalities, growth inhibition in children, decreased resistance to infection, weight gain. May decrease effects of insulin or antidiabetic medicine. May induce edema.

E

(continued)

■ TABLE E–1B
Administration and Common Nutrition-Related Side Effects of Selected Drugs   (continued)

Drug Classification and Name	Administration	Common Side Effects That May Influence Nutrition Status
Immunosuppressants (continued)		
Prednisone (continued)		Alters protein and carbohydrate metabolism. Decreases absorption of calcium and phosphorus.
Laxatives		
Bisacodyl	Do not give with milk or antacids.	Nausea, vomiting, abdominal cramps.
Castor oil	Give with juice or carbonated beverages to mask taste.	Nausea, abdominal cramps. May reduce absorption of fat-soluble vitamins.
Lactulose		Nausea, constipation, abdominal cramps.
Mineral oil	Give with juice or carbonated beverages to mask taste. Do not give with meals.	Nausea, abdominal cramps. May reduce absorption of fat-soluble vitamins.
Miscellaneous		
Colchicine	Give with meals to decrease GI distress.	Nausea, vomiting, diarrhea, abdominal pain.
Lithium carbonate	Give with food. Maintain consistent sodium intake daily.	Thirst, metallic taste.
Oral contraceptives	Give with food.	Nausea, edema, weight changes. May cause hyperglycemia, hypercalcemia, or folate deficiency.

Sources: *Nursing 91 Drug Handbook,* (Springhouse, PA: Springhouse Corporation, 1991) and D. E. Powers and A. O. Moore, *Food Medication Interaction,* (Phoenix, AR: Food Medication Interactions, 1989).
Note: The multitude of drugs and nutrients that interact are far too numerous to list in a nutrition textbook like this one. Indeed, whole books are available to cover the subject. The side effects shown in this table are common side effects. Other side effects can and do occur. This table provides only a sampling of interactions. More detailed texts should be consulted for the drugs you encounter in clinical practice.

■ *Growth Charts and Anthropometric Data*

Growth charts allow health care professionals to evaluate the growth and development of children from birth to 18 years of age. Chapter 19 (pp. 616–617) gives an example of how to use a growth chart. To assess parameters of growth and development for various gender and age groups, use the charts shown in Figures E-1 through E-6.

■ FIGURE E–1A
Girls: Birth to 36 Months Physical Growth NCHS Percentiles—Length and Weight for Age

**GIRLS: BIRTH TO 36 MONTHS
PHYSICAL GROWTH
NCHS PERCENTILES***

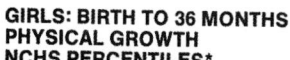

NAME _____   RECORD # _____

E

Adapted from: Hamill PVV, Drizd TA, Johnson CL, Reed RB, Roche AF, Moore WM: Physical growth: National Center for Health Statistics percentiles. AM J CLIN NUTR 32:607-629, 1979. Data from the Fels Longitudinal Study, Wright State University School of Medicine, Yellow Springs, Ohio.

© 1982 Ross Laboratories

DATE	AGE	LENGTH	WEIGHT	HEAD CIRC.	COMMENT

SIMILAC® WITH IRON
Infant Formula

ISOMIL®
Soy Protein Formula with Iron

Reprinted with permission
of Ross Laboratories

■ **FIGURE E–1B**

Girls: Birth to 36 Months Physical Growth NCHS Percentiles—Head Circumference for Age and Weight for Length

E

GIRLS: BIRTH TO 36 MONTHS PHYSICAL GROWTH NCHS PERCENTILES*

NAME _____ RECORD # _____

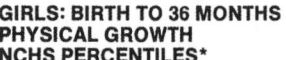

* Adapted from: Hamill PVV, Drizd TA, Johnson CL, Reed RB, Roche AF, Moore WM: Physical growth: National Center for Health Statistics percentiles. AM J CLIN NUTR 32:607-629, 1979. Data from the Fels Longitudinal Study, Wright State University School of Medicine, Yellow Springs, Ohio.

© 1982 Ross Laboratories

■ FIGURE E–2A
Boys: Birth to 36 Months Physical
Growth NCHS Percentiles—Length
and Weight for Age

**BOYS: BIRTH TO 36 MONTHS
PHYSICAL GROWTH
NCHS PERCENTILES***

NAME _____   RECORD # _____

*Adapted from: Hamill PVV, Drizd TA, Johnson CL, Reed RB,
Roche AF, Moore WM: Physical growth: National Center for Health
Statistics percentiles. AM J CLIN NUTR 32:607-629, 1979. Data
from the Fels Longitudinal Study, Wright State University School of
Medicine, Yellow Springs, Ohio.

© 1982 Ross Laboratories

■ FIGURE E-2B

Boys: Birth to 36 Months Physical Growth NCHS Percentiles—Head Circumference for Age and Weight for Length

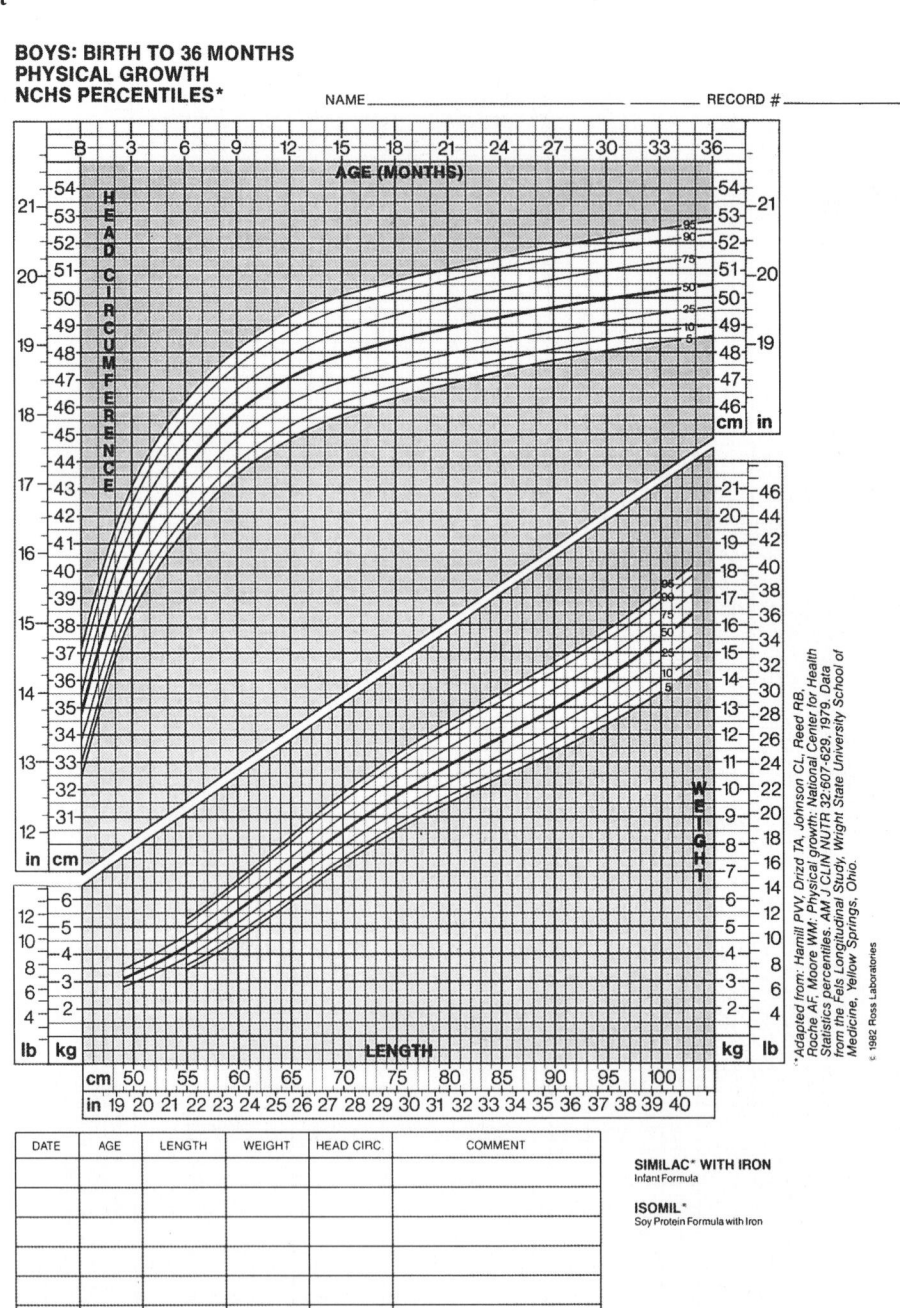

■ FIGURE E-3
Girls: 2 to 18 Years Physical Growth
NCHS Percentiles—Height and
Weight for Age

GIRLS: 2 TO 18 YEARS
PHYSICAL GROWTH
NCHS PERCENTILES*

E

■ **FIGURE E–4**
Boys: 2 to 18 Years Physical Growth
NCHS Percentiles—Height and
Weight for Age

E

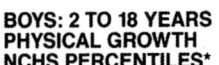

BOYS: 2 TO 18 YEARS
PHYSICAL GROWTH
NCHS PERCENTILES*

■ **FIGURE E–5**
Girls: Prepubescent Physical Growth
NCHS Percentiles—Weight for Height

GIRLS: PREPUBESCENT PHYSICAL GROWTH NCHS PERCENTILES*

NAME _____ RECORD # _____

DATE	AGE	STATURE	WEIGHT	COMMENT

Adapted from: Hamill PVV, Drizd TA, Johnson CL, Reed RB, Roche AF, Moore WM. Physical growth: National Center for Health Statistics percentiles. AM J CLIN NUTR 32:607-629, 1979 Data from the National Center for Health Statistics (NCHS) Hyattsville, Maryland.

© 1982 Ross Laboratories

■ **FIGURE E–6**
Boys: Prepubescent Physical Growth
NCHS Percentiles—Weight for Height

E

■ TABLE E-2
How to Determine Body Frame by Elbow Breadth

To make a simple approximation of frame size, do the following. Extend the arm, and bend the forearm upward at a 90° angle. Keep the fingers straight, and turn the inside of the wrist away from the body. Place the thumb and index finger on the two prominent bones on *either side* of the elbow. Measure the space between the fingers against a ruler or a tape measure.[a] Compare the measurements with the following standards.

These standards represent the elbow measurements for medium-framed men and women of various heights. Measurements smaller than those listed indicate a small frame, and larger measurements indicate a large frame.

Men		**Women**	
Height in 1-Inch Heels	Elbow Breadth	Height in 1-Inch Heels	Elbow Breadth
5 ft 2 inches to 5 ft 3 inches	2½ to 2⅞ inches	4 ft 10 inches to 4 ft 11 inches	2¼ to 2½ inches
5 ft 4 inches to 5 ft 7 inches	2⅝ to 2⅞ inches	5 ft 0 inches to 5 ft 3 inches	2¼ to 2½ inches
5 ft 8 inches to 5 ft 11 inches	2¾ to 3 inches	5 ft 4 inches to 5 ft 7 inches	2⅜ to 2⅝ inches
6 ft 0 inches to 6 ft 3 inches	2¾ to 3⅛ inches	5 ft 8 inches to 5 ft 11 inches	2⅜ to 2⅝ inches
6 ft 4 inches and over	2⅞ to 3¼ inches	6 ft 0 inches and over	2½ to 2¾ inches

[a]For the most accurate measurement, measure elbow breadth with a caliper.

Source: Metropolitan Life Insurance Company.

■ TABLE E-3
Frame Size from Height-Wrist Circumference Ratios (r)[a]

Frame Size	Male r Values	Female r Values
Small	>10.4	>11.0
Medium	9.6–10.4	10.1–11.0
Large	<9.6	<10.1

[a]$r = \dfrac{\text{height (cm)}}{\text{wrist circumference (cm)}^b}$.

[b]The wrist is measured where it bends (distal to the styloid process), on the right arm (see Figure E-7).

Source: Adapted from J. P. Grant, Patient selection, *Handbook of Total Parenteral Nutrition* (Philadelphia: Saunders, 1980), p. 15.

■ FIGURE E-7
Wrist Circumference

place tape here

Styloid process ("wristbone")

In adults, assessors evaluate weight for height. To use most height-weight tables, the assessor must determine the client's frame size. Tables E-2 and E-3 present two methods of determining frame size, and Figure E-7 shows how to measure the wrist when it is used to determine frame size. Another method of assessing body weight in adults is the body mass index (BMI). Figure E-8 (on the next page) presents a nomogram for BMI.

Fatfold measurements assist health care professionals in evaluating the composition of body weight. As already explained in Chapter 19, a lean tissue measure can be computed from the triceps fatfold measurement together with the midarm circumference measurement: the midarm muscle circumference (see pp. 621–622). Table E-4 gives triceps fatfold percentile standards, Table E-5 shows the midarm muscle circumference percentile standards, and Figure E-9 illustrates a nomogram method for determining midarm muscle circumference from these two measures (see pp. E-23 and E-24).

E

■ **FIGURE E–8**

Nomogram for Body Mass Index (BMI)

Weights and heights are without clothing. With clothes, add 5 lb for men or 3 lb for women, and 1 inch in height for shoes. Draw a straight line, or place a ruler, from your height (left) to your weight (right). At the point where it crosses the BMI line, read you BMI. The accompanying table in the margin indicates the BMI used to define cutoff points and the inside back covers present this information graphically.

Source: From the 1983 Metroplitan Life Insurance Company tables, designed by B. T. Burton and W. R. Roster, Health implications of obesity, and NIH Consensus Development Conference, *Journal of the American Dietetic Association* 85 (1985): 1117–1121.

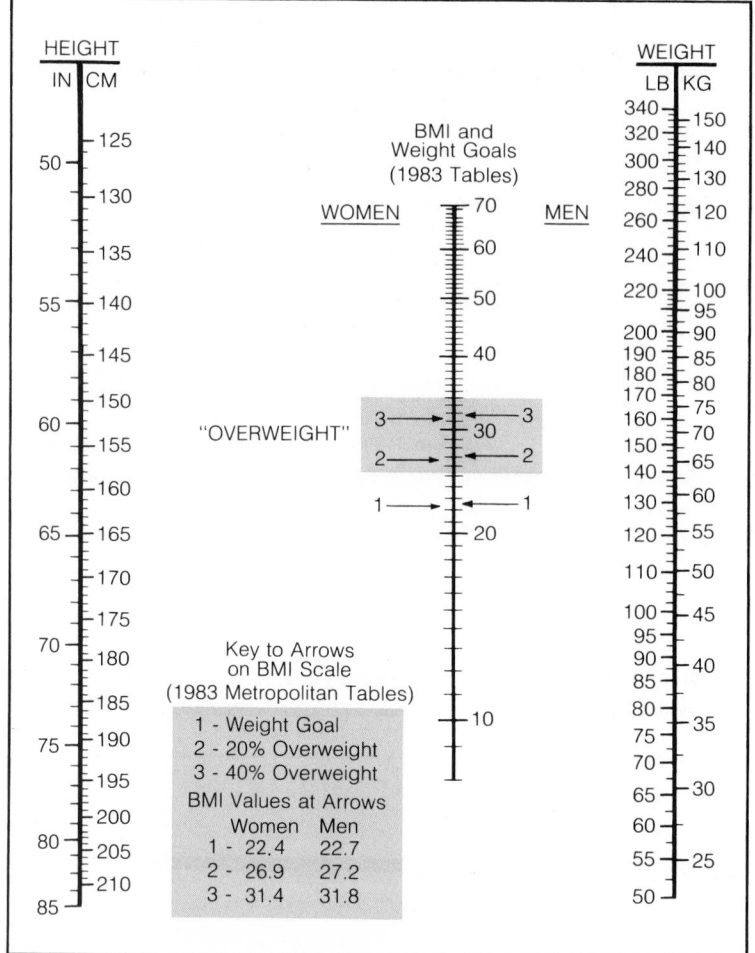

	Men	Women
Underweight	<20.7	<19.1
Acceptable weight	20.7 to 27.8	19.1 to 27.3
Overweight	≥27.8	≥27.3
Severe overweight	≥31.1	≥32.3
Morbid obesity	≥45.4	≥44.8

■ TABLE E-4
Triceps Fatfold Percentiles (millimeters)

	Male					Female				
Age	5th	25th	50th	75th	95th	5th	25th	50th	75th	95th
1-1.9	6	8	10	12	16	6	8	10	12	16
2-2.9	6	8	10	12	15	6	9	10	12	16
3-3.9	6	8	10	11	15	7	9	11	12	15
4-4.9	6	8	9	11	14	7	8	10	12	16
5-5.9	6	8	9	11	15	6	8	10	12	18
6-6.9	5	7	8	10	16	6	8	10	12	16
7-7.9	5	7	9	12	17	6	9	11	13	18
8-8.9	5	7	8	10	16	6	9	12	15	24
9-9.9	6	7	10	13	18	8	10	13	16	22
10-10.9	6	8	10	14	21	7	10	12	17	27
11-11.9	6	8	11	16	24	7	10	13	18	28
12-12.9	6	8	11	14	28	8	11	14	18	27
13-13.9	5	7	10	14	26	8	12	15	21	30
14-14.9	4	7	9	14	24	9	13	16	21	28
15-15.9	4	6	8	11	24	8	12	17	21	32
16-16.9	4	6	8	12	22	10	15	18	22	31
17-17.9	5	6	8	12	19	10	13	19	24	37
18-18.9	4	6	9	13	24	10	15	18	22	30
19-24.9	4	7	10	15	22	10	14	18	24	34
25-34.9	5	8	12	16	24	10	16	21	27	37
35-44.9	5	8	12	16	23	12	18	23	29	38
45-54.9	6	8	12	15	25	12	20	25	30	40
55-64.9	5	8	11	14	22	12	20	25	31	38
65-74.9	4	8	11	15	22	12	18	24	29	36

Note: Measurements sometimes fall between the percentiles shown here and require you to estimate the percentile given the information provided in this table. For example, a measurement of 7 mm for a 27-year-old male would be about the 20th percentile.

Source: Adapted from A. R. Frisancho, New norms of upper limb fat and muscle areas for assessment of nutritional status, *American Journal of Clinical Nutrition* 34 (1981): 2540-2545.

■ TABLE E-5
Midarm Muscle Circumference Percentiles (centimeters)

	Male					Female				
Age	5th	25th	50th	75th	95th	5th	25th	50th	75th	95th
1-1.9	11.0	11.9	12.7	13.5	14.7	10.5	11.7	12.4	13.9	14.3
2-2.9	11.1	12.2	13.0	14.0	15.0	11.1	11.9	12.6	13.3	14.7
3-3.9	11.7	13.1	13.7	14.3	15.3	11.3	12.4	13.2	14.0	15.2
4-4.9	12.3	13.3	14.1	14.8	15.9	11.5	12.8	13.6	14.4	15.7
5-5.9	12.8	14.0	14.7	15.4	16.9	12.5	13.4	14.2	15.1	16.5
6-6.9	13.1	14.2	15.1	16.1	17.7	13.0	13.8	14.5	15.4	17.1
7-7.9	13.7	15.1	16.0	16.8	19.0	12.9	14.2	15.1	16.0	17.6
8-8.9	14.0	15.4	16.2	17.0	18.7	13.8	15.1	16.0	17.1	19.4
9-9.9	15.1	16.1	17.0	18.3	20.2	14.7	15.8	16.7	18.0	19.8
10-10.9	15.6	16.6	18.0	19.1	22.1	14.8	15.9	17.0	18.0	19.7
11-11.9	15.9	17.3	18.3	19.5	23.0	15.0	17.1	18.1	19.6	22.3
12-12.9	16.7	18.2	19.5	21.0	24.1	16.2	18.0	19.1	20.1	22.0
13-13.9	17.2	19.6	21.1	22.6	24.5	16.9	18.3	19.8	21.1	24.0
14-14.9	18.9	21.2	22.3	24.0	26.4	17.4	19.0	20.1	21.6	24.7
15-15.9	19.9	21.8	23.7	25.4	27.2	17.5	18.9	20.2	21.5	24.4
16-16.9	21.3	23.4	24.9	26.9	29.6	17.0	19.0	20.2	21.6	24.9
17-17.9	22.4	24.5	25.8	27.3	31.2	17.5	19.4	20.5	22.1	25.7
18-18.9	22.6	25.2	26.4	28.3	32.4	17.4	19.1	20.2	21.5	24.5
19-24.9	23.8	25.7	27.3	28.9	32.1	17.9	19.5	20.7	22.1	24.9
25-34.9	24.3	26.4	27.9	29.8	32.6	18.3	19.9	21.2	22.8	26.4
35-44.9	24.7	26.9	28.6	30.2	32.7	18.6	20.5	21.8	23.6	27.2
45-54.9	23.9	26.5	28.1	30.0	32.6	18.7	20.6	22.0	23.8	27.4
55-64.9	23.6	26.0	27.8	29.5	32.0	18.7	20.9	22.5	24.4	28.0
65-74.9	22.3	25.1	26.8	28.4	30.6	18.5	20.8	22.5	24.4	27.9

Source: Adapted from A. R. Frisancho, New norms of upper limb fat and muscle areas for assessment of nutritional status, *American Journal of Clinical Nutrition* 34 (1981): 2540-2545.

E

E

■ **FIGURE E–9**

Nomograms for Determination of Midarm Muscle Circumference

To obtain arm muscle circumference using either nomogram, lay a ruler between values of arm circumference and fatfold, and read off arm muscle circumference.

Source: Reproduced with permission from J. Gurney and D. Jelliffe, Arm anthropometry in nutritional assessment; nomogram for rapid calculation of muscle circumference and cross-sectional muscle and fat areas, *American Journal of Clinical Nutrition* 26 (1973): 912, as adapted by A. Grant, *Nutritional Assessment Guidelines*, 2nd ed., 1979 (available from Anne Grant, Box 25057, Northgate Station, Seattle, WA 98125).

■ *Functional Tests of Nutrition Status*

Nutrition assessors sometimes use functional tests of nutrition status to identify nutrient deficiencies. One such test uses a dynamometer (described in Chapter 19) to measure hand grip strength (see p. 625). Like all assessment methods, following instructions carefully helps to ensure accurate measures. To measure hand grip strength, the assessor asks the client to squeeze the dynamometer as tightly as possible, takes three or four measurements, and records the highest value measured. Measurements can be taken on either the dominant or nondominant arm. Table E-6 shows the lower limits of acceptable hand grip strength in males and females based on age.

■ *Laboratory Tests of Nutrition Status*

As Chapter 19 pointed out, urine and blood tests provide valuable information in a nutrition assessment. Two urine tests—creatinine excretion and urine urea nitrogen—require a 24-hour urine collection, and, therefore, are not routinely used.

Collecting a 24-hour urine sample presents many problems. Much effort is wasted if everyone involved does not conscientiously follow proper techniques. The collection of urine and recording of food intake data requires client cooperation. The client must receive thorough instructions on how to collect and save all urine samples, and must be advised to call for help if needed. If even one urine sample is spilled or discarded, the test is invalid.

Most hospitals have a standard time for beginning urinary collections (often, between 6:00 AM and 6:00 PM). For nitrogen balance studies, food intake must also be recorded during the exact same time period. All nurses caring for the client on all shifts must record, or ensure that the client records, food intake data carefully. Each urine sample is added to the collection container and refrigerated until the collection is complete.

To calculate the creatinine-height index (CHI) from the measured urinary creatinine and the client's height, use the following equation:

$$CHI = \frac{\text{Measured urinary creatinine (24-hour sample)}}{\text{Standard creatinine excretion for height and sex}} \times 100.$$

For example, to calculate the CHI in a man of medium frame, 5 ft 8 inches tall, who excretes 1,090 mg of creatinine in 24 hours, follow these steps:

■ Look up the standard creatinine excretion (Table E-7).

In this example, the standard creatinine excretion is 1.56 g or 1,560 mg.

■ Use this information to complete the CHI equation:

$$CHI = \frac{1,090 \text{ mg}}{1,560 \text{ mg}} \times 100 = 70\%.$$

Based on the CHI, the man in this example has a skeletal muscle mass 70 percent of that considered typical for a man of his height. Table E-8 shows the standard creatinine excretions for women.

■ **TABLE E–6**
Lower Limits of Acceptable Grip Strength

Age	Female grip strength (kg)	Male grip strength (kg)
15	28	42
20	29	43
25	30	44
30	30	45
35	30	45
40	30	45
45	30	45
50	29	45
55	28	44
60	27	43
65	25	41
70	23	39
75	20	37
80	18	35
85	15	32
90	11	29
95	8	26

Source: Reprinted by permission of the American Society of Parenteral and Enteral Nutrition, Silver Spring, MD 20879, from A. R. Webb, L.A. Newman, M. Taylor, and J. B. Keogh, Hand grip dynamometry as a predicator of postoperative complications: Reappraisal using age standardized grip strengths, *Journal of Parenteral and Enteral Nutrition* 13 (1989): 30–33.

Note: The figures shown in this table represent 85% of the standard for each age and gender category.

E

■ TABLE E–7
Creatinine-Height Index Standards for Men

Height		Small Frame			Medium Frame			Large Frame		
			Creatinine			Creatinine			Creatinine	
in	cm	Ideal Weight (kg)	(g/24 h)	(mmol/d)[a]	Ideal Weight (kg)	(g/24 h)	(mmol/d)[a]	Ideal Weight (kg)	(g/24 h)	(mmol/d)[a]
61	154.9	52.7	1.21	10.7	56.1	1.29	11.4	60.7	1.40	12.4
62	157.5	54.1	1.24	11.0	57.7	1.33	11.8	62.0	1.43	12.6
63	160.0	55.4	1.27	11.2	59.1	1.36	12.0	63.6	1.46	12.9
64	162.5	56.8	1.31	11.6	60.4	1.39	12.3	65.2	1.50	13.3
65	165.1	58.4	1.34	11.8	62.0	1.43	12.6	66.8	1.54	13.6
66	167.6	60.2	1.39	12.3	63.9	1.47	13.0	68.9	1.59	14.1
67	170.2	62.0	1.43	12.6	65.9	1.52	13.4	71.1	1.64	14.5
68	172.7	63.9	1.47	13.0	67.7	1.56	13.8	72.9	1.68	14.9
69	175.3	65.9	1.52	13.4	69.5	1.60	14.1	74.8	1.72	15.2
70	177.8	67.7	1.56	13.8	71.6	1.65	14.6	76.8	1.77	15.6
71	180.3	69.5	1.60	14.1	73.6	1.69	14.9	79.1	1.82	16.1
72	182.9	71.4	1.64	14.5	75.7	1.74	15.4	81.1	1.87	16.5
73	185.4	73.4	1.69	14.9	77.7	1.79	15.8	83.4	1.92	17.0
74	187.9	75.2	1.73	15.3	80.0	1.85	16.4	85.7	1.97	17.4
75	190.5	77.0	1.77	15.6	82.3	1.89	16.7	87.7	2.02	17.9

[a]To convert urinary creatinine measures (g/24 h) to standard international units (mmol/d) multiply by 8.840.

Source: A. Grant and S. DeHoog, *Nutritional Assessment and Support,* 3rd ed., 1985 (available from P.O. Box 25057, Northgate Station, Seattle, WA 98125).

■ TABLE E–8
Creatinine-Height Index Standards for Women

Height		Small Frame			Medium Frame			Large Frame		
			Creatinine			Creatinine			Creatinine	
in	cm	Ideal Weight (kg)	(g/24 h)	(mmol/d)[a]	Ideal Weight (kg)	(g/24 h)	(mmol/d)[a]	Ideal Weight (kg)	(g/24 h)	(mmol/d)[a]
56	142.2	43.2	0.79	7.0	46.1	0.83	7.3	50.7	0.91	8.0
57	144.8	44.3	0.80	7.1	47.3	0.85	7.5	51.8	0.93	8.2
58	147.3	45.4	0.82	7.2	48.6	0.88	7.8	53.2	0.96	8.5
59	149.8	46.8	0.84	7.4	50.0	0.90	8.0	54.5	0.98	8.7
60	152.4	48.2	0.87	7.7	51.4	0.93	8.2	55.9	1.01	8.9
61	154.9	49.5	0.89	7.9	52.7	0.95	8.4	57.3	1.03	9.1
62	157.5	50.9	0.92	8.1	54.3	0.98	8.7	58.9	1.06	9.4
63	160.0	52.3	0.94	8.3	55.9	1.01	8.9	60.6	1.09	9.6
64	162.5	53.9	0.97	8.6	57.9	1.04	9.2	62.5	1.13	10.0
65	165.1	55.7	1.00	8.8	59.8	1.08	9.5	64.3	1.16	10.3
66	167.6	57.5	1.04	9.2	61.6	1.11	9.8	66.1	1.19	10.5
67	170.2	59.3	1.07	9.5	63.4	1.14	10.1	67.9	1.22	10.8
68	172.7	61.4	1.11	9.8	65.2	1.17	10.3	70.0	1.26	11.1
69	175.2	63.2	1.14	10.1	67.0	1.21	10.7	72.0	1.30	11.5
70	177.8	65.0	1.17	10.3	68.9	1.24	11.0	74.1	1.33	11.8

[a]To convert urinary creatinine measures (g/24 h) to standard international units (mmol/d) multiply by 8.840.

Source: A. Grant and S. DeHoog, *Nutritional Assessment and Support,* 3rd ed., 1985 (available from P.O. Box 25057, Northgate Station, Seattle, WA 98125).

E

Other laboratory tests help detect iron deficiency. Chapter 19 (pp. 631–634) describes the tests used in assessing iron status and provides standard values for hemoglobin and hematocrit. Tables E-9 through E-12 provide standards for other measures of iron status: serum ferritin, serum iron, transferrin saturation, erythrocyte protoporphyrin, and mean corpuscular volume.

■ *Physical Findings*

Finally, the nutrition assessor uses physical examinations to search for signs of nutrient deficiency or toxicity. Table 19–13 in Chapter 19 presents a summary of physical findings organized by body system; Table E-13 presents a summary of symptoms of vitamin and mineral imbalances organized by nutrients.

Nutrition assessments vary in their depth and accuracy. While for some cases, minimal measures may be all that is necessary, but for clients who are very ill or who show signs of nutrition problems, thorough tests must be conducted.

■ TABLE E–9
Standards for Serum Ferritin

Group	Deficient (ng/ml)
Children (3 – 14 yr)	<10
Adolescents and adults	<12
Pregnant women	<10

■ TABLE E–10
Standards for Serum Iron

Age	Sex	Deficient		Acceptable	
		(μg/100 ml)	(μmol/L)	(μg/100 ml)	(μmol/L)
< 2 yr	(M-F)	< 30	< 5.3	30 or >	5.3 or >
2 – 5 yr	(M-F)	< 40	< 7.1	40 or >	7.1 or >
6 – 12 yr	(M-F)	< 50	< 8.9	50 or >	8.9 or >
> 12 yr	(M)	< 60	< 10.7	60 or >	10.7 or >
	(F)	< 40	< 7.1	40 or >	7.1 or >

Note: To convert serum iron values (μg/100 ml) to international standard units, (μmol/L), multiply by 0.1791.

■ TABLE E–11
Standards for Percent Transferrin Saturation

Age	Sex	Deficient	Acceptable
< 2 yr	(M-F)	< 15	15 or >
2–12 yr	(M-F)	< 20	20 or >
> 13 yr	(M)	< 20	20 or >
	(F)	< 15	15 or >

E

■ TABLE E–12
Standards for Erythrocyte Protoporphyrin and Mean Corpuscular Volume

Age	Erythrocyte Protoporphyrin (μg/dL RBC)	MCV (fL)
1–2 yr	> 80	< 73
3–4 yr	> 75	< 75
5–10 yr	> 70	< 76
11–14 yr	> 70	< 78
15–74 yr	> 70	< 80

■ TABLE E–13
Symptoms of Vitamin and Mineral Imbalances

Vitamin Name	Deficiency Disease Name	Deficiency Symptoms	Toxicity Symptoms
		Bones/Teeth[a]	
Vitamin A	Hypovitaminosis A	Cessation of bone growth, change in shapes of bones, painful joints; malfunctioning of enamel-forming cells, development of cracks in teeth and tendency to decay, atrophy of dentin-forming cells	Increased activity of osteoclasts[b] causing decalcification, joint pain, fragility, stunted growth, and thickening of long bones; increase of pressure inside skull, mimicking brain tumor; headaches
		Blood	
		Microcytic anemia, often masked by dehydration	Loss of hemoglobin and potassium by red blood cells, cessation of menstruation, slowed clotting time, easily induced bleeding
		Eyes[c]	
		Night blindness, change in epithelial tissue caused by failure to secrete mucopolysaccharide (hyperkeratinization), drying (xerosis), triangular gray spots on eye (Bitot's spots), irreversible drying (keratomalacia), and degeneration of the cornea causing blindness (most severe)	
		Skin[d]	
		Plugging of hair follicles with keratin, forming white lumps (hyperkeratosis)	Dryness; itching; peeling; rashes; dry, scaling lips; cracking and bleeding of lips; nosebleeds; loss of hair; brittle nails
		Digestive System	
		Changes in lining, diarrhea	Nausea, vomiting, abdominal pain, diarrhea, weight loss
		Immune System	
		Depression of immune reactions	Stimulation of immune reactions
		Nervous/Muscular System	
		Brain and spinal cord growth too fast for stunted skull and spine, paralysis caused by injury to brain and nerves	Loss of appetite, irritability, fatigue, insomnia, restlessness, headache, blurred vision, nausea, vomiting, muscle weakness, interference with thyroxin

■ **TABLE E–13**
Symptoms of Vitamin and Mineral Imbalances   (continued)

Vitamin Name	Deficiency Disease Name	Deficiency Symptoms	Toxicity Symptoms

Respiratory Tract

Vitamin A
(continued)

Changes in lining, infections

Urogenital Tract

Changes in lining that favor calcium deposition, resulting in kidney stones and bladder disorders; infections of bladder and kidney; infections of vagina

Reproductive System

Amenorrhea[e]

Liver[f]

Jaundice,[g] enlargement, massive accumulation of fat and vitamin A

Spleen

Enlargement

Bones/Teeth

Vitamin D	Rickets, osteomalacia	*Rickets* Faulty calcification, resulting in misshapen bones (bowing of legs) and retarded growth; enlargement of ends of long bones (knees, wrists); deformities of ribs (bowed, with beads or knobs);[h] delayed closing of fontanel, resulting in rapid enlargement of head (see accompanying figure); slow eruption of teeth; teeth not well formed, with a tendency to decay	*Osteomalacia* Softening effect; deformities of limbs, spine, thorax, and pelvis; demineralization; pain in pelvis, lower back, and legs; bone fractures

Increased calcium withdrawal

Fontanel
A fontanel is the open space in the top of a baby's skull before the bones have grown to-gether. In rick-ets, closing of the fontanel is delayed.

Posterior fontanel normally closes by the end of the first year.

Anterior fontanel normally closes by the end of the second year.

Blood

Decreased calcium and/or phosphorus	Decreased calcium and/or phosphorus, increased alkaline phosphatase[i]	Increased calcium and phosphorus concentrations

Nervous/Muscular Systems

Lax muscles resulting in protrusion of abdomen; muscle spasms	Involuntary twitching, muscle spasms	Loss of appetite, headache, weakness, fatigue, excessive thirst, irritability, apathy

E

(continued)

■ TABLE E–13
Symptoms of Vitamin and Mineral Imbalances   (continued)

Vitamin Name	Deficiency Disease Name	Deficiency Symptoms	Toxicity Symptoms
		Excretory System	
Vitamin D (continued)		Increased calcium in stools, decreased calcium in urine	Increased excretion of calcium in urine, kidney stones, irreversible renal damage
		Other	
		Abnormally high secretion of parathormone	Calcification of soft tissues (blood vessels, kidneys, heart, lungs, tissues around joints), death
		Blood/Circulatory System	
Vitamin E		Red blood cell breakage,[j] anemia	Augments effects of anticlotting medication
		Digestive System	
			General discomfort
		Nervous/Muscular Systems	
		Degeneration, weakness, difficulty walking, severe pain in calf muscles	Headache, weakness, dizziness, fatigue, visual abnormalties
		Other	
		Fibrocystic breast disease	
		Blood/Circulatory System	
Vitamin K		Hemorrhaging	Interference with anticlotting medication, possible jaundice caused by vitamin K analogues
		Blood/Circulatory System	
Thiamin	Beriberi	Edema, enlarged heart, abnormal heart rhythms, heart failure	Rapid pulse
		Nervous/Muscular Systems	
		Degeneration, wasting, weakness, painful calf muscles, low morale, difficulty walking, loss of ankle and knee jerk reflexes, mental confusion, paralysis	Weakness, headaches, insomnia, irritability
		Mouth, Gums, Tongue	
Riboflavin	Ariboflavinosis	Cracks at corners of mouth,[k] magenta tongue	
		Nervous System and Eyes	
		Hypersensitivity to light,[l] reddening of cornea	
		Other	
		Skin rash	Interference with anticancer medication

■ **TABLE E–13**
Symptoms of Vitamin and Mineral Imbalances   (continued)

Vitamin Name	Deficiency Disease Name	Deficiency Symptoms	Toxicity Symptoms
Niacin	Pellagra	**Digestive System**	
		Diarrhea	Diarrhea, heartburn, nausea, ulcer irritation, vomiting
		Mouth, Gums, Tongue	
			Inflamed, swollen, smooth tongue[m]
		Nervous System	
		Irritability, loss of appetite, weakness, dizziness, mental confusion progressing to psychosis or delirium	
		Skin	
		Bilateral symmetrical dermatitis, especially on areas exposed to sun	Painful flush and rash, itching, burning, excessive sweating
		Other	
			Abnormal liver function, low blood pressure
Vitamin B$_6$		**Blood/Circulatory System**	
		Microcytic anemia	Bloating
		Mouth, Gums, Tongue	
		Smooth tongue,[m] cracked corners of the mouth[k]	
		Nervous/Muscular Systems	
		Abnormal brain wave pattern, irritability, muscle twitching, convulsions	Depression, fatigue, irritability, headaches, numbness, damage to nerves leading to loss of reflexes and sensation, difficulty walking
		Skin	
		Irritation of sweat glands, dermatitis	
		Other	
		Kidney stones	
Folate		**Blood/Circulatory System**	
		Macrocytic or megaloblastic anemia	
		Digestive System	
		Heartburn, diarrhea (loss of villi and their enzymes), constipation	Diarrhea
		Immune System	
		Suppression, frequent infections	
		Mouth, Gums, Tongue	
		Smooth, red tongue[m]	
		Nervous System	
		Depression, mental confusion, fainting, fatigue	Insomnia, irritability

(continued)

■ **TABLE E–13**
Symptoms of Vitamin and Mineral Imbalances   (continued)

Vitamin Name	Deficiency Disease Name	Deficiency Symptoms	Toxicity Symptoms
Folate (continued)			**Other** Masking of vitamin B_{12}– deficiency symptoms
Vitamin B_{12}	Pernicious anemia[n]	**Blood/Circulatory System** Macrocytic or megaloblastic anemia	
		Mouth, Gums, Tongue Smooth tongue[m]	
		Nervous System Fatigue, degeneration of peripheral nerves progressing to paralysis	
		Skin Hypersensitivity	
Pantothenic acid		**Digestive System** Vomiting, intestinal distress	Occasional diarrhea
		Nervous System Insomnia, fatigue	
			Other Water retention (infrequent)
Biotin		**Blood/Circulatory System** Abnormal heart action	
		Digestive System Loss of appetite, nausea	
		Nervous/Muscular Systems Depression, muscle pain, weakness, fatigue	
		Skin Drying, scaly dermatitis, loss of hair	
Vitamin C	Scurvy	**Blood/Circulatory System** Microcytic anemia, atherosclerotic plaques, pinpoint hemorrhages	Blood cell breakage in certain racial groups[o]
			Digestive System Nausea, abdominal cramps, diarrhea
		Immune System Depression, frequent infections	
		Mouth, Gums, Tongue Bleeding gums, loosened teeth	
		Nervous/Muscular Systems Muscle degeneration and pain, hysteria, depression	Headache, fatigue, insomnia

■ TABLE E–13
Symptoms of Vitamin and Mineral Imbalances   (continued)

Vitamin/Mineral Name	Deficiency Symptoms	Toxicity Symptoms
	Skeletal System	
Vitamin C (continued)	Bone fragility, joint pain	
	Skin	
	Rough skin, blotchy bruises	Hot flashes, rashes
	Other	
	Failure of wounds to heal	Interference with medical tests, aggravation of gout symptoms, excessive urination, kidney stones,[p] (deficiency symptoms may appear at first on withdrawal of high doses)
Major Minerals		
Calcium	Stunted growth in children, implicated in bone loss (osteoporosis) in adults	Excess calcium is excreted except in hormonal imbalance states (not caused by nutritional deficiency)
Phosphorus	Deficiency unknown	
Magnesium	Weakness; confusion; depressed pancreatic hormone secretion; if extreme, convulsions, bizarre muscle movements (especially of the eye and facial muscles), hallucinations, and difficulty in swallowing;[q] in children, growth failure	Not known; large doses have been taken in the form of the laxative Epsom salts without ill effects except diarrhea
Sodium	Muscle cramps, mental apathy, loss of appetite	Hypertension[r]
Chloride	Growth failure in children; muscle cramps, mental apathy, loss of appetite	Vomiting
Potassium	Deficiency accompanies dehydration; causes muscular weakness, paralysis, and confusion	Muscular weakness; vomiting; if given into a vein, can stop the heart
Sulfur	None known; protein deficiency would occur first	Would occur only if sulfur amino acids were eaten in excess; this (in animals) depresses growth
Trace Minerals		
	Eyes	
Iron	Blue sclerae	
	GI Tract	
⟨	Lactose intolerance, and possibly intolerance to other sugars; increased risk of lead and cadmium poisoning	
	Immune System	
	Reduced resistance to infection (lowered immunity)	Infections

(continued)

■ TABLE E–13
Symptoms of Vitamin and Mineral Imbalances   (continued)

Mineral Name	Deficiency Symptoms	Toxicity Symptoms
	Nervous/Muscular Systems	
Iron (continued)	Reduced work productivity, tolerance to work, and voluntary work; reduced physical fitness; weakness; fatigue; impaired cognitive function (children); reduced learning ability; increased distractibility (inability to pay attention); impaired visual discrimination; impaired reactivity and coordination (infants)	
	Skin	
	Itching; pale nailbeds, eye membranes, and palm creases; concave nails; impaired wound healing	
	General	
	Reduced resistance to cold, inability to regulate body temperature, pica (clay eating, ice eating)	
	Blood	
Zinc	Tendency to atherosclerosis, elevated ammonia levels, decreased alkaline phosphatase, decreased insulin concentration	Anemia: reduced hemoglobin production
	Bones	
	Growth retardation, abnormal collagen synthesis	Growth in length, but without normal zinc content
	Cells/Metabolism	
	Decreased DNA synthesis, impaired cell division and protein synthesis	Raised LDL, lowered HDL
	Digestive System	
	Diarrhea, vomiting, decreased calcium and copper absorption	Reduced sense of smell, reduced sensitivity to the taste of salt, weight loss, delayed glucose absorption, diarrhea, nausea, impaired folate absorption
	Eyes	
	Night blindness	

E

■ TABLE E–13
Symptoms of Vitamin and Mineral Imbalances   (continued)

Mineral Name	Deficiency Symptoms	Toxicity Symptoms
Glandular System		
Zinc (continued)	Delayed onset of puberty, small gonads in males, decreased synthesis and release of testosterone, abnormal glucose tolerance, reduced synthesis of adrenocortical hormones, altered thyroid function	
Immune System		
	Altered skin test responses, reduced numbers of white blood cells and antibody-forming cells, thymus atrophy, increased susceptibility to infection	Fever, elevated white blood cell count
Kidney		
		Renal failure
Liver/Spleen		
	Enlargement	
Nervous/Muscular Systems		
	Anorexia (poor appetite), mental lethargy, irritability	Muscular pain and incoordination, heart muscle degeneration, exhaustion, dizziness, drowsiness
Reproductive System		
	Impaired reproductive function (rats), low sperm counts	Reproductive failure
Skin		
	Generalized hair loss; lesions; rough, dry appearance; slow healing of wounds and burns	
Iodine	Enlargement of the thyroid gland, weight gain, mental and physical retardation of an infant	Enlargement of the thyroid gland, depressed thyroid activity
Copper	Anemia, bone changes (rare in human beings)	Vomiting, diarrhea
Fluoride	Susceptibility to tooth decay	Fluorosis (discoloration of teeth), nausea, diarrhea, chest pain, itching, vomiting
Selenium	Anemia (rare); heart disease	Digestive system disorders, loss of hair and nails, skin lesions, nervous system disorders, tooth damage

E

(continued)

■ TABLE E–13
Symptoms of Vitamin and Mineral Imbalances   (continued)

Mineral Name	Deficiency Symptoms	Toxicity Symptoms
Chromium	Diabetes-like condition marked by an inability to use glucose normally; associated with coronary artery disease	Unknown as a nutrition disorder; occupational exposures damage skin and kidneys
Cobalt	Unknown in human beings except in vitamin B_{12} deficiency	Unknown as a nutrition disorder; occupational exposures damage skin and red blood cells
Molybdenum	Unknown	Enzyme inhibition
Manganese	(In animals): poor growth, nervous system disorders, reproductive abnormalities	Nervous system disorders

[a]Highlight 10 describes vitamin A's role in tooth formation in more detail.
[b]Osteoclasts are the cells that destroy bone during its growth. Those that build bone are osteoblasts.
[c]The eyes' symptoms of vitamin A deficiency are collectively known as *xerophthalmia*.
[d]A related toxicity condition, hypercarotenemia, is caused by the accumulation of too much of the vitamin A precursor beta-carotene in the blood, which turns the skin noticeably yellow. Hypercarotenemia is not, strickly speaking, a toxicity symptom.
[e]Elevated serum carotene concentrations are associated with amenorrhea.
[f]If liver impairment is severe, the "classic" signs seen in skin and hair may be masked.
[g]A symptom of liver disease, in which bile and related pigments spill into the bloodstream and the skin yellows, is *jaundice* (JAWN-diss).
[h]Bowing of the ribs causes the symptom known as *pigeon breast*. The beads that form on the ribs resemble rosary beads; thus this symptom is known as *rachitic* (ra-KIT-ik) *rosary* ("the rosary of rickets").
[i]Alkaline phosphatase is an enzyme in the blood that rises during bone resorption.
[j]The breaking of red blood cells is called *erythrocyte hemolysis*.
[k]Cracks at the corners of the mouth are termed *cheilosis* (kee-LOH-sis).
[l]Hypersensitivity to light is *photophobia*.
[m]Smoothness of the tongue is caused by loss of its surface structures and is termed *glossitis* (gloss-EYE-tis).
[n]The name *pernicious anemia* refers to the vitamin B_{12} deficiency caused by lack of intrinsic factor, but not to that caused by inadequate dietary intake.
[o]Groups susceptible to vitamin C toxicity are Sephardic Jews, black Americans and Africans, and Asians.
[p]People who have a tendency toward gout and those who have a genetic abnormality that alters the break down of vitamin C are prone to forming kidney stones. Vitamin C is inactivated and degraded by several routes, and sometimes a product along the way is oxalate, which can form stones in the kidneys. People can also have oxalate crystals in their kidneys that are not due to vitamin C overdoses.
[q]A still more severe deficiency causes.tetany, an extreme, prolonged contraction of the muscles similar to that caused by low blood calcium.
[r]Chapter 28 describes the role of sodium in the development of hypertension.

E

Nutrition Resources

People interested in nutrition often want to know where, in their own town or county, they can find reliable nutrition information. Wherever you live, there are several sources you can turn to:

- The Department of Health may have a nutrition expert.
- The local extension agent is often an expert.
- The food editor of your local paper may be well informed.
- The dietitian at the local hospital had to fulfill a set of qualifications before he or she became an R.D. (see Highlight 2).
- There may be knowledgeable professors of nutrition or biochemistry at a nearby college or university.

The syndicated column on nutrition by J. Mayer and J. Dwyer, which appears in many newspapers, presents well-researched, reliable answers to current questions. The column by R. Alfin-Slater and D.B. Jelliffe is also accurate and trustworthy. In addition, you may be interested in building a nutrition library of your own. Books you can buy, journals you can subscribe to, and addresses you can write to for general information are given below.

■ Books

A 54-page list of references with critiques of each, *Nutrition References and Book Reviews*, is available for purchase from the Chicago Nutrition Association. (See "Addresses," below).

This 900-page paperback has a chapter on each of 58 topics, including energy, obesity, 32 nutrients, several diseases, malnutrition, growth and its assessment, immunity, alcohol, fiber, dental health, drugs, and toxins. The only major omissions seem to be nutrition and food intake and national nutrition status surveys. Watch for an update; these come out every several years. The most recent update is:

- *Nutrition Reviews' Present Knowledge in Nutrition*, 5th ed. (Washington, D.C.: Nutrition Foundation, 1984).

A scholarly 592-page volume originally printed as a special supplement to the *Journal of Nutrition* is:

- *Nutritional Requirements of Man: A Conspectus of Research* (New York: Nutrition Foundation, 1980).

The *Conspectus* has major review articles on human requirements for protein, amino acids, vitamin A, calcium, zinc, vitamin C, iron, folate, and copper.

This 1,694-page volume is a major technical reference book on nutrition topics. It contains encyclopedic articles on the nutrients, foods, the diet, metabolism, malnutrition, age-related needs, and nutrition in disease.

- R. S. Goodhart, M. E. Shils, and V. R. Young, eds., *Modern Nutrition in Health and Disease*, 7th ed. (Philadelphia: Lea and Febiger, 1988).

Another book that readers may wish to add to their libraries is the latest edition of *Recommended Dietary Allowances*, available from the National Academy of Sciences (see "Addresses," below). The Canadian equivalent is *Recommended Nutrient Intakes for Canadians*, available by mail from the Canadian Government Publishing Centre, Supply and Services Canada, Ottowa, Ontario K1A 0S9, Canada.

We also recommend our own book that explores current nutrition topics other than those treated here. The 5th edition is slated for publication in 1990:

- E. M. N. Hamilton, E. N. Whitney, and F. S. Sizer, *Nutrition: Concepts and Controversies*, 4th ed. (St. Paul, Minn.: West, 1988).

Another of our books provides information pertinent to each stage of life:

- L. K. DeBruyne and S. R. Rolfes, *Life Cycle Nutrition: Conception through Adolescence*, ed. E. N. Whitney (St. Paul, Minn.: West, 1989).

■ *Journals*

Nutrition Today, the publication of the Nutrition Today Society, is an excellent magazine for the interested layperson. It makes a point of raising controversial issues and providing a forum for conflicting opinions. References are seldom printed in the magazine but are available on request. Six issues per year are published. Order from the Director of Membership Services, Nutrition Today Society. (See "Addresses," below.)

The *Journal of the American Dietetic Association,* the official publication of the ADA, contains articles of interest to dietitians and nutritionists, news of legislative action on food and nutrition, and a very useful section of abstracts of articles from many other journals of nutrition and related areas. There are twelve issues per year, available from the American Dietetic Association. (See "Addresses," below.)

Nutrition Reviews, a publication of the Nutrition Foundation, Inc., does much of the work for the library researcher, compiling recent evidence on current topics and presenting extensive bibliographies. Twelve issues per year are available from the Nutrition Foundation. (See "Addresses," below.)

Nutrition and the M.D. is a monthly newsletter that provides up-to-date, easy-to-read, and practical information on nutrition for health care providers. It is available from PM, Inc. (See "Addresses," below.)

Other journals that deserve mention here are *Food Technology, Journal of Nutrition, American Journal of Clinical Nutrition,* and *Journal of Nutrition Education. FDA Consumer,* a government publication with many articles of interest to the consumer, is available from the Food and Drug Administration. (See "Addresses," below.) Many other journals of value are referred to throughout this book.

Some of this book's highlights, as well as other articles of interest to consumers, are available as individual booklets called *Nutrition Clinics.* You can write for a free publication list from the J. B. Lippincott Company. (See "Addresses," below.) Many of the other organizations listed below will also provide publication lists free on request.

■ *Addresses*

U.S. Government

The U.S. Department of Agriculture (USDA) has several divisions. The USDA's Food Safety and Inspection Service (FSIS) inspects and analyzes domestic and imported meat, poultry, and meat and poultry food products; establishes standards for, and approves recipes and labels of, processed meat and poultry products; and monitors the meat and poultry industries for violations of inspection laws. To obtain publications or ask questions, write or call:

- FSIS Consumer Inquiries
  USDA
  Washington, DC 20250
  (202) 472-4485
  USDA also maintains a Meat and Poultry Hotline:
  1-800-535-4555

The USDA's Agricultural Research Service (ARS) conducts research to fulfill the diverse needs of agricultural users—from farmers to consumers—in the areas of crop and animal production, protection, processing, and distribution; food safety and quality; and natural resources conservation. Write to the Information Division, ARS, USDA (same address).

The USDA's Human Nutrition Information Service (HNIS) maintains the USDA's Nutrient Data Bank; conducts the Nationwide Food Consumption Survey; monitors the nutrient content of the U.S. food supply; provides nutrition guidelines for education and action programs; collects and disseminates food and nutrition materials; and conducts nutrition education research. Write to:

- HNIS, USDA
  6505 Belcrest Road
  Federal Building No. 1, Room 325-A
  Hyattsville, MD 20782

The USDA's Food and Nutrition Service (FNS) administers the Food Stamp Program; the national School Lunch and School Breakfast programs; the Special Supplemental Food Program for Women, Infants, and Children (WIC); and the food distribution, Child Care Food, summer food service, and special milk programs. Write to:

- FNS, USDA
  500 12th Street SW
  Washington, DC 20250

The USDA's Agricultural Marketing Service (AMS) operates a variety of marketing programs and services—several of interest to consumers—that include developing grades and standards for the trading of food and other farm products and carrying out grading services on request from packers and processors; inspecting egg products for wholesomeness; administering marketing orders that aid in the marketing of milk, fruits, vegetables, and related specialty crops like nuts; and administering truth-in-seed labeling and other regulatory programs. Write to:

- Information Division
  AMS, USDA
  Washington, DC 20250

The USDA's *Food News for Consumers,* a quarterly newsletter, is available from the U.S. Government Printing Office (address below).

Other U.S. Government addresses are:

- Food and Drug Administration (FDA)
  5600 Fishers Lane
  Rockville, MD 20852
- The Food and Nutrition Information Education Resources Center (FNIERC)
  National Agriculture Library
  10301 Baltimore Boulevard, Room 304
  Beltsville, MD 20705
  (301) 344–3719
- National Academy of Sciences/National Research Council (NAS/NRC)
  2101 Constitution Avenue NW
  Washington, DC 20418
- National Center for Health Statistics (NCHS)
  U.S. Department of Health and Human Services (USDHHS)
  Public Health Service
  3700 East-West Highway
  Hyattsville, MD 20782
- U.S. Government Printing Office
  The Superintendent of Documents
  Washington, DC 20402

Canadian Government

- Department of Community Health
  1075 Ste-Foy Road, 7th Floor
  Quebec, Quebec G1S 2M1, Canada
- Home Economics Directorate
  880 Portage Avenue, 2nd Floor
  Winnipeg, Manitoba R3G 0P1, Canada
- Nutrition Programs
  446 Jeanne Mance Building
  Tunney's Pasture
  Ottawa, Ontario K1A 1B4, Canada
- Nutrition Services
  P.O. Box 488
  Halifax, Nova Scotia B3J 3R8, Canada
- Nutrition Services
  P.O. Box 6000
  Fredericton, New Brunswick E3B 5H1, Canada
- Public Health Resource Service
  15 Overlea Boulevard, 5th Floor
  Toronto, Ontario M4H 1A9, Canada

Consumer and Advocacy Groups

- Action for Children's Television (ACT)
  46 Austin Street
  Newtonville, MA 02160
- Center for Science in the Public Interest (CSPI)
  1755 S Street NW
  Washington, DC 20009
- Children's Foundation
  1420 New York Avenue NW, Suite 800
  Washington, DC 20005
- Community Nutrition Institute
  1146 19th Street NW
  Washington, DC 20036
- The Consumer Information Center
  Department 609K
  Pueblo, CO 81009
- Food Research and Action Center (FRAC)
  2011 I Street NW
  Washington, DC 20006
- National Council against Health Fraud, Inc.
  P.O. Box 1276
  Loma Linda, CA 92354
- National Self-Help Clearinghouse
  33 West 42nd Street, Room 1227
  New York, NY 10036
- Nutrition Information Service
  234 Webb Building
  Birmingham, AL 35294

Professional and Service Organizations

- Al-Anon Family Group Headquarters
  P.O. Box 182
  Madison Square Station
  New York, NY 10010
- Alcoholics Anonymous World Services
  P.O. Box 459
  Grand Central Station
  New York, NY 10017
- American Academy of Pediatrics
  P.O. Box 1034
  Evanston, IL 60204
- American College of Nutrition
  100 Manhattan Avenue #1606
  Union City, NJ 07087
- American Council on Science and Health
  1995 Broadway
  New York, NY 10023
- American Dental Association
  211 East Chicago Avenue
  Chicago, IL 60611
- American Diabetes Association
  1660 Duke Street
  Alexandria, VA 22314
  (800) 232–3472
- American Dietetic Association
  216 West Jackson Boulevard, Suite 800
  Chicago, IL 60606
  (312) 899–0040

F

- American Heart Association
  7320 Greenville Avenue
  Dallas, TX 75231
- American Home Economics Association
  2010 Massachusetts Avenue NW
  Washington, DC 20036
- American Institute for Cancer Research
  803 West Broad Street
  Falls Church, VA 22046
- American Institute of Nutrition
  9650 Rockville Pike
  Bethesda, MD 20014
- American Medical Association
  Nutrition Information Section
  535 North Dearborn Street
  Chicago, IL 60610
- American National Red Cross
  Food and Nutrition Consultant
  National Headquarters
  Washington, DC 20006
- American Public Health Association
  1015 Fifteenth Street NW
  Washington, DC 20005
- American Society for Clinical Nutrition
  9650 Rockville Pike
  Bethesda, MD 20014
- Canadian Diabetes Association
  78 Bond Street
  Toronto, Ontario M5B 2J8, Canada
  (416) 362–4440
- Canadian Dietetic Association
  480 University Avenue, Suite 601
  Toronto, Ontario M3G IV2, Canada
  (416) 596–0857
- Chicago Nutrition Association
  8158 Kedzie Avenue
  Chicago, IL 60652
- High Blood Pressure Information Center
  120/80, National Institutes of Health (NIH)
  Bethesda, MD 20205
  (703) 558–4880
- Institute of Food Technologists
  221 North LaSalle Street
  Chicago, IL 60601
- La Leche League International, Inc.
  9616 Minneapolis Avenue
  Franklin Park, IL 60131
- J. B. Lippincott Company
  East Washington Square
  Philadelphia, PA 19105
- March of Dimes Birth Defects Foundation (National Headquarters)
  1275 Mamaroneck Avenue
  White Plains, NY 10605

- National Clearinghouse for Alcohol Information
  Box 2345
  Rockville, MD 20850
- National Council on Alcoholism
  733 Third Avenue
  New York, NY 10017
- National Nutrition Consortium
  1635 P Street NW, Suite 1
  Washington, DC 20036
- National Osteoporosis Foundation
  2100 M Street NW, Suite 602
  Washington, DC 20037
  (202) 223–2226
- Nutrition Foundation, Inc.
  1126 Sixteenth Street NW, Suite 111
  Washington, DC 20036
- Nutrition Today Society
  428 East Preston Street
  Baltimore, MD 21202
- Overeaters Anonymous (OA)
  2190 190th Street
  Torrance, CA 90504
  (213) 320–7941
- PM, Inc. (Publisher of *Nutrition and the M.D.*)
  14545 Friar, #106
  Van Nuys, CA 91411
- Society for Nutrition Education
  1700 Broadway, Suite 300
  Oakland, CA 94612
- Technical Information Center
  Office on Smoking and Health
  5600 Fishers Lane, Room 1–16
  Rockville, MD 20857

Trade Organizations

Trade organizations produce many excellent free materials on nutrition and provide nutrition information about their products. Naturally, they also promote their own products. The student must learn to differentiate between slanted and valid information. We find the brief reviews in *Contemporary Nutrition* (General Mills), *Dairy Council Digest*, Ross Laboratories' *Dietetic Currents*, and R. A. Seelig's reviews from the United Fresh Fruit and Vegetable Association to be generally reliable and very useful.

- ABC Corporation
  1330 Avenue of the Americas
  New York, NY 10019
- American Egg Board
  1460 Renaissance Street
  Park Ridge, IL 60068

- American Meat Institute
  P.O. Box 3556
  Washington, DC 20007
- Beech-Nut Nutrition Hotline
  (800) 523-6633
- Best Foods
  Division of CPC International
  Consumer Service Department
  Internation Plaza
  Englewood Cliffs, NJ 07623
- Biosearch Medical Products, Inc.
  P.O. Box 1700
  Somerville, NJ 08876
- Borden Farm Products
  Borden Company, Consumer Affairs
  180 East Broad Street
  Columbus, OH 43215
- Campbell Soup Company
  Food Service Products Division
  375 Memorial Avenue
  Camden, NJ 08101
- Del Monte Teaching Aids
  P.O. Box 9075
  Clinton, IA 52736
- Egg Nutrition Center
  2501 M Street NW, Suite 410
  Washington, DC 20037
- Fleischmann's Margarines
  Standard Brands, Inc.
  625 Madison Avenue
  New York, NY 10022
- General Foods Consumer Center
  250 North Street
  White Plains, NY 10625
- General Mills
  P.O. Box 113
  Minneapolis, MN 55440
- Gerber Products Company
  445 State Street
  Fremont, MI 49412
- H. J. Heinz
  Consumer Relations
  P.O. Box 57
  Pittsburgh, PA 15230
- Hunt-Wesson Foods
  Educational Services
  1645 West Valencia Drive
  Fullerton, CA 92634
- Kellogg Company
  Department of Home Economics Services
  Battle Creek, MI 49016
- Kendall-McGaw Laboratories, Inc.
  2525 McGaw Avenue
  Irvine, CA 92714

- McGraw-Hill Films
  Association Films, Inc.
  600 Grand Avenue
  Ridgefield, NJ 07657
- Mead Johnson Nutritionals
  2404 Pennsylvania Avenue
  Evansville, IN 47721
- Meat and Poultry Hotline
  (800) 535-4555
- National Dairy Council
  6300 North River Road
  Rosemont, IL 60018
- Nestlé Company
  Home Economics Division
  100 Bloomingdale Road
  White Plains, NY 10605
- Norwich-Eaton Pharmaceuticals
  17 Eaton Avenue
  Norwich, NY 13815
- NutraSweet Company
  P.O. Box 830
  Deerfield, IL 60015
- Nutrex Corporation
  1168 Aster Avenue, Bldg. C
  Sunnyvale, CA 94086
- Oscar Mayer Company
  Consumer Service
  P.O. Box 1409
  Madison, WI 53701
- Pillsbury Company
  1177 Pillsbury Building
  608 Second Avenue South
  Minneapolis, MN 55402
- The Potato Board
  1385 South Colorado Boulevard, Suite 512
  Denver, CO 80222
- Procter and Gamble Company
  One Procter and Gamble Plaza
  Cincinnati, OH 45202
- Rice Council
  P.O. Box 22802
  Houston, TX 77027
- Ross Laboratories
  Director of Professional Services
  625 Cleveland Avenue
  Columbus, OH 43216
- Sandoz Nutrition
  5320 West 23rd Street
  P.O. Box 370
  Minneapolis, MN 55440
- Sherwood Medical, Inc.
  1831 Olive Street
  St. Louis, MO 63103

F

- Sister Kenny Institute
  Chicago Avenue at 27th Street
  Minneapolis, MN 55407
- Soy Protein Council
  1800 M Street NW
  Washington, DC 20036
- Sunkist Growers
  Consumer Service, Division BB
  P.O. Box 7888, Valley Annex
  Van Nuys, CA 91409
- Travenol Laboratories
  1425 Lake Cook Road
  Deerfield, IL 60015
- United Fresh Fruit and Vegetable Association
  727 North Washington Street
  Alexandria, VA 22314
- Vitamin Information Bureau
  383 Madison Avenue
  New York, NY 10017
- Vitamin Nutrition Information Service (VNIS)
  Hoffmann-LaRoche
  340 Kingsland Avenue
  Nutley, NJ 07110
- Wheat Flour Institute
  600 Maryland Avenue
  Washington, DC 20024

Organizations Concerned with World Hunger

- Bread for the World
  802 Rhode Island Avenue NE
  Washington, DC 20018

- The Hunger Project
  2015 Steiner Street
  San Francisco, CA 94115
- Institute for Food and Development Policy
  1885 Mission Street
  San Francisco, CA 94103
- Interreligious Taskforce on U.S. Food Policy
  110 Maryland Avenue NE
  Washington, DC 20002
- Meals for Millions/Freedom from Hunger Foundation
  1800 Olympic Boulevard
  P.O. Drawer 680
  Santa Monica, CA 90406
- Oxfam America
  115 Broadway
  Boston, MA 02116
- Worldwatch Institute
  1776 Massachusetts Avenue NW
  Washington, DC 20036

United Nations

- Food and Agriculture Organization (FAO)
  North American Regional Office
  1325 C Street SW
  Washington, DC 20025
- World Health Organization (WHO)
  1211 Geneva 27
  Switzerland

F

Food Exchange Systems

Contents

For an introduction to the use of food group plans and exchange systems, see Chapter 2. The details of the U.S. Four Food Group Plan, the U.S. Exchange System, and the Canadian Food Group System are presented here.

■ TABLE G–1
Servings in the U.S. Four Food Group Plan

Food Group	Servings (adult)	Food Item	Serving Size
Meat and meat alternates	2	Cheese	2 oz
		Cooked lean meat, poultry, or fish	2 oz
		Dried beans or peas	1 c
		Eggs	2
		Lunch meats	2 oz
		Nuts	½ c
		Peanut butter	4 tbsp
		Sunflower seeds	½ c
		Tofu	1 c
		Tuna	2 oz
Milk and milk products	2	Cheese	1 to 1½ oz
		Cottage cheese[a]	1½ to 2 c
		Ice cream[a]	1¾ c
		Milk	1 c
		Pudding or custard	1 c
		Yogurt	1 c
Fruits and vegetables	4[b]	Most vegetables and fruits, including canned:	½ c
		Sources of vitamin A:	
		Apricots	
		Broccoli[c]	
		Cantaloupe[c]	
		Carrots	
		Greens	
		Spinach	
		Sweet potatoes[c]	
		Sources of vitamin C:	
		Cabbage	
		Grapefruit	
		Green peppers	
		Oranges	
		Potatoes	
		Strawberries	
		Tomatoes	

■ TABLE G–1
Servings in the U.S. Four Food Group Plan   (continued)

Food Group	Servings (adult)	Food Item	Serving Size
		Apples, bananas, oranges, pears, potatoes, tomatoes	1 medium
		Cantaloupe	¼ medium
		Chili peppers	¼ c
		Corn	1 medium
		Grapefruit	½ medium
		Green peppers	½ medium
		Lettuce/salad greens	1 c
		Vegetable-base soups	1 c
		Vegetable/fruit juices	½ c
Grains (bread and cereal products)	4[d]	Bagels	½ (3″)
		Biscuits	1 (2″)
		Bread	1 slice
		Buns (hamburger/hot dog)	½
		Crackers	6
		Dinner rolls	1-oz roll
		Dry cereal	1 oz
		English muffins	½
		Pancakes	1 (4″)
		Pasta	½ c (cooked)
		Pita pocket bread	½ (6″)
		Rice, oatmeal, grits	½ c (cooked)
		Tortillas	1 (7″)

[a]The amount of a nutritional serving is much larger than an average serving.
[b]One serving should be rich in vitamin C; at least one every other day should be rich in vitamin A.
[c]Good sources of both vitamins A and C.
[d]Enriched or whole-grain products only.

G

The U.S. Exchange System

The U.S. Exchange System divides the foods suitable for use in planning a healthy diet into six lists—the starch/bread, meat/meat alternate, vegetable, fruit, milk, and fat lists.[1] These lists are shown in Tables G-2 through G-7. Following these lists are three other sets of foods: free foods, combination foods, and foods for occasional use (Tables G-8, G-9, and G-10).

■ TABLE G-2
Starch/Bread List

(15 g carbohydrate, 3 g protein, trace fat, 80 kcal)

Amount	Food
Cereals/Grains/Pasta	
⅓ c	Bran cereals, concentrated
½ c	Bran cereals, flaked
½ c	Bulgur, cooked
½ c	Cooked cereals
2½ tbsp	CornMeal, dry
3 tbsp	Grape-Nuts
½ c	Grits, cooked
¾ c	Other ready-to-eat unsweetened cereals
½ c	Pasta, cooked
1½ c	Puffed cereals
⅓ c	Rice, white or brown, cooked
½ c	Shredded Wheat
3 tbsp	Wheat germ
Dried Beans/Peas/Lentils	
¼ c	Baked beans
⅓ c	Beans and peas, cooked, such as kidney, white, split, black-eyed
⅓ c	Lentils, cooked
Starchy Vegetables	
½ c	Corn
1 cob	Corn, on the cob, 6″ long
½ c	Lima beans
½ c	Peas, green, canned or frozen
½ c	Plantains
1 small (3 oz)	Potatoes, baked
½ c	Potatoes, mashed
¾ c	Squash, winter (acorn, butternut)
⅓ c	Yams, sweet potatoes, plain
Bread	
½ (1 oz)	Bagels
2 (⅔ oz)	Bread sticks, crisp, 4″ × ½″
1 c	Croutons, low-fat
½	English muffins
½ (1 oz)	Frankfurter or hamburger buns
½ loaf	Pita, 6″ across

■ TABLE G-2
Starch/Bread List   (continued)

Amount	Food
1 (1 oz)	Plain rolls, small
1 slice (1 oz)	Raisin, unfrosted
1 slice (1 oz)	Rye, pumpernickel
1	Tortillas, 6″ across
1 slice (1 oz)	White (including French, Italian)
1 slice (1 oz)	Whole-wheat
Crackers/Snacks	
8	Animal crackers
3	Graham crackers, 2½″ square
¾ oz	Matzoth
5 slices	Melba toast
24	Oyster crackers
3 c	Popcorn, popped, no fat added
¾ oz	Pretzels
4	Rye crisp, 2″ × 3½″
6	Saltine-type crackers
2 to 4 (¾ oz)	Whole-wheat crackers, no fat added (crisp breads)
Starch Foods Prepared with Fat	

(Count as 1 starch/bread serving, plus 1 fat serving.)

Amount	Food
1	Biscuits, 2½″ across
½ c	Chow mein noodles
1 (2 oz)	Corn bread, 2″ cube
6	Crackers, round butter type
10 (1½ oz)	French fries, 2″ to 3 ½″ long
1	Muffins, plain, small
2	Pancakes, 4″ across
¼ c	Stuffing, bread, prepared
2	Taco shells, 6″ across
1	Waffles, 4½″ square
4 to 6 (1 oz)	Whole-wheat crackers, fat added

3 g or more dietary fiber per serving. Average fiber contents of whole-grain products is 2 g/serving. For starch foods not on this list, the general rule is that ½ c cereal, grain, or pasta is 1 serving; 1 oz of a bread product is 1 serving.

■ TABLE G-3
Meat/Meat Alternate Lists

(Lean meat = 7 g protein, 3 g fat, 55 kcal. Medium-fat meat = 7 g protein, 5 g fat, 75 kcal. High-fat meat = 7 g protein, 8 g fat, 100 kcal.)

Lean Meat and Alternates

Category	Amount	Food
Beef:	1 oz	USDA Good or Choice grades of lean beef, such as round, sirloin, and flank steak; tenderloin; chipped beef
Pork:	1 oz	Lean pork, such as fresh ham; canned, cured, or boiled ham; Canadian bacon, tenderloin

G

■ TABLE G–3
Meat/Meat Alternate Lists   (continued)

(Lean meat = 7 g protein, 3 g fat, 55 kcal. Medium-fat meat = 7 g protein, 5 g fat, 75 kcal. High-fat meat = 7 g protein, 8 g fat, 100 kcal.)

Lean Meat and Alternates

Category	Amount	Food
Veal:	1 oz	All cuts are lean except for veal cutlets (ground or cubed); examples of lean veal: chops and roasts
Poultry:	1 oz	Chicken, turkey, Cornish hen (without skin)
Fish:	1 oz	All fresh and frozen fish
	2 oz	Crab, lobster, scallops, shrimp, clams (fresh or canned in water)
	6 medium	Oysters
	¼ c	Tuna , canned in water
	1 oz	Herring, uncreamed or smoked
	2 medium	Sardines, canned
Wild Game:	1 oz	Venison, rabbit, squirrel
	1 oz	Pheasant, duck, goose (without skin)
Cheese:	¼ c	Any cottage cheese
	2 tbsp	Grated Parmesan
	1 oz	Diet cheeses (with less than 55 kcal/oz)
Other:	1 oz	95% fat-free lunch meats
	3 whites	Egg whites
	¼ c	Egg substitutes with less than 55 kcal per ¼ c

Medium-Fat Meat and Alternates

Category	Amount	Food
Beef:	1 oz	Most beef products fall into this category; examples: all ground beef, roasts (rib, chuck, rump), steak (cubed, porterhouse, T-bone), meatloaf
Pork:	1 oz	Most pork products fall into this category; examples: chops, loin roast, Boston butt, cutlets
Lamb:	1 oz	Most lamb products fall into this category; examples: chops, leg, roast
Veal:	1 oz	Cutlet, ground or cubed, unbreaded
Poultry:	1 oz	Chicken (with skin), domestic duck or goose (well-drained of fat), ground turkey
Fish:	¼ c	Tuna, canned in oil and drained
	¼ c	Salmon, canned
Cheese:		Skim or part-skim milk cheeses, such as:
	¼ c	Ricotta
	1 oz	Mozzarella
	1 oz	Diet cheeses (with 56 to 80 kcal/oz)
Other:	1 oz	86% fat-free lunch meat
	1	Eggs (high in cholesterol, limit to 3 per week)
	¼ c	Egg substitutes with 56 to 80 kcal per ¼ c
	4 oz	Tofu, 2 ½″ × 2¾″ × 1″
	1 oz	Liver, hearts, kidneys, sweetbreads (high in cholesterol)

■ TABLE G–3
Meat/Meat Alternate Lists   (continued)

Category	Amount	Food

High-Fat Meat and Alternates[a]

Beef:	1 oz	Most USDA Prime cuts of beef, such as ribs, corned beef
Pork:	1 oz	Spareribs, ground pork, pork sausages (patties or links)
Lamb:	1 oz	Patties, ground lamb
Fish:	1 oz	Any fried fish product
Cheese:	1 oz	All regular cheeses, such as American, blue, Cheddar, Monterey, Swiss
Other:	1 oz	Lunch meats, such as bologna, salami, pimento loaf
	1 oz	Sausage, such as Polish, Italian
	1 oz	Knockwurst, smoked
	1 oz	Bratwurst
	1 (10/lb)	Frankfurters (turkey or chicken)
	1 tbsp	Peanut butter (contains unsaturated fat)

Count as 1 high-fat meat plus 1 fat exchange:

1 frank	(10/lb)	Frankfurters (beef, pork, or combination)

400 mg or more sodium per exchange. Meats contribute no fiber to the diet.
[a]These items are high in saturated fat, cholesterol, and kcalories, and should be used no more than three times per week.

■ TABLE G–4
Vegetable List

(5 g carbohydrate, 2 g protein, 25 kcal)
All portion sizes, except as otherwise noted, are ½ c of any cooked vegetable or vegetable juice, 1 c of any raw vegetable

Artichokes, ½ medium	Mushrooms, cooked
Asparagus	Okra
Bean sprouts	Onions
Beans (green, wax, Italian)	Pea pods
Beets	Rutabagas
Broccoli	Sauerkraut
Brussels sprouts	Spinach, cooked
Cabbage, cooked	Summer squash (crookneck)
Carrots	Tomatoes, 1 large
Cauliflower	Tomato/vegetable juice
Eggplant	Turnips
Green peppers	Water chestnuts
Greens (collard, mustard, turnip)	Zucchini, cooked
Kohlrabi	
Leeks	

Starchy vegetables such as corn, peas, and potatoes are found on the Starch/Bread List.
For free vegetables, see the Free Food List (Table G–8).

400 mg or more sodium per serving. Most vegetable servings contain 2 to 3 g dietary fiber.

G

■ TABLE G–5
Fruit List

(15 g carbohydrate, 60 kcal)
All portion sizes, unless otherwise noted, are ½ c fresh fruit or fruit juice, ¼ c dried fruit.

Amount	Food
Fresh, Frozen, and Unsweetened Canned Fruit	
1	Apples, raw, 2″ across
½ c	Applesauce, unsweetened
4	Apricots, medium, raw
½ c (4 halves)	Apricots, canned
½	Bananas, 9″ long
¾ c	Blackberries, raw
¾ c	Blueberries, raw
⅓	Cantaloupe, 5″ across
1 c	Cantaloupe, cubes
12	Cherries, large, raw
½ c	Cherries, canned
2	Figs, raw, 2″ across
½ c	Fruit cocktail, canned
½	Grapefruit, medium
¾ c	Grapefruit, segments
15	Grapes, small
⅛	Honeydew melon, medium
1	Honeydew melon, cubes
1	Kiwis, large
¾ c	Mandarin oranges
½	Mangoes, small
1	Nectarines, 1½″ across
1	Oranges, 2½″ across
1 c	Papayas
1 peach (¾ c)	Peaches, 2¾″ across
½ c (2 halves)	Peaches, canned
½ large or 1 small	Pears
½ c (2 halves)	Pears, canned
2	Persimmons, medium, native
¾ c	Pineapple, raw
⅓ c	Pineapple, canned
2	Plums, raw, 2″ across
½	Pomegranates
1 c	Raspberries, raw
1¼ c	Strawberries, raw, whole
2	Tangerines, 2½″ across
1¼ c	Watermelon, cubes
Dried Fruit	
4 rings	Apples
7 halves	Apricots
2½ medium	Dates
1½	Figs
3 medium	Prunes
2 tbsp	Raisins
Fruit Juice	
½ c	Apple juice/cider
⅓ c	Cranberry juice cocktail
⅓ c	Grape juice
½ c	Grapefruit juice
½ c	Orange juice
½ c	Pineapple juice
⅓ c	Prune juice

3 g or more dietary fiber per serving. Average fiber contents of fresh, frozen, and dry fruits: 2 g/serving.

■ TABLE G–6
Milk List

(Nonfat and very low-fat milk = 12 g carbohydrate, 8 g protein, trace fat, 90 kcal. Low-fat milk = 12 g carbohydrate, 8 g protein, 5 g fat, 120 kcal. Whole milk = 12 g carbohydrate, 8 g protein, 8 g fat, 150 kcal.)

Amount	Food
Nonfat and Very Low-Fat Milk	
1 c	Nonfat milk
1 c	½% milk
1 c	1% milk
⅓ c	Dry nonfat milk
½ c	Evaporated nonfat milk
1 c	Low-fat buttermilk
8 oz	Plain nonfat yogurt
Lowfat Milk	
1 c fluid	2% milk
8 oz	Plain low-fat yogurt, with added nonfat milk solids
Whole Milk	
1 c	Whole milk
½ c	Evaporated whole milk
8 oz	Whole plain yogurt

■ TABLE G–7
Fat List (5 g fat, 45 kcal)

Amount	Food
Unsaturated Fats	
⅛ medium	Avocados
1 tsp	Margarine
1 tbsp	Margarine, diet[a]
1 tsp	Mayonnaise
1 tbsp	Mayonnaise, reduced kcalorie[a]
	Nuts and seeds:
6 whole	Almonds, dry roasted
1 tbsp	Cashews, dry roasted
20 small or 10 large	Peanuts
2 whole	Pecans
2 tsp	Pumpkin seeds
1 tbsp	Other nuts
1 tbsp	Seeds, pine nuts, sunflower seeds (without shells)
2 whole	Walnuts
1 tsp	Oil (corn, cottonseed, safflower, soybean, sunflower, olive, peanut)
10 small or 5 large	Olives[a]
1 tbsp	Salad dressing, all varieties[a]
2 tsp	Salad dressing, mayonnaise type
1 tbsp	Salad dressing, mayonnaise type, reduced kcalorie
2 tbsp	Salad dressing, reduced kcalorie[b]

G

■ TABLE G–7
Fat List (5 g fat, 45 kcal)   (continued)

Amount	Food
Saturated Fats	
1 slice	Bacon[a]
1 tsp	Butter
½ oz	Chitterlings
2 tbsp	Coconut, shredded
2 tbsp	Coffee whitener, liquid
4 tsp	Coffee whitener, powder
1 tbsp	Cream (heavy, whipping)
2 tbsp	Cream (light, coffee, table)
2 tbsp	Cream (sour)
1 tbsp	Cream cheese
¼ oz	Salt pork[a]

(Two tablespoons of low-kcalorie salad dressing is a free food.)

[a]If more than one or two servings are eaten, these foods provide 400 mg or more sodium.

 400 mg or more sodium per serving.

■ TABLE G–8
Free Foods

A free food is any food or drink that contains less than 20 kcal/serving. People with diabetes are advised to eat as much as they want of those items that have no serving size specified. They may eat two or three servings per day of those items that have a specific serving size. It is suggested that they spread them out through the day.

Amount	Food
Drinks	Bouillon, low-sodium
	Bouillon or broth without fat
	Carbonated drinks, sugar-free
	Carbonated water
	Club soda
1 tbsp	Cocoa powder, unsweetened
	Coffee/tea
	Drink mixes, sugar-free
	Tonic water, sugar-free
Nonstick Pan Spray	
Fruit:	
½ c	Cranberries, unsweetened
½ c	Rhubarb, unsweetened
Vegetables (raw, 1 c)	Cabbage
	Celery
	Chinese cabbage
	Cucumbers
	Green onions
	Hot peppers
	Mushrooms
	Radishes
	Zucchini
Salad Greens	Endive
	Escarole
	Lettuce
	Romaine
	Spinach

■ TABLE G–8
Free Foods   (continued)

Amount	Food
Sweet Substitutes	Candy, hard, sugar-free
	Gelatin, sugar-free
	Gum, sugar-free
2 tsp	Jam/jelly, sugar-free
1 to 2 tbsp	Pancake syrup, sugar-free
	Sugar substitutes (saccharin, aspartame)
2 tbsp	Whipped topping
Condiments	
1 tbsp	Catsup
	Horseradish
	Mustard
	Pickles, dill, unsweetened
2 tbsp	Salad dressing, low-kcalorie
1 tbsp	Taco sauce
	Vinegar
Seasonings	Basil, fresh
	Celery seeds
	Chili powder
	Chives
	Cinnamon
	Curry
	Dill
	Flavoring extracts (almond, butter, lemon, peppermint, vanilla, walnut, etc.)
	Garlic
	Garlic powder
	Herbs
	Hot pepper sauce
	Lemon
	Lemon juice
	Lemon pepper
	Lime
	Lime juice
	Mint
	Onion powder
	Oregano
	Paprika
	Pepper
	Pimento
	Soy sauce
	Soy sauce, low-sodium ("lite")
	Spices
¼ c	Wine, used in cooking
	Worcestershire sauce

 3 g or more dietary fiber per serving.
 400 mg or more sodium per serving.

■ **TABLE G–9**
Combination Foods

Much of the food we eat is mixed together in various combinations. These combination foods do not fit into only one exchange list. It can be quite hard to tell what is in a certain casserole dish or baked food item. This is a list of average values for some typical combination foods. This list will help you fit these foods into your meal plan. Ask your dietitian for information about any other foods you'd like to eat. The *American Diabetes Association/American Dietetic Association Family Cookbooks* and the *American Diabetes Association Holiday Cookbook* have many recipes and further information about many foods, including combination foods. Check your library or local bookstore.

Food	Amount	Exchanges
Casseroles, homemade	1 c (8 oz)	2 starch, 2 medium-fat meat, 1 fat
Cheese pizza, thin crust	¼ of 15 oz, or ¼ of 10″	2 starch, 1 medium-fat meat, 1 fat
Chili with beans, commercial	1 c (8 oz)	2 starch, 2 medium-fat meat, 2 fat
Chow mein, without noodles or rice	2 c (16 oz)	1 starch, 2 vegetable, 2 lean meat
Macaroni and cheese	1 c (8 oz)	2 starch, 1 medium-fat meat, 2 fat
Soups:		
Bean	1 c (8 oz)	1 starch, 1 vegetable, 1 lean meat
Chunky, all varieties	10¾-oz can	1 starch, 1 vegetable, 1 medium-fat meat
Cream, made with water	1 c (8 oz)	1 starch, 1 fat
Vegetable or broth	1 c (8 oz)	1 starch
Spaghetti and meatballs, canned	1 c (8 oz)	2 starch, 1 medium-fat meat, 1 fat
Sugar-free pudding, made with nonfat milk	½ c	1 starch

If beans are used as a meat substitute:

Dried beans, peas, lentils	1 c (cooked)	2 starch, 1 lean meat

400 mg or more sodium per serving.
3 g or more dietary fiber per serving

■ **TABLE G–10**
Foods for Occasional Use

The following list includes average exchange values for some foods high in sugar and fat. People are advised to use them only occasionally and in moderate amounts.

Food	Amount	Exchanges
Angel food cake	1/12 cake	2 starch
Cake, no icing	1/12 cake, or a 3″ square	2 starch, 2 fat
Cookies	2 small, 1¾″ across	1 starch, 1 fat
Frozen fruit yogurt	⅓ c	1 starch
Gingersnaps	3	1 starch
Granola	¼ c	1 starch, 1 fat
Granola bars	1 small	1 starch, 1 fat
Ice cream, any flavor	½ c	1 starch, 2 fat
Ice milk, any flavor	½ c	1 starch, 1 fat
Sherbet, any flavor	¼ c	1 starch
Snack chips, all varieties	1 oz	1 starch, 2 fat
Vanilla wafers	6 small	1 starch, 1 fat

If more than one serving is eaten, these foods have 400 mg or more sodium.

■ *The Canadian Food Group System*

The Canadian Food Group System is similar to the U.S. Exchange System, but the serving sizes and some of the foods listed are different. This food group system, as explained in the handbook *Good Health Eating Guide*, is a revision of the Canadian exchange system of meal planning.[2] Features of the new system similar to those of the exchange system include the following:

- Foods are divided into six groups according to carbohydrate, protein, and fat content.
- Foods are interchangeable within a group.
- Most foods are eaten in measured amounts.
- An energy value is given for each food group.

Additional features of the food group system include the following:

- Protein foods low in fat are emphasized in the protein foods group. Protein foods containing extra fat are identified.
- The user is able to distinguish between complex and simple carbohydrates (starches and sugars).

Tables G–11 through G–17 present the Canadian Food Group System.

■ **TABLE G–11**
Protein Foods Group

(7 g protein, 3 g fat, 55 kcal)

Food	Measure	Mass (weight)
Cheese		
All types, made from partly skim milk (e.g., mozzarella, part-skim)	1 piece, 5 cm × 2 cm × 2 cm (2″ × ¾″ × ¾″)	25 g
Cottage cheese, all types	50 ml (¼ c)	55 g
Fish		
Anchovies (see ''Extras,'' Table G–17)		
Canned, drained (e.g., chicken haddie, mackerel, salmon, tuna)	50 ml (¼ c)	30 g
Cod tongues/cheeks	75 ml (⅓ c)	50 g
Fillet or steak (e.g., Boston blue, cod, flounder, haddock, halibut, perch, pickerel, pike, salmon, shad, sole, trout, whitefish)	1 piece, 6 cm × 2 cm × 2 cm (2½″ × ¾″ × ¾″)	30 g
Herring	⅓ fish	30 g
Octopus	50 ml (¼ c)	40 g
Sardines	2 medium or 3 small	30 g
Seal, walrus	1 slice, 6 cm × 4 cm × 1 cm (2½″ × 1½″ × ½″)	25 g
Smelts	2 medium	30 g
Squid	50 ml (¼ c)	40 g
Shellfish		
Clams, mussels, oysters, scallops, snails	3 medium	30 g
Crab, lobster, flaked	50 ml (¼ c)	30 g
Shrimp, fresh	5 large	30 g
Frozen	10 medium	30 g
Canned	18 small	30 g
Dry pack	50 ml (¼ c)	30 g
Meat and Poultry (e.g., beef, chicken, ham, lamb, pork, turkey, veal, wild game)		
Back bacon	3 slices, thin	25 g
Chop	½ chop, with bone	35 g
Minced or ground, lean	30 ml (2 tbsp)	25 g
Sliced, lean	1 slice, 10 cm × 5 cm × 5 mm (4″ × 2″ × ¼″)	25 g
Steak, lean	1 piece, 4 cm × 3 cm × 2 cm (1½″ × 1¼″ × ¾″)	25 g
Organ Meats		
Hearts, liver	1 slice, 5 cm × 5 cm × 1 cm (2″ × 2″ × ½″)	25 g
Kidneys, sweetbreads, chopped	50 ml (¼ c)	25 g
Tongue	1 slice, 80 cm × 6 cm × 5 mm (3¼″ × 2½″ × ¼″)	25 g
Tripe, 1 piece = 4 cm × 4 cm × 8 mm (1½″ × 1½″ × ⅜″)	5 pieces	50 g
Soyabean		
Bean curd or tofu, 1 block = 6 cm × 6 cm × 4 cm (2½″ × 2 ½″ × 1½″)	½ block	70 g
The following choices contain extra fat, so use them less often.		
Cheese		
Cheeses, all types made from whole milk (e.g., brick, Brie, Camembert, Cheddar, Edam, Tilsit)	1 piece, 5 cm × 2 cm × 2 cm (2″ × ¾″ × ¾″)	25 g
Cheese, coarsely grated (e.g., Cheddar)	75 ml (⅓ c)	25 g
Cheese, dry, finely grated (e.g., Parmesan)	45 ml (3 tbsp)	15 g
Cheese, ricotta	50 ml (¼ c)	55 g

G

■ TABLE G–11
Protein Foods Group   (continued)

Food	Measure	Mass (weight)
Eggs		
Eggs, in shell, raw or cooked	1 medium	50 g
Eggs, without shell, cooked or poached in water	1 medium	45 g
Eggs, scrambled	50 ml (¼ c)	55 g
Fish		
Eel	5 cm, 4-cm diameter (2″, 1½″ diameter)	50 g
Meat		
Bologna	1 slice, 5 mm, 10-cm diameter (¼″, 4″ diameter)	40 g
Canned lunch meats	1 slice, 85 mm × 45 mm × 10 mm (3½″ × 1¾″ × ½″)	40 g
Corned beef, canned	1 slice, 75 mm × 55 mm × 5 mm (3″ × 2¼″ × ¼″)	25 g
Corned beef, fresh	1 slice, 10 cm × 5 cm × 5 mm (4″ × 2″ × ¼″)	25 g
Ground beef, medium-fat	30 ml (2 tbsp)	25 g
Meat spreads, canned	45 ml (3 tbsp)	35 g
Pâté (see ''Fats and oils group,'' Table G–16)		
Sausages, garlic, Polish or knockwurst	1 slice, 1 cm, 5-cm diameter (½″, 2″ diameter)	50 g
Sausages, pork, links	1 link	25 g
Spareribs or shortribs, with bone	10 cm × 6 cm (4″ × 2½″)	65 g
Stewing beef	1 cube, 25 mm (1″)	25 g
Summer sausage or salami	1 slice, 5 mm, 10-cm diameter (¼″, 4″ diameter)	40 g
Wieners	½ medium	25 g
Miscellaneous		
Blood pudding	1 slice, 5 cm × 1 cm (2″ × ½″)	25 g
Peanut butter, all kinds	15 ml (1 tbsp)	15 g

■ TABLE G–12
Starchy Foods Group

(15 g carbohydrate (starch), 2 g protein, 68 kcal)

Food	Measure	Mass (weight)
Breads		
Bagels	½	25 g
Bread crumbs	50 ml (¼ c)	25 g
Bread cubes	250 ml (1 c)	25 g
Bread sticks, 11 cm × 1 cm (4½″ × ½″)	2	20 g
Brewis, cooked	50 ml (¼ c)	45 g
English muffins, crumpets	½	25 g
Flour	40 ml (2½ tbsp)	20 g
Hamburger buns	½	30 g
Hot dog buns	½	30 g
Kaiser rolls	½	25 g
Matzoth, 15 cm (6″) square	1	20 g
Melba toast, rectangular	4	15 g
Pita, 20-cm (8″) diameter	¼	25 g
Plain rolls	1 small	25 g
Raisin	1 slice	25 g
Rusks	2	20 g
Rye, coarse or pumpernickel, 10 cm × 10 cm × 8 mm (4″ × 4″ × ⅜″)	½ slice	25 g

G

■ TABLE G–12
Starchy Foods Group   (continued)

Food	Measure	Mass (weight)
Tortillas, 15 cm (6″)	1	20 g
White (French and Italian)	1 slice	25 g
Whole-wheat, cracked wheat, rye, white enriched	1 slice	25 g
Cereals		
Bran flakes, 40% bran	125 ml (½ c)	20 g
Cooked cereals, cooked	125 ml (½ c)	125 g
Dry	30 ml (2 tbsp)	20 g
Cornmeal, cooked	125 ml (½ c)	125 g
Dry	30 ml (2 tbsp)	20 g
Ready-to-eat unsweetened cereal	250 ml (1 c)	20 g
Shredded Wheat, biscuits, bite size	125 ml (½ c)	20 g
Shredded Wheat biscuits, rectangular or round	1	20 g
Wheat germ	75 ml (⅓ c)	30 g
Cookies and Biscuits		
See ''Prepared Foods'' (below).		
Grains		
Barley, cooked	125 ml (½ c)	120 g
Dry	30 ml (2 tbsp)	20 g
Bulgur, kasha, cooked, moist	125 ml (½ c)	70 g
Cooked, crumbly	75 ml (⅓ c)	40 g
Dry	30 ml (2 tbsp)	20 g
Rice, cooked, loosely packed	125 ml (½ c)	105 g
cooked, tightly packed	75 ml (⅓ c)	70 g
Tapioca, pearl and granulated, quick cooking, dry	30 ml (2 tbsp)	15 g
Pastas		
Macaroni, cooked	125 ml (½ c)	70 g
Noodles, cooked	125 ml (½ c)	80 g
Spaghetti, cooked	125 ml (½ c)	70 g
Starchy Vegetables		
Beans and peas, dried, cooked	125 ml (½ c)	80 g
Breadfruit	1 slice	75 g
Corn, canned, whole kernel	125 ml (½ c)	85 g
Canned, creamed	75 ml (⅓ c)	60 g
Corn, on the cob, 13 cm, 4-cm diameter (5″, 1½″ diameter)	1 small cob	140 g
Cornstarch	30 ml (2 tbsp)	15 g
Plantains	⅓ small	50 g
Popcorn, unbuttered, large kernel	750 ml (3 c)	20 g
Potatoes, whipped	125 ml (½ c)	105 g
Potatoes, whole, 13 cm, 5-cm diameter (5″, 2″ diameter)	½	95 g
Yams, sweet potatoes, 13 cm, 5-cm diameter (5″, 2″ diameter)	½	75 g
Prepared Foods		
Baking powder biscuits, 5-cm diameter (2″ diameter)	1	30 g
Cookies, plain (e.g., digestive, oatmeal)	2	20 g
Cupcake, un-iced, 5-cm diameter (2″ diameter)	1 small	35 g
Doughnuts, cake type, plain, 7-cm diameter (2 ¾″ diameter)	1	30 g
Muffins, plain, 6-cm diameter (2 ½″ diameter)	1 small	40 g
Pancakes, homemade using 50 ml (¼ c) batter	1 small	50 g
Potatoes, french fries, 5 cm × 9 cm (2″ × 3 ½″)	10	65 g
Soup, canned, prepared with equal volume of water	250 ml (1 c)	260 g
Waffles, homemade, using 50 ml (¼ c) batter	1 small	35 g

■ TABLE G-13
Milk Group

Type of Milk	Carbohydrate	Protein	Fat	Energy
Nonfat	6 g	4 g	0 g	40 kcal
2%	6 g	4 g	2 g	58 kcal
Whole	6 g	4 g	4 g	76 kcal

Food	Measure	Mass (weight)
Buttermilk	125 ml (½ c)	125 g
Evaporated milk	50 ml (¼ c)	50 g
Milk	125 ml (½ c)	125 g
Powdered milk, regular	30 ml (2 tbsp)	15 g
Instant	50 ml (¼ c)	15 g
Unflavoured yogurt	125 ml (½ c)	125 g

■ TABLE G-14
Fruits and Vegetables Group

(10 g carbohydrate (simple sugar), 1 g protein, 44 kcal)

Food	Measure	Mass (weight)
Fruits (fresh, frozen without sugar, canned in water)		
Apples, raw	½ medium	75 g
Raw, without skin and core	½ medium	65 g
Sauce	125 ml (½ c)	120 g
Apricots, raw	2 medium	115 g
Canned, in water	4 halves, plus 30 ml (2 tbsp) liquid	110 g
Bake-apples (cloudberries), raw	125 ml (½ c)	120 g
Bananas, 15 cm (6"), with peel	½ small	75 g
Peeled	½ small	50 g
Blackberries, raw	125 ml (½ c)	70 g
Canned, in water	125 ml (½ c), includes 30 ml (2 tbsp) liquid	100 g
Blueberries, raw	125 ml (½ c)	120 g
Boysenberries, raw	125 ml (½ c)	70 g
Canned, in water	125 ml (½ c), includes 30 ml (2 tbsp) liquid	100 g
Cantaloupe, wedge with rind, 13-cm (5") diameter	¼	240 g
Cubed or diced	250 ml (1 c)	160 g
Cherries, raw, with pits	10	75 g
Raw, without pits	10	70 g
Canned, in water, with pits	75 ml (⅓ c), includes 30 ml (2 tbsp) liquid	90 g
Canned, in water, without pits	75 ml (⅓ c), includes 30 ml (2 tbsp) liquid	85 g
Crabapples, raw	1 small	55 g
Cranberries, raw	250 ml (1 c)	100 g
Figs, raw	1 medium	50 g
Canned, in water	3 medium, plus 30 ml (2 tbsp) liquid	100 g
Foxberries, raw	250 ml (1 c)	100 g
Fruit, mixed, cut up	125 ml (½ c)	120 g
Fruit cocktail, canned, in water	125 ml (½ c), includes 30 ml (2 tbsp) liquid	120 g
Gooseberries, raw	250 ml (1 c)	150 g
Canned, in water	250 ml (1 c), includes 30 ml (2 tbsp) liquid	230 g
Grapefruit, raw, with rind	½ small	185 g
Raw, sectioned	125 ml (½ c)	100 g
Canned, in water	125 ml (½ c), includes 30 ml (2 tbsp) liquid	120 g
Grapes, raw, slip skin	125 ml (½ c)	75 g
Raw, seedless	125 ml (½ c)	75 g
Canned, in water	75 ml (⅓ c), includes 30 ml (2 tbsp) liquid	115 g
Guavas, raw	½	50 g
Honeydew melon, raw, with rind	¹⁄₁₀	225 g
Cubed or diced	250 ml (1 c)	170 g
Huckleberries, raw	125 ml (½ c)	70 g
Kiwis, raw, with skin	2	155 g

G

■ **TABLE G–14**
Fruits and Vegetables Group   (continued)

Food	Measure	Mass (weight)
Kumquats, raw	3	60 g
Loganberries, raw	125 ml (½c)	70 g
Loquats, raw	8	130 g
Lychee fruit, raw	8	120 g
Mandarin oranges, raw, with rind	1	135 g
Raw, sectioned	125 ml (½ c)	100 g
Canned, in water	125 ml (½ c), includes 30 ml (2 tbsp) liquid	100 g
Mangoes, raw, without skin and seed	⅓	65 g
Diced	75 ml (⅓ c)	65 g
Nectarines	½ medium	75 g
Oranges, raw, with rind	1 small	90 g
Raw, sectioned	125 ml (½ c)	90 g
Papayas, raw, with skin and seeds	¼ medium	150 g
Raw, without skin and seeds	¼ medium	100 g
Cubed or diced	125 ml (½ c)	100 g
Peaches, raw, with seed and skin, 6-cm (2½) diameter	1 large	130 g
Raw, sliced, diced	125 ml (½ c)	100 g
Canned, in water, halves or slices	125 ml (½ c), includes 30 ml (2 tbsp) liquid	120 g
Pears, raw, with skin and core	½	90 g
Raw, without skin and core	½	85 g
Canned, in water, halves	2 halves, plus 30 ml (2 tbsp) liquid	90 g
Persimmons, raw, native	1	30 g
Raw, Japanese	¼	50 g
Pineapple, raw, sliced	1 slice, 8-cm diameter, 2 cm thick (3⅓" diameter, ¾" thick)	75 g
Raw, diced	125 ml (½ c)	75 g
Canned, in juice, diced	75 ml (⅓ c), includes 15 ml (1 tbsp) liquid	55 g
Canned, in juice, sliced	1 slice, plus 15 ml (1 tbsp) liquid	55 g
Canned, in water, diced	125 ml (½ c), includes 30 ml (2 tbsp) liquid	100 g
Canned, in water, sliced	2 slices, plus 15 ml (1 tbsp) liquid	100 g
Plums, raw, prune type	2	60 g
Damson	6	65 g
Japanese	1	70 g
Canned, in apple juice	2, plus 30 ml (2 tbsp) liquid	70 g
Canned, in water	3, plus 30 ml (2 tbsp) liquid	100 g
Pomegranates, raw	½	140 g
Raspberries, raw, black or red	125 ml (½ c)	65 g
Canned, in water	125 ml (½ c), includes 30 ml (2 tbsp) liquid	100 g
Saskatoons (see Blueberries)	250 ml (1 c)	150 g
Strawberries, raw	250 ml (1 c)	150 g
Canned, in water	250 ml (1 c), includes 30 ml (2 tbsp) liquid	240 g
Tangelos, raw	1	205 g
Tangerines, raw	1	115 g
Raw, sectioned	125 ml (½ c)	100 g
Watermelon, raw, with rind	1 wedge, 125-mm triangle, 22 mm thick (5" triangle, 1" thick)	310 g
Cubed or diced	250 ml (1 c)	160 g
Dried Fruit		
Apples	5 pieces	15 g
Apricots	4 halves	15 g
Banana flakes	30 ml (2 tbsp)	15 g
Currants	30 ml (2 tbsp)	15 g
Dates, without pits	2	15 g
Peaches	½	15 g
Pears	½	15 g
Prunes, raw, with pits	2	15 g
Raw, without pits	2	10 g
Stewed, no liquid	2	20 g
Stewed, with liquid	2, plus 15 ml (1 tbsp) liquid	35 g
Raisins	30 ml (2 tbsp)	15 g

G

■ TABLE G–14
Fruits and Vegetables Group   (continued)

Food	Measure	Mass (weight)
Juices (no sugar added or unsweetened)		
Apricot, grape, guava, mango, prune	50 ml (¼ c)	55 g
Apple, carrot, papaya, pear, pineapple, pomegranate	75 ml (⅓ c)	80 g
Grapefruit, loganberry, orange, raspberry, tangelo, tangerine	125 ml (½ c)	130 g
Tomato, tomato-based mixed vegetables	250 ml (1 c)	255 g
Vegetables (fresh, frozen, or canned)		
Artichokes, Jerusalem, mature or late season[a]	2 small	50 g
Beets, diced or sliced	125 ml (½ c)	85 g
Carrots, diced	125 ml (½ c)	75 g
Parsnips, mashed	125 ml (½ c)	80 g
Peas, fresh or frozen	125 ml (½ c)	80 g
Canned	75 ml (⅓ c)	55 g
Pumpkin, mashed	125 ml (½ c)	45 g
Rutabagas, mashed	125 ml (½ c)	85 g
Sauerkraut	250 ml (1 c)	235 g
Snow peas	10 pods	100 g
Squash, yellow or winter, mashed	125 ml (½ c)	115 g
Succotash	75 ml (⅓ c)	55 g
Tomatoes, canned	250 ml (1 c)	240 g
Turnips, mashed	125 ml (½ c)	115 g
Vegetables, mixed	125 ml (½ c)	90 g
Water chestnuts	8 medium	50 g

[a]Jerusalem artichokes contain inulin, which converts to carbohydrate during storage, in or out of the ground. Jerusalem artichokes in early season (autumn) are low in carbohydrate, but in late season (winter/spring) they become a fruits and vegetables choice.

G

■ TABLE G—15
Extra Vegetables Group

(½ c = 3.5 g carbohydrate, 14 kcal.)

Artichokes, globe or French
Artichokes, Jerusalem, early season[a]
Asparagus
Bamboo shoots
Bean sprouts, mung or soyabean
Beans, string, green, or yellow
Bitter melon (balsam pear)
Bok choy
Broccoli
Brussels sprouts
Cabbage
Cauliflower
Celery
Chard
Cucumbers
Eggplant
Endive
Fiddleheads
Greens: beet, collard, dandelion, mustard, turnip, etc.
Kale
Kohlrabi
Leeks
Lettuce
Mushrooms
Okra
Onions, green or mature
Parsley
Peppers, green or red
Radishes
Rhubarb
Shallots
Spinach
Sprouts: alfalfa radish, etc.
Tomatoes, raw
Vegetable marrow
Watercress
Zucchini

If eaten in large amounts, the following foods must be counted as 1 fruits and vegetables choice:

Brussels sprouts, cooked, 250 ml (1 c)	155 g
Eggplant, cooked, diced, 250 ml (1 c)	200 g
Kohlrabi, cooked, diced, 250 ml (1 c)	140 g
Leeks, cooked, edible parts of 4 leeks	100 g
Okra, cooked, sliced, 250 ml (1 c)	160 g
Onion, mature, cooked, 250 ml (1 c)	210 g
Rhubarb, cooked, no sugar added, 250 ml (1 c)	244 g
Tomatoes, raw, 2 medium (6-cm, or 2½", diameter) *or* 1 large (13-cm, or 5", diameter)	270 g

[a]Jerusalem artichokes contain inulin, which converts to carbohydrate during storage, in or out of the ground. Jerusalem artichokes in early season (autumn) are low in carbohydrate, but in late season (winter/spring) they become a fruits and vegetables choice.

■ TABLE G—16
Fats and Oils Group

(5 g fat, 45 kcal)

Food	Measure	Mass (Weight)
Avocado pears	⅛	30 g
Bacon, side, crisp	1 slice	5 g
Butter	5 ml (1 tsp)	5 g
Cheese spread	15 ml (1 tbsp)	15 g
Coconut, fresh	45 ml (3 tbsp)	15 g
Dried	15 ml (1 tbsp)	10 g
Cream, half and half (cereal), 10%	30 ml (2 tbsp)	30 g
Light (coffee), 20%	15 ml (1 tbsp)	15 g
Sour, 12 to 14%	45 ml (3 tbsp)	35 g
Whipping, 32 to 37%	15 ml (1 tbsp)	15 g
Cream cheese	15 ml (1 tbsp)	15 g
Gravy	30 ml (2 tbsp)	30 g
Lard	5 ml (1 tsp)	5 g
Margarine	5 ml (1 tsp)	5 g
Nuts, shelled:		
Almonds	8	20 g
Brazil nuts	2	5 g
Cashews	5	10 g
Filberts, hazelnuts	5	10 g
Macadamia	3	5 g
Peanuts	10	10 g
Pecans	5 halves	5 g
Pignolias, pine nuts	25 ml (5 tsp)	10 g
Pistachios, shelled	20	10 g
In shell	20	20 g
Pumpkin and squash seeds	20 ml (4 tsp)	10 g
Sesame seeds	15 ml (1 tbsp)	10 g
Sunflower seeds, shelled	15 ml (1 tbsp)	10 g
In shell	45 ml (3 tbsp)	15 g
Walnuts	4 halves	10 g
Oil, cooking and salad	5 ml	5 g
Olives, green	10	45 g
Ripe	7	40 g
Pâté, liverwurst, meat spreads	15 ml (1 tbsp)	15 g
Salad dressing: blue, French, Italian, mayonnaise, Thousand Island	5 ml (1 tsp)	5 g
Salt pork, raw or cooked	5 ml	5 g
Sesame oil	5 ml	5 g

■ TABLE G–17
Extras

(may be used without measuring)

Beverages
Bouillon from cube, powder or liquid
Bouillon or clear broth
Coffee, clear
Consommé
Herbal teas, unsweetened
Mineral water
Soda water, club soda
Sugar-free soft drinks
Tea, clear
Water

Condiments
Chowchow, unsweetened tomato pickles
Garlic
Gelatin, unsweetened
Ginger root
Horseradish, uncreamed
Lemon juice or lemon wedges
Lime juice or lime wedges
Mustard
Parsley
Pickles, unsweetened dill pickles or sour cucumber pickles
Pimentos
Soya sauce
Vinegar
Worcestershire sauce

Herbs and spices
Cinnamon, marjoram, pepper, salt, thyme, etc.

Miscellaneous
Artificial sweetener, such as cyclamate or saccharin
Baking powder, baking soda
Dulse
Flavorings and extracts (e.g., vanilla)
Rennet

■ TABLE G–17
Extras (continued)

(2.5 g carbohydrate, 15 kcal, limited to amount indicated)

Food	Measure
Anchovies	2 fillets
Barbecue sauce	15 ml (1 tbsp)
Bran, natural	30 ml (2 tbsp)
Brewer's yeast	5 ml (1 tsp)
Carob powder	5 ml (1 tsp)
Catsup	5 ml (1 tsp)
Chili sauce	5 ml (1 tsp)
Cocoa powder	5 ml (1 tsp)
Cranberry sauce, unsweetened	15 ml (1 tbsp)
Dietetic fruit spreads	5 ml (1 tsp)
Marschino cherries	1
Nondiary coffee whitener	5 ml (1 tsp)
Nuts, chopped pieces	5 ml (1 tsp)
Relishes	5 ml (1 tsp)
Sugar substitutes, granular	5 ml (1 tsp) (3 to 4 packages)
Whipped toppings	15 ml (1 tbsp)
Yogurt, plain	30 ml (2 tbsp)

▨ *Notes*

1. The U.S. Exchange System presented here is based on material in *Exchange Lists for Meal Planning,* 1986, prepared by committees of the American Diabetes Association and the American Dietetic Association, with permission of both organizations.
2. The tables for the Canadian Food Group System are taken from *Good Health Eating Guide* (Toronto: Canadian Diabetes Association, 1981), and are used with the association's permission.

G

Table of Food Composition

This table of food composition is not the standard table found in most nutrition textbooks. The list of foods chosen is an expanded version of that presented in the 1986 edition of the USDA *Home and Garden Bulletin Number 72, Nutritive Value of Foods*. The *Bulletin*, however, does not contain the values for dietary fiber, vitamin B_6, folate, magnesium, or zinc. Also, many additional foods have been added (such as frozen yogurt, canola oil, and imitation seafood items) to reflect current food patterns. The latest data for beef is also included. It is from the USDA data tapes and reflects the leaner cuts of beef now sold.

To achieve a complete and reliable listing of nutrients for all the foods, many sources of information had to be researched. Government sources of information are the primary base for all the data: USDA *Handbooks 8–1* through *8–18*; *Handbook 8–21*; prepublication material on cereals, grains, and pasta; and current supplemental data on vegetables and other foods. In addition, provisional USDA information of nutrient values—both published and unpublished—and many conversations with the staff members at the USDA Human Nutrition Information Service in Hyattsville, Maryland, have provided professional assistance to refine the data.

Even with all the government sources available, there are still many missing nutrient values; and as the various government data are updated, conflicting values are reported from the USDA for the same items. To fill in the missing values and resolve discrepancies, other sources of information were used. These reliable sources include refereed journal articles, food composition tables from Canada and England, information from other nutrient data banks and publications, unpublished scientific data, and manufacturers' data.

Estimates of nutrient amounts for foods and nutrients include all possible adjustments in the interest of accuracy. When multiple values were reported for a nutrient, the numbers were averaged and weighted with consideration of the original number of samples in the separate sources. Whenever water percentages were available, estimates of nutrient amounts were adjusted for water content. When no water was given, water percentage was assumed to be that shown in the table. Whenever a reported weight appeared inconsistent (cooked eggplant and collards, for example), many kitchen tests were made, and the average weight of the typical product was given as tested.

When estimates of nutrient amounts in cooked foods were derived from reported amounts in raw foods, published retention factors were applied. Some reported data for combination foods were modified in this table to include newer data available for major ingredients. For example, since the "pies" were analyzed and reported, newer data on fruits have been published. Older reported data on certain bakery items were updated for the new enrichment levels for certain nutrients.

Considerable effort has been made to report the most accurate data available and to eliminate missing values. There will always be changes in the future, and the authors welcome any suggestions or comments for the future.

■ It is important to know

that there can be many different nutrient values reported for foods. Many factors influence the amounts of nutrients in foods, including the mineral content of the soil, the method of processing, genetics, the diet of the animal or the fertilizer of the plant, the season of the year, methods of analysis, the difference in moisture content of the samples analyzed, the length and method of storage, and methods of cooking the food.

As a result, different nutrient values for the same food item are reported, even by reliable sources. Although each nutrient from USDA government data is presented as a single number in some USDA publications, each number is actually an average of a range of data. In the more detailed reports (Handbook 8 series), the number of samples is identified, and the standard deviation of the data is also noted. USDA data will have different reported values for foods as well, as older information is replaced with newer data in the more recent publications. Therefore, nutrient data should be viewed and used only as a guide, a close approximation of nutrient content.

Dietary fiber deserves a special word. Estimates of dietary fiber are included for all the foods in this table. The sources of this information are primarily extensive published and unpublished information from the USDA Human Nutrition Information Service in Hyattsville, Maryland; *Composition of Foods by Southgate* (England); and many journal articles.

It is important to know that this is emerging data on dietary fiber, and to expect additional research and refinement of analytical techniques to modify the data in the future. Dietary fiber is composed of cellulose, hemicellulose, lignin, pectin, gums, and mucilages. Very little data are yet available on the gum and mucilage components in foods, but there is considerable data on the other components.

Many different analytical techniques are used to measure various components of fiber, and these methods are undergoing their own review of accuracy in the scientific community. In this table, either an estimate of the total dietary fiber (a specific analytical technique) or a combination of measures for the insoluble components and pectin, when available, are used.

Vitamin A is reported in retinol equivalents. The amount of this vitamin can vary by the season of the year. Reported values in both dairy products and plants are higher in summer and early fall than in winter. The values reported here represent year-round averages. In the organ meats of all animal products (liver especially), there are large amounts of vitamin A, and these amounts vary widely, depending on the background of the animal. The vitamin is present in very small amounts in regular meat and is often reported as a trace.

Newer reported vitamin A values for some plant foods have increased significantly due to additional information and sometimes to newer plant genetics. New vitamin A values for canned pumpkin, for example, are 3.5 times greater than the previously reported values. This information was used to modify the vitamin A value of pumpkin pie, which had not yet been updated.

The energy and nutrients in recipes and combination foods vary widely, depending on the ingredients. The various fatty acids and cholesterol are influenced by the type of fat used (the specific type of oil, vegetable shortening, butter, margarine, etc.).

Total fats, as well as the breakdown of total fats to saturated, monounsaturated, and polyunsaturated fats, are listed in the table. The fatty acids seldom add up exactly to the total. This is due to rounding and to the existence of small amounts of other fatty acid components that are not included in the three basic categories.

Niacin values are for preformed niacin and do not include additional niacin that may form in the body from the conversion of tryptophan.

The items in this table have been organized into several categories, which are listed at the head of each right-hand page. As the key shows, each group has a number and that number is indicated in the first column. For ease in paging through this table, the category listed on the page you are on is highlighted in color. Thus if 7-GRAIN is colored and you are looking for dairy foods, turn back a few pages; if you are looking for sweets, turn forward.

This table has been prepared for West Publishing Company and is copyrighted by ESHA Research in Salem, Oregon—the developer and publisher of ''The Food Processor®'' computerized nutrition systems. The major sources for the data from the U.S. Department of Agriculture are supplemented by over 450 additional sources of information. Because the list of references is so extensive, it is not provided here, but it is available from the publisher.

H

Table H–1 Food Composition

Grp	Computer Code No.	Food Description	Measure	Wt (g)	H$_2$O (%)	Ener (kcal)	Prot (g)	Carb (g)	Dietary Fiber (g)	Fat (g)	Fat Breakdown (g) Sat	Mono	Poly
BEVERAGES													
		Alcoholic:											
		Beer:											
1	1	Regular (12 fl oz)	1½ c	356	92	146	1	13	1	0	0	0	0
1	2	Light (12 fl oz)	1½ c	354	95	100[1]	1	5	1	0	0	0	0
		Gin, rum, vodka, whiskey:											
1	3	80 proof	1½ fl oz	42	67	97	0	<.1	0	0	0	0	0
1	4	86 proof	1½ fl oz	42	64	105	0	<.1	0	0	0	0	0
1	5	90 proof	1½ fl oz	42	62	110	0	<.1	0	0	0	0	0
		Liqueur:											
1	1359	Coffee Liqueur, 53 proof	1½ fl oz	52	31	174	0	24	0	<1	.1	t	.1
1	1360	Coffee & cream liqueur, 34 proof	1½ fl oz	47	47	154	1	10	0	7	4.5	2.1	.3
1	1361	Creme de menthe, 72 proof	1½ fl oz	50	28	186	0	21	0	<1	t	t	.1
		Wine:											
1	6	Dessert (4 fl oz)	½ c	118	72	181[2]	<1	14[2]	0	0	0	0	0
1	7	Red	3½ fl oz	103	88	74	<1	2	0	0	0	0	0
1	8	Rosé	3½ fl oz	103	89	73	<1	2	0	0	0	0	0
1	9	White medium	3½ fl oz	103	90	70	<1	1	0	0	0	0	0
		Carbonated[3]:											
1	10	Club soda (12 fl oz)	1½ c	355	100	0	0	0	0	0	0	0	0
1	11	Cola beverage (12 fl oz)	1½ c	370	89	151	0	39	0	0	0	0	0
1	12	Diet cola (12 fl oz)	1½ c	355	100	2	0	<1	0	0	0	0	0
1	13	Diet soda pop–average (12 fl oz)	1½ c	355	100	2	0	<1	0	0	0	0	0
1	14	Ginger ale (12 fl oz)	1½ c	366	91	124	0	32	0	0	0	0	0
1	15	Grape soda (12 fl oz)	1½ c	372	89	161	0	42	0	0	0	0	0
1	16	Lemon-lime (12 fl oz)	1½ c	368	90	149	0	38	0	0	0	0	0
1	17	Orange (12 fl oz)	1½ c	372	88	177	0	46	0	0	0	0	0
1	18	Pepper-type soda (12 fl oz)	1½ c	368	89	151	0	38	0	0	0	0	0
1	19	Root beer (12 fl oz)	1½ c	370	89	152	<1	39	0	0	0	0	0
		Coffee[3]:											
1	20	Brewed	1 c	240	99	2[4]	<1	1	<1	0	0	0	0
1	21	Prepared from instant	1 c	240	99	2[4]	<1	1	0	0	0	0	0
		Fruit drinks, noncarbonated[5]:											
1	22	Fruit punch drink, canned	1 c	253	88	118	<1	30	0	<1	t	t	t
1	1358	Gatorade	1 c	230	99	39	0	11	0	0	0	0	0
1	23	Grape drink, canned	1 c	250	88	112	0	35	<1	<1	t	t	t
1	1304	Koolade, sweetened with sugar	1 c	240	100	100	0	25	0	0	0	0	0
1	1356	Koolade, sweetened with nutrasweet	1 c	240	100	4	0	0	0	0	0	0	0
		Lemonade, frozen:											
1	26	Concentrate (6-oz can)	¾ c	219	52	397	1	103	1	<1	.1	t	.1
1	27	Lemonade prepared from frozen concentrate	1 c	248	89	100	<1	26	<1	<1	t	t	t
		Limeade, frozen:											
1	28	Concentrate (6-oz can)	¾ c	218	50	408	<1	108	1	<1	t	t	.1
1	29	Limeade prepared from frozen concentrate	1 c	247	89	102	<1	27	<1	<1	t	t	t
1	24	Pineapple grapefruit, canned	1 c	250	88	117	1	29	0	<1	t	t	.1
1	25	Pineapple orange, canned	1 c	250	87	125	3	29	0	<1	t	t	.1
		Fruit and vegetable juices: see Fruit and Vegetable sections											

[1]kCalories can vary from 78 to 131 for 12 fl oz.
[2]Values are for sweet dessert wine. Dry dessert wines contain 149 kcal and 5 g of carbohydrate.
[3]Mineral content varies depending on water source.
[4]kCalorie values from USDA vary from 1 to 4 kcalories per cup.
[5]Usually less than 10% fruit juice.

(Computer code number is for West Diet Analysis program)

GRP KEY: 1 = BEV 2 = DAIRY 3 = EGGS 4 = FAT/OIL 5 = FRUIT 6 = BAKERY 7 = GRAIN 8 = FISH 9 = BEEF 10 = POULTRY
11 = SAUSAGE 12 = MIXED/FAST 13 = NUTS/SEEDS 14 = SWEETS 15 = VEG/LEG 16 = MISC 22 = SOUP/SAUCE

Chol (mg)	Calc (mg)	Iron (mg)	Magn (mg)	Phos (mg)	Pota (mg)	Sodi (mg)	Zinc (mg)	VT-A (RE)	Thia (mg)	Ribo (mg)	Niac (mg)	V-B6 (mg)	Fola (µg)	VT-C (mg)
0	18	.11	23	44	89	19	.07	0	.02	.09	1.61	.18	21	0
0	18	.14	18	43	64	10	.11	0	.03	.11	1.39	.12	15	0
0	0	.02	0	2	1	<1	.02	0	<.01	<.01	<.01	t	0	0
0	0	.02	0	2	1	<1	.02	0	<.01	<.01	<.01	0	0	0
0	0	.02	0	2	1	<1	.02	0	<.01	<.01	<.01	0	0	0
0	1	.03	1	3	15	4	.01	0	<.01	.01	.08	—	0	0
—	7	.06	1	23	15	43	.08	—	0	.03	.04	—	0	0
0	0	.04	0	0	0	3	—	0	0	0	<.01	0	0	—
0	9	.24	11	11	109	11	.08	0	.02	.02	.25	0	<1	0
0	8	.44	13	14	115	6	.10	0	<.01	.03	.08	.04	2	0
0	9	.39	10	15	102	5	.06	0	<.01	.02	.08	.03	1	0
0	9	.33	11	14	82	5	.07	0	<.01	<.01	.07	.01	<1	0
0	17	.15	4	0	6	75	.36	0	0	0	0	0	0	0
0	9	.13	3	46	4	15	.05	0	0	0	0	0	0	0
0	12	.11	4	30	0	21[6]	.28	0	.02	.08	0	0	0	0
0	14	.14	3	38	7	21[6]	.10	0	0	0	0	0	0	0
0	12	.66	3	1	5	25	.18	0	0	0	0	0	0	0
0	12	.31	4	0	3	57	.26	0	0	0	0	0	0	0
0	9	.25	2	1	4	41	.18	0	0	0	.06	0	0	0
0	19	.23	4	4	9	46	.38	0	0	0	0	0	0	0
0	12	.14	1	41	2	38	.15	0	0	0	0	0	0	0
0	19	.19	4	2	3	49	.26	0	0	0	0	0	0	0
0	4	.12	14	3	130	5	.08	0	0	.02	.53	0	<1	0
0	8	.12	9	8	87	8	.07	0	0	<.01	.69	0	0	0
0	19	.52	5	3	64	56	.31	4	.06	.06	.05	0	3	75
0	23	—	—	0	23	123	—	0	—	—	—	—	—	—
0	3	.41	5	3	13	16	.28	<1	.08	.02	.07	.02	1	85
0	0	0	0	0	0	0	0	0	0	0	0	0	0	6
0	0	0	0	0	0	0	0	0	0	0	0	0	0	6
0	15	1.58	11	19	148	8	.17	21	.06	.21	.16	.06	22	39[7]
0	4	.41	3	5	38	8	.05	5	.02	.05	.04	.02	6	10[7]
0	11	.22	60	13	129	<1	.11	<1	.02	.02	.22	.11	25	26
0	3	.06	15	3	33	<1	.03	<1	<.01	<.01	.05	.03	6	7
0	18	.77	15	14	154	34	.15	9	.08	.04	.67	.10	26	115
0	13	.67	14	10	116	9	.14	133	.08	.05	.52	.12	27	56

H

[6]Value for product sweetened with aspartame only; sodium is 32 mg if a blend of aspartame and sodium saccharin is used; 75 mg if just sodium saccharin is used.
[7]Vitamin C can range from 5 to 72 mg in a small can of frozen concentrate, and from 1 to 18 mg in l c of prepared lemonade.

(For purposes of calculations, use "0" for t, <1, <.1, <.01, etc.)

Table H–1 Food Composition

Grp	Computer Code No.	Food Description	Measure	Wt (g)	H₂O (%)	Ener (kcal)	Prot (g)	Carb (g)	Dietary Fiber (g)	Fat (g)	Sat	Mono	Poly
BEVERAGES—Con.													
1	1357	Perrier® bottled water, 6.5 fl oz bottle	1 ea	192	100	0	0	0	0	0	0	0	0
		Tea[8]:											
1	30	Brewed	1 c	240	100	2	<.01	1	0	0	0	0	0
1	31	From instant, unsweetened	1 c	237	100	2	0	<1	0	0	0	0	0
1	32	From instant, sweetened	1 c	262	91	86	0	22	0	0	0	0	0
DAIRY													
		Butter: see Fats and Oils, #158, 159, 160											
		Cheese, natural:											
2	33	Blue	1 oz	28	42	100	6	1	0	8	5.3	2.2	.2
2	34	Brick	1 oz	28	41	105	6	1	0	8	5.3	2.4	.2
2	35	Brie	1 oz	28	48	95	6	<1	0	8	5.0	2.3	.3
2	36	Camembert	1 oz	28	52	85	6	<1	0	7	4.3	2.0	.2
		Cheddar:											
2	37	Cut pieces	1 oz	28	37	114	7	<1	0	9	6.0	2.7	.3
2	38	1″ cube	1 ea	17	37	69	4	<1	0	6	3.6	1.6	.2
2	39	Shredded	1 c	113	37	455	28	1	0	37	24	11	1
		Cottage:											
2	40	Creamed, large curd	1 c	225	79	235	28	6	0	10	6.4	3.0	.3
2	41	Creamed, small curd	1 c	210	79	215	26	6	0	9	6.0	2.7	.3
2	42	With fruit	1 c	226	72	279	22	30	0	8	4.9	2.2	.3
2	43	Low fat 2%	1 c	226	79	205	31	8	0	4	2.8	1.2	.1
2	44	Low fat 1%	1 c	226	82	164	28	6	0	2	1.5	.7	.1
2	45	Dry curd	1 c	145	80	123	25	3	0	1	.4	.2	<.1
2	46	Cream	1 oz	28	54	99	2	1	0	10	6.2	2.8	.4
2	47	Edam	1 oz	28	42	101	7	<1	0	8	5.0	2.3	.2
2	48	Feta	1 oz	28	55	75	5	1	0	6	4.2	1.3	.2
2	49	Gouda	1 oz	28	42	101	7	1	0	8	5.0	2.2	.2
2	50	Gruyère	1 oz	28	33	117	8	<1	0	9	5.4	2.9	.5
2	51	Gorgonzola	1 oz	28	39	111	7	0	0	9	5.5	2.4	.5
2	52	Liederkranz	1 oz	28	53	87	5	0	0	8	5.3	2.2	.2
2	53	Monterey jack	1 oz	28	41	106	7	<1	0	9	5.4	2.4	.2
		Mozzarella, made with:											
2	54	Whole milk	1 oz	28	54	80	5	1	0	6	3.7	1.9	.2
2	55	Part skim milk, low moisture	1 oz	28	49	80	8	1	0	5	3.1	1.4	.1
2	56	Muenster	1 oz	28	42	104	6	<1	0	8	5.4	2.5	.2
		Parmesan, grated:											
2	57	Cup, not pressed down	1 c	100	18	455	42	4	0	30	19	8.7	.7
2	58	Tablespoon	1 tbsp	5	18	23	2	<1	0	2	1	.4	<.1
2	59	Ounce	1 oz	28	18	129	12	1	0	9	5.4	2.5	.2
2	60	Provolone	1 oz	28	41	100	7	1	0	8	4.8	2.1	.2
		Ricotta, made with:											
2	61	Whole milk	1 c	246	72	428	28	7	0	32	20	8.9	1
2	62	Part skim milk	1 c	246	74	340	28	13	0	19	12	5.7	.6
2	63	Romano	1 oz	28	31	110	9	1	0	8	4.9	2.2	.2
2	64	Swiss	1 oz	28	37	107	8	1	0	8	5.0	2.1	.3
		Pasteurized processed cheese products:											
2	65	American	1 oz	28	39	106	6	<1	0	9	5.6	2.5	.3
2	66	Swiss	1 oz	28	42	95	7	1	0	7	4.6	2.0	.2
2	67	American cheese food	1 oz	28	44	93	6	2	0	7	4.4	2.0	.2
2	68	American cheese spread	1 oz	28	48	82	5	2	0	6	3.8	1.8	.2

[8]Mineral content varies depending on water source.

(Computer code number is for West Diet Analysis program)

GRP KEY: 1 = BEV   2 = DAIRY   3 = EGGS   4 = FAT/OIL   5 = FRUIT   6 = BAKERY   7 = GRAIN   8 = FISH   9 = BEEF   10 = POULTRY
11 = SAUSAGE   12 = MIXED/FAST   13 = NUTS/SEEDS   14 = SWEETS   15 = VEG/LEG   16 = MISC   22 = SOUP/SAUCE

Chol (mg)	Calc (mg)	Iron (mg)	Magn (mg)	Phos (mg)	Pota (mg)	Sodi (mg)	Zinc (mg)	VT-A (RE)	Thia (mg)	Ribo (mg)	Niac (mg)	V-B6 (mg)	Fola (µg)	VT-C (mg)
0	26	0	1	0	0	3	0	0	0	0	0	0	0	0
0	0	.05	7	1	89	7	.05	0	0	.03	.1	0	12	0
0	5	.05	5	3	47	8	.07	0	0	<.01	<.01	<.09	1	0
0	1	.04	3	3	49	1	.06	0	0	.04	.09	0	5	0
21	150	.09	7	110	73	396	.75	65	.01	.11	.29	.05	10	0
27	191	.13	7	128	38	159	.73	86	<.01	.1	.03	.02	6	0
28	52	.14	6	53	43	178	.7	57	.02	.15	.11	.07	18	0
20	110	.09	6	98	53	236	.68	71	.01	.14	.18	.06	18	0
30	204	.20	8	146	28	176	.92	86	.01	.11	.02	.02	5	0
18	124	.12	5	88	17	107	.54	52	<.01	.07	.01	.01	3	0
119	815	.77	31	579	111	701	3.51	342	.03	.42	.09	.08	21	0
34	135	.26	11	297	190	911	.8	108	.05	.37	.30	.14	27	<1
31	126	.30	11	277	177	850	.8	101	.04	.34	.27	.14	26	<1
25	108	.25	9	236	151	915	.66	81	.04	.29	.23	.12	22	<1
19	155	.36	14	340	217	918	.95	45	.05	.42	.33	.17	30	0
10	138	.32	12	302	193	918	.86	25	.05	.37	.29	.15	28	t
10	46	.33	6	151	47	19	.68	12	.04	.21	.23	.12	21	0
31	23	.34	2	30	34	84	.33	124	<.01	.06	.03	.01	4	0
25	207	.13	8	152	53	274	1.06	72	.01	.11	.02	.02	5	0
25	140	.18	5	96	18	316	.81	36	.04	.23	.29	.02	3	0
32	198	.07	8	155	34	232	1.1	49	<.01	.10	.02	.02	6	0
31	287	.06	4	172	23	95	1	98	.02	.08	.03	.02	3	0
25	149	.12	8	121	26	513	.57	103	.01	.09	.2	.04	9	0
21	110	.12	7	100	68	390	.7	91	.01	.18	.1	.04	34	0
26	212	.2	8	126	23	152	.85	81	<.01	.11	.02	.02	3	0
22	147	.05	5	105	19	106	.7	68	<.01	.07	.02	.02	2	0
15	207	.08	8	149	27	150	.83	54	<.01	.1	.03	.02	3	0
27	203	.13	8	133	38	178	.84	90	<.01	.09	.03	.02	3	0
79	1376	.95	51	807	107	1862	3.19	173	.04	.39	.32	.11	8	0
4	69	.05	3	40	5	93	.16	9	<.01	.02	.02	<.01	<1	0
22	390	.27	14	229	30	528	1	49	.01	.11	.09	.03	2	0
20	214	.15	8	141	39	248	.89	75	<.01	.09	.04	.02	3	0
124	509	.94	28	389	257	207	2.85	330	.03	.48	.26	.11	14	0
76	669	1.09	4	449	307	307	3.29	278	.05	.46	.19	.05	14	0
29	302	.23	12	215	26	340	1	40	.01	.11	.02	.03	2	0
26	272	.05	10	171	31	74	1.1	72	<.01	.1	.03	.02	2	0
27	174	.11	6	211	46	406	.93	82	.01	.1	.02	.02	2	0
24	219	.17	8	216	61	388	1.02	65	<.01	.08	.01	.01	2	0
18	163	.24	9	130	79	337	.85	62	.01	.13	.04	.02	2	0
16	159	.09	8	201	69	381	.78	54	.01	.12	.04	.03	2	0

H

(For purposes of calculations, use "0" for t, <1, <.1, <.01, etc.)

Table H–1 Food Composition

Grp	Computer Code No.	Food Description	Measure	Wt (g)	H₂O (%)	Ener (kcal)	Prot (g)	Carb (g)	Dietary Fiber (g)	Fat (g)	Fat Breakdown (g) Sat	Mono	Poly
DAIRY—Con.													
		Cream, sweet:											
		Half and half (cream and milk):											
2	69	Cup	1 c	242	81	315	7	10	0	28	17	8	1
2	70	Tablespoon	1 tbsp	15	81	20	<1	1	0	2	1.1	.5	.1
		Light, coffee or table:											
2	71	Cup	1 c	240	74	469	6	9	0	46	29	13	1.7
2	72	Tablespoon	1 tbsp	15	74	30	<1	1	0	3	1.8	.8	.1
		Light whipping cream, liquid:											
2	73	Cup	1 c	239	64	699	5	7	0	74	46	22	2.1
2	74	Tablespoon	1 tbsp	15	64	44	<1	<1	0	5	2.9	1.4	.1
		Heavy whipping cream, liquid[9]:											
2	75	Cup	1 c	238	58	821	5	7	0	88	55	25	3.3
2	76	Tablespoon	1 tbsp	15	58	51	<1	<1	0	6	3.5	1.6	.2
		Whipped cream, pressurized[9]:											
2	77	Cup	1 c	60	61	154	2	7	0	13	8.3	3.9	.5
2	78	Tablespoon	1 tbsp	4	61	10	<1	<1	0	1	.5	.2	<.1
		Cream, sour, cultured:											
2	79	Cup	1 c	230	71	493	7	10	0	48	30	14	1.8
2	80	Tablespoon	1 tbsp	14	71	30	<1	1	0	3	1.8	.9	.1
		Cream products—imitation and part dairy:											
		Coffee whitener:											
2	81	Frozen or liquid	1 tbsp	15	77	20	<1	2	0	2	1.4	t	t
2	82	Powdered	1 tsp	2	2	11	<1	1	0	1	.6	t	t
		Dessert topping, frozen:											
2	83	Cup	1 c	75	50	239	1	17	0	19	16	1.2	.4
2	84	Tablespoon	1 tbsp	5	50	15	<1	1	0	1	1.0	.1	t
		Dessert topping from mix:											
2	85	Cup	1 c	80	67	151	3	13	0	10	8.6	.7	.2
2	86	Tablespoon	1 tbsp	5	67	9	<1	1	0	1	.5	<.1	t
		Dessert topping, pressurized:											
2	87	Cup	1 c	70	60	185	1	11	0	16	13	1.4	.2
2	88	Tablespoon	1 tbsp	4	60	11	<1	1	0	1	.8	.1	t
		Sour cream imitation:											
2	91	Cup	1 c	230	71	479	6	15	0	45	41	1.4	.1
2	92	Tablespoon	1 tbsp	14	71	29	<1	1	0	3	2.5	.1	t
		Sour dressing, part dairy:											
2	89	Cup	1 c	235	75	416	8	11	0	39	31	4.6	1.1
2	90	Tablespoon	1 tbsp	15	75	25	<1	1	0	2	2.0	.3	.1
		Milk, fluid:											
2	93	Whole milk	1 c	244	88	150	8	11	0	8	5.1	2.4	.3
2	94	2% low-fat milk	1 c	244	89	121	8	12	0	5	2.9	1.4	.2
2	95	2% milk solids added[10]	1 c	245	89	125	9	12	0	5	2.9	1.4	.2
2	96	1% low-fat milk	1 c	244	90	102	8	12	0	3	1.6	.8	.1
2	97	1% milk solids added[10]	1 c	245	90	105	9	12	0	2	1.5	.7	.1
2	98	Skim milk	1 c	245	91	86	8	12	0	<1	.3	.1	t
2	99	Skim milk solids added[10]	1 c	245	90	91	9	12	0	1	.4	.2	t
2	100	Buttermilk	1 c	245	90	99	8	12	0	2	1.3	.6	.1

[9] For whipped cream, (non-pressurized), double the liquid cream volume of codes 75,76 or 73,74. One tablespoon liquid cream becomes 2 Tablespoons when "whipped".

[10] Milk solids added, label claims less than 10 g protein per cup.

(Computer code number is for West Diet Analysis program)

GRP KEY: 1 = BEV 2 = DAIRY 3 = EGGS 4 = FAT/OIL 5 = FRUIT 6 = BAKERY 7 = GRAIN 8 = FISH 9 = BEEF 10 = POULTRY
11 = SAUSAGE 12 = MIXED/FAST 13 = NUTS/SEEDS 14 = SWEETS 15 = VEG/LEG 16 = MISC 22 = SOUP/SAUCE

Chol (mg)	Calc (mg)	Iron (mg)	Magn (mg)	Phos (mg)	Pota (mg)	Sodi (mg)	Zinc (mg)	VT-A (RE)	Thia (mg)	Ribo (mg)	Niac (mg)	V-B6 (mg)	Fola (µg)	VT-C (mg)
89	254	.17	25	230	314	98	1.23	259	.09	.36	.19	.09	6	2
6	16	.01	2	14	20	6	.08	16	.01	.02	.01	<.01	<1	<1
159	231	.1	21	192	292	95	.65	437	.08	.36	.14	.08	6	2
10	14	.01	1	12	18	6	.04	27	<.01	.02	.01	<.01	<1	<1
265	166	.07	17	146	231	82	.60	705	.06	.30	.1	.07	9	1
17	10	<.01	1	9	15	5	.04	44	<.01	.02	.01	<.01	1	<1
326	154	.07	17	149	179	89	.55	1002	.05	.26	.09	.06	10	1
20	10	<.01	1	9	11	6	.03	63	<.01	.02	.01	<.01	1	<1
46	61	.03	6	54	88	78	.22	124	.02	.04	.04	.03	1	0
3	4	<.01	<1	3	5	5	.01	8	<.01	<.01	<.01	<.01	<1	0
102	268	.14	26	195	331	123	.69	448	.08	.34	.15	.04	25	2
6	16	.01	2	12	20	7	.04	27	<.01	.02	.01	<.01	2	<1
0	1	<.01	<1	10	29	12	<.01	1[10]	0	0	0	0	0	0
0	<1	.02	<1	8	16	4	.01	<1[10]	0	<.01	0	0	0	0
0	5	.09	1	6	14	19	.03	65[11]	0	0	0	0	0	0
0	<1	.01	<1	<1	1	1	<.01	4[11]	0	0	0	0	0	0
8	72	.03	8	69	121	53	.22	39[11]	.02	.09	.05	.02	3	1
<1	5	<.01	<1	4	8	3	.14	3[11]	<.01	<.01	<.01	<.01	<1	<1
0	4	.01	1	13	13	43	.01	33[11]	0	0	0	0	0	0
0	<1	<.01	<1	1	1	3	<.01	2[11]	0	0	0	0	0	0
0	6	.01	—	102	369	235	0	0	0	0	0	0	0	0
0	<1	<.01	—	6	23	14	0	0	0	0	0	0	0	0
213	266	.07	23	205	381	113	.87	5[11]	.09	.38	.17	.04	28	2
1	17	<.01	2	13	24	7	.05	<1[11]	.01	.02	.01	<.01	2	<1
33	291	.12	33	228	370	120	.94	76	.09	.4	.2	.1	12	2
22	297	.12	33	232	377	122	.96	140	.1	.4	.21	.1	12	2
18	314	.12	35	245	397	128	.98	140	.1	.42	.22	.11	12	2
10	300	.12	34	235	381	123	.96	145	.1	.41	.21	.11	12	2
10	314	.12	35	245	397	128	.98	145	.1	.42	.22	.11	12	2
4	302	.1	28	247	406	126	.92	149	.09	.34	.22	.1	14	2
5	316	.12	37	255	419	130	1	149	.1	.43	.22	.11	12	2
9	285	.12	26	219	371	257	1.03	20	.08	.38	.14	.08	12	2

[11]Vitamin A value is from beta-carotene used for coloring.

H

(For purposes of calculations, use "0" for t, <1, <.1, <.01, etc.)

Table H–1 Food Composition

Grp	Computer Code No.	Food Description	Measure	Wt (g)	H₂O (%)	Ener (kcal)	Prot (g)	Carb (g)	Dietary Fiber (g)	Fat (g)	Fat Breakdown (g) Sat	Mono	Poly
DAIRY—Con.													
		Milk, canned:											
2	101	Sweetened condensed	1 c	306	27	982	24	166	0	27	17	7.4	1
2	102	Evaporated, whole	1 c	252	74	340	17	25	0	20	12	5.9	.6
2	103	Evaporated, skim	1 c	255	79	200	19	29	0	1	.3	.2	t
		Milk, dried:											
2	104	Buttermilk	1 c	120	3	464	41	59	0	7	4.3	2.0	.3
		Instant, nonfat:											
2	105	Envelope[12]	1 ea	91	4	326	32	48	0	1	.4	.2	t
2	106	Cup	1 c	68	4	244	24	36	0	1	.3	.1	t
2	107	Goat milk	1 c	244	87	168	9	11	0	10	6.5	2.7	.4
2	108	Kefir[13]	1 c	233	82	122	9	9	0	5	2.9	1.2	.1
		Milk beverages and powdered mixes:											
		Chocolate:											
2	109	Whole	1 c	250	82	210	8	26	4	8	5.3	2.5	.3
2	110	2% fat	1 c	250	84	180	8	26	4	5	3.1	1.5	.2
2	111	1% fat	1 c	250	84	160	8	26	4	3	1.5	.8	.1
		Chocolate-flavored beverages:											
2	112	Powder containing nonfat dry milk:	1 oz	28	1	100	4	23	<1	1	.7	.4	t
2	113	Drink prepared with water	¾ c	206	86	100	4	23	<1	1	.7	.4	t
2	114	Powder without nonfat dry milk:	¾ oz	22	<1	75	1	20	<1	1	.4	.2	t
2	115	Drink prepared with whole milk	1 c	266	81	226	9	31	<1	9	5.5	2.6	.3
2	116	Eggnog, commercial	1 c	254	74	342	10	34	0	19	11	5.7	.9
		Instant Breakfast:											
2	1027	Envelope, dry powder only	1 ea	37	3	130	7	23	0	0	0	0	0
2	1028	Prepared with whole milk	1 c	281	87	280	15	34	0	8	5.1	2.4	.3
2	1029	Prepared with 2% milk	1 c	281	88	251	15	35	0	5	2.9	1.4	.2
2	1283	Prepared with 1% milk	1 c	281	89	232	15	35	0	3	1.5	.7	.1
2	1284	Prepared with skim milk	1 c	282	89	216	15	35	0	<1	.3	.1	t
		Malted milk, chocolate flavor:											
2	117	Powder[14], 3 heaping tsp:	¾ oz	21	1	79	1	18	<1	1	.5	.2	.1
2	118	Drink prepared with whole milk	1 c	265	81	229	9	30	<1	9	5.2	2.6	.4
		Malted milk, natural flavor:											
2	119	Powder[14], 3 heaping tsp:	¾ oz	21	2	87	2	16	<1	2	.9	.4	.3
2	120	Drink prepared with whole milk	1 c	265	81	237	10	27	<1	10	6.0	2.8	.6
		Milk shakes:											
2	121	Chocolate (10 fl oz)	1¼ c	283	72	360	10	58	<1	11	6.6	3.0	.4
2	122	Vanilla (10 fl oz)	1¼ c	283	75	314	10	51	<1	8	5.3	2.4	.3
		Milk desserts:											
2	134	Custard, baked	1 c	265	77	305	14	29	0	15	6.8	5.4	.7
		Ice cream, regular vanilla (about 11% fat):											
		Hardened:											
2	123	½ gallon	½ gal	1064	61	2153	38	254	0	115	71	33	4
2	124	Cup	1 c	133	61	269	5	32	0	14	8.3	4.1	.5
2	125	Fluid ounces	3 oz	50	61	101	2	12	0	5	3.3	1.6	.2
2	126	Soft serve	1 c	173	60	377	7	38	0	22	14	6.7	1.0
		Ice cream, rich vanilla (about 16% fat):											
		Hardened:											
2	127	½ gallon	½ gal	1188	59	2805	33	256	0	190	118	55	7
2	128	Cup	1 c	148	59	349	4	32	0	24	15	6.8	.9

[12]Yields 1 qt fluid milk when reconstituted according to package directions.

[13]Most values provided by product labeling.

[14]The latest USDA data from *Handbook 8–14* on beverages updates previous USDA data.

(Computer code number is for West Diet Analysis program)

GRP KEY: 1 = BEV 2 = DAIRY 3 = EGGS 4 = FAT/OIL 5 = FRUIT 6 = BAKERY 7 = GRAIN 8 = FISH 9 = BEEF 10 = POULTRY
11 = SAUSAGE 12 = MIXED/FAST 13 = NUTS/SEEDS 14 = SWEETS 15 = VEG/LEG 16 = MISC 22 = SOUP/SAUCE

Chol (mg)	Calc (mg)	Iron (mg)	Magn (mg)	Phos (mg)	Pota (mg)	Sodi (mg)	Zinc (mg)	VT-A (RE)	Thia (mg)	Ribo (mg)	Niac (mg)	V-B6 (mg)	Fola (µg)	VT-C (mg)
104	868	.58	78	775	1136	389	2.88	248	.28	1.27	.64	.16	34	8
74	657	.48	60	510	764	267	1.94	136	.12	.8	.49	.13	18	5
10	738	.7	68	497	845	293	2.18	300	.11	.8	.4	.14	22	3
83	1421	.36	131	1119	1910	621	4.82	65	.47	1.9	1.05	.41	57	7
16	1120	.28	107	896	1552	500	4.01	646[15]	.38	1.59	.81	.31	45	5
12	837	.21	80	670	1160	373	3.06	483[15]	.28	1.19	.61	.24	34	4
28	326	.12	34	270	499	122	.73	137	.12	.34	.68	.11	2	3
10	350	.5	28	319	205	50	.9	155	.45	.44	.3	.09	20	6
31	280	.6	33	251	417	149	1.02	73	.09	.41	.31	.1	12	2
17	284	.6	33	254	422	151	.91	143	.09	.41	.32	.1	12	2
7	287	.6	33	256	425	152	1.02	148	.1	.42	.32	.1	12	2
1	89	.29	23	88	223	139	1.26	1	.03	.17	.18	.04	3	1
1	89	.29	23	88	223	139	1.26	1	.03	.17	.18	.04	3	1
0	8	.68	21	28	128	45	.33	1	.01	.03	.11	<.01	4	<1
33	300	.8	54	256	498	165	1.26	76	.1	.43	.32	.1	12	3
149	330	.51	47	278	420	138	1.17	203	.09	.48	.27	.13	2	4
0	10	7.9	80	15	0	166	3.00	175	.30	.07	5.00	.40	100	27
33	301	8.0	113	243	370	286	3.95	251	.39	.46	5.20	.50	112	29
18	307	8.0	113	247	377	289	3.96	315	.40	.47	5.21	.51	112	29
10	310	8.0	124	250	381	289	3.96	315	.40	.48	5.21	.51	112	29
4	312	8.0	108	262	406	292	3.96	327	.39	.41	5.22	.50	113	29
1	13	.48	15	37	130	53	.17	4	.04	.04	.42	.03	4	<1
34	304	.6	47	265	499	172	1.09	80	13	.44	.63	.14	16	3
4	63	.16	20	75	159	103	.21	19	.11	.19	1.1	.09	10	1
37	354	.27	52	303	529	223	1.14	94	.2	.59	1.31	.19	22	3
37	319	.88	47	288	567	273	1.15	64	.16	.69	.46	.14	10	1
32	344	.26	35	289	492	232	1.01	90	.13	.52	.52	.15	9	2
213	297	1.1	37	310	387	209	1.53	146	.11	.5	.3	.13	24	1
478	1405	.96	149	1075	2053	926	11.3	1064	.42	2.63	1.08	.49	22	6
59	176	.12	18	134	257	116	1.41	133	.05	.33	.13	.06	3	1
23	66	.05	7	50	97	44	.53	50	.02	.12	.05	.02	1	<1
153	236	.43	25	199	338	153	1.99	199	.08	.45	.18	.1	9	1
701	1212	.83	131	927	1770	867	9.74	1758	.36	2.27	.93	.43	23	5
88	151	.1	16	115	221	108	1.21	219	.04	.28	.12	.05	2	1

[15] With added vitamin A.

H

(For purposes of calculations, use "0" for t, <1, <.1, <.01, etc.)

Table H–1 Food Composition

Grp	Computer Code No.	Food Description	Measure	Wt (g)	H₂O (%)	Ener (kcal)	Prot (g)	Carb (g)	Dietary Fiber (g)	Fat (g)	Fat Breakdown (g) Sat	Mono	Poly
DAIRY—Con.													
		Milk Desserts—Con.											
		Ice milk, vanilla (about 4% fat):											
		Hardened:											
2	129	½ gallon	½ gal	1048	69	1467	41	232	0	45	28	13	1.7
2	130	Cup	1 c	131	69	184	5	29	0	6	3.5	1.6	.2
2	131	Soft serve (about 3% fat)	1 c	175	70	223	8	38	0	5	2.9	1.3	.2
		Pudding, canned, 5 oz can = .55 cup:											
2	135	Chocolate	1 ea	142	68	205	3	30	<1	11	9.5	.5	.1
2	136	Tapioca	1 ea	142	74	160	3	28	0	5	4.8	t	t
2	137	Vanilla	1 ea	142	69	220	2	33	0	10	9.5	.3	.1
		Puddings, prepared from dry mix with whole milk:											
2	138	Chocolate, instant	1 c	260	71	310	8	54	<1	8	4.6	2.2	.4
2	139	Chocolate, regular, cooked	½ c	130	73	150	4	25	<1	4	2.4	1.1	.1
2	140	Rice, cooked	½ c	132	73	155	4	27	<1	4	2.3	1.1	.1
2	141	Tapioca, cooked	½ c	130	75	145	4	25	0	4	2.3	1.1	.1
2	142	Vanilla, instant	½ c	130	73	150	4	27	0	4	2.2	1.1	.2
2	143	Vanilla, regular, cooked	½ c	130	74	145	4	25	0	4	2.3	1	.1
		Sherbet (2% fat):											
2	132	½ gallon	½ gal	1542	66	2158	17	469	0	31	19	8.8	1.1
2	133	Cup	1 c	193	66	270	2	59	0	4	2.4	1.1	.1
2	144	Soy milk	1 c	240	93	79	7	4	0	5	.5	.8	2.0
2	1584	Yogurt, frozen, low fat[16]	½ c	87	70	110	4	17	0	2	1.1	.5	<1
		Yogurt, low fat:											
2	145	Fruit added[17]	1 c	227	74	231	10	43	<1	2	1.6	.7	.1
2	146	Plain	1 c	227	85	144	12	16	0	3	2.3	1.0	.1
2	147	Vanilla or coffee flavor	1 c	227	79	193	11	31	0	3	1.8	.8	.1
2	148	Yogurt, made with nonfat milk (<.1% fat)	1 c	227	85	127	13	17	0	<1	.3	.1	t
2	149	Yogurt, made with whole milk (3.3% fat)	1 c	227	88	138	8	11	0	7	4.8	2.0	.2
EGGS[18]													
		Raw, large:											
3	150	Whole, without shell	1 ea	50	75	75	6	1	0	5	1.6	1.6	.7
3	151	White	1 ea	33.4	88	17	4	<1	0	0	0	0	0
3	152	Yolk	1 ea	16.6	49	59	3	<1	0	5	1.6	1.9	.7
		Cooked:											
3	153	Fried in margarine	1 ea	46	69	91	6	1	0	7	1.9	2.7	1.3
3	154	Hard-cooked, shell removed	1 ea	50	75	79	6	1	0	5	1.6	2.0	.7
3	155	Hard-cooked, chopped	1 c	136	75	211	17	2	0	14	4.5	5.5	2.0
3	156	Poached, no added salt	1 ea	50	75	75	6	1	0	5	1.5	1.9	.7
3	157	Scrambled with milk and margarine	1 ea	61	73	100	7	1	0	7	2.2	2.9	1.3
FATS and OILS													
		Butter:											
4	158	Stick	½ c	113	16	813	1	<1	0	92	57	27	3.4
4	159	Tablespoon	1 tbsp	14	16	100	<1	<1	0	12	7.2	3.3	.4
4	160	Pat (about 1 tsp)[19]	1 ea	5	16	34	<1	<1	0	4	2.5	1.2	.2

[16] Data is a composite of USDA information and several manufacturers.

[17] Carbohydrate and kcalories vary widely—consult label if more precise values are needed.

[18] This data is newest revised information from the USDA with 24% less cholesterol.

[19] Pat is 1″ square, ⅓″ thick; about 1 tsp; 90 per lb.

(Computer code number is for West Diet Analysis program)

GRP KEY: 1 = BEV 2 = DAIRY 3 = EGGS 4 = FAT/OIL 5 = FRUIT 6 = BAKERY 7 = GRAIN 8 = FISH 9 = BEEF 10 = POULTRY
11 = SAUSAGE 12 = MIXED/FAST 13 = NUTS/SEEDS 14 = SWEETS 15 = VEG/LEG 16 = MISC 22 = SOUP/SAUCE

Chol (mg)	Calc (mg)	Iron (mg)	Magn (mg)	Phos (mg)	Pota (mg)	Sodi (mg)	Zinc (mg)	VT-A (RE)	Thia (mg)	Ribo (mg)	Niac (mg)	V-B6 (mg)	Fola (µg)	VT-C (mg)
146	1404	1.47	147	1035	2117	838	4.40	419	.61	2.78	.94	.68	21	6
18	176	.18	19	129	265	105	.55	52	.08	.35	.12	.09	3	1
13	274	.28	29	202	412	163	.86	44	.12	.54	.18	.13	5	1
1	74	1.2	24	117	254	285	.70	31	.04	.17	.6	.03	3	<1
1	119	.3	24	113	212	252	.70	<1	.03	.14	.4	.03	3	<1
1	79	.2	24	94	155	305	.70	<1	.03	.12	.6	.03	3	<1
28	260	.6	48	658	352	880	1.18	66	.08	.36	.22	.13	10	2
15	146	.2	24	120	190	167	.59	34	.05	.2	.13	.06	4	1
15	133	.5	16	110	165	140	.60	33	.10	.18	.6	.05	6	1
15	131	.1	16	103	167	152	.50	34	.04	.18	.1	.05	6	1
15	129	.1	16	273	164	375	.50	33	.04	.17	.1	.05	6	1
15	132	.1	16	102	166	178	.50	34	.04	.18	.1	.05	6	1
113	827	2.47	124	594	1588	709	10.6	308	.26	.71	1.05	.2	108	31
14	103	.31	15	74	198	88	1.33	39	.03	.09	.13	.03	14	4
0	10	1.38	45	117	338	30	.54	8	.39	.17	.35	.10	4	0
7	120	.05	5	980	148	45	.56	17	.03	.14	.07	.03	7	<1
10	345	.16	31	325	442	125	1.68	25	.08	.4	.22	.09	21	2
14	415	.18	40	326	531	159	2.02	36	.10	.49	.26	.11	25	2
11	388	.16	36	306	497	150	1.88	30	.10	.46	.24	.10	23	2
4	452	.2	43	354	579	173	2.20	5	.11	.53	.28	.12	28	2
30	275	.11	27	216	352	104	1.34	68	.07	.32	.17	.07	16	1
213	25	.72	5	89	60	61	.55	97	.03	.25	.04	.07	25	0
0	2	.01	4	4	48	55	<.1	0	<.01	.15	.03	<.01	1	0
213	23	.7	1	81	16	7	.54	97	.03	.11	.01	.07	24	0
211	25	.72	5	89	61	162	.55	114	.03	.24	.04	.07	18	0
212	25	.72	5	86	63	62	.55	84	.03	.26	.03	.06	22	0
574	68	1.95	14	233	171	169	1.5	227	.09	.70	.09	.16	61	0
212	25	.72	5	89	60	61	.55	95	.03	.22	.03	.06	18	0
215	44	.72	7	104	84	171	.6	119	.03	.26	.05	.07	18	0
247	27	.18	2	26	29	933[20]	.06	852[21]	.01	.04	.05	<.01	3	0
31	3	.02	<1	3	4	116[20]	.01	106[21]	<.01	<.01	.01	t	<1	0
11	1	.01	<1	1	1	41[20]	<.01	38[21]	t	<.01	<.01	t	<1	0

[20] For salted butter; unsalted butter contains 12 mg sodium per stick or ½ c, 1.5 mg/tbsp, or .5 mg/pat.
[21] Values for vitamin A are a year-round average.

(For purposes of calculations, use "0" for t, <1, <.1, <.01, etc.)

H

Table H–1 Food Composition

Grp	Computer Code No.	Food Description	Measure	Wt (g)	H$_2$O (%)	Ener (kcal)	Prot (g)	Carb (g)	Dietary Fiber (g)	Fat (g)	Fat Breakdown (g)		
											Sat	Mono	Poly
FATS and OILS—Con.													
		Fats, cooking:											
4	1363	Bacon fat	1 tbsp	14	<1	126	0	0	0	14	5.0	6.7	1.7
4	1362	Beef fat/tallow	1 c	205	0	1837	0	0	0	205	102	85.6	8.2
4	1364	Chicken fat	1 c	205	<1	1846	0	0	0	205	61.2	92.0	43.0
		Vegetable shortening:											
4	161	Cup	1 c	205	0	1812	0	0	0	205	51	91	54
4	162	Tablespoon	1 tbsp	13	0	15	0	0	0	13	3.3	5.8	3.4
		Lard:											
4	163	Cup	1 c	205	0	1849	0	0	0	205	80	93	23
4	164	Tablespoon	1 tbsp	13	0	115	0	0	0	13	5.1	5.9	1.5
		Margarine:											
		Imitation (about 40% fat), soft:											
4	165	8-oz container	8 oz	227	58	785	1	1	0	88	18	36	31
4	166	Tablespoon	1 tbsp	14	58	50	<.1	<.1	0	6	1.1	2.2	2.0
		Regular, hard (about 80% fat):											
4	167	Cup	½ c	113	16	812	1	1	0	91	18	41	29
4	168	Tablespoon	1 tbsp	14	16	100	<1	<1	0	11	2.3	5.1	3.6
4	169	Pat[19]	1 ea	5	16	36	<.1	<.1	0	4	.8	1.8	1.3
		Regular, soft (about 80% fat):											
4	170	8-oz container	8 oz	227	16	1626	2	1	0	183	31	65	79
4	171	Tablespoon	1 tbsp	14	16	100	1	<.1	0	11	2.0	4.0	4.9
		Spread (about 60% fat), hard:											
4	172	Cup	½ c	113	37	610	1	0	0	69	16	29	20
4	173	Tablespoon	1 tbsp	14	37	75	<.1	0	0	9	2.0	3.6	2.5
4	174	Pat[19]	1 ea	5	37	25	<.1	0	0	3	.7	1.3	.9
		Spread (about 60% fat), soft:											
4	175	8 oz container	8 oz	227	37	1225	1	0	0	138	29	72	31
4	176	Tablespoon	1 tbsp	14	37	75	<.1	0	0	9	1.8	4.4	1.9
		Oils:											
		Canola:											
4	1585	Cup	1 c	218	0	1927	0	0	0	218	13.1	128	65
4	1586	Tablespoon	1 tbsp	14	0	125	0	0	0	14	.8	8.2	4.1
		Corn:											
4	177	Cup	1 c	218	0	1927	0	0	0	218	28	53	128
4	178	Tablespoon	1 tbsp	14	0	125	0	0	0	14	1.8	3.4	8.2
		Olive:											
4	179	Cup	1 c	216	0	1909	0	0	0	216	29	159	18
4	180	Tablespoon	1 tbsp	14	0	125	0	0	0	14	1.9	10	1.2
		Peanut:											
4	181	Cup	1 c	216	0	1909	0	0	0	216	36	100	69
4	182	Tablespoon	1 tbsp	14	0	125	0	0	0	14	2.4	6.5	4.5
		Safflower:											
4	183	Cup	1 c	218	0	1927	0	0	0	218	20	26	162
4	184	Tablespoon	1 tbsp	14	0	125	0	0	0	14	1.3	1.7	10
		Soybean:											
4	185	Cup	1 c	218	0	1927	0	0	0	218	33	94	82
4	186	Tablespoon	1 tbsp	14	0	125	0	0	0	14	2	6	5
		Soybean/cottonseed:											
4	187	Cup	1 c	218	0	1927	0	0	0	218	39	64	105
4	188	Tablespoon	1 tbsp	14	0	125	0	0	0	14	2.5	4	7

[19]Pat is 1″ square, ⅓″ thick; about 1 tsp; 90 per lb.

(Computer code number is for West Diet Analysis program)

GRP KEY: 1 = BEV   2 = DAIRY   3 = EGGS   4 = FAT/OIL   5 = FRUIT   6 = BAKERY   7 = GRAIN   8 = FISH   9 = BEEF   10 = POULTRY
11 = SAUSAGE   12 = MIXED/FAST   13 = NUTS/SEEDS   14 = SWEETS   15 = VEG/LEG   16 = MISC   22 = SOUP/SAUCE

Chol (mg)	Calc (mg)	Iron (mg)	Magn (mg)	Phos (mg)	Pota (mg)	Sodi (mg)	Zinc (mg)	VT-A (RE)	Thia (mg)	Ribo (mg)	Niac (mg)	V-B6 (mg)	Fola (µg)	VT-C (mg)
84	—	—	—	—	—	140	—	<1	—	—	—	0	—	—
223	2	.41	—	27	0	0	—	<1	<.01	<.01	<.01	<.01	<1	0
174	—	—	—	—	—	—	—	350	—	—	—	0	0	0
0	0	0	0	0	0	0	.10	0	0	0	0	0	0	0
0	0	0	0	0	0	0	0	0	0	0	0	0	0	0
195	<1	0	<1	6	<1	<1	.23	0	0	0	0	0	0	0
12	<1	0	<1	<1	<1	<1	.01	0	0	0	0	0	0	0
0	40	0	3	31	57	2178[22]	.23	2254[23]	.01	.05	.03	.01	2	<1
0	3	0	<1	2	4	136[22]	.03	141[23]	<.01	<.01	<.01	<.01	<1	<1
0	34	.07	3	26	48	1066[22]	.23	1122[23]	.01	.04	.03	.01	1	<1
0	4	.01	<1	3	6	133[22]	.03	139[23]	<.01	<.01	<.01	<.01	<1	<1
0	2	.01	<1	1	2	47[22]	.01	50[23]	t	<.01	<.01	t	<1	<1
0	60	0	5	46	86	2448[22]	.46	2254[23]	.02	.07	.05	.02	2	<1
0	4	0	<1	3	5	153[22]	.03	140[23]	<.01	<.01	<.01	<.01	<1	<1
0	24	0	2	18	34	1123[22]	.17	1122[23]	<.01	.03	.02	.01	1	<1
0	3	0	<1	2	4	139[22]	.02	139[23]	<.01	<.01	<.01	<.01	<1	<1
0	1	0	<1	1	2	50[22]	.01	50[23]	t	<.01	<.01	t	<1	<1
0	47	0	4	37	68	2256[22]	.35	2254[23]	.16	.06	.04	.01	2	<1
0	3	0	<1	2	4	139[22]	.02	139[23]	.01	<.01	<.01	<.01	<1	<1
0	0	0	0	0	0	0	—	0	0	0	0	0	0	0
0	0	0	0	0	0	0	—	0	0	0	0	0	0	0
0	0	.01	0	2	0	0	.02	0	0	0	0	0	<1	0
0	0	0	0	0	0	0	.03	0	0	0	0	0	0	0
0	<1	.83	<1	3	0	0	.13	0	0	0	0	0	<1	0
0	<1	.05	<1	<1	0	0	.01	0	0	0	0	0	0	0
0	t	.06	<1	0	0	0	.02	t	0	0	0	0	<1	0
0	t	<.01	<1	0	0	0	<.01	t	0	0	0	0	0	0
0	0	0	—	0	0	0	.41	0	0	0	0	0	0	0
0	0	0	—	0	0	0	.03	0	0	0	0	0	0	0
0	<1	.05	<1	1	0	0	.4	0	0	0	0	0	<1	0
0	t	0	<1	t	0	0	.03	0	0	0	0	0	t	0
0	0	0	—	0	0	0	.4	0	0	0	0	0	<1	0
0	0	0	—	0	0	0	.03	0	0	0	0	0	0	0

[22] For salted margarine.
[23] Based on average vitamin A content of fortified margarine. Federal specifications require a minimum of 15,000 IU/lb.

(For purposes of calculations, use "0" for t, <1, <.1, <.01, etc.)

H

Table H–1 Food Composition

Grp	Computer Code No.	Food Description	Measure	Wt (g)	H₂O (%)	Ener (kcal)	Prot (g)	Carb (g)	Dietary Fiber (g)	Fat (g)	Fat Breakdown (g) Sat	Mono	Poly
FATS and OILS—Con.													
		Oils—Con.											
		Sunflower:											
4	189	Cup	1 c	218	0	1927	0	0	0	218	23	43	143
4	190	Tablespoon	1 tbsp	14	0	125	0	0	0	14	1.4	2.7	9.2
		Salad dressings/ sandwich spreads:											
4	191	Blue cheese salad dressing	1 tbsp	15	32	75	1	1	<1	8	1.5	1.9	4.3
		French salad dressing:											
4	192	Regular	1 tbsp	16	35	85	<.1	1	<1	9	1.4	4	3.5
4	193	Low calorie	1 tbsp	16	75	24	<.1	2	<1	2	.2	.3	1
		Italian salad dressing:											
4	194	Regular	1 tbsp	14	34	80	<1	1	<1	9	1.3	3.7	3.2
4	195	Low calorie	1 tbsp	15	86	5	<.1	1	<1	1.5	.2	.3	.9
		Mayonnaise:											
4	196	Regular	1 tbsp	14	15	100	<1	<1	0	11	1.7	3.2	5.8
4	197	Imitation, low calorie	1 tbsp	15	63	35	0	2	0	3	.5	.7	1.6
4	198	Ranch style salad dressing	½ c	119	35	435	4	6	0	45	6.7	19	17
		Mayo type salad dressing:											
4	199	Regular	1 tbsp	15	40	58	<1	4	0	5	.7	1.4	2.7
4	1030	Low calorie	1 tbsp	15	63	35	<1	2	0	3	.5	.8	1.4
4	200	Tartar sauce	1 tbsp	14	34	74	<1	1	<1	8	1.2	2.6	3.9
		Thousand Island salad dressing:											
4	201	Regular	1 tbsp	16	46	60	<1	2	<1	6	1.0	1.3	3.2
4	202	Low calorie	1 tbsp	15	69	25	<1	2	<1	2	.2	.4	.9
		Salad dressings, prepared from home recipe:											
4	203	Cooked type[24]	1 tbsp	16	69	25	1	2	0	2	.5	.6	.3
4	204	Vinegar and oil	1 tbsp	16	47	70	0	0	0	8	1.5	2.4	3.9
FRUITS and FRUIT JUICES													
		Apples:											
		Fresh, raw, with peel:											
5	205	2¾″ diam (about 3 per lb with cores)	1 ea	138	84	80	<1	21	3	<1	.1	t	.1
5	206	3¼″ diam (about 2 per lb with cores)	1 ea	212	84	125	<1	32	5	1	.1	t	.2
5	207	Raw, peeled slices	1 c	110	84	65	<1	16	3	<1	.1	t	.1
5	208	Dried, sulfured	10 ea	64	32	155	1	42	8	<1	t	t	.1
5	209	Apple juice, bottled or canned	1 c	248	88	116	<1	29	<1	<1	.1	t	.1
		Applesauce:											
5	210	Sweetened	1 c	255	80	195	<1	51	4	<1	<.1	t	.1
5	211	Unsweetened	1 c	244	88	106	<1	28	4	<1	<.1	t	<.1
		Apricots:											
5	212	Raw, without pits (about 12 per lb with pits)	3 ea	106	86	51	1	12	2	<1	t	.2	.1
		Canned (fruit and liquid):											
5	213	Heavy syrup	1 c	258	78	214	1	55	4	<1	t	.1	t
5	214	Halves	3 ea	85	78	70	<1	18	1	<.1	t	t	t
5	215	Juice pack	1 c	248	87	119	2	31	4	<.1	t	t	t
5	216	Halves	3 ea	84	87	40	1	10	1	<.1	t	t	t
		Dried:											
5	217	Dried halves	10 ea	35	31	83	1	22	3	<1	t	.1	t
5	218	Cooked, unsweetened, with liquid	1 c	250	75	210	3	55	7	<1	t	.2	.1
5	219	Apricot nectar, canned	1 c	251	85	141	1	36	2	<1	t	.1	t

[24] Fatty acid values apply to product made with regular margarine.

(Computer code number is for West Diet Analysis program)

GRP KEY: 1=BEV 2=DAIRY 3=EGGS 4=FAT/OIL 5=FRUIT 6=BAKERY 7=GRAIN 8=FISH 9=BEEF 10=POULTRY
11=SAUSAGE 12=MIXED/FAST 13=NUTS/SEEDS 14=SWEETS 15=VEG/LEG 16=MISC 22=SOUP/SAUCE

Chol (mg)	Calc (mg)	Iron (mg)	Magn (mg)	Phos (mg)	Pota (mg)	Sodi (mg)	Zinc (mg)	VT-A (RE)	Thia (mg)	Ribo (mg)	Niac (mg)	V-B6 (mg)	Fola (µg)	VT-C (mg)
0	0	0	0	0	0	0	—	0	0	0	0	0	0	0
0	0	0	0	0	0	0	—	0	0	0	0	0	0	0
3	12	.03	11	11	6	164	.04	10	<.01	.02	.01	<.01	4	t
0	2	.06	<1	1	2	188	.01	t	t	t	t	<.01	0	t
0	6	.07	—	5	3	306	.03	t	t	t	t	0	t	t
0	1	.03	<1	1	5	162	.02	3	t	t	t	.03	0	t
0	1	.03	<1	1	4	136	0	t	t	t	t	0	t	t
8	2	.07	<1	4	5	80	.02	12	<.01	<.01	<.01	<.01	<1	0
4	0	0	—	0	2	75	—	0	0	0	0	0	t	0
47	119	.31	12	100	158	522	.43	86	.04	.17	08	.05	6	1
4	2	.03	<1	4	1	105	0	13	<.01	<.01	t	<.01	t	0
4	3	.03	—	4	1	75	.02	10	.03	t	t	—	t	—
4	3	.1	<1	4	11	182	.02	9	<.01	<.01	<.01	<.01	<1	t
4	2	.09	<1	3	18	110	.03	15	<.01	<.01	.03	<.01	6	t
2	2	.09	<1	3	17	153	0	14	<.01	<.01	.03	<.01	<1	t
9	13	.08	—	14	19	117	0	20	.01	.02	.04	0	<1	t
0	0	0	—	0	1	0	—	0	0	0	0	0	—	0
0	10	.25	6	10	159	1	.05	7	.02	.02	.11	.07	4	8
0	15	.38	9	23	244	1	.08	11	.04	.03	.16	.1	6	12
0	4	.1	3	8	124	1	.04	5	.02	.01	.1	.05	<1	4
0	9	.9	10	24	288	56[25]	.13	0	0	.1	.59	.08	1	3
0	17	.92	8	17	295	7	.07	<1	.05	.04	.25	.07	1	2[26]
0	10	1	7	18	156	8	.1	3	.03	.07	.50	.07	2	4[26]
0	7	.29	7	18	183	5	.06	7	.03	.06	.46	.06	2	3[26]
0	15	.58	8	21	313	1	.28	166	.03	.04	.64	.06	9	11
0	23	.77	18	33	361	10	.27	317	.05	.06	.97	.14	4	8
0	7	.26	6	10	119	3	.09	105	.02	.02	.32	.05	1	3
0	30	.74	24	50	409	9	.27	419	.05	.05	.85	.18	5	12
0	10	.25	8	17	139	3	.1	142	.02	.02	.29	.06	2	4
0	16	1.65	16	41	482	4	.26	253	<.01	.05	1.05	.06	4	1
0	40	4.2	42	103	1222	8	.66	591	.02	.08	2.36	.28	0	4
0	18	.96	13	23	286	8	.23	330	.02	.04	.65	.16	3	2[27]

[25] Sodium bisulfite used to preserve color; unsulfured product would contain lower levels of sodium.

[26] Value based on products without added vitamin C. Bottled apple juice with added vitamin c usually contains 41.6 mg/100 g, or 103 mg per cup. Check label for specific vitamin C values.

[27] Without added vitamin C. Products with added vitamin c contain 136 mg per cup. Check label.

(For purposes of calculations, use "0" for t, <1, <.1, <.01, etc.)

H

Table H–1 Food Composition

Grp	Computer Code No.	Food Description	Measure	Wt (g)	H₂O (%)	Ener (kcal)	Prot (g)	Carb (g)	Dietary Fiber (g)	Fat (g)	Sat	Mono	Poly
											Fat Breakdown (g)		

FRUITS and JUICES—Con.

Grp	No.	Food Description	Measure	Wt (g)	H₂O (%)	Ener (kcal)	Prot (g)	Carb (g)	Dietary Fiber (g)	Fat (g)	Sat	Mono	Poly
		Avocados, raw, edible part only:											
5	220	California (½ lb with refuse)	1 ea	173	73	305	4	12	17	30	4.5	19	3.5
5	221	Florida (1 lb with refuse)	1 ea	304	80	340	5	27	29	27	5	15	5
5	222	Mashed, fresh, average	1 c	230	74	370	5	17	22	35	6	22	5
		Bananas, raw, without peel:											
5	223	Whole, 8¾" long (weighs 175 g w/peel)	1 ea	114	74	105	1	27	2	1	.2	<.1	.1
5	224	Slices	1 c	150	74	138	2	35	3	1	.3	.1	.1
5	1285	Bananas, dehydrated slices	1 c	100	3	346	4	88	8	2	.7	.2	.3
5	225	Blackberries, raw	1 c	144	86	74	1	18	10	1	.3	.1	.1
		Blueberries:											
5	226	Fresh	1 c	145	85	82	1	21	4	1	<.1	.2	.3
		Frozen, sweetened:											
5	227	10-oz container	10 oz	284	77	230	1	62	7	<1	.1	.1	.2
5	228	Cup	1 c	230	77	185	1	51	5	<1	.1	.1	.2
		Cherries:											
5	229	Sour, red pitted, canned water pack	1 c	244	90	90	2	22	3	<1	.1	.1	.1
5	230	Sweet, raw, without pits	10 ea	68	81	49	1	11	1	1	.1	.2	.2
5	231	Cranberry juice cocktail[28]	1 c	253	85	145	<1[29]	36	1	<1	t	t	.1
5	232	Cranberry-apple juice	1 c	253	86	169	<1	43	1	1[30]	.2	.1	.4
5	233	Cranberry sauce, canned, strained	1 c	277	61	419	1	108	6	<1	<.1	.1	.2
		Dates:											
5	234	Whole, without pits	10 ea	83	22	228	2	61	7	<1	.2	.1	t
5	235	Chopped	1 c	178	22	489	4	131	15	1	.3	.2	.1
5	236	Figs, dried	10 ea	187	28	477	6	122	21	2	.4	.5	1.1
		Fruit cocktail, canned, fruit and liquid:											
5	237	Heavy syrup pack	1 c	255	80	185	1	48	3	<1	<.1	<.1	.1
5	238	Juice pack	1 c	248	87	115	1	29	3	<1	t	t	t
		Grapefruit:											
		Raw 3¾" diam-weight with rind is 241g for one-half											
5	239	Pink/red, half fruit, edible part	1 half	123	91	37	1	9	2	<1	t	t	<.1
5	240	White, half fruit, edible part	1 half	118	90	39	1	10	2	<1	t	t	<.1
5	241	Canned sections with liquid	1 c	254	84	152	1	39	3	<1	<.1	<.1	.1
		Grapefruit juice:											
5	242	Fresh, raw	1 c	247	90	96	1	23	1	<1	<.1	<.1	.1
		Canned:											
5	243	Unsweetened	1 c	247	90	93	1	22	1	<1	<.1	<.1	.1
5	244	Sweetened	1 c	250	87	115	1	28	1	<1	<.1	<.1	.1
		Frozen concentrate, unsweetened:											
5	245	Undiluted, 6-fl-oz can	¾ c	207	62	300	4	72	3	1	.2	.2	.3
5	246	Diluted with 3 cans water	1 c	247	89	102	1	24	1	<1	<.1	<.1	.1
		Grapes, raw, European type (adherent skin):											
5	247	Thompson seedless	10 ea	50	81	35	<1	9	1	<1	.1	t	.1
5	248	Tokay/Emperor, seeded types	10 ea	57	81	40	<1	10	1	<1	.1	t	.1
		Grape juice:											
5	249	Bottled or canned	1 c	253	84	155	1	38	1	<1	.1	t	.1
		Frozen concentrate, sweetened:											
5	250	Undiluted, 6-fl-oz can	¾ c	216	54	385	1	96	4	1	.2	<.1	.2
5	251	Diluted with 3 cans water	1 c	250	87	128	<1	32	1	<1	.1	t	.1

[28]Data here are from the newest USDA *Handbook 8–14* on beverages. These data are somewhat different from that presented in *Handbook 8–9* on fruits and fruit juices.

[29]The newest USDA *Handbook 8–14* data on beverages indicates "0" for protein.

[30]The newest USDA *Handbook 8–14* data on beverages indicates "0" for fat.

(Computer code number is for West Diet Analysis program)

GRP KEY: 1 = BEV   2 = DAIRY   3 = EGGS   4 = FAT/OIL   5 = FRUIT   6 = BAKERY   7 = GRAIN   8 = FISH   9 = BEEF   10 = POULTRY
11 = SAUSAGE   12 = MIXED/FAST   13 = NUTS/SEEDS   14 = SWEETS   15 = VEG/LEG   16 = MISC   22 = SOUP/SAUCE

Chol (mg)	Calc (mg)	Iron (mg)	Magn (mg)	Phos (mg)	Pota (mg)	Sodi (mg)	Zinc (mg)	VT-A (RE)	Thia (mg)	Ribo (mg)	Niac (mg)	V-B6 (mg)	Fola (µg)	VT-C (mg)
0	19	2.04	70	73	1097	21	.73	106	.19	.21	3.32	.48	113	14
0	33	1.6	104	119	1484	14	1.28	186	.33	.37	5.84	.85	162	24
0	25	2.3	90	95	1378	24	.97	141	.25	.28	4.42	.64	142	18
0	7	.35	32	22	451	1	.19	9	.05	.11	.62	.66	24	10
0	9	.46	43	29	593	1	.25	12	.07	.15	.81	.87	31	14
0	22	1.15	108	74	1491	3	.61	31	.18	.24	2.80	.54	40	7
0	46	.8	29	30	282	0	.39	24	.04	.06	.58	.08	49	30
0	9	.24	7	15	129	9	.16	15	.07	.07	.7	.05	9	20
0	16	1.11	7	20	169	4	.14	12	.06	.15	.72	.17	19	3
0	13	.9	6	16	138	3	.14	10	.05	.12	.58	.14	16	2
0	27	3.34	15	25	240	17	.17	184	.04	.1	.43	.11	20	5
0	10	.3	8	13	152	0	.04	15	.03	.04	.3	.02	3	5
0	8	.38	5	5	45	5	.18	1	.02	.02	.09	.05	<1	90[31]
0	18	.15	5	7	68	5	.1	<1	.01	.05	.15	.06	<1	81[31]
0	11	.61	8	17	72	80	.09	6	.04	.06	.28	.05	3	6
0	27	1	29	33	541	2	.24	4	.08	.08	1.83	.16	14	0
0	58	2.14	63	70	1161	5	.52	9	.16	.18	3.92	.34	29	0
0	269	4.18	111	128	1331	21	.94	25	.13	.17	1.3	.42	16	1
0	16	.73	14	28	224	15	.21	52	.05	.05	.95	.11	1	5
0	20	.53	17	34	235	10	.21	76	.03	.04	0	.13	2	7
0	13	.15	10	11	158	0	.09	32[32]	.04	.03	.24	.05	15	47
0	14	.07	11	9	175	0	.08	1	.04	.02	.32	.05	12	39
0	36	1.02	25	25	328	4	.21	0	.1	.05	.62	.05	22	54
0	22	.49	30	37	400	2	.13	2[33]	.1	.05	.49	.11	52	94
0	17	.49	24	27	378	2	.22	2	.1	.05	.57	.05	26	72
0	20	.9	24	28	405	5	.15	2	.1	.06	.8	.05	26	67
0	56	1.02	78	101	1002	6	.38	6	.3	.16	1.6	.32	26	248
0	20	.34	26	34	337	2	.12	2	.1	.05	.54	.11	52	83
0	5	.13	3	7	92	1	.03	4	.05	.03	.15	.06	4	5
0	6	.15	4	8	105	1	.03	4	.05	.03	.17	.06	4	6
0	22	.61	24	27	334	8	.13	2	.07	.09	.66	.16	7	<1
0	28	.78	32	32	160	15	.28	6	.11	.2	.93	.32	9	179[34]
0	10	.26	11	11	53	5	.10	2	.04	.07	.31	.11	4	60[34]

[31]Nutrient added.
[32]Vitamin A in Texas red grapefruit would be 74 RE.
[33]This is Vitamin A for white grapefruit juice; pink or red grapefruit juice = 109 RE per cup.
[34]With added Vitamin C (ascorbic acid).

(For purposes of calculations, use "0" for t, <1, <.1, <.01, etc.)

Table H–1 Food Composition

Grp	Computer Code No.	Food Description	Measure	Wt (g)	H₂O (%)	Ener (kcal)	Prot (g)	Carb (g)	Dietary Fiber (g)	Fat (g)	Fat Breakdown (g) Sat	Mono	Poly
		FRUITS and FRUIT JUICES—Con.											
5	252	Kiwi fruit, raw, peeled (88g with peel)	1 ea	76	83	46	1	11	3	<1	t	.2	.2
5	253	Lemons, raw, without peel and seeds (about 4 per lb whole)	1 ea	58	89	17	1	5	1	<1	t	t	.1
		Lemon juice:											
		Fresh:											
5	254	Cup	1 c	244	91	60	1	21	1	t	t	t	t
5	255	Tablespoon	1 tbsp	15	91	4	<.1	1	<1	t	t	t	t
		Canned or bottled, unsweetened:											
5	256	Cup	1 c	244	92	52	1	16	1	<1	.1	<.1	.2
5	257	Tablespoon	1 tbsp	15	92	3	<1	1	<1	<.1	t	t	t
		Frozen, single strength, unsweetened:											
5	258	Cup	1 c	244	92	54	1	16	1	<1	.1	<.1	.2
5	259	Tablespoon	1 tbsp	15	92	3	<1	1	<1	<.1	t	t	t
		Lime juice:											
		Fresh:											
5	260	Cup	1 c	246	90	65	1	22	1	<1	<.1	<.1	.1
5	261	Tablespoon	1 tbsp	15	90	4	<1	1	<1	<.1	t	t	t
5	262	Canned or bottled, unsweetened	1 c	246	92	50	1	16	1	1	.1	.1	.2
5	263	Mangos, raw, edible part (weighs 300 g with skin and seeds)	1 ea	207	82	135	1	35	7	1	.1	.2	.1
		Melons, raw, without rind and cavity contents:											
5	264	Cantaloupe, 5″ diam (2⅓ lb whole with refuse), orange flesh	½ ea	267	90	94	2	22	3	1	.1	.1	.2
5	265	Honeydew, 6½″ diam (5¼ lb whole with refuse), slice = 1/10 melon	1 slice	129	90	45	1	12	1	<1	t	t	<.1
5	266	Nectarines, raw, without pits, 2½″ diam	1 ea	136	86	67	1	16	3	1	.1	.2	.3
		Oranges, raw:											
5	267	Whole without peel and seeds, 2⅝″ dm. (weighs 180 g with peel and seeds)	1 ea	131	87	60	1	15	3	<1	t	<.1	<.1
5	268	Sections, without membranes	1 c	180	87	85	2	21	4	<1	<.1	<.1	<.1
		Orange juice:											
5	269	Fresh, all varieties	1 c	248	88	111	2	26	1	<1	.1	.1	.1
5	270	Canned, unsweetened	1 c	249	89	105	1	25	<1	<1	<.1	.1	.1
5	271	Chilled	1 c	249	88	110	2	25	<1	1	.1	.1	.2
		Frozen concentrate:											
5	272	Undiluted (6-oz can)	¾ c	213	58	339	5	81	2	<1	.1	.1	.1
5	273	Diluted with 3 parts water by volume	1 c	249	88	110	2	27	<1	<1	t	<.1	<.1
5	1345	Orange juice, from dry crystals	1 c	248	89	114	2	27	0	<1	.1	.1	.1
5	274	Orange and grapefruit juice, canned	1 c	247	89	105	1	25	<1	<1	<.1	<.1	.1
		Papayas, raw:											
5	275	½″ slices	1 c	140	89	60	1	14	2	<1	.1	.1	<.1
5	276	Whole fruit, 3½″ diam by 5⅛″, without seeds and skin (1 lb with refuse)	1 ea	304	89	117	2	30	5	<1	.1	.1	.1
5	1031	Papaya nectar, canned	1 c	250	85	142	<1	36	2	<1	.1	.1	.1
		Peaches:											
5	277	Raw, whole, 2½″ diam, peeled, pitted (about 4 per lb whole)	1 ea	87	88	37	1	10	2	<1	t	<.1	<.1

(Computer code number is for West Diet Analysis program)

GRP KEY: 1=BEV 2=DAIRY 3=EGGS 4=FAT/OIL 5=FRUIT 6=BAKERY 7=GRAIN 8=FISH ` ᴰᴱᴱᴱ  `=POULTRY
11=SAUSAGE 12=MIXED/FAST 13=NUTS/SEEDS 14=SWEETS 15=VEG/LEG 16=MISL   E

Chol (mg)	Calc (mg)	Iron (mg)	Magn (mg)	Phos (mg)	Pota (mg)	Sodi (mg)	Zinc (mg)	VT-A (RE)	Thia (mg)	Ribo (mg)	Niac (mg)		Fola (µg)	VT-C (mg)
0	20	.3	23	30	252	4	.08[35]	13	.02	.04	.4		17[35]	75
0	15	.35	2	9	80	1	.06	2	.02	.01	.06		7	31
0	18	.08	16	14	303	2	.12	5	.07	.02	.24	.12	32	112
0	1	<.01	1	1	19	<1	.01	<1	<.01	<.01	.02	.01	2	7
0	26	.31	22	21	248	50[36]	.15	4	.10	.02	.48	.11	25	61
0	2	.02	1	1	15	3[36]	.01	<1	.01	<.01	.03	.01	2	4
0	19	.30	20	20	218	4	.12	4	.14	.03	.33	.15	23	77
0	1	.02	1	1	14	<1	.01	<1	.01	<.01	.02	.01	1	5
0	22	.08	14	18	268	2	.15	3	.05	.03	.25	.11	21	72
0	1	<.01	1	1	17	<1	.01	<1	<.01	<.01	.02	.08	1	5
0	30	.6	16	25	185	39[36]	.15	4	.08	.01	.4	.07	20	16
0	21	2.6	18	22	323	4	.07	806	.12	.12	1.21	.28	39	57
0	29	.56	19	45	825	24	.43	861	.1	.06	1.53	.31	80	113
0	8	.09	9	13	350	13	.11	5	.1	.02	.77	.08	39	32
0	6	.21	11	22	288	0	.12	100	.02	.06	1.35	.03	5	7
0	52	.14	13	18	237	<1	.09	27	.11	.05	.37	.08	40	70
0	72	.19	18	25	326	<1	.4	37	.16	.07	.51	.11	83	96
0	27	.50	27	42	496	2	.12	50	.22	.07	.99	.1	109	124
0	20	1.1	27	35	436	5	.17	44	.15	.04	.4	.1	15	86
0	25	.42	28	27	473	2	.11	19[37]	.28	.05	.7	.13	45[37]	82[37]
0	68	.75	73	121	1436	6	.38	59	.6	.14	1.53	.33	331	294
0	22	.27	24	40	474	2	.13	19	.2	.04	.5	.11	109	97
0	40	.02	5	31	50	1	—	.50	.20	.07	1.00	0	0	80
0	20	1.1	24	35	390	7	.18	29	.14	.07	.83	.06	20	72
0	33	.3	14	12	247	9	.10	282	.04	.05	.47	.03	26	92
0	72	.3	31	16	780	8	.22	612	.08	.10	1.03	.06	48	188
0	24	.86	8	1	78	14	.38	28	.02	.01	.38	.02	5	8
0	4	.1	6	10	171	0	.12	47	.02	.04	.86	.02	3	6

[35]Data are estimated from other fruit data.
[36]Sodium benzoate and sodium bisulfite added as preservatives.
[37]Values for juice from California oranges indicate the following values for 1 c: 36 RE of vitamin A, 72µg of folacin, and 106 mg of vitamin C.

(For purposes of calculations, use "0" for t, <1, <.1, <.01, etc.)

H

Table H–1 Food Composition

Grp	Computer Code No.	Food Description	Measure	Wt (g)	H₂O (%)	Ener (kcal)	Prot (g)	Carb (g)	Dietary Fiber (g)	Fat (g)	Fat Breakdown (g) Sat	Mono	Poly
		FRUITS and FRUIT JUICES—Con.											
		Peaches—Con.											
5	278	Raw, sliced	1 c	170	88	73	1	19	3	<1	t	.1	.1
		Canned, fruit and liquid:											
		Heavy syrup pack:											
5	279	Cup	1 c	256	79	190	1	51	3	<1	<.1	.1	.1
5	280	Half	1 ea	81	79	60	<1	16	1	<1	t	<.1	<.1
		Juice pack:											
5	281	Cup	1 c	248	88	109	2	29	3	<1	t	<.1	<.1
5	282	Half	1 ea	77	88	34	<1	9	1	<1	t	t	t
		Dried:											
5	283	Uncooked	10 ea	130	32	311	5	80	11	1	.1	.4	.5
5	284	Cooked, fruit and liquid	1 c	258	78	200	3	51	4	1	.1	.2	.3
		Frozen, sliced, sweetened:											
5	285	10-oz package	1 ea	284	75	267	2	68	6	<1	<.1	.1	.2
5	286	Cup, thawed measure	1 c	250	75	235	2	60	4	<1	<.1	.1	.2
5	1032	Peach nectar, canned	1 c	249	86	134	1	35	1	<1	t	<.1	<.1
		Pears:											
		Fresh, with skin, cored:											
5	287	Bartlett, 2½″ diam (about 2½ per lb)	1 ea	166	84	98	1	25	5[38]	1	<.1	.1	.2
5	288	Bosc, 2½″ diam (about 3 per lb)	1 ea	141	84	85	1	21	4[38]	1	<.1	.1	.1
5	289	D'Anjou, 3″ diam (about 2 per lb)	1 ea	200	84	120	1	30	6[38]	1	<.1	.2	.2
		Canned, fruit and liquid:											
		Heavy syrup pack:											
5	290	Cup	1 c	255	80	188	1	49	4[38]	<1	t	.1	.1
5	291	Half	1 ea	79	80	59	<1	15	1[38]	<1	t	t	t
		Juice pack:											
5	292	Cup	1 c	248	86	123	1	32	4[38]	<1	t	<.1	<.1
5	293	Half	1 ea	77	86	38	<1	10	1[38]	<1	t	t	t
5	294	Dried halves	10 ea	175	27	459	3	122	19	1	.1	.2	.3
5	1033	Pear nectar, canned	1 c	250	84	149	<1	39	2	<1	t	t	t
		Pineapple:											
5	295	Fresh chunks, diced	1 c	155	86	76	1	19	2	1	<.1	<.1	.2
		Canned, fruit and liquid:											
		Heavy syrup pack:											
5	296	Crushed, chunks, tidbits	1 c	255	79	199	1	52	2	<1	t	<.1	.1
5	297	Slices	1 ea	58	79	45	<1	12	1	<.1	t	t	<.1
		Juice Pack:											
5	298	Crushed, chunks, tidbits	1 c	250	84	150	1	39	2	<1	t	<.1	.1
5	299	Slices	1 ea	58	84	35	<1	9	1	<.1	t	t	t
5	300	Pineapple juice, canned, unsweetened	1 c	250	86	140	1	34	1	<1	t	t	.1
		Plantains, without peel:											
5	301	Raw slices (one whole plantain weighs 179 g without peel)	1 c	148	65	181	2	47	7[39]	1	.2	.1	.1
5	302	Cooked, boiled, sliced	1 c	154	67	179	1	48	7	<1	.1	<.1	.1
		Plums, canned:											
		Fresh:											
5	303	Medium 2⅛″ diam	1 ea	66	85	36	1	9	1	<1	<.1	.3	.1
5	304	Small, 1½″ diam	1 ea	28	85	15	<1	4	1	<1	t	.1	<.1

[38] Dietary fiber data vary 2.4 to 3.4 g/100 g for fresh pears; 1.6 to 2.6 g/100 g for canned pears.
[39] Dietary fiber value partially derived from data for bananas.

(Computer code number is for West Diet Analysis program)

GRP KEY: 1 = BEV   2 = DAIRY   3 = EGGS   4 = FAT/OIL   5 = FRUIT   6 = BAKERY   7 = GRAIN   8 = FISH   9 = BEEF   10 = POULTRY
11 = SAUSAGE   12 = MIXED/FAST   13 = NUTS/SEEDS   14 = SWEETS   15 = VEG/LEG   16 = MISC   22 = SOUP/SAUCE

Chol (mg)	Calc (mg)	Iron (mg)	Magn (mg)	Phos (mg)	Pota (mg)	Sodi (mg)	Zinc (mg)	VT-A (RE)	Thia (mg)	Ribo (mg)	Niac (mg)	V-B6 (mg)	Fola (µg)	VT-C (mg)
0	9	.19	11	20	335	1	.18	91	.03	.07	1.68	.03	6	11
0	8	.69	13	29	235	16	.22	85	.03	.06	1.57	.05	8	7
0	3	.22	4	9	75	5	.07	27	.01	.02	.5	.01	3	2
0	15	.72	18	43	317	11	.26	94	.02	.04	1.44	.05	8	9
0	5	.21	6	13	98	3	.09	29	.01	.01	.45	.02	3	3
0	37	5.28	54	155	1295	9	.74	281	<.01	.28	5.69	.09	6	6
0	23	3.37	35	99	825	6	.46	51	.01	.05	3.92	.1	<1	10
0	9	1.05	14	31	369	17	.14	81	.04	.10	1.9	.05	9	268[40]
0	8	.93	12	28	325	16	.13	71	.03	.09	1.63	.04	8	236[40]
0	13	.47	11	16	101	10	.20	64	.01	.04	.72	.03	2	13
0	19	.42	9	18	208	1	.20	3	.03	.07	.17	.03	12	7
0	16	.40	8	16	176	<1	.17	3	.03	.06	.1	.03	10	6
0	22	.50	11	22	250	<1	.24	4	.04	.08	.2	.04	14	8
0	13	.56	11	18	166	13	.21	1	.03	.06	.62	.04	3	3
0	4	.17	3	5	51	4	.06	<1	.01	.02	.19	.01	1	1
0	22	.71	17	29	238	10	.22	1	.03	.03	.5	.04	5	4
0	7	.22	5	9	74	3	.07	<1	.01	.01	.15	.01	2	1
0	59	3.68	58	103	932	10	.68	1	.01	.25	2.4	.01	21	12
0	11	.65	6	7	33	8	.16	<1	<.01	.03	.32	.03	2	3
0	11	.57	21	11	175	2	.12	4	.14	.06	.65	.14	16	24
0	36	.97	40	18	265	3	.31	4	.23	.06	.73	.19	12	19
0	8	.22	9	4	60	1	.70	1	.05	.02	.17	.04	3	4
0	35	.70	35	15	305	3	.25	10	.24	.05	.71	.19	12	24
0	8	.16	8	4	71	1	.06	2	.06	.02	.17	.04	3	6
0	43	.65	34	20	335	3	.28	1	.14	.06	.64	.24	58	27[41]
0	4	.89	55	50	739	6	.27	167[42]	.08	.08	1.02	.44	33	27
0	3	.89	49	43	716	8	.21	140	.07	.08	1.16	.37	40	17
0	3	.07	4	7	114	<1	.07	21	.03	.06	.33	.05	3	6
0	1	.03	2	3	48	<1	.03	9	.01	.03	.14	.02	1	3

[40]With added vitamin C (ascorbic acid).
[41]If vitamin C is added, it contains 96 mg per cup.
[42]Vitamin A values range from 1.5 RE for white-fleshed varieties to 178 RE for yellow-fleshed varieties.

(For purposes of calculations, use "0" for t, <1, <.1, <.01, etc.)

H

Table H–1   Food Composition

Grp	Computer Code No.	Food Description	Measure	Wt (g)	H₂O (%)	Ener (kcal)	Prot (g)	Carb (g)	Dietary Fiber (g)	Fat (g)	Sat	Mono	Poly
											Fat Breakdown (g)		

FRUITS—Con.
Plums—Con.
Canned, purple, with liquid:
Heavy Syrup pack:

Grp	No.	Food Description	Measure	Wt (g)	H₂O (%)	Ener (kcal)	Prot (g)	Carb (g)	Dietary Fiber (g)	Fat (g)	Sat	Mono	Poly
5	305	Cup	1 c	258	76	230	1	60	4	<1	t	.2	.1
5	306	Plums	3 ea	110	76	98	<1	25	2	<1	t	.1	t
		Juice pack:											
5	307	Cup	1 c	252	84	146	1	38	4	<.1	t	<.1	t
5	308	Plums	3 ea	95	84	55	<1	14	2	<.1	t	t	t
		Prunes, dried, pitted:											
5	309	Uncooked (10 prunes weigh 97 g with pits, 84 g without pits.)	10 ea	84	32	201	2	53	8[43]	<1	<.1	.3	.1
5	310	Cooked, unsweetened, fruit and liquid (250 g with pits)	1 c	212	70	227	2	60	9	<1	<.1	.3	.1
5	311	Prune juice, bottled or canned	1 c	256	81	181	2	45	3	<.1	t	<.1	t
		Raisins, seedless:											
5	312	Cup, not pressed down	1 c	145	15	435	5	115	9	1	.2	<.1	.2
5	313	One packet, ½ oz	½ oz	14	15	41	<1	11	1	<.1	t	t	t
		Raspberries:											
5	314	Fresh	1 c	123	87	60	1	14	8	1	t	.1	.4
		Frozen, sweetened:											
5	315	10-oz container	10 oz	284	73	293	2	74	15	<1	t	<.1	.3
5	316	Cup, thawed measure	1 c	250	73	255	2	65	12	<1	t	<.1	.2
5	317	Rhubarb, cooked, added sugar	1 c	240	68	279	1	75	5	<1	t	t	.1
		Strawberries:											
5	318	Fresh, whole, capped	1 c	149	92	45	1	11	4	1	<.1	.1	.3
		Frozen, sliced, sweetened:											
5	319	10-oz container	10 oz	284	73	273	2	74	6	<1	t	.1	.2
5	320	Cup, thawed measure	1 c	255	73	245	1	66	8	<1	t	.1	.2
		Tangerines, without peel and seeds:											
5	321	Fresh (2⅜″ whole) 116g with refuse	1 ea	84	88	37	1	9	2	<1	t	<.1	<.1
5	322	Canned, light syrup, fruit and liquid	1 c	252	83	154	1	41	4	<1	<.1	<.1	.1
5	323	Tangerine juice, canned, sweetened	1 c	249	87	125	1	30	1	<1	<.1	<.1	.1
		Watermelon, raw, without rind and seeds:											
5	324	Piece, 1″ thick by 10″ diam (weighs 2 lb with refuse or 926g)	1 pce	482	92	152	3	35	2	2	.3	.2	1
5	325	Diced	1 c	160	92	50	1	12	1	1	.1	.1	.4

BAKED GOODS:
BREADS, CAKES, COOKIES, CRACKERS, PIES, PANCAKES, TORTILLAS

Grp	No.	Food Description	Measure	Wt (g)	H₂O (%)	Ener (kcal)	Prot (g)	Carb (g)	Dietary Fiber (g)	Fat (g)	Sat	Mono	Poly
6	326	Bagels, plain, enriched, 3½″ diam	1 ea	68	32	180	7	35	1	1	.2	.3	.4
		Biscuits:											
6	327	From home recipe	1 ea	28	28	100	2	13	1	5	1.2	2	1.3
6	328	From mix	1 ea	28	29	94	2	14	1	3	.8	1.4	.9
6	329	From refrigerated dough	1 ea	20	30	65	1	10	<1	2	.6	.9	.6
6	330	Bread crumbs, dry grated (see 364, 365 for soft crumbs)	1 c	100	7	390	13	73	4	5	1.5	1.6	1
		Breads:											
6	331	Boston brown bread, canned, 3¼″ slice	1 pce	45	45	95	2	21	2	1	.26	.13	.14
		Cracked wheat bread (¼ cracked-wheat flour, ¾ enr wheat flour):											
6	332	1-lb loaf	1 ea	454	35	1190	42	227	23	16	3.1	4.3	5.7
6	333	Slice (18 per loaf)	1 pce	25	35	65	2	13	1	1	.2	.2	.3
6	334	Slice, toasted	1 pce	21	26	65	2	13	1	1	.2	.2	.3

[43]Dietary fiber data can vary between 8 and 13 g for 10 prunes.

(Computer code number is for West Diet Analysis program)

GRP KEY: 1 = BEV   2 = DAIRY   3 = EGGS   4 = FAT/OIL   5 = FRUIT   6 = BAKERY   7 = GRAIN   8 = FISH   9 = BEEF   10 = POULTRY
11 = SAUSAGE   12 = MIXED/FAST   13 = NUTS/SEEDS   14 = SWEETS   15 = VEG/LEG   16 = MISC   22 = SOUP/SAUCE

Chol (mg)	Calc (mg)	Iron (mg)	Magn (mg)	Phos (mg)	Pota (mg)	Sodi (mg)	Zinc (mg)	VT-A (RE)	Thia (mg)	Ribo (mg)	Niac (mg)	V-B6 (mg)	Fola (µg)	VT-C (mg)
0	23	2.17	13	34	235	49	.18	67	.04	.1	.75	.07	7	1
0	10	.92	6	14	100	21	.08	29	.02	.04	.32	.03	3	<1
0	25	.86	20	38	388	3	.28	254	.06	.15	1.19	.1	8	7
0	10	.32	8	15	147	1	.11	96	.02	.06	.45	.04	3	3
0	43	2.08	38	66	626	3	.45	167	.07	.14	1.65	.22	3	3
0	49	2.35	43	74	708	4	.51	65	.05	.21	1.53	.46	<1	6
0	31	3.02	36	64	707	10	.54	1	.04	.18	2.01	.56	1	11
0	71	3.02	48	140	1089	17	.46	1	.23	.13	1.19	.36	5	5
0	7	.29	5	14	105	2	.05	<1	.02	.01	.12	.04	1	<1
0	27	.7	22	15	187	0	.57	16	.04	.11	1.11	.07	32	31
0	43	1.85	37	48	324	3	.51	17	.05	.13	.65	.1	74	47
0	38	1.62	32	43	285	3	.45	15	.05	.11	1.5	.09	65	41
0	348	.5	30	19	230	2	.19	17	.04	.06	.48	.05	13	8
0	21	.57	16	28	247	2	.19	4	.03	.1	.34	.09	28	85
0	31	1.7	20	37	278	9	.17	7	.05	.14	1.1	.09	47	118
0	28	1.5	18	33	250	8	.15	6	.04	.13	1.02	.08	42	106
0	12	.08	10	8	132	1	.38	77	.09	.02	.13	.06	17	26
0	18	.93	19	25	197	15	.60	212	.13	.11	1.1	.11	34	50
0	45	.5	20	35	443	2	.08	105	.15	.05	.25	.08	8	55
0	38	.82	52	41	560	10	.34	176	.39	.1	.96	.69	10	47
0	13	.27	17	14	186	3	.11	59	.13	.03	.32	.23	3	15
0	20	2.1	15	61	65	300	.61	0	.26	.20	2.4	.03	16	0
t	48	.7	6	36	32	195	.15	3	.08	.08	.8	.01	2	t
t	59	.58	7	129	57	265	.18	4	.12	.11	.85	.01	2	t
1	4	.47	4	78	18	249	.09	0	.08	.05	.67	.01	1	0
5	122	4.1	31	141	152	736	.50	0	.35	.35	4.8	.02	28	0
3	41	.90	40	72	131	113	.35	0	.06	.04	.7	.06	8	0
0	295	12.1	218	581	608	1966	6.36	0	1.73	1.73	15.3	.42	218	t
0	16	.67	12	32	34	106	.35	0	.1	.1	.84	.02	12	t
0	16	.67	12	32	34	106	.35	0	.07	.1	.84	.02	9	t

H

(For purposes of calculations, use "0" for t, <1, <.1, <.01, etc.)

Table H–1   Food Composition

Grp	Computer Code No.	Food Description	Measure	Wt (g)	H₂O (%)	Ener (kcal)	Prot (g)	Carb (g)	Dietary Fiber (g)	Fat (g)	Fat Breakdown (g) Sat	Mono	Poly
		BAKED GOODS—Con.											
		Breads—Con.											
		French/Vienna bread, enriched:											
6	335	1-lb loaf	1 ea	454	34	1270	43	230	8	18	4	6	6
6	336	French, slice, 5 × 2½ × 1″	1 pce	35	34	100	3	18	1	1	.3	.4	.5
6	337	Vienna, slice 4¾ × 4 × ½″	1 pce	25	34	70	2	13	1	1	.2	.3	.3
		French toast: see Mixed Dishes, and Fast Foods, code # 691											
		Italian bread, enriched:											
6	338	1-lb loaf	1 ea	454	32	1255	41	256	5	4	.6	.3	1.6
6	339	Slice, 4½ × 3¼ × ¾″	1 pce	30	32	83	3	17	<1	<1	<.1	t	.1
		Mixed grain bread, enriched:											
6	340	1-lb loaf	1 ea	454	37	1165	45	212	18	17	3	4	7
6	341	Slice (18 per loaf)	1 pce	25	37	65	2	12	2	1	.2	.2	.4
6	342	Slice, toasted	1 pce	23	27	65	2	12	2	1	.2	.2	.4
		Oatmeal bread, enriched:											
6	343	1-lb loaf	1 ea	454	37	1145	38	212	16	20	4	7	8
6	344	Slice (18 per loaf)	1 pce	25	37	65	2	12	1	1	.2	.4	.5
6	345	Slice, toasted	1 pce	23	30	65	2	12	1	1	.2	.4	.5
6	346	Pita pocket bread, enr, 6½″ round	1 ea	60	31	165	6	33	1	1	.1	.1	.4
		Pumpernickel bread (⅔ rye flour, ⅓ enr. wheat flour):											
6	347	1-lb loaf	1 ea	454	37	1160	42	218	19	16	3	4	6
6	348	Slice, 5 × 4 × ⅜″	1 pce	32	37	80	3	15	2	1	.2	.3	.5
6	349	Slice, toasted	1 pce	29	28	80	3	15	1	1	.2	.3	.5
		Raisin bread, enriched:											
6	350	1-lb loaf	1 ea	454	33	1260	37	239	12	18	4	7	7
6	351	Slice (18 per loaf)	1 pce	25	33	68	2	13	1	1	.2	.4	.4
6	352	Slice, toasted	1 pce	21	24	68	2	13	1	1	.2	.4	.4
		Rye bread, light (⅓ rye flour, ⅔ enr. wheat flour):											
6	353	1-lb loaf	1 ea	454	37	1190	38	218	30	17	3.3	5.2	5.5
6	354	Slice, 4¾ × 3¾ × ⁷⁄₁₆″	1 pce	25	37	65	2	12	2	1	.2	.3	.3
6	355	Slice, toasted	1 pce	22	28	65	2	12	2	1	.2	.3	.3
		Wheat bread (blend of enr. wheat flour and whole-wheat flour):[44]											
6	356	1-lb loaf	1 ea	454	37	1160	43	213	25	19	3.9	7.3	4.5
6	357	Slice (18 per loaf)	1 pce	25	37	65	2	12	1	1	.2	.4	.3
6	358	Slice, toasted	1 pce	23	28	65	2	12	1	1	.2	.4	.3
		White bread, enriched:											
6	359	1-lb loaf	1 ea	454	37	1210	38	222	12	18	5.6	6.5	4.2
6	360	Slice (18 per loaf)	1 pce	25	37	65	2	12	<1	1	.3	.4	.2
6	361	Slice, toasted	1 pce	22	28	65	2	12	<1	1	.3	.4	.2
6	362	Slice (22 per loaf)	1 pce	20	37	55	2	10	<1	1	.2	.3	.2
6	363	Slice, toasted	1 pce	17	28	55	2	10	<1	1	.2	.3	.2
		White bread cubes, crumbs:											
6	364	Cubes, soft	1 c	30	37	80	2	15	1	1	.4	.4	.3
6	365	Crumbs, soft	1 c	45	37	120	4	22	1	2	.6	.6	.4
		Whole-wheat bread:											
6	366	1-lb loaf	1 ea	454	38	1110	44	206	51	20	6	7	5
6	367	Slice (16 per loaf)	1 pce	28	38	70	3	13	2	1	.4	.4	.3
6	368	Slice, toasted	1 pce	25	29	70	3	13	2	1	.4	.4	.3

[44]A blend of white and whole-wheat flour—no official ratio specified.

(Computer code number is for West Diet Analysis program)

GRP KEY: 1 = BEV 2 = DAIRY 3 = EGGS 4 = FAT/OIL 5 = FRUIT 6 = BAKERY 7 = GRAIN 8 = FISH 9 = BEEF 10 = POULTRY
11 = SAUSAGE 12 = MIXED/FAST 13 = NUTS/SEEDS 14 = SWEETS 15 = VEG/LEG 16 = MISC 22 = SOUP/SAUCE

Chol (mg)	Calc (mg)	Iron (mg)	Magn (mg)	Phos (mg)	Pota (mg)	Sodi (mg)	Zinc (mg)	VT-A (RE)	Thia (mg)	Ribo (mg)	Niac (mg)	V-B6 (mg)	Fola (µg)	VT-C (mg)
0	499	14	91	386	409	2633	2.9	0	2.09	1.59	18.2	.24	168	t
0	39	1.08	7	30	32	203	.22	0	.16	.12	1.4	.02	13	t
0	28	.77	5	21	23	145	.16	0	.12	.09	1	.01	9	t
0	77	12.7	106	350	336	2656	3.1	0	1.86	1.06	15.1	.24	160	0
0	5	.8	7	23	22	176	.21	0	.12	.07	1	.02	11	0
0	472	14.8	222	962	990	1870	5.45	t	1.77	1.73	18.9	.47	295	
0	27	.8	12	55	56	106	.3	t	.1	.1	1.1	.03	16	t
0	27	.8	12	55	56	106	.3	t	.08	.1	1.1	.02	12	t
0	267	12	154	563	707	2231	4.45	0	2.09	1.2	15.4	.07	15	0
0	15	.7	9	31	39	124	.25	0	.12	.07	.85	<.01	1	0
0	15	.7	9	31	39	124	.25	0	.09	.07	.85	<.01	1	0
0	49	1.45	16	60	71	339	.50	0	.27	.13	2.32	.01	12	0
0	322	12.4	309	990	1966	2461	5.18	0	1.54	2.36	15	.72	222	0
0	23	.88	22	71	141	177	.4	0	.11	.17	1.06	.05	16	0
0	23	.88	22	71	141	177	.4	0	.09	.17	1.06	.05	12	0
0	463	14.1	114	395	1058	1657	2.81	1	1.5	2.81	18.6	.15	159	t
0	25	.78	6	22	59	92	.16	t	.08	.16	1.02	.01	9	t
0	25	.80	6	22	59	92	.16	t	.06	.16	1.02	.01	8	t
0	363	12.3	109	658	926	3164	5.77	0	1.86	1.45	15	.43	177	0
0	20	.68	8	36	51	175	.38	0	.1	.08	.83	.02	10	0
0	20	.68	6	36	51	175	.38	0	.08	.08	.83	.02	8	0
0	572	15.8	209	835	627	2447	4.77	t	2.09	1.45	20.5	.50	204	t
0	32	.87	12	47	35	135	.26	t	.12	.08	1.13	.03	11	t
0	32	.87	12	47	35	135	.26	t	.10	.08	1.20	.02	8	t
0	572	12.9	95	490	508	2334	2.81	t	2.13	1.41	17.0	.15	159	t
0	32	.71	5	27	28	129	.16	t	.12	.08	.94	.01	9	t
0	32	.71	5	27	28	129	.16	t	.09	.08	.94	.01	9	t
0	25	.57	4	22	22	103	.12	t	.09	.06	.75	.01	7	t
0	25	.6	4	21	22	103	.12	t	.07	.06	.75	.01	7	t
0	38	.85	6	32	34	154	.19	t	.14	.09	1.13	.01	11	t
0	57	1.28	9	49	50	231	.28	t	.21	.14	1.69	.02	16	t
0	327	15.5	422	1180	799	2887	7.63	t	1.59	.95	17.4	.85	250	t
0	20	.97	26	74	50	180	.50	t	.10	.06	1.09	.05	16	t
0	20	.97	26	74	50	180	.50	t	.08	.06	1.08	.05	12	t

H

(For purposes of calculations, use "0" for t, <1, <.1, <.01, etc.)

Table H–1   Food Composition

Grp	Computer Code No.	Food Description	Measure	Wt (g)	H₂O (%)	Ener (kcal)	Prot (g)	Carb (g)	Dietary Fiber (g)	Fat (g)	Fat Breakdown (g) Sat	Mono	Poly
BAKED GOODS—Con.													
		Bread stuffing, prepared from mix:											
6	369	Dry type	1 c	140	33	500	9	50	4	31	6	13	10
6	370	Moist type, with egg	1 c	203	61	420	9	40	4	26	5	11	8
		Cakes, prepared from mixes:[45]											
		Angel food cake:											
6	371	Whole cake, 9 ¾″ diam tube	1 ea	635	38	1510	38	342	3	2	.4	.2	1
6	372	Piece, 1/12 of cake	1 pce	53	38	125	3	29	<1	<1	t	t	.1
6	373	Boston cream pie, 1/8 of cake	1 pce	120	35	260	3	44	1	8	2.8	3.1	1.5
		Coffee cake:											
6	374	Whole cake, 7¾ × 5⅛ × 1¼″	1 ea	430	30	1385	27	225	3	41	12	17	10
6	375	Piece, 1/6 of cake	1 pce	72	30	230	5	38	2	7	2.0	2.8	1.6
		Devil's food with chocolate frosting:											
6	376	Whole cake, 2 layer, 8 or 9″ diam	1 ea	1107	24	3755	49	645	5	136	56	51	20
6	377	Piece, 1/16 of cake	1 pce	69	24	235	3	40	1	8	3.5	3.2	1.2
6	378	Cupcake, 2½″ diam	1 ea	42	24	143	2	25	<1	5	2.1	2.0	.7
		Gingerbread:											
6	379	Whole cake, 8″ square	1 ea	570	37	1575	18	291	3	39	10	16	11
6	380	Piece, 1/9 of cake	1 pce	63	37	174	2	32	2	4	1.1	1.8	1.2
		Yellow, with chocolate frosting, 2 layer:											
6	381	Whole cake, 8 or 9″ diam	1 ea	1108	26	3735	45	638	5	125	48	49	22
6	382	Piece, 1/16 of cake	1 pce	69	26	235	3	40	<1	8	3	3.1	1.4
		Cakes from home recipes with enriched flour:											
		Carrot cake, cream cheese frosting:[46]											
6	383	Whole, 9 × 13″ cake	1 ea	1792	23	6496	63	832	20	328	69	135	114
6	384	Piece, 1/16 of 9 × 13″ cake 2¼ × 3¼″	1 pce	112	23	406	4	52	1	21	4.3	8.5	7.1
		Fruitcake, dark, 7½″ diam tube, 2¼″ high:[46]											
6	385	Whole cake	1 ea	1361	18	5185	74	783	38	228	48	113	52
6	386	Piece, 1/32 of cake, ⅔″ arc	1 pce	43	18	165	2	25	2	7	1.5	3.6	1.6
		Sheet cake, plain, no frosting:[47]											
6	387	Whole cake, 9″ square	1 ea	777	25	2830	35	434	3	108	30	45	26
6	388	Piece, 1/9 of cake	1 pce	86	25	315	4	48	<1	12	3.3	5	2.8
		Sheet cake, plain, uncooked white frosting:[48]											
6	389	Whole cake, 9″ square	1 ea	1096	21	4020	37	694	3	129	42	50	26
6	390	Piece, 1/9 of cake	1 pce	121	21	445	4	77	<1	14	5	6	3
		Pound cake:[48]											
6	391	Loaf, 8½ × 3½ × 3¼″	1 ea	514	22	2025	33	265	4	94	21	41	27
6	392	Piece, 1/17 of loaf, ½″ slice	1 pce	30	22	120	2	15	<1	5	1.2	2.4	1.6
		Cakes, commercial:											
		Pound cake:											
6	393	Loaf, 8½ × 3½ × 3″	1 ea	500	24	1935	26	257	4	94	52	30	4
6	394	Slice, 1/17 of loaf, ½″ slice	1 pce	29	24	110	2	15	<1	5	3.0	1.7	.2
		Snack cakes:											
6	395	Chocolate w/creme filling, 2 small cakes per package	1 ea	28	20	105	1	17	<1	4	1.7	1.5	.6
6	396	Sponge cake w/creme filling, 2 small cakes per package	1 ea	42	19	155	1	27	<1	5	2.3	2.1	.5

[45]Excepting angel food cake, cakes were made from mixes containing vegetable shortening, and frostings were made with margarine. All mixes use enriched flour.
[46]Made with vegetable oil.
[47]Cake made with vegetable shortening.
[48]Made with margarine.

(Computer code number is for West Diet Analysis program)

GRP KEY: 1 = BEV   2 = DAIRY   3 = EGGS   4 = FAT/OIL   5 = FRUIT   6 = BAKERY   7 = GRAIN   8 = FISH   9 = BEEF   10 = POULTRY
11 = SAUSAGE   12 = MIXED/FAST   13 = NUTS/SEEDS   14 = SWEETS   15 = VEG/LEG   16 = MISC   22 = SOUP/SAUCE

Chol (mg)	Calc (mg)	Iron (mg)	Magn (mg)	Phos (mg)	Pota (mg)	Sodi (mg)	Zinc (mg)	VT-A (RE)	Thia (mg)	Ribo (mg)	Niac (mg)	V-B6 (mg)	Fola (µg)	VT-C (mg)
0	92	2.2	30	136	126	1254	.55	273	.17	.20	2.50	.02	14	0
67	81	2.03	45	134	118	1023	.78	256	.10	.18	1.62	.04	20	t
0	527	2.73	51	1086	845	3226	.82	0	.32	1.27	1.6	.08	51	0
0	44	.23	4	91	71	269	.07	0	.03	.11	.13	.01	4	0
20	26	.6	11	70	40	225	.23	70	.01	.18	.7	.05	7	0
279	262	7.30	27	748	469	1853	3.70	194	.82	.90	7.70	.12	30	1
47	44	1.22	5	125	78	310	.62	32	.14	.15	1.29	.02	5	t
598	653	22.1	200	1162	1439	2900	7.95	498	1.11	1.66	10	.32	82	1
37	41	1.40	12	72	90	181	.53	31	.07	.1	.6	.02	1	t
23	25	.85	7	44	55	110	.40	19	.04	.06	.37	.01	3	t
6	513	10.8	41	570	1562	1733	5.52	0	.86	1.03	7.4	.07	36	1
1	57	1.20	5	63	173	192	.61	0	.10	.11	.82	.01	4	t
576	1008	15.5	72	2017	1208	2515	3.31	465	1.22	1.66	11.1	.45	80	1
36	63	.97	5	126	75	157	.21	29	.08	.10	.69	.03	5	t
912	440	20	185	1040	1856	2336	7.2	10,600	1.92	1.97	15.0	1.12	192	23
57	27	1.2	12	65	116	146	.45	663	.11	.14	1.0	.06	12	1
640	1293	37.6	340	1592	6138	2123	6.8	422	2.41	2.55	17	1.72	54	504
20	41	1.2	11	50	194	67	.22	13	.08	.08	.5	.05	2	16
552	497	11.7	108	793	614	2331	2.75	373	1.24	1.40	10.1	.26	54	2
61	55	1.3	12	88	68	258	.31	41	.14	.15	1.1	.03	15	t
636	548	11	108	822	669	2488	2.90	647	1.21	1.42	9.9	.27	110	2
70	61	1.2	12	91	74	275	.32	71	.13	.16	1.1	.03	12	t
555	339	9.3	48	473	483	1645	2.69	1033	.93	1.08	7.8	.39	55	1
32	20	.5	3	28	28	98	.16	60	.05	.06	.5	.02	3	t
1100	146	9.3	48	517	443	1857	1.95	715	.96	1.12	8.1	.38	55	1
64	8	.5	3	30	26	108	.11	41	.06	.06	.5	.02	3	t
15	21	1.0	3	26	34	105	.17	4	.06	.09	.7	.01	3	0
7	14	.6	3	44	37	155	.21	9	.07	.06	.6	.02	4	0

H

(For purposes of calculations, use "0" for t, <1, <.1, <.01, etc.)

Table H–1   Food Composition

Grp	Computer Code No.	Food Description	Measure	Wt (g)	H₂O (%)	Ener (kcal)	Prot (g)	Carb (g)	Dietary Fiber (g)	Fat (g)	Fat Breakdown (g) Sat	Mono	Poly
		BAKED GOODS—Con.											
		Cakes—Con.											
		White cake with white frosting, 2-layer:											
6	397	Whole cake, 8 or 9″ diam	1 ea	1140	24	4170	43	670	5	148	33	62	42
6	398	Piece, ¹⁄₁₆ of cake	1 pce	71	24	260	3	42	<1	9	2.1	3.8	2.6
		Yellow cake with chocolate frosting, 2-layer:											
6	399	Whole cake, 8 or 9″ diam	1 ea	1108	23	3895	40	620	5	175	92	59	10
6	400	Piece, ¹⁄₁₆ of cake	1 pce	69	23	245	3	39	<1	11	5.7	3.7	.6
		Cheesecake:											
6	401	Whole cake, 9″ diam	1 ea	1110	46	3350	60	317	5	213	120	66	15
6	402	Piece, ¹⁄₁₂ of cake	1 pce	92	46	278	5	26	1	18	9.9	5.4	1.2
6	1035	Cheese puffs/Cheetos®	1 oz	28.4	1	158	2	14	<1	10	4.8	3.4	.6
		Cookies made with enriched flour:											
		Brownies with nuts:											
6	403	Commercial with frosting, 1½ × 1¾ × 7⁄8	1 ea	25	13	100	1	16	<1	4	1.6	2	.8
6	404	Home recipe, 1¾ × 1¾ × 7⁄8″[49]	1 ea	20	10	95	1	11	<1	6	1.4	2.8	1.2
		Chocolate chip cookies:											
6	405	Commercial, 2¼″ diam	4 ea	42	4	180	2	28	<1	9	2.9	3.1	2.6
6	406	Home recipe, 2¼″ diam[50]	4 ea	40	3	185	2	26	1	11	3.9	4.3	2
6	407	From refrigerated dough, 2¼″ diam	4 ea	48	5	225	2	32	1	11	4	4.4	2
6	408	Fig bars	4 ea	56	12	210	2	42	3	4	1	1.5	1
6	409	Oatmeal raisin cookies, 2⅝″ diam	4 ea	52	4	245	3	36	1	10	2.5	4.5	2.8
6	410	Peanut butter cookies, home recipe, 2⅝″ diam[50]	4 ea	48	3	245	4	28	1	14	4	5.8	2.8
6	411	Sandwich-type cookies, all	4 ea	40	2	195	2	29	<1	8	2	3.6	2.2
		Shortbread cookies:											
6	412	Commercial, small	4 ea	32	6	155	2	20	1	8	2.9	3	1.1
6	413	From home recipe, large[51]	2 ea	28	3	145	2	17	1	8	1.3	2.7	3.4
6	414	Sugar cookies from refrigerated dough, 2½″ diam	4 ea	48	4	235	2	31	<1	12	2.3	5	3.6
6	415	Vanilla wafers	10 ea	40	4	185	2	29	<1	7	1.8	3	1.8
6	416	Corn chips	1 oz	28	1	155	2	16	1	9	1.8	3.4	3.7
		Crackers:[52]											
6	1034	Armenian cracker bread	4 pce	28.4	4	117	5	19	4	2	.4	.7	1.1
6	417	Cheese crackers	10 ea	10	4	50	1	5	<1	3	.9	1.2	.3
6	418	Cheese crackers with peanut butter	4 ea	30	3	150	4	19	<1	8	1.6	3.2	1.2
6	419	Graham crackers	2 ea	14	4	60	1	11	<1	1	.4	.6	.4
6	420	Melba toast, plain	1 pce	5	4	20	1	4	<1	<1	.1	.1	.1
6	421	Rye wafers, whole grain	2 ea	14	5	55	1	10	2	1	.3	.4	.3
6	422	Saltine® crackers[53]	4 ea	12	4	50	1	9	<1	1	.5	.4	.2
6	423	Snack-type crackers, round	3 ea	9	3	45	1	6	<1	3	.6	1.2	.3
6	424	Wheat crackers, thin	4 ea	8	3	35	1	5	1	1	.4	.5	.4
6	425	Whole wheat wafers	2 ea	8	4	35	1	5	1	2	.5	.6	.4
6	426	Croissants, 4½ × 4 × 1¾″	1 ea	57	22	235	5	27	1	12	3.5	6.7	1.4
		Danish pastry											
6	427	Packaged ring, plain, 12 oz	1 ea	340	27	1305	21	152	3	71	22	29	16
6	428	Round piece, plain, 4¼″ diam 1″ high	1 ea	57	27	220	4	26	1	12	3.6	4.8	2.6

[49]Made with vegetable oil.
[50]Made with vegetable shortening.
[51]Made with margarine.
[52]Crackers made with enriched white (wheat) flour except for rye wafers and whole-wheat wafers.
[53]Made with lard.

H

GRP KEY: 1 = BEV 2 = DAIRY 3 = EGGS 4 = FAT/OIL 5 = FRUIT 6 = BAKERY 7 = GRAIN 8 = FISH 9 = BEEF 10 = POULTRY
11 = SAUSAGE 12 = MIXED/FAST 13 = NUTS/SEEDS 14 = SWEETS 15 = VEG/LEG 16 = MISC 22 = SOUP/SAUCE

Chol (mg)	Calc (mg)	Iron (mg)	Magn (mg)	Phos (mg)	Pota (mg)	Sodi (mg)	Zinc (mg)	VT-A (RE)	Thia (mg)	Ribo (mg)	Niac (mg)	V-B6 (mg)	Fola (µg)	VT-C (mg)
46	536	15.5	60	1585	832	2827	1.77	194	3.19	2.05	27.6	.16	64	0
3	33	1	4	99	52	176	.11	12	.2	.13	1.7	.01	4	0
609	366	19.9	72	1884	1972	3080	3.3	488	.78	2.22	10	.45	80	0
38	23	1.24	5	117	123	192	.21	30	.05	.14	.62	.03	5	0
2053	622	5.33	111	977	1088	2464	4.66	833	.33	1.44	5.11	.71	200	56
170	52	.44	9	81	90	204	.39	69	.03	.12	.42	.06	17	5
5	18	.20	7	29	23	344	—	26	.01	.03	.20	—	—	0
14	13	.61	14	26	50	59	.36	18	.08	.07	.33	.04	5	t
18	9	.40	11	26	35	51	.31	6	.05	.05	.3	.04	4	t
5	16	.8	10	41	56	140	.3	15	.1	.23	.9	.02	4	t
18	13	1	14	34	82	82	.22	5	.06	.06	.58	.03	4	0
22	13	1.04	10	34	62	173	.24	8	.06	.10	.89	.01	4	0
27	40	1.36	15	34	162	180	.36	6	.08	.07	.73	.07	4	t
2	18	1.1	26	58	90	148	.53	12	.09	.08	1	.03	6	0
22	21	1.1	19	60	110	142	.36	5	.07	.07	1.9	.04	12	0
0	12	1.4	15	40	66	189	.21	0	.09	.07	.8	.01	1	0
27	13	.8	4	39	38	123	.15	8	.10	.09	.9	.01	3	0
0	6	.55	4	31	18	125	.13	89	.08	.06	.71	.01	2	t
29	50	.9	8	91	33	261	.24	11	.09	.06	1.1	.02	4	0
25	16	.8	6	36	50	150	.12	14	.07	.1	1	.01	4	0
0	35	.5	21	52	52	233	.44	11	.04	.05	.4	.04[54]	3[55]	1
0	21	.45	41	1	77	—	.90	1	.06	.04	1.05	.03	12	2
6	11	.35	3	17	17	112	.07	5	.05	.04	.4	.01	—	0
4	26	1.2	2	94	64	338	.06	3	.16	.12	2.4	.03	—	0
0	6	.37	6	20	36	86	.11	0	.02	.03	.6	.01	2	0
0	6	.1	1	10	11	44	—	0	.01	.01	.1	.01	.7	0
0	7	.5	16	44	65	115	1.60	0	.06	.03	.5	.03	10	0
4	3	.5	3	12	17	165	.09	0	.06	.05	.6	<.01	2	0
0	9	.3	2	18	12	90	.05	t	.03	.03	.3	<.01	1	0
.6	3	.25	6[56]	15	17	69	.24[56]	t	.04	.03	.4	.01	3[55]	0
0	3	.24	8[56]	22	31	59	.23	0	.02	.03	.4	.01	3[55]	0
13	20	2.1	9	64	68	452	.32	13	.17	.13	1.3	.03	18	0
292	360	6.5	68	347	316	1302	2.86	99	.95	1.02	8.5	.12	84	t
49	60	1.1	11	58	53	218	.48	17	.16	.17	1.4	.02	14	t

[54] B6 values vary from 0 to .04 g between various brands—check label.
[55] Folacin values estimated and derived from values for cornmeal and corn tortillas.
[56] Values derived from whole-wheat recipes and retention values.

(For purposes of calculations, use "0" for t, <1, <.1, <.01, etc.)

H

Table H–1 Food Composition

Grp	Computer Code No.	Food Description	Measure	Wt (g)	H₂O (%)	Ener (kcal)	Prot (g)	Carb (g)	Dietary Fiber (g)	Fat (g)	Fat Breakdown (g) Sat	Mono	Poly
		BAKED GOODS—Con.											
		Danish Pastry—Con.											
6	429	Ounce, plain	1 oz	28	28	110	2	13	<1	6	1.8	2.4	1.3
6	430	Round piece with fruit	1 pce	65	30	235	4	28	1	13	3.9	5.2	2.9
		Desserts, 3 × 3 inch piece:											
6	1348	Apple crisp	1 pce	78	58	146	1	25	1	5	1.0	2.3	1.7
6	1353	Apple cobbler	1 pce	104	56	201	2	35	2	6	1.4	2.7	1.9
6	1349	Cherry crisp	1 pce	138	73	157	2	27	2	5	1.0	2.3	1.7
6	1352	Cherry cobbler	1 pce	129	65	199	2	34	1	6	1.4	2.7	1.9
6	1350	Peach crisp	1 pce	139	72	166	2	30	2	5	1.0	2.3	1.7
6	1351	Peach cobbler	1 pce	130	64	130	2	37	2	6	1.4	2.7	1.9
		Doughnuts:											
6	431	Cake type, plain, 3¼″ diam	1 ea	50	21	210	2	25	1	12	3.4	5.8	2
6	432	Yeast-leavened, glazed, 3¾″ diam	1 ea	60	27	235	4	26	1	13	5.2	5.5	.9
		English muffins:											
6	433	Plain, enriched	1 ea	57	42	140	5	26	2	1	.3	.2	.3
6	434	Toasted	1 ea	50	29	140	5	26	2	1	.3	.2	.3
		Muffins, 2½″ diam, 1½″ high:											
		From home recipe:											
6	435	Blueberry[57]	1 ea	45	37	135	3	20	2	5	1.5	2.1	1.2
6	436	Bran, wheat[58]	1 ea	45	35	125	3	19	3	6	1.4	1.6	2.3
6	437	Cornmeal	1 ea	45	33	145	3	21	2	5	1.5	2.2	1.4
		From commercial mix:											
6	438	Blueberry	1 ea	45	33	140	3	22	2	5	1.4	2	1.2
6	439	Bran	1 ea	45	28	140	3	24	3	4	1.3	1.6	1
6	440	Cornmeal	1 ea	45	30	145	3	22	2	6	1.7	2.3	1.4
		Pancakes, 4″ diam:											
6	441	Buckwheat, from mix with egg and milk	1 ea	27	58	55	2	6	1	2	.9	.9	.5
6	442	Plain, from home recipe	1 ea	27	50	60	2	9	1	2	.5	.8	.5
6	443	Plain, from mix; egg, milk, oil added	1 ea	27	54	60	2	8	1	2	.5	.9	.5
		Piecrust, with enriched flour, vegetable shortening, baked:											
6	444	Home recipe, 9″ shell	1 ea	180	15	900	11	79	4	60	15	26	16
		From mix:											
6	445	Piecrust for 2-crust pie	1 ea	320	19	1485	21	141	6	93	23	41	25
6	446	1 pie shell	1 ea	180	19	835	12	79	4	52	13	23	14
		Pies, 9″ diam; pie crust made with vegetable shortening, enriched flour:											
		Apple pie:[59]											
6	447	Whole pie	1 ea	945	48	2420	22	360	19	105	25	46	29
6	448	Piece, ⅙ of pie	1 pce	158	48	405	4	60	3	18	4.1	7.6	4.9
		Banana cream pie:[60]											
6	449	Whole pie	1 ea	1190	66	1915	38	282	10	77	27	29	15
6	450	⅙ of pie	1 pce	198	66	319	6	47	2	13	4.5	4.9	2.5
		Blueberry pie:[59]											
6	451	Whole pie	1 ea	945	51	2285	23	330	22	102	24	45	28
6	452	Piece, ⅙ of pie	1 pce	158	51	380	4	55	4	17	4.0	7.5	4.7

[57] Made with vegetable shortening.
[58] Made with vegetable oil.
[59] Recipes updated for latest USDA values for fruits/nuts/fruit juice.
[60] Recipe based on pie crust, cooked vanilla pudding, 2 bananas.

(Computer code number is for West Diet Analysis program)

GRP KEY: 1 = BEV   2 = DAIRY   3 = EGGS   4 = FAT/OIL   5 = FRUIT   6 = BAKERY   7 = GRAIN   8 = FISH   9 = BEEF   10 = POULTRY
11 = SAUSAGE   12 = MIXED/FAST   13 = NUTS/SEEDS   14 = SWEETS   15 = VEG/LEG   16 = MISC   22 = SOUP/SAUCE

Chol (mg)	Calc (mg)	Iron (mg)	Magn (mg)	Phos (mg)	Pota (mg)	Sodi (mg)	Zinc (mg)	VT-A (RE)	Thia (mg)	Ribo (mg)	Niac (mg)	V-B6 (mg)	Fola (μg)	VT-C (mg)
24	30	.55	6	29	27	109	.24	9	.08	.09	.7	.01	7	t
56	17	1.3	13	80	57	233	.55	11	.16	.14	1.4	.02	16	t
0	20	.77	12	15	112	66	.09	65	.05	.04	.41	.03	3	4
1	32	.76	7	42	86	305	.17	76	.08	.07	.70	.04	3	<1
0	29	2.16	16	22	163	73	.14	144	.06	.08	.56	.05	10	3
1	39	1.78	10	46	113	311	.21	135	.09	.10	.81	.05	9	2
0	24	.00	18	30	197	71	.19	104	.05	.05	1.01	.03	5	5
1	35	.90	11	52	139	309	.24	105	.08	.08	1.15	.03	5	3
20	23	.8	12	111	58	192	.25	5	.12	.12	1.1	.02	4	t
21	17	1.4	13	55	64	222	.30	<1	.28	.12	1.8	.28	13	0
0	96	1.7	11	67	331	378	.41	0	.26	.18	2.14	.02	18	0
0	96	1.7	11	67	331	378	.41	0	.23	.18	2.14	.02	15	0
19	54	.9	11	46	47	198	.29	9	.10	.11	.9	<.01	12	1
24	60	1.4	34	125	99	189	.37	30	.11	.13	1.3	.01	9	3
23	66	.9	11	59	57	169	.31	15	.11	.11	.9	.04	5	t
45	15	.9	7	90	54	225	.21	11	.11	.13	1.17	<.01	14	<1
28	27	1.7	28	182	50	385	.95	14	.08	.12	1.9	.12	19	0
42	30	1.3	11	128	31	291	.34	16	.09	.09	.8	.04	5	t
20	59	.4	18	91	66	125	.5	17	.04	.05	.2	.06	6	t
16	27	.5	7	38	33	115	.23	10	.06	.07	.5	.02	4	t
16	36	.7	7	71	43	160	.23	7	.09	.12	.8	.01	3	t
0	25	4.5	31	90	90	1100	1.50	0	.54	.40	5.0	.17	32	0
0	131	9.3	44	272	179	2600	1.19	0	1.07	.79	9.89	.27	57	0
0	74	5.23	25	153	101	1462	.79	0	.60	.44	5.57	.15	32	0
0	170	10	69	300	600	2844	1.6	28	1.04	.76	9.5	.5	48	2
0	28	1.67	12	50	100	476	.27	5	.18	.13	1.6	.08	8	<1
90	880	6.54	186	809	2000	2532	4.17	222	.94	1.75	7.40	1.77	116	26
15	147	1.09	31	135	333	422	.69	37	.16	.29	1.23	.30	19	4
0	155	12.3	60	274	756	2533	1.68	85	1.04	.85	10.4	.43	84	36
0	26	2.1	10	46	126	423	.28	14	.17	.14	1.73	.07	14	6

(For purposes of calculations, use "0" for t, <1, <.1, <.01, etc.)

H

Table H–1 Food Composition

Grp	Computer Code No.	Food Description	Measure	Wt (g)	H₂O (%)	Ener (kcal)	Prot (g)	Carb (g)	Dietary Fiber (g)	Fat (g)	Fat Breakdown (g) Sat	Mono	Poly
		BAKED GOODS—Con.											
		Pies—Con.											
		Cherry pie:[59]											
6	453	Whole pie	1 ea	945	47	2465	26	363	15	107	25	47	30
6	454	Piece, ⅙ of pie	1 pce	158	47	410	4	61	2	18	4.2	7.8	4.9
		Chocolate cream pie:[61]											
6	455	Whole pie	1 ea	1051	63	1863	45	255	4	76	27	30	15
6	456	Piece, ⅙ of pie	1 pce	175	63	311	7	42	1	13	4.5	5.0	2.5
		Custard pie:											
6	457	Whole pie	1 ea	910	58	1760	46	204	4	84	28	35	17
6	458	Piece, ⅙ of pie	1 pce	152	58	293	8	34	1	13	.9	5.8	2.8
		Lemon meringue pie:[59]											
6	459	Whole Pie	1 ea	840	47	2140	31	317	5	84	21	37	22
6	460	Piece, ⅙ of pie	1 pce	140	47	355	5	53	1	14	3.5	6.2	3.7
		Peach pie:[59]											
6	461	Whole pie	1 ea	945	48	2410	24	361	17	105	25	46	29
6	462	Piece, ⅙ of pie	1 pce	158	48	405	4	61	3	17	4.1	7.7	4.8
		Pecan pie:[59]											
6	463	Whole pie	1 ea	825	20	3500	38	551	10	142	24	75	34
6	464	Piece, ⅙ of pie	1 pce	138	20	583	6	92	5	24	3.9	13	5.7
		Pumpkin pie:[59]											
6	465	Whole Pie	1 ea	910	59	2200	54	308	15	94	34	37	17
6	466	Piece, ⅙ of pie	1 pce	152	59	367	9	51	5	16	5.7	6.1	2.8
		Pies, fried, commercial:											
6	467	Apple	1 ea	85	43	255	2	32	2	14	5.8	6.6	.6
6	468	Cherry	1 ea	85	43	250	2	32	1	14	5.8	6.7	.6
		Pretzels, made with enriched flour:											
6	469	Thin sticks, 2¼″ long	10 ea	3	2	10	<1	2	<1	<1	t	<.1	<.1
6	470	Dutch twists, 2¾ × 2⅝″	1 ea	16	2	65	2	13	<1	1	.1	.2	.2
6	471	Thin twists, 3¼ × 2¼ × ¼″	10 ea	60	3	240	6	48	2	2	.4	.8	.6
		Rolls and buns, enriched:											
		Commercial:											
6	472	Cloverleaf rolls, 2½″ diam, 2″ high	1 ea	28	32	85	2	14	1	2	.5	.8	.6
6	473	Hotdog buns	1 ea	40	34	115	3	20	1	2	.5	.8	.6
6	474	Hamburger buns	1 ea	45	34	129	4	23	1	2	.6	.9	.7
6	475	Hard rolls, white, 3¾″ diam, 2″ high	1 ea	50	25	155	5	30	1	2	.4	.5	.6
6	476	Submarine rolls or hoagies, 11½ × 3 × 2½	1 ea	135	31	400	11	72	2	8	1.8	3	2.2
		From home recipe:											
6	477	Dinner rolls 2½″ diam, 2″ high	1 ea	35	26	120	3	20	1	3	.8	1.2	.9
6	478	Toaster pastries, fortified	1 ea	54	13	210	2	38	1	6	1.7	3.6	.4
		Tortilla chips:											
6	1271	Plain	1 oz	28	4	139	2	17	1	8	1.1	3.1	3.1
6	1036	Nacho flavor	1 oz	28	1	139	2	18	1	7	1.4	2.5	2.8
6	1037	Taco flavor	1 oz	28	1	140	3	18	1	7	1.4	2.5	2.7
		Tortillas:											
6	479	Corn, enriched, 6″ diam	1 ea	30	45	65	2	13	2	1	.1	.3	.6
6	480	Flour, 8″ diam	1 ea	35	27	105	3	19	1	3	.4	1.2	1.0
6	1301	Flour tortilla, 10.5″ diam.	1 ea	57	27	168	4	31	2	4	.6	1.9	1.6
6	481	Taco shells	1 ea	14	4	59	1	9	1	2	.2	.6	1.2

[59] Recipes updated for latest USDA values for fruits/nuts/fruit juice.
[61] Based on value for pie crust, cooked chocolate pudding with meringue.

H

(Computer code number is for West Diet Analysis program)

GRP KEY: 1 = BEV 2 = DAIRY 3 = EGGS 4 = FAT/OIL 5 = FRUIT 6 = BAKERY 7 = GRAIN 8 = FISH 9 = BEEF 10 = POULTRY
11 = SAUSAGE 12 = MIXED/FAST 13 = NUTS/SEEDS 14 = SWEETS 15 = VEG/LEG 16 = MISC 22 = SOUP/SAUCE

Chol (mg)	Calc (mg)	Iron (mg)	Magn (mg)	Phos (mg)	Pota (mg)	Sodi (mg)	Zinc (mg)	VT-A (RE)	Thia (mg)	Ribo (mg)	Niac (mg)	V-B6 (mg)	Fola (µg)	VT-C (mg)
0	220	19	91	350	920	2873	1.87	416	1.13	.85	9.50	.50	93	5
0	37	3.17	15	58	153	480	.31	70	.19	.14	1.58	.08	16	1
90	958	6.46	176	881	1332	2565	4.46	204	.91	1.80	6.38	.54	66	3
15	160	1.08	29	147	222	427	.74	34	.15	.30	1.06	.09	11	<1
705	742	8.64	110	880	1040	2000	4.75	573	.82	1.60	5.50	.51	91	1
118	124	1.44	18	147	173	333	.79	96	.14	.27	.92	.08	15	4
822	150	8.4	54	412	420	2369	3.06	395	.59	.84	.50	.30	78	25
137	25	1.4	9	69	70	395	.51	66	.10	.14	.83	.05	13	4
0	160	11.3	98	332	1408	2533	2.11	690	1.04	.93	13.9	.39	72	28
0	27	1.90	16	55	235	423	.35	115	.18	.16	2.30	.07	12	5
822	210	12.0	192	777	781	1823	8.8	248	1.63	.99	6.6	.51	110	0
137	35	1.85	32	130	130	304	1.47	41	.22	.17	1.1	.08	18	0
655	1273	15.8	240	1269	2400	2029	5.96	11170[62]	.82	1.76	7.3	.64	120	6
109	212	2.63	40	211	400	338	.99	1861[62]	.14	.29	1.22	.11	20	1
14	12	.94	6	34	42	326	.14	3	.09	.06	1.0	.03	4	1
13	11	.70	7	41	61	371	.15	19	.06	.06	.60	.04	8	1
0	1	.06	1	3	3	48	.03	0	.01	.01	.13	<.01	<1	0
0	4	.32	4	15	16	258	.17	0	.05	.04	.70	<.01	3	0
0	16	1.2	15	55	61	966	.42	0	.19	.15	2.6	.01	10	0
t	33	.81	6	44	36	155	.22	t	.14	.09	1.10	.01	11	<1
0	54	1.19	8	44	56	241	.36	t	.20	.13	1.58	.01	15	<1
0	61	1.34	9	50	63	271	.41	t	.22	.15	1.78	.02	17	<1
0	24	1.40	14	46	49	313	.44	0	.20	.12	1.70	.02	17	0
0	100	3.80	31	115	128	683	1.17	0	.54	.33	4.50	.09	49	0
12	16	1.10	10	36	41	98	.32	8	.12	.12	1.20	.01	12	0
0	104	2.16	10	104	91	248	.31	150[63]	.17	.18	2.27	.2	43	4
0	82	1.00	22	74	30	140	.42	1	.01	.02	.20	.08	<1	<1
0	17	.40	13	98	109	107	.42	13	.04	.03	.40	.10	—	0
0	45	.70	27	91	72	191	.42	15	.08	.09	.80	.10	—	0
0	42	.60	19	55	43	1	.36	8	.05	.03	.40	.09	6	0
0	21	.55	12	59	35	134	.27	0	.13	.08	1.20	.01	16	0
0	34	.88	19	94	56	215	.43	0	.21	.13	1.93	.02	25	0
0	26	.26	9	33	25	62	.22	1	<.01	.01	.25	.02	2	0

[62] Latest USDA values of Vitamin A for canned pumpkin are almost 3.5 times greater than previously published values. Canned pumpkin is usually a blend of pumpkin and winter squash.
[63] Vitamin A values from label declaration varies from 100 to 150 RE for major brands.

(For purposes of calculations, use "0" for t, <1, <.1, <.01, etc.)

Table H–1 Food Composition

Grp	Computer Code No.	Food Description	Measure	Wt (g)	H$_2$O (%)	Ener (kcal)	Prot (g)	Carb (g)	Dietary Fiber (g)	Fat (g)	Fat Breakdown (g) Sat	Mono	Poly
		BAKED GOODS—Con.											
		Waffles, 7″ diam:											
6	482	From home recipe	1 ea	75	37	245	7	26	1	13	4	4.9	2.6
6	483	From mix, egg/milk added	1 ea	75	42	205	7	27	1	8	2.7	2.9	1.5
		GRAIN PRODUCTS: CEREAL, FLOUR, GRAIN, PASTA and NOODLES, POPCORN											
		Barley, pearled:											
7	484	Dry, uncooked	1 c	200	11	700	16	158	31	2	.4	.3	1.1
7	485	Cooked	1 c	157	69	193	4	44	4	1	.1	.1	.3
		Breakfast cereals, hot, cooked:											
		Corn grits (hominy) enriched cooked:											
7	486	Regular and quick, prepared	1 c	242	85	146	4	31	5	<1	t	.1	.3
7	487	Instant, prepared from packet, white	1 pkt	137	85	80	2	18	3	<1	t	.1	.1
		Cream of Wheat®, cooked:											
7	488	Regular, quick, instant	1 c	244	86	140	4	29	3	1	.1	.1	.2
7	489	Mix and eat, plain, packet	1 ea	142	82	100	3	21	2	<1	<.1	<.1	.1
7	490	Malt-O-Meal® cereal, cooked	1 c	240	88	122	4	26	3	<1	<.1	<.1	.1
		Oatmeal or rolled oats, cooked:											
7	491	Regular, quick, instant, nonfortified	1 c	234	85	145	6	25	4	2	.4	.8	1
		Instant, fortified:											
7	492	Plain, from packet	¾ c	177	86	104	4	18	3	2	.3	.6	.7
7	493	Flavored, from packet	¾ c	164	76	160	5	31	3	2	.3	.7	.8
7	494	Whole wheat cereal, cooked	1 c	242	84	150	5	33	4	1	.1	.1	.3
		Breakfast cereals, ready to eat:											
7	495	All-Bran®	⅓ c	28	3	70	4	22	9	<1	.1	.1	.3
7	1306	Alpha Bits®	1 c	28	1	111	2	25	1	1	.1	.2	.3
7	1307	Apple Jacks®	1 c	28	2	110	2	26	<1	<1	<.1	<.1	<.1
7	1308	Bran Buds®	1 c	84	3	217	12	64	23	2	.4	.3	1.1
7	1305	Bran Chex®	1 c	49	2	156	5	39	9	1	.2	.2	.8
7	1309	Buc Wheats®	¾ c	28	3	110	2	24	2	1	.1	.1	.5
7	1310	C.W. Post® plain	1 c	97	2	432	9	69	2	15	11.3	1.7	1.4
7	1311	C.W. Post® with raisins	1 c	103	4	446	9	74	2	15	11.0	1.7	1.4
7	496	Cap'n Crunch®	1 c	37	2	156	2	30	1	3	2.2	.4	.5
7	1312	Cap'n Crunchberries®	1 c	35	3	146	2	29	<1	3	1.9	.4	.5
7	1313	Cap'n Crunch®, peanut butter	1 c	35	2	154	3	27	<1	5	1.9	1.4	1.0
7	497	Cheerios®	1 c	23	5	89	3	16	2	1	.3	.5	.6
7	1314	Cocoa Krispies®	1 c	36	3	139	2	32	<1	<1	.2	.2	.2
7	1316	Cocoa Pebbles®	⅔ c	21	2	87	1	18	<1	1	<.1	<.1	<.1
7	1315	Corn Bran®	1 c	36	3	124	3	30	7	1	.2	.3	.7
7	1317	Corn Chex®	1 c	28	2	111	2	25	<1	<1	.1	.3	.6
7	498	Corn Flakes, Kellogg's®	1¼ c	28	3	110	2	24	1	<1	t	t	.1
7	499	Corn Flakes, Post Toasties®	1¼ c	28	3	110	2	24	1	<1	t	t	.1
7	1318	Cracklin' Oat Bran®	1 c	60	4	229	6	41	9	9	2.1	2.3	3.5
7	1038	Crispy Wheat 'N Raisins®	1 c	43	7	150	3	35	2	1	.1	.1	.4
7	1319	Fortified oat flakes	1 c	48	3	177	9	35	1	1	.1	.3	.3
7	500	40% Bran Flakes, Kellogg's®	1 c	39	3	125	5	35	5	1	.14	.14	.4
7	501	40% Bran Flakes, Post®	1 c	47	3	152	5	37	6	1	.2	.2	.3
7	502	Froot Loops®	1 c	28	2	111	2	25	<1	1	.2	.1	.1

(Computer code number is for West Diet Analysis program)

H

GRP KEY: 1=BEV 2=DAIRY 3=EGGS 4=FAT/OIL 5=FRUIT 6=BAKERY 7=GRAIN 8=FISH 9=BEEF 10=POULTRY 11=SAUSAGE 12=MIXED/FAST 13=NUTS/SEEDS 14=SWEETS 15=VEG/LEG 16=MISC 22=SOUP/SAUCE

Chol (mg)	Calc (mg)	Iron (mg)	Magn (mg)	Phos (mg)	Pota (mg)	Sodi (mg)	Zinc (mg)	VT-A (RE)	Thia (mg)	Ribo (mg)	Niac (mg)	V-B6 (mg)	Fola (µg)	VT-C (mg)
102	154	1.50	17	135	129	445	.65	39	.18	.24	1.50	.03	13	t
59	179	1.20	14	257	146	515	.52	49	.14	.23	.90	.03	4	t
0	32	4.2	51	378	320	6	4.47	0	.24	.1	7.9	.45	40	0
0	17	2.1	35	85	146	5	1.29	0	.13	.1	3.2	.18	25	0
0	1	1.55[64]	11	29	54	0[65]	.18	15[66]	.24[64]	.15[64]	1.96[64]	.06	2	0
0	7	1[64]	5	16	29	343	.08	0	.18[64]	.08[64]	1.3[64]	.03	1	0
0	54[64]	10.9[64]	12	43[67]	46	5[67,68]	.35	0	.24[64]	.07[64]	1.5[64]	.02	9	0
0	20[64]	8.10[64]	7	20[64]	38	241	.20	376[64]	.43[64]	.28[64]	5.0[64]	.01	5	0
0	5	9.6[64]	14	24[64]	31	2[68]	.17	0	.48[64]	.24[64]	5.8[64]	.02	5	0
0	19	1.59	56	178	131	2[68]	1.15	5	.26	.05	.3	.05	9	0
0	163[64]	6.32[64]	51	133	99	285[64]	1	453[64]	.53[64]	.29[64]	5.49[64]	.74	150	0
0	168[64]	6.7[64]	51	148	137	254[64]	1	460[64]	.53[64]	.38[64]	5.9[64]	.77	150	<1
0	17	1.5	53	168	171	3	1.16	0	.17	.12	2.13	.07	25	0
0	23	4.5[64]	106	264	320	260	3.7	375[64]	.37[64]	.43[64]	5.0[64]	.5	100	15[64]
0	8	1.80	17	51	100	219	1.50	375	.40	.40	5.0	.50	100	—
0	3	4.50	6	30	23	125	3.70	375	.40	.40	5.0	.50	100	15
0	56	13.4	267	729	930	516	11.1	1112	1.10	1.30	14.8	1.50	297	45
0	29	7.80	126	327	394	455	2.14	11	.60	.26	8.6	.90	173	26
0	60	8.10	24	60	—	235	.30	682	.68	.77	9.0	.90	—	27
0	47	15.4	67	224	198	167	1.64	1284	1.30	1.50	17.1	1.70	342	—
0	51	16.4	74	232	260	160	1.64	1364	1.30	1.50	18.1	1.90	364	—
0	6	9.83[64]	15	47	48	278	4.01	5[64]	.66[64]	.71[64]	8.64[64]	1	238	0
0	11	9.04	14	47	49	243	3.56	0	.59	.67	8.14	.93	128	—
0	7	9.10	19	49	57	268	3.79	0	.60	.70	8.97	1.04	244	—
0	38	3.6[64]	31	109	82	246	.63	304[64]	.32[64]	.32[64]	4.0[64]	.4	5	12[64]
0	6	2.30	12	47	53	275	1.90	477	.50	.50	6.3	.60	127	19
0	4	1.30	9	16	35	102	1.10	282	.30	.30	3.7	.40	75	—
0	41	12.2	18	52	70	310	4.00	—	.38	.70	10.9	.86	232	—
0	3	1.80	4	11	23	271	.10	14	.40	.07	5.0	.50	100	15
0	1	1.8[64]	3	18	26	351	.06	375[64]	.37[64]	.43[64]	5.0[64]	.51	100	15[64]
0	1	.7[64]	3	12	33	297	.06	375[64]	.37[64]	.43[64]	5.0[64]	.51	100	0
0	40	3.80	116	241	355	402	3.20	794	.80	.90	10.6	1.10	212	32
0	71	6.80	35	117	174	204	.51	569	.60	.60	7.6	.80	40	—
0	68	13.7	58	176	343	429	1.50	636	.60	.70	.39	.90	169	—
0	19	11.2[64]	71	192	248	363	5.15	522[64]	.51[64]	.59[64]	6.86[64]	.7	138	0
0	21	7.47[64]	102	296	251	431	2.5	629[64]	.62[64]	.72[64]	8.3[64]	.85	166	0
0	3	4.5[64]	9	28	30	125	3.7	225[64]	.4[64]	.4[64]	5.0[64]	.5	100	15[64]

[64] Nutrient added (values sometimes based on label declaration).

[65] Cooked without salt. If salt is added according to label recommendation, sodium content is 540 mg.

[66] Value for yellow corn grits; cooked white corn grits contain 0 RE of Vitamin A.

[67] Values for regular and instant cereal. For quick cereal, phosphorus is 102 mg, and sodium is 142 mg.

[68] Cooked without salt. If added according to label recommendations, sodium content is 390 mg for Cream of Wheat; 324 mg for Malt-O-Meal; 374 mg for oatmeal.

(For purposes of calculations, use "0" for t, <1, <.1, <.01, etc.)

H

Table H–1 Food Composition

Grp	Computer Code No.	Food Description	Measure	Wt (g)	H₂O (%)	Ener (kcal)	Prot (g)	Carb (g)	Dietary Fiber (g)	Fat (g)	Fat Breakdown (g)		
											Sat	Mono	Poly
GRAIN PRODUCTS—Con.													
		Cereals—Con.											
7	1320	Frosted Mini-Wheats®	4 ea	31	5	111	3	26	2	<1	.1	<.1	.2
7	1321	Frosted Rice Krispies®	1 c	28	3	109	1	26	1	<1	<.1	<.1	<.1
7	1323	Fruit & Fiber® w/apples	½ c	28	2	90	3	22	4	1	.2	.2	.6
7	1324	Fruit & Fiber® w/dates	½ c	28	2	90	3	21	4	1	.2	.2	.6
7	1325	Fruitful Bran® cereal	¾ c	34	3	110	3	27	5	0	0	0	0
7	1322	Fruity Pebbles® cereal	⅞ c	28	3	113	1	24	<1	2	.3	.2	.4
7	503	Golden Grahams®	1 c	39	2	156	2	33	2	2	1.0	.1	.2
7	504	Granola, homemade	1 c	122	3	595	15	67	13	33	5.8	9.4	17
7	505	Grape Nuts®	½ c	57	3	210	6	46	5	<1	t	t	.2
7	1326	Grape Nuts® flakes	⅞ c	28	3	102	3	23	2	<1	<.1	<.1	.1
7	1327	Honey & Nut Corn flakes	¾ c	28	4	113	2	23	<1	2	.2	.5	.7
7	506	Honey Nut Cheerios®	1 c	33	3	127	4	27	1	1	.2	.4	.5
7	1328	Honey Bran	1 c	35	3	119	3	29	4	1	.1	.1	.4
7	1329	Honeycomb®	1 c	22	1	86	1	20	<1	<1	.1	.1	.2
7	1330	King Vitamin® cereal	1 c	21	2	85	1	18	<1	1	.7	.2	.2
7	1039	Kix®	1 c	19	3	73	2	16	<1	<1	.1	.1	.2
7	1331	Life®	1 c	44	5	162	8	32	1	1	.1	.2	.4
7	507	Lucky Charms®	1 c	32	3	125	3	26	1	1	.2	.4	.5
7	508	Nature Valley® Granola	1 c	113	4	503	12	76	12	20	13	2.8	2.8
7	1332	Nutri-Grain™—Barley	1 c	41	3	153	5	34	2	<1	<.1	<.1	.1
7	1333	Nutri-Grain™—Corn	1 c	42	3	160	3	36	3	1	.1	.3	.6
7	1334	Nutri-Grain™—Rye	1 c	40	3	144	4	34	3	<1	.1	.1	.1
7	1335	Nutri-Grain™—Wheat	1 c	44	3	158	4	37	3	<1	.1	.1	.3
7	1336	100% Bran	1 c	66	3	178	8	48	20	3	.6	.6	1.9
7	509	100% Natural® cereal, plain	¼ c	28	2	135	3	18	3	6	4.1	1.2	.5
7	1337	100% Natural® with apples	1 c	104	2	478	11	70	5	20	15.5	1.8	1.3
7	1338	100% Natural® with raisins & dates	1 c	100	4	496	11	72	4	20	13.7	3.7	1.7
7	510	Product 19®	1 c	33	3	126	3	27	<1	<1	t	t	.1
7	1339	Quisp®	1 c	30	2	124	2	25	<1	2	1.5	.3	.3
7	511	Raisin Bran, Kellogg's®	1 c	49	8	158	5	37	6	1	.2	.1	.4
7	512	Raisin Bran, Post®	1 c	56	9	170	5	42	6	1	.2	.2	.4
7	1040	Raisins, Rice & Rye™	1 c	46	9	155	3	39	<1	<1	<.1	<.1	<.1
7	1041	Rice Chex®	¾ c	19	3	75	1	17	1	1	.2	.2	.3
7	513	Rice Krispies, Kellogg's®	1 c	29	2	112	2	25	<1	<1	t	t	.1
7	514	Rice, puffed	1 c	14	3	55	1	13	<1	<1	t	t	<.1
7	515	Shredded Wheat®	¾ c	32	5	115	3	25	4	1	.1	.1	.3
7	516	Special K®	1½ c	32	2	125	6	24	<1	<1	t	t	t
7	1340	Sugar Corn Pops®	1 c	28	3	108	1	26	<1	<1	t	<.1	.1
7	518	Sugar Frosted Flakes®	1 c	35	3	133	2	32	1	<1	t	t	t
7	517	Super Sugar Crisp®	1 c	33	2	123	2	30	<1	<1	t	t	.1
7	519	Sugar Smacks®	¾ c	28	3	106	2	25	<1	<1	.1	.1	.2
7	1341	Tasteeos®	1 c	24	2	94	3	19	1	1	.2	.2	.3
7	1342	Team®	1 c	42	4	164	3	36	<1	1	.2	.2	.3
7	520	Total®, wheat, with added calcium	1 c	33	4	122	3	26	2	1	.1	.1	.4
7	521	Trix®	1 c	28	2	109	1	25	<1	1	.2	.1	.1
7	1042	Wheat & Raisin Chex®	1 c	54	7	185	5	43	4	<1	.1	.1	.2
7	1344	Wheat Chex®	1 c	46	3	169	5	38	3	1	.2	.2	.6
7	1043	Wheat, puffed	1 c	12	3	44	2	10	2	<1	t	t	.1
7	522	Wheaties®	1 c	29	5	101	3	23	3	1	.1	.1	.2

GRP KEY: 1 = BEV   2 = DAIRY   3 = EGGS   4 = FAT/OIL   5 = FRUIT   6 = BAKERY   7 = GRAIN   8 = FISH   9 = BEEF   10 = POULTRY
11 = SAUSAGE   12 = MIXED/FAST   13 = NUTS/SEEDS   14 = SWEETS   15 = VEG/LEG   16 = MISC   22 = SOUP/SAUCE

Chol (mg)	Calc (mg)	Iron (mg)	Magn (mg)	Phos (mg)	Pota (mg)	Sodi (mg)	Zinc (mg)	VT-A (RE)	Thia (mg)	Ribo (mg)	Niac (mg)	V-B6 (mg)	Fola (µg)	VT-C (mg)
0	10	2.00	26	81	106	9	1.60	410	.40	.50	5.5	.60	109	16
0	1	1.80	5	27	21	240	.31	375	.40	.40	5.0	.50	100	15
0	10	4.50	60	150	168	195	1.50	375	.38	.43	5.0	.50	100	0
0	10	4.50	60	100	168	170	1.50	378	.38	.43	5.0	.50	100	0
0	10	8.10	60	150	150	240	3.75	378	.38	.43	5.0	.50	100	0
0	4	1.80	6	16	22	157	2	375	.40	.40	5.0	.50	100	0
0	24	6.2[64]	16	56	82	476	.34	521[64]	.5[64]	.6[64]	6.9[64]	.7	136	21[64]
0	76	4.84	141	494	612	12	4.47	4	.73	.31	2.14	.43	99	1
0	20	16	52	153	183	341	2	753[64]	.7[64]	.9[64]	10.0[64]	1	200	0
0	11	4.50	31	84	99	218	.57	375	.40	.40	5.0	.50	100	—
0	3	1.80	6	13	36	225	.11	375	.40	.40	5.0	.50	100	15
0	23	5.2[64]	39	122	115	299	.87	437[64]	.4[64]	.5[64]	5.8[64]	.6	4	17[64]
0	16	5.60	46	132	151	202	.90	463	.50	.50	6.2	.60	23	19
0	4	1.40	8	22	70	166	1.20	291	.30	.30	3.9	.40	78	—
0	—	12.7	7	—	26	161	.16	717	.09	1.06	12.9	1.18	286	33
0	23	5.40	8	26	29	226	.17	250	.27	.27	3.33	.33	2	10
0	154	11.6	55	238	197	229	1.55	0	.95	1.00	11.6	.05	37	—
0	36	5.1[64]	27	88	66	227	.56	424[64]	.4[64]	.5[64]	5.6[64]	.6	—	17[64]
0	71	3.78	116	354	389	232	2.19	8	.39	.19	.83	.32	85	0
0	11	1.45	32	126	108	277	5.40	540	.50	.60	7.2	.70	145	22
0	1	.89	27	120	98	276	5.50	556	.50	.60	7.4	.75	148	22
0	8	1.13	31	104	72	272	5.30	530	.50	.60	7.0	.70	141	21
0	12	1.24	34	164	120	299	5.80	583	.60	.70	7.7	.80	155	23
0	46	8.12	312	801	824	457	5.74	0	1.60	1.80	20.9	2.10	200	63
0	49	.83	34	104	138	12	.63	2	.09	.15	.6	.64	8	0
0	157	2.89	71	350	513	52	2.00	8	.33	.58	1.88	.11	17	—
0	160	3.12	124	347	538	47	2.11	8	.30	.64	2.08	.17	45	—
0	4	21[64]	12	47	51	378	.5	1769[64]	1.7[64]	2[64]	23.3[64]	2.3	466	70[64]
0	9	6.31	12	25	45	241	.18	—	.54	.76	5.80	.91	8	—
0	25	24[64]	73	200	307	293	5.0	500[64]	.51[64]	.57[64]	6.67[64]	.67	133	0
0	27	9.01[64]	96	237	349	370	3.01	750[64]	.74[64]	.85[64]	10[64]	1.02	200	0
0	10	5.60	20	50	144	350	4.70	467	.50	.60	6.30	.60	125	0
0	3	1.20	5	19	22	158	.26	1	.27	.20	3.34	.33	67	10
0	4	1.8[64]	10	34	30	340	.48	388[64]	.4[64]	.4[64]	5.0[64]	.5	100	15[64]
0	1	.15[64]	4	14	16	<1	.14	0	.02[64]	.01[64]	.42[64]	.01	3	0
0	12	1.35	42	112	115	3	1.05	0	.08	.09	1.67	.08	16	0
0	9	5.06[64]	18	62	55	298	4.16	429[64]	.45[64]	.45[64]	5.63[64]	.56	112	17[64]
0	2	1.80	2	8	20	90	1.50	225	.40	.40	5.00	.50	100	15
0	1	2.2[64]	3	26	22	284	.05	463[64]	.5[64]	.5[64]	6.2[64]	.6	124	19[64]
0	7	2.1[64]	20	60	123	29	1.7	437[64]	.4[64]	.5[64]	5.8[64]	.6	116	0
0	3	1.8[64]	13	31	42	75	.28	375[64]	.37[64]	.43[64]	5[64]	.5	100	15[64]
0	11	3.80	26	96	71	183	.69	318	.30	.40	4.20	.40	9	13
0	6	2.57	19	65	71	259	.58	556	.55	.63	7.40	.80	—	22
0	200	21[64]	34	137	123	330	.15	1769[64]	1.7[64]	2[64]	23.3[64]	2.3	400	70[64]
0	6	4.5[64]	6	22	27	169	.13	379[64]	.4[64]	.4[64]	4.9[64]	.5	99	15[64]
0	—	7.70	53	163	174	306	1.19	<1	.50	.60	7.10	.70	143	2
0	18	7.30	58	182	174	308	1.23	0	.60	.17	8.10	.80	162	24
0	3	.57	17	43	42	0	.30	0	.02	.03	1.30	.02	4	0
0	44	4.6[64]	32	100	108	363	.65	388[64]	.4[64]	.4[64]	5.1[64]	.5	9	15[64]

[64] Nutrient added (values sometimes based on label declaration).

(For purposes of calculations, use "0" for t, <1, <.1, <.01, etc.)

Table H–1 Food Composition

Grp	Computer Code No.	Food Description	Measure	Wt (g)	H₂O (%)	Ener (kcal)	Prot (g)	Carb (g)	Dietary Fiber (g)	Fat (g)	Fat Breakdown (g)		
											Sat	Mono	Poly
GRAIN PRODUCTS—Con.													
		Buckwheat:											
		Flour:											
7	523	Dark	1 c	98	12	338	12	71	8	3	.5	.8	.9
7	524	Light	1 c	98	12	340	6	78	6	1	.2	.4	.4
7	525	Whole grain, dry	1 c	175	11	586	23	128	16	4	.8	1.4	1.5
		Bulgar:											
7	526	Dry, uncooked	1 c	140	9	479	17	106	31	2	.3	.2	.8
7	527	Cooked	1 c	182	78	151	6	34	11	<1	.1	.1	.2
		Cornmeal:											
7	528	Whole-ground, unbolted, dry	1 c	122	10	442	10	94	13	4	.6	1.2	2
7	529	Bolted, nearly whole, dry	1 c	122	10	441	10	91	12	4	.6	1.2	2
7	530	Degermed, enriched, dry	1 c	138	12	505	12	107	10	2	.3	.6	1
7	531	Degermed, enriched, cooked	1 c	240	88	120	3	26	3	<1	.1	.1	.3
		Macaroni, cooked:											
7	532	Enriched	1 c	140	66	197	7	40	2	1	.1	.1	.4
7	533	Vegetable, enriched	1 c	134	68	172	6	36	2	.1	<.1	<.1	<.1
7	534	Whole wheat	1 c	140	67	174	8	37	2	1	.1	.1	.3
7	535	Millet, cooked	½ c	120	71	143	4	28	1	1	.2	.2	.6
		Noodles:											
7	536	Egg noodles, cooked	1 c	160	69	213	8	40	4	2	.5	.7	.6
7	537	Chow mein, dry	1 c	45	.73	237	4	26	2	14	2	4	8
7	538	Spinach noodles, dry	3½ oz	100	8	372	13	75	7	2	1.0	1.1	1.1
7	1343	Oat bran, dry	¼ c	25	6	61	4	17	4	2	.3	.6	.7
		Popcorn:											
7	539	Air popped, plain	1 c	8	4	30	1	6	1	<1	t	.1	.2
7	540	Popped in veg oil/salted	1 c	11	3	55	1	6	1	3	.5	1.4	1.2
7	541	Sugar-syrup coated	1 c	35	4	135	2	30	1	1	.1	.3	.6
		Rice:											
7	542	Brown rice, cooked	1 c	195	73	217	5	45	3	2	.3	.6	.6
		White, enriched, all types:											
7	543	Regular/long grain, dry	1 c	185	12	675	13	148	2	1	.3	.4	.3
7	544	Regular/long grain, cooked	1 c	205	69	264	6	57	1	<1	.2	.2	.2
7	545	Instant, prepared without salt	1 c	165	76	162	3	35	1	<1	.1	.1	.1
		Parboiled/converted rice:											
7	546	Raw, dry	1 c	185	10	686	13	151	4	1	.3	.3	.3
7	547	Cooked	1 c	175	73	200	4	43	1	<1	.1	.2	<.1
7	548	Wild rice, cooked	1 c	164	74	166	4	35	3	<1	.1	.1	<.1
7	549	Rye flour, medium	1 c	102	10	361	10	79	15	2	.2	.2	.8
7	1044	Soy flour, low fat	1 c	88	3	370	51	34	12	6	.9	1.3	3.3
		Spaghetti, cooked:											
7	550	without salt, enriched	1 c	140	66	197	7	40	2	1	.5	.1	.4
7	551	with salt, enriched	1 c	140	66	197	7	40	2	1	.5	.1	.4
7	552	Whole wheat spaghetti, cooked	1 c	140	94	174	7	37	5	1	.1	.1	.3
7	1302	Tapioca, dry	1 c	152	11	518	.3	135	2	<.1	<.1	<.1	<.1
7	553	Wheat bran	½ c	30	10	65	5	19	8	1	.2	.2	.7
		Wheat germ:											
7	554	Raw	1 c	100	11	360	23	52	12	10	1.7	1.4	6
7	555	Toasted	1 c	113	6	432	33	56	16	12	2.1	1.7	7.5
7	556	Rolled wheat, cooked	1 c	240	80	142	4	32	5	1	.1	.1	.3
7	557	Whole-grain wheat, cooked	⅓ c	50	86	28	1	7	1	<1	<.1	<.1	.1

(Computer code number is for West Diet Analysis program)

GRP KEY: 1 = BEV 2 = DAIRY 3 = EGGS 4 = FAT/OIL 5 = FRUIT 6 = BAKERY 7 = GRAIN 8 = FISH 9 = BEEF 10 = POULTRY
11 = SAUSAGE 12 = MIXED/FAST 13 = NUTS/SEEDS 14 = SWEETS 15 = VEG/LEG 16 = MISC 22 = SOUP/SAUCE

Chol (mg)	Calc (mg)	Iron (mg)	Magn (mg)	Phos (mg)	Pota (mg)	Sodi (mg)	Zinc (mg)	VT-A (RE)	Thia (mg)	Ribo (mg)	Niac (mg)	V-B6 (mg)	Fola (µg)	VT-C (mg)
0	32	2.5	135	298	490	1	2.65	0	.58	.16	2.75	.41	125	0
0	11	1	47	86	314	1	2.56	0	.09	.05	.47	.09	100	0
0	200	6.7	335	560	740	3	4.4	0	1.05	.26	7.7	.37	53	0
0	49	3.4	230	420	574	24	2.7	0	.33	.16	7.2	.48	38	0
0	18	1.8	58	73	124	9	1.04	0	.1	.05	1.8	.15	33	0
0	7	4.2	155	294	350	43	2.22	57	.47	.25	4.4	.37	31	0
0	21	4.2	154	272	303	43	2.22	57	.37	.1	2.3	.56	29	0
0	7	5.7	55	116	224	4	1	57	1	1	7	.35	66	0
0	2	1.48	17	34	38	1	.23	14	.14	.1	1.2	.06	6	0
0	10	2	25	76	43	1	.74	0	.29	.14	2.34	.05	10	0
0	15	1	26	67	42	8	.59	7	.15	.08	1.4	.03	4	0
0	21	1.5	42	125	62	4	1.1	0	.2	.1	1	.11	7	0
0	4	1	53	120	74	2	1.1	0	.1	.1	1.6	.13	23	0
50	19	2.5	30	110	45	11	1	10	.3	.13	2.4	.06	11	0
0	14	2.1	23	72	54	197	1	4	.3	.2	3	.05	10	0
0	58	2.1	174	322	376	36	2.8	46	.37	.2	4.6	.32	48	0
0	15	1.4	59	184	142	1	.78	0	.29	.05	.23	.04	13	—
0	1	.2	23	22	20	<1	.22	1	.03	.01	.2	.02	3	0
0	3	.27	25	31	19	86	.28	2	.01	.02	.1	.02	3	0
0	2	.5	29	47	90	<1	.29	3	.13	.02	.4	.03	3	0
0	20	1	84	162	84	10	1.23	0	.19	.05	3	.28	8	0
0	52	8	46	213	213	9	2.02	0	1	1	7.76	.3	15	0
0	23	2.3	27	96	80	4	.94	0	.33	.03	3.03	.19	6	0
0	13	1.04	8	23	6.6	5[69]	.4	0	.12	.08	1.45	.017	6.6	0
0	111	7	57	252	222	9.3	1.78	0	1.1	.13	6.7	.65	32	0
0	33	2	21	74	65	5	.54	0	.44	.03	2.5	.03	7	0
0	5	1	53	135	166	5	2.2	0	.1	.14	2.1	.221	43	0
0	25	2.16	77	211	347	3	2	0	.29	.11	1.76	.273	38	0
0	165	5.27	202	522	2262	16	1.04	4	.33	.25	1.90	.46	361	0
0	10	2.00	25	76	43	1	.74	0	.29	.14	2.34	.05	10	0
0	10	2	25	76	43	140	.74	0	.29	.14	2.34	.05	10	0
0	21	1.5	42	125	62	4	1.14	0	.15	.06	1	.11	7	0
0	30	2.4	1.5	10.6	17	2	.182	0	.01	.15	0	0	6	0
0	22	3.2	183	304	355	.6	2.18	0	.16	.17	4.07	.39	24	0
0	39	6.3	239	842	892	12	12	0	1.88	.5	6	1.3	281	0
0	51	10.3	362	1295	1070	5	18.9	0	1.89	.93	6.32	1.11	398	0
0	17	1.5	58	130	165	2	1.22	0	.17	.06	2.2	.08	27	0
0	3	.3	12	26	33	<1	.24	0	.04	.01	.5	.03	4	0

[69]If prepared with salt according to label recommendation, sodium would be 608 mg.

(For purposes of calculations, use "0" for t, <1, <.1, <.01, etc.)

H

Table H–1   Food Composition

Grp	Computer Code No.	Food Description	Measure	Wt (g)	H₂O (%)	Ener (kcal)	Prot (g)	Carb (g)	Dietary Fiber (g)	Fat (g)	Sat	Mono	Poly
		GRAIN PRODUCTS—Con.											
		Wheat flour (unbleached):											
		All-purpose white flour, enriched:											
7	558	Sifted	1 c	115	12	419	12	88	3	1	.2	.1	.5
7	559	Unsifted	1 c	125	12	455	13	95	3	1	.2	.1	.5
7	560	Cake or pastry flour, enriched, sifted	1 c	96	12	348	8	75	3	1	.1	.1	.4
7	561	Self-rising, enriched, unsifted	1 c	125	11	442	12	93	3	1	.2	.1	.5
7	562	Whole wheat, from hard wheats	1 c	120	10	407	16	87	15	2	.4	.3	1
		MEATS: FISH and SHELLFISH											
8	1045	Bass, baked or broiled	3.5 oz.	100	70	125	24	0	0	4	.9	1.6	1.2
		Bluefish:											
8	1046	Baked or broiled	3.5 oz.	100	68	159	26	0	0	5	1.1	2.1	1.3
8	1047	Fried in bread crumbs	3.5 oz.	100	61	205	23	5	0	10	2.1	4.3	2.5
		Clams:											
8	563	Raw meat only	3 oz	85	82	63	11	2	<1	1	.1	.1	.2
8	564	Canned, drained	3 oz	85	64	126	22	4	t	2	.2	.2	.5
8	1290	Steamed, meat only	20 ea	90	64	133	23	5	<1	2	.2	.2	.5
		Cod:											
8	565	Baked with butter	3½ oz	100	75	132	23	0	0	3	.4	.3	.5
8	566	Batter fried	3½ oz	100	61	199	20	8	0	10	3.9	5.5	.9
8	567	Poached, no added fat	3½ oz	100	76	102	22	0	0	1	.2	.1	.3
		Crab, meat only:											
8	1048	Blue crab, cooked	1 c	135	77	138	27	0	0	2	.3	.4	.9
8	1049	Dungeness Crab, cooked	.75 c	101	74	85	18	<1	0	2	.3	.6	1.1
8	568	Canned	1 c	135	76	133	28	0	0	2	.3	.3	.6
8	1587	Crab, imitation, from surimi	3 oz	85	74	87	10	9	0	1	—	—	—
8	569	Fish sticks, breaded pollock	2 ea	57	46	155	9	14	<1	7	1.8	2.9	1.8
		Flounder/sole, baked with lemon juice:											
8	570	With butter	3 oz	85	73	120	16	<1	0	6	3.2	1.5	.5
8	571	With margarine	3 oz	85	73	120	16	<1	0	6	1.2	2.3	1.9
8	572	Without added fat	3 oz	85	78	99	21	0	0	1	.3	.3	.4
		Haddock:											
8	573	Breaded, fried[70]	3 oz	85	61	175	17	7	<1	9	2.4	3.9	2.4
8	1050	Smoked	3.5 oz	100	72	116	25	0	0	1	.2	.2	.3
8	574	Broiled with butter and lemon juice	3 oz	85	72	140	23	0	0	6	3.3	1.6	.7
8	1051	Smoked	3.5 oz	100	49	224	21	0	0	15	2.5	4.8	6.9
8	1054	Raw	3.5 oz	100	78	110	21	0	0	2	.3	.7	.8
8	575	Herring, pickled	3 oz	85	55	223	12	8	0	15	2.0	10	1.4
8	1052	Lobster meat, cooked w/ moist heat	1 c	145	77	142	30	2	0	1	.2	.2	1
8	576	Ocean perch, breaded/fried	3 oz	85	59	185	16	7	<1	11	3	5	3
8	1056	Octopus, raw	3.5 oz.	100	80	82	15	2	0	1	.2	.2	.2
		Oysters:											
8	577	Raw, Eastern	1 c	248	85	170	18	10	0	6	1.6	.6	1.8
8	578	Raw, Pacific	1 c	248	82	200	23	12	0	6	1.3	.9	2.2
		Cooked:											
8	579	Eastern, breaded, fried, medium	6 ea	88	65	173	8	10	<1	11	2.8	4.1	2.9
8	580	Western, simmered	3½ oz	100	71	135	19	7	0	2	.5	.4	.9
		Pollock, cooked:											
8	581	Baked or broiled	3 oz	85	74	96	20	0	0	1	.2	.1	.6
8	1055	Moist heat, poached	3.5 oz	100	72	128	23	0	0	1	.2	.1	.6

[70]Dipped in egg, milk and bread crumbs; fried in vegetable shortening.

(Computer code number is for West Diet Analysis program)

GRP KEY: 1=BEV   2=DAIRY   3=EGGS   4=FAT/OIL   5=FRUIT   6=BAKERY   7=GRAIN   8=FISH   9=BEEF   10=POULTRY
11=SAUSAGE   12=MIXED/FAST   13=NUTS/SEEDS   14=SWEETS   15=VEG/LEG   16=MISC   22=SOUP/SAUCE

Chol (mg)	Calc (mg)	Iron (mg)	Magn (mg)	Phos (mg)	Pota (mg)	Sodi (mg)	Zinc (mg)	VT-A (RE)	Thia (mg)	Ribo (mg)	Niac (mg)	V-B6 (mg)	Fola (μg)	VT-C (mg)
0	17	5.34	25	124	123	2	.8	0	.90	.57	6.8	.05	30	0
0	19	5.8	28	135	134	3	.88	0	1.0	.62	7.4	.06	33	0
0	13	7	15	82	101	2	.6	0	.90	.41	6.5	.032	18	0
0	423	5.8	24	744	155	1587	.78	0	.80	.50	7.29	.06	53	0
0	41	4.7	166	415	486	6	3.52	0	.54	.26	7.6	.41	53	0
80	86	1.61	32	216	385	75	.70	35	.10	.03	2.40	.35	9	0
63	9	.62	42	290	477	77	1.04	127	.08	.11	7.78	.53	2	<1
60	8	.53	37	285	413	67	.90	120	.06	.08	5.50	.37	2	<1
29	39	11.9	8	144	267	47	1.16	77	.09	.18	1.5	.07	13	9
57	78	23.8	16	287	534	95	2.32	145	.01	.36	2.85	.07	4	3
60	83	25.2	17	304	565	100	2.46	154	.01	.38	3.02	.08	4	4
60	20	.49	42	140	245	224	.58	30	.09	.08	2.51	.28	10	<1
55	80	.5	36	200	370	100	.5	26	.04	.04	2.2	.24	9	<1
55	14	.49	42	138	244	78	.58	14	.09	.08	2.51	.28	11	<1
135	140	1.22	45	278	437	376	5.70	20	.14	.12	3.00	.33	20	2
64	46	.37	46	184	359	299	4.33	14	.04	.16	2.92	.33	20	2
120	137	1.13	52	351	505	450	5.42	14	.11	.11	1.85	.41	22	0
17	11	.33	—	—	77	715	—	—	—	.02	.15	—	—	—
64	11	.42	14	103	149	332	.38	18	.07	.1	1.21	.03	10	0
68	16	.28	50	187	272	145	.53	54	.07	.1	1.85	.20	10	1
55	16	.28	50	187	273	151	.53	69	.07	.1	1.85	.20	10	1
58	16	.28	50	246	292	89	.53	10	.07	.1	1.85	.20	10	1
55	34	1.15	26	183	270	123	.85	20	.06	.1	2.9	.13	14	0
77	49	1.40	54	251	415	763	.50	22	.05	.05	5.07	.40	3	<1
45	51	.91	91	242	490	100	.43	174	.06	.08	6.06	.34	6	<1
100	48	.84	83	222	450	480	.42	45	.05	.07	5.80	.33	5	<1
32	47	.84	83	222	450	54	.42	47	.06	.08	5.85	.34	12	<1
11	65	1.04	8	76	59	740	.45	219	.03	.12	2.8	.11	2	0
104	88	.57	51	268	510	551	4.23	38	<1	1	1.55	.112	16	t
46	92	1.2	26	191	241	138	.41	20	.10	.11	2	.22	6	0
48	53	5.30	—	186	—	—	1.68	<1	.03	.04	2.10	.36	—	<1
136	111	16.6	135	344	568	277	226[71]	223	.34	.41	3.3	.12	25	24
136	20	12.7	55	402	417	262	41.2[71]	223	.17	.58	5	.12	25	72
72	54	6.12	51	140	215	367	76.7[71]	86	.13	.18	1.45	.06	12	7
48	16	10.2	44	322	334	210	33[71]	81	.14	.46	3.82	.10	17	7
82	5	.24	31	250	329	98	.51	19	.06	.07	1.4	.06	4	t
70	60	.53	1	252	400	98	.54	9	.04	.18	3.14	.27	12	0

(For purposes of calculations, use "0" for t, <1, <.1, <.01, etc.)

Table H–1 Food Composition

Grp	Computer Code No.	Food Description	Measure	Wt (g)	H₂O (%)	Ener (kcal)	Prot (g)	Carb (g)	Dietary Fiber (g)	Fat (g)	Fat Breakdown (g) Sat	Mono	Poly
		MEATS: FISH and SHELLFISH—Con.											
		Salmon:											
8	582	Canned pink, solids and liquid	3 oz	85	69	118	17	0	0	5	1.3	1.5	1.7
8	583	Broiled or baked	3 oz	85	62	183	23	0	0	9	1.6	4.5	2.1
8	584	Smoked	3 oz	85	72	99	16	0	0	4	.8	1.7	.8
8	585	Atlantic sardines, canned, drained, 2 = 24 g	3 oz	85	60	177	21	0	0	11	1.4	3.6	4.7
8	586	Scallops, breaded, cooked from frozen	6 ea	93	59	200	17	9	<1	10	2.5	4.2	2.7
8	1588	Scallops, imitation, from surimi	3 oz	85	74	84	11	9	0	<1	—	—	—
		Shrimp:											
8	587	Cooked, boiled, 18 large shrimp	3½ oz	100	77	99	21	0	0	1	.3	.2	.4
8	588	Canned, drained	⅔ c	85	73	102	20	1	0	2	.3	.3	.6
8	589	Fried, 4 large = 30g[70]	12 ea	90	53	218	19	10	<1	11	1.9	3.4	4.6
8	1057	Raw, large, about 7 g each	14 ea	100	76	106	20	1	0	2	.3	.3	.7
8	1589	Shrimp, imitation, from surimi	3 oz	85	75	86	11	8	0	1	—	—	—
8	1053	Snapper, baked or broiled	3.5 oz	100	70	128	26	0	0	2	.4	.3	.6
8	1060	Squid, fried in flour[72]	3 oz	85	65	149	15	7	<1	6	1.6	2.3	1.8
8	1590	Surimi[73]	3 oz	85	76	84	13	6	0	1	—	—	—
		Swordfish:											
8	1058	Baked or broiled	3.5 oz	100	76	121	20	0	0	4	1.1	1.6	.9
8	1059	Raw	3.5 oz	100	69	155	25	0	0	5	1.4	2.0	1.2
8	590	Trout, baked or broiled	3 oz	85	63	129	22	<1	0	4	.7	1.1	1.3
		Tuna, light, canned, drained solids:											
8	591	Oil pack	3 oz	85	60	163	25	0	0	7	1.2	1.4	3.1
8	592	Water pack	3 oz	85	71	111	25	0	0	1	.2	.1	.3
8	1061	Tuna, raw, average	3.5 oz	100	68	144	23	0	0	5	1.3	1.4	1.7
		MEATS: BEEF, LAMB, PORK and others											
		BEEF, cooked:[74]											
		Braised, simmered, pot roasted:											
		Relatively fat, like choice chuck blade:											
9	593	Lean and fat, piece 2½ × 2½ × ¾″	3 oz	85	43	309	22	0	0	24	9	10	.8
9	594	Lean only	3 oz	85	53	224	26	0	0	12	5	5	.4
		Relatively lean, like choice round:											
9	595	Lean and fat, piece 4⅛ × 2¼ × ¾″	3 oz	85	54	242	24	0	0	15	6	7	1
9	596	Lean only	3 oz	85	57	187	27	0	0	8	2.7	3.5	.3
		Ground beef, broiled, patty 3 × ⅝″:											
9	597	Extra lean, about 16% fat	3 oz	85	57	225	24	0	0	13	5.3	6.0	.5
9	598	Lean, 21% fat	3 oz	85	54	238	24	0	0	15	6	6.7	.6
		Roasts, oven cooked, no added liquid:											
		Relatively fat, prime rib:											
9	601	Lean and fat, piece 4⅛ × 2¼ × ½″	3 oz	85	46	348	19	0	0	30	12	13	1
9	602	Lean only	3 oz	61	58	248	23	0	0	17	7	7	.5
		Relatively lean, choice round:											
9	603	Lean and fat, piece 2½ × 2½ × ¾″	3 oz	85	57	242	24	0	0	15	6	7	.6
9	604	Lean only	3 oz	75	63	187	27	0	0	8	3	4	.3
		Steak, broiled, relatively lean, choice sirloin:											
9	605	Lean and fat, piece 2½ × 2½ × ¾″	3 oz	85	54	229	24	0	0	14	6	6	.6
9	606	Lean only	3 oz	72	60	172	26	0	0	7	3.0	3	.3

[70]Dipped in egg, bread crumbs, and flour; fried in vegetable shortening.
[72]Recipe is 94.6% squid, 4.9% flour, and 0.6% salt.
[73]Surimi is processed from Walleye (Alaska) pollock. Also see Imitation crab, shrimp, scallops.
[74]Outer layer of fat removed to about 1/2″ of the lean. Deposits of fat within the cut remain.

(Computer code number is for West Diet Analysis program)

GRP KEY: 1 = BEV 2 = DAIRY 3 = EGGS 4 = FAT/OIL 5 = FRUIT 6 = BAKERY 7 = GRAIN 8 = FISH 9 = BEEF 10 = POULTRY
11 = SAUSAGE 12 = MIXED/FAST 13 = NUTS/SEEDS 14 = SWEETS 15 = VEG/LEG 16 = MISC 22 = SOUP/SAUCE

Chol (mg)	Calc (mg)	Iron (mg)	Magn (mg)	Phos (mg)	Pota (mg)	Sodi (mg)	Zinc (mg)	VT-A (RE)	Thia (mg)	Ribo (mg)	Niac (mg)	V-B6 (mg)	Fola (μg)	VT-C (mg)
37	181[75]	.72	29	279	277	471	.78	14	.02	.16	5.6	.10	13	0
74	6	.47	26	234	319	56	.43	53	.18	.14	5.67	.19	14	0
20	9	.72	15	139	149	666	.26	22	.02	.09	4.01	.24	2	0
121	325[75]	2.5	33	417	337	429	1.11	57	.07	.19	4.5	.14	10	0
57	39	.76	55	219	310	431	.99	21	.04	.10	1.4	.18	11	0
18	7	.26	—	—	88	676	—	—	.01	.01	.26	—	—	—
195	39	3.09	34	137	182	224	1.56	18	.03	.03	2.59	.13	4	<1
147	50	2.32	35	198	179	143	1.07	15	.02	.03	2.34	.09	2	0
159	60	1.13	36	196	213	310	1.24	50	.12	.12	2.76	.09	7	1.4
152	52	2.41	37	205	185	148	1.11	3	.03	.03	2.55	.10	3	2
31	16	.51	—	—	76	599	—	—	.02	.03	.15	—	—	—
47	40	.24	37	201	522	57	.44	12	.05	.08	3.46	.27	9	<1
221	33	.86	33	213	237	260	1.5	0	.05	.39	2.21	.05	—	4
25	7	.22	—	—	95	122	—	—	.02	.02	.19	—	—	—
39	4	.81	27	263	288	90	1.15	36	.04	.10	9.68	.33	14	1
50	6	1.04	34	337	369	115	1.47	41	.04	.12	11.8	.38	16	1
62	73	2.07	33	272	539	29	1.18	19	.07	.19	2.3	.42	6	3
27	11	1.2	26	265	176	301	.77	20	.03	.09	10.1	.32	5	0
28	10	2.7	26	158	267	303	.77	20	.03	.10	13.2	.32	5	0
38	16	1.02	38	191	252	39	.60	18	.24	.25	8.65	.46	25	0
87	11	2.52	16	168	194	54	6.92	<1	.06	.20	2.0	.21	4.25	0
90	11	3.13	19	200	224	60	8.73	<1	.07	.24	2.27	.25	5	0
82	5	2.65	19	208	240	43	4.18	<1	.06	.21	3.17	.28	9	0
82	4	2.94	21	231	262	43	4.66	<1	.06	.22	3.47	.31	9	0
84	8	2.36	21	162	314	70	5.47	<1	.06	.27	5	.27	9	0
86	10	2.08	20	155	297	76	5.27	<1	.05	.2	5	.27	9	0
72	9	1.8	16	146	254	54	4.5	<1	.06	.15	2.8	.22	6	0
69	9	2.2	21	181	320	63	5.90	<1	.07	.18	3.5	.26	7	0
82	5	2.6	19	208	240	42	4.2	<1	.06	.20	3.17	.28	9	0
82	4	3	21	231	262	43	5	<1	.06	.22	3.5	.31	9	0
77	9	2.6	23	187	309	53	5	<1	1	.23	3.3	.34	8	0
76	9	3	27	208	343	56	6	<1	.1	.25	3.6	.38	9	0

[75]If bones are discarded, calcium value is greatly reduced.

H

(For purposes of calculations, use "0" for t, <1, <.1, <.01, etc.)

Table H–1   Food Composition

Grp	Computer Code No.	Food Description	Measure	Wt (g)	H₂O (%)	Ener (kcal)	Prot (g)	Carb (g)	Dietary Fiber (g)	Fat (g)	Sat	Mono	Poly
		MEATS: BEEF, LAMB, PORK and others—Con.											
		BEEF, Cooked—Con.											
		Steak, broiled, relatively fat, choice T-bone:											
9	1063	Lean and fat	3 oz	85	50	253	21	0	0	18	7	7.5	.7
9	1064	Lean only	3 oz	85	60	182	24	0	0	9	3.5	3.5	.3
		Variety meats:											
9	1086	Brains, pan fried	3 oz	85	71	167	11	0	0	13	3.2	3.4	2.0
9	599	Heart, simmered	3 oz	85	64	149	25	<1	0	5	1.4	1.1	1.2
9	600	Liver, fried	3 oz	85	56	185	23	7	0	7	2.3	1.4	1.5
9	1062	Tongue, cooked	3 oz	85	56	241	19	<1	0	18	7.6	8.1	.7
9	607	Beef, canned, corned	3 oz	85	58	213	23	0	0	13	5	5	.5
9	608	Beef, dried, cured	1 oz	28	57	47	8	<1	0	1	.4	.5	.1
		LAMB, domestic, cooked:											
		Chop, arm, braised (5.6 oz raw with bone):											
9	609	Lean and fat	2.5 oz	70	44	244	21	0	0	17	7	7	1
9	610	Lean part of #609	1.9 oz	55	49	152	19	0	0	8	2.8	3.4	.5
		Chop, loin, broiled (4.2 oz raw with bone):											
9	611	Lean and fat	2.3 oz	64	52	201	16	0	0	15	6	6	1
9	612	Lean part of #611	1.6 oz	46	61	100	14	0	0	5	1.6	2.0	.3
9	1067	Cutlet, avg of lean cuts, cooked	3 oz	85	62	175	24	0	0	8	2.9	3.6	.5
		Leg, roasted, 3 oz piece = 4⅛ × 2¼ × ½":											
9	613	Lean and fat	3 oz	85	57	219	22	0	0	14	5.9	5.9	1.0
9	614	Lean only	3 oz	85	64	162	24	0	0	7	2.4	2.9	.4
		Rib, roasted, 3 oz piece = 2½ × 2½ × ¾":											
9	615	Lean and fat	3 oz	85	48	305	18	0	0	25	11	11	1.9
9	616	Lean only	3 oz	85	60	197	22	0	0	11	4	5	1
		Shoulder, roasted:											
9	1065	Lean and fat	3 oz	85	56	235	19	0	0	17	7.4	7.1	1.4
9	1066	Lean only	3 oz	85	64	163	22	0	0	8	3.1	3.2	.7
		Variety meats:											
9	1069	Brains, pan-fried	3 oz	85	61	232	14	0	0	19	4.8	3.4	1.9
9	1068	Heart, braised	3 oz	85	64	158	22	2	0	7	2.7	1.9	.66
9	1070	Sweetbreads, cooked	3 oz	85	62	196	16	0	0	13	6.3	5.1	.7
9	1071	Tongue, cooked	3 oz	85	58	234	18	0	0	17	6.7	8.5	1.1
		PORK, CURED, cooked (see also #669–672):											
9	617	Bacon, medium slices	3 pce	19	13	109	6	<1	0	9	3.3	4.5	1.1
9	1087	Breakfast strips, cooked	3 pce	34	27	156	10	<1	0	13	4.3	5.6	1.9
9	618	Canadian-style bacon	2 pce	47	62	86	11	1	0	4	1.3	1.9	.4
		Ham, roasted:											
9	619	Lean and fat, 2 pieces 4⅛ × 2¼ × ¼"	3 oz	85	58	207	18	0	0	14	5.1	7	2
9	620	Lean only	3 oz	85	66	133	21	0	0	5	1.6	2.2	.5
9	621	Ham, canned, roasted	3 oz	85	66	140	18	<1	0	7	2.4	3.5	.8
		PORK, fresh, cooked:											
		Chops, loin (cut 3 per lb with bone):											
		Braised:											
9	1291	Lean and fat	1 ea	71	44	261	19	0	0	20	7.2	9.1	2.2
9	1292	Lean only	1 ea	55	51	150	18	0	0	8	2.8	3.6	.0
		Broiled:											
9	622	Lean and fat	3.1 oz	87	50	275	24	0	0	19	7	9	2
9	623	Lean only from #622	2.5 oz	72	57	166	23	0	0	8	2.6	3.4	.9

(Computer code number is for West Diet Analysis program)

GRP KEY: 1 = BEV   2 = DAIRY   3 = EGGS   4 = FAT/OIL   5 = FRUIT   6 = BAKERY   7 = GRAIN   8 = FISH   9 = BEEF   10 = POULTRY
11 = SAUSAGE   12 = MIXED/FAST   13 = NUTS/SEEDS   14 = SWEETS   15 = VEG/LEG   16 = MISC   22 = SOUP/SAUCE

Chol (mg)	Calc (mg)	Iron (mg)	Magn (mg)	Phos (mg)	Pota (mg)	Sodi (mg)	Zinc (mg)	VT-A (RE)	Thia (mg)	Ribo (mg)	Niac (mg)	V-B6 (mg)	Fola (µg)	VT-C (mg)
71	7	2.3	21	156	302	52	3.98	<1	.09	.19	3.47	.29	6	0
68	6	2.55	25	177	346	56	4.59	<1	.09	.21	3.94	.33	7	0
1697	8	1.89	12	328	301	134	1.15	0	.11	.22	3.21	.33	5	3
164	5	6.39	21	213	198	54	2.66	0	.12	1.31	3.46	.18	2	1
410	9	5.34	20	392	310	90	4.63	9126[76]	.18	3.52	12.3	1.22	187	20
91	6	2.88	14	121	153	51	4.08	0	.03	.30	1.83	.14	4	<1
73	10	1.77	12	94	116	856	3.04	0	.02	.13	2.07	.11	8	1
12	2	1.28	9	49	126	984	1.49	0	.02	.06	1.6	1	3	4.2
84	18	1.7	18	145	216	51	4.28	2	.05	.18	4.7	.08	13	0
66	14	1.5	16	127	185	41	4.0	1	.04	.15	3.5	.07	12	0
64	13	1.15	15	125	209	49	2.22	2	.07	.16	4.5	.08	12	0
44	9	.93	13	105	175	39	1.91	1	.05	.13	3.2	.07	11	0
78	13	1.74	22	179	293	64	4.48	<1	.09	.24	5.37	.14	19	0
79	9	1.69	20	162	266	56	3.74	2	.09	.23	5.6	.13	17	0
76	7	1.81	22	175	287	58	4.2	1	.09	.25	5.4	.14	20	0
82	19	1.4	17	141	231	62	2.96	2	.07	.18	5.7	.10	13	0
74	18	1.5	20	165	268	69	3.8	<1	.08	.20	5.24	.13	19	0
78	15	1.72	19	155	220	55	3.81	<1	.08	.21	5.66	.10	17	0
73	14	1.9	22	172	236	57	4.46	<1	.08	.23	5.39	.12	21	0
2128	18	1.73	18	421	304	133	1.70	0	.14	.31	3.87	.20	6	20
212	12	4.70	21	216	160	54	3.13	0	.14	1.01	3.71	.25	2	6
347	29	1.53	20	357	221	179	1.79	0	.03	.2	1.79	.02	12	15
161	8	2.24	14	114	134	57	2.54	0	.07	.36	3.14	.14	2	6
16	2	.32	5	64	92	303	.62	0	.13	.05	1.39	.05	1	6[77]
36	5	.67	9	90	158	714	1.25	0	.25	.13	2.58	.12	1	15
27	5	.38	10	138	181	719	.79	0	.38	.09	3.22	.21	2	10[77]
53	6	.74	16	182	243	1009	1.97	0	.51	.19	3.8	.32	3	0
47	6	.8	19	193	269	1128	2.19	0	.58	.22	4.27	.4	3	0
35	6	.91	16	188	298	908	1.97	0	.82	.21	4.27	.33	4	19[77]
73	6	.82	14	141	245	46	2.15	2	.43	.21	4.24	.26	3	<1
58	5	.77	13	131	230	41	2.05	2	.38	.20	3.82	.25	3	<1
84	4	.71	22	184	312	61	1.68	3	.87	.24	4.35	.35	4	<1
71	4	.66	22	176	302	56	1.61	2	.83	.22	3.99	.34	4	<1

[76] Value varies widely.
[77] Values based on products containing added ascorbic acid or sodium ascorbate. If none added, ascorbic acid content would be negligible.

(For purposes of calculations, use "0" for t, <1, <.1, <.01, etc.)

H

Table H–1   Food Composition

Grp	Computer Code No.	Food Description	Measure	Wt (g)	H₂O (%)	Ener (kcal)	Prot (g)	Carb (g)	Dietary Fiber (g)	Fat (g)	Fat Breakdown (g) Sat	Mono	Poly
		MEATS: BEEF, LAMB, PORK and others—Con.											
		PORK, Fresh Cooked—Con.											
		Pan fried:											
9	624	Lean and fat	3.1 oz	89	45	334	21	0	0	27	10	13	3
9	625	Lean only from #624	2.4 oz	67	54	178	19	0	0	11	3.7	4.8	1.3
		Leg, roasted:											
9	626	Lean and fat, piece 2½ × 2½ × ¾″	3 oz	85	53	250	21	0	0	18	6	8	2
9	627	Lean only from #626	3 oz	85	60	187	24	0	0	9	3.2	4.2	1.1
		Rib, roasted:											
9	628	Lean and fat, piece 2½ × 2½ × ¾″	3 oz	85	51	270	21	0	0	20	7	9	2
9	629	Lean only	3 oz	85	57	210	24	0	0	12	4.1	5.3	1.4
		Shoulder, braised:											
9	630	Lean and fat, 3 pieces 2½ × 2½ × ¼″	3 oz	85	47	293	23	0	0	22	8	10	2
9	631	Lean only	3 oz	85	54	208	27	0	0	10	4	5	1.3
9	1088	Spareribs, cooked, yield from 1 lb raw with bone	6.25 oz	177	40	703	51	0	0	54	20.8	25.1	6.2
9	1095	Rabbit, roasted (1 cup meat = 140g)	3 oz	85	59	175	26	0	0	7	2.1	1.9	1.4
		VEAL, cooked:											
9	632	Veal cutlet, braised or broiled, 4⅛ × 2¼ × ½″	3 oz	85	60	166	27	0	0	6	1.6	2.0	.5
9	633	Veal rib roasted, lean, 2 pieces 4⅛ × 2¼ × ¼″	3 oz	85	65	151	22	0	0	6	1.8	2.3	.6
9	634	Veal liver, pan-fried	3 oz	85	53	208	25	3	0	10	3.6	1.6	1.5
9	1096	Venison (Deer meat) roasted	3.5 oz	100	65	158	30	0	0	3	1.3	.9	.6
		MEATS: POULTRY and POULTRY PRODUCTS											
		CHICKEN, cooked:											
		Fried, batter dipped:[78]											
10	635	Breast (5.6 oz with bones)	1 ea	140	52	364	35	13	<1	19	5	8	4
10	636	Drumstick (3.4 oz with bones)	1 ea	72	53	193	16	6	<1	11	3	5	3
10	637	Thigh	1 ea	86	52	238	19	8	<1	14	4	6	3
10	638	Wing	1 ea	49	46	159	10	5	<1	11	3	4	3
		Fried, flour coated:[78]											
10	639	Breast (4.2 oz with bones)	1 ea	98	57	218	31	2	<1	9	2.4	3.4	1.9
10	1212	Breast, without skin	1 ea	86	60	161	29	<1	0	4	1.1	1.5	.9
10	640	Drumstick (2.6 oz with bones)	1 ea	49	57	120	13	1	<1	7	1.8	2.7	1.6
10	641	Thigh	1 ea	62	54	162	17	2	<1	9	2.5	3.6	2.1
10	1099	Thigh, without skin	1 ea	52	59	113	15	1	<1	5	1.5	2.0	1.3
10	642	Wing	1 ea	32	49	103	8	1	<1	7	1.9	2.8	1.6
		Roasted:											
10	643	All types of meat	1 c	140	64	266	41	0	0	10	2.9	3.7	2.4
10	644	Dark meat	1 c	140	63	286	38	0	0	14	3.7	5.0	3.2
10	645	Light meat	1 c	140	65	242	43	0	0	6	1.8	2.2	1.4
10	646	Breast, without skin	½ ea	86	65	142	27	0	0	3	.9	1.1	.7
10	647	Drumstick	1 ea	44	67	76	13	0	0	2	.7	.8	.6
10	648	Thigh	1 ea	62	59	153	16	0	0	10	2.9	3.8	2.1
10	1100	Thigh, without skin	1 ea	52	63	109	14	0	0	6	1.6	2.2	1.3
		Stewed, all types:											
10	649		1 c	140	67	248	38	0	0	9	2.6	3.3	2.2
10	656	Canned, boneless chicken	5 oz	142	69	235	31	0	0	11	3.1	4.5	2.5
10	1102	Chicken gizzards, simmered	1 ea	22	67	34	6	<1	0	1	.2	.2	.2
10	1101	Chicken hearts, simmered	1 ea	3.3	65	6	1	<1	0	<1	.1	.1	.1
10	650	Chicken liver, simmered	1 ea	20	68	30	5	2	0	1	.4	.3	.2

[78]Fried in vegetable shortening.

(Computer code number is for West Diet Analysis program)

GRP KEY: 1 = BEV 2 = DAIRY 3 = EGGS 4 = FAT/OIL 5 = FRUIT 6 = BAKERY 7 = GRAIN 8 = FISH 9 = BEEF 10 = POULTRY
11 = SAUSAGE 12 = MIXED/FAST 13 = NUTS/SEEDS 14 = SWEETS 15 = VEG/LEG 16 = MISC 22 = SOUP/SAUCE

Chol (mg)	Calc (mg)	Iron (mg)	Magn (mg)	Phos (mg)	Pota (mg)	Sodi (mg)	Zinc (mg)	VT-A (RE)	Thia (mg)	Ribo (mg)	Niac (mg)	V-B6 (mg)	Fola (µg)	VT-C (mg)
92	4	.75	23	190	323	64	1.74	3	.91	.25	4.58	.35	4	<1
71	3	.67	21	178	305	57	1.61	2	.84	.22	4.03	.34	4	<1
79	5	.85	18	210	280	50	2.43	2	.54	.27	3.89	.33	9	<1
80	6	.95	21	239	317	54	2.77	2	.59	.3	4.2	.38	10	<1
69	9	.76	16	190	313	37	1.67	3	.5	.24	4.17	.3	7	<1
67	10	.85	18	218	360	40	1.9	3	.54	.26	4.6	.34	7	<1
93	6	1.4	16	162	286	74	3.43	3	.46	.26	4.43	.23	3	<1
95	6	1.64	19	189	339	85	4.16	3	.5	.3	5	.35	4	<1
214	83	3.27	43	462	566	165	8.14	5	.72	.68	9.69	.62	7	0
73	17	2.02	17	192	255	31	2.02	2	.05	.14	6.09	.29	8	0
100	20	.99	24	213	288	76	4.33	t	.05	.29	7.16	.28	13	0
97	10	.82	20	176	264	82	3.81	t	.05	.25	6.4	.23	12	0
280	10	4.45	22	373	372	112	6.69	4784[79]	.21	2.86	14.4	.73	272	18
112	7	4.47	24	226	335	54	2.75	0	.18	.60	6.71	.32[80]	4[80]	0
119	28	1.75	34	258	282	385	1.33	28	.16	.2	14.7	.6	8	0
62	12	.97	14	106	134	194	1.67	19	.08	.16	3.67	.2	6	0
80	16	1.24	18	134	165	248	1.75	25	.1	.2	4.92	.23	8	0
39	10	.63	8	59	68	157	.67	17	.05	.07	2.58	.15	3	0
88	16	1.17	29	228	253	74	1.07	15	.08	.13	13.5	.57	4	0
78	14	.98	27	212	237	68	.93	6	.07	.11	12.7	.55	4	0
44	6	.66	11	86	112	44	1.42	12	.04	.11	2.96	.17	4	0
60	8	.93	15	116	147	55	1.56	18	.06	.15	4.31	.21	5	0
53	7	.76	14	103	134	49	1.45	11	.05	.13	3.70	.20	4	0
26	5	.4	6	48	57	25	.56	12	.02	.04	2.14	.13	1	0
125	21	1.69	35	273	340	120	2.94	22	.1	.25	12.8	.65	8	0
130	21	1.86	33	250	336	130	3.92	30	.1	.32	9.17	.5	11	0
118	21	1.49	38	302	345	108	1.73	12	.09	.16	17.4	.84	5	0
73	13	.89	25	196	220	64	.86	5	.06	.1	11.8	.52	3	0
41	5	.57	11	81	108	42	1.4	8	.03	.1	2.67	.17	4	0
58	8	.83	14	108	137	52	1.46	30	.04	.13	3.95	.19	4	0
49	6	.68	12	95	124	46	1.34	10	.04	.12	3.39	.18	4	0
116	20	1.63	29	210	252	98	2.79	21	.07	.23	8.56	.37	8	0
88	20	2.2	17	158	196	714	2.13	48	.02	.18	8.99	.5	4	3
43	2	.91	4	34	39	15	.96	12	.01	.05	.87	.03	12	<1
8	1	.30	1	7	4	2	.24	<1	<.01	.02	.09	.01	3	<1
126	3	1.7	2	62	28	10	.87	983	.03	.35	.89	.12	154	3

[79] Value varies widely.
[80] Values estimated from other game meat.

(For purposes of calculations, use "0" for t, <1, <.1, <.01, etc.)

Table H–1   Food Composition

Grp	Computer Code No.	Food Description	Measure	Wt (g)	H₂O (%)	Ener (kcal)	Prot (g)	Carb (g)	Dietary Fiber (g)	Fat (g)	Fat Breakdown (g) Sat	Mono	Poly
MEATS: POULTRY and POULTRY PRODUCTS—Con.													
		DUCK, roasted:											
10	1293	Meat with skin, about 2.7 cups	½ duck	382	52	1287	73	0	0	108	37	49	14
10	651	Meat only, about 1.5 cups	½ duck	221	64	445	52	0	0	25	9.2	8.2	3.2
		GOOSE, domesticated, roasted:											
10	1294	Meat only, 4.2 cups	½ goose	591	57	1406	171	0	0	75	27	26	9
10	1295	Meat w/skin, about 5.5 cups	½ goose	774	52	2362	195	0	0	170	53	79	20
		TURKEY, roasted, meat only:											
10	652	Dark meat	3 oz	85	63	159	24	0	0	6	2.1	1.4	1.8
10	653	Light meat	3 oz	85	66	133	25	0	0	3	.9	.5	.7
10	654	All types, chopped or diced	1 c	140	65	238	41	0	0	7	2.3	1.5	2.0
10	655	All types, sliced	3 oz	85	65	145	25	0	0	4	1.4	.9	1.2
10	1103	Ground turkey, cooked	3.5 oz	100	60	229	24	0	0	14	3.8	5.0	3.3
		Turkey breast:											
10	1104	Barbecued	1 oz	28	70	40	6	0	0	1	.4	.5	.3
10	1105	Hickory smoked	1 oz	28	70	35	6	1	0	1	.3	.3	.3
10	1106	Gizzard, cooked	1 ea	67	65	109	20	<1	0	3	.7	.5	.7
10	1107	Heart, cooked	1 ea	16	64	28	4	<1	0	1	.3	.2	.3
10	1108	Liver, cooked	1 ea	75	66	127	18	3	0	4	1.4	1.1	1.1
		Poultry food products (see also items in sausages and lunchmeats section):											
10	658	Chicken roll, light meat	2 pce	57	69	90	11	1	0	4	1.2	1.7	.9
10	659	Gravy and turkey, frozen package	5 oz	142	85	95	8	7	<1	4	1.2	1.4	.7
10	660	Turkey loaf, breast meat	2 pce	42	72	46	10	0	0	1	.2	.2	.1
10	661	Turkey patties, breaded, fried	1 ea	64	50	181	9	10	<1	12	3	4.8	3
10	662	Turkey, frozen, roasted, seasoned	3 oz	85	68	130	18	3	0	5	1.6	1	1.4
MEATS: SAUSAGES and LUNCHMEATS (see also Poultry food products)													
		Beerwurst/beer salami:											
11	1072	Beef	1 pce	23	54	75	3	<1	0	7	2.8	3.3	.2
11	1074	Pork	1 pce	23	62	55	3	<1	0	4	1.4	2.1	.5
11	1075	Berliner	1 pce	23	61	53	4	1	0	4	1.4	1.8	.4
		Bologna:											
11	1297	Beef	1 pce	23	55	72	3	<1	0	7	2.7	3.1	.2
11	663	Beef and pork	1 pce	28	54	89	3	1	0	8	3.0	3.8	.7
65	1298	Pork	1 pce	23	61	57	4	<1	0	5	1.6	2.3	.5
11	664	Turkey	1 pce	28	66	56	4	<1	0	4	1.5	1.9	1.2
11	665	Braunschweiger sausage	2 pce	57	48	205	8	2	0	18	6.2	8.5	2.1
11	1073	Brotwurst, link	1 ea	70	51	226	10	2	0	20	7.0	9.3	2.0
11	666	Brown-and-serve sausage links, cooked	1 ea	13	45	50	2	<1	0	5	1.7	2.2	.5
11	1089	Cheesefurter/cheese smokie	1 ea	43	53	141	6	1	0	13	4.5	5.9	1.3
11	1090	Corned beef loaf, jellied	1 pce	28	67	46	7	0	0	2	.8	.9	.1
		Frankfurters (see also #657):											
11	1077	Beef, large link, 8/pkg.	1 ea	57	54	184	6	1	0	17	6.8	8.2	.7
11	1078	Beef and pork, large link, 8/pkg.	1 ea	57	54	183	6	1	0	17	6.1	7.8	1.6
11	667	Beef and pork, smaller link, 10/pkg.	1 ea	45	54	145	5	1	0	13	4.8	6.2	1.2
10	657	Chicken frankfurter, 10/pkg.	1 ea	45	58	115	6	3	0	9	2.5	3.8	1.8
11	668	Turkey, smaller link, 10/pkg.	1 ea	45	63	102	6	1	0	8	2.7	3.3	2.1
		Ham:											
11	669	Ham lunchmeat, canned, 3 x 2 x ½"	1 pce	21	52	70	3	<1	0	6	2.3	3.0	.8
11	670	Chopped ham, packaged	2 pce	22	61	98	7	<1	0	8	2.6	3.9	.9

(Computer code number is for West Diet Analysis program)

GRP KEY: 1=BEV   2=DAIRY   3=EGGS   4=FAT/OIL   5=FRUIT   6=BAKERY   7=GRAIN   8=FISH   9=BEEF   10=POULTRY
11=SAUSAGE   12=MIXED/FAST   13=NUTS/SEEDS   14=SWEETS   15=VEG/LEG   16=MISC   22=SOUP/SAUCE

Chol (mg)	Calc (mg)	Iron (mg)	Magn (mg)	Phos (mg)	Pota (mg)	Sodi (mg)	Zinc (mg)	VT-A (RE)	Thia (mg)	Ribo (mg)	Niac (mg)	V-B6 (mg)	Fola (µg)	VT-C (mg)
320	43	10.3	62	595	780	227	7.12	241	.67	1.03	18.4	.70	25	0
198	26	5.97	44	449	557	143	5.75	51	.57	1.04	11.3	.55	22	0
569	84	17.0	148	1828	2291	447	16.0	71	.54	2.31	24.1	2.75	13	0
708	104	21.9	169	2091	2546	543	16.0	162	.60	2.50	32.3	2.89	17	0
72	27	1.99	21	174	247	67	3.8	0	.05	.21	3.1	.3	8	0
59	16	1.14	24	186	259	54	1.73	0	.05	.12	5.81	.46	5	0
107	35	2.49	37	298	418	99	4.34	0	.09	.26	7.62	.64	10	0
64	21	1.51	23	181	254	60	2.64	0	.05	.16	4.63	.39	6	0
69	25	1.93	24	196	270	83	2.86	0	.05	.17	4.82	.39	7	0
16	2	.12	7	74	57	156	.35	0	.01	.03	2.73	.11	1	<1
13	1	.20	7	79	59	208	.30	0	.01	.03	2.75	.11	1	<1
155	10	3.64	13	86	141	37	2.79	37	.02	.22	2.06	.08	36	1
36	2	1.10	4	33	29	9	.84	1	.01	.14	.52	.05	13	<1
469	8	5.85	11	204	146	48	2.32	2806	.04	1.07	4.46	.39	499	1
28	24	.55	10	89	129	331	.41	14	.04	.07	3	.31	2	0
26	20	1.32	11	115	87	787	.99	18	.03	.18	2.55	.14	2	0
17	3	.17	9	97	118	608	.48	0	.02	.05	3.54	.15	2	0[81]
40	9	1.41	12	173	176	512	1.5	7	.06	.12	1.47	.13	3	0
45	4	1.4	20	207	253	578	2.37	0	.04	.14	5.3	.24	5	0
13	2	.31	3	24	42	214	.61	0	.03	.03	.66	.05	1	3
13	2	.17	3	24	58	285	.40	0	.13	.04	.75	.08	1	7
11	3	.27	3	30	65	298	.57	0	.09	.05	.72	.05	1	2
13	3	.32	2	19	36	230	.46	0	.01	.03	.61	.04	1	4
16	3	.43	3	26	51	289	.55	0	.05	.04	.73	.05	1	6[82]
14	3	.18	3	33	65	272	.47	0	.12	.04	.90	.06	1	8
28	23	.43	4	37	56	248	.49	0	.02	.05	1.04	.05	1	<1
89	6	5.32	6	96	113	652	1.62	2406	.14	.87	4.78	.19	57	5[82]
44	34	.72	11	94	197	778	1.47	0	.18	.16	2.31	.09	2	20
9	1	.1	2	14	25	105	.15	0	.05	.02	.40	.03	1	0
29	25	.46	5	76	89	465	.97	3	.11	.07	1.25	.05	1	8
12	3	.58	3	18	25	294	1.08	0	<.01	.03	.46	.04	1	2
27	7	.76	7	47	90	584	1.21	0	.03	.06	1.44	.06	2	14
29	6	.66	7	49	95	639	1.05	0	.11	.07	1.50	.08	2	15
23	5	.52	6	39	75	504	.83	0	.09	.05	1.18	.06	2	12[82]
45	43	.9	8	48	38	616	1	17	.03	.05	1.39	.09	2	0
39	58	.77	8	83	88	454	1	17	.04	.08	1.7	.10	2	<1
13	1	.15	2	17	45	271	.31	0	.08	.04	.66	.04	1	<1
21	3	.4	5	58	119	573	.77	0	.23	.07	1.4	.13	2	1[82]

[81] If sodium ascorbate is added, product contains 11 mg ascorbic acid.
[82] Values based on products containing added ascorbic acid or sodium ascorbate. If none added, ascorbic acid content would be negligible.

H

(For purposes of calculations, use "0" for t, <1, <.1, <.01, etc.)

Table H–1 Food Composition

Grp	Computer Code No.	Food Description	Measure	Wt (g)	H₂O (%)	Ener (kcal)	Prot (g)	Carb (g)	Dietary Fiber (g)	Fat (g)	Fat Breakdown (g) Sat	Mono	Poly
		MEATS: SAUSAGES and LUNCHMEATS—Con.											
		Ham—Con.											
11	671	Ham lunchmeat, regular	2 pce	57	65	103	10	2	0	6	1.9	2.8	.7
11	672	Ham lunchmeat, extra lean	2 pce	57	70	75	11	1	0	3	.9	1.3	.3
11	673	Turkey ham	2 pce	57	72	73	11	1	0	3	1.0	.8	.8
11	1091	Keilbasa sausage	1 pce	26	54	81	3	1	0	7	2.6	3.4	.8
11	1092	Knockwurst sausage-link	1 ea	68	56	209	8	1	0	19	6.9	8.7	2.0
11	1093	Mortadella lunchmeat	1 pce	15	52	47	2	<1	0	4	1.4	1.7	.5
11	1097	Olive loaf lunchmeat	2 pce	57	58	133	7	5	<1	9	3.3	4.5	1.1
11	1080	Pastrami, turkey	2 pce	57	72	74	11	1	0	4	1.0	1.2	.9
11	1081	Pepperoni sausage, small slices	4 pce	22	27	109	5	1	0	10	3.6	4.6	1
11	1094	Pickle & pimento loaf	2 pce	57	57	149	7	3	<1	12	4.5	5.4	1.5
11	1082	Polish sausage	1 oz.	28	53	92	4	<1	0	8	2.9	3.8	.9
		Pork sausage, cooked:[83]											
11	674	Link, small	1 ea	13	45	48	3	<1	0	4	1.4	1.8	.5
11	1079	Patty	1 pce	27	45	100	5	<1	0	8	2.9	3.8	1.0
		Salami:											
11	675	Pork and beef	2 pce	57	60	143	8	1	0	11	4.6	5.2	1.1
11	676	Turkey	2 pce	57	66	111	9	<1	0	8	2.3	2.6	2.0
11	677	Dry, beef and pork	2 pce	20	35	85	5	1	0	7	2.4	3.4	.6
		Sandwich spreads:											
11	1300	Ham salad	1 c	240	63	518	21	26	<1	37	12.1	17.3	6.5
11	678	Pork and beef	1 tbsp	15	60	35	1	2	0	3	.9	1.1	.4
10	1296	Poultry sandwich spread	1 tbsp	13	60	25	2	1	0	2	.5	.4	.8
		Smoked link sausage:											
11	1083	Beef and pork	1 ea	68	39	265	15	1	0	22	7.7	10.0	2.6
11	1084	Pork	1 ea	68	52	229	9	1	0	21	7.2	9.7	2.2
11	1085	Summer sausage	1 pce	23	48	80	4	1	0	7	2.8	3.2	.4
11	1076	Turkey breakfast sausage	1 pce	28	60	65	6	0	0	4	1.6	1.8	1.2
11	679	Vienna sausage, canned	1 ea	16	60	45	2	<1	0	4	1.5	2.0	.3
		MIXED DISHES and FAST FOODS											
		MIXED DISHES:											
		Beef stew with vegetables:											
12	680	Homemade	1 c	245	82	220	16	15	3	11	4.4	4.5	.5
12	1109	Canned	1 c	245	83	194	14	18	1	8	3.1	3.1	.4
12	1116	Beef, macaroni & tomato sauce casserole	1 c	226	80	189	10	25	2	6	2.1	2.3	.4
12	681	Beef pot pie, homemade[84]	1 pce	210	55	515	21	39	1	30	8	13	7
12	682	Chicken à la king, home recipe	1 c	245	68	470	27	12	1	34	13	13	6
12	683	Chicken and noodles, home recipe	1 c	240	71	365	22	26	1	18	5	7	4
12	684	Chicken chow mein, canned	1 c	250	89	95	7	18	5	1	.1	.1	.8
12	685	Chicken chow mein, home recipe	1 c	250	78	255	23	10	4	11	4	4	3
12	686	Chicken pot pie, home recipe[84]	1 pce	232	57	545	23	42	2	31	10	16	7
12	1112	Chicken salad w/celery	.5 c	78	53	266	11	1	<1	25	4.1	7.2	12.0
12	687	Chili with beans, canned	1 c	255	76	286	15	30	8	14	6	6	1
12	688	Chop suey with beef and pork	1 c	250	75	300	26	13	2	17	4	7	4
12	689	Corn pudding[85]	1 c	250	76	271	11	32	9	13	6.3	4.3	1.7
12	690	Cole slaw[86]	1 c	120	82	84	2	15	2	3	.5	.9	1.6
12	1110	Corned beef hash-canned	1 c	220	67	382	18	22	1	10	4.2	4.9	.5
12	1113	Egg salad	1 c	183	66	438	19	3	<1	39	8.4	13.2	13.5

[83] Cooked weight is half the weight of raw sausage.

[84] Crust made with vegetable shortening and enriched flour.

[85] Recipe: 55% yellow corn, 23% whole milk, 14% egg, 4% sugar, 3% salt, and 1% pepper.

[86] Recipe: 41% cabbage; 12% celery; 12% table cream; 12% sugar; 7% green pepper; 6% lemon juice; 4% onion; 3% pimento; 3% vinegar; 2% each for salt, dry mustard, and white pepper.

(Computer code number is for West Diet Analysis program)

GRP KEY: 1 = BEV 2 = DAIRY 3 = EGGS 4 = FAT/OIL 5 = FRUIT 6 = BAKERY 7 = GRAIN 8 = FISH 9 = BEEF 10 = POULTRY
11 = SAUSAGE 12 = MIXED/FAST 13 = NUTS/SEEDS 14 = SWEETS 15 = VEG/LEG 16 = MISC 22 = SOUP/SAUCE

Chol (mg)	Calc (mg)	Iron (mg)	Magn (mg)	Phos (mg)	Pota (mg)	Sodi (mg)	Zinc (mg)	VT-A (RE)	Thia (mg)	Ribo (mg)	Niac (mg)	V-B6 (mg)	Fola (µg)	VT-C (mg)
32	4	.56	11	140	188	746	1.21	0	.49	.14	2.98	.19	2	16[82]
27	4	.43	10	124	198	810	1.09	0	.53	.13	2.74	.26	2	15[82]
32	5	1.56	12	138	163	548	1.58	0	.04	.15	2.72	.16	4	0
17	11	.38	4	38	70	280	.52	0	.06	.06	.75	.05	1	6
39	7	.62	8	67	136	687	1.13	0	.23	.10	1.86	.11	2	18
8	3	.21	2	15	24	187	.32	0	.02	.02	.40	.02	<1	4
22	62	.31	11	72	169	842	.78	0	.17	.15	1.04	.13	1	5
30	5	.81	10	142	155	569	1.46	0	.05	.15	2.48	.16	4	<1
8	2	.31	4	26	76	449	.55	0	.07	.06	1.09	.06	—	<1
21	54	.58	10	79	193	787	.79	<1	.17	.14	1.16	.11	1	8
20	3	.41	4	39	67	248	.55	0	.14	.04	.98	.05	1	0
11	4	.16	2	24	47	168	.33	0	.1	.03	.59	.04	1	<1
22	9	.34	5	50	97	349	.68	0	.20	.07	1.22	.09	2	<1
37	7	1.51	9	65	112	604	1.21	0	.14	.21	2.02	.12	1	7[82]
46	11	.93	9	73	125	535	1.25	0	.06	.15	2.23	.14	5	<1
16	2	.3	4	28	76	372	.64	0	.12	.06	.97	.1	0	6[82]
88	19	1.42	23	286	359	2187	2.64	42	1.04	.29	5.02	.36	3	14
6	2	.12	1	9	16	152	.15	1	.03	.02	.26	.02	<1	0
4	1	.08	3	4	24	49	.25	6	<.01	.01	.22	.01	1	<1
46	20	.79	13	110	228	1020	1.92	0	.48	.18	3.08	.24	2	1
48	7	.99	8	73	129	642	1.44	0	.18	.12	2.19	.12	2	13
16	2	.47	3	23	53	334	.47	0	.04	.07	.94	.07	1	5
23	5	.52	6	52	76	191	.97	0	.03	.08	1.42	.08	1	—
8	2	.14	1	8	16	152	.26	0	.01	.02	.26	.02	<1	0
71	29	2.9	40	184	613	292	5.3	569	.15	.17	4.7	.28	37	17
15	23	3.18	39	56	417	992	4.23	262	.07	.12	2.43	.20	31	7
22	30	2.39	37	118	562	974	2.07	111	.19	.17	3.51	.30	23	16
42	29	3.8	6	149	334	596	3.17	517	.29	.29	4.8	.24	29	6
221	127	2.5	20	358	404	760	1.8	272	.1	.42	5.4	.23	11	12
103	26	2.4	37	247	211	600	2.14	130	.05	.17	4.3	.16	9	1
8	45	1.3	14	85	418	725	1.3	28	.05	.1	1	.09	12	13
75	58	2.50	28	293	473	718	2.12	50	.08	.23	4.3	.41	19	10
56	70	3.0	25	232	343	594	2.0	735	.32	.32	4.9	.46	29	5
48	16	.66	11	80	137	199	.80	31	.03	.08	3.25	.17	4	1
43	119	8.75	115	393	932	1330	5.10	86	.12	.27	.91	.34	41	4
68	60	4.80	32	248	425	1053	3.58	60	.28	.38	5.0	.32	22	33
230	100	1.40	38	143	402	138	1.26	89	1.03	.32	2.47	.30	63	7
10[87]	54	.70	12	38	218	28	.24	98	.08	.07	.33	.18	32	39
132	29	4.40	3	147	440	1354	4.38	0	.12	.40	4.60	.41	15	8
629	94	3.39	21	282	211	428	2.24	300	.12	.45	.16	.18	74	0

[82] Values based on products containing added ascorbic acid or sodium ascorbate. If none added, ascorbic acid content would be negligible.
[87] From dairy cream in recipe.

(For purposes of calculations, use "0" for t, <1, <.1, <.01, etc.)

H

Table H–1 Food Composition

Grp	Computer Code No.	Food Description	Measure	Wt (g)	H₂O (%)	Ener (kcal)	Prot (g)	Carb (g)	Dietary Fiber (g)	Fat (g)	Fat Breakdown (g) Sat	Mono	Poly
MIXED DISHES and FAST FOODS—Con.													
		MIXED DISHES—Con.											
12	691	French toast, home recipe[88]	1 pce	65	53	123	5	15	1	4	1.1	1.4	1.1
12	1355	Green pepper, stuffed	1 ea	172	76	217	10	16	1	13	5.3	5.2	.6
		Lasagna:											
12	1346	With meat	1 pce	245	64	398	26	30	2	20	9.2	7.2	1.5
12	1111	Without meat	1 pce	218	64	316	20	30	2	14	6.9	4.7	1.3
12	1117	Frozen entree	1 pce	205	73	275	17	19	1	12	6.3	4.2	1.2
		Macaroni and cheese:											
12	692	Canned[89]	1 c	240	80	230	9	26	1	10	5	3	1
12	693	Home recipe[90]	1 c	200	58	430	17	40	1	22	10	7	4
12	1115	Macaroni salad-no cheese	1 c	141	61	371	3	18	1	33	5.1	9.5	17.2
		Meat loaf:											
12	1120	Beef	1 pce	87	62	193	16	4	<1	12	4.8	5.2	.6
12	1119	Beef and pork (1/3)	1 pce	87	59	212	15	5	<1	15	5.5	6.3	1.2
12	1303	Moussaka (lamb and eggplant)	1 c	250	79	250	21	16	6	11	3.6	4.3	1.9
12	715	Potato salad with mayonnaise and egg[91]	1 c	250	76	358	7	28	4	21	4	6	9
12	694	Quiche lorraine, ⅛ of 8″ quiche[84]	1 pce	176	47	600	13	29	1	48	23	18	4
		Spaghetti (enriched) in tomato sauce:											
		With cheese:											
12	695	Canned	1 c	250	80	190	6	39	3	2	.4	.4	.5
12	696	Home recipe	1 c	250	77	260	9	37	3	9	3	3.6	1.2
		With meatballs:											
12	697	Canned	1 c	250	78	260	12	39	3	10	2	4	3
12	698	Home recipe	1 c	248	70	330	19	39	3	12	4	4	2
12	716	Spinach soufflé[92]	1 c	136	74	218	11	3	4	18	7	7	3
12	717	Tuna salad[93]	1 c	205	63	383	33	19	2	19	3	6	9
12	1121	Tuna noodle casserole, recipe	1 c	202	73	251	21	24	<1	7	2.0	1.5	3.2
12	1270	Waldorf salad	1 c	142	58	424	4	13	4	42	5.6	11.2	23.1
		FAST FOODS and SANDWICHES: see end of this appendix for additional Fast Foods.											
		Burrito:[94]											
12	699	Beef and bean	1 ea	175	54	390	21	40	5	18	7	7	2
12	700	Bean	1 ea	174	55	322	13	47	8	10	4	3	2
		Cheeseburger:											
12	701	Regular	1 ea	112	46	300	15	28	1	15	7	6	1
12	702	4-oz patty	1 ea	194	46	524	30	40	2	31	15	12	1
12	703	Chicken patty sandwich	1 ea	157	52	436	25	34	1	22	6	10	5
12	704	Corn dog	1 ea	111	45	330	10	27	<1	20	8	10	1
12	705	Enchilada, cheese	1 ea	163	63	320	10	29	3	19	11	6	.8
12	706	English muffin with egg, cheese, bacon	1 ea	138	49	360	18	31	2	18	8	8	.7
		Fish sandwich:											
12	707	Regular, with cheese	1 ea	140	43	420	16	39	1	23	6	7	8
12	708	Large, without cheese	1 ea	170	48	470	18	41	1	27	6	9	10

[84]Crust made with vegetable shortening and enriched flour.
[88]Recipe: 35% whole milk, 32% white bread, 29% egg, and cooked in 4% margarine.
[89]Made with corn oil.
[90]Made with margarine.
[91]Recipe: 62% potatoes; 12% egg; 8% mayonnaise; 7% celery; 6% sweet pickle relish; 2% onion; 1% each for green pepper, pimiento, salt, and dry mustard.
[92]Recipe: 29% whole milk, 26% spinach, 13% egg white, 13% cheddar cheese, 7% egg yolk, 7% butter, 4% flour, 1% salt and pepper.
[93]Made with drained chunk light tuna, celery, onion, pickle relish, and mayonnaise-type salad dressing.
[94]Made with a 10½″-diameter flour tortilla.

(Computer code number is for West Diet Analysis program)

GRP KEY: 1 = BEV   2 = DAIRY   3 = EGGS   4 = FAT/OIL   5 = FRUIT   6 = BAKERY   7 = GRAIN   8 = FISH   9 = BEEF   10 = POULTRY
11 = SAUSAGE   12 = MIXED/FAST   13 = NUTS/SEEDS   14 = SWEETS   15 = VEG/LEG   16 = MISC   22 = SOUP/SAUCE

Chol (mg)	Calc (mg)	Iron (mg)	Magn (mg)	Phos (mg)	Pota (mg)	Sodi (mg)	Zinc (mg)	VT-A (RE)	Thia (mg)	Ribo (mg)	Niac (mg)	V-B6 (mg)	Fola (µg)	VT-C (mg)
73	79	1.08	12	82	96	189	.47	57	.15	.17	1.09	.04	18	<1
38	15	2.32	23	91	227	210	2.58	29	.11	.10	2.96	.22	14	83
56	460	3.08	41	393	507	783	3.23	168	.22	.33	3.64	.35	16	7
30	457	2.38	35	345	424	760	1.93	168	.21	.28	2.01	.22	14	7
90	246	2.48	52	253	437	967	1.25	97	.19	.33	2.70	.29	25	6
24	199	1.0	31	182	139	730	1.20	72	.12	.24	1.0	.02	8	<1
24	27	1.14	23	50	162	315	.34	40	.10	.07	.67	.07	7	3
98	29	1.90	19	123	227	340	3.50	26	.06	.18	3.19	.18	8	1
97	33	1.39	18	128	238	392	2.86	26	.19	.19	3.07	.19	8	1
143	129	2.75	44	245	695	485	3.29	125	.25	.32	4.78	.35	44	7
170	48	1.63	39	130	635	1323	.78	83	.19	.15	2.23	.35	17	25
44	362	1.8	37	322	240	1086	1.20	232	.20	.40	1.8	.05	10	1
285	211	1.4	23	276	283	653	1.95	454	.11	.32	1.2	.15	17	<1
3	40	2.8	21	88	303	955	1.12	120	.35	.28	4.5	.13	6	10
8	80	2.3	26	135	408	955	1.3	140	.25	.18	2.3	.20	8	13
23	53	3.3	20	113	245	1220	2.39	100	.15	.18	2.3	.12	5	5
89	124	3.7	40	236	665	1009	2.45	159	.25	.30	.4	.20	10	22
184	230	1.34	37	231	202	763	1.29	675	.09	.31	.48	.12	62	3
27	35	2.0	40	365	365	824	1.15	55	.06	.14	13.3	.17	15	5
52	37	1.94	31	182	224	869	.97	34	.14	.17	8.59	.24	13	1
22	44	.98	41	88	279	246	.69	41	.10	.06	.37	.16	19	6
52	165	2.7	61	274	388	516	3.30	58	.26	.29	4.36	.73	48	5
15	181	2.53	76	243	427	1030	2.37	58	.26	.23	2.40	1.01	55	5
44	135	2.30	22	174	219	672	2.53	65	.26	.24	3.70	.11	20	1
104	236	4.45	43	320	407	1224	5.27	128	.33	.49	7.37	.23	23	3
68	44	1.87	30	173	194	2732	1.00	16	.29	.26	9.21	.37	18	4
37	34	1.94	22	303	164	1252	1.44	<1	.28	.17	3.27	.11	2	3
44	324	1.31	50	133	240	784	2.51	186	.09	.42	1.91	.39	34	1
213	197	3.10	28	290	201	832	1.86	160	.46	.50	3.71	.15	35	1
56	132	1.85	29	223	274	667	.95	25	.32	.27	3.30	.10	24	3
90	61	2.23	34	246	375	621	.88	15	.35	.24	3.52	.12	43	1

H

(For purposes of calculations, use "0" for t, <1, <.1, <.01, etc.)

Table H–1 Food Composition

Grp	Computer Code No.	Food Description	Measure	Wt (g)	H₂O (%)	Ener (kcal)	Prot (g)	Carb (g)	Dietary Fiber (g)	Fat (g)	Fat Breakdown (g) Sat	Mono	Poly
		MIXED DISHES and FAST FOODS—Con.											
		FAST FOODS and SANDWICHES—Con.											
		Hamburger with bun:											
12	709	Regular	1 ea	98	46	245	12	28	1	11	4	5	1
12	710	4-oz patty	1 ea	174	50	445	25	38	1	21	7	12	1
12	711	Hotdog/frankfurter and bun	1 ea	85	53	260	8	21	1	15	5	7	2
12	712	Cheese pizza, ⅛ of 15″ round[95]	1 pce	120	46	290	15	39	2	9	4	3	1
		SANDWICHES:											
		Avocado, cheese, tomato & lettuce:											
12	1276	On white bread, firm	1 ea	205	59	464	15	39	7	29	9.1	11.8	6.0
12	1278	On part whole wheat	1 ea	195	60	432	14	33	8	29	8.7	11.8	6.0
12	1277	On whole wheat	1 ea	209	58	459	16	39	13	29	9.1	11.9	6.2
		Bacon, lettuce & tomato sandwich:											
12	1137	On white bread, soft	1 ea	135	54	333	11	30	2	19	5.2	7.4	5.5
12	1139	On part whole wheat	1 ea	135	54	327	12	28	3	19	4.9	7.5	5.5
12	1138	On whole wheat	1 ea	149	53	355	13	34	8	20	5.4	7.7	5.7
		Cheese sandwich, grilled:											
12	1140	On white bread, soft	1 ea	117	37	399	17	28	1	24	12.7	7.6	2.3
12	1142	On part whole wheat	1 ea	117	37	393	18	27	3	24	12.5	7.7	2.3
12	1141	On whole wheat	1 ea	131	38	420	20	33	7	25	12.9	7.9	2.6
		Chicken salad sandwich:											
12	1143	On white bread, soft	1 ea	99.7	44	300	10	28	1	16	3.0	4.9	7.5
12	1145	On part whole wheat	1 ea	99.7	44	294	11	27	3	16	2.8	5.0	7.5
12	1144	On whole wheat	1 ea	114	44	321	12	33	8	17	3.2	5.2	7.8
12	1146	Corned beef & swiss cheese on rye	1 ea	147	45	429	27	25	5	24	9.4	8.2	5.0
		Egg salad sandwich:											
12	1147	On white bread, soft	1 ea	111	47	325	9	28	1	19	3.9	6.2	7.7
12	1149	On part whole wheat	1 ea	111	47	319	10	27	3	19	3.7	6.3	7.7
12	1148	On whole wheat	1 ea	125	47	346	12	33	7	20	4.1	6.4	8.0
		Ham sandwich:											
12	1279	On rye bread	1 ea	116	55	242	16	25	5	9	1.9	3.2	2.8
12	1151	On white bread, soft	1 ea	122	54	262	16	28	1	9	2.2	3.4	2.7
12	1153	On part whole wheat	1 ea	122	54	256	17	27	3	9	2.0	3.5	2.7
12	1152	On whole wheat	1 ea	136	53	283	18	33	7	10	2.4	3.7	3.0
		Ham & cheese sandwich:											
12	1280	On soft white bread	1 ea	151	51	369	22	29	1	18	7.8	6.0	3.0
12	1282	On part whole wheat bread	1 ea	151	51	363	23	28	3	18	7.6	6.1	3.0
12	1281	On whole wheat	1 ea	165	50	390	25	33	7	19	8.0	6.2	3.3
12	1150	Ham & swiss on rye	1 ea	145	51	350	24	26	5	17	7.0	5.3	3.1
		Ham salad sandwich:											
12	1154	On white bread, soft	1 ea	125	48	345	10	34	1	19	4.8	7.2	5.9
12	1156	On part whole wheat	1 ea	125	48	339	11	33	3	19	4.6	7.3	6.0
12	1155	On whole wheat	1 ea	139	47	366	12	38	7	20	5.0	7.5	6.2
12	1157	Patty melt sandwich: ground beef & cheese on rye:	1 ea	177	45	567	32	25	5	38	14.1	13.9	6.5
		Peanut butter & jam sandwich:											
12	1158	On soft white bread	1 ea	100	27	347	12	45	3	15	2.8	6.8	4.3
12	1160	On part whole wheat	1 ea	100	27	341	12	44	5	15	2.5	6.9	4.3
12	1159	On whole wheat	1 ea	114	29	368	14	50	9	16	3.0	7.1	4.6
12	1161	Reuben sandwich, grilled: corned beef, swiss cheese, sauerkraut on rye:	1 ea	233	61	480	28	29	7	28	10.2	10.0	6.2
		Roast beef sandwich:											
12	713	On a bun	1 ea	150	52	345	22	34	1	13	4	7	2
12	1162	On soft white bread	1 ea	122	51	286	17	28	1	11	2.5	3.7	4.4

[95]Crust made with vegetable shortening and enriched flour.

(Computer code number is for West Diet Analysis program)

GRP KEY: 1 = BEV   2 = DAIRY   3 = EGGS   4 = FAT/OIL   5 = FRUIT   6 = BAKERY   7 = GRAIN   8 = FISH   9 = BEEF   10 = POULTRY
11 = SAUSAGE   12 = MIXED/FAST   13 = NUTS/SEEDS   14 = SWEETS   15 = VEG/LEG   16 = MISC   22 = SOUP/SAUCE

Chol (mg)	Calc (mg)	Iron (mg)	Magn (mg)	Phos (mg)	Pota (mg)	Sodi (mg)	Zinc (mg)	VT-A (RE)	Thia (mg)	Ribo (mg)	Niac (mg)	V-B6 (mg)	Fola (µg)	VT-C (mg)
32	56	2.20	19	107	202	463	2.0	14	.23	.24	3.80	.12	16	1
71	75	4.84	38	225	404	763	5.01	28	.38	.38	7.85	.28	24	2
23	59	1.71	13	83	113	745	1.19	<1	.29	.19	2.48	.07	17	12
56	220	1.60	36	216	230	699	1.81	106	.34	.29	4.20	.04	40	2
32	312	3.02	54	242	557	556	1.69	160	.41	.43	3.98	.25	74	11
32	299	3.09	66	274	562	518	1.87	160	.36	.40	4.02	.29	76	11
32	279	3.52	105	353	608	660	2.46	160	.35	.37	4.18	.36	91	11
21	81	2.22	22	138	253	647	1.06	50	.42	.25	3.71	.10	35	13
21	80	2.57	36	181	269	661	1.30	50	.42	.26	4.13	.15	41	13
21	60	3.00	76	260	315	803	1.89	50	.41	.23	4.29	.21	55	13
55	424	1.82	25	489	158	1155	2.24	214	.28	.38	2.14	.06	25	<1
55	424	2.17	39	531	174	1169	2.49	214	.28	.38	2.56	.10	30	<1
55	404	2.61	78	610	219	1311	3.07	214	.26	.35	2.72	.17	45	<1
25	80	1.94	18	102	136	401	.76	18	.28	.21	3.73	.11	22	1
25	79	2.30	32	144	152	415	.00	18	.28	.22	4.15	.15	28	1
25	59	2.73	71	223	197	557	1.59	18	.27	.19	4.31	.22	43	1
85	331	3.98	32	310	174	1045	4.37	85	.23	.41	3.65	.14	25	0
164	96	2.49	17	133	119	447	.92	90	.29	.29	2.14	.07	38	<1
164	95	2.85	31	176	135	461	1.16	90	.29	.29	2.56	.11	44	<1
164	75	3.28	71	255	180	603	1.75	90	.28	.26	2.72	.18	59	<1
29	49	1.94	25	203	311	1261	1.91	4	.74	.30	4.50	.32	23	14
29	80	2.17	25	191	271	1199	1.50	4	.80	.31	4.94	.29	23	14
29	79	2.52	39	234	287	1213	1.74	4	.80	.32	5.36	.33	29	14
29	59	2.96	78	313	333	1355	2.33	4	.79	.29	5.52	.40	44	14
56	256	2.28	31	405	318	1610	2.44	88	.81	.42	4.96	.31	26	14
56	256	2.64	45	447	334	1624	2.69	88	.81	.42	5.38	.35	31	14
56	236	3.07	84	526	379	1766	3.27	88	.79	.39	5.54	.42	46	14
55	325	1.99	35	376	342	1336	3.03	77	.75	.40	4.52	.34	25	14
27	77	2.00	18	134	156	887	1.02	19	.52	.25	3.36	.11	21	4
27	77	2.36	32	177	172	901	1.26	19	.52	.25	3.78	.15	26	4
27	57	2.79	71	256	217	1043	1.85	19	.51	.22	3.94	.22	41	4
107	228	3.33	40	423	410	923	6.63	139	.25	.45	6.08	.31	26	<1
0	83	2.23	55	153	246	403	1.06	1	.30	.21	5.39	.12	42	<1
0	82	2.59	69	195	262	417	1.30	1	.30	.21	5.81	.16	47	<1
0	62	3.02	108	274	308	559	1.89	1	.28	.18	5.97	.23	62	<1
85	358	5.20	44	328	313	1642	4.55	133	.25	.43	3.80	.24	27	12
55	60	4.04	38	222	338	757	3.66	32	.39	.33	6.02	.28	42	2
30	80	2.86	23	157	298	757	2.63	8	.31	.29	5.10	.21	23	<1

(For purposes of calculations, use "0" for t, <1, <.1, <.01, etc.)

Table H–1   Food Composition

Grp	Computer Code No.	Food Description	Measure	Wt (g)	H$_2$O (%)	Ener (kcal)	Prot (g)	Carb (g)	Dietary Fiber (g)	Fat (g)	Fat Breakdown (g) Sat	Mono	Poly
MIXED DISHES and FAST FOOD—Con.													
SANDWICHES—Con.													
Roast Beef—Con.													
12	1164	On part whole wheat bread	1 ea	122	51	280	18	27	3	11	2.3	3.8	4.4
12	1163	On whole wheat bread	1 ea	136	50	307	19	32	7	12	2.7	3.9	4.7
		Tuna salad sandwich:											
12	1165	On soft white	1 ea	116	47	309	13	32	2	14	2.6	4.1	6.6
12	1167	On part whole wheat bread	1 ea	116	47	303	14	31	3	14	2.4	4.2	6.7
12	1166	On whole wheat bread	1 ea	130	47	331	15	37	8	15	2.8	4.4	6.9
		Turkey sandwich:											
12	1168	On soft white bread	1 ea	122	52	277	18	28	1	10	2.1	3.2	4.5
12	1170	On part whole wheat	1 ea	122	52	271	18	26	3	11	1.9	3.3	4.5
12	1169	On whole wheat	1 ea	136	51	298	20	32	7	11	2.3	3.4	4.8
		Turkey ham sandwich:											
12	1272	On rye bread	1 ea	116	55	239	15	25	5	9	1.9	2.6	3.3
12	1273	On soft white bread	1 ea	122	55	259	16	29	1	9	2.2	2.8	3.2
12	1275	On part whole wheat	1 ea	122	54	253	16	28	3	9	2.0	2.9	3.2
12	1274	On whole wheat	1 ea	136	53	281	18	33	7	10	2.4	3.1	3.5
12	714	Taco, corn tortilla, beef filling	1 ea	78	52	207	14	10	1	13	5	5	2
		Tostada:											
12	1114	With refried beans	1 ea	157	69	212	10	26	7	9	3.6	2.5	2.3
12	1118	With beans & beef	1 ea	192	67	332	18	20	4	21	9.4	7.2	2.6
12	1354	With beans & chicken	1 ea	157	67	249	19	19	4	11	4.4	3.5	2.9
		Vegetarian Foods:											
12	1175	Nuteena	1 ea	34	52	89	7	3	1	6	—	—	—
12	1171	Proteena	1 pce	67	58	160	8	5	1	12	—	—	—
12	1172	Redi-burger	1 pce	71	56	140	17	5	2	6	—	—	—
12	1173	Vege-Burger	1 pce	68	57	130	14	5	1	6	—	—	—
12	1174	Breakfast links	.5 c	108	73	110	22	4	1	1	—	—	—
NUTS, SEEDS and PRODUCTS													
		Almonds:											
13	1365	Dry roasted, salted	1 c	138	3	810	23	33	18	71	6.8	46.2	15.0
13	718	Slivered, packed, unsalted	1 c	135	4	795	27	28	15[96]	70	7	46	15
		Whole, dried, unsalted:											
13	719	Cup	1 c	142	4	837	28	29	17[96]	74	7	48	16
13	720	Ounce	1 oz	28	4	167	6	6	3[96]	15	1	10	3
13	721	Almond butter	1 tbsp	16	1	101	2	3	1	9	1	6	2
13	722	Brazil nuts, dry (about 7)	1 oz	28	3	186	4	4	3	19	5	7	7
		Cashew nuts:											
		Dry roasted, salted											
13	723	Cup	1 c	137	2	787	21	45	8	63	13	37	11
13	724	Ounce	1 oz	28	2	163	4	9	2	13	3	8	2
		Oil roasted, salted:											
13	725	Cup	1 c	130	4	748	21	37	8	63	12	37	11
13	726	Ounce	1 oz	28	4	163	5	8	2	14	3	8	2

[96]Values reported for dietary fiber in almonds vary from 7.0 to 14.3g/100g.

(Computer code number is for West Diet Analysis program)

GRP KEY: 1 = BEV   2 = DAIRY   3 = EGGS   4 = FAT/OIL   5 = FRUIT   6 = BAKERY   7 = GRAIN   8 = FISH   9 = BEEF   10 = POULTRY
11 = SAUSAGE   12 = MIXED/FAST   13 = NUTS/SEEDS   14 = SWEETS   15 = VEG/LEG   16 = MISC   22 = SOUP/SAUCE

Chol (mg)	Calc (mg)	Iron (mg)	Magn (mg)	Phos (mg)	Pota (mg)	Sodi (mg)	Zinc (mg)	VT-A (RE)	Thia (mg)	Ribo (mg)	Niac (mg)	V-B6 (mg)	Fola (µg)	VT-C (mg)
30	79	3.22	37	200	314	771	2.87	8	.31	.29	5.52	.25	29	<1
30	59	3.65	76	279	359	912	3.46	8	.29	.26	5.68	.32	44	<1
25	80	2.27	23	133	199	559	.65	22	.28	.21	5.43	.14	30	2
25	80	2.63	37	176	215	573	.89	22	.28	.22	5.85	.19	36	2
25	60	3.06	76	255	260	715	1.48	22	.26	.19	6.01	.25	51	2
29	76	1.87	23	192	223	1151	1.00	8	.29	.24	6.82	.23	23	<1
29	76	2.23	37	235	239	1165	1.24	8	.28	.24	7.24	.27	28	<1
29	56	2.66	77	314	285	1307	1.83	8	.27	.21	7.40	.34	43	<1
35	50	3.04	27	214	273	986	2.37	4	.25	.32	4.46	.21	24	0
35	81	3.28	26	203	233	924	1.96	5	.31	.34	4.90	.18	24	<1
35	80	3.63	40	245	249	938	2.20	5	.30	.34	5.32	.23	29	<1
35	60	4.06	80	324	295	1080	2.79	5	.29	.31	5.48	.29	44	<1
45	85	1.29	23	141	183	141	2.89	27	.03	.13	2.49	.16	13	1
15	177	1.93	62	195	422	618	1.55	74	.06	.14	.85	1.01	47	6
62	186	2.16	52	247	442	483	3.57	132	.08	.24	2.94	.67	37	6
53	162	1.69	48	242	358	474	1.94	81	.07	.19	4.53	.73	34	3
<1	11	1.96	—	—	43	203	—	<1	1.65	.17	3.77	.20	—	<1
0	21	1.20	40	111	200	120	.87	10	.47	.58	.14	.45	60	—
0	22	1.60	31	99	280	460	1.20	26	.64	.50	7.80	.50	23	—
0	19	1.40	13	56	120	370	1.20	10	.60	.40	6.70	.80	17	—
0	32	2.70	24	105	110	190	1.10	10	.53	.68	5.00	.56	27	—
0	389	5.25	419	756	1063	1076	6.76	0	.18	.83	3.89	.10	88	1
0	359	4.94	400	702	988	15	3.94	0	.28	1.05	4.54	.15	79	1
0	378	5.20	420	738	1034	15[97]	4.15	0	.30	1.11	4.77	.16	83	1
0	75	1.04	84	147	208	3[97]	.83	0	.06	.22	.96	.03	17	<1
0	43	.59	49	84	121	2[98]	.49	0	.02	.1	.46	.01	0	<1
0	50	.97	64	170	170	<1	1.30	t	.28	.04	.46	.07	1	<1
0	62	8.22	356	671	774	877[99]	7.67	0	.27	.27	1.92	.35	95	0
0	13	1.70	74	139	160	181[99]	1.59	0	.06	.06	.4	.07	20	0
0	53	5.33	332	554	689	814[100]	6.18	0	.55	.23	2.34	.33	88	0
0	12	1.16	72	121	151	177[100]	1.35	0	.12	.05	.51	.07	19	0

[97]Salted almonds contain 1108 mg sodium per cup, 221 mg per ounce.
[98]Salted almond butter contains 72 mg sodium per tablespoon.
[99]Dry-roasted cashews without salt contain 21 mg sodium per cup, or 4 mg per ounce.
[100]Oil-roasted cashews without salt contain 22 mg sodium per cup, or 5 mg per ounce.

H

(For purposes of calculations, use "0" for t, <1, <.1, <.01, etc.)

Table H–1 Food Composition

Grp	Computer Code No.	Food Description	Measure	Wt (g)	H$_2$O (%)	Ener (kcal)	Prot (g)	Carb (g)	Dietary Fiber (g)	Fat (g)	Sat	Mono	Poly
		NUTS, SEEDS and PRODUCTS—Con.											
		Cashew nuts, unsalted:											
13	1366	Dry roasted	1 c	137	2	787	21	45	8	64	12.6	37.4	10.7
13	1367	Oil roasted	1 c	130	4	748	21	37	8	63	12.4	36.9	10.6
13	727	Cashew butter	1 tbsp	16	3	94	3	4	1	8	2	5	1
13	728	European chestnuts, roasted, 1 c = approx 17 kernels	1 c	143	40	350	5	76	19	3	.6	1.1	1.2
		Coconut:											
		Raw:											
13	729	Piece 2 × 2 × ½″	1 pce	45	47	159	2	7	5	15	13	.6	.2
13	730	Shredded/grated, unpacked[101]	1 c	80	47	283	3	12	9	27	24	1	.3
		Dried, shredded/grated:											
13	731	Unsweetened	1 c	78	3	515	5	19	12	50	45	2	.6
13	732	Sweetened	1 c	93	16	466	3	44	9	33	29	1	.4
		Filberts (hazelnuts), chopped:											
13	733	Cup	1 c	115	5	727	15	18	7	72	5	57	7
13	734	Ounce	1 oz	28	5	179	4	4	2	18	1	14	2
		Macadamia nuts, oil roasted:											
		Salted:											
13	735	Cup	1 c	134	2	962	10	17	7	103	15	81	2
13	736	Ounce	1 oz	28	2	204	2	4	1	22	3	17	.4
13	1368	Unsalted	1 c	134	2	962	10	17	7	103	15.4	80.9	1.8
		Mixed nuts:											
13	737	Dry roasted, salted	1 c	137	2	814	24	35	12	70	10	43	15
13	738	Oil roasted, salted	1 c	142	2	876	24	30	13	80	12	45	19
13	1369	Oil roasted, unsalted	1 c	142	2	876	24	30	13	80	12.4	45.0	18.9
		Peanuts:											
		Oil roasted, salted:											
13	739	Cup	1 c	144	2	837	38	27	13	71	10	35.2	22.4
13	740	Ounce	1 oz	28	2	163	7	5	2	14	2	7	4
13	1370	Oil roasted, unsalted	1 c	144	2	837	38	27	13	71	9.9	35.2	22.4
		Dried, unsalted:											
13	741	Cup	1 c	146	7	827	38	24	13	72	10	36	23
13	742	Ounce	1 oz	28	7	161	7	5	3	14	2	7	4
13	743	Peanut butter	1 tbsp	16	2	94	4	3	1	8	1.5	4.0	2.3
		Pecans, halves:											
		Dried, unsalted:											
13	744	Cup	1 c	108	5	720	8	20	7[102]	73	6	46	18
13	745	Ounce	1 oz	28	5	190	2	5	2[102]	19	1.5	12	5
13	1372	Dry roasted, salted	¼ c	28	1	187	2	6	2	18	1.5	11.5	4.6
13	746	Pine nuts/piñons, dried	1 oz	28	6	161	3	5	2	17	3	7	7
		Pistachio nuts:											
13	747	Dried, shelled	1 oz	28	4	164	6	7	1	14	2	9	2
13	1373	Dry roasted, salted, shelled	1 c	128	2	776	19	35	14	68	8.6	45.7	10.3

[101] 1 c packed = 130 g.
[102] Dietary fiber data calculated/derived from data on other nuts.

(Computer code number is for West Diet Analysis program)

GRP KEY: 1 = BEV 2 = DAIRY 3 = EGGS 4 = FAT/OIL 5 = FRUIT 6 = BAKERY 7 = GRAIN 8 = FISH 9 = BEEF 10 = POULTRY
11 = SAUSAGE 12 = MIXED/FAST 13 = NUTS/SEEDS 14 = SWEETS 15 = VEG/LEG 16 = MISC 22 = SOUP/SAUCE

Chol (mg)	Calc (mg)	Iron (mg)	Magn (mg)	Phos (mg)	Pota (mg)	Sodi (mg)	Zinc (mg)	VT-A (RE)	Thia (mg)	Ribo (mg)	Niac (mg)	V-B6 (mg)	Fola (µg)	VT-C (mg)
0	62	8.22	356	671	774	21	7.67	0	.27	.27	1.92	.35	95	0
0	53	5.33	332	554	689	22	6.18	0	.55	.23	2.34	.33	88	0
0	7	.09	41	73	87	2[103]	.83	0	.05	.03	.26	.04	11	0
0	42	1.30	47	153	846	3	.82	4	.35	.25	1.92	.71	100	37
0	6	1.09	14	51	160	9	.50	0	.03	.01	.24	.02	12	2
0	12	1.94	26	90	285	16	.88	0	.05	.02	.43	.04	21	3
0	20	2.59	70	161	423	29	1.57	0	.05	.08	.47	2.34	7	1
0	14	1.79	47	100	313	244	1.69	0	.03	.02	.44	.29	9	1
0	216	3.76	328	359	512	3	2.76	8	.57	.13	1.31	.7	83	1
0	53	.93	81	89	126	1	.68	2	.14	.03	.32	.17	20	<1
0	60	2.41	157	268	441	348[104]	1.47	1	.28	.15	2.71	.33	79	0
0	13	.51	33	57	94	74[104]	.31	<1	.06	.03	.57	.07	17	0
0	60	2.41	157	268	441	9	1.47	1	.28	.15	2.71	.33	79	0
0	96	5.07	308	596	817	917[105]	5.21	2	.27	.27	6.44	.41	69	1
0	153	4.56	334	659	825	926[105]	7.22	3	.71	.32	7.19	.34	118	1
0	153	4.56	334	659	825	16	7.22	3	.71	.32	7.19	.34	118	1
0	126	2.63	266	744	982	624[106]	9.55	0	.364	.156	20.6	.367	181	0
0	24	.51	52	145	191	121[106]	1.86	0	.07	.03	4	.07	35	0
0	126	2.63	266	744	982	8.6	9.55	0	.364	.156	20.6	.367	181	0
0	85	4.72	263	559	1047	23	4.78	0	.97	.19	20.7	.43	153	0
0	17	.92	51	109	204	5	.93	0	.19	.04	4.02	.08	30	0
0	5.5	.27	25	52	115	77[107]	.4	0	.02	.02	2.1	.06	13	0
0	39	2.30	138	314	423	1[108]	5.91	14	.92	.14	.96	.20	42	1
0	10	.61	36	83	111	<1	1.55	4	.24	.04	.25	.05	11	1
0	10	.62	38	86	105	221	1.61	4	.09	.04	.26	.05	12	1
0	2	.87	67	10	178	20	1.22	1	.35	.06	1.24	.08	19	<1
0	38	1.93	45	143	310	2[109]	.38	7	.22	.05	.31	.06	17	<1
0	90	4.06	166	609	1242	998	1.74	30	.54	.32	1.80	.27	74	0

[103] Salted cashew butter contains 98 mg sodium per tablespoon.
[104] Macadamia nuts without salt contain 9 mg sodium per cup, or 2 mg per ounce.
[105] Mixed nuts without salt contain about 15 mg sodium per cup.
[106] Peanuts without salt contain 22 mg sodium per cup, or 4 mg per ounce.
[107] Peanut butter without added salt contains 3 mg sodium per tablespoon.
[108] Salted pecans contain 816 mg sodium per cup, or 214 mg per ounce.
[109] Salted pistachios contain approx 221 mg sodium per ounce.

(For purposes of calculations, use "0" for t, <1, <.1, <.01, etc.)

Table H–1 Food Composition

Grp	Computer Code No.	Food Description	Measure	Wt (g)	H₂O (%)	Ener (kcal)	Prot (g)	Carb (g)	Dietary Fiber (g)	Fat (g)	Fat Breakdown (g) Sat	Mono	Poly
		NUTS, SEEDS and PRODUCTS—Con.											

Grp	Code No.	Food Description	Measure	Wt (g)	H₂O (%)	Ener (kcal)	Prot (g)	Carb (g)	Dietary Fiber (g)	Fat (g)	Sat	Mono	Poly
NUTS, SEEDS and PRODUCTS—Con.													
		Pumpkin kernels:											
13	748	Dried, unsalted	1 oz	28	7	154	7	5	2	13	2.5	4	6
13	1374	Roasted, salted	1 c	227	7	1185	75	31	9	96	18.1	29.7	43.6
13	749	Sesame seeds, hulled, dried	¼ c	38	5	221	10	4	6	21	3	8	9
		Sunflower seed kernels:											
13	750	Dry	¼ c	36	5	205	8	7	2	18	2	3	12
13	751	Oil roasted	¼ c	34	3	208	7	5	2	19	2	4	13
13	752	Tahini (sesame butter)	1 tbsp	15	3	91	3	3	2	8	1	3	4
		Black walnuts, chopped:											
13	753	Cup	1 c	125	4	759	30	15	7	71	5	16	47
13	754	Ounce	1 oz	28	4	172	7	3	2	16	1	4	11
		English walnuts, chopped:											
13	755	Cup	1 c	120	4	770	17	22	7	74	7	17	47
13	756	Ounce	1 oz	28	4	182	4	5	2	18	2	4	11
SWEETENERS and SWEETS: see also Dairy (milk desserts) and Baked Goods													
14	757	Apple butter	2 tbsp	35	52	66	<1	17	<1	<1	.1	<.1	.1
14	1124	Butterscotch topping	3 tbsp	50	33	156	1	41	0	<1	—	—	—
		Cake frosting:											
14	1127	Canned, average of all types	2.5 tbsp	39	15	160	0	24	0	7	1.7	2.9	1.7
14	1123	Prepared from mix	2.5 tbsp	39	15	167	0	28	0	6	—	—	—
		Candy:											
14	1128	Almond Joy® candy bar	1 oz	28	7	151	2	19	1.9	8	6.7	.6	.1
14	758	Caramel, plain or chocolate	1 oz	28	8	115	1	22	<1	3	2.2	.3	.1
		Chocolate (see also, #784, 785, 971):											
		Milk chocolate:											
14	759	Plain	1 oz	28	1	145	2	16	1	9	5.4	3	.3
14	760	With almonds	1 oz	28	2	150	3	15	1	10	4.4	4.7	1.0
14	761	With peanuts	1 oz	28	1	155	5	10	2	12	3.5	5.2	2.7
14	762	With rice cereal	1 oz	28	2	140	2	18	1	7	4.4	2.5	.2
14	763	Semisweet chocolate chips	1 c	170	1	860	7	97	5	61	36	20	2
14	764	Sweet dark chocolate	1 oz	28	1	150	1	16	1	10	5.9	3.3	.3
14	1133	English toffee candy bar	1 ea	32	2	220	1	11	<1	19	7	7	2
14	765	Fondant candy, uncoated (mints, candy corn, other)	1 oz	28	3	105	0	27	0	0	0	0	0
14	766	Fudge, chocolate	1 oz	28	8	115	1	21	2	3	2.1	1	.1
14	767	Gum drops	1 oz	28	12	98	0	25	0	<1	t	t	.1
14	768	Hard candy, all flavors	1 oz	28	1	109	0	28	0	0	0	0	0
14	769	Jelly beans	1 oz	28	6	104	t	26	0	<.1	t	t	.1
14	1134	M&M's Plain choc. candies®	48 grm	48	1	237	3	33	<1	10	5	3	3
14	1135	M&M's Peanut choc. candies®	47 grm	47.3	2	240	5	28	1	12	5	5	2
14	1130	MARS® bar	1 ea	50	7	240	4	30	1	11	4.8	4.4	.8
14	1129	MILKY WAY® candy bar	1 ea	60	7	260	3	43	<1	9	5.4	3.0	.3
14	1132	REESE's® peanut butter cup	2 ea	45	4	240	6	22	2	14	5.2	5.4	2.4
14	1131	SNICKERS® candy bar, 2.2oz size	1 ea	61.2	7	290	7	37	2	14	—	—	—
14	1125	Caramel topping	3 tbsp	50	31	155	1	39	<1	—	—	—	—
14	771	Gelatin salad/dessert	½ c	120	84	70	2	17	<1	0	0	0	0
		Honey:											
14	772	Cup	1 c	339	17	1030	1	279	0	0	0	0	0
14	773	Tablespoon	1 tbsp	21	17	65	<.1	17	0	0	0	0	0

(Computer code number is for West Diet Analysis program)

GRP KEY: 1=BEV 2=DAIRY 3=EGGS 4=FAT/OIL 5=FRUIT 6=BAKERY 7=GRAIN 8=FISH 9=BEEF 10=POULTRY 11=SAUSAGE 12=MIXED/FAST 13=NUTS/SEEDS 14=SWEETS 15=VEG/LEG 16=MISC 22=SOUP/SAUCE

Chol (mg)	Calc (mg)	Iron (mg)	Magn (mg)	Phos (mg)	Pota (mg)	Sodi (mg)	Zinc (mg)	VT-A (RE)	Thia (mg)	Ribo (mg)	Niac (mg)	V-B6 (mg)	Fola (µg)	VT-C (mg)
0	12	4.25	152	333	229	5[110]	2.12	11	.06	.09	.50	.03	26	<1
0	98	33.9	1212	2600	1830	1305	16.9	88	.25	.66	3.60	.20	115	0
0	49	2.93	130	291	153	15	2.23	<1	.27	.03	1.76	.30	38	0
0	42	2.44	128	254	248	1	1.82	2	.83	.10	1.62	.46	85	<1
0	19	2.26	43	385	163	205[111]	1.76	2	.11	.10	1.40	.40	79	<1
0	21	.83	53	119	69	5	1.57	1	.24	.02	.85	.06	15	1
0	73	3.84	253	580	655	1	4.28	37	.27	.14	.86	.70	83	1
0	16	.87	57	132	149	0	.97	8	.06	.03	.20	.16	19	<1
0	113	2.93	203	380	602	12	3.28	15	.46	.18	1.25	.67	79	4
0	27	.69	48	90	142	3	.78	4	.11	.04	.30	.16	19	1
0	5	.25	2	13	89	1	.01	0	<.01	.01	.08	.01	<1	1
14	56	.10	3	23	34	66	.12	<1	0	.04	0	<.01	.06	0
0	—	—	—	—	—	91	—	0	—	—	—	—	—	—
0	—	—	—	—	—	84	—	0	—	—	—	—	—	—
0	20	.5	16	42	92	48	.43	3	.01	.05	.14	.05	2.1	.1
1	42	.4	6	35	54	64	.15	<1	.01	.05	.1	<.01	0	t
6	50	.4	16	61	96	23	.37	10	.02	.1	.1	.02	<1	t
5	61	.56	33	77	125	23	.48	8	.03	.13	.31	.02	4	t
3	32	.68	35	87	155	19	.68	8	.11	.07	2.2	.05	16	t
6	48	.2	13	57	100	46	.29	8	.01	.08	.1	.01	<1	t
0	51	5.8	230	178	593	24	2.39	3	.1	.14	.9	.04	22	t
0	7	.6	32	41	86	5	.42	1	.01	.04	.1	.01	5	t
0	0	.20	11.5	0	50	90	.24	5	.053	.05	.10	.04	1	0
0	2	.1	—	2	1	57	.1	0	<.01	<.01	.01	.01	0	0
1	22	.3	14	24	42	54	.16	16	.01	.03	.1	.01	2	t
0	2	.1	—	—	1	10	0	5	0	<.01	.01	0	0	0
0	6	.1	<1	2	1	7	0	0	0	0	0	0	0	0
0	1	.30	—	1	11	7	0	0	0	<.01	.01	—	0	0
0	79	.76	30	65	171	41	.57	13	.03	.12	.27	.01	5	—
0	59	.67	38	64	162	29	.66	<1	.03	.09	1.48	.03	5	—
0	85	.55	37	63	176	85	.59	<1	.02	.16	.48	.01	5	—
14	86	.49	22	80	167	140	.45	25	.03	.15	.20	.01	7	1
3	35	.68	47	87	168	92	.9	8	.03	.05	2.12	.06	17	—
0	70	.49	39	75	209	170	.69	5	.03	.11	1.84	.02	6	—
0	28	.10	3	23	33	152	—	<1	0	.05	0	—	—	0
0	2	.10	<1	23	91	55	.03	0	.01	.01	.20	<.01	0	0
0	17	1.70	7	20	173	17	.40	0	.02	.14	1.0	.06	32	3
0	1	.11	<1	1	11	1	.02	0	<.01	.01	.06	<.01	2	<1

[110] Salted pumpkin/squash kernels contain approximately 163 mg sodium per ounce.

[111] Unsalted sunflower seeds contain 1 mg sodium per ¼ cup.

(For purposes of calculations, use "0" for t, <1, <.1, <.01, etc.)

Table H–1 Food Composition

Grp	Computer Code No.	Food Description	Measure	Wt (g)	H₂O (%)	Ener (kcal)	Prot (g)	Carb (g)	Dietary Fiber (g)	Fat (g)	Fat Breakdown (g) Sat	Mono	Poly
SWEETENERS and SWEETS—Con.													
		Jams or preserves:											
14	774	Tablespoon	1 tbsp	20	29	54	<1	14	<1	<.1	0	t	t
14	775	Packet	1 ea	14	29	38	<.1	10	<1	<.1	0	t	t
		Jellies:											
14	776	Tablespoon	1 tbsp	18	28	49	<.1	13	<1	<.1	t	t	t
14	777	Packet	1 ea	14	28	39	<.1	10	<1	<.1	t	t	t
14	1136	Marmalade	1 tbsp	20	29	52	<1	14	<1	0	0	0	0
14	770	Marshmallows	4 ea	28	17	90	t	23	0	0	0	0	0
14	1126	Marshmallow creme topping	3 tbsp	50	20	158	<1	40	0	0	0	0	0
14	778	Popsicles, 3 oz when fluid	1 ea	95	80	70	0	18	0	0	0	0	0
		Sugars:											
14	779	Brown sugar	1 c	220	2	820	0	212	0	0	0	0	0
		White sugar, granulated:											
14	780	Cup	1 c	200	1	770	0	199	0	0	0	0	0
14	781	Tablespoon	1 tbsp	12	1	45	0	12	0	0	0	0	0
14	782	Packet	1 ea	6	1	25	0	6	0	0	0	0	0
14	783	White sugar, powdered, sifted	1 c	100	<1	385	0	99	0	0	0	0	0
		Syrups:											
		Chocolate:											
14	784	Thin type	2 tbsp	38	37	85	1	22	1	<1	.2	.1	.1
14	785	Fudge type	2 tbsp	38	25	125	2	21	1	5	3	2	.2
14	786	Molasses, blackstrap[112]	2 tbsp	40	24	85	0	22	0	0	0	0	0
14	787	Pancake table syrup (corn and maple)	¼ c	84	25	244	0	64	0	0	0	0	0
VEGETABLES AND LEGUMES													
15	788	Alfalfa seeds, sprouted	1 c	33	91	10	1	1	1	<1	t	t	.1
15	789	Artichokes, cooked globe (300 g with refuse)	1 ea	120	84	60	4	13	10	<1	<.1	t	.1
		Artichoke hearts:											
15	1177	Cooked from frozen	9 oz	240	87	108	7	22	18	1	.3	<.1	.5
15	1176	Marinated	6 oz	170	59	168	4	13	11	14	2.0	3.0	7.7
		Asparagus, green, cooked:											
		From raw:											
15	790	Cuts and tips	½ c	90	92	23	2	4	2	<1	.1	t	.1
15	791	Spears, ½″ diam at base	4 spears	60	92	15	2	3	1	<1	<.1	t	.1
		From frozen:											
15	792	Cuts and tips	1 c	180	91	50	5	9	3	1	.2	t	.3
15	793	Spears, ½″ diam at base	4 spears	60	91	17	2	3	1	<1	.1	t	.1
15	794	Canned, spears, ½″ diam at base	4 spears	80	95	11	2	2	1	1	.1	t	.2
15	795	Bamboo shoots, canned, drained slices	1 c	131	94	25	2	4	3	1	.1	t	.2
		Beans (see also Great northern, #855; Kidney beans, #860; Navy beans, #876; Pinto beans, #898; Refried beans, #921; Soybeans, #925):											
15	796	Black beans, cooked	1 c	172	66	227	15	41	15	1	.2	.1	.4
		Canned beans (white/navy):											
15	803	Beans w/pork and tomato sauce	1 c	253	73	247	13	49	14	3	1.0	1.1	.3
15	804	Beans w/pork and sweet sauce	1 c	253	71	282	13	53	14	4	1.4	1.6	.5
15	805	Beans with frankfurters	1 c	257	70	366	17	40	18	17	6	7	2
		Lima beans:											
15	797	Thick seeded (Fordhooks), cooked from frozen	½ c	85	74	85	5	16	5	<1	.1	t	.1

[112]Light molasses would contain about 66 mg calcium, 2.1 mg iron, 18 mg magnesium, and 366 mg potassium for 2 tbsp.

(Computer code number is for West Diet Analysis program)

GRP KEY: 1=BEV 2=DAIRY 3=EGGS 4=FAT/OIL 5=FRUIT 6=BAKERY 7=GRAIN 8=FISH 9=BEEF 10=POULTRY
11=SAUSAGE 12=MIXED/FAST 13=NUTS/SEEDS 14=SWEETS 15=VEG/LEG 16=MISC 22=SOUP/SAUCE

Chol (mg)	Calc (mg)	Iron (mg)	Magn (mg)	Phos (mg)	Pota (mg)	Sodi (mg)	Zinc (mg)	VT-A (RE)	Thia (mg)	Ribo (mg)	Niac (mg)	V-B6 (mg)	Fola (µg)	VT-C (mg)
0	4	.20	1	2	18	2	.01	t	<.01	.01	.04	<.01	2	<1
0	3	.14	<1	1	13	1	<.01	t	<.01	.01	.03	<.01	1	<1
0	2	.12	<1	1	16	4	0	t	<.01	<.01	.04	<.01	2	1
0	1	.09	<1	1	12	3	0	t	<.01	<.01	.03	<.01	2	1
0	7	.12	1	3	12	4	—	1	<.01	<.01	1.08	<.01	1	1.2
0	1	.45	1	2	2	25	<.01	0	0	<.01	.01	<.01	0	0
0	16	.8	2	6	16	29	<.01	0	0	<.01	.02	—	0	2
0	0	.01	—	0	4	11	0	0	0	0	0	0	0	0
0	187	4.80	135	56	757	97	.08	0	.02	.07	.20	0	0	0
0	3	.10	<1	.1	7	5	.04	0	0	0	0	0	0	0
0	<1	.01	<1	t	t	t	<.01	0	0	0	0	0	0	0
0	<1	<.01	<1	t	t	t	<.01	0	0	0	0	0	0	0
0	0	.08	<1	0	4	2	<.01	0	0	0	0	0	0	0
0	6	.75	26	49	85	36	.39	1	.02	.02	.11	<.01	3	0
0	38	.50	18	60	82	42	.39	13	.08	.08	.08	<.01	3	0
0	274[112]	10.1[112]	103[112]	34	1171[112]	38	0	0	.08	.08	.80	.11	6	0
0	2	.06	2	8	14	38	.08	0	0	0	0	t	<1	0
0	11	.32	9	23	26	2	.30	5	.03	.04	.16	.01	12	3
0	54	1.55	72	103	425	114	.59	22	.08	.08	1.20	.13	61	12
0	50	1.34	74	146	634	127	.86	39	.15	.38	2.20	.21	285	12
0	39	1.62	48	102	438	900	.54	28	.06	.17	1.38	.15	149	52
0	22	.59	17	55	279	4	.43	75	.09	.11	.95	.13	88	25
0	14	.4	11	37	186	2	.29	50	.06	.07	.63	.09	59	16
0	41	1.15	23	99	392	7	1.01	147	.12	.19	1.87	.16	176	44
0	14	.38	8	33	131	2	.34	49	.04	.06	.62	.06	59	15
0	11	.5	8	30	122	278[113]	.32	38	.05	.07	.7	.04	69	13
0	10	.42	6	33	105	9	.30	1	.03	.03	.18	—	40	1
0	47	3.60	121	241	611	1	1.92	1	.42	.10	.87	.12	256	0
17	141	8.30	88	297	759	45	2.60	31	.13	.12	1.26	.18	57	8
17	155	4.20	87	266	673	1113	3.80	29	.12	.15	.89	.22	95	8
15	123	4.45	71	267	604	849	4.79	40	.15	.14	2.32	.12	77	6
0	19	1.16	29	54	347	1105	.37	16	.06	.05	.91	.10	55	11

[112] Light molasses would contain about 66 mg calcium, 2.1 mg iron, 18 mg magnesium, and 366 mg potassium for 2 tbsp.
[113] Special dietary pack contains 3 mg sodium.

(For purposes of calculations, use "0" for t, <1, <.1, <.01, etc.)

H

Table H–1 Food Composition

Grp	Computer Code No.	Food Description	Measure	Wt (g)	H₂O (%)	Ener (kcal)	Prot (g)	Carb (g)	Dietary Fiber (g)	Fat (g)	Sat	Mono	Poly

Fat Breakdown (g): Sat, Mono, Poly

Grp	No.	Food Description	Measure	Wt (g)	H₂O (%)	Ener (kcal)	Prot (g)	Carb (g)	Dietary Fiber (g)	Fat (g)	Sat	Mono	Poly
VEGETABLES and LEGUMES—Con.													
		Lima Beans—Con.											
15	798	Thin seeded (baby), cooked from frozen	½ c	90	72	94	6	18	8	<1	.1	t	.1
15	799	Cooked from dry, drained	1 c	188	70	217	15	39	18	1	.2	.1	.3
		Snap beans/green beans, cuts and french style:											
15	800	Cooked from raw	1 c	125	89	44	2	10	3	<1	.1	t	.2
15	801	Cooked from frozen	1 c	135	92	36	2	8	4	<1	<.1	t	.1
15	802	Canned, drained	1 c	136	93	26	2	6	2	<1	<.1	t	.1
		Bean sprouts (mung):											
15	806	Raw	1 c	104	90	31	3	6	3	<1	<.1	t	.1
15	807	Cooked, stir fried	1 c	124	84	62	5	13	3	<1	<.1	.1	.1
15	808	Cooked, boiled, drained	1 c	124	93	26	3	5	3	<1	<.1	t	<.1
		Beets:											
		Cooked from fresh:											
15	809	Sliced or diced	½ c	85	91	26	1	6	2	<.1	t	t	t
15	810	Whole beets, 2″ diam	2 beets	100	91	31	1	7	2	<.1	t	t	t
		Canned:											
15	811	Sliced or diced	½ c	85	91	27	1	6	2	<1	t	t	<.1
15	812	Pickled slices	½ c	114	82	74	1	19	2	<1	t	t	<.1
15	813	Beet greens, cooked, drained	1 c	144	89	40	4	8	3	<1	<.1	.1	.1
		Black-eyed peas: see Peas											
		Broccoli:											
15	817	Raw, chopped	1 c	88	91	24	3	5	3	<1	.1	t	.1
15	818	Raw, spears	1 spear	151	91	42	5	8	6	1	.1	<.1	.3
		Cooked from raw:											
15	819	Spears	1 spear	180	91	50	5	9	7	<1	.1	<.1	.3
15	820	Chopped	1 c	156	91	44	5	8	6	<1	.1	<.1	.3
		Cooked from frozen:											
15	821	Spear, small piece	1 spear	30	91	8	1	2	1	<.1	t	t	t
15	822	Chopped	1 c	184	91	51	6	10	6	<1	<.1	t	<.1
		Brussels sprouts:											
15	823	Cooked from raw	1 c	156	87	60	6	14	6	1	.2	.1	.4
15	824	Cooked from frozen	1 c	155	87	65	6	13	5	1	.1	.1	.3
		Cabbage, common varieties:											
15	825	Raw, shredded or chopped	1 c	70	92	16	1	4	2	<1	t	t	.1
15	826	Cooked, drained	1 c	150	94	32	1	7	4	<1	.1	<.1	.2
		Chinese cabbage:											
15	1178	Bok-choy, raw, shredded	1 c	70	95	9	1	2	1	<1	t	t	.1
15	827	Bok choy, cooked, drained	1 c	170	96	20	3	3	3	<1	<.1	t	.1
15	828	Pe-Tsai, raw, chopped	1 c	76	94	11	1	2	2	<1	<.1	t	.1
		Cabbage, red, coarsely chopped:											
15	829	Raw	1 c	70	92	19	1	4	2	<1	t	t	.1
15	830	Cooked	½ c	75	94	16	1	3	4	<1	t	t	.1
15	831	Savoy cabbage, coarsely chopped, raw	1 c	70	91	20	1	4	2	<.1	t	t	<.1

GRP KEY: 1 = BEV 2 = DAIRY 3 = EGGS 4 = FAT/OIL 5 = FRUIT 6 = BAKERY 7 = GRAIN 8 = FISH 9 = BEEF 10 = POULTRY
11 = SAUSAGE 12 = MIXED/FAST 13 = NUTS/SEEDS 14 = SWEETS 15 = VEG/LEG 16 = MISC 22 = SOUP/SAUCE

Chol (mg)	Calc (mg)	Iron (mg)	Magn (mg)	Phos (mg)	Pota (mg)	Sodi (mg)	Zinc (mg)	VT-A (RE)	Thia (mg)	Ribo (mg)	Niac (mg)	V-B6 (mg)	Fola (µg)	VT-C (mg)
0	25	1.76	50	101	370	26	.50	15	.06	.05	.69	.11	58	5
0	32	4.50	82	208	955	4	1.79	0	.30	.10	.79	.30	156	0
0	58	1.60	32	48	373	4	.45	83[114]	.09	.12	.77	.07	42	12
0	61	1.11	29	33	151	17	.84	71[115]	.07	.10	.56	.08	42	11
0	36	1.22	18	26	147	339[116]	.39	47[117]	.02	.08	.27	.05	43	6
0	14	.95	22	56	154	6	.43	2	.09	.13	.78	.09	63	14
0	16	2.40	38	70	200	14	1.12	3	.17	.22	1.49	.10	72	20
0	15	.81	18	34	125	12	.58	2	.06	.13	1.01	.05	35	14
0	9	.53	31	26	266	42	.21	1	.03	.01	.23	.03	49	5
0	11	.62	37	31	312	49	.25	1	.03	.01	.27	.03	86	6
0	13	1.55	13	15	126	233[118]	.18	1	.01	.04	.15	.05	22	4
0	13	.47	17	19	169	301	.30	1	.03	.06	.29	.03	35	3
0	165	2.74	97	58	1308	346	.72	734	.17	.42	.72	.19	47	36
0	42	.78	22	58	286	24	.36	136[119]	.06	.10	.56	.14	62	82
0	72	1.33	38	99	490	41	.60	233[119]	.10	.18	.96	.24	107	141
0	83	1.51	43	106	525	47	.68	250[119]	.10	.2	1.03	.26	90	134
0	72	1.24	37	92	456	40	.59	217[119]	.09	.18	.90	.22	78	116
0	15	.18	6	16	54	7	.09	57[119]	.02	.02	.14	.04	9	12
0	94	1.12	37	101	331	44	.55	348[119]	.10	.15	.84	.19	55	74
0	56	1.88	32	87	491	17	.50	112	.17	.12	.95	.31	94	97
0	38	1.15	37	84	504	36	.55	91	.16	.18	.83	.27	157	71
0	32	.40	10	16	172	12	.12	9	.04	.02	.21	.07	40	33
0	50	.59	23	38	308	29	.24	13	.09	.08	.34	.10	31	36
0	74	.56	13	26	176	<1	.29	210	.03	.05	.35	.07	57	32
0	158	1.77	18	49	630	57	.43	437	.05	.11	.73	.30	32	44
0	59	.23	10	22	181	7	.17	91	.03	.04	.30	.18	60	21
0	36	.35	11	29	144	8	.15	3	.05	.02	.21	.15	19	40
0	28	.27	8	21	105	6	.11	2	.03	.01	.15	.11	9	26
0	25	.28	20	29	161	20	.26	70	.05	.02	.21	.13	32	22

[114]Data is for green varieties; yellow beans contain 10 RE per cup.
[115]Data is for green varieties; yellow beans contain 15 RE per cup.
[116]Dietary pack contains 3 mg sodium per cup.
[117]For green varieties; yellow beans contain 14 RE per cup.
[118]Dietary pack contains 39 mg sodium.
[119]Vitamin A for whole plant: leaves are 1600 RE/100 g raw; flower clusters are 300/100 g raw; stalks are 40 RE/100 g raw.

(For purposes of calculations, use "0" for t, <1, <.1, <.01, etc.)

Table H-1 Food Composition

Grp	Computer Code No.	Food Description	Measure	Wt (g)	H₂O (%)	Ener (kcal)	Prot (g)	Carb (g)	Dietary Fiber (g)	Fat (g)	Fat Breakdown (g) Sat	Mono	Poly
		VEGETABLES and LEGUMES—Con.											
		Carrots:											
		Raw:											
15	832	Whole, 7½ × 1⅛″	1 carrot	72	88	31	1	7	2	<1	t	t	.1
15	833	Grated	½ c	55	88	24	1	6	2	<1	t	t	<.1
		Cooked, sliced, drained:											
15	834	Cooked from raw	½ c	78	87	35	1	8	3	<1	<.1	t	.1
15	835	Cooked from frozen	½ c	73	90	26	1	6	3	<.1	t	t	<.1
15	836	Canned, sliced, drained	½ c	73	93	17	<1	4	1	<1	<.1	t	.1
15	837	Carrot juice	½ c	123	89	49	1	11	2	<1	<.1	t	.1
		Cauliflower:											
15	838	Raw, flowerets	½ c	50	92	12	1	2	1	<.1	t	t	<.1
		Cooked, drained, flowerets:											
15	839	From raw	½ c	62	92	15	1	3	1	<1	t	t	.1
15	840	From frozen	1 c	180	94	34	3	7	3	<1	.1	<.1	.2
		Celery, pascal type, raw:											
15	841	Large outer stalk, 8 × 1½″ (at root end)	1 stalk	40	95	6	<1	1	1	<.1	t	t	t
15	842	Diced	½ c	60	95	11	<1	2	1	<.1	t	t	<.1
		Chard, swiss:											
15	1179	Raw, chopped	1 c	36	93	7	1	1	1	<1	t	t	<.1
15	1180	Cooked	1 c	175	93	35	3	7	4	<1	<.1	t	.1
		Chick-peas (see Garbanzo, #854)											
		Collards, cooked, drained:											
15	843	From raw	1 c	128	92	35	2	8	4	<1	.1	<.1	.1
15	844	From frozen	1 c	170	88	63	3	14	6	1	.1	.1	.3
		Corn:											
		Cooked, drained:											
15	845	From raw, on cob, 5″ long	1 ear	77	70	83	3	19	3	1	.2	.3	.5
15	846	From frozen, on cob, 3½″ long	1 ear	63	73	59	2	14	3	<1	.1	.1	.2
15	847	Kernels, cooked from frozen	½ c	82	76	67	2	17	3	<.1	t	t	<.1
		Canned:											
15	848	Cream style	½ c	128	79	93	2	23	2	<1	.1	.2	.3
15	849	Whole kernel, vacuum pack	1 c	210	77	166	5	41	3	1	.2	.3	.5
		Cowpeas; (see Black-eyed peas, #814–816)											
15	850	Cucumbers with peel, ⅛″ thick, 2⅛″ diam	6 slices	28	96	4	<1	1	<1	<.1	t	t	t
		Dandelion greens:											
15	851	Raw	1 c	55	86	25	1	5	1	<1	<.1	<.1	.2
15	852	Chopped, cooked, drained	1 c	105	90	35	2	7	1	1	.2	<.1	.4
15	853	Eggplant, cooked	1 c	160	92	45	1	11	6	<1	.1	<.1	.2
15	854	Garbanzo beans (chick-peas), cooked	1 c	164	60	269	15	45	11	4	.4	1.0	2.0
15	855	Great northern beans, cooked	1 c	177	69	210	15	37	11	1	.3	<.1	.3
15	856	Escarole/curly endive, chopped	1 c	50	94	9	1	2	1	<1	t	t	<.1
15	857	Jerusalem artichokes, raw slices	1 c	150	78	114	3	26	2	<.1	—	t	t
		Kale, cooked, drained:											
15	858	From raw	1 c	130	91	42	3	7	4	1	.1	<.1	.3
15	859	From frozen	1 c	130	90	39	4	7	3	1	.1	<.1	.3
15	860	Kidney beans, canned	1 c	256	77	216	13	39	19	<1	.1	.1	.4
		Kohlrabi:											
15	1181	Raw slices	1 c	140	91	38	2	9	2	<1	t	t	.1
15	861	Cooked	1 c	165	90	48	3	11	2	<1	t	t	.1

(Computer code number is for West Diet Analysis program)

GRP KEY: 1=BEV 2=DAIRY 3=EGGS 4=FAT/OIL 5=FRUIT 6=BAKERY 7=GRAIN 8=FISH 9=BEEF 10=POULTRY
11=SAUSAGE 12=MIXED/FAST 13=NUTS/SEEDS 14=SWEETS 15=VEG/LEG 16=MISC 22=SOUP/SAUCE

Chol (mg)	Calc (mg)	Iron (mg)	Magn (mg)	Phos (mg)	Pota (mg)	Sodi (mg)	Zinc (mg)	VT-A (RE)	Thia (mg)	Ribo (mg)	Niac (mg)	V-B6 (mg)	Fola (µg)	VT-C (mg)
0	19	.36	11	32	233	25	.14	2025	.07	.04	.67	.11	10	7
0	15	.28	8	24	178	19	.11	1547	.05	.03	.51	.08	8	5
0	24	.48	10	24	177	52	.23	1915	.03	.04	.40	.19	11	2
0	21	.35	7	19	115	43	.18	1292	.02	.03	.32	.09	8	2
0	19	.47	6	17	131	176[120]	.19	1006	.01	.02	.40	.08	7	2
0	29	.56	17	51	358	36	.22	3159	.11	.07	.47	.27	5	11
0	14	.29	7	23	178	7	.09	1	.04	.03	.32	.12	33	36
0	17	.26	7	22	200	4	.15	1	.04	.04	.34	.13	32	34
0	31	.74	16	43	250	33	.23	4	.07	.10	.56	.16	74	56
0	16	.16	5	10	115	35	.05	5	.02	.02	.13	.04	11	3
0	25	.25	7	15	170	55	.08	8	.03	.03	.19	.06	13	4
0	18	.65	29	17	136	77	.16	259	.01	.03	.14	.03	20	11
0	102	3.96	150	58	961	313	.59	1198	.06	.15	.63	.12	57	32
0	29	.21	9	10	168	21	.14	349	.03	.07	.37	.07	8	16
0	54	.38	16	19	307	37	.26	638	.05	.12	.68	.12	129	28
0	2	.47	25	79	192	13	.37	17[121]	.17	.06	1.24	.18	36	5
0	2	.38	18	47	158	3	.40	13[121]	.11	.04	.96	.14	19	3
0	2	.25	15	39	114	4	.29	20[121]	.06	.06	1.05	.18	19	2
0	4	.49	22	65	172	365[122]	.68	12[121]	.03	.07	1.23	.08	57	6
0	11	.88	48	134	390	572[123]	.97	51[121]	.09	.15	2.46	.12	104	17
0	4	.08	3	5	42	1	.07	1	.01	.01	.09	.02	4	1
0	103	1.71	20	36	218	42	.62	770	.11	.14	.39	.02	64	19
0	147	1.89	26	44	244	46	.80	1229	.14	.18	.50	.04	82	19
0	10	.56	21	35	397	5	.24	10	.12	.03	.96	.14	23	2
0	80	4.74	78	275	477	11	2.51	4	.19	.10	.86	.23	282	2
0	121	3.77	88	293	692	4	1.55	<1	.28	.10	1.21	.21	181	2
0	26	.42	8	14	157	11	.40	103	.04	.04	.20	.01	71	3
0	21	5.10	26	117	644	6	.11	3	.30	.09	1.95	.11	15	6
0	94	1.17	23	36	296	30	.31	962	.07	.09	.70	.18	30	53
0	179	1.22	23	36	417	20	.23	826	.06	.15	.87	.11	31	33
0	62	3.22	73	240	658	873	1.41	0	.27	.23	1.17	.06	129	3
0	34	.56	27	64	490	28	.32	5	.07	.03	.56	.21	14	87
0	41	.66	31	74	561	34	.32	6	.07	.03	.64	.18	13	89

[120]Dietary pack contains 31 mg sodium.
[121]For yellow varieties; white varieties contain only a trace of vitamin A.
[122]Dietary pack contains 4 mg sodium per ½ cup.
[123]Dietary pack contains 6 mg sodium per cup.

(For purposes of calculations, use "0" for t, <1, <.1, <.01, etc.)

Table H–1 Food Composition

Grp	Computer Code No.	Food Description	Measure	Wt (g)	H₂O (%)	Ener (kcal)	Prot (g)	Carb (g)	Dietary Fiber (g)	Fat (g)	Fat Breakdown (g) Sat	Mono	Poly
		VEGETABLES and LEGUMES—Con.											
		Leeks:											
15	1183	Raw, chopped	1 c	104	83	63	2	15	2	<1	.1	<.1	.4
15	1182	Cooked, chopped	.5 c	52	91	16	<1	4	2	<1	t	t	.1
15	862	Lentils, cooked from dry	1 c	198	70	230	18	40	10	1	.1	.1	.4
		Lentils, sprouted:											
15	1288	Stir fried	3.5 oz	100	69	101	9	21	4	<1	.1	.1	.2
15	1289	Raw	1 c	77	67	81	7	17	3	<1	<.1	.1	.2
		Lettuce:											
		Butterhead/Boston types:											
15	863	Head, 5″ diam	1 head	163	96	21	2	4	3	<1	<.1	t	.2
15	864	Leaves, 2 inner or outer	2 leaves	15	96	2	<1	<1	<1	<.1	t	t	t
		Iceberg/crisphead:											
15	865	Head, 6″ diam	1 head	539	96	70	5	11	9	1	.1	<.1	.5
15	866	Wedge, ¼ of head	1 wedge	135	96	18	1	3	2	<1	<.1	t	.1
15	867	Chopped or shredded	1 c	56	96	7	1	1	1	<1	t	t	.1
15	868	Loose leaf, chopped	1 c	56	94	10	1	2	1	<1	t	t	.1
		Romaine:											
15	869	Chopped	1 c	56	95	9	1	1	1	<1	t	t	.1
15	870	Inner leaf	1 leaf	10	95	2	<1	<1	<1	<.1	t	t	t
		Mushrooms:											
15	871	Raw, sliced	½ c	35	92	9	1	2	1	<1	t	t	.1
15	872	Cooked from raw, pieces	½ c	78	91	21	2	4	2	<1	<.1	t	.1
15	873	Canned, drained	½ c	78	91	19	1	4	2	<1	<.1	t	.1
		Mustard greens:											
15	874	Cooked from raw	1 c	140	94	21	3	3	3	<1	t	.2	.1
15	875	Cooked from frozen	1 c	150	94	29	3	5	3	<1	t	.2	.1
15	876	Navy beans, cooked from dry	1 c	182	63	259	16	48	16	1	.3	.1	.4
		Okra, cooked:											
15	877	From fresh pods	8 pods	85	90	27	2	6	2	<1	<.1	t	<.1
15	878	From frozen slices	½ c	92	91	34	2	8	2	<1	.1	.1	.1
		Onions:											
15	879	Raw, chopped	1 c	160	90	61	2	14	3	<1	<.1	<.1	.1
15	880	Raw, sliced	1 c	115	90	44	1	10	2	<1	<.1	<.1	.1
15	881	Cooked, drained, chopped	½ c	105	88	46	1	11	2	<1	<.1	<.1	.1
15	882	Dehydrated flakes	¼ c	14	4	45	1	12	1	<.1	t	t	<.1
		Spring onions:											
15	883	Chopped, bulb and top	½ c	50	90	16	1	4	1	.1	t	t	<.1
15	1185	Green tops only, chopped	1 c	100	92	34	2	6	3	<1	.1	.1	.2
15	1184	White part only, chopped	1 c	100	92	50	1	10	3	<1	<.1	t	.1
15	884	Onion rings, breaded, prepared f/frozen	2 rings	20	29	81	1	8	<1	5	1.7	2.2	1
		Parsley:											
15	885	Raw, chopped	½ c	30	88	10	1	2	2	<.1	t	t	<.1
15	886	Raw, sprigs	10 sprigs	10	88	3	<1	1	1	<.1	t	t	t
15	887	Freeze dried	¼ c	1	2	4	<1	1	1	<.1	t	t	<.1
15	888	Parsnips, sliced, cooked	1 c	156	78	125	2	30	5	1	.1	.2	.1
		Peas:											
		Black-eyed peas, cooked:											
15	814	From dry, drained	1 c	171	70	198	13	36	21	1	.2	.1	.4
15	815	From fresh, drained	1 c	165	76	160	5	33	12	1	.2	<.1	.3
15	816	From frozen, drained	1 c	170	66	224	14	40	14	1	.3	.1	.5
15	889	Edible-pod, peas, cooked	1 c	160	89	67	5	11	4	<1	.1	<.1	.2

(Computer code number is for West Diet Analysis program)

GRP KEY: 1=BEV 2=DAIRY 3=EGGS 4=FAT/OIL 5=FRUIT 6=BAKERY 7=GRAIN 8=FISH 9=BEEF 10=POULTRY
11=SAUSAGE 12=MIXED/FAST 13=NUTS/SEEDS 14=SWEETS 15=VEG/LEG 16=MISC 22=SOUP/SAUCE

Chol (mg)	Calc (mg)	Iron (mg)	Magn (mg)	Phos (mg)	Pota (mg)	Sodi (mg)	Zinc (mg)	VT-A (RE)	Thia (mg)	Ribo (mg)	Niac (mg)	V-B6 (mg)	Fola (µg)	VT-C (mg)
0	61	2.18	29	36	187	21	.17	10	.06	.03	.42	.24	67	13
0	16	.57	7	9	45	5	.12	2	.01	.01	.10	.08	16	2
0	37	6.59	71	356	731	4	2.50	2	.34	.14	2.10	.35	358	3
0	14	3.10	35	153	284	9	1.60	4	.22	.09	1.20	.16	84	13
0	19	2.47	28	133	248	8	1.16	4	.18	.10	.87	.15	77	13
0	52	.49	18	38	419	8	.42	158	.10	.10	.49	.11	119	13
0	5	.05	2	3	39	1	.04	15	.01	.01	.05	.01	11	1
0	102	2.70	49	108	852	48	1.19	178	.25	.16	1.01	.22	302	21
0	26	.68	12	27	213	12	.30	45	.06	.04	.25	.05	76	5
0	11	.28	5	11	89	5	.12	19	.03	.02	.11	.02	31	2
0	38	.78	6	14	148	5	.19	106	.03	.04	.22	.03	60	10
0	20	.62	3	25	162	4	.19	146	.06	.06	.28	.03	76	13
0	4	.11	1	5	29	1	.03	26	.01	.01	.05	.06	14	2
0	2	.43	4	36	130	1	.30	0	.04	.16	1.44	.03	7	1
0	5	1.36	9	68	278	2	.68	0	.06	.23	3.48	.07	14	3
0	9	.62	6	52	101	332	.56	0	.05	.17	1.25	.06	10	0
0	104	1.56	21	57	283	22	.30	424	.06	.09	.61	.18	20	35
0	152	1.68	20	36	209	38	.30	671	.06	.08	.39	.16	20	21
0	128	4.5	107	285	669	2	1.93	<1	.37	.11	.97	.30	255	1
0	54	.38	48	48	274	4	.47	49	.11	.05	.74	.16	39	14
0	88	.62	47	42	215	3	.57	47	.09	.11	.72	.04	134	11
0	32	.35	16	53	251	5	.30	0	.07	.03	.24	.19	30	10
0	23	.25	12	38	181	3	.22	0	.05	.02	.17	.13	22	7
0	23	.25	12	37	174	3	.22	0	.04	.02	.17	.14	16	5
0	36	.22	13	42	227	3	.26	0	.01	.01	.03	.22	23	11
0	36	.74	10	19	138	8	.20	20	.03	.04	.26	.03	32	9
0	56	2.20	21	39	260	7	.22	400	.07	.10	.60	0	80	51
0	40	.89	16	40	230	7	.25	<1	.07	.03	.33	.10	36	27
0	6	.34	4	16	26	75	.08	5	.06	.03	.72	.02	3	<1
0	39	1.86	13	12	161	12	.22	156	.02	.03	.21	.05	55	27
0	13	.62	4	4	54	4	.07	52	.01	.01	.07	.02	18	9
0	2	.75	5	8	88	5	.09	89	.02	.03	.15	.02	22	2
0	58	.90	46	108	573	16	.40	0	.13	.08	1.10	.15	91	20[124]
0	42	4.30	91	266	476	6	2.20	3	.35	.1	.85	.17	356	1
0	211	1.85	86	84	690	7	1.7	131	.17	.24	2.3	.11	210	4
0	40	3.60	85	208	638	9	2.42	13	.42	.11	1.24	.16	240	5
0	67	3.15	42	89	383	6	.60	30	.21	.12	.86	.23	48	77

[124]Value for Vitamin C is highest right after harvest and drops after that.

(For purposes of calculations, use "0" for t, <1, <.1, <.01, etc.)

Table H–1 Food Composition

Grp	Computer Code No.	Food Description	Measure	Wt (g)	H₂O (%)	Ener (kcal)	Prot (g)	Carb (g)	Dietary Fiber (g)	Fat (g)	Sat	Mono	Poly
	VEGETABLES and LEGUMES—Con.
		Peas—Con.											
		Green peas:											
15	890	Canned, drained	½ c	85	82	59	4	11	4	<1	.1	<.1	.1
15	891	Cooked from frozen	½ c	80	80	63	4	11	4	<1	<.1	t	.1
15	892	Split, green, cooked from dry	1 c	196	69	231	16	41	10	1	.1	.2	.3
		Peas and carrots:											
15	1187	Cooked from frozen	½ c	80	86	38	2	8	3	<1	.1	<.1	.2
15	1186	Canned, with liquid	½ c	128	88	48	3	11	4	<1	.1	<.1	.2
		Peppers, hot:											
15	893	Hot green chili, canned	½ c	68	92	17	1	4	1	<.1	t	t	<.1
15	894	Hot green chili, raw	1 pepper	45	88	18	1	4	1	<.1	t	t	<.1
15	895	Jalapenos, chopped, canned	½ c	68	90	17	1	3	2	<1	.4	t	.2
		Peppers, sweet, green:											
15	896	Whole pod (90 g with refuse), raw	1 pod	74	92	20	1	5	1	<1	.1	t	.1
15	897	Cooked, chopped (1 pod cooked = 73 g)	½ c	68	92	19	1	5	1	<1	<.1	t	.1
		Peppers, sweet, red:											
15	1286	Raw, chopped	½ c	50	92	14	<1	3	1	<1	<.1	t	.1
15	1287	Cooked, chopped	½ c	68	92	19	1	5	1	<1	<.1	t	.1
15	898	Pinto beans, cooked from dry	1 c	171	64	235	14	44	20	1	.2	.2	.3
15	1191	Poi - two finger	1 c	240	72	269	1	65	6	<1	.1	<.1	.1
		Potatoes:[125]											
		Baked in oven, 4¾ × 2⅓″ diam:											
15	899	With skin	1 potato	202	71	220	5	51	5	<1	.1	t	.1
15	900	Flesh only	1 potato	156	75	145	3	34	2	<1	<.1	t	.1
15	901	Skin only	1 ea	58	47	115	2	27	2	<.1	t	t	<.1
		Baked in microwave, 4¾ × 2⅓″ diam:											
15	902	With skin	1 potato	202	72	212	5	49	5	<1	.1	t	.1
15	903	Flesh only	1 potato	156	74	156	3	36	2	<1	<.1	t	.1
15	904	Skin only	1 ea	58	64	77	3	17	2	<.1	t	t	<.1
		Boiled, about 2½″ diam:											
15	905	Peeled after boiling	1 potato	136	77	119	3	27	2	<1	<.1	t	.1
15	906	Peeled before boiling	1 potato	135	78	116	2	27	2	<1	<.1	t	.1
		French fried, strips 2-3½″ long, frozen:											
15	907	Oven heated	10 strips	50	53	111	2	17	1	4	2.1	1.8	.3
15	908	Fried in veg oil	10 strips	50	38	158	2	20	1	8	2.5	1.6	3.8
15	1188	Fried in veg. and animal oil	10 strips	50	38	158	2	20	1	8	3.4	4.0	.5
15	909	Hashed brown, from frozen	1 c	156	56	340	5	44	3	18	7	8	2
		Mashed:											
15	910	Home recipe with milk[126]	1 c	210	78	162	4	37	3	1	.7	.3	.1
15	911	Home recipe with milk and margarine	1 c	210	76	222	4	35	3	9	2.2	3.7	2.5
15	912	Prepared from flakes; water, milk, margarine, salt added	1 c	215	76	239	4	28	2	13	3.0	5.4	3.7
		Potato products, prepared:											
		Au gratin:											
15	913	From dry mix	1 c	245	79	228	6	32	4	10	6.3	3	.3
15	914	From home recipe[127]	1 c	245	74	322	12	28	4	19	12	5	1

[125] Vitamin C varies with length of storage. After 3 months of storage approximately two-thirds of the ascorbic acid remains; after 6 to 7 months, about one-third remains.

[126] Recipe: 84% potatoes, 15% whole milk, 1% salt.

[127] Recipe: 55% potatoes, 30% whole milk, 9% cheddar cheese, 3% butter, 2% flour, 1% salt.

(Computer code number is for West Diet Analysis program)

GRP KEY:　1 = BEV　2 = DAIRY　3 = EGGS　4 = FAT/OIL　5 = FRUIT　6 = BAKERY　7 = GRAIN　8 = FISH　9 = BEEF　10 = POULTRY
11 = SAUSAGE　12 = MIXED/FAST　13 = NUTS/SEEDS　14 = SWEETS　15 = VEG/LEG　16 = MISC　22 = SOUP/SAUCE

Chol (mg)	Calc (mg)	Iron (mg)	Magn (mg)	Phos (mg)	Pota (mg)	Sodi (mg)	Zinc (mg)	VT-A (RE)	Thia (mg)	Ribo (mg)	Niac (mg)	V-B6 (mg)	Fola (μg)	VT-C (mg)
0	17	.81	15	57	147	186[128]	.60	65	.10	.07	.62	.05	38	8
0	19	1.25	23	72	134	70	.75	77	.23	.14	1.18	.09	47	8
0	26	2.52	71	195	710	4	1.96	1	.37	.11	1.74	.09	127	1
0	18	.75	13	39	127	55	.36	621	.18	.06	.92	.07	21	7
0	29	.97	18	58	128	332	.74	739	.10	.07	.74	.11	24	8
0	5	.34	8	12	143	10	.02	42[129]	.01	.03	.54	.08	35	46
0	8	.54	11	21	153	3	.14	35[129]	.04	.04	.43	.13	11	109
0	18	1.90	8	12	92	995	.13	116	.02	.03	.34	.14	35	9
0	7	.34	7	14	131	1	.09	47	.05	.02	.38	.18	16	66
0	6	.31	7	12	113	1	.08	40	.04	.02	.32	.16	10	51
0	5	.23	5	10	89	1	.06	285	.03	.02	.26	.12	11	95
0	6	.31	7	12	113	1	.08	256	.04	.02	.32	.16	11	116
0	82	4.47	95	273	800	3	1.85	<1	.32	.16	.68	.27	294	4
0	37	2.11	58	94	439	28	2.04	5	.31	.10	2.64	—	—	10
0	20	2.75	55	115	844	16	.65	0	.22	.07	3.32	.70	22	26
0	8	.55	39	78	610	8	.45	0	.16	.03	2.18	.47	14	20
0	20	2.20	25	59	332	12	.28	0	.07	.07	1.78	.35	13	8
0	22	2.50	54	212	903	16	.73	0	.24	.07	3.46	.70	24	31
0	8	.64	39	170	641	11	.51	0	.20	.04	2.54	.50	19	24
0	27	3.44	22	48	377	9	.30	0	.04	.04	1.29	.28	10	9
0	7	.42	30	60	515	6	.41	0	.14	.03	1.96	.41	14	18
0	10	.42	26	54	443	7	.37	0	.13	.03	1.77	.36	12	10
0	4	.67	11	43	229	15	.21	0	.06	.02	1.15	.12	8	6
0	10	.38	17	47	366	108	.19	0	.09	.01	1.63	.12	15	5
0	10	.38	17	47	366	108	.19	0	.09	.01	1.63	.12	15	5
0	24	2.36	27	112	680	53	.50	0	.17	.03	3.78	.20	26	10
4	55	.57	39	100	628	636	.60	12	.19	.08	2.35	.49	17	14
4[130]	54	.55	37	97	607	619	.58	41	.18	.11	2.27	.47	17	13
4[130]	92	.40	30	108	428	733	.51	176	.30	.14	1.91	.26	15	25
12	203	.78	37	233	537	1076	.59	76	.05	.20	2.30	.10	3	8
56[131]	292	1.56	48	277	970	1064	1.69	93	.16	.28	2.43	.43	25	24

[128] Dietary pack contains 1.7 mg sodium.

[129] Data is for green chili peppers; red varieties contain 809 RE vitamin A per ½ cup; 484 RE per whole pepper.

[130] Data is for margarine; if butter is used, cholesterol = 25 mg for 29 total mg.

[131] Data is for butter; if margarine is used, cholesterol = 37 mg.

(For purposes of calculations, use "0" for t, <1, <.1, <.01, etc.)

Table H–1 Food Composition

Grp	Computer Code No.	Food Description	Measure	Wt (g)	H₂O (%)	Ener (kcal)	Prot (g)	Carb (g)	Dietary Fiber (g)	Fat (g)	Fat Breakdown (g) Sat	Mono	Poly
		VEGETABLES and LEGUMES—Con.											
		Potato Products—Con.											
		Potato salad (see Mixed Dishes #715)											
		Scalloped:											
15	915	From dry mix	1 c	245	79	228	5	31	3	11	6.5	3.0	.5
15	916	Home recipe[132]	1 c	245	81	210	7	26	3	9	5.5	2.6	.4
15	1192	Potato puffs, cooked from frozen	.5 c	62	53	138	2	19	1	7	3.2	2.7	.5
15	917	Potato chips (14 chips = about 1 oz)	14 chips	28	2	148	2	15	1	10	2.6	1.8	5.2
		Pumpkin:											
15	918	Cooked from raw, mashed	1 c	245	94	50	2	12	4	<1	.1	t	t
15	919	Canned	1 c	245	90	83	3	20	5	1	.4	.1	<.1
15	920	Red radishes	10 radishes	45	95	7	<1	2	1	<1	t	t	t
15	921	Refried beans, canned	1 c	253	72	270	16	47	22	3	1	1.2	.4
15	1375	Rutabaga, cooked cubes	.5 c	85	90	29	1	7	1	<1	<.1	<.1	.1
15	922	Sauerkraut, canned with liquid	1 c	236	92	44	2	10	4	<1	.1	<.1	.1
		Seaweed:											
15	923	Kelp, raw	1 oz	28	82	12	1	3	1	<1	.1	<.1	t
15	924	Spirulina, dried	1 oz	28	5	82	16	7	1	2	.8	.2	.6
15	925	Soybeans, cooked from dry	1 c	172	63	298	29	17	5	15	2.2	3.4	8.7
		Soybean products:											
15	926	Miso	½ c	138	46	283	16	39	7	8	1.2	1.9	4.7
15	927	Tofu	½ c	124	85	94	10	2	2	6	.9	1.3	3.4
		Spinach:											
15	928	Raw, chopped	1 c	56	92	12	2	2	2	<1	<.1	t	.1
		Cooked, drained:											
15	929	From raw	1 c	180	91	41	5	7	4	<1	.1	t	.2
15	930	From frozen (leaf)	1 c	190	90	53	6	10	5	<1	.1	t	.2
15	931	Canned, drained solids	1 c	214	92	50	6	7	6	1	.2	<.1	.5
		Spinach soufflé (Mixed Dishes)											
		Squash, summer varieties, cooked slices:											
15	932	Varieties averaged	1 c	180	94	36	2	8	3	1	.1	<.1	.2
15	933	Crookneck	1 c	180	94	36	2	8	3	1	.1	<.1	.2
15	934	Zucchini	1 c	180	95	29	1	7	4	<.1	t	t	<.1
		Squash, winter varieties, cooked:											
		Average of all varieties, baked:											
15	935	Mashed	1 c	245	89	96	2	21	7	2	.3	.1	.7
15	936	Baked cubes	1 c	205	89	79	2	18	6	1	.3	.1	.5
		Acorn squash:											
15	937	Baked, mashed	1 c	245	83	137	3	36	7	<1	<.1	t	.1
15	1218	Boiled, mashed	1 c	245	90	83	2	22	6	<1	<.1	t	.1
15	938	Butternut, baked cubes	1 c	205	88	83	2	22	6	<1	<.1	t	.1
		Butternut squash:											
15	1219	Baked, mashed	1 c	245	88	99	2	26	7	<1	<.1	t	.1
15	1193	Cooked from frozen	1 c	240	88	94	3	24	7	<1	<.1	t	.1
		Hubbard squash:											
15	1194	Baked, mashed	1 c	240	85	120	6	26	6	1	.3	.1	.6
15	1195	Boiled, mashed	1 c	236	91	70	4	15	7	1	.2	.1	.4
15	1196	Spaghetti squash, baked or boiled	1 c	155	92	45	1	10	4	<1	.1	<.1	.2
15	1189	Succotash, cooked from frozen	1 c	170	74	158	7	34	9	2	.3	.3	.7

[132]Recipe: 59% potatoes, 36% whole milk, 2% butter, 2% flour, 1% salt.

GRP KEY: 1 = BEV   2 = DAIRY   3 = EGGS   4 = FAT/OIL   5 = FRUIT   6 = BAKERY   7 = GRAIN   8 = FISH   9 = BEEF   10 = POULTRY
11 = SAUSAGE   12 = MIXED/FAST   13 = NUTS/SEEDS   14 = SWEETS   15 = VEG/LEG   16 = MISC   22 = SOUP/SAUCE

Chol (mg)	Calc (mg)	Iron (mg)	Magn (mg)	Phos (mg)	Pota (mg)	Sodi (mg)	Zinc (mg)	VT-A (RE)	Thia (mg)	Ribo (mg)	Niac (mg)	V-B6 (mg)	Fola (µg)	VT-C (mg)
27	88	.93	34	137	497	835	.61	51	.05	.14	2.52	.10	3	8
29[133]	140	1.41	46	154	926	821	.98	46	.17	.23	2.58	.44	21	26
0	19	.97	12	30	236	462	.19	1	.12	.05	1.34	.14	.10	4
0	7	.34	17	43	369	133[134]	.30	0	.04	.01	1.19	.14	13	12
0	37	1.40	22	74	564	3	.45	265	.08	.19	1.01	.16	33	12
0	64	3.41	56	85	504	12	.42	5404	.06	.13	.9	.14	30	10
0	9	.13	4	8	104	11	.13	t	<.01	.02	.14	.03	12	10
0	118	4.5	99	214	994	1071	3.45	0	.12	.14	1.23	.28	150	15
0	36	.40	18	42	244	15	.26	0	.06	.03	.54	.08	13	19
0	72	3.47	31	46	401	1561	.44	4	.05	.05	.34	.31	4	35
0	48	.81	34	12	25	66	.35	3	.01	.04	.13	—	51	—
0	34	8.08	55	33	386	297	—	16	.68	1.04	3.63	.10	—	3
0	175	8.84	148	421	886	1	1.98	2	.27	.49	.69	.40	93	3
0	92	3.78	58	211	226	5032	4.58	12	.13	.35	1.19	.3	46	0
0	130	6.65	127	120	150	9	1.00	11	.10	.06	.24	.06	19	<1
0	55	1.52	44	27	312	44	.30	448	.04	.11	.41	.11	109	16
0	244	6.42	157	100	838	126	1.37	1750	.17	.43	.88	.44	262	40
0	277	2.89	131	91	566	163	1.33	1756	.11	.32	.80	.28	204	23
0	271	4.92	162	94	740	683[135]	.99	1878	.03	.30	.83	.21	209	31
0	48	.64	44	69	346	2	.71	52[136]	.08	.07	.92	.12	36	9
0	48	.64	44	69	346	2	.71	52[136]	.09	.09	.92	.17	36	10
0	23	.63	40	72	455	5	.32	43[136]	.07	.07	.77	.14	30	8
0	34	.81	20	49	1071	2	.64	872	.21	.06	1.72	.18	69	24
0	28	.67	16	41	895	3	.54	730	.17	.05	1.43	.15	57	20
0	108	2.28	104	111	1071	11	.42	105	.41	.03	2.16	.48	46	26
0	65	1.37	63	67	645	6	.27	63	.25	.02	1.30	.29	28	16
0	84	1.23	59	55	582	7	.27	1435	.15	.04	1.99	.25	39	31
0	100	1.47	71	66	697	8	.32	1715	.18	.04	2.38	.30	47	37
0	46	1.40	22	34	319	4	.29	801	.12	.09	1.11	.17	29	8
0	41	1.13	53	55	859	19	.36	1450	.18	.11	1.34	.41	39	23
0	23	.67	32	33	504	12	.22	945	.10	.07	.79	.24	23	15
0	33	.52	17	21	182	28	.31	17	.06	.03	1.26	.15	12	6
0	25	1.51	39	119	451	77	.76	39	.13	.12	2.22	.16	57	10

[133]Data is for butter; if margarine is used cholesterol = 15 mg.
[134]If no salt added, sodium = 2 mg.
[135]Dietary pack contains 58 mg sodium.
[136]Applies to squash including skin; flesh has no appreciable vitamin A value.

H

(For purposes of calculations, use "0" for t, <1, <.1, <.01, etc.)

Table H–1   Food Composition

Grp	Computer Code No.	Food Description	Measure	Wt (g)	H$_2$O (%)	Ener (kcal)	Prot (g)	Carb (g)	Dietary Fiber (g)	Fat (g)	Fat Breakdown (g) Sat	Mono	Poly
VEGETABLES and LEGUMES—Con.													
		Sweet potatoes:											
		Cooked, 5 × 2″ diam:											
15	939	Baked in skin, peeled	1 potato	114	73	118	2	28	3	<1	<.1	t	.1
15	940	Boiled without skin	1 potato	151	73	160	2	37	5	<1	.1	t	.2
15	941	Candied, 2½ × 2″	1 pce	105	67	144	1	29	2	3	1.4	.7	.2
		Canned:											
15	942	Solid pack, mashed	1 c	265	74	258	5	59	6	<1	.1	t	.2
15	943	Vacuum pack, mashed	1 c	255	76	233	4	54	5	1	.1	t	.2
15	944	Vacuum pack, 2¾ × 1″	1 pce	40	76	36	1	8	1	<1	t	t	<.1
		Tomatoes:											
15	945	Raw, whole, 2⅗″ diam	1 tomato	123	94	26	1	6	2	<1	<.1	<.1	.2
15	946	Raw, chopped	1 c	180	94	38	2	8	3	<1	.1	.1	.2
15	947	Cooked from raw	1 c	240	92	65	3	14	4	1	.1	.2	.4
15	948	Canned, solids and liquid	1 c	240	94	47	2	10	3	1	.1	.1	.2
15	949	Tomato juice, canned	1 c	244	94	42	2	10	2	<1	t	t	.1
		Tomato products, canned:											
15	950	Paste	1 c	262	74	220	10	49	11	2	.3	.4	.9
15	951	Puree	1 c	250	87	102	4	25	6	<1	<.1	<.1	.1
15	952	Sauce	1 c	245	89	74	3	18	4	<1	.1	.1	.2
15	953	Turnips, cubes, cooked from raw	½ c	78	94	14	1	4	2	<1	t	t	<.1
		Turnip greens, cooked:											
15	954	From raw (leaves and stems)	1 c	144	94	29	2	6	4	<1	.1	t	.1
15	955	From frozen (chopped)	½ c	82	90	24	3	4	4	<1	.1	t	.1
15	956	Vegetable juice cocktail, canned	1 c	242	94	46	2	11	2	<1	<.1	<.1	.1
		Vegetables, mixed:											
15	957	Canned, drained	1 c	163	87	77	4	15	6	<1	.1	<.1	.2
15	958	Frozen, cooked, drained	1 c	182	83	107	5	24	7	<1	.1	t	.1
		Water chestnuts, canned:											
15	959	Slices	½ c	70	86	35	1	9	2	<.1	t	t	t
15	960	Whole	4 ea	28	86	14	<1	4	1	<1	t	t	t
15	1190	Watercress, fresh, chopped	.5 c	17	95	2	<1	<1	<1	<1	t	t	t
MISCELLANEOUS													
		Baking powders for home use:											
		Sodium aluminum sulfate:											
16	962	With monocalcium phosphate monohydrate	1 tsp	3	2	5	t	1	0	0	0	0	0
16	963	With monocalcium phosphate monohydrate, calcium sulfate	1 tsp	3	1	5	t	1	0	0	0	0	0
16	964	Straight phosphate	1 tsp	4	2	5	t	1	0	0	0	0	0
16	965	Low sodium	1 tsp	4	1	5	t	1	0	0	0	0	0
16	1204	Baking soda	1 tsp	3	1	0	0	0	0	0	0	0	0
16	966	Basil, ground	1 tbsp	5	6	11	1	3	1	<1	—	—	—
16	961	Carob flour	1 c	103	3	185	5	92	34	1	.1	.2	.2

H

GRP KEY: 1 = BEV   2 = DAIRY   3 = EGGS   4 = FAT/OIL   5 = FRUIT   6 = BAKERY   7 = GRAIN   8 = FISH   9 = BEEF   10 = POULTRY
11 = SAUSAGE   12 = MIXED/FAST   13 = NUTS/SEEDS   14 = SWEETS   15 = VEG/LEG   16 = MISC   22 = SOUP/SAUCE

Chol (mg)	Calc (mg)	Iron (mg)	Magn (mg)	Phos (mg)	Pota (mg)	Sodi (mg)	Zinc (mg)	VT-A (RE)	Thia (mg)	Ribo (mg)	Niac (mg)	V-B6 (mg)	Fola (µg)	VT-C (mg)
0	32	.52	23	63	397	12	.33	2488	.08	.14	.7	.28	26	28
0	32	.8	15	41	278	20	.4	2575	.08	.21	1	.36	22	26
0[137]	27	1.2	12	27	198	73	.16	440	.02	.04	.41	.17	12	7
0	77	3.4	61	133	536	191	.54	3857	.07	.23	2.4	.48	42	13
0	56	2.27	57	125	796	136	.46	2036	.09	.14	1.89	.49	42	67
0	9	.36	9	20	125	21	.07	319	.02	.02	.3	.08	7	11
0	6	.55	14	30	273	11	.11	77	.07	.06	.77	.10	18	22[138]
0	9	.81	20	43	400	16	.16	112	.11	.09	1.13	.14	27	34[138]
0	14	1.34	34	74	670	26	.26	178	.17	.14	1.80	.23	31	55
0	63[139]	1.45	29	46	529	390[140]	.38	145	.11	.07	1.76	.22	35	36
0	22	1.41	27	46	537	881[141]	.34	136	.12	.08	1.64	.27	49	45
0	92	7.84	134	207	2442	170[142]	2.1	647	.41	.5	8.44	1	40	111
0	37	2.32	60	99	1051	49[143]	.54	340	.18	.14	4.29	.38	39	88
0	34	1.88	46	78	908	1481[144]	.6	240	.16	.14	2.82	.33	39	32
0	18	.17	6	15	106	39	.16	0	.02	.02	.23	.05	7	9
0	198	1.15	32	41	293	41	.29	792	.07	.1	.59	.26	171	40
0	125	1.59	21	27	184	12	.34	654	.04	.06	.38	.06	32	18
0	27	1.02	27	41	467	883	.48	283	.1	.07	1.76	.34	38	67
0	44	1.71	26	68	474	243	.67	1899	.07	.08	.94	.13	39	8
0	46	1.49	40	93	308	64	.89	779	.13	.22	1.55	.14	35	6
0	3	.61	3	14	82	6	.27	t	.01	.02	.25	—	8	1
0	1	.25	1	5	33	2	.11	t	<.01	.01	.1	—	3	<1
0	20	.03	4	10	56	7	.03	80	.02	.02	.03	.02	34	7
0	58	0	t	87	5	329	0	0	0	0	0	0	0	0
0	183	0	—	45	4	290	0	0	0	0	0	0	0	0
0	239	0	—	359	6	312	0	0	0	0	0	0	0	0
0	207	0	—	314	891	t	0	0	0	0	0	0	0	0
0	0	—	—	—	—	821	—	0	0	0	0	0	0	0
0	95	1.89	18	22	154	2	.26	42	.01	.01	.31	—	—	3
0	359	3.03	56	81	852	36	.94	2	.06	.48	1.95	.38	30	<1

[137] For recipe using margarine; if butter is used, cholesterol = 8 mg.

[138] Year-round average. From June through October, ascorbic acid is approximately 32 mg and 47 mg, respectively, for one tomato and 1 c chopped tomato. From November through May, market samples average around 12 and 18 mg, respectively.

[139] Calcium is added as a firming agent.

[140] Dietary pack contains 31 mg sodium.

[141] If no salt is added, sodium content is 24 mg.

[142] If salt is added, sodium content is 2070 mg.

[143] If salt is added, sodium content is 998 mg.

[144] With salt added.

(For purposes of calculations, use "0" for t, <1, <.1, <.01, etc.)

H

Table H–1 Food Composition

Grp	Computer Code No.	Food Description	Measure	Wt (g)	H₂O (%)	Ener (kcal)	Prot (g)	Carb (g)	Dietary Fiber (g)	Fat (g)	Fat Breakdown (g) Sat	Mono	Poly
MISCELLANEOUS—Con.													
		Catsup:											
16	967	Cup	1 c	245	67	255	4	67	4	1	.2	.2	.4
16	968	Tablespoon	1 tbsp	15	67	16	<1	4	<1	<.1	t	t	t
16	1200	Cayenne (red pepper)	1 tbsp	5.3	8	17	1	3	2	1	.2	.2	.4
16	969	Celery seed	1 tsp	2	6	9	<1	1	<1	1	<.1	.3	.1
16	970	Chili powder	1 tsp	3	8	8	<1	1	1	<1	.1	.1	.2
		Chocolate:											
16	971	Baking, unsweetened For other chocolate items, see Sweeteners and Sweets	1 oz	28	2	145	4	7	4	15	9	5	.5
16	972	Coriander, fresh	¼ c	4	93	<1	<1	<1	<1	<.1	<.01	<.01	.01
16	1197	Cornstarch	1 tbsp	8	8	20	<.1	5	<.1	<.1	t	t	t
16	973	Cinnamon	1 tsp	2	10	6	<1	2	1	<.1	t	t	t
16	974	Curry powder	1 tsp	2	10	6	<1	1	<1	<1	t	.2	<.1
16	1202	Dill weed, dried	1 tbsp	3.1	7	8	1	2	<1	<1	—	—	—
		Garlic:											
16	975	Cloves	4 cloves	12	59	18	1	4	<1	<.1	t	t	<.1
16	976	Powder	1 tsp	3	6	9	<1	2	<1	<.1	t	t	t
16	977	Gelatin, dry, plain	1 envelope	7	13	25	6	0	1	0	0	0	0
16	978	Ginger root, raw, sliced	5 slices	11	87	8	<1	2	<1	<1	t	t	t
16	1198	Horseradish, prepared	1 tbsp	15	87	6	<1	1	<1	<1	t	t	t
16	1199	Hummous/Humous	1 c	246	65	420	33	50	4	21	3.1	8.8	7.8
16	979	Mustard, prepared, (1 packet = 1 tsp) Miso (see #926 under Vegetables and Legumes, Soybean products)	1 tsp	5	80	4	<1	<1	<1	<1	t	.2	t
		Olives:											
16	980	Green	10 olives	39	78	45	<1	<1	1	6	.6	3.6	.3
16	981	Ripe, pitted	10 olives	45	80	52	<1	3	1.5	5	.6	3.6	.4
16	982	Onion powder	1 tsp	2.1	5	5	<1	2	<1	<.1	t	t	t
16	983	Oregano, ground	1 tsp	2	7	5	<1	1	<1	<1	t	t	.1
16	984	Paprika	1 tsp	2	10	6	<1	1	<1	<1	t	t	.2
16	985	Pepper, black	1 tsp	2	11	5	<1	1	<1	<.1	<.1	<.1	<.1
		Pickles:											
16	986	Dill, medium, 3¾ × 1¼″ diam	1 pickle	65	92	12	<1	3	1	<1	<.1	t	<.1
16	987	Fresh pack, slices, 1½″ diam × ¼″	4 slices	30	79	20	<1	5	<1	<.1	t	t	t
16	988	Sweet, medium	1 pickle	35	65	41	<1	11	<1	.1	t	t	<.1
16	989	Pickle relish, sweet	1 tbsp	15	63	20	<.1	5	<1	<.1	t	t	<.1
16	1201	Sage, ground Popcorn (see Grain Products, #539-541)	1 tbsp	2	8	6	<1	1	<1	<1	.1	<.1	<.1
22	1347	Salsa, from recipe	.85 c	184	91	79	2	9	3	5	.7	3.4	.5
16	990	Salt	1 tsp	6	0	0	0	0	0	0	0	0	0
		Salt substitute:											
16	1205	Morton Salt Substitute	1 tbsp	6	0	0	0	<1	0	0	0	0	0
16	1206	No Salt, packet, Norcliff Thayer	1 packet	.75	0	0	0	0	0	0	0	0	0
16	1207	Light Salt, Morton	1 tsp	6	0	0	0	0	0	0	0	0	0
16	991	Vinegar, cider	1 tbsp	15	94	2	0	1	0	0	0	0	0
		Yeast:											
16	992	Baker's, dry, active, package	1 package	7	5	20	3	3	2	<1	t	.1	t
16	993	Brewer's, dry	1 tbsp	8	5	25	3	3	3	<.1	t	t	0

(Computer code number is for West Diet Analysis program)

H

GRP KEY: 1 = BEV   2 = DAIRY   3 = EGGS   4 = FAT/OIL   5 = FRUIT   6 = BAKERY   7 = GRAIN   8 = FISH   9 = BEEF   10 = POULTRY
11 = SAUSAGE   12 = MIXED/FAST   13 = NUTS/SEEDS   14 = SWEETS   15 = VEG/LEG   16 = MISC   22 = SOUP/SAUCE

Chol (mg)	Calc (mg)	Iron (mg)	Magn (mg)	Phos (mg)	Pota (mg)	Sodi (mg)	Zinc (mg)	VT-A (RE)	Thia (mg)	Ribo (mg)	Niac (mg)	V-B6 (mg)	Fola (µg)	VT-C (mg)
0	47	1.72	54	96	1178	2906	.56	250	.22	.18	3.3	.44	37	37
0	3	.11	3	6	72	178	.04	15	.01	.01	.21	.03	2	2
0	8	.41	8	16	107	7	.13	221	.02	.05	.46	—	—	4
0	38	.90	10	11	30	4	.14	<1	.01	.01	.1	—	—	<1
0	7	.37	4	8	50	26	.07	91	.01	.02	.21	—	1	2
0	22	1.9	82	109	235	1	1.01	1	.02	.1	.38	.01	18	0
0	4	.08	1	1	22	1	—	11	<.01	<.01	.03	<.01	.4	<1
0	.12	.08	.16	.7	.16	.5	<.01	0	0	0	0	0	0	0
0	28	.86	1	1	11	1	.05	1	<.01	<.01	.03	.02	—	1
0	10	.59	5	7	31	1	.08	2	<.01	<.01	.07	—	—	<1
0	50	1.50	13	16	110	6	.10	—	.01	.01	.09	.05	—	—
0	22	.2	3	18	48	2	1.06	0	.02	.01	.08	.40	<1	4
0	2	.08	2	12	31	1	.07	0	.01	<.01	.02	.57	2	<1
0	1	0	2	0	2	6	0	0	0	0	0	<.01	0	0
0	2	.05	5	3	46	1	.22	0	<.01	<.01	.08	.02	2	1
0	9	.10	4	5	44	14	.18	0	.01	<.01	.06	.01	2	1
0	124	3.87	71	275	427	599	2.70	6	.23	.13	1.01	.98	146	19
0	4	.1	3	4	7	63	.03	0	<.01	.01	.07	<.01	0	<1
0	24	.6	9	6	21	936	.03	12	<.01	<.01	.01	.01	<1	<1
0	40	1.49	2	1	4	392	.10	18	<.01	<.01	.02	<.01	.3	.4
0	8	.06	3	7	20	1	.05	0	01	<.01	.01	.03	3	<1
0	24	.66	4	3	25	<1	.07	10	<.01	t	.09	—	—	1
0	4	.50	4	7	49	1	.09	127	.01	.04	.32	—	—	2
0	9	.61	4	4	26	1	.03	<1	<.01	<.01	.02	0	—	0
0	6	.34	7	14	199	833	.09	21	.01	.02	.04	<.01	1	1
0	3	.20	2	6	20	201	.02	4	t	.01	.02	<.01	0	1
0	1	.21	1	4	11	329	.03	4	<.01	.01	.06	.01	<1	<1
0	3	.13	1	2	30	107	.01	2	t	t	<.01	0	0	1
0	33	.56	9	2	21	0	.09	12	.02	.01	.11	—	—	1
0	18	.86	19	41	347	191	.20	150	.09	.07	.93	.16	28	39
0	14	<.01	2	3	.3	2132	t	0	0	0	0	0	0	0
0	30	0	t	28	2800	t	0	0	0	0	0	0	0	0
0	—	—	—	—	385	0	—	0	0	0	0	0	0	0
0	<1	0	4	0	1500	1100	0	0	0	0	0	0	0	0
0	1	.09	<1	1	15	t	02	0	0	0	0	0	0	0
0	4	1.1	16	90	140	4	.43	t	.17	.38	2.7	.14	266	t
0	17[145]	1.39	18	140	152	10	.63	t	1.25	.34	3.16	.4	313	t

[145]Value varies from 6 to 60 mg.

(For purposes of calculations, use "0" for t, <1, <.1, <.01, etc.)

Table H–1 Food Composition

Grp	Computer Code No.	Food Description	Measure	Wt (g)	H₂O (%)	Ener (kcal)	Prot (g)	Carb (g)	Dietary Fiber (g)	Fat (g)	Sat	Mono	Poly
SOUPS, SAUCES, AND GRAVIES													
		SOUPS, canned, condensed:											
		Unprepared, condensed:											
22	1210	Cream of celery	1 c	251	85	180	3	18	1	11	2.8	2.6	5.0
22	1215	Cream of chicken	1 c	251	82	233	7	19	<1	15	4.2	.8	3.0
22	1216	Cream of mushroom	1 c	251	81	257	4	19	<1	19	5.2	3.6	8.9
22	1220	Onion	1 c	246	86	114	8	16	1	3	.5	1.5	1.3
		Prepared with equal volume of whole milk:											
22	994	Clam chowder, New England	1 c	248	85	163	9	17	1	7	3.0	2.3	1.1
22	1209	Cream of celery	1 c	248	87	165	6	15	<1	10	4.0	2.5	2.7
22	995	Cream of chicken	1 c	248	85	191	7	15	<1	12	5	4	2
22	996	Cream of mushroom	1 c	248	85	205	6	15	<1	14	5	3	5
22	1214	Cream of potato	1 c	248	87	148	6	17	<1	6	3.8	1.7	.6
22	1213	Oyster stew	1 c	245	89	134	6	10	0	8	5.1	2.1	.3
22	997	Tomato	1 c	248	85	160	6	22	<1	6	2.9	1.6	1.1
		Prepared with equal volume of water:											
22	998	Bean with bacon	1 c	253	84	173	8	23	3	6	1.5	2.2	1.8
22	999	Beef broth, bouillon, consommé	1 c	240	98	16	3	<1	0	1	.3	.2	t
22	1000	Beef noodle	1 c	244	92	84	5	9	<1	3	1.2	1.2	.5
22	1001	Chicken noodle	1 c	241	92	75	4	9	1	2	.7	1.1	.6
22	1002	Chicken rice	1 c	241	94	60	4	7	1	2	.5	.9	.4
22	1208	Chili beef soup	1 c	250	85	169	7	22	1	7	3.3	2.8	.3
22	1003	Clam chowder, Manhatten	1 c	244	92	78	2	12	1	2	.4	.4	1.3
22	1004	Cream of chicken	1 c	244	91	115	3	9	<1	7	2.1	3.3	1.5
22	1005	Cream of mushroom	1 c	244	90	130	2	9	1	9	2.4	1.7	4.2
22	1006	Minestrone	1 c	241	91	80	4	11	1	3	.5	.7	1.1
22	1211	Onion soup	1 c	241	93	57	4	8	<1	2	.3	.8	.7
22	1007	Split pea with ham	1 c	253	82	189	10	28	1	4	1.8	1.8	.6
22	1008	Tomato	1 c	244	90	86	2	17	<1	2	.4	.4	1.0
22	1009	Vegetable beef	1 c	244	92	79	6	10	1	2	.9	.8	.1
22	1010	Vegetarian vegetable	1 c	241	92	70	2	12	2	2	.3	.8	.7
		SOUPS, dehydrated:											
		Unprepared, dry products:											
22	1011	Bouillon	1 packet	6	3	14	1	1	<1	1	.3	.2	t
22	1012	Onion	1 packet	7	4	20	1	4	<1	<1	.1	.2	.1
		Prepared with water:											
22	1299	Beef broth/bouillon	1 c	244	97	20	1	2	<1	1	.3	.3	<.1
22	1376	Chicken broth/bouillon	1 c	244	97	21	1	1	<1	1	.3	.4	.4
22	1013	Chicken noodle	¾ c	188	94	40	2	6	<1	1	.2	.4	.3
22	1122	Cream of chicken	1 c	261	91	107	2	13	1	5	3.4	1.2	.4
22	1014	Onion	¾ c	184	96	20	1	4	<1	<1	.1	.3	.1
22	1217	Split pea	1 c	255	87	133	8	23	1	2	.4	.7	.3
22	1015	Tomato vegetable	¾ c	189	94	41	1	8	<1	1	.3	.3	.1
		SAUCES											
		From dry mixes, prepared with milk:											
22	1016	Cheese sauce	1 c	279	77	305	16	23	<1	17	9	5	2
22	1017	Hollandaise	1 c	259	84	240	5	14	—	20	12	6	1
22	1019	White sauce	1 c	264	81	240	10	21	<1	13	6	5	2
		From home recipe:											
22	1019	White sauce, medium[146]	1 c	250	73	395	10	24	<1	30	9	12	7
		Ready to serve:											
22	1020	Barbeque sauce	1 tbsp	16	81	10	<1	2	<1	<1	<.1	.1	.1
22	1021	Soy sauce	1 tbsp	18	71	9	1	2	0	t	0	0	0

[146] Made with enriched flour, margarine, and whole milk.

(Computer code number is for West Diet Analysis program)

GRP KEY: 1 = BEV 2 = DAIRY 3 = EGGS 4 = FAT/OIL 5 = FRUIT 6 = BAKERY 7 = GRAIN 8 = FISH 9 = BEEF 10 = POULTRY
11 = SAUSAGE 12 = MIXED/FAST 13 = NUTS/SEEDS 14 = SWEETS 15 = VEG/LEG 16 = MISC 22 = SOUP/SAUCE

Chol (mg)	Calc (mg)	Iron (mg)	Magn (mg)	Phos (mg)	Pota (mg)	Sodi (mg)	Zinc (mg)	VT-A (RE)	Thia (mg)	Ribo (mg)	Niac (mg)	V-B6 (mg)	Fola (µg)	VT-C (mg)
28	80	1.25	13	75	246	1899	.30	61	.06	.10	.67	.03	5	<1
20	68	1.21	5	75	174	1973	1.26	112	.06	.12	1.64	.03	3	<1
3	64	1.05	9	84	167	2032	1.19	0	.06	.17	1.62	.03	7	2
0	53	1.35	5	22	138	2116	1.23	0	.07	.05	1.21	.10	31	3
22	187	1.48	23	157	300	992	1.3	40	.07	.24	1.03	.13	12	4
32	186	.69	22	151	309	1010	.20	68	.07	.25	.44	.06	9	1
27	180	.67	18	152	273	1046	.68	94	.07	.26	.92	.07	8	1
20	178	.59	20	156	270	1076	.64	38	.08	.28	.81	.06	15	2
22	166	.54	17	160	323	1060	.68	67	.08	.24	.64	.09	9	1
32	167	1.04	21	162	235	1040	10.3	45	.07	.23	.34	.06	7	4
17	159	1.82	23	148	450	932	.29	109	.13	.25	1.52	.16	21	68
3	81	2.05	44	132	403	952	1.03	89	.09	.03	.57	.04	32	2
1	15	.41	9	31	130	782	.6	0	<.01	.05	1.87	.07	2	0
5	15	1.1	6	46	100	952	1.54	63	.07	.06	1.07	.04	4	<1
7	17	.78	7	36	55	900	.55	71	.05	.06	1.39	.01	2	<1
7	17	.75	1	22	101	815	.26	66	.02	.02	1.13	.02	1	<1
12	43	2.40	30	148	525	1035	1.40	503	.06	.08	1.07	.16	10	4
2	27	1.64	10	41	188	578	.98	98	.03	.04	.82	.10	10	4
10	34	.61	3	37	88	986	.63	56	.03	.06	.82	.02	2	<1
2	46	.5	5	49	100	1032	.59	0	.05	.09	.7	.02	3	1
2	34	.92	7	56	312	911	.74	234	.05	.04	.94	.10	16	1
0	26	.67	2	11	69	1053	.61	0	.03	.02	.60	.05	15	1
8	22	2.28	48	213	399	1008	1.32	44	.15	.08	1.48	.07	3	1
0	13	1.76	8	34	263	872	.24	69	.09	.05	1.42	.11	15	67
5	17	1.11	6	41	173	956	2	189	.04	.05	1.03	.08	11	2
0	21	1.08	7	35	209	823	.46	301	.05	.05	.92	.06	11	1
1	4	.06	3	19	27	1019	0	<1	<.01	.02	.27	.01	2	0
<1	10	.14	3	23	47	627	.06	<1	.02	.04	.4	.01	2	<1
0	10	.02	7	24	37	1362	.07	.5	<.01	.02	.36	0	0	.01
1	15	.08	4	13	25	1484	.01	4	.01	.03	.20	.02	—	<1
2	24	.37	5	24	23	957	.15	5	.05	.04	.66	.01	1	<1
3	76	—	—	96	215	1184	—	—	—	.20	—	.05	—	—
0	9	.14	6	22	48	635	.06	<1	.02	.04	.36	<.01	2	<1
3	22	1.01	46	134	238	1220	.59	5	.22	.15	1.34	.05	15	—
0	6	.47	15	23	78	856	.13	15	.04	.03	.59	.04	2	5
53	569	.3	32	438	552	1565	.95	117	.15	.56	.3	.1	12	2
52	124	.9	—	127	124	1564	—	220	.05	.18	.1	.5	—	t
34	425	.3	30	256	444	797	1.15	92	.08	.45	.5	.06	16	3
32	292	.9	35	238	381	888	1.05	340	.15	.43	.8	.1	12	2
0	3	.13	1	3	27	128	.03	14	<.01	<.01	.06	.02	1	1
0	3	.36	6	20	32	1029	.07	0	.01	.02	.61	.03	3	0

(For purposes of calculations, use "0" for t, <1, <.1, <.01, etc.)

H

Table H–1 Food Composition

Grp	Computer Code No.	Food Description	Measure	Wt (g)	H$_2$O (%)	Ener (kcal)	Prot (g)	Carb (g)	Dietary Fiber (g)	Fat (g)	Fat Breakdown (g) Sat	Mono	Poly
		SOUPS, SAUCES and GRAVIES—Con.											
		SAUCES—Con.											
		Spaghetti sauce: canned:											
22	1377	Plain	1 c	249	75	272	5	40	3	12	1.7	6.1	3.3
22	1378	With meat	.8 c	206	75	220	8	27	1	10	2.5	4.5	1.5
22	1379	With mushrooms	.75 c	185	75	162	2	9	2	5	.6	2.3	1.2
22	1380	Teriyaki sauce	1 tbsp	18	84	15	1	3	0	<1	t	t	<.1
		GRAVIES:											
		Canned:											
22	1022	Beef	1 c	233	87	123	9	11	<1	5	2.7	2.2	.2
22	1023	Chicken	1 c	238	85	189	5	13	<1	14	3.4	6.1	3.6
22	1024	Mushroom	1 c	238	89	120	3	13	<1	6	1	3	2.4
		From dry mix:											
22	1025	Brown	1 c	258	92	75	2	13	<1	2	.8	.7	.1
22	1026	Chicken	1 c	260	91	85	3	14	<1	2	.5	.9	.4

(Computer code number is for West Diet Analysis program)

GRP KEY: 1=BEV 2=DAIRY 3=EGGS 4=FAT/OIL 5=FRUIT 6=BAKERY 7=GRAIN 8=FISH 9=BEEF 10=POULTRY
11=SAUSAGE 12=MIXED/FAST 13=NUTS/SEEDS 14=SWEETS 15=VEG/LEG 16=MISC 22=SOUP/SAUCE

Chol (mg)	Calc (mg)	Iron (mg)	Magn (mg)	Phos (mg)	Pota (mg)	Sodi (mg)	Zinc (mg)	VT-A (RE)	Thia (mg)	Ribo (mg)	Niac (mg)	V-B6 (mg)	Fola (μg)	VT-C (mg)
0	70	1.62	60	90	957	1236	.53	306	.14	.15	3.75	.40	39	28
17	36	2.80	15	106	444	1045	1.05	189	.20	.16	3.40	.27	13	2
0	22	1.50	22	45	500	744	.51	362	.12	.12	1.40	.24	19	14
0	4	.31	11	28	41	690	.02	0	<.01	.01	.23	.02	4	0
7	14	1.63	5	70	189	1305	2.33	0	.07	.08	1.54	.02	5	0
5	48	1.1	5	69	260	1375	1.91	264	.04	.1	1.06	.02	3	0
0	17	1.6	—	36	252	1357	1.66	0	.08	.15	1.6	.05	0	0
3	67	.2	10	44	57	1076	.31	0	.04	.09	.8	0	0	0
3	39	.3	—	47	62	1134	.32	0	.05	.15	.8	.03	—	3

(For purposes of calculations, use "0" for t, <1, <.1, <.01, etc.)

H

Table H–1 Food Composition

	Computer Code								Dietary		Fat Breakdown (g)		
Grp	No.	Food Description	Measure	Wt (g)	H₂O (%)	Ener (kcal)	Prot (g)	Carb (g)	Fiber (g)	Fat (g)	Sat	Mono	Poly

Grp	No.	Food Description	Measure	Wt (g)	H$_2$O (%)	Ener (kcal)	Prot (g)	Carb (g)	Dietary Fiber (g)	Fat (g)	Sat	Mono	Poly
ARBY'S													
12	1402	Bac'n Cheddar, deluxe	1 ea	229	56	532	29	35	<1	33	8	14	11
		Roast beef sandwiches:											
12	1403	Regular	1 ea	147	51	353	22	32	<1	15	7	5	2
12	1404	Junior	1 ea	85	48	218	13	21	<1	71	4	5	2
12	1405	Super	1 ea	246	58	529	33	46	<1	29	3	11	9
12	1406	Deluxe	1 ea	247	62	486	26	43	<1	23	9	8	5
12	1407	Beef 'n Cheddar	1 ea	198	57	451	25	42	<1	20	7	8	4
		Chicken sandwiches:											
12	1408	Chicken breast sandwich	1 ea	184	52	489	23	48	<1	26	4	8	14
12	1409	Chicken salad sandwich	1 ea	156	53	386	18	33	<1	20	—	—	—
12	1410	Chicken salad & croissant	1 ea	150	50	472	22	16	<1	36	—	—	—
12	1411	Chicken club sandwich	1 ea	234	44	513	31	40	<1	29	5	8	14
12	1412	Hot ham and cheese sandwich	1 ea	162	62	330	23	33	<1	15	4	7	3
12	1413	Turkey deluxe sandwich	1 ea	221	61	399	27	36	<1	20	4	4	12
		Baked potatoes:											
12	1414	Plain	1 ea	241	75	240	6	50	6	<2	0	.5	1
12	1415	Deluxe, w/butter & sour cream	1 ea	312	74	463	8	53	6	25	12	8	3
12	1416	W/broccoli & cheese	1 ea	340	70	417	11	85	6	18	7	7	8
12	1417	W/mushrooms & cheese	1 ea	347	70	515	15	58	6	27	6	11	9
12	1418	Taco	1 ea	425	70	619	23	73	6	27	11	9	3
		Milkshakes:											
12	1419	Chocolate	1 ea	340	74	451	10	77	<1	12	3	7	2
12	1420	Jamocha	1 ea	326	75	368	9	59	0	11	3	6	2
12	1421	Vanilla	1 ea	312	75	330	11	46	0	12	4	5	2

Source: Arby's Inc., Atlanta Georgia for the basic nutrients. Values for dietary fiber, magnesium, phosphorus, potassium, zinc, vitamin A (in RE's), B6, folacin, some of the fatty acids, and percent water are estimates calculated from known values for major ingredients.

Grp	No.	Food Description	Measure	Wt (g)	H$_2$O (%)	Ener (kcal)	Prot (g)	Carb (g)	Dietary Fiber (g)	Fat (g)	Sat	Mono	Poly
BURGER KING													
		Croissant sandwiches:											
12	1422	With egg, bacon & cheese	1 ea	119	49	335	15	20	<1	24	13	8	2
12	1423	With egg, sausage & cheese	1 ea	163	49	538	19	20	<1	41	20	12	3
12	1424	With egg, ham & cheese	1 ea	145	58	335	18	20	<1	20	12	7	1
		Whopper sandwiches:											
12	1425	Whopper	1 ea	265	57	640	27	42	<1	41	16	19	4
12	1426	Whopper w/cheese	1 ea	289	57	723	31	43	<1	48	20	20	3
12	1427	Double beef	1 ea	351	56	850	46	52	<1	52	20	24	5
12	1428	Double w/cheese	1 ea	374	55	950	51	54	<1	60	24	28	4
12	1429	Whopper, Junior	1 ea	136	52	370	15	31	<1	17	6	8	1
12	1430	Whopper, Junior w/cheese	1 ea	158	55	420	17	32	<1	20	9	8	1
12	1431	Hamburger	1 ea	109	46	275	15	29	<1	12	5	6	<1
12	1432	Cheeseburger	1 ea	120	45	317	17	30	<1	15	7	6	1
12	1433	Bacon double cheeseburger	1 ea	159	41	510	33	27	<1	31	14	15	2
12	1434	Chicken sandwich	1 ea	230	46	688	26	56	<1	40	11	17	10
12	1435	Chicken tenders	1 ea	95	50	204	20	10	0	10	3	4	2
12	1436	Ham & cheese sandwich	1 ea	230	59	471	24	44	<1	23	10	8	4
12	1437	Whaler fish sandwich	1 ea	189	45	488	19	45	<1	27	6	9	10
12	1438	Whaler sandwich w/cheese	1 ea	201	45	530	21	46	<1	30	7	9	10
12	1439	French fries, regular	1 svg	74	37	227	3	24	<1	13	5	4	1
12	1440	Onion rings, regular	1 svg	79	37	274	4	28	<1	16	5	7	4
		Milkshakes:											
12	1441	Chocolate, medium	1 ea	273	76	320	8	46	<1	12	—	—	—
12	1442	Vanilla, medium	1 ea	273	74	321	9	49	<1	10	—	—	—

GRP KEY: 1 = BEV   2 = DAIRY   3 = EGGS   4 = FAT/OIL   5 = FRUIT   6 = BAKERY   7 = GRAIN   8 = FISH   9 = BEEF   10 = POULTRY
11 = SAUSAGE   12 = MIXED/FAST   13 = NUTS/SEEDS   14 = SWEETS   15 = VEG/LEG   16 = MISC   22 = SOUP/SAUCE

Chol (mg)	Calc (mg)	Iron (mg)	Magn (mg)	Phos (mg)	Pota (mg)	Sodi (mg)	Zinc (mg)	VT-A (RE)	Thia (mg)	Ribo (mg)	Niac (mg)	V-B6 (mg)	Fola (µg)	VT-C (mg)
83	120	2.5	—	—	422	1672	3	85	.4	.48	7	—	—	1
39	32	2	16	120	368	588	3	t	.27	.43	6.23	.20	14	0
23	16	1	8	60	197	345	1.5	t	.13	.24	4	.10	7	0
47	48	2.5	25	190	503	798	3.8	60	.34	.4	7	.30	21	1.2
59	100	6.30	25	190	500	1288	3.8	10	.30	.34	5	.30	22	t
52	76	2	24	260	335	955	3	60	.27	.4	6	.22	19	0
45	64	2	30	180	330	1099	1.5	0	.2	.5	7	.38	18	5
30	—	—	—	—	—	630	—	—	—	—	—	—	—	—
12	—	—	—	—	—	725	—	—	—	—	—	—	—	—
75	120	2	—	—	430	1423	2.3	—	.47	.57	8	—	—	0
45	80	1.5	31	405	312	1350	.9	60	.4	.32	4	.31	26	24
39	64	1.5	30	250	346	1047	1.5	91	.27	.4	7	.52	20	5
0	0	1.80	80	175	1333	58	0	0	.08	.13	2.7	1.08	30	33
40	520	1.5	83	200	1420	203	0	60	.08	.13	2.7	1.10	33	33
22	80	1.5	97	400	1455	361	0	60	.08	.16	2.7	1.15	60	45
47	200	1.5	91	440	1445	923	9	227	.13	.24	2.7	1.25	36	33
145	450	3.60	105	530	1425	1065	4.7	860	.38	.26	8	1.40	38	63
36	200	.4	48	350	410	341	1.5	91	.11	.65	.7	.14	14	0
35	200	0	36	350	525	262	1.5	91	.11	.65	.7	.14	14	0
32	240	0	36	350	686	281	1.5	91	.11	.65	0	.14	37	0
249	136	2.00	20	249	182	762	1.5	150	.32	.30	2	.06	24	t
293	145	2.90	19	292	284	1042	2.4	150	.36	.32	4	.06	24	t
262	136	2.20	24	317	256	987	1.9	150	.49	.32	3	.06	24	t
94	80	4.90	43	237	547	842	4.5	60	.33	.41	7	.40	35	14
117	210	4.90	47	360	570	1126	5.1	85	.34	.48	7	.40	35	14
188	91	7.30	60	387	760	1080	8.5	60	.34	.56	10	.50	45	14
211	222	7.30	65	510	730	1535	9.1	85	.35	.63	10	.50	45	14
41	40	2.80	24	127	275	486	2.3	30	.23	.25	4	.20	17	6
52	105	2.80	27	189	287	628	2.6	85	.23	.29	4	.20	17	6
37	37	2.70	23	124	235	509	2.4	15	.23	.25	4	.12	18	3
48	102	3.80	26	186	247	651	2.6	70	.23	.29	4	.13	24	3
104	168	3.80	37	328	363	728	5.1	85	.31	.42	6	.30	30	t
82	79	3.30	54	274	375	1423	1.2	13	.45	.31	10	.40	18	t
47	18	.70	24	236	200	636	.6	5	.08	.08	7	.34	10	t
70	195	3.20	42	384	419	1534	2.4	85	.87	.42	6	.31	25	7
84	t	2.20	40	249	366	592	.1	20	.28	.21	4	.13	3	t
95	112	2.20	43	311	378	734	1.1	40	.27	.24	4	.13	3	t
14	t	.50	21	114	360	160	.3	0	.10	.30	7.5	.23	20	t
0	124	.80	18	195	173	665	.4	—	t	t	t	.07	8	t
—	260	1.60	46	262	567	202	1.0	—	.13	.55	t	—	—	t
—	295	t	32	284	505	205	1.0	—	.11	.57	t	—	—	t

Table H–1 Food Composition

Grp	Computer Code No.	Food Description	Measure	Wt (g)	H$_2$O (%)	Ener (kcal)	Prot (g)	Carb (g)	Dietary Fiber (g)	Fat (g)	Fat Breakdown (g) Sat	Mono	Poly
BURGER KING—Con.													
		Pies:											
12	1443	Apple pie	1 ea	125	51	305	3	44	<1	12	—	—	—
12	1444	Cherry pie	1 ea	128	42	357	4	55	<1	13	—	—	—
12	1445	Pecan pie	1 ea	113	20	459	5	64	1	20	3	11	5

Source: Burger King Corporation for basic nutrients. Values for dietary fiber and percent water, calculated from known values for major ingredients.

Grp	No.	Food Description	Measure	Wt (g)	H$_2$O (%)	Ener (kcal)	Prot (g)	Carb (g)	Dietary Fiber (g)	Fat (g)	Sat	Mono	Poly
DAIRY QUEEN													
		Ice cream cones:											
12	1446	Small	1 ea	85	65	140	3	22	0	4	2	1	<1
12	1447	Regular	1 ea	142	65	240	6	38	0	7	—	—	—
12	1448	Large	1 ea	213	65	340	9	57	0	10	—	—	—
		Dipped ice cream cones:											
12	1449	Small	1 ea	92	58	190	3	25	<1	9	—	—	—
12	1450	Regular	1 ea	156	58	340	6	42	<1	16	—	—	—
12	1451	Large	1 ea	234	58	510	9	64	<1	24	—	—	—
		Sundaes:											
12	1452	Small	1 ea	106	60	190	3	33	<1	4	—	—	—
12	1453	Regular	1 ea	177	60	310	5	56	<1	8	—	—	—
12	1454	Large	1 ea	248	60	440	8	78	<1	10	—	—	—
12	1455	Banana split	1 ea	383	67	540	9	103	<1	11	—	—	—
12	1456	Peanut buster parfait	1 ea	305	52	740	16	94	<1	34	—	—	—
12	1457	Hot fudge brownie delight	1 ea	266	55	600	9	85	<1	25	—	—	—
12	1458	Strawberry shortcake	1 ea	312	61	540	10	100	<1	11	—	—	—
12	1459	Buster bar	1 ea	149	45	460	10	41	<1	29	—	—	—
12	1460	Dilly bar	1 ea	85	55	210	3	21	<1	13	—	—	—
12	1461	DQ ice cream sandwich	1 ea	60	47	140	3	24	<1	4	—	—	—
		Milkshakes:											
12	1462	Small	1 ea	291	63	490	10	82	<1	13	—	—	—
12	1463	Regular	1 ea	418	63	710	14	120	<1	19	—	—	—
12	1464	Large	1 ea	489	63	831	16	140	<1	22	—	—	—
		Malted milkshakes:											
12	1465	Small	1 ea	291	60	520	10	91	<1	13	—	—	—
12	1466	Regular	1 ea	418	60	760	14	134	<1	18	—	—	—
12	1467	Large	1 ea	489	60	889	16	157	<1	21	—	—	—
12	1468	Float	1 ea	397	76	410	5	82	0	7	—	—	—
12	1469	Freeze	1 ea	397	72	500	9	89	0	12	—	—	—
		Mr. Misty:											
12	1470	Regular	1 ea	330	81	250	0	63	0	0	0	0	0
12	1471	Kiss	1 ea	89	81	70	0	17	0	0	0	0	0
12	1472	Freeze	1 ea	411	72	500	9	91	0	12	—	—	—
12	1473	Float	1 ea	411	78	390	5	74	0	7	—	—	—
12	1474	Chicken sandwich	1 ea	202	46	608	27	46	<1	34	8	15	17
12	1475	Fish fillet sandwich	1 ea	177	52	430	20	45	<1	18	4	6	6
12	1476	Fish fillet sandwich w/cheese	1 ea	191	51	483	23	46	<1	22	7	7	6
		Hamburgers:											
12	1477	Single	1 ea	148	51	360	21	33	<1	16	6	7	1
12	1478	Double	1 ea	210	52	530	36	33	<1	28	10	13	2
12	1479	Triple	1 ea	272	52	710	51	33	<1	45	17	21	4
		Cheeseburgers:											
12	1480	Single	1 ea	162	51	410	24	33	<1	20	8	8	1
12	1481	Double	1 ea	239	51	650	43	34	<1	37	15	14	2
12	1482	Triple	1 ea	301	52	820	58	34	<1	50	20	20	3

GRP KEY: 1 = BEV 2 = DAIRY 3 = EGGS 4 = FAT/OIL 5 = FRUIT 6 = BAKERY 7 = GRAIN 8 = FISH 9 = BEEF 10 = POULTRY
11 = SAUSAGE 12 = MIXED/FAST 13 = NUTS/SEEDS 14 = SWEETS 15 = VEG/LEG 16 = MISC 22 = SOUP/SAUCE

Chol (mg)	Calc (mg)	Iron (mg)	Magn (mg)	Phos (mg)	Pota (mg)	Sodi (mg)	Zinc (mg)	VT-A (RE)	Thia (mg)	Ribo (mg)	Niac (mg)	V-B6 (mg)	Fola (µg)	VT-C (mg)
4	t	1.20	t	31	122	412	.2	4	.27	.16	.6	.03	7	5
6	t	1.10	12	37	166	204	.2	15	.24	.16	.5	.03	4	8
4	24	1.10	16	84	204	374	<1	16	.28	.18	.6	.06	15	t
10	100	.40	13	100	134	45	.47	25	.03	.17	t	.04	2	t
15	150	.70	20	200	220	80	.49	49	.06	.34	t	.06	3	t
25	250	1.40	30	300	330	115	1.0	98	.12	.51	t	.09	4	t
10	100	.40	13	100	134	55	.47	25	.03	.17	t	.04	2	t
20	150	.70	20	200	220	100	.70	49	.06	.34	t	.06	3	t
30	250	1.40	30	300	330	145	1.0	98	.12	.51	t	.09	4	t
10	100	.40	13	150	145	75	.45	25	.03	.17	.17	.03	2	t
20	200	1.10	26	200	290	120	.90	49	.06	.34	.3	.06	4	t
30	250	1.40	40	300	435	165	1.35	98	.12	.43	.4	.09	6	t
30	250	1.80	60	350	670	150	2.1	160	.15	.51	.4	.80	9	15
30	250	1.80	50	450	500	250	1.5	74	.15	.43	2	.10	7	t
20	200	1.80	30	300	300	225	.90	74	.12	.34	.3	.06	4	t
25	250	1.80	—	300	—	215	—	98	.23	.51	t	—	—	12
10	100	1.10	—	250	—	175	—	25	.12	.17	2	—	—	t
10	100	.40	—	100	—	50	—	25	.03	.17	t	—	—	t
5	60	.04	—	60	—	40	—	15	.03	.07	.4	—	—	t
35	350	1.80	30	400	480	180	.10	123	.15	.60	.3	.14	3	t
50	450	2.70	43	500	690	260	.14	184	.23	.77	.4	.20	4	t
60	550	3.60	60	600	960	304	.20	200	.30	.94	.4	.28	6	t
35	350	2.70	30	400	480	180	.10	123	.15	.60	.4	.14	3	t
50	450	4.50	43	600	690	260	.14	184	.30	.85	.8	.20	4	t
60	550	5.40	60	700	960	304	.20	200	.37	.90	.8	.28	6	t
20	200	1.10	—	200	—	85	—	40	.06	.26	t	—	—	t
30	300	1.80	—	350	—	180	—	98	.15	.51	t	—	—	t
0	t	t	—	t	—	10	—	0	t	t	t	—	—	t
0	t	t	—	t	—	10	—	—	t	t	t	—	—	t
30	300	1.40	—	200	—	140	—	98	.12	.51	t	—	—	t
20	200	.70	—	200	—	95	—	49	.06	.26	t	—	—	t
78	150	5.4	15	250	200	725	.5	20	.6	.59	.8	.16	9	2.4
40	150	3.6	20	150	370	674	.3	<1	.6	.42	8	.16	40	<1
49	250	3.6	22	200	370	870	.3	100	.67	.51	8	.16	20	<1
45	100	3.60	33	150	290	630	4.5	10	.30	.17	5	.18	16	t
85	100	6.30	45	300	410	660	6.4	20	.45	.34	9	.28	23	t
135	100	9.00	60	450	532	690	8.2	28	.60	.51	14	.33	29	t
50	200	3.60	35	250	300	790	5.0	110	.30	.17	5	.20	20	t
95	350	6.30	50	500	443	980	7.3	160	.45	.43	9	.30	30	t
145	350	9.00	65	700	550	1010	9.2	200	.60	.60	14	.55	37	t

H

Table H–1 Food Composition

Grp	Computer Code No.	Food Description	Measure	Wt (g)	H₂O (%)	Ener (kcal)	Prot (g)	Carb (g)	Dietary Fiber (g)	Fat (g)	Sat	Mono	Poly
											Fat Breakdown (g)		
DAIRY QUEEN—Con.													
		Hotdogs:											
12	1483	Regular	1 ea	100	50	280	11	21	<1	16	6	7	2
12	1484	With cheese	1 ea	114	49	330	15	21	<1	21	8	8	2
12	1485	With chili	1 ea	128	55	320	13	23	2	20	8	8	2
		Super hotdogs:											
12	1486	Regular	1 ea	175	48	520	17	44	<1	27	9	12	3
12	1487	With cheese	1 ea	196	48	580	22	45	<1	34	11	13	3
12	1488	With chili	1 ea	218	53	570	21	47	2	32	11	13	3
12	1489	French fries, small	1 svg	71	47	200	2	25	<1	10	4	3	<1
12	1490	French fries, large	1 svg	113	47	320	3	40	<1	16	7	5	1
12	1491	Onion Rings	1 svg	85	28	280	4	31	<1	16	5	7	4

Source: International Dairy Queen Inc., Minneapolis, MN for basic nutrients. Values for dietary fiber, magnesium, potassium, zinc, fatty acids, vitamin A (RE's), B6, folacin and percent water, calculated from known values for the major ingredients.

Grp	Computer Code No.	Food Description	Measure	Wt (g)	H₂O (%)	Ener (kcal)	Prot (g)	Carb (g)	Dietary Fiber (g)	Fat (g)	Sat	Mono	Poly
JACK IN THE BOX													
12	1492	Breakfast Jack sandwich	1 ea	126	49	307	18	30	<1	13	—	—	—
12	1493	Canadian crescent	1 ea	134	42	472	19	25	<1	31	—	—	—
12	1494	Sausage crescent	1 ea	156	38	584	22	28	<1	43	—	—	—
12	1495	Supreme crescent	1 ea	146	38	547	20	27	<1	40	—	—	—
12	1496	Pancakes breakfast platter	1 ea	231	45	612	15	87	<1	22	8.6	7.6	3.5
12	1497	Scrambled egg breakfast platter	1 ea	249	51	662	24	52	<1	40	17.1	16	4.7
12	1498	Hamburger	1 ea	98	44	276	13	30	<1	12	—	—	—
12	1499	Cheeseburger	1 ea	113	44	323	16	32	<1	15	—	—	—
12	1500	Jumbo Jack	1 ea	205	57	485	26	38	<1	26	—	—	—
12	1501	Jumbo Jack w/cheese	1 ea	246	56	630	32	45	<1	35	—	—	—
12	1502	Bacon cheeseburger supreme	1 ea	231	45	724	34	44	<1	46	—	—	—
12	1503	Swiss & baconburger	1 ea	231	52	643	33	31	<1	43	—	—	—
12	1504	Ham & swiss burger	1 ea	203	44	638	36	37	<1	39	—	—	—
12	1505	Chicken supreme	1 ea	228	52	601	31	39	<1	36	—	—	—
12	1506	Moby Jack sandwich	1 ea	137	40	444	16	39	<1	25	—	—	—
12	1583	Double cheeseburger	1 ea	149	64	467	21	33	—	27	12.3	11.6	3.1
		Tacos:											
12	1508	Regular	1 ea	81	57	191	8	16	<1	11	—	—	—
12	1509	Super	1 ea	135	63	288	12	21	<1	17	—	—	—
12	1513	Taco salad	1 ea	358	81	377	31	10	1	24	—	—	—
12	1516	French fries	1 svg	68	40	221	2	27	<1	12	—	—	—
12	1517	Hash brown potatoes	1 svg	62	60	116	2	11	<1	7	3.6	3.2	.4
12	1518	Onion rings	1 svg	108	28	382	5	39	<1	23	—	—	—
		Milkshakes:											
12	1519	Chocolate	1 ea	322	77	330	11	55	0	7	—	—	—
12	1520	Strawberry	1 ea	328	77	320	10	55	0	7	—	—	—
12	1521	Vanilla	1 ea	317	76	320	10	57	0	6	—	—	—
12	1522	Apple turnover	1 ea	119	38	410	4	45	<1	24	—	—	—

Source: Jack in the Box Restaurants, Foodmaker, Inc., San Diego, CA for basic nutrients. Some values for dietary fiber, magnesium, phosphorus, potassium, zinc, vitamin A (RE's), B6, folacin, and fatty acids calculated from known values for major ingredients.

H

GRP KEY: 1 = BEV   2 = DAIRY   3 = EGGS   4 = FAT/OIL   5 = FRUIT   6 = BAKERY   7 = GRAIN   8 = FISH   9 = BEEF   10 = POULTRY
11 = SAUSAGE   12 = MIXED/FAST   13 = NUTS/SEEDS   14 = SWEETS   15 = VEG/LEG   16 = MISC   22 = SOUP/SAUCE

Chol (mg)	Calc (mg)	Iron (mg)	Magn (mg)	Phos (mg)	Pota (mg)	Sodi (mg)	Zinc (mg)	VT-A (RE)	Thia (mg)	Ribo (mg)	Niac (mg)	V-B6 (mg)	Fola (µg)	VT-C (mg)
45	80	1.40	21	100	130	830	1.4	t	.12	.14	3	.08	20	<1
55	150	1.40	24	200	140	990	1.9	85	.12	.17	3	.08	24	<1
55	80	1.80	38	150	170	985	1.8	60	.15	.26	4	.17	30	<1
80	150	2.70	24	150	210	1365	2.8	t	.23	.26	5	.14	35	<1
100	250	1.40	38	300	220	1605	2.5	100	.23	.26	5	.16	39	<1
100	150	2.70	48	250	250	1595	2.5	60	.23	.43	6	.25	45	<1
10	t	.34	16	60	450	115	t	0	.06	t	.8	.16	15	9
15	t	1.08	24	100	700	185	.3	0	.09	.03	1.2	.30	25	15
15	20	.72	16	60	110	140	.3	15	.09	t	.4	.08	10	2
203	170	3.10	24	310	190	871	1.8	120	.47	.41	3	.11	—	<1
226	125	3.40	—	—	—	851	—	135	.50	.40	3.6	—	—	3
187	170	2.90	—	—	—	1012	—	—	.60	.51	4.6	—	—	t
178	150	2.70	—	—	—	1053	—	—	.64	.54	4.2	—	—	t
99	100	1.8	36	633	237	888	1.9	69	.03	.75	7	.19	3	6
354	200	5.4	55	483	635	1188	3.0	252	.3	.77	5	.34	30	4.8
29	70	2.70	20	115	165	521	1.8	9	.36	.24	3.2	.10	—	1
42	160	2.70	22	194	177	749	2.3	57	.36	.27	3.3	.10	—	1
64	97	6.90	35	208	390	905	3.7	—	.51	.21	7	.25	—	5
110	250	4.50	49	411	499	1665	4.8	—	.53	.34	12	.31	—	5
70	310	4.90	—	—	—	1307	—	—	.56	.51	8.8	—	—	3
99	230	4.70	—	—	—	1354	—	—	.45	.41	6.8	—	—	3
117	268	6.10	—	—	—	1330	—	—	.76	.48	7.6	—	—	10
60	240	3.00	—	—	—	1582	—	—	.52	.37	10.6	—	—	4
47	160	2.20	30	263	246	820	1.1	—	.40	.25	2.8	.08	—	<1
72	400	2.7	—	—	—	842	—	—	.15	.34	6	—	—	—
21	100	1.10	35	146	257	460	1.2	—	.07	.17	1.0	.13	—	<1
37	150	1.60	45	198	347	765	1.8	—	.12	.08	1.4	.18	—	2
102	280	4.30	—	—	—	1436	—	141	.18	.53	6	—	—	7
8	10	.50	23	75	360	164	.26	<1	.07	.03	1.20	.18	—	3
3	40	.36	—	—	—	211	—	0	.06	.03	1.2	—	—	4
27	30	1.40	16	69	109	407	.40	<1	.21	.12	1.80	.06	—	3
25	350	.70	55	330	650	270	1.20	—	.15	.59	.60	.18	—	3
25	350	.40	40	328	613	240	1.10	—	.15	.43	.40	.16	—	3
25	350	.30	38	312	599	230	1.00	<1	.15	.34	.40	.20	—	<1
15	11	1.40	10	33	69	350	.20	—	.23	.12	2.50	.03	—	<1

H

Table H–1 Food Composition

Grp	Computer Code No.	Food Description	Measure	Wt (g)	H₂O (%)	Ener (kcal)	Prot (g)	Carb (g)	Dietary Fiber (g)	Fat (g)	Fat Breakdown (g)		
											Sat	Mono	Poly
KENTUCKY FRIED CHICKEN													
		Original Recipe:											
12	1253	Center breast	1 ea	95	52	236	24	7	<1	14	4	7	2
12	1251	Side breast	1 ea	69	39	199	16	7	<1	12	3	5	3
12	1250	Drumstick	1 ea	47	53	117	12	3	<1	7	2	3	2
12	1252	Thigh	1 ea	88	49	257	18	7	<1	18	4	7	4
12	1249	Wing	1 ea	42	44	136	10	4	<1	9	2	4	2
		Dinners:											
12	1254	2 pce dinner, white	1 ea	322	64	604	30	48	1	32	7	12	10
12	1255	2 pce dinner, dark	1 ea	346	65	643	35	46	1	35	8	13	11
12	1256	2 pce dinner, combination	1 ea	341	63	661	33	48	1	38	8	14	11
		Extra crispy recipe:											
12	1261	Center breast	1 ea	104	39	297	24	14	<1	16	4	7	4
12	1259	Side breast	1 ea	84	39	286	17	14	<1	18	5	7	4
12	1258	Drumstick	1 ea	58	51	155	13	5	<1	9	2	4	2
12	1260	Thigh	1 ea	107	45	343	20	13	<1	23	6	10	6
12	1257	Wing	1 ea	53	36	201	11	9	<1	14	4	6	3
		Dinners:											
12	1262	2 pce dinner, white	1 ea	348	60	755	33	60	1	43	10	16	12
12	1263	2 pce dinner, dark	1 ea	375	62	765	38	55	1	54	11	16	13
12	1264	2 pce dinner, combination	1 ea	371	60	902	36	58	1	48	12	18	14
12	1265	Mashed potatoes	⅓ c	80	81	60	2	12	<1	1	<1	<1	<1
12	1266	Chicken gravy	⅓ c	78	76	59	2	4	<1	4	1	2	<1
12	1267	Dinner roll	1 ea	21	31	61	2	11	<1	1	<1	<1	<1
12	1268	Corn on the cob	1 ea	143	70	176	5	32	2	3	<1	1	1
12	1269	Coleslaw	⅓ c	79	76	103	1	12	<1	6	1	2	3
12	1381	Kentucky nuggets	1 ea	16	44	46	3	2	<1	3	1	2	<1
		Kentucky nugget sauces:											
12	1382	Barbeque	2 tbsp	30	51	35	<1	7	—	1	<1	<1	<1
12	1383	Sweet & sour	2 tbsp	30	50	58	<1	13	—	1	<1	<1	<1
12	1384	Honey	1 tbsp	15	50	49	0	12	—	<1	—	—	—
12	1385	Mustard	2 tbsp	30	52	36	1	6	—	1	—	—	—
12	1386	Kentucky fries	1 svg	119	45	268	5	33	<1	13	3	8	1
12	1387	Mashed potatoes & gravy	⅓ c	86	80	62	2	10	<1	1	<1	<1	<1
12	1388	Buttermilk biscuit	1 ea	75	27	269	5	32	<1	14	4	8	1
12	1389	Potato salad	⅓ c	90	76	141	2	13	1	9	1	3	5
12	1390	Baked beans	⅓ c	89	71	105	5	18	6	1	<1	<1	<1
12	1391	Chicken Little sandwich	1 ea	57	52	177	6	17	1	9	2	3	3

Source: Kentucky Fried Chicken Corporation

Grp	Computer Code No.	Food Description	Measure	Wt (g)	H₂O (%)	Ener (kcal)	Prot (g)	Carb (g)	Dietary Fiber (g)	Fat (g)	Sat	Mono	Poly
LONG JOHN SILVER'S													
		Fish, batter fried:											
12	1523	Fish & fryes, 3 pce	1 ea	350	55	853	43	64	<1	48	—	—	—
12	1524	Fish & fryes, 2 pce	1 ea	260	53	651	30	53	<1	36	—	—	—
12	1525	Fish dinner, 3 pce	1 ea	540	60	1180	47	93	<1	70	—	—	—
		Fish, breaded & fried:											
12	1526	Fish dinner, 3 pce	1 ea	450	60	940	35	84	<1	52	—	—	—
12	1527	Fish dinner, 2 pce	1 ea	400	60	818	26	76	<1	46	—	—	—
		Chicken:											
12	1528	Chicken plank dinner, 3 pce	1 ea	370	60	885	32	72	<1	51	—	—	—
12	1529	Chicken plank dinner, 4 pce	1 ea	440	60	1037	41	82	<1	59	—	—	—
12	1530	Chicken nugget dinner, 6 pce	1 ea	300	60	699	23	54	<1	45	—	—	—
12	1531	Clam chowder	1 svg	185	85	128	7	15	<1	5	—	—	—
12	1532	Clam dinner	1 ea	460	60	955	22	100	<1	58	—	—	—
12	1533	Fish & chicken dinner	1 ea	460	60	935	36	73	<1	55	—	—	—

GRP KEY: 1 = BEV   2 = DAIRY   3 = EGGS   4 = FAT/OIL   5 = FRUIT   6 = BAKERY   7 = GRAIN   8 = FISH   9 = BEEF   10 = POULTRY
11 = SAUSAGE   12 = MIXED/FAST   13 = NUTS/SEEDS   14 = SWEETS   15 = VEG/LEG   16 = MISC   22 = SOUP/SAUCE

Chol (mg)	Calc (mg)	Iron (mg)	Magn (mg)	Phos (mg)	Pota (mg)	Sodi (mg)	Zinc (mg)	VT-A (RE)	Thia (mg)	Ribo (mg)	Niac (mg)	V-B6 (mg)	Fola (µg)	VT-C (mg)
87	30	1.17	28	205	267	631	.72	6	.08	.11	7.57	.31	8	2
70	50	.98	19	151	176	558	.77	4	.06	.08	5.66	.20	6	1
63	12	.80	13	95	122	207	1.29	3	.04	.09	2.38	.09	4	1
109	34	1.45	22	169	217	566	1.65	5	.08	.16	4.03	.17	9	2
55	22	.68	10	76	86	302	.58	3	.03	.04	2.28	.10	4	1
133	142	3.31	61	326	643	1528	1.88	77	.22	.19	10.0	.50	39	37
180	116	3.90	66	363	720	1441	3.47	77	.25	.32	8.46	.46	42	37
172	126	3.78	64	344	684	1536	2.76	77	.24	.27	8.36	.47	41	37
79	62	1.29	29	218	244	584	.77	6	.11	.11	7.89	.30	11	2
65	57	1.12	21	157	188	564	.88	5	.12	.13	5.37	.24	9	2
66	11	.95	14	100	147	263	1.32	4	.07	.11	3.07	.16	6	1
109	49	1.49	24	185	228	549	1.73	7	.12	.19	5.35	.17	11	2
59	16	.65	12	77	100	312	.67	3	.06	.09	2.94	.11	5	1
132	143	6.03	65	333	689	1544	2.08	77	.31	.29	10.4	.56	43	37
183	130	4.09	70	383	776	1480	3.58	77	.32	.38	10.4	.54	46	37
176	135	6.40	68	361	729	1529	2.93	77	.31	.35	10.3	.49	45	37
<1	21	.28	14	41	218	228	.16	5	.01	.04	.96	.11	7	5
2	9	.48	2	10	21	398	.04	1	.01	.03	.47	<.01	2	<1
1	21	.53	6	28	29	118	.20	1	.10	.04	.98	.01	7	<1
<1	7	.79	53	134	323	12	.99	27	.14	.11	1.80	.22	71	2
4	29	.19	9	20	115	171	.13	28	.03	.03	.20	.07	10	19
12	2	.13	4	29	33	140	.22	30	.02	.03	1.00	.04	1	2
1	6	.24	5	10	75	450	.05	37	.01	.01	.19	.02	3	<1
1	5	.16	2	5	39	148	.02	6	.01	.02	.04	.01	1	<1
t	1	.11	<1	<1	6	10	<.01	0	.01	<.01	.04	t	1	3
1	10	.26	6	15	23	346	.09	1	.02	.01	.16	.02	3	1
1	24	.94	28	78	606	81	.31	0	.17	.06	2.70	.18	20	3
1	19	.35	9	28	137	297	.11	5	.01	.04	1.00	.08	8	1
1	77	1.22	9	264	95	521	.29	30	.28	.13	1.80	.03	8	<1
11	10	.32	15	32	256	396	.29	27	.07	.02	.60	.19	7	3
1	54	1.43	29	90	229	387	1.29	10	.06	.04	.50	.07	32	2
20	39	1.40	10	105	114	398	.93	6	.15	.14	1.65	.07	11	<1
106	—	—	—	—	—	2025	—	—	—	—	—	—	—	—
75	—	—	—	—	—	1352	—	—	—	—	—	—	—	—
119	—	—	—	—	—	2797	—	—	—	—	—	—	—	—
101	—	—	—	—	—	1900	—	—	—	—	—	—	—	—
76	—	—	—	—	—	1526	—	—	—	—	—	—	—	—
25	—	—	—	—	—	1918	—	—	—	—	—	—	—	—
25	—	—	—	—	—	2433	—	—	—	—	—	—	—	—
25	—	—	—	—	—	853	—	—	—	—	—	—	—	—
17	—	—	—	—	—	611	—	—	—	—	—	—	—	—
27	—	—	—	—	—	1543	—	—	—	—	—	—	—	—
56	—	—	—	—	—	2076	—	—	—	—	—	—	—	—

H

Table H–1   Food Composition

Grp	Computer Code No.	Food Description	Measure	Wt (g)	H₂O (%)	Ener (kcal)	Prot (g)	Carb (g)	Dietary Fiber (g)	Fat (g)	Fat Breakdown (g) Sat	Mono	Poly
LONG JOHN SILVER'S—Con.													
12	1534	Oyster dinner	1 ea	360	60	789	17	78	<1	45	—	—	—
12	1535	Scallop dinner	1 ea	320	60	747	17	66	<1	45	—	—	—
12	1536	Seafood platter	1 ea	410	60	976	29	85	<1	58	—	—	—
12	1537	Batter fried shrimp dinner	1 ea	300	60	711	17	60	<1	45	—	—	—
12	1538	Fish sandwich platter	1 ea	400	60	835	30	84	<1	42	—	—	—
		Salads:											
12	1539	Ocean chef	1 ea	320	85	229	27	13	2	8	—	—	—
12	1540	Seafood	1 ea	480	85	426	19	22	2	30	—	—	—
12	1541	Cole slaw	1 svg	98	70	182	1	11	<1	15	—	—	—
12	1542	Fries	1 svg	85	42	247	4	31	<1	12	—	—	—
12	1543	Hush puppies	1 ea	47	37	145	3	18	<1	7	—	—	—

Source: Long John Silver's Inc., Lexington, KY.

Grp	Computer Code No.	Food Description	Measure	Wt (g)	H₂O (%)	Ener (kcal)	Prot (g)	Carb (g)	Dietary Fiber (g)	Fat (g)	Sat	Mono	Poly
McDONALD'S													
		Sandwiches:											
12	1221	Big Mac	1 ea	215	48	560	25	43	1	32	10	21	2
12	1591	McDLT Sandwich	1 ea	234	59	580	26	36	1.4	42	12	17	9
12	1222	Quarter Pounder	1 ea	166	49	410	23	34	1	21	8	11	1
12	1223	Quarter Pounder w/cheese	1 ea	194	48	520	29	35	1	29	11	16	1
12	1224	Filet-O-Fish sandwich	1 ea	142	44	440	14	38	<1	26	5	10	11
12	1225	Hamburger	1 ea	102	46	260	12	31	<1	10	4	5	1
12	1226	Cheeseburger	1 ea	116	45	310	15	31	<1	14	5	8	1
12	1227	French fries-small serving	1 svg	68	37	220	4	26	1	12	3	8	5
12	1228	Chicken McNuggets	6 ea	112	49	270	20	17	<1	16	4	10	2
		Sauces (packet):											
12	1229	Barbeque	1 ea	30	51	70	<1	8	<1	<1	<1	1	1
12	1230	Hot Mustard	1 ea	30	53	70	1	8	<1	4	<1	1	2
12	1231	Sweet & sour	1 ea	32	50	60	<1	14	<1	<1	<1	<1	<1
		Lowfat Milkshakes:											
12	1232	Chocolate	10 fl oz	293	70	320	12	66	<1	2	.8	.9	<1
12	1233	Strawberry	10 fl oz	293	72	320	11	67	<1	1	.6	.6	<1
12	1234	Vanilla	10 fl oz	293	73	290	11	60	<1	1	.63	.67	<1
		Sundaes:											
12	1235	Hot fudge	1 ea	169	60	240	7	51	<1	3	2	1	<1
12	1236	Strawberry	1 ea	171	62	210	6	49	<1	1	1	.4	<1
12	1237	Hot Caramel	1 ea	174	57	270	7	59	<1	3	2	1	<1
12	1238	Vanilla cone	1 ea	80	65	100	4	22	<1	1	<1	<1	4
		Pies:											
12	1239	Apple pie	1 ea	83	45	260	2	30	<1	15	5	9	1
12	1240	Apple Bran Muffin	1 ea	85	44	190	5	46	3	0	0	0	0
		Cookies, package:											
12	1241	McDonaldland cookies	1 pkg	56	3	290	4	47	<1	9	2	7	<1
12	1242	Chocolate chip cookies	1 pkg	56	3	330	4	42	2	16	5	10	<1
		Breakfast items:											
12	1243	English muffin, w/butter	1 ea	59	42	170	5	27	<1	5	2	2	1
12	1244	Egg McMuffin	1 ea	138	51	290	8.2	28	<1	11	4	6	1
12	1245	Hot cakes w/butter & syrup	1 ea	176	46	410	8	74	<1	9	4	3	3
12	1246	Scrambled eggs	1 ea	100	70	140	12	1	<1	10	3	5	1
12	1247	Pork Sausage	1 svg.	48	43	180	8	0	<1	16	6	9	2
12	1248	Hash brown potato patty	1 ea	53	56	130	1	15	1	7	3	4	<1
12	1392	Sausage McMuffin	1 ea	117	38	370	17	27	<1	22	8	12	2
12	1393	Sausage McMuffin w/egg	1 ea	167	47	440	23	28	<1	27	9	15	3
12	1394	Biscuit with spread	1 ea	75	27	260	5	32	<1	13	3	9	1

GRP KEY: 1 = BEV   2 = DAIRY   3 = EGGS   4 = FAT/OIL   5 = FRUIT   6 = BAKERY   7 = GRAIN   8 = FISH   9 = BEEF   10 = POULTRY
11 = SAUSAGE   12 = MIXED/FAST   13 = NUTS/SEEDS   14 = SWEETS   15 = VEG/LEG   16 = MISC   22 = SOUP/SAUCE

Chol (mg)	Calc (mg)	Iron (mg)	Magn (mg)	Phos (mg)	Pota (mg)	Sodi (mg)	Zinc (mg)	VT-A (RE)	Thia (mg)	Ribo (mg)	Niac (mg)	V-B6 (mg)	Fola (µg)	VT-C (mg)
55	—	—	—	—	—	763	—	—	—	—	—	—	—	—
37	—	—	—	—	—	1579	—	—	—	—	—	—	—	—
95	—	—	—	—	—	2161	—	—	—	—	—	—	—	—
127	—	—	—	—	—	1297	—	—	—	—	—	—	—	—
75	—	—	—	—	—	1402	—	—	—	—	—	—	—	—
64	—	—	—	—	—	986	—	—	—	—	—	—	—	—
113	—	—	—	—	—	1086	—	—	—	—	—	—	—	—
12	—	—	—	—	—	367	—	—	—	—	—	—	—	—
13	—	—	—	—	—	.6	—	—	—	—	—	—	—	—
—	—	—	—	—	—	405	—	—	—	—	—	—	—	—
103	256	4	41	338	268	950	5.04	88	.48	.41	6.81	.285	23	2
109	225	4	45	321	414	990	6	188	.39	.36	7	.26	30	7
86	142	4	38	258	334	660	5.3	45	.36	.29	6.7	.28	24	3
118	296	3.7	42	315	356	1150	6	190	.37	.39	6.7	.24	24	3
50	165	1.8	27	227	149	1030	.88	36	.30	.15	3.00	.10	20	.1
37	122	2.29	20	129	145	500	2.13	15	.28	.16	3.84	.12	17	2
53	197	2.3	23	205	157	750	2.60	112	.30	.21	3.86	.12	21	2
0	9	.61	27	101	564	70	.32	0	.13	0	1.8	.22	19	2
56	14	1	27	293	313	580	.923	0	.12	.12	8.3	.394	11	0
0	15	—	6	15	23	250	.09	15	.01	.01	.15	.01	3	.45
5	15	.22	6	15	23	250	.09	2	.01	.01	.15	.01	3	.45
0	11	.17	2	5	39	190	.02	32	0	.01	.08	.01	.6	.64
10	322	.84	47	319	555	240	1.21	92	.13	.52	.41	.148	15	0
10	327	.1	36	302	509	170	1.07	92	.13	.48	.31	.148	11	0
10	327	.10	35	339	521	170	1.09	92	.13	.48	.31	.148	36	0
6	235	.48	36	243	422	170	1.01	65	.08	.35	.30	.138	11	0
5	191	.16	29	188	302	95	.838	65	.07	.29	.25	.056	21	1
13	222	.1	31	243	356	180	.916	88	.08	.35	.26	.054	14	0
3	112	.23	13	120	136	70	.482	87	.04	.18	.37	.046	2	0
0	11	.71	6	26	38	240	.16	0	.06	.02	.32	.02	5	11
0	31	.6	—	—	—	230	—	.7	.02	.08	.4	—	—	.7
0	9	2.1	11	72	50	300	.325	0	.25	.18	2.54	.03	6	0
4	24	2.2	27	102	160	280	.50	0	.18	.21	2.47	.03	6	0
9	151	1.61	13	69	66	270	.50	31	.33	.14	2.47	.04	16	0
226	256	2.77	26	322	168	740	1.92	151	.47	.33	3.71	.21	30	0
21	114	2.08	23	412	154	640	.56	52	.32	.33	2.82	.099	7	0
399	57	2.08	13	269	138	290	1.69	157	.07	.26	.05	.20	66	0
48	8	.67	8	86	115	350	1.33	0	.27	.10	2.31	.165	1	0
9	6	.27	13	65	238	330	.164	0	.06	.02	.85	.124	6	2
64	235	2.3	24	189	219	830	1.71	72	.60	.29	4.8	.15	23	0
263	263	3.34	30	291	298	980	2.39	150	.64	.42	4.8	.20	33	0
1	75	1.31	9	264	95	730	.292	0	.23	.11	1.65	.03	8	0

H

Table H–1   Food Composition

Grp	Computer Code No.	Food Description	Measure	Wt (g)	H₂O (%)	Ener (kcal)	Prot (g)	Carb (g)	Dietary Fiber (g)	Fat (g)	Fat Breakdown (g) Sat	Mono	Poly
McDONALD'S—Con.													
		Breakfast Items—Con.											
12	1395	Biscuit w/sausage	1 ea	123	32	440	13	32	<1	29	9	17	3
12	1396	Biscuit w/sausage & egg	1 ea	180	43	529	20	33	<1	35	11	20	3
12	1397	Biscuit w/bacon, egg & cheese	1 ea	156	41	440	18	33	<1	26	8	16	2
		Salads:											
12	1398	Chef salad	1 ea	283	84	230	21	8	2	13	6	7	1
12	1399	Shrimp salad	1 ea	262	88	104	14	6	2	3	1	2	<1
12	1400	Garden salad	1 ea	213	91	110	7	6	2	7	3	3	<1
12	1401	Chunky chicken salad	1 ea	250	88	140	23	5	2	3	1	2	1

Source: McDonald's Corporation, Oak Brook, Illinois. Some values for Salads estimated from known values for major ingredients.

Grp	Computer Code No.	Food Description	Measure	Wt (g)	H₂O (%)	Ener (kcal)	Prot (g)	Carb (g)	Dietary Fiber (g)	Fat (g)	Sat	Mono	Poly
TACO BELL													
		Burritos:											
12	1544	Bean	1 ea	191	58	357	13	54	8	10	3	5	2
12	1545	Beef	1 ea	191	58	403	22	39	2	17	7	7	2
12	1546	Bean & beef	1 ea	191	58	381	17	46	5	14	7	6	1
12	1547	Burrito supreme	1 ea	241	66	413	18	46	5	18	8	8	2
12	1548	Double beef supreme	1 ea	255	66	457	24	42	2	22	10	10	2
12	1549	Enchirito	1 ea	213	61	382	20	31	5	20	9	8	1
12	1550	Fajita (steak taco)	1 ea	135	65	234	15	20	2	11	5	4	1
		Tacos:											
12	1551	Regular	1 ea	78	55	183	10	11	1	11	5	3	1
12	1552	Taco bellgrande	1 ea	163	63	355	18	18	2	23	11	6	1
12	1553	Taco light	1 ea	170	59	410	19	18	2	29	12	8	5
12	1554	Soft taco	1 ea	92	52	228	12	18	2	12	5	4	1
		Tostadas:											
12	1555	Regular	1 ea	156	67	243	10	27	7	11	4	4	1
12	1556	Beefy tostada	1 ea	198	69	322	15	22	4	20	10	8	1
12	1557	Bellbeefer	1 ea	177	63	312	17	32	<1	13	6	4	2
12	1558	Mexican pizza	1 ea	223	55	575	21	40	5	48	31	14	2
12	1559	Taco salad with salsa	1 ea	595	73	941	36	63	5	61	19	18	12
		Nachos:											
12	1560	Regular	1 ea	106	40	356	7	38	<1	19	12	5	1
12	1561	Bellgrande	1 ea	287	58	649	22	61	6	35	12	20	3
12	1562	Pintos & cheese	1 ea	128	69	190	9	19	7	9	4	4	1
12	1563	Taco sauce	1 ea	3.7	96	2	<1	<1	<1	<1	<1	<1	<1
12	1564	Salsa	1 ea	9.7	95	18	1	4	1	<1	<1	<1	<1
12	1565	Cinnamon Crispas	1 ea	47.3	1	259	3	27	<1	15	4	2	1

Source: Taco Bell Corporation, California for most nutrient values. Values for Dietary fiber, mono-unsaturated fat, magnesium, phosphorus, zinc, folacin, Vitamin B6, Vitamin A in REs, and percentage water are estimates calculated from known values of major ingredients.

Grp	Computer Code No.	Food Description	Measure	Wt (g)	H₂O (%)	Ener (kcal)	Prot (g)	Carb (g)	Dietary Fiber (g)	Fat (g)	Sat	Mono	Poly
WENDY's													
		Hamburgers:											
12	1566	Single, on white bun, no toppings	1 ea	119	41	350	21	29	<1	16	7	9	1
12	1568	Double, on white bun, no toppings	1 ea	197	44	560	41	32	<1	34	7	13	8
12	1569	Big classic	1 ea	241	63	470	26	36	2	25	7	10	5
		Cheeseburgers:											
12	1570	Bacon cheeseburger	1 ea	147	46	460	29	23	<1	28	13	13	2
12	1571	Single, w/all toppings	1 ea	215	50	548	30	32	2	33	13	12	5
12	1572	Double, w/all toppings	1 ea	291	50	735	48	27	2	48	18	18	6

GRP KEY: 1 = BEV 2 = DAIRY 3 = EGGS 4 = FAT/OIL 5 = FRUIT 6 = BAKERY 7 = GRAIN 8 = FISH 9 = BEEF 10 = POULTRY
11 = SAUSAGE 12 = MIXED/FAST 13 = NUTS/SEEDS 14 = SWEETS 15 = VEG/LEG 16 = MISC 22 = SOUP/SAUCE

Chol (mg)	Calc (mg)	Iron (mg)	Magn (mg)	Phos (mg)	Pota (mg)	Sodi (mg)	Zinc (mg)	VT-A (RE)	Thia (mg)	Ribo (mg)	Niac (mg)	V-B6 (mg)	Fola (μg)	VT-C (mg)
49	83	1.98	18	359	235	1080	1.33	0	.49	.21	3.96	.12	12	0
275	116	3.16	25	490	321	1250	3.16	88	.53	.35	3.99	.199	36	0
253	185	2.56	21	496	250	1230	1.67	162	.36	.33	2.47	.11	47	0
128	256	1.51	35	200	400	490	1.40	514	.31	.29	3.6	.04	60	14
193	65	1.33	60	180	420	480	1.90	372	.13	.10	1.08	.06	60	13
83	149	1.26	18	80	280	160	.40	391	.10	.16	.59	.06	60	14
78	24	1	20	140	350	230	.66	458	.22	.17	8.5	.34	61	20
9	147	3.47	65	210	428	888	2.05	65	.037	2.02	1.98	1.00	55	53
57	114	3.73	35	225	313	1051	4.00	100	.398	2.14	3.44	.23	27	2
36	111	2.15	50	220	370	958	2.67	80	.49	.42	3.09	.59	38	2
33	153	3.6	50	227	432	921	3.00	185	.41	2.12	2.89	.52	40	27
57	145	4	52	230	431	1053	4.00	200	.43	2.2	3.68	.30	30	9
54	269	2.84	61	263	423	1243	3.51	157	.256	.418	2.3	.61	29	28
14	117	3.03	24	150	207	485	3.18	133	.403	.341	3.71	.17	15	3
32	84	1.10	16	100	159	276	2.12	42	.05	.142	1.07	.12	10	1
56	182	1.91	18	100	334	472	2.12	132	.11	.29	2.02	.12	13	5
56	155	2.4	18	100	316	594	2.12	128	.2	.33	2.5	.12	13	5
32	116	2.27	18	100	178	516	2.12	42	.39	.22	2.74	.12	10	1
16	179	1.53	62	195	401	596	1.55	84	.061	.169	.626	1.01	47	45
40	185	1.96	43	206	408	764	2.97	152	.24	.29	1.61	.56	31	6
39	174	2.36	22	125	299	855	2.10	121	.16	.30	1.73	.12	<1	5
81	453	3.08	80	400	449	1364	5.40	355	.36	.39	2.00	1.11	60	7
80	398	7.1	130	460	1212	1662	5.59	450	.51	.75	4.8	1.30	140	77
9	178	.99	40	200	158	423	.80	27	.03	.16	.09	.14	4	2
36	297	3.48	100	400	674	997	4.30	280	.104	.34	2.17	.98	33	58
16	156	1.42	110	156	385	642	2.17	87	.05	.146	.396	.21	68	52
0	2	.07	—	—	13	126	—	19	<.01	<.01	.06	—	—	<1
0	36	.60	—	—	376	376	—	112	.02	.14	—	—	—	2
1	37	1.26	—	—	36	127	—	<1	.138	.084	.966	—	—	<1
65	100	4.50	20	118	265	420	2.10	—	.38	.34	6	.12	<1	<1
125	48	6.30	42	339	431	575	8.35	—	.22	.43	9.00	.47	29	<1
80	40	4.55	34	200	470	900	5.11	60	.26	.25	4.80	.25	30	12
65	136	3.60	33	296	332	860	5.14	82	.27	.28	5.70	.24	25	1
84	177	4.00	33	339	430	864	4.41	111	.34	.35	5.29	.25	28	6
165	180	5.40	50	470	620	883	8.80	112	.36	.53	10.0	.46	31	6

H

Table H-1　Food Composition

Grp	Computer Code No.	Food Description	Measure	Wt (g)	H₂O (%)	Ener (kcal)	Prot (g)	Carb (g)	Dietary Fiber (g)	Fat (g)	Fat Breakdown (g)		
											Sat	Mono	Poly
		WENDY'S—Con.											
		Baked potatoes:											
12	1573	Plain	1 ea	250	75	250	6	52	5	<1	<1	<1	<1
12	1574	W/bacon & cheese	1 ea	350	71	570	19	57	5	30	12	11	6
12	1575	W/broccoli & cheese	1 ea	365	74	500	13	54	5	25	9	8	5
12	1576	W/cheese	1 ea	350	71	590	17	55	5	34	13	13	7
12	1577	W/chili & cheese	1 ea	400	72	510	22	63	8	20	13	7	<1
12	1578	W/sour cream & chives	1 ea	310	71	460	7	53	5	24	10	8	3
12	1579	Chili	1 c	256	77	230	21	16	5	9	3	4	<1
12	1580	French fries	1 svg	106	43	306	4	38	<1	15	7	5	2
12	1581	Frosty dairy dessert	1 c	216	35	354	7	53	0	13	5	3	2
12	1582	Chocolate chip cookie	1 ea	64	5	320	3	40	1	17	6	6	5

Source: Wendy's International, for most nutrient values. Some of the values for Dietary fiber, the types of fatty acids, magnesium, phosphorus, zinc, Vitamin B6, Vitamin A in REs, and percentage water for estimates calculated from known values of major ingredients.

H

GRP KEY: 1 = BEV　2 = DAIRY　3 = EGGS　4 = FAT/OIL　5 = FRUIT　6 = BAKERY　7 = GRAIN　8 = FISH　9 = BEEF　10 = POULTRY
11 = SAUSAGE　12 = MIXED/FAST　13 = NUTS/SEEDS　14 = SWEETS　15 = VEG/LEG　16 = MISC　22 = SOUP/SAUCE

Chol (mg)	Calc (mg)	Iron (mg)	Magn (mg)	Phos (mg)	Pota (mg)	Sodi (mg)	Zinc (mg)	VT-A (RE)	Thia (mg)	Ribo (mg)	Niac (mg)	V-B6 (mg)	Fola (μg)	VT-C (mg)
0	40	2.7	67	169	1360	60	.65	0	.28	.10	3.82	.70	68	36
22	200	3.7	80	406	1380	180	2.53	150	.225	.17	4.64	.866	33	36
22	250	3.6	83	373	1550	2.19	.865	350	.31	.255	4	.861	66	90
22	350	3.6	78	49.7	1380	2.22	.609	200	.225	.255	3.3	.80	33	36
22	250	6.1	111	498	1590	810	3.78	172	.32	.26	4.1	.9	50	36
15	40	2.7	70	185	1420	230	.9	100	.225	.13	3	.79	32	36
30	60	4.50	60	320	565	960	3.78	200	.12	.17	3.00	.26	40	9
15	13	1.02	45	197	689	105	.51	0	.15	.04	2.96	.27	33	12
45	257	.86	43	238	518	194	.92	143	.11	.45	.31	.12	17	<1
5	10	1.09	15	62	100	235	.46	0	.06	.07	.4	.03	6	0

H

Recommended Nutrient Intakes (RDA, RNI)

Some of the U.S. recommendations for nutrient intakes appear in the RDA table on the inside front cover, left. The remaining RDA are here, in Tables I–1, I–2, and I–3. The U.S. RDA used on food labels are on the inside front cover, right. The Canadian recommendations are in Tables I–4 and I–5.

◼ TABLE I–1
Estimated Safe and Adequate Daily Dietary Intakes of Additional Selected Vitamins and Minerals (United States)[a]

Age (years)	Vitamins	
	Biotin (µg)	Pantothenic Acid (mg)
Infants		
0–0.5	10	2
0.5–1	15	3
Children		
1–3	20	3
4–6	25	3–4
7–10	30	4–5
11 +	30–100	4–7
Adults	30–100	4–7

Age (years)	Trace Elements[b]				
	Chromium (µg)	Molybdenum (µg)	Copper (mg)	Manganese (mg)	Fluoride (mg)
Infants					
0–0.5	10–40	15–30	0.4–0.6	0.3–0.6	0.1–0.5
0.5–1	20–60	20–40	0.6–0.7	0.6–1.0	0.2–1.0
Children					
1–3	20–80	25–50	0.7–1.0	1.0–1.5	0.5–1.5
4–6	30–120	30–75	1.0–1.5	1.5–2.0	1.0–2.5
7–10	50–200	50–150	1.0–2.0	2.0–3.0	1.5–2.5
11 +	50–200	75–250	1.5–2.5	2.0–5.0	1.5–2.5
Adults	50–200	75–250	1.5–3.0	2.0–5.0	1.5–4.0

[a]Because there is less information on which to base allowances, these figures are not given in the main table of the RDA and are provided here in the form of ranges of recommended intakes.
[b]Because the toxic levels for many trace elements may be only several times usual intakes, the upper levels for the trace elements given in this table should not be habitually exceeded.

Source: *Recommended Dietary Allowances*, © 1989 by the National Academy of Sciences, National Academy Press, Washington D.C.

■ TABLE I–2
Estimated Minimum Requirements of Sodium, Chloride, and Potassium

Age (years)	Sodium[a] (mg)	Chloride (mg)	Potassium[b] (mg)
Infants			
0.0–0.5	120	180	500
0.5–1.0	200	300	700
Children			
1	225	350	1,000
2–5	300	500	1,400
6–9	400	600	1,600
Adolescents	500	750	2,000
Adults	500	750	2,000

[a]Sodium requirements are based on estimates of needs for growth and for replacement of obligatory losses. They cover a wide variation of physical activity patterns and climatic exposure but do not provide for large, prolonged losses from the skin through sweat.
[b]Dietary potassium may benefit the prevention and treatment of hypertension and recommendations to include many servings of fruits and vegetables would raise potassium intakes to about 3,500 mg/day.

Source: *Recommended Dietary Allowances*, © 1989 by the National Academy of Sciences, National Academy Press, Washington, D.C.

I

■ TABLE I-3
Median Heights and Weights and Recommended Energy Intakes (United States)

Age	Weight		Height		Average Energy Allowance			
(years)	(kg)	(lb)	(cm)	(inches)	REE[a] (kcal/day)	Multiples of REE[b]	kcal per kg	kcal per day[c]
Infants								
0.0–0.5	6	13	60	24	320		108	650
0.5–1.0	9	20	71	28	500		98	850
Children								
1–3	13	29	90	35	740		102	1,300
4–6	20	44	112	44	950		90	1,800
7–10	28	62	132	52	1,130		70	2,000
Males								
11–14	45	99	157	62	1,440	1.70	55	2,500
15–18	66	145	176	69	1,760	1.67	45	3,000
19–24	72	160	177	70	1,780	1.67	40	2,900
25–50	79	174	176	70	1,800	1.60	37	2,900
51 +	77	170	173	68	1,530	1.50	30	2,300
Females								
11–14	46	101	157	62	1,310	1.67	47	2,200
15–18	55	120	163	64	1,370	1.60	40	2,200
19–24	58	128	164	65	1,350	1.60	38	2,200
25–50	63	138	163	64	1,380	1.55	36	2,200
51 +	65	143	160	63	1,280	1.50	30	1,900
Pregnant (2nd and 3rd trimesters)								+300
Lactating								+500

[a]REE (resting energy expenditure) represents the energy expended by a person at rest under normal conditions.
[b]Recommended energy allowances assume light to moderate activity and were calculated by multiplying the REE by an activity factor.
[c]Average energy allowances have been rounded.

Source: *Recommended Dietary Allowances*, © 1989 by the National Academy of Sciences, National Academy Press, Washington, D.C.

I

■ TABLE I–4
Recommended Nutrient Intakes for Canadians, 1990

Age	Sex	Weight (kg)	Protein (g/day)[a]	Fat-Soluble Vitamins Vitamin A (RE/day)[b]	Vitamin D (μg/day)[c]	Vitamin E (mg/day)[d]
Months						
0–4	Both	6.0	12[b]	400	10	3
5–12	Both	9.0	12	400	10	3
Years						
1	Both	11	13	400	10	3
2–3	Both	14	16	400	5	4
4–6	Both	18	19	500	5	5
7–9	M	25	26	700	2.5	7
	F	25	26	700	2.5	6
10–12	M	34	34	800	2.5	8
	F	36	36	800	2.5	7
13–15	M	50	49	900	2.5	9
	F	48	46	800	2.5	7
16–18	M	62	58	1,000	2.5	10
	F	53	47	800	2.5	7
19–24	M	71	61	1,000	2.5	10
	F	58	50	800	2.5	7
25–49	M	74	64	1,000	2.5	9
	F	59	51	800	2.5	6
50–74	M	73	63	1,000	5	7
	F	63	54	800	5	6
75+	M	69	59	1,000	5	6
	F	64	55	800	5	5
Pregnancy (additional amount needed)						
1st trimester			5	0	2.5	2
2nd trimester			15	0	2.5	2
3rd trimester			24	0	2.5	2
Lactation (additional amount needed)			20	400	2.5	3

Recommended intakes of energy and of certain nutrients are not listed in this table because of the nature of the variables upon which they are based. The figures for energy are estimates of average requirements for expected patterns of activity (see Table I–5). For nutrients not shown, the following amounts are recommended based on at least 2,000 kcal/day and body weights as given: thiamin, 0.4 mg/1,000 kcal (0.48/5,000 kJ); riboflavin, 0.5 mg/1,000 kcal (0.6 mg/5,000 kJ); niacin, 7.2 NE/1,000 kcal (8.6 NE/5,000 kJ); vitamin B_6, 15 μg, as pyridoxine, per gram of protein. Recommended intakes during periods of growth are taken as appropriate for individuals representative of the midpoint in each age group. All recommended intakes are designed to cover individual variations in essentially all of a healthy population subsisting upon a variety of common foods available in Canada.

Source: Health and Welfare Canada, *Nutrition Recommendations: The Report of the Scientific Review Committee,* (Ottawa: Canadian Government Publishing Centre, 1990), Table 20, p. 204.

I

Water-Soluble Vitamins			Minerals					
Vitamin C (mg/day)[e]	Folate (μg/day)	Vitamin B$_{12}$ (μg/day)	Calcium (mg/day)	Phosphorus (mg/day)	Magnesium (mg/day)	Iron (mg/day)	Iodine (μg/day)	Zinc (mg/day)
20	25	0.3	250	150	20	0.3[g]	30	2[h]
20	40	0.4	400	200	32	7	40	3
20	40	0.5	500	300	40	6	55	4
20	50	0.6	550	350	50	6	65	4
25	70	0.8	600	400	65	8	85	5
25	90	1.0	700	500	100	8	110	7
25	90	1.0	700	500	100	8	95	7
25	120	1.0	900	700	130	8	125	9
25	130	1.0	1,100	800	135	8	110	9
30	175	1.0	1,100	900	185	10	160	12
30	170	1.0	1,000	850	180	13	160	9
40	220	1.0	900	1,000	230	10	160	12
30	190	1.0	700	850	200	12	160	9
40	220	1.0	800	1,000	240	9	160	12
30	180	1.0	700	850	200	13	160	9
40	230	1.0	800	1,000	250	9	160	12
30	185	1.0	700	850	200	13[i]	160	9
40	230	1.0	800	1,000	250	9	160	12
30	195	1.0	800	850	210	8	160	9
40	215	1.0	800	1,000	230	9	160	12
30	200	1.0	800	850	210	8	160	9
0	200	0.2	500	200	15	0	25	6
10	200	0.2	500	200	45	5	25	6
10	200	0.2	500	200	45	10	25	6
25	100	0.2	500	200	65	0	50	6

[a]The primary units are expressed per kilogram of body weight. The figures shown here are examples.
[b]One retinol equivalent (RE) corresponds to the biological activity of 1 μg of retinol, 6 μg of beta-carotene, or 12 μg of other carotenes.
[c]Expressed as cholecalciferol or ergocalciferol.
[d]Expressed as δ-α-tocopherol equivalents, relative to which β- and γ-tocopherol and α-tocotrienol have activities of 0.5, 0.1, and 0.3, respectively.
[e]Cigarette smokers should increase intake by 50 percent.
[f]The assumption is made that the protein is from breast milk or is of the same biological value as that of breast milk, and that between 3 and 9 months, adjustment for the quality of the protein is made.
[g]Based on the assumption that breast milk is the source of iron.
[h]Based on the assumption that breast milk is the source of zinc.
[i]After menopause, the recommended intake is 8 mg/day.

I

■ TABLE I–5
Average Energy Requirements for Canadians

Age	Sex	Average Height (cm)	Average Weight (kg)	Requirements[a] (kcal/kg)[b]	(MJ/kg)[b]	(kcal/day)	(MJ/day)	(kcal/cm)	(MJ/cm)
Months									
0–2	Both	55	4.5	120–100	0.50–0.42	500	2.0	9	0.04
3–5	Both	63	7.0	100–95	0.42–0.40	700	2.8	11	0.05
6–8	Both	69	8.5	95–97	0.40–0.41	800	3.4	11.5	0.05
9–11	Both	73	9.5	97–99	0.41	950	3.8	12.5	0.05
Years									
1	Both	82	11	101	0.42	1,100	4.8	13.5	0.06
2–3	Both	95	14	94	0.39	1,300	5.6	13.5	0.06
4–6	Both	107	18	100	0.42	1,800	7.6	17	0.07
7–9	M	126	25	88	0.37	2,200	9.2	17.5	0.07
	F	125	25	76	0.32	1,900	8.0	15	0.06
10–12	M	141	34	73	0.30	2,500	10.4	17.5	0.07
	F	143	36	61	0.25	2,200	9.2	15.5	0.06
13–15	M	159	50	57	0.24	2,800	12.0	17.5	0.07
	F	157	48	46	0.19	2,200	9.2	14	0.06
16–18	M	172	62	51	0.21	3,200	13.2	18.5	0.08
	F	160	53	40	0.17	2,100	8.8	13	0.05
19–24	M	175	71	42	0.18	3,000	12.6		
	F	160	58	36	0.15	2,100	8.8		
25–49	M	172	74	36	0.15	2,700	11.3		
	F	160	59	32	0.13	1,900	8.0		
50–74	M	170	73	31	0.13	2,300	9.7		
	F	158	63	29	0.12	1,800	7.6		
75+	M	168	69	29	0.12	2,000	8.4		
	F	155	64	23	0.10	1,500	6.3		

[a]Requirements can be expected to vary within a range of ±30%.
[b]First and last figures are averages at the beginning and at the end of the 3-month period.

Source: Health and Welfare Canada, *Nutrition Recommendations: The Report of the Scientific Review Committee,* (Ottawa: Canadian Government Publishing Centre, 1990), Tables 5 and 6, pp. 25, 27.

I

Measures of Protein Quality

Contents

Chapter 6 describes protein quality. This appendix explains the different measures researchers use to assess the quality of a food protein.

◼ Chemical Scoring

The simplest way to evaluate a food protein's quality is to study the amino acid composition of the protein itself, in the laboratory. The amino acid composition of a test protein can be compared with the composition of egg protein (the reference protein), and a chemical score can be derived to express the theoretical value of the test protein. A test protein with a limiting amino acid (see p. 140) that is present in only 70 percent of the amount found in egg protein, for example, would receive a chemical score of 70. If you fed the test protein to human beings under carefully controlled conditions in which the total protein fed was just enough to meet the requirements, you would expect that nitrogen would be excreted in the urine equal in quantity to 30 percent of the nitrogen fed. Table J–1 shows how to use a reference pattern for the nine essential amino acids.

chemical score: a rating of the quality of a test protein arrived at by comparing its amino acid pattern with that of a reference protein.

In a world where food is scarce and where many people's diets contain marginal or inadequate amounts of protein, it is important to know which foods contain the highest-quality protein. It is possible to determine the amino acid composition of any protein relatively inexpensively, but unfortunately, chemical scoring does not always reflect accurately the way the body will use a protein. The advantages of chemical scoring are that it is simple and inexpensive, it identifies in one step the limiting amino acid, and it can be used to score mixtures of different proportions of two or more proteins mathematically without having to make up a mixture and test it. Its chief weaknesses are that it fails to predict the digestibility of a protein, which may strongly affect its quality; it relies on a chemical procedure in which certain amino acids may be destroyed, so that the pattern that is analyzed may lack accuracy; and it is blind to other features of the protein (such as the presence of substances that may inhibit the digestion or utilization of the protein) that would only be revealed by a test in living animals.

◼ Biological Value

To determine the actual value of a protein as it is used by the body, it is necessary to measure not only urinary, but also fecal, losses of nitrogen when that protein is actually fed to human beings under test conditions. (Even then, small additional losses from sweat, shed skin, hair, and fingernails will be missed.) This kind of experiment determines the biological value (BV) of proteins, a measure used internationally.

biological value: see p. 141.

■ TABLE J–1
A Reference Pattern for Chemical Scoring of Proteins

Essential Amino Acids	Whole Egg Mg Amino Acid per G Nitrogen
Histidine	145
Isoleucine	340
Leucine	540
Lysine	440
Methionine + cystine[a]	355
Phenylalanine + tyrosine[b]	580
Threonine	294
Tryptophan	106
Valine	410
Total	3,210

[a]Methionine is essential and is also used to make cystine. Thus the methionine requirement is lower if cystine is supplied.
[b]Phenylalanine is essential and is also used to make tyrosine if there is not enough of the latter. Thus the phenylalanine requirement is lower if tyrosine is also supplied.

Note: To interpret the table, read, "For every 3,210 units of essential amino acids, 145 must be histidine, 340 must be isoleucine, 540 must be leucine," and so on. To compare a test protein with the reference protein, the experimenter would first obtain a chemical analysis of the test protein's amino acids. Then, taking 3,210 units of the amino acids, the experimenter would compare the amount of each amino acid to the amount found in 3,210 units of essential amino acids in egg protein. For example, suppose the test protein contained (per 3,210 units) 360 units of isoleucine; 500 units of leucine; 350 of lysine; and for each of the other amino acids, more units than egg protein contains. The two amino acids that are low are leucine (500 as compared with 540 in egg) and lysine (350 versus 440 in egg). The ratio, amino acid in the test protein divided by amino acid in egg, is 500/540 (or about 0.93) for leucine and 350/440 (or about 0.80) for lysine. Lysine is the limiting amino acid (lowest ratio compared with egg), so the test protein receives a chemical score of 80.

In a test of biological value, two nitrogen balance studies are done. In the first, no protein is fed, and nitrogen (N) excretions in the urine and feces are measured. It is assumed that under these conditions, N lost in the urine is the amount the body always necessarily loses by filtration into the urine each day, regardless of what protein is fed (endogenous N). The N lost in the feces (called metabolic N in the equation) is the amount the body invariably loses into the intestine each day, whether or not food protein is fed. (To help you remember terms: endogenous N is "urinary N on a zero-protein diet"; metabolic N is "fecal N on a zero-protein diet.")

In the second study, an amount of protein slightly below the requirement is fed. Intake and losses are measured. The BV is then derived using this formula:

$$BV = \frac{\text{food N} - (\text{fecal N} - \text{metabolic N}) - (\text{urinary N} - \text{endogenous N})}{\text{food N} - (\text{fecal N} - \text{metabolic N})} \times 100.$$

The denominator of this equation expresses the amount of nitrogen *absorbed:* food N minus fecal N (excluding the N the body would lose in the feces anyway, even without food). The numerator expresses the amount of N *retained* from the N absorbed: absorbed N (as in the denominator) minus the N excreted in the urine (excluding the N the body would lose in the urine anyway, even without food). Thus it can be more simply expressed:

$$BV = \frac{\text{N retained}}{\text{N absorbed}} \times 100.$$

This method has the advantages of being based on experiments with human beings (it can be done with animals, too, of course) and of measuring actual nitrogen retention. But it is also cumbersome, expensive, and often impractical, and it is based on several assumptions that may not be valid. For example, the subjects used for testing may not be similar physiologically or in terms of their normal environment or typical food intake to those for whom the test protein may ultimately be used. For another example, that protein is retained in the body does not necessarily mean that it is being well utilized. There is considerable exchange of protein among tissues (protein turnover) that is hidden from view when only N intake and output are measured. One tissue could be shorted, and the test of biological value wouldn't detect this.

Net Protein Utilization

Like measurements of BV, determinations of net protein utilization (NPU) involve two balance studies: one on zero, and the other on submaximal, nitrogen intake. The formula for NPU is:

net protein utilization (NPU): the amount of protein nitrogen that is retained from a given amount of protein nitrogen eaten; a measure of protein quality.

$$NPU = \frac{\text{food N} - (\text{fecal N} - \text{metabolic N}) - (\text{urinary N} - \text{endogenous N})}{\text{food N}} \times 100.$$

The numerator is the same as it is for BV, but the denominator represents food N intake only—not absorbed N. More simply expressed:

$$NPU = \frac{\text{N retained}}{\text{N intake}} \times 100.$$

This method has advantages similar to those of BV determinations and is more frequently used, employing animals as the test subjects. A drawback is that if a low NPU is obtained, the test results offer no help in distinguishing between two possible causes: a poor amino acid composition of the test protein or poor digestibility. There is also a limit to the extent to which animal test results can be assumed to be applicable to human beings.

Protein Efficiency Ratio

The protein efficiency ratio (PER) is the best-known procedure for evaluating protein quality and is used in the United States as the basis for regulations regarding food labeling and for the protein RDA. Young rats are fed a measured amount of protein and weighed periodically as they grow. The PER is expressed as:

protein efficiency ratio (PER): the grams of weight gained by growing animals per gram of protein fed; a measure of protein quality.

$$PER = \frac{\text{weight gain (g)}}{\text{protein intake (g)}}.$$

This method has the virtues of economy and simplicity, but it also has many drawbacks. The experiments are time-consuming; the amino acid needs of rats are not the same as those of human beings; and the amino acid needs for growth are not the same as for the maintenance of adult animals (growing animals need more lysine, for example).

J

The PER is used to qualify statements about daily protein requirements in the United States. You are assumed to eat protein with a PER equal to, or better than, that of the milk protein casein; if the protein's PER is lower, you need more of the protein. Food labels have to take protein quality into consideration, using the PER of casein as a reference point. If the protein in the package has a PER as great as, or greater than, that of casein, then 45 grams of that protein is considered to be 100 percent of the U.S. RDA. If its PER is less than that of casein, then there have to be 65 grams of it to meet 100 percent of the U.S. RDA.

J

Self-Study Forms

This appendix contains the forms needed to complete the self-study exercises presented throughout the book. For reasons of space, Form 4 appears first, followed by Forms 1 through 3 and 5 through 7.

■ FORM 4
Percentage of kCalories from Protein, Fat, Carbohydrate, and Alcohol

From Form 3:

Protein:	_____g/day × 4 kcal/g	= (P) _____	kcal/day.
Fat:	_____g/day × 9 kcal/g	= (F) _____	kcal/day.
Carbohydrate:	_____g/day × 4 kcal/g	= (C) _____	kcal/day.
Alcohol:		(A) _____	kcal/day.[a]
	Total kcal/day	= (T) _____	kcal/day.

Percentage of kcalories from protein:

$\dfrac{\text{(P)}}{\text{(T)}}$ × 100 = _____% of total kcalories.

Percentage of kcalories from fat:

$\dfrac{\text{(F)}}{\text{(T)}}$ × 100 = _____% of total kcalories.

Percentage of kcalories from carbohydrate:

$\dfrac{\text{(C)}}{\text{(T)}}$ × 100 = _____% of total kcalories.

Percentage of kcalories from alcohol:

$\dfrac{\text{(A)}}{\text{(T)}}$ × 100 = _____% of total kcalories.

Note: The four percentages can total 99, 100, or 101, depending on the way in which figures were rounded off earlier.

[a]To find out how many kcalories in a beverage are from alcohol, look up the beverage in Appendix H. Figure out how many kcalories are from carbohydrate (multiply carbohydrate grams times 4), fat (fat grams times 9), and protein (protein grams times 4). The remaining kcalories are from alcohol.

■ FORM 1
Nutrient Intakes (Use One Form for Each Day)

Food	Approximate Measure or Weight	Energy[a] (kcal)	Prot[b] (g)	Carb[b] (g)	Fiber[b] (g)	Fat[b] (g)	Fat Breakdown Sat (g)	Mono (g)	Poly (g)	Chol[a] (mg)	Calcium[a] (mg)	Iron[c] (mg)	Magn[a] (mg)	Phos[a] (mg)	Potas[a] (mg)	Sodium[a] (mg)	Zinc[b] (mg)	Vit A[a] (RE)	Thia[c] (mg)	Ribo[c] (mg)	Niac[b] (mg)	V B$_6$[b] (mg)	Fol[a] (µg)	Vit C[b] (mg)
Total																								

[a]Compute these values to the nearest whole number.
[b]Compute these values to one decimal place.
[c]Compute these values to two decimal places.

■ **FORM 2**
Average Daily Energy and Nutrient Intakes

Day	Energy (kcal)	Protein (g)	Carb (g)	Fiber (g)	Fat (g)	**Fat Breakdown** Sat (g)	Mono (g)	Poly (g)	Chol (mg)	Calcium (mg)	Iron (mg)	Magn (mg)	Phos (mg)	Potas (mg)	Sodium (mg)	Zinc (mg)	Vit A (RE)	Thia (mg)	Ribo (mg)	Niac (mg)	V B$_6$ (mg)	Fol (µg)	Vit C (mg)
1																							
2																							
3																							
Total																							
Average daily intake (divide total by 3)																							

■ **FORM 3**
Comparison with a Standard Intake

Day	Energy (kcal)	Protein (g)	Fat (g)	Carb (g)	Fiber (g)	Chol (mg)	Calcium (mg)	Iron (mg)	Magn (mg)	Phos (mg)	Potas (mg)	Sodium (mg)	Zinc (mg)	Vit A (RE)	Thia (mg)	Ribo (mg)	Niac (mg)	V B$_6$ (mg)	Fol (µg)	Vit C (mg)
Average daily intake (from Form 2)																				
Standard[a]																				
Intake as percentage of standard[b]																				

[a]Taken from RDA tables (inside front cover, left) and Appendix I or *Recommended Nutrient Intakes for Canadians* (Appendix I).
[b]For example, if your intake of protein was 50 g and the standard for a person your age and sex was 46 g, then you consumed (50 ÷ 46) × 100, or 109 percent of the standard.

K

K

■ FORM 5
Food Selection Scorecard

Food Group and Recommended Intake	Your Intake from Group (Specify Food and Amount)	Your Score
Fruits and vegetables—4 or more portions (½ c cooked edible portion or 3 to 4 oz raw); at least 1 raw daily.		
1 portion vitamin A–rich dark green or deep orange fruit or vegetable (any food with more than your RDA) = 10 points (no more than 10 points allowed).		
1 portion vitamin C–rich fruit or vegetable (any food with more than your RDA) = 10 points (no more than 10 points allowed).		
Other fruits and vegetables, including potatoes = 2.5 points each.		
Subtotal (no more than 25 points allowed)		
Breads and cereals—4 or more portions of whole-grain or enriched (1 oz dry-weight cereal or 1-oz slice bread or equivalent grain product).		
1 portion cereal or 2 bread equivalents = 10 points (no more than 10 points allowed).		
Other bread equivalents = 5 points each.		
Subtotal (no more than 25 points allowed)		
Milk and milk products—2 or more portions (8 oz fluid milk; calcium equivalents are 1⅓ oz hard cheese, 1⅓ c cottage cheese, 1 pint ice milk or ice cream).		
1 portion = 12.5 points.		
Subtotal (no more than 25 points allowed)		
Meat and meat substitutes—2 or more portions of meat (2 to 3 oz cooked lean meat, fish, poultry; protein equivalents are 2 eggs, 2 oz hard cheese, or ½ c cottage cheese) and 2 portions legumes or nuts (¾ c cooked legumes, 4 tbsp peanut butter, 1 oz nuts or sunflower seeds); count cheese either in milk group or in meat group, not both.		
2 portions meat = 12.5 points.		
2 portions legumes = 12.5 points.		
Subtotal (no more than 25 points allowed)		
Grand total (no more than 100 points)		

The above are foundation foods. Additional foods are those that do not fit into the above groupings but add flavor, interest, variety, and (often) kcalories. List those eaten:

■ FORM 6
Diet Planning by Exchange Groups

Amounts to Be Delivered[a]

Exchange List	Number of Exchanges[b]	Carbohydrate ___g	Protein ___g	Fat ___g	Energy ___kcal
Starch/bread					
Meat					
Vegetable					
Fruit					
Milk					
Fat					
	Total actually delivered[c]				

[a]From step 3, Chapter 12 self study exercise.
[b]From steps 4, 5, 6, Chapter 12 self study exercise.
[c]From step 7, Chapter 12 self study exercise.

■ FORM 7
Meal patterns

Exchange List	Total Exchanges to Be Consumed Daily[a]	Exchanges Consumed at Each Meal				
		Breakfast	Lunch	Snack	Dinner	Snack
Starch/bread						
Meat						
Vegetable						
Fruit						
Milk						
Fat						

[a]From Form 6, column 2.

K

Enteral Formulas

The availability of a staggering number of enteral formulas complicates the decision of selecting an appropriate formula. The formulas shown in this Appendix provide some examples, but the list is by no means complete. Furthermore, be aware that the composition of formulas changes periodically. Health care providers must consult with manufacturers' current literature before selecting a formula. Addresses of formula manufacturers listed in this Appendix can be found in Appendix F (see Trade Organizations).

■ TABLE L–1
Enteral Formulas

Product	Manufacturer	Form	Volume to meet 100% U.S. RDA	kCal/ ml	Protein g/ 1,000 ml	Carbohydrate g/ 1,000 ml	Fat g/ 1,000 ml	mOsm/ kg	Notes
Intact Formulas: Isotonic or Near-Isotonic Formulas									
Compleat® Modified	Sandoz Nutrition	liquid	1,500 ml	1.07	43	140	37	300	Lactose-free
Entrition®	aBiosearch	liquid	2,000 ml	1.00	35	136	35	300	Lactose-free, low-residue
Fortison®	Sherwood Medical	liquid	2,000 ml	1.00	35	125	40	300	Lactose-free
Isocal®	Mead Johnson	liquid	1,900 ml	1.06	34	135	44	270	Lactose-free, low-residue
Isocal® HN	Mead Johnson	liquid	1,800 ml	1.06	44	124	45	270	Lactose-free, 40% fat from MCT oil
Isosource®	Sandoz Nutrition	liquid	1,500 ml	1.20	43	170	41	360	Lactose-free, low-residue, 50% fat from MCT oil
Isosource® HN	Sandoz Nutrition	liquid	1,500 ml	1.20	53	160	41	360	Lactose-free, low-residue, 50% fat from MCT oil
Isotein® HN	Sandoz Nutrition	powder	1,770 ml	1.20	68	160	34	300	Lactose-free
Jevity®	Ross	liquid	1,325 ml	1.00	42	144	35	300	Lactose-free, 14 g fiber/1,000 ml, 50% fat from MCT
Osmolite®	Ross	liquid	2,000 ml	1.00	35	137	36	300	Lactose-free, low-residue
Osmolite® HN	Ross	liquid	1,400 ml	1.06	44	141	37	300	Lactose-free, low-residue, 50% fat from MCT
PediaSure®	Ross	liquid	1,100	1.00	30	110	50	325	Intended for use with children; nearly lactose-free
Travasorb® MCT	Travenol	powder, liquid	2,000	1.00	49	123	33	312	Lactose-free, low-residue, 80% fat from MCT oil
Ultracal®	Mead Johnson	liquid	1,180	1.06	44	123	45	310	Lactose-free, 13.6 g fiber/1,000 ml, 40% fat from MCT
Intact Formulas: Standard, Low- to Moderate-Residue Formulas[a]									
Ensure®	Ross	liquid	2,000	1.06	37	145	37	470	Lactose-free
Meritene®	Sandoz Nutrition	liquid	1,250	0.96	58	110	32	510[b]	Contains lactose

(continued)

■ TABLE L–1
Enteral Formulas (continued)

Product	Manufacturer	Form	Volume to meet 100% U.S. RDA	kCal/ml	Protein g/1,000 ml	Carbohydrate g/1,000 ml	Fat g/1,000 ml	mOsm/kg	Notes
Nutrex Besure®	Nutrex	powder	1,900	1.06	37	144	35	450	Lactose-free
Resource®	Sandoz Nutrition	liquid	1,900	1.06	37	140	37	430	Lactose-free
Sustacal®	Mead Johnson	liquid	1,100	1.01	61	140	23	650[c]	Lactose-free
Intact Formulas: Standard, Fiber-Containing Formulas									
Compleat® Regular	Sandoz Nutrition	liquid	1,500	1.07	43	130	43	450	Blenderized formula, contains lactose, 4.3 g fiber/1,000 ml
Enrich®	Ross	liquid	1,530	1.10	40	162	37	480	Lactose-free, 14 g fiber/1,000 ml
Fibersource®	Sandoz Nutrition	liquid	1,500	1.20	43	170	41	390	Lactose-free, 10 g fiber/1,000 ml
Fibersource® HN	Sandoz Nutrition	liquid	1,500	1.20	53	160	41	390	Lactose-free, 7 g fiber/1,000 ml
Jevity® (see "Intact Formulas: Isotonic or Near-Isotonic Formulas")									
Nutrex Encare with Fiber®	Nutrex	powder	1,200	1.46	40	241	37	460	Lactose-free, 17 g fiber/1,000 ml
Sustacal with Fiber®	Mead Johnson	liquid	1,400	1.06	46	140	35	480	Lactose-free, 8 g fiber/1,000 ml
Ultracal® (see "Intact Formulas: Isotonic or Near-Isotonic Formulas")									
Hydrolyzed Formulas[d]									
Criticare HN®	Mead Johnson	liquid	1,900	1.06	38	220	53	650	Lactose free, low-residue
Stresstein®	Sandoz Nutrition	powder	2,000	1.20	70	170	28	910	Lactose-free, low-residue
Traum-Aid HBC®	Kendall McGaw	powder	3,000	1.00	56	166	12.4	675	Lactose-free, low-residue, 50% of protein from branched-chain amino acids
Travasorb Standard®	Travenol	liquid	1,900	1.06	35	136	35	488	Lactose-free, low-residue

(continued)

L

■ TABLE L-1
Enteral Formulas   (continued)

Product	Manufacturer	Form	Volume to meet 100% U.S. RDA	kCal/ ml	Protein g/ 1,000 ml	Carbohydrate g/ 1,000 ml	Fat g/ 1,000 ml	mOsm/ kg	Notes
Hydrolyzed Formulas[d]									
Vital HN®	Ross	powder	1,500	1.00	42	185	11	500	Lactose-free, low-residue
Vivonex®	Norwich Eaton	powder	1,800	1.00	20	231	2	550	Lactose-free, low-residue
Vivonex HN®	Norwich Eaton	powder	3,000	1.00	46	210	1	810	Lactose-free, low-residue
Vivonex T.E.N.®	Norwich Eaton	powder	2,000	1.00	38	206	3	630	Lactose-free, low-residue, 33% of protein from branched-chain amino acids
Special-Use Formulas: High-kCalorie Formulas (see also "Special Use Formulas: High-kCalorie, High-Protein Formulas")									
Ensure Plus®	Ross	liquid	1,400	1.50	55	200	53	690	Lactose-free
Resource Plus®	Sandoz Nutrition	liquid	1,600	1.50	55	200	53	600	Lactose-free
Sustacal HC®	Mead Johnson	liquid	1,800	1.50	61	190	58	650	Lactose-free
Special-Use Formulas: High-Nitrogen (Protein) Formulas									
Ensure HN®	Ross	liquid	1,400	1.06	44	139	35	470	Lactose-free
Fibersource HN®	Sandoz Nutrition	liquid	1,500	1.20	53	160	41	390	Lactose-free, 7 g fiber/1,000 ml
Isocal HN®	Mead Johnson	liquid	1,250	1.06	44	124	45	270	Lactose-free
Isosource HN®	Sandoz Nutrition	liquid	1,500	1.20	43	170	41	360	Lactose-free
Isotein HN	Sandoz Nutrition	powder	1,800	1.20	68	160	34	300	Lactose-free
Special-Use Formulas: High-kCalorie, High-Protein Formulas									
Isocal HCN®	Mead Johnson	liquid	1,000	2.00	75	200	102	640	Lactose-free
Magnacal®	Sherwood Medical	liquid	1,000	2.00	70	250	80	590	Lactose-free
TraumaCal®	Mead Johnson	liquid	1,500	1.50	82	142	68	490	Lactose-free
TwoCal HN®	Ross	liquid	1,000	2.00	84	217	91	690	Lactose-free
Special-Use Formulas: Other									
Amin-Aid®	Kendall McGaw	powder	—	2.00	19	366	46	700	Hydrolyzed formula, lactose-free, no added vitamins or electrolytes; intended for use in renal failure

(continued)

TABLE L–1
Enteral Formulas (continued)

Product	Manufacturer	Form	Volume to meet 100% U.S. RDA	kCal/ ml	Protein g/ 1,000 ml	Carbohydrate g/ 1,000 ml	Fat g/ 1,000 ml	mOsm/ kg	Notes
Hepatic-Aid II®	Kendall McGaw	powder	—	1.10	44	169	36	560	Hydrolyzed formula with 46% of protein as branched-chained amino acids, lactose-free, no added vitamins or electrolytes; intended for use in liver failure
Impact®	Sandoz Nutrition	liquid	1,500	1.00	56	132	28	375	Lactose-free: enriched with arginine, RNA, and omega-3 fatty acids; intended to improve immune competence
Pediasure	Ross	liquid	1,100	1.00	30	108	49	310	Virtually lactose-free; intended for use with children ages 1 to 6
Pulmocare®	Ross	liquid	950	1.50	63	106	92	490	Lactose-free; intended for use in respiratory insufficiency
Replena®	Ross	liquid	—	2.00	30	253	95	615	Lactose-free; low in electrolytes; intended for use in renal disease before dialysis is instituted
Travasorb Hepatic®	Travenol	powder	2,100	1.10	29	209	14	690	Hydrolyzed formula with 50% of protein from branched-chained amino acids; lactose-free; intended for use in liver failure

(continued)

L

TABLE L-1
Enteral Formulas (continued)

Product	Manufacturer	Form	Volume to meet 100% U.S. RDA	kCal/ ml	Protein g/ 1,000 ml	Carbohydrate g/ 1,000 ml	Fat g/ 1,000 ml	mOsm/ kg	Notes
Travasorb Renal®	Travenol	powder	—	1.35	23	271	18	590	Hydrolyzed formula; lactose-free; does not contain fat-soluble vitamins or electrolytes; intended for use in renal failure

[a]With the exception of Ultracal, all formulas listed under "Intact Formulas: Isotonic or Near-Isotonic Formulas" can be used as a standard, low- to moderate-residue formula.
[b]Vanilla flavor.
[c]Vanilla and strawberry flavors.
[d]Many special-use formulas are also hydrolyzed (see "Special Use Formulas: Other").

TABLE L-2
Enteral Formulas—Protein Modules

Product	Manufacturer	Form	Major Protein Source	kCal/g	Protein (g/100 kcal)	Carbohydrate (g/100 kcal)	Fat (g/100 kcal)	Notes
Casec®	Mead Johnson	powder	Calcium caseinate	3.7	23.8	—	2.0	
Nutrisource Amino Acids®	Sandoz Nutrition	powder	Free amino acids	3.9	24.9	—	—	
Nutrisource Amino Acids-High Branched Chain®	Sandoz Nutrition	powder	Free amino acids	3.8	24.9	—	—	44% branched-chain amino acids
Nutrisource Protein®	Sandoz Nutrition	powder	Delactosed lactalbumin, egg white solids	4.0	18.8	1.7	2.1	
Pro Mod®	Ross	powder	Whey protein and soy lecithin	5.6	18.9	2.4	2.0	
Propac®	Sherwood Medical	powder	Whey protein	4.0	19.2	1.3	20	

Index

This index lists primarily topics that received significant mention in the text. Pages inclusive (for example, 53–56) indicate major discussions; pages in **bold face** refer to defined terms; pages in *italics* refer to figures, diagrams, or chemical structures; pages followed by a "t" (for example, 5t) refer to tables; letter-number combinations (such as C-23) refer to appendixes.

PHOTO CREDITS (CONTINUED)

Kidd & Company; **197** Courtesy of Dr. Samuel Dreizen, D.D.S., M.D.; **204** © *Nutrition Today*, C. Butterworth & G. Blackburn, Hospital Nutrition and How to Access the Nutritional Status of a Patient. Nutrition Today Teaching Aid #18 (Nutrition Today: Annapolis, MD); **214 (left)** © Lester Bergman and Associates, Inc.; **(right)** © Michael Abbey/Science Soource/Photo Researchers Inc.; **222** © Lester Bergman and Associates, Inc.; **225** © *Nutrition Today*, H. Sandstead, J. Carter, and W. Darby, Nutritional Deficiencies, Nutrition Today Teaching Aid #5 (Nutrition Today, Annapolis, MD), 1975; **227** From C. Conn, The Specialist in General Practice, 2nd ed. (Philadelphia: Saunders, 1957); **229** Ray Stanyard; **237, 238** Sandra Silvers, Electron Microscopist at Florida State University Electron Microscope Facility, color by Kidd & Company; **246** David Farr; **247** © *Nutrition Today*, H. Sandstead, J. Carter, and W. Darby, Nutritional Deficiencies, Nutrition Today Teaching Aid #5 (Nutrition Today, Annapolis, MD), 1975; **251** Ray Stanyard; **254** © Owen Franken/Stock, Boston; **256** Courtesy of Parke-Davis and Company; **257** © Alan Oddie/PhotoEdit; **271, 272** From D.W. Fawcett, *The Cell*, 2nd ed. (Philadelphia: Saunders, 1981); color by Kidd & Company; **272** © Anthony Vannelli; **274** © Mark A. Mittelman/Taurus Photos; **285** © Leslye Borden/PhotoEdit; **288** Courtesy of U.S. Department of Agriculture; **295(a)** Courtesy of Gjon Mill; **(b)** © Nutrition Today; **306** © Tony Freeman/PhotoEdit; **314, 315** From D. W. Fawcett, *The Cell*, 2nd ed. (Philadelphia: Saunders, 1982); color by Kidd & Company; **316** Courtesy of Dr. M. F. Pertuz; **319(a)** © Lester Bergman & Associates, Inc.; **(b)** Michael Abbey/Science Source/Photo Researchers; **324** Ray Stanyard; **329** Reproduced with permission of *Nutrition Today* Magazine, P.O. Box 1829, Annapolis, MD, 21404, March 1968; **331** Ray Stanyard; **333** © Lester Bergman and Associates Inc.; **348, 349** From D.W. Fawcett, *The Cell*, 2nd ed. (Philadelphia: Saunders, 1981); color by Kidd & Company; **350, 351** Ray Stanyard; **358** © Roger Miller/The Image Bank; **365** © Tony Freeman/PhotoEdit; **366** © Lawrence Migdale/Stock, Boston; **370** © Frank Whitney/The Image Bank; **379** © Richard Hutchings/PhotoEdit; **389** © George S. Zimbel/Monkmeyer Press; **392** © Bill Stanton/International Stock Photography; **395, 396** From

D. W. Fawcett, *The Cell*, 2nd. ed. (Philadelphia: Saunders, 1981); color by Kidd & Company; **399** © Tony Freeman/PhotoEdit; **402** © Peter Menzel; **403** © A. Tannenbaum/Sygma; **407** © Patrick Wood/Stock, Boston; **412** © Peter Menzel; **418** © Patrick J. LaCroix/The Image Bank; **421** Felicia Martinez/PhotoEdit; **425** © Daemmrich/Stock, Boston; **429, 430** From D. W. Fawcett, *The Cell*, 2nd. ed. (Philadelphia: Saunders, 1981); color by Kidd & Company; **432 (top left and right, bottom left)** Petit Format/Nestle/ Photo Researchers, Inc. **(bottom right)** © Anthony Vannelli; **436** © Robert McElroy/Woodfin Camp and Associates; **439** Robert Brenner/PhotoEdit; **441** © Francis Wardle; **442** © Pascale/Photo Researchers, Inc.; **445** © Anthony Vannelli; **453** Streissguth, A. P., Clarren, S. K., & Jones, K. L. (1985, July). Natural History of the Fetal Alcohol Syndrome: A ten-year follow-up of eleven patients. *Lauret, II*, 89–92; **455, 456** From D. W. Fawcett, *The Cell*, 2nd. ed. (Philadelphia: Saunders, 1981); color by Kidd & Company; **456** © Anthony Vannelli; **458** © Francis Wardle; **466** © Tony Freeman/PhotoEdit; **473** © Martha Bates/Stock, Boston; **479** © Richard Hutchings/PhotoEdit; **483** © Owen Franken/Stock/Boston; **494, 495** From D. W. Fawcett, *The Cell*, 2nd. ed. (Philadelphia: Saunders, 1981); color by Kidd & Company; **495, 506** Courtesy of U.S. Department of Agriculture; **515** © Steven M. Stone/The Picture Cube; **517, 518** Felicia Martinez/PhotoEdit; **526** © Juan-Pablo Lira/The Image Bank; **528, 529** Sandra Silver, Electron Microscopist at Florida State University Microscope Facility, color by Kidd & Company; **530(a)** © Rick Browne/Stock, Boston; **(b)** © Cary Wolinsky/Stock, Boston; **541** © Daemmrich/Stock, Boston; **548** *Seeds* Magazine: Ending U.S. World Hunger, 222 East Lake Drive, Decatur, GA 30030; **550** © Ira Kirschenbaum/Stock, Boston; **551** © Alan Oddie/PhotoEdit; **552** © Diane M. Lowe/Stock, Boston; **561** NASA; **565** (top) © Tony Freeman/PhotoEdit; (bottom) © Alan Oddie/PhotoEdit; **573, 574** © Richard Megna, 1988/ Fundamental Photographs; **599** © Stephen McBrady/PhotoEdit; **601** © Steve Hansen/Stock, Boston; **602, 603** © Charles Gellis/Photo Researchers, Inc.; **603 (margin)** © Jeff Dunn/The Picture Cube; **613** © Frank Siteman/ The Picture Cube; **614** © Mary Kaye Denny/PhotoEdit; **615 (bottom left)** © Ulrike

Welsch/Photo Researchers; **(bottom right)** © Charles Gumpton/Stock, Boston; **(margin)** © Tony Freeman/PhotoEdit; **624 (top)** © Frank Siteman/ The Picture Cube; **(bottom), 625 (top)** © David Young-Wolff/PhotoEdit; **(bottom)** © MacDonald Photo/The Picture Cube; **629** © Susan Leavines/Photo Researchers, Inc.; **634** © Robert Brenner/PhotoEdit; **643** © David Young-Wolff/PhotoEdit; **647, 648** © Torre Johnson/WoodfinCamp and Associates; **651** © Gary Bistram/The Image Bank; **653** © Mary Kaye Denny/PhotoEdit; **657** © Charles Gumpton/Stock, Boston; **658** © David Young-Wolff/PhotoEdit; **659** © Richard Pasley/Stock, Boston; **661** © Jay Freis/The Image Bank; **667 (top)** © Jay Brousseau/The Image Bank; **(bottom)** © Jan Halaska/Photo Researchers, Inc.; **669** © Custom Medical Stock Photo; **672, 673** © Manfred Kage/Peter Arnold, Inc.; **674** © Tony Freeman/ PhotoEdit; **685** © Simon Fraser/Princess Mary Hospital, Newcastle/Science Photo Library; Photo Researchers, Inc.; **692** © Tony Freeman/PhotoEdit; **703, 704** © Philip A. Harrington/The Image Bank; **711** © Custom Medical Stock Photo; **717 (left)** Pharmacia Deltec Inc., St. Paul, Minnesota; **(right)** Courtesy of Abbott Laboratories; **719, 720** Sandra Silvers, Electron Microscopist at Florida State University Electron Microscope Facility, Color by Kidd & Company; **725** © Junebug Clark/Science Source; **740** © Herb Snitzer/Stock, Boston; **747, 748** B. F. King, University of California School of Medicine/BPS; **749** © Anthony Vannelli; **752** © Roger Miller/The Image Bank; **771, 772** Sandra Silvers, Electron Microscopist at Florida State University Electron Microscope Facility, Color by Kidd & Company; **774** Murray Alcosser/The Image Bank; **800, 801** © The Image Bank; **821, 822** © John Walsh/Science Photo Library/Photo Researchers, Inc.; **827** © L. V. Bergman & Associates, Inc.; **830** Jean Claude LeJeune/Stock, Boston; **841 , 851** © Tony Freeman/PhotoEdit; **853, 854** Sandra Silvers, Electron Microscopist at Forida State University Electron Microscope Facility, Color by Kidd & Company; **855** Reproduced by Permission of ICI Pharmaceuticals Division, Cheshirs, England; **886** © Tony Freeman/ PhotoEdit; **893, 894, 923, 924** Sandra Silvers, Electron Microscopist at Florida Sate University Electron Microscope Facility, color by Kidd & Company; **948** © Michael Skott/The Image Bank; **952** Peter Menzel/Stock, Boston.

West's NutriPro™

You can purchase your West's **NutriPro**™ Software Package using the order form below. It is available through West Publishing Company. The package was developed by ESHA Research and consists of one 5-1/4" or 3-1/2" disk and *The Student Manual to Accompany West's NutriPro*™.

NutriPro™ runs on IBM PC, PS/2 and compatible machines (minimum of 512K). It is a menu-driven program that allows you to analyze your nutritional and health status. Using the computer, you can plan a diet and exercise program to achieve or maintain your desired weight and nutrient intake. NutriPro™ is a fast, flexible program filled with diet analysis and planning options.

To order by phone, call: 1-800-328-9352.
Specify 5-1/4" disk: 0-314-85178-X
3-1/2" disk: 0-314-85161-5.

ORDER FORM

Complete form and return with payment to:
West Publishing Company
C.O.P. Department
P.O. Box 64833
St. Paul, MN 55164-1803

❏ Send one West's NutriPro™ manual and 3-1/2" disk (ISBN: 0-314-85161-5).
❏ Send one West's NutriPro™ manual and 5-1/4" disk (ISBN: 0-314-85178-X).
I have enclosed a check payable to West Publishing Company for **$29.95 plus** the local tax of $_____. Total amount $_____.

Or, charge to: ❏ Master Card ❏ VISA. Credit Card #: _____
Expiration Date: _____

Name:_____

Street Address:_____

City_____ State _____ Zip _____

Order subject to approval of vendor. Applicable local tax to be added.
Price subject to change without notice.

Please allow 6 to 8 weeks for delivery.

Acceptable Weight for Height Based on Body Mass Index (BMI)

To determine your acceptable weight range, find your height in the top line. Look down the column below it and find the range represented by the color blue. Look to the left column to see what weights are acceptable for you.

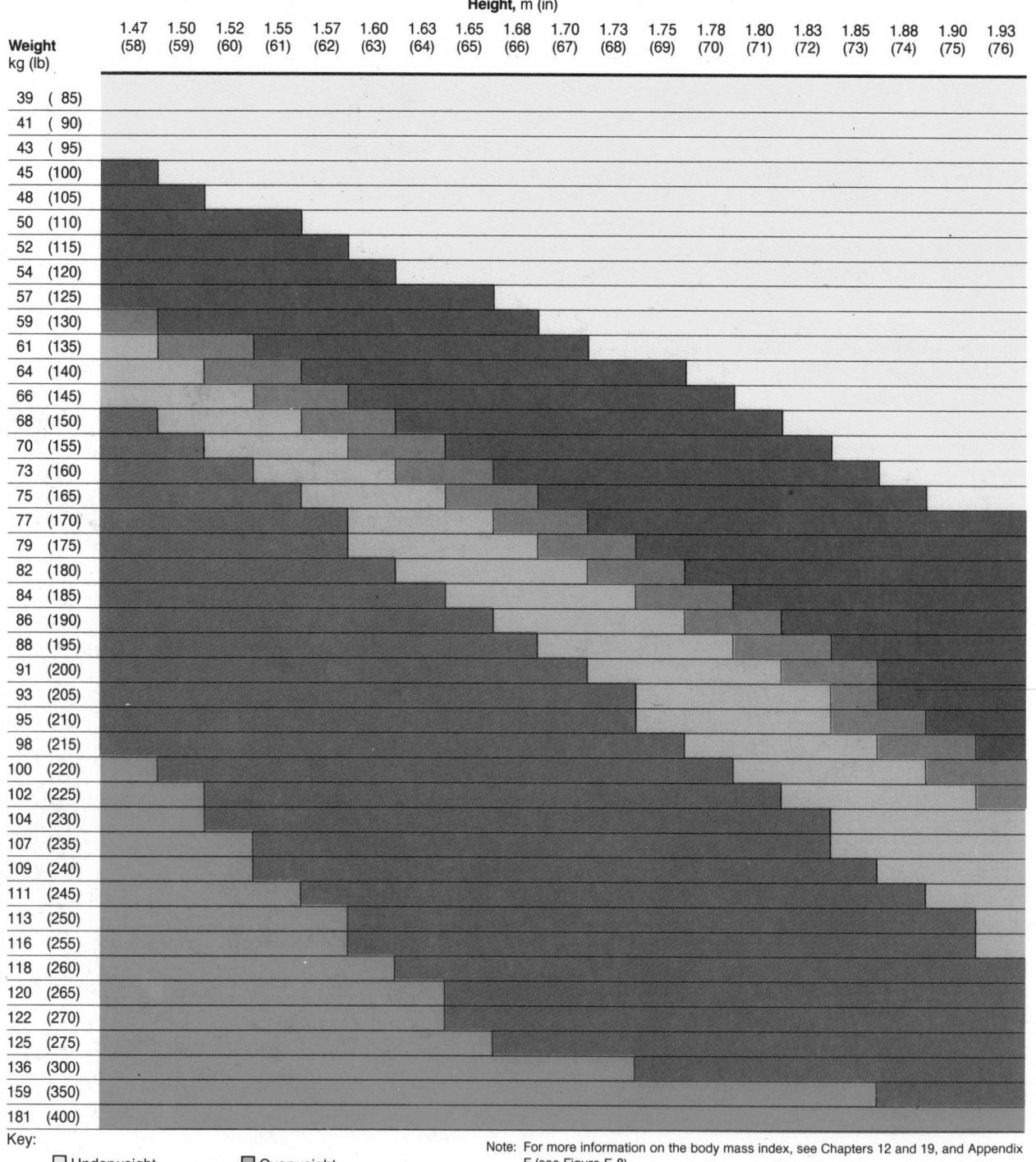

Men
Height, m (in)

Key:

- ☐ Underweight
- ■ Acceptable weight
- ■ Marginal overweight
- ☐ Overweight
- ■ Severe overweight
- ☐ Morbid obesity

Note: For more information on the body mass index, see Chapters 12 and 19, and Appendix E (see Figure E-8).

Source: Adapted from M. I. Rowland, A nomogram for computing body mass index, Dietetic Currents 16 (1989): 9, used and reprinted with permission of Ross Laboratories, Columbus, OH 43216. Copyright 1989 Ross Laboratories.